THE MARATHON:
PHYSIOLOGICAL, MEDICAL, EPIDEMIOLOGICAL, AND PSYCHOLOGICAL STUDIES

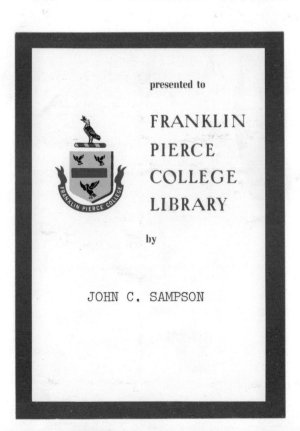

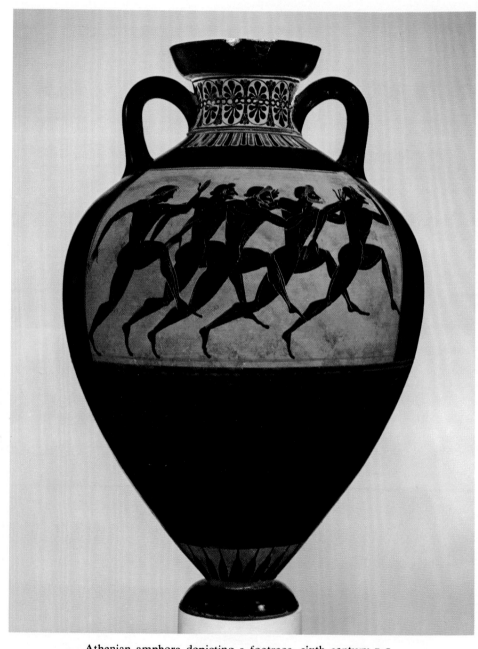

Athenian amphora depicting a footrace, sixth century B.C.
Courtesy of the Metropolitan Museum of Art, Rodgers Fund, 1914

ANNALS OF THE NEW YORK ACADEMY OF SCIENCES

Volume 301

THE MARATHON: PHYSIOLOGICAL, MEDICAL, EPIDEMIOLOGICAL, AND PSYCHOLOGICAL STUDIES

Edited by Paul Milvy

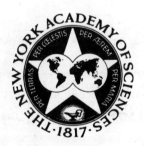

The New York Academy of Sciences
New York, New York
1977

Library of Congress Cataloging in Publication Data

Main entry under title:

The Marathon.

(Annals of the New York Academy of Sciences; v. 301)
Papers of a conference held by the New York Academy of Sciences, October 25-28, 1976.
Includes index.
1. Marathon running—Physiological effect—Congresses.   2. Heart—Congresses.
3. Physical fitness—Congresses. I. Milvy, Paul. II. New York Academy of Sciences.
III. Series: New York Academy of Sciences. Annals; v. 301. [DNLM: 1. Exertion—
Congresses. 2. Running—Congresses. W1 AN626YL v. 301/QT260 M311 1976]
Q11.N5   vol. 301   [RC1220.M35]   508'.1s   [612'.044]
ISBN 0–89072–047–9   77–14583

PCP
Printed in the United States of America
ISBN 0-89072-047-9

ANNALS OF THE NEW YORK ACADEMY OF SCIENCES

VOLUME 301

October 31, 1977

THE MARATHON: PHYSIOLOGICAL, MEDICAL, EPIDEMIOLOGICAL,
AND PSYCHOLOGICAL STUDIES *

Editor and Conference Chairman
PAUL MILVY

CONTENTS

* This series of papers is the result of a conference entitled The Marathon: Physiological, Medical, Epidemiological, and Psychological Studies, held by The New York
Academy of Sciences on October 25-28, 1976.

Financial assistance was received from:

- AGFA-GEVAERT, INC.
- AIR FORCE OFFICE OF SCIENTIFIC RESEARCH
- W. A. BAUM CO., INC.
- WARREN E. COLLINS, INC.
- EXXON CORPORATION
- NEW YORK ROAD RUNNERS CLUB
- OFFICE OF NAVAL RESEARCH
- QUINTON INSTRUMENTS
- A. H. ROBINS COMPANY
- ROSS LABORATORIES
- SANDOZ, INC.
- E. R. SQUIBB AND SONS, INC.
- TROTTER TREADMILLS
- UPJOHN COMPANY

IN SPECIAL RECOGNITION

DAVID BRUCE DILL

Dr. D. B. Dill has been making important contributions to both applied and theoretical physiology for over fifty years. Perhaps the exciting developments in the early stages of Dr. Dill's career at the Fatigue Laboratory at Harvard University gave him the impetus to produce over 300 publications including two books.

Seldom can the well-defined study of an entire discipline be completely attributed to a single body of workers. The Fatigue Laboratory of Harvard University, which existed from 1926 to 1946, is an instance where a group of researchers made lasting contributions toward a comprehensive study of man's adaptation to his surroundings. The principal directors were L. J. Henderson (theoretical research) and D. B. Dill (research and administration). Under their leadership over 50 individuals conducted research related to the physiology of individuals and their environment. The work included studies of construction workers at Boulder Dam in the heat of the Nevada desert, farm workers in the humid delta lands in Mississippi, and miners at 17,500-foot elevation enduring cold weather conditions of the Andes mountain. Dr. Dill and others from the lab, including Ancel Keys, S. Robinson, A. V. Bock, and J. H. Talbott, were pioneers in conducting experiments of subjects living under these extreme conditions. Their classic procedures serve as a prototype for today's sophisticated experimenters.

In another phase of testing at Harvard, Dr. Dill supervised experiments involving exercise physiology. Dogs were used quite frequently in experiments. As part of an investigation of fatigue in dogs, a treadmill test was performed on a remarkable dog, Sally, who ran, without food, for 27 hours including 5 minutes of rest per hour. Sally ran a total of 111 miles, experiencing a climb of 18.2 miles. A well-known athlete who participated in Harvard experiments was the famous marathoner Clarence De Mar, who participated in 32 Boston marathons and won several times. He was the first runner to undergo stress testing, and the procedures and discoveries made at that time are very much relevant to the many experiments being conducted on runners today.

Dr. Dill's background before going to Harvard is interesting. He was born on April 22, 1891 in Eskridge, Kansas. He graduated from high school in 1908 at Santa Ana, California, received a BS at Occidental College in 1913 and an MS in chemistry in 1914 at Stanford. After teaching high school for several years, he worked for the Bureau of Chemistry, now known as the Food and Drug Administration. Dr. Carl Alsburg was the Bureau director at that time. He and Dill left the Bureau when Alsburg became director of the Stanford Food Research Institute and Dill became his student to work on a Ph.D. Dill finished in 1925 and went on to establish his prominence in Physiology.

The history and contributions of the Harvard Fatigue Laboratory can be found in the book *The Harvard Fatigue Laboratory: Its History and Contributions,* written by Dr. Dill's son-in-law and daughter, Dr. and Mrs. S. Horvath. Dr. Horvath was one of two successful Ph.D. students who studied under Dr. Dill at the lab. Horvath later helped to develop the successful University of California at Santa Barbara Institute of Environmental Stress. Incidentally, the other student was S. Robinson, who founded the Human Physiology Laboratory at Indiana University.

Although Dill's accomplishments at Harvard in the 1930s would exceed the aspirations of many young scientists, his activities were far from over. At the age of 50, D. B. Dill was commissioned as a major in the Army Air Force. Dill's original service time was to have been a 6-month tour, but he wound up serving from 1941 to 1946. It was Dill's job to help coordinate efforts of physiologists with those of the military. As a result nearly 180 papers were contributed by the Harvard group alone. Dr. Dill and his collaborators issued reports that were basically concerned with important concepts in human physiology; however, much was imparted concerning the diet, food, and clothing needed by combat soldiers.

The demise of the Harvard lab brought Dill to the position of director of medical research for the Army Chemical Research and Development Laboratories. He served in this capacity from 1947 to 1961.

After leaving this job at age 70, Dr. Dill joined his erstwhile student Sid Robinson at Indiana. They collaborated on a book *Adaptation to the Environment*, which serves as a reference to the physiology of aging and environmental adaptation.

In 1966 Dr. Dill's idea of retirement was to help establish the University of Nevada Laboratory of Environmental Pathology and Physiology at Boulder City under an NSF grant with the Desert Research Institute. He has efficiently and effectively worked with high school students in conducting research experiments. Dill's current projects include physiological studies on burros and kangaroo rats. In addition, Dill continues working with elderly people and the intricate problems of aging.

Dr. Dill continues to add to his imposing list of publications. He lives with his wife Chloris and has two children, Elizabeth Dill Horvath and D. B. Dill, Jr. Dr. Dill's contributions and achievements are recognized all over the world and are an inspiration to mankind. Dill has the remarkable ability to make friends with anyone and seems at home just as well with fledgling physiologists as he does with mathematical statisticians.

A. Goldman

INTRODUCTION AND WELCOME

Paul Milvy

Environmental Sciences Laboratory
Mount Sinai School of Medicine
New York, New York 10029

The marathon is a 26-mile 385-yard (42.195 km) running race that taxes the participant to the extreme. By virtue of this fact, the marathoner's body and mind must be conditioned to an exceptional degree to prepare, endure, and master this race. The human discipline brought to bear in this endeavor has medical, physiological, and psychological consequences. Just as the understanding of the body in health may be deepened by the study of its pathology, so too, it seems reasonable to infer, may increased understanding of the human body under normal conditions of life be achieved by the study of the body under conditions of special stress and prolonged exertion.

This conference will address itself to the scientific and medical disciplines involved in the research of prolonged yet intense exercise. It will emphasize long distance running, although not be limited to it. The modern marathon has been run at an average rate of just under 5 minutes per mile for its entire length. Physical activity of this quantity and quality requires an energy expenditure that is both intense and prolonged, and consequently an enormous stress is placed upon the body and its organ systems. Cardiovascular, metabolic, gastrointestinal, and possibly pulmonary changes, as well as changes in the muscular and skeletal systems, are all involved in the training, the running, and the recovery phases of long distance running at this rate. For this reason alone we feel that a scientific and medical conference devoted to these aspects of the body and its functioning is of real merit.

But there are other reasons, more general in nature, that suggest that such a conference is very appropriate. Sports medicine and the science of exercise physiology have developed at a rapid rate during the last decade in this country. This has been a result of several factors. It has been a response to our ignorance as well as to our knowledge. In terms of the former we know too little about the fundamental changes in the human body that occur as a result of athletic training and participation and exposure of the body to athletic stress. That there are changes that are beneficial as well as deleterious is recognized although the general principles required to maximize the one and minimize the other are not well understood from a fundamental medical and scientific point of view. The growth of the disciplines of sports medicine and exercise physiology has also been a response to our knowledge, for, from a perspective that is relative rather than absolute, we have accumulated a great deal of applied and basic knowledge in this field when contrasted to just a decade ago. New knowledge feeds upon itself, exposing areas of ignorance and engendering new and more fundamental questions that beg for answers. It is appropriate at this time to convene a conference that can attempt to integrate and correlate some of the diverse findings as well as to confront some of the problems and uncertainties that remain extant.

In the last decade, with the growth of participation in sports by our population, with the popularity of "jogging," and with the concern for exercise in

1

general, there has developed an extensive and growing body of scientific literature devoted to sports in general, and running and jogging in particular. Reasons may be advanced for the increasing participation of the general population in the specific areas of aerobic jogging and long distance running. The expansion of leisure time and the decrease in hard physical work that are concomitant with the increased efficiency of our country's industrial and technological capacities has led to the growing mass participation in sports that we refer to above. It has probably also in part been responsible for a population that is sedentary and overweight, that overconsumes the foods that are nutritionally ill-advised, that smokes too much, and that is just beginning to acknowledge the pernicious medical consequences of this life-style. And this awareness has catalyzed many to try to alter these trends, as individuals, by taking up jogging, running, and other physically demanding activities.

Only a small but growing corpus of fundamental research is devoted to endurance sports, and this material although available, is often scattered in a variety of scientific and medical journals. One can also venture to suggest that the research that is published is often too applied and phenomenological and too little scientific and fundamental. It is too fragmented and dispersed, too little integrated and cohesive. Meetings held in this field are too often popularizations of science and medicine for the athletic coach and the runner and are not really forums for scientists to talk science with their colleagues. Often these meetings emphasize sports injuries and training and the more applied and less fundamental aspects of sports medicine and the physiology of exercise. Scientifically and medically competent research in this field is conducted and reported in the literature, but an effort to synthesize and integrate these studies by the mechanism of a conference, where original state-of-the-art papers are presented and scrutinized by the conferees, and finally published, has never been forthcoming.

May I welcome all of you to the conference with the ancient greeting, "Joy to you," * and to paraphrase Pheidippides, "Rejoice, we commence." †

---

* LUCION, trans. by K. Kilburn. 1959. Vol. **6**: 177. Harvard University Press. Cambridge, Mass.

† BROWNING, ROBERT. 1898. Pheidippides. *In* The Complete Works of Robert Browning. Charlotte Porter & Helen A. Clarke, Eds. **2**: 117–124. George D. Sproul, Publisher, New York, N.Y.

FIBER TYPES AND METABOLIC POTENTIALS OF SKELETAL MUSCLES IN SEDENTARY MAN AND ENDURANCE RUNNERS *

Bengt Saltin, Jan Henriksson, Else Nygaard, and Per Andersen

August Krogh Institute
Copenhagen University
DK-2100 Copenhagen Ø
Denmark

Eva Jansson

Department of Clinical Physiology
Karolinska Hospital
Stockholm, Sweden

During the last decade the needle biopsy technique has been widely applied for obtaining samples from the skeletal muscle of healthy people. In the early exercise studies the metabolic response of whole muscle was the focus of attention.[1,2] More recently, histochemical techniques have been applied to identify different fiber types in human skeletal muscle and to relate their contractile characteristics to their function and metabolism in exercise. The metabolic potential of muscle tissue has also been evaluated by determining different substrate and enzyme activities. In this paper these latter reports will be reviewed. Special attention will be given to the adaptations that take place as a result of physical inactivity and activity.

Classification of Skeletal Muscle Fibers in Man

The smallest unit that can be activated in a muscle contraction is the motor unit. The muscle fibers within that unit appear to have identical characteristics,[3,4] although a few exceptions have been described.[5] The most frequently used method to distinguish among different muscle fiber types is based on single or multiple stains of freeze-sectioned muscle samples. The number of stains available for classifying muscle fibers is overwhelming. This explains the existence of the great number of different systems employed to classify and name muscle fiber types. In TABLE 1 a summary is presented of some of the commonly used stains and the nomenclature applied. The classical terminology of red and white muscle fibers was based on the color of the fibers, which in turn was related to the myoglobin content.[7] The activities of the mitochondrial enzymes are related to the myoglobin content, while the content of sarcoplasmatic, glycolytic enzymes usually are inversely related to the oxidative enzymes and myoglobin content.[8,9] Stains for glycolytic or oxidative enzymes as well as for myoglobin give rise to a variety of staining intensities. Fibers can be divided into different classes, but the boundaries between these classes are

* The papers cited in this article that were written by the authors (August Krogh Institute) have been sponsored by grants from the Danish Natural Science Research Council and the Research Council of the Danish Sports Federation.

3

TABLE 1

A SUMMARY OF SOME OF THE MORE FREQUENTLY USED STAINS AND NOMENCLATURE TO DESIGNATE FIBER TYPES *

Base for Classification	Reference	Nomenclature		
1. Myoglobin	7, 9	Red	Intermediate	White
2. Mitochondrial enzymes	11, 21	High Oxidative (HO)	Oxidative (O)	Low Oxidative (LO)
3. Glycolytical enzymes	11, 21	Low glycolytic (LG)	Glycolytic (G)	High Glycolytic (HG)
4. Lipids	17, 19, 22	High content (C)	Intermediate content (B)	Low content (A)
5. Myofibrillar ATPase † (preincubations pH 10.3, 4.6–4.8)	10, 14, 15	Slow twitch (ST) (type I)	Fast twitch (FT$_a$) (type IIA)	Fast twitch (FT$_b$) (type IIB)
Combination of 2, 3, and 5	9	SO	FOG	FG

* A general reference for the stains applied is Reference 6.
† This stain for classification gives a fourth fiber type (IIC) staining dark at preincubations of pH 10.3 and 4.3. This fiber is rarely seen in normal adult human muscles.

unclear. This is true for skeletal muscle of most species, including man. In 1962 Engel suggested the use of a stain for myofibrillar ATPase after alkaline preincubation.[10] This method separates muscle fibers into two well-defined groups. He proposed the names type I and II fibers for those fibers staining light and dark, respectively. The type I fibers were supposed to have slow contraction times, and the type II fibers, fast. By adding a stain for a mito-chondrial enzyme, a subdivision of the type II fibers is sometimes possible: One type of fiber can be found with a high oxidative potential, and another, low.[11] Thus, in many species two rather distinctly different subgroups of type II muscle fibers are present. Using these same two stains on the skeletal muscle of man, Edgerton *et al.*[12] and Prince *et al.*[13] also found different types of fibers, which they accepted as being clearly separated into three groups. We do not find this procedure satisfactory (FIGURE 1) as we do not see clear-cut boundaries between the two groups of type II fibers.

In man, a subdivision of the type II fibers can be made by the use of the different sensitivities for acid pH that the type II fibers have. Some of them lose activity (and thereby their dark color) at a pH of 4.6–4.8, whereas other type II fibers maintain color until a pH of 4.5 (FIGURE 1). Brooke and Kaiser named the latter subgroup IIB, and the former, type IIA.[14, 15]

At this point it is worth emphasizing that it appears as if the subdivision of type II fibers as done by Edgerton *et al.*[12] and Prince *et al.*[13] on the one hand, and by Brooke and Kaiser on the other,[14, 15] do not give rise to identical sub-groups of the type II fibers. With a mitochondrial stain, a larger number of type IIB (fast twitch glycolytic) fibers are identified as compared to the use of the stain for myofibrillar ATPase after an alkaline (pH 10.3) and an acid preincubation (pH 4.6–4.8). Before a more firm conclusion can be reached on this particular point a comparative study is necessary of the two different methods to classify the skeletal muscle fibers of man.

Muscle Fiber Nomenclature

In the preceding discussion, different names have been used to designate the different fiber types (TABLE 1). We have neutral names like type I and IIA and IIB fibers or A, B, and C fibers, as others prefer to call them.[16, 17] However, the disadvantage with neutral names is that the names do not indicate any of the characteristics of the different fiber types. Peter *et al.* favor a nomenclature that includes both contractile and metabolic characteristics of the different fibers.[9] This nomenclature is based upon the close correlation between enzyme activity levels and the contractile characteristics, as well as the specific metabolism of the fibers.

Good experimental evidence is available revealing a close coupling between the characteristics of a fiber and its function in many species.[1, 8, 9] In man, such a complete validation is still lacking. However, contractile characteristics of the fibers [18, 19, 20] together with quantitative data of the metabolic profile [21] give a good base for the assumption that a coupling between the characteristics of a fiber and its function also exists in man.[22] With this background we find that it is valid to use descriptive terms when naming the fibers. However, we will not go further than to designate the two main types as slow (ST) and fast twitch (FT) fibers, and add an "a" (FT$_a$) and a "b" (FT$_b$) for the subgroups of the fast twitch fibers. The reason for this is as follows: It is true that in

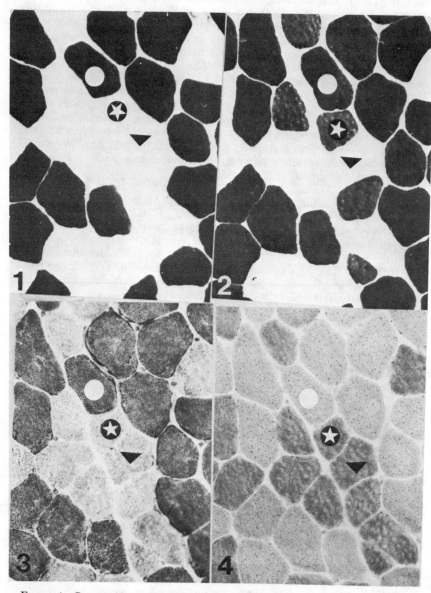

FIGURE 1. Cross-sections of human skeletal muscle (vastus lateralis) are stained for myofibrillar ATPase after preincubations in (1) pH 4.3, (2) 4.6, (3) NADH-diaphorase, and (4) α-glycerophosphate dehydrogenase. Of note is the fact that classification of the different fiber types is solely based on the stains for myofibrillar ATPase.

sedentary subjects a difference can be observed in metabolic potentials, both with histochemical and quantitative biochemical techniques, when one compares the different fiber types (TABLES 1, 2, FIGURE 2). However, the absolute level for the activities of oxidative and glycolytic enzymes is, in all fiber types in human skeletal muscle, large enough to accommodate a rather substantial aerobic and anaerobic metabolism. Moreover, with endurance training, for example, the enhancement of the oxidative potential of FT_a and FT_b fibers is very impressive, resulting in a potential for oxidation in these fibers markedly surpassing the aerobic capacity of ST fibers of untrained subjects.[21, 23] Thus we feel that it is wrong to include abbreviations for the metabolic potentials in the names as these, in some cases, can be very misleading. The subscripts "a" and "b" indicate that there are certain differences in the population of FT fibers most likely related to differences in the myosin molecules.[15] When this

TABLE 2

A SUMMARY OF MEAN VALUES FOR DIFFERENT VARIABLES MEASURED
ON HUMAN SKELETAL MUSCLE TO CHARACTERIZE THE DIFFERENT FIBER TYPES *

Characteristics	Muscle Fiber Types			
	ST	FT_a	FT_b	References
Contractile characteristics				
Ca²⁺ act. myosin ATPase				
(mmoles/min·mg myosin)	0.16	0.48		21
Mg²⁺ act. actomyosin ATPase				
(mmoles/min·g protein)	0.30	0.84		27
"Time to peak tension" (msec)	80	30		18, 19
Enzymes				
Creatine phosphokinase				
(mmoles/min·g protein)	13.1	16.6		27
Phosphofructokinase				
(mmoles/kg·min, wet weight)	9.4	14.0	20.0	21
Succinate dehydrogenase				
(mmoles/kg·min, wet weight)	11.5	9.0	6.5	21

* Values for substrate concentrations can be found in Reference 22.

point has been more completely clarified and possibly found to be correlated to different contractile characteristics, it will be time to exchange the neutral subscripts to more descriptive terms.

In connection with these problems it may be worthwhile to consider the question as to whether the previously described fiber types in human skeletal muscles are similar to those found in the muscle fiber types of other species. To a certain extent it may be true for the ST fiber of man, which should be equivalent with the SO fiber of other species, as well as for the human FT_b being similar to the FG fibers (TABLE 1). The FT_a fiber and the FOG fiber may be the fiber that is most different both in character and function, when comparing man with other species such as the cat, rat, guinea pig.[8]

Besides the difference in staining intensity for oxidative enzymes, it appears that in such species as rats and guinea pigs the FOG fibers are more easily recruited in muscle contractions than the FOG fibers in human muscles.[8] Moreover, Thorstensson and Karlsson [24] have provided some indirect evidence that the fatigability of human FT fibers is different from that of the fast-twitching fibers in cat gastrocnemius muscle.[25]

A study comparing the staining profiles and physiological properties of fiber types in the same muscles of different species, ranging from lower vertebrates to primates and man, with the known physical activity levels would constitute an extremely valuable contribution at this time. Until such a study becomes available, caution is recommended regarding the application of conclusions to more than the species studied.

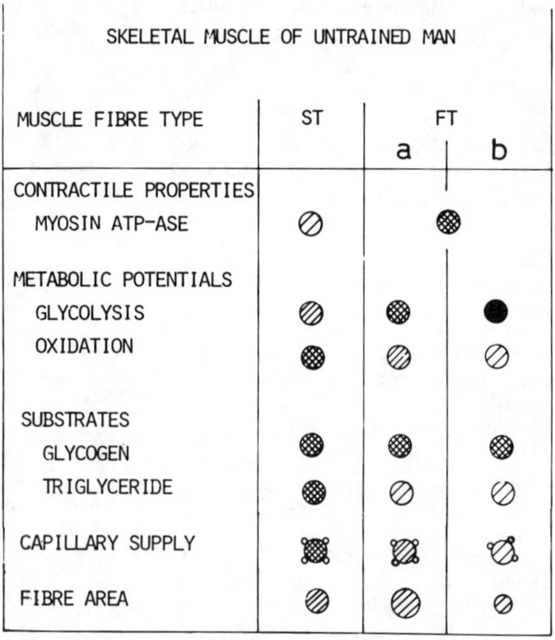

FIGURE 2. A schematic summary of some characteristics observed for the three major types of fiber found in skeletal muscle of sedentary subjects. The results are primarily based on histochemical findings, but the results in TABLE 2 have also been used.

Quantitative Measures of Contractile and Metabolic Characteristics of Different Muscle Fiber Types

Histochemical techniques can at best give a semiquantitative estimation of the metabolic profile of a certain fiber type and its twitch characteristics. Reliable quantitative data exist on muscle from cats, guinea pigs, and rats,[8] and are now becoming available for muscle from man (TABLE 2).

The muscles of man are mixed in regard to fiber composition and the fiber types exist in a mosaic pattern. To determine quantitatively the metabolic profile one has to use a method where fibers are dissected out, typed, and analyzed for content of a substrate or an enzyme.[21] By adding the information on twitch characteristics obtained *in vivo*[19] or *in vitro*[18, 20] contraction times for FT and ST fibers are also available. In many aspects these quantitative data confirm what has been postulated from the histochemical work on muscle from man. Nevertheless, it is important to point out that the activity of succinate dehydrogenase is considerably higher in ST fibers than in FT_a and FT_b fibers in muscles of sedentary men (TABLE 2). The reverse pattern is true for phosphofructokinase. It is also of note that the glycolytic potential is considerable in the ST fiber and that the oxidative potential is substantial in the FT_b fiber.

There has been some argument about a lower glycogen content in the ST fibers compared to the FT fibers,[8, 26] but direct measurements of the glycogen content of the different fiber types clearly demonstrate that at rest after a mixed diet no significant differences between fiber types can be detected in man. In contrast, the other major intramuscular substrate, the triglyceride pool, is much larger in the ST fibers than in the FT fibers. Whether this is different in the subgroups of FT fibers is not known, although staining with Sudan black or oil red for lipids does indicate that this is the case.[17, 22] The Ca^{++}-activated myosin ATPase is approximately 2.5 times higher in FT than ST fibers, which matches well with the data on contraction times.[18, 20] Whether FT_a fibers have a higher myosin ATPase activity or a faster time to peak tension than FT_b fibers cannot be settled either by our work[21] or other data.[19, 27] In rat soleus muscle Kugelberg found a close relationship between histochemical staining intensity for myofibrillar ATPase and contraction times.[5] Based on these results Prince *et al.*[13] have suggested that the FG (FT_b) fibers have slower contraction times than the FOG (FT_a) fibers in man. This may be true, but with the existing large variation between species, we need more direct evidence before any firm conclusions can be drawn on this particular point. Moreover, Burke's data on cat muscle point to the possibility of quite different contraction times, although histochemical staining properties are the same or very similar.[4, 25]

Muscle Fiber Composition in Human Skeletal Muscle

The most commonly studied muscle in man is the lateral portion of the thigh (vastus lateralis). In a recent study of 70 men and 45 women—all 16-years-old—representing an unselected group of individuals at this age, a mean value of 52% of total fibers as being ST fibers was found for both sexes[28] (FIGURE 3). Within the FT fibers, the FT_a fibers were approximately twice as common as the FT_b fibers, the mean values being 33% and 14% of total fibers, respectively. Similar mean values for the percentage of ST, FT_a, and FT_b fibers were observed in a study of 54 adult women.[29] Thus, ample evidence is available suggesting that no difference exists between males and females in this respect. For both sexes a wide variation in fiber composition between individuals is present, which is most pronounced for the males. Whether this is due to a sex difference cannot be fully answered today. However, all available reports on muscle fiber composition in man indicate that greater extremes in fiber composition are found in males.[26, 28-33]

Another difference between the sexes is found in the size of the fibers. In general, cross-sectional areas of fibers are larger in male than in female muscle (TABLE 3). In men the mean cross-sectional area of the FT fibers of the thigh (FT_a being larger than FT_b fibers) is larger than the mean area of ST fiber,

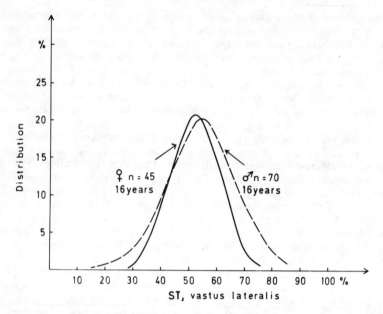

FIGURE 3. The distribution of relative occurrence of ST fibers in vastus lateralis in men and women.[28]

TABLE 3

CROSS-SECTIONAL AREAS (μm^2) OF SKELETAL MUSCLE FIBERS
IN THE VASTUS LATERALIS MUSCLE FROM NOT SPECIALLY TRAINED SUBJECTS *

Fiber Type	Male		Female	
	16 yrs	20–30 yrs	16 yrs	20–30 yrs
ST	4880 (1200)	5310 (1210)	4310 (1270)	3948 (740)
FT$_a$	5500 (1390)	6110 (1200)	4310 (1300)	3637 (820)
FT$_b$	4900 (1590)	5600 (1450)	3920 (910)	2235 (605)
n	70	10	45	25
References	28	36, 53, 81	28	29

* Mean values ($\pm$ standard deviations). The increase in muscle fiber size after the age of 16 in males is most likely related to the fact that they are still growing. Females do not grow much after the age of 16. The reduction in muscle fiber may be related to less physical activity later in life.

whereas in sedentary women the ST fiber is larger than the FT_a. In both sexes the FT_b fiber is the smallest fiber. One possible explanation for the difference between fiber areas in the two sexes may be related to differences in the physical activity pattern. All fiber types can respond to increased activity with some enlargement of the size of the fiber.[34-36] In particular, the FT fibers can markedly increase their size.[37] The small-sized FT fibers in the thigh muscles of sedentary women may be related to the fact that only a few daily life activities involve the FT fibers. In favor of such a hypothesis is the finding that the FT fibers are larger than the ST fibers in the deltoid muscle of females with small children or among groups of females playing team handball,[29] and also the fact that 16-year-old girls who are still quite active physically have the same size FT_a and ST fibers.[28] Brooke and Kaiser [38] have reached a similar conclusion when comparing mothers having severely handicapped children with mothers having children with no disabilities. The former had larger FT fibers than the latter.

One of the problems encountered when muscle fiber composition is determined on small muscle samples (<200 fibers) is whether there exists a large variation in fiber composition and fiber sizes within a muscle. In post mortem studies it has been shown that little or no variation exists between different parts of the muscle.[39, 40] If there is a difference, a mean value of 5%-10% higher content of ST fibers is found in the center of the muscle.[40] These findings may partly explain why the coefficient of variation for the fiber composition is reported to be between 5%-8% when repeated sampling from the deltoid or vastus lateralis muscle of an individual is performed.[29, 31, 33]

Muscle Fiber Composition in Different Muscles

There is a large interindividual variation in muscle fiber composition, but what about the fiber composition in different muscles of the same subject? Post mortem studies of muscle fiber composition indicate that a certain relationship exists (FIGURE 4). The available data also demonstrate that there are rather close similarities between some muscles whereas other muscles have a more pronounced predominance of one fiber type. The vastus lateralis, rectus femoris, and gastrocnemius muscles of the lower extremity and the deltoid and biceps muscles of the upper extremity appear to contain approximately 50% ST and 50% FT fibers. On the other hand, the soleus muscle has 25%-40% more ST fibers than the other leg muscles, and the triceps muscle 10%-30% more FT fibers than the other arm muscles. It might be expected that the postural muscles around the spine and the intercostal muscles would be predominantly made up of ST fibers. This, however, is not the case.[20, 40] One explanation for the fact that most skeletal muscles of man are so homogenously mixed is that although they may have special functions demanding a special fiber type all muscles are also involved in other activities where the characteristics of the different fiber types are needed.

Muscle Fiber Composition of Athletes

During recent years it has been very popular to determine muscle fiber composition of elite athletes in different types of events. In regard to the rela-

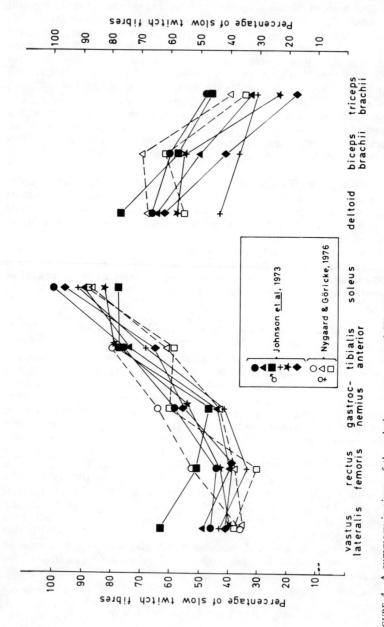

FIGURE 4. A summary is given of the relative occurrence of ST fibers in some muscles of the body.[29, 40] The muscle samples are obtained post mortem, within 24 hours after the death of the person. The death has in all cases occurred suddenly and no known diseases of muscles were present.

tive distribution of ST and FT fibers, the most interesting findings are that sprinters have a marked predominance of FT fibers in their leg muscles, and long distance runners, the opposite (FIGURE 5). It is of note also that throwers, weight-lifters, and high-jumpers generally have an even distribution of fiber types in their leg and arm muscles. Both sexes are similar in this respect.[29, 37, 41] The findings on distance runners and sprinters fit with what is known about the special characteristics of the different fibers. However, it is more difficult to understand why sprinters have a predominance of FT fibers, while athletes in more explosive events such as high-jumping and shot-putting do not. One explanation may be that in sprinting there is a greater demand on FT fibers as they fatigue so quickly.[24, 33] The possibility also exists that in athletic performances where a single contraction of one or two groups of muscles is of

TABLE 4

A SUMMARY OF RELATIVE OCCURRENCE OF DIFFERENT FIBER TYPES IN MUSCLES FROM ORIENTEERS (CROSS-COUNTRY RUNNERS), TRACK-RUNNERS (5,000 m OR LONGER DISTANCES), AND CONTROL SUBJECTS *

Male	ST	FT_a	FT_b	Unclassified
Orienteers, n=8, Reference 23				
Vastus lateralis	68.1± 8.4	24.8±10.4	3.3±4.0	4.2±4.7
Gastrocnemius	67.1± 8.7	28.9± 8.9	1.9±4.3	2.1±3.1
Deltoid	68.1±14.4	13.7± 7.9	18.2±7.9	0.0±0.0
Runners, n=10, Reference 81				
Gastrocnemius	61.4± 4.6	36.9± 5.6	0.5±0.8	1.2±1.1
Control, n=70, Reference 70				
Vastus lateralis	54.0±12.2	32.3± 9.1	13.0±7.6	0.9±2.1

* Of note is the fact that the control subjects are 16 years old, and although they are not specially trained, these boys are more physically active than 20–30-year-old men. It is unlikely that the percentage of ST fibers would be different in untrained subjects but the percentage of FT_a fibers may be a few percent too high and the FT_b fibers correspondingly too low. Mean values ± standard deviation.

importance for success, a high degree of synchronous activation of fibers is required. Such a synchronous firing pattern may be easier to establish in motor units made up of ST fibers.

Studies involving the subgrouping of FT fibers are less common, and almost all of them have involved middle and long distance runners or swimmers.[23, 42, 43] The only exceptions are some studies on three weight-lifters[13] and female[29] as well as male[44] team handball players. The occurrence of FT_a fibers was quite normal in these groups, but the size of the FT_b fibers was quite pronounced and up to twice as large as found in sedentary subjects.

Endurance-trained subjects have a high occurrence of FT_a fibers and few or no FT_b fibers in the muscles involved in the training, whereas muscle groups only partially or not at all engaged in the exercise have some or a normal content of FT_b fibers (TABLE 4). Both sexes are similar in this regard. As the

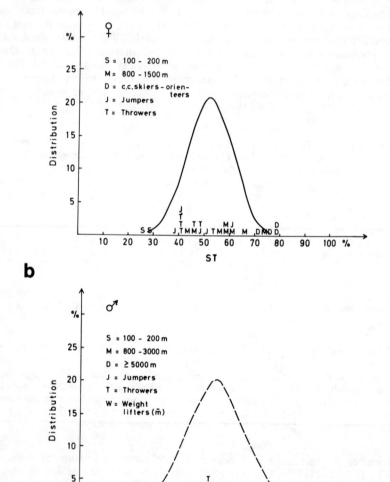

FIGURE 5. To the data in FIGURE 3 we added individual values for the relative occurrence of ST fibers in athletes performing well in different sport events.[23, 29, 31, 37, 41] (a) Female. (b) Male.

untrained muscles in endurance-trained subjects contain a normal number of FT_b fibers and since we know from studies where the activity pattern has been varied that the percentage of FT_b fibers also changes,[15, 46] it is suggested that the lack of FT_b fibers is part of an adaptive response to the endurance training. At this point it is worth emphasizing that all fiber typing on the endurance-trained muscles in our studies has been based on the stain for myofibrillar ATPase, and not on stains for any oxidative enzymes.

Metabolic Profile of Skeletal Muscles of Endurance Athletes

Frequent reports are available on enzyme activities and substrate contents of skeletal muscles of athletes. It is difficult, however, to compare enzyme data of different studies as different methods have been used and different muscles have been sampled. The problem may be partially overcome if control subjects are included. However, all too often little concern has been devoted to the problem of whether the subjects of the control group are representative or not. This is a general question in exercise physiology as so many of those who volunteer as normal or sedentary subjects very often are considerably more active than the average man. This constitutes a major problem when evaluating the oxidative potential of muscles as the mitochondrial enzymes are so closely related to the activity level. In the study of muscle fiber composition in 16-year-old boys and girls the activity of several enzymes were also measured.[28] These values cannot be used as control values, as at this age the subjects, especially the boys, but also the girls, are more physically active than people a few years older.[47] The values reported for the SDH activity in the leg muscles of the boys and girls were 10.4 ± 2.6 and 7.9 ± 2.4 mM/kg·min, respectively. Gollnick *et al.*[31] reported SDH activity for untrained men to be 8–9 mM/kg·min whereas Costill *et al.*[37, 41] found values around 6–7 mM/kg·min, and for sedentary females a mean value of 7 mM/kg·min has been reported.[29] Based on these observations it may be appropriate to consider an SDH activity in the vastus lateralis of approximately 7 mM/kg·min as a normal value for sedentary subjects, with females having slightly lower values than men.[29, 37]

Elite distance runners and swimmers have SDH activities of 20–25 mM/kg·min.[23, 42, 43] As physical inactivity results in a pronounced decrease in the SDH activity, down to levels approximately 3–4 mM/kg·min (see below), the range for the aerobic potential of the muscle cell appears to be quite large; in fact, two to three times larger than the maximal variation seen for maximal oxygen uptake, which between extremes may vary by a factor of 2–3. For the muscles of sedentary subjects the highest oxidative potential is always observed in the ST fibers. In highly trained orienteers (cross-country runners) with SDH activity levels around 21 mM/kg·min in their gastrocnemius muscles, the SDH activity of the FT fibers is as high as the ST fibers.[23] The finding indicates that it is not only the ST but also the FT_a and the FT_b fibers that can adapt and increase their oxidative capacity. In fact, on a percentage basis the FT fibers have increased the most in these subjects.

In the muscles of endurance athletes the glycolytic enzymes appear to have the same or a slightly reduced activity as compared with untrained subjects.[37, 41] The activities of the LDH isozymes 1 and 2 (and probably also hexokinase) are exceptions.[49] Both of these enzymes appear to follow the profile of the oxidative enzymes. Glycogen content is usually somewhat higher in trained than untrained muscles [50] with no demonstrated difference between fiber types. It is not known whether the triglyceride storage in skeletal muscles also is increased with training.

Capillary Supply of Skeletal Muscle

In most species skeletal muscle capillaries can easily be identified by different techniques. The capillarization of human skeletal muscle is more difficult to study, but histochemical staining [51] as well as electron microscopy [52] have been used. The following data were obtained with an ordinary PAS-stain, in which the glycogen in the muscles had been removed by preincubation of the cross-section in α-amylase,[53] thereby making the capillaries around the fibers more easily visible (FIGURE 6). In sedentary men and women the mean number of capillaries around ST and FT$_a$ fiber types is 4, and for FT$_b$ fibers, 3 (TABLE 5). When the cross-sectional area of the fiber types is taken into consideration, a significant difference in capillarization between ST fibers and the FT fibers is found for the men. For females, with rather small FT fibers in their leg muscles, this difference is insignificant.

The reason for taking the area of a fiber into account when expressing the capillary supply is that it will serve as an indication of diffusion distances. The validity of this concept can be questioned in view of our present knowledge of mitochondrial distribution [54, 55] and the function of myoglobin as a facilitator for the diffusion of oxygen within a muscle cell.[56] These factors plus the observation of a highly selective muscle fiber recruitment in different types of muscle contractions [22, 57, 58] may invalidate the use of the classical Krogh concept [59] of diffusing distances in the tissue and suggest that other measures of expressing capillary supply of muscle tissue would provide better information. The total or average number of capillaries around a muscle fiber might be more representative.

In subjects of both sexes with various aerobic power capacities, there is a close correlation between the oxygen uptake, expressed in ml/kg·min, and the mean number of capillaries per fiber (FIGURE 7). Preliminary results from longitudinal training studies indicate that the capillary supply of skeletal muscle can easily be increased, and that the increase is closely related to the activity level of the muscle.[36]

In the above, support has been presented for the concept that the size of a fiber and the diffusion distances were of lesser importance than the absolute number of capillaries around a muscle fiber. In disagreement with such a concept is the finding of surprisingly small fibers in the shoulder muscles of elite swimmers and the gastrocnemius muscles of elite orienteers.[29, 29, 43] Furthermore, they have 5–6 capillaries around each fiber (TABLE 5). When compared with untrained muscles in their own bodies or with sedentary subjects, it is striking how small the unit area per capillary is in the trained muscles of endurance athletes. The basic principles, in Krogh's view, of the importance of the diffusing distances within the tissue thus appears to be important. The functional significance could be that the level of oxygenation of all parts of a muscle cell can be kept high in a trained muscle. This would be important in the trained muscles as the intramyofibrillar content of mitochondria can be high.[54, 55]

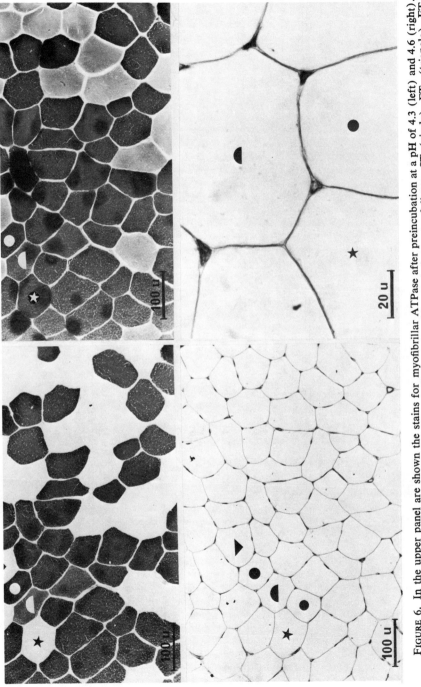

FIGURE 6. In the upper panel are shown the stains for myofibrillar ATPase after preincubation at a pH of 4.3 (left) and 4.6 (right). The lower panel shows the modified PAS-stain (two magnifications). The symbols are as follows: ST (circle), FT_a (triangle), FT_b (star), and unclassified (=IIc, half circle).

TABLE 5

CAPILLARY SUPPLY OF HUMAN SKELETAL MUSCLE FIBERS

| | Number of Capillaries Around Fiber Types | | | | | | Fiber Type Area (μm^2) per Capillary | | | | | |
| | Vastus Lateralis | | | Deltoid | | | Vastus Lateralis | | | Deltoid | | |
	ST	FT$_a$	FT$_b$	ST	FT$_a$	FT$_b$	ST	FT$_a$	FT$_b$	ST	FT$_a$	FT$_b$
Sedentaries												
Male												
$n=3$, Reference 53	4.2	4.0	3.2				1014	1335	1338			
Female												
$n=8$, Reference 29	4.6 (1.1)*	3.7 (1.1)	2.9 (0.9)	3.7	3.2	2.5	1034 (263)	1062 (301)	878 (312)	1339	1966	1956
Endurance trained												
Male (runners)												
$n=3$, Reference 53	5.9	5.2	4.3				997	1213	1235			
$n=3$, Reference 23	5.9	5.4	—									
Female (runners)												
$n=4$, Reference 29	5.1 (0.8)	4.8 (0.9)	3.6 (0.5)	5.2 (0.9)	5.4 (1.0)	—	901 (308)	871 (194)	840 (176)	635 (77)	719 (38)	—

* Numbers in parentheses indicate standard deviations.

Adaptations to Endurance Training

Earlier, some indications were given about the responses seen in skeletal muscle as a result of endurance training. This discussion has mainly been based on cross-sectional studies of subjects with well-established differences in physical activity pattern for extended periods of time. In this section we will examine the same problems but to a larger extent will rely upon longitudinal studies. In rats, a variation in the activity level causes the oxidative potential of muscle

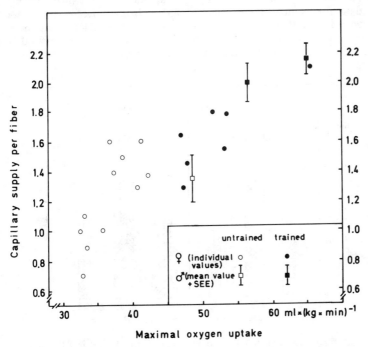

FIGURE 7. Mean number of capillaries per muscle fiber (vastus lateralis) in relation to the maximal oxygen uptake (bicycle exercise). Observations on extremely well-trained subjects (the deltoid and the gastroc muscles) indicate that the mean number of capillaries per fiber in these subjects is above the value presented in the graph.[23, 29, 36, 43, 53]

to vary.[60] The situation is quite similar in man. When a leg is immobilized in a cast for 4 weeks the activity of SDH drops to half of its initial value, and intense retraining for 4–6 weeks returns the enzyme activity to a normal level.[46] When sedentary subjects participate in a conditioning program the activity of both citric acid cycle (SDH) and respiratory chain enzymes (cytochrome oxidase) are enhanced.[61] During the first 4 weeks no difference between the increase of these two enzymes and the increase in maximal oxygen uptake is found. After the first month of training the rate of enhancement of maximal oxygen uptake is less than that of the oxidative enzymes. Following the termination of the training program the maximal oxygen uptake returns much more slowly to pretraining levels than do the oxidative enzymes. This augmentation of the oxidative potential of the muscle is localized in the fibers most actively involved in the training regimen.[62] Thus low-medium intensity training, mainly involving ST fibers during the training sessions, only gave rise to a significant increase in the SDH activity of the ST fibers (FIGURE 8). On the other hand, after high intensity interval training, the largest increase in SDH activity was found in the FT fibers.

These findings complement the cross-sectional data and show that skeletal muscle of man has a wide capacity for adaptation of its oxidative potential. These data also point to the possibility of their being different stimuli for the oxidative potential of the muscle cells and for the factors determining the whole body's capacity to consume oxygen as the time course for changes is so different during the later phases of the training and in the period after the training.[61]

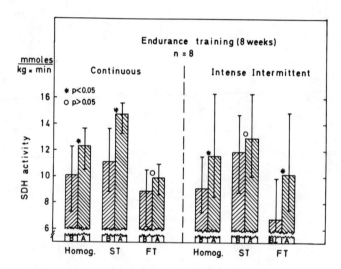

FIGURE 8. The activity of SDH in homogenate of muscle and in ST and FT fibers before and after continuous and interval type training.[62]

Our results may also give some insight into the factors regulating the synthesis and degradation of the oxidative enzymes. It has been suggested that intracellular hypoxia is the trigger for the changes observed in training.[63] The marked enhancement of the oxidative capacity of the muscle cells during chronic submaximal exercise argues against hypoxia being a factor of importance. Recently Harri and Valtola [64] put forward the idea of a specific activation of the β-receptors of the muscle fibers when they are involved in this muscular activity. This latter possibility fits well with the present finding of the importance of the fibers being activated for a change to take place. We cannot, however, distinguish between an eventual role for the activation of β-receptors, trophic or acetylcholine activity mediated by the motor nerve,[65] or any metabolic factor closely linked to the metabolic status of the cell or to the flux of oxygen.

The same type of muscular activity that gave rise to an increased oxidative capacity of the muscle has little or no effect on the glycolytic potential when judged from cross-sectional studies.[37] In fact, elite distance runners usually have a low level of glycolytic enzymes.[23, 37, 41] Longitudinal studies do not offer a clear-cut picture. In training studies aimed at an improvement of the maximal oxygen capacity of the body, both an increase in phosphofructokinase [34, 66] and no increase has been observed.[62] In a study where leg muscle strength was improved, no change in phosphofructokinase activity was found.[67, 68] At the moment no studies are available where the aim has been to improve the local anaerobic potential. Most likely the glycolytic potential can be enhanced by training, but the stimulus for this to occur is very specific and different from what enhances aerobic potential and strength.

It was mentioned above that in the endurance-trained muscles few or no FT$_b$ fibers were present (TABLE 4). Moreover, in some of these muscles as high as 10%–12% of the fibers were darkly stained at both acid and alkaline preincubations (type IIC fibers in the Brooke and Kaiser scheme,[14, 15] but probably better named unclassified).[23, 43] These facts bring us back to the question of whether a physiological stimulus such as extreme endurance training can result in a conversion of fiber types? Burke and Edgerton [8] are convinced that this does not take place if the fiber typing is based on "the property of contraction time and associated myosin ATPase activity." It is true that no direct measurements of these kinds are available on skeletal muscle from man in connection with endurance training, but as pointed out above, there is already a change in sensitivity for an acid pH after some weeks of moderate endurance training.[15] In fact, having a leg in a cast for 4 weeks and then resuming training for another 4-week period causes the same changes to occur.[46] That is, the number of fibers with increased sensitivity for pH 4.6–4.8 (FT$_a$ fibers) is reduced with the immobilization and increased in the retraining period.[46] Since Brooke and Kaiser have shown that the difference in pH sensitivity is related to the reactivity of sulfhydryl groups of the myosin molecule,[15] it is conceivable that the lack of FT$_b$ fibers in the endurance-trained muscles reflects a change in the structure of the myosin molecules. It should be quite clear, however, that the present results do not prove that a "true" interconversion of fibers occurs but they are indicative of this possibility. Further studies with more extreme training and measurement of Ca^{++}-activated myosin ATPase or Mg^{++}-activated actomyosin ATPase are needed.

In none of the longitudinal studies, where there was an observed change in the ratio of FT$_a$ to FT$_b$ fibers, has a significant change in the number of unclassified (type IIC) fibers been detected. Again it must be emphasized that the intensity, and especially the duration of the training, are very small in these longitudinal studies as compared with what today's elite distance runners undertake. Thus, the lack of an increase in the number of unclassified (type IIC) fibers in the longitudinal studies is no proof that endurance training is not able to cause it. Moreover, the unclassified fibers are there in some of the very best endurance-trained runners, and their presence requires an explanation.

The only time in life when there normally is a high percentage of unclassified (type IIC) fibers is after birth when the muscles may contain 10%–50% of these fibers.[69] They are thought of as being undifferentiated muscle fibers.[70, 71] The content of these fibers is reduced to less than 2% within a year after birth.[69] Do these unclassified fibers found in endurance-trained muscles constitute fibers in a stage of development waiting for the nerve to establish the contact? This question cannot be answered.

It can be said that fiber splitting can occur as a result of a physiological overload. In cats trained to lift larger and larger weights the number of fibers increase considerably.[72] To what extent can results from strength training of cat forearm flexor muscles help explain our present problem is not known. There are some facts arguing against a hypothesis of fiber splitting with extreme endurance training, one being that most unclassified fibers are of similar sizes to the ST fibers, although some few fibers can be quite small. Another fact is that no contact with a mother cell appears to be present. On the other hand, the finding of small fibers in the bulky muscles of endurance-trained swimmers [24, 43] implies a need for new fibers to be developed at some stage of the training. The finding by Pette and associates [73] of a reduction in fiber size as a function of prolonged tonic stimulation is, in this connection, of interest.

Another explanation for the high percentage of type IIC fibers found in orienteers' trained muscles put forward by Jansson and Kaijser [23] is that it is related to a degenerative-regenerative process continuously going on in these heavily overloaded muscles. It is known that satelite cells in necrotic fibers develop.[74] It is difficult to see, however, why muscle fibers of the vastus and the gastrocnemius muscles should become necrotic. Moreover, this explanation also lacks the support of a histochemical picture of fibers in various stages of development. A third possibility could be that the functional contact between the motor nerve and some of the muscle fibers in the unit is momentarily lost, and later re-established. Such an explanation is very similar to the concept of sick motorneurons put forward by McComas and associates [75] in explaining some muscular disorders.

Whether or not any of the proposed explanations can be proved to be right the observation of a varying number of unclassified fibers with extreme endurance training is a challenging one, and the problem deserves to be studied in great depth.

Importance of Local Adjustment

There appears to be no question about the importance of the enhancement of the oxidative potential and the capillarization of the muscle cell for its capacity to perform endurance work and to utilize oxygen,[35, 76] although the time course for these changes to take place may not be directly related, nor may they, from a quantitative standpoint, match each other.[61] Further, females have a lower oxidative potential than males in their muscle at a given maximal oxygen uptake.[28, 37] Some of these aspects are dealt with elsewhere.[46] Here, more attention will be focused upon the changes in the metabolic response to exercise that accompany the enhanced aerobic potential of the muscle cell.

In studies where only one leg has been trained, the local adaptation can be proven to occur only in the trained leg.[35, 76] When regular two-legged submaximal exercise is performed after training, significantly less lactate is accumulated in the trained leg (FIGURE 9). The release of lactate from the trained leg during a 1-hour exercise period decreases until there is no release or an uptake during the latter phases of the exercise period. The untrained limb releases lactate throughout the exercise period. Utilization of substrate during the 1-hour exercise period is also changed towards a significantly higher rate of oxidation of lipids in the trained as compared to the untrained leg.[76] That these changes take place with training has been known for a long time. The present results may add to our understanding of the metabolism taking place during exercise in terms of the regulatory mechanisms involved.

Since the arterial blood supply is the same to the two legs during the exercise,[35, 76] the supply of substrate or the presence of hormones must be similar and can be excluded as being important for the observed differences. Instead, the results point to the overall enhancement of the aerobic potential (including capillarization) of the muscle cell as being crucial.

The possible regulatory mechanisms involved range from a change in the number of receptor places or proteins of the muscle fibers to simple factors such as reduced diffusing distances for substrates furnished by the blood. It is

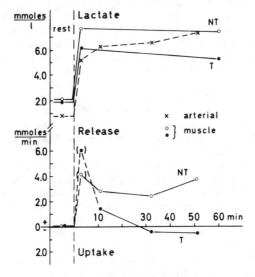

FIGURE 9. Lactate concentrations in muscle and blood when performing two-legged bicycle exercise for 1 hour at about 70% of maximal oxygen uptake, and the release of lactate from untrained and trained leg.[35]

well documented that the uptake and oxidation of free fatty acids (FFA) by the muscle is a function of the arterial FFA concentration, and that during exercise only a small fraction of what is offered the exercising muscles is utilized.[77] The major limitation in the transport of FFA from the capillary to the cell is the diffusion of the albumin-bound FFA molecule in the capillaries. There is a very low percentage of the FFA as the free form in the plasma and interstitial fluid. Any reduction in the diffusion distance between capillaries and muscle cells facilitates FFA uptake and enhances its utilization. As an augmentation of both capillaries and mitochondrial oxidative enzymes is found with training, not only of ST but also of the two types of FT fibers an enhancement of the oxidation of FFA may occur in all types of fibers. In turn, citrate concentration can be raised in these fibers thus having an inhibitory influence on the activity of phosphofructokinase, retarding glycolysis and lactate formation.[22, 78]

Some Practical Implications

In FIGURE 10 a schematic and in part hypothetical summary is given for the adaptive responses with training seen for some of the variables discussed above. Maximal oxygen uptake may increase 15%–30% during the first 2–3 months of training, and a further improvement to 40%–50% may occur over the next 9–24 months. After a termination of the training, maximal oxygen uptake will rather slowly return to the pretraining level. The concomitant changes in citric acid cycle and respiratory chain enzymes are more vivid, as these enzymes may have rather short turnover times, with half-lives on the order of 1 to 3 weeks.[61] Less precise is the information about the time course for and the magnitude of the conversion of FT_b to FT_a fibers and degree of capillarization. Transition of fiber types may be quite labile in a manner similar to the oxidative enzymes, whereas the capillarization especially after a training period may change at a slower rate. Of note is the fact that data on man for this particular point is almost completely lacking. From a practical standpoint, these differences in time courses for the adaptive response of the muscle can have some interest. After 8–10 weeks of a conditioning program, the time where so many longitudinal studies are terminated, no difference between the relative changes in any of the variables studied is significant. Thus a good relationship is found between all indices of the training response.

After half a year or more of uninterrupted training, the situation may be quite different. The metabolic capacity of the tissue may be enhanced to a much larger extent than the circulatory capacity and the capacity of the body to utilize oxygen. In this phase lactate production and lactate accumulation in muscle and blood during exercise may be lower than expected from the relative exercise intensity. Moreover, the glycogen-saving effect, which training brings about, is probably most pronounced at this stage of the training. A practical consequence of this could be that the capacity to perform prolonged exercise is also augmented; i.e., the well-trained person can work closer to his maximal oxygen uptake for a longer period of time. In the two studies available on the relationship between short-term and long-term work capacity with training, no significant differences could be established comparing untrained subjects with endurance athletes[79] or before and after the participation in a conditioning program.[80] The explanation for the inability to demonstrate a difference could be that in the cross-sectional study the exercise tests were performed on a bicycle ergometer and the trained subjects were runners.[79] In the longitudinal study the training period may have been too short to reach the point of demarcation between maximal oxygen uptake and the metabolic capacity of the muscle tissue.[80] During the time of peak performance capacity the level of adaptation is maximal, resulting in a lowered rate of glycogen utilization and a high rate of lipid oxidation. Both of these metabolic factors are of primary importance for the observed enhanced work capacity, especially the capacity to perform intense exercise for an extended period of time (>30 min). During the detraining period a reverse situation may be present; a rapidly declining content of mitochondrial enzymes with a more slowly decreasing level of maximal oxygen uptake. Thus, a comparison of the circulatory and metabolic

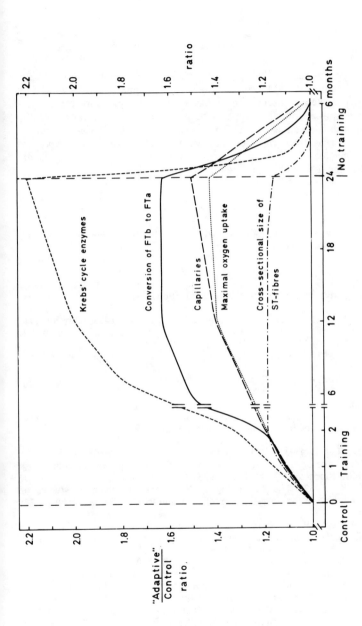

FIGURE 10. A schematic, and in part, hypothetical summary of some of the adaptations taking place in active muscle with endurance training (bicycling or running). The graph is based on longitudinal and cross-sectional studies of man. When there is a complete lack of data from man (as in the case for the capillarization after training) results from other species have been used. It should be pointed out that in endurance trained muscles the ST fibers can be smaller than what is observed in the same muscle of sedentary people (c.f. the deltoid muscle of female swimmers). For further explanation see the text.

capacities associated with peak performance and some weeks of detraining may more fully elucidate the factors related to the capacity to perform prolonged work.

Summary

This description of some of the present knowledge on skeletal muscle fibers, their metabolic potentials, and their interplay with the degree of physical activity has revealed that skeletal muscle of man has a very large capacity for adaptation. Moreover, this adaptability appears to be of utmost importance for the metabolic response as well as for performance. Although all this is true, it should not distract us from the fact that we are lacking the most important information. The questions that need to be answered are: What triggers the changes to take place? Which are the regulatory mechanisms?

References

1. PERNOW, B. & B. SALTIN, Eds. 1971. Muscle metabolism during exercise. Vol. 11. Plenum Press. New York.
2. HOWALD, H. & J. POORTMANS, Eds. 1975. Metabolic adaptation to prolonged physical exercise. Birkhäuser Verlag. Basel, Switzerland.
3. EDSTRÖM, L. & E. KUGELBERG. 1968. Histochemical composition, distribution of fibers and fatiguability of single motor units. J. Neurol. Psychiat. 31: 424–433.
4. BURKE, R. E., D. N. LEVINE, P. TSAIRIS & F. E. ZAJAC. 1973. Physiological types and histochemical profiles in motor units of the cat gastrocnemius. J. Physiol. 234: 723–748.
5. KUGELBERG, E. 1973. Histochemical composition, contraction speed and fatiguability of rat soleus motor units. J. Neurol. Sci. 20: 177–198.
6. PEARSE, A. G. E. 1961. Histochemistry—Theoretical and Applied. 1st edit. (And 1968. 2nd edit.) Churchill. London.
7. NEEDHAM, D. M. 1926. Red and white muscle. Physiol. Rev. 6: 1.
8. BURKE, E. & V. R. EDGERTON. 1975. Motor unit properties and selective involvement in movement. In "Exercise and Sport Sciences Reviews" Vol. 3, pp. 31–81.
9. PETER, J. B., R. J. BARNARD, V. R. EDGERTON, C. A. GILLESPIE & K. E. STEMPEL. 1972. Metabolic profiles of three fibre types of skeletal muscle in guinea pigs and rabbits. Biochemistry. 11: 2627–2633.
10. ENGEL, W. K. 1962. The essentiality of histo- and cytochemical studies of skeletal muscle in the investigation of neuromuscular disease. Neurol. 12: 778–784.
11. BARNARD, R. J., V. R. EDGERTON, T. FURUKAWA & J. B. PETER. 1971. Histochemical biochemical, and contractile properties of red, white and intermediate fibres. Amer. J. Physiol. 220: 410–414.
12. EDGERTON, V. R., B. SALTIN, B. ESSEN & D. R. SIMPSON. 1975. Glycogen depletion in specific types of human skeletal fibers in intermittent and continuous exercise. In Metabolic Adaptations to Prolonged Physical Exercise. H. Howald & J. Poortmans, Eds. Birkhäuser Verlag. Basel, Switzerland.
13. PRINCE, F. P., R. S. HIKIDA & F. C. HAGERMAN. 1976. Human muscle fibre types in power lifters, distance runners, and untrained subjects. Pflügers Arch. 363: 19–26.
14. BROOKE, M. H. & K. K. KAISER. 1970. Muscle fibre types: how many and what kind? Arch. of Neurol. (Chicago) 23: 369–379.

15. BROOKE, M. H. & K. K. KAISER. 1970. Three "myosin ATPase" systems: the nature of their pH liability and sulphydryl dependence. J. Histochem. Cytochem. **18:** 670–672.
16. GUTH, L. & F. J. SAMAHA. 1969. Qualitative differences between actomyosin ATPase of slow and fast mammalian muscle. Exp. Neurol. **25:** 138–152.
17. SCHMALBRUCH, H. & Z. KAMIENIECKA. 1974. Fibre types in the human brachial biceps muscle. Exp. Neurol. **44:** 313–328.
18. EBERSTEIN, A. & J. GOODGOLD. 1968. Slow and fast twitch fibres in human skeletal muscle. Amer. J. Physiol. **215:** 535–541.
19. BUCHTHAL, F. & H. SCHMALBRUCH. 1970. Contraction times and fibre types in intact human muscle. Acta Physiol. Scand. **79:** 435–452.
20. HANSON, J. 1974. Effects of repetitive stimulation on membrane potentials and twitch in human and rat muscle fibres. Acta Physiol. Scand. **92:** 238–248.
21. ESSÉN, B., E. JANSSON, J. HENRIKSSON, A. W. TAYLOR & B. SALTIN. 1975. Metabolic characteristics of fibre types in human skeletal muscles. Acta Physiol. Scand. **95:** 153–165.
22. ESSÉN, B. 1977. Ann. N.Y. Acad. Sci. This volume.
23. WAHREN, J., P. FELIG, G. AHLBORG & L. JORFELDT. 1971. Glucose metabolism Acta Physiol. Scand. **99.** To be published.
24. THORSTENSSON, A. & J. KARLSSON. 1976. Fatigability and fibre composition of human skeletal muscle. Acta Physiol. Scand. **98:** 318–322.
25. BURKE, R. E. & P. TSAIRIS. 1974. The corrleation of physiological properties with histochemical characteristics in single muscle units. Ann. N.Y. Acad. Sci. **228:** 145–159.
26. EDSTRÖM, L. & B. NYSTRÖM. 1969. Histochemical types and sizes of fibres in normal human muscles. Acta Neurol. Scand. **45:** 257–269.
27. THORSTENSSON, A., P. TESCH, B. SJÖDIN & J. KARLSSON. 1977. Actomyosin ATPase, myokinase, CPK, and LDH in human fast and slow twitch muscle fibres. Acta Physiol. Scand. **99:** 225–229.
28. HEDBERG, G. & E. JANSSON. 1976. Skelettmuskelfiberkomposition. Kapacitet och intresse för olika fysiska aktiviteter bland elever i gymnasieskolan. Rapport 54, Pedagogiska Inst., Umeå.
29. NYGAARD, E. & T. GØRICKE. 1976. Morphological studies of skeletal muscles in women. Report No. 99 (in Danish). August Krogh Institute. Copenhagen.
30. BROOKE, M. & W. ENGEL. 1969. The histographic analysis of human muscle biopsies with regard to fibre types. Neurology (Minneapolis) **19:** 221–233.
31. GOLLNICK, P. D., R. B. ARMSTRONG, C. W. SAUBERT IV, K. PIEHL & B. SALTIN. 1972. Enzyme activity and fiber composition in skeletal muscle of untrained and trained men. J. Appl. Physiol. **33:** 312–314.
32. EDSTRÖM, L. & B. EKBLOM. 1972. Differences in sizes of red and white muscle fibres in vastus lateralis of muscle quadriceps femoris or normal individuals and athletes. Scand. J. Clin. Lab. Invest. **30:** 175–181.
33. THORSTENSSON, A., L. LARSSON, P. TESCH & J. KARLSSON. 1976. Muscle strength and fiber composition in athletes and sedentary men. Med. Sci. Sports. To be published.
34. GOLLNICK, P. D., R. B. ARMSTRONG, B. SALTIN, C. W. SAUBERT IV, W. L. SEMBROWICH & R. E. SHEPHERD. 1973. Effect of training on enzyme activity and fibre composition of human skeletal muscle. J. Appl. Physiol. **34:** 107–111.
35. SALTIN, B., K. NAZAR, D. L. COSTILL, E. STEIN, E. JANSSON, B. ESSÉN & P. D. GOLLNICK. 1976. The nature of the training response, peripheral and central adaptations to one-legged exercise. Acta Physiol. Scand. **96:** 289–305.
36. ANDERSEN, P. & J. HENRIKSSON. 1977. Capillary supply of the quadriceps femoris muscle of man: Adaptive response to exercise. J. Physiol. To be published.
37. COSTILL, D. L., J. DANIELS, W. EVANS, W. FINK, G. KRAHENBUHL & B. SALTIN. 1976. Skeletal muscle enzymes and fibre composition in male and female and track athletes. J. Appl. Physiol. **90:** 149–154.

38. BROOKE, M. H. & K. K. KAISER. 1974. The use and abuse of muscle histochemistry. Ann. N.Y. Acad. Sci. **228:** 121–144.
39. EDGERTON, V. R., J. L. SMITH & D. R. SIMPSON. 1975. Muscle fibre type populations of human leg muscles. Histochem. J. **7:** 259–266.
40. JOHNSON, M. A., J. POLGAR, D. WEIGHTMAN & D. APPLETON. 1973. Data on distribution of fibre types in thirty-six human muscles. An autopsy study. J. Neurol. Sci. **18:** 111–129.
41. COSTILL, D. L., W. J. FINK & M. L. POLLOCK. 1976. Muscle fiber composition and ezyme activities of elite distance runners. Med. Sci. Sports. **8:** 96–100.
42. JANSSON, E. 1975. Type II fibers in human skeletal muscle: Biochemical characteristics and distribution. Acta Physiol. Scand. **95:** 47A.
43. NYGAARD, E. 1976. Adaptational changes in human skeletal muscle with different levels of physical activity. Acta Physiol. Scand. Suppl. **440:** 291.
44. MIKKELSEN, F. & M. OLESEN. 1976. Handboll, idrottsfysiologisk rapport nr. 118, Trygg-Hansa, Stockholm.
45. ANDERSEN, P. & J. HENRIKSSON. 1977. Training induced changes in the subgroups of human Type II skeletal muscle fibres. Acta Physiol. Scand. **99:** 123–125.
46. SALTIN, B. 1977. The interplay between peripheral and central factors in the adaptive response to exercise and training. Ann. N.Y. Acad. Sci. This volume.
47. ENGSTRÖM, L. M. 1975. Fysisk Aktivitet under Ungdomsåren (In Swedish). Pedagogiska Institutionen, Lärarhögskolan i Stockholm.
48. SJÖDIN, B. 1976. Lactate dehydrogenase in human skeletal muscle. Acta Physiol. Scand. Suppl. 436.
49. BASS, A., K. VONDRA, R. RATH & V. VITEK. 1975. M. quadriceps femoris of man, a muscle with an unusual enzyme activity pattern of energy supplying metabolism in mammals. Pflügers Arch. **354:** 249–255.
50. HERMANSEN, L., E. HULTMAN & B. SALTIN. 1967. Muscle glycogen during prolonged severe exercise. Acta Physiol. Scand. **71:** 129–139.
51. HERMANSEN, L. & M. WACHTLOVA. 1971. Capillary density of skeletal muscle in well-trained and untrained men. J. Appl. Physiol. **30:** 860–863.
52. BRODAL, P., F. INGJER & L. HERMANSEN. 1976. Capillary supply of skeletal muscle fibers in untrained and endurance trained men. Acta Physiol. Scand. Suppl. **440:** 178.
53. ANDERSEN, P. 1975. Capillary density in skeletal muscle of man. Acta Physiol. Scand. **95:** 203–205.
54. KIESSLING, K. H., K. PIEHL & C. G. LUNDQUIST. 1971. Effect of physical training on ultrastructural features in human skeletal muscle. In Muscle Metabolism during Exercise. B. Pernow & B. Saltin, Eds. Vol. 11. Plenum Press. New York, N.Y.
55. HOWALD, H. 1975. Ultrastructural adaptation of skeletal muscle to prolonged physical exercise. In Metabolic Adaptation to Prolonged Physical Exercise. Eds.: H. Howald & J. R. Poortmans, Eds. Vol. 8. Birkhäuser Verlag. Basel, Switzerland.
56. WITTENBERG, J. B. 1970. Myoglobin-facilitated oxygen diffusion: Role of myoglobin in oxygen entry into muscle. Physiol. Rev. **50:** 560–656.
57. GOLLNICK, P. D., K. PIEHL & B. SALTIN. 1974. Selective glycogen depletion pattern in human skeletal muscle fibres after exercise of varying intensity and at varying pedalling rates. J. Physiol. **241:** 45–57.
58. GOLLNICK, P. D., J. KARLSSON, K. PIEHL & B. SALTIN. 1974. Selective glycogen depletion in skeletal muscle fibres of man following sustained contractions. J. Physiol. **241:** 59–67.
59. KROGH, A. 1918/19. The number and distribution of capillaries in muscles with calculations of the oxygen pressure head necessary for supplying the tissue. J. Physiol. **52:** 409–415.
60. HOLLOSZY, J. O. & F. W. BOOTH. 1976. Biochemical adaptations to endurance training in muscle. Amer. Rev. Physiol. **38:** 273–291.

61. HENRIKSSON, J. & J. S. REITMAN. 1977. Time course of activity changes in human skeletal muscle succinate dehydrogenase and cytochrome oxidase activities and maximal oxygen uptake with physical activity and inactivity. Acta Physiol. Scand. **99**: 91–97.

62. HENRIKSSON, J. & J. S. REITMAN. 1976. Quantitative measures of enzyme activities in type I and type II muscle fibres of man after training. Acta Physiol. Scand. **97**: 392–397.

63. HOLM, J. & T. SCHERSTÉN. 1974. Metabolic changes in skeletal muscles after physical conditioning and in peripheral arterial insufficiency. Swedish J. Defence Med. **10**: 71.

64. HARRI, M. N. E. & J. VALTOLA. 1975. Comparison of the effects of physical exercise, cold acclimation and repeated injections of isoprenaline on rat muscle enzymes. Acta Physiol. Scand. **95**: 391–399.

65. GUTMAN, E. 1976. Neurotrophic relations. *In* Ann. Review Physiol. **38**: 177–216.

66. ERIKSSON, B., P. D. GOLLNICK & B. SALTIN. 1973. Muscle metabolism and enzyme activities after training in boys 11–13 years old. Acta Physiol. Scand. **87**: 485–497.

67. THORSTENSSON, A., B. SJÖDIN & J. KARLSSON. 1975. Enzyme activities and muscle strength after "sprint training" in man. Acta Physiol. Scand. **94**: 313–318.

68. THORSTENSSON, A., B. HULTÉN, W. VON DÖBELN & J. KARLSSON. 1976. Effect of strength training on enzyme activities and fibre characteristics in human skeletal muscle. Acta Physiol. Scand. **96**: 392–398.

69. COLLING-SALTIN, A. S. 1977. Enzyme histochemistry of developing skeletal muscle in the fetus. To be published.

70. DUBOWITZ, V. 1967. Infantile muscular atrophy—a broad spectrum. Clinical Proceedings of the Children's Hospital (Washington) **23**: 223.

71. DUBOWITZ, V. & M. H. BROOKE. 1973. "Muscle Biopsy: a Modern Approach," In: "Major Problems in Neurology," Vol. 2. W. B. Saunders Co., Ltd., London.

72. GONYEA, W. J., E. G. ERICSON & F. BONDE-PETERSEN. 1976. Fibre splitting in skeletal muscle induced by weight lifting exercise in cats. Acta Physiol. Scand. **99**: 105–109.

73. PETTE, D., B. U. RAMIREZ, W. MÜLLER, R. SIMON, G. U. EXNER & R. HILDEBRAND. 1975. Influence of intermittent long-term stimulation on contractile, histochemical and metabolic properties of fibre populations in fast and slow rabbit muscles. Pflügers Arch. **361**: 1–7.

74. SCHMALBRUCH, H. & U. HELLHAMMER. 1976. The number of satellite cells in normal human muscle. The anatomical record. **185**: 229–288.

75. McCOMAS, A. J., R. E. P. SICA, A. R. M. UPTON & F. PETITO. 1974. Sick motoneurons and muscle disease. Ann. N.Y. Acad. Sci. **228**: 261–270.

76. HENRIKSSON, J. 1977. Training induced adaptation of skeletal muscle and metabolism during submaximal exercise. J. Physiol. To be published.

77. GOLLNICK, P. D. 1970. Ann. N.Y. Acad. Sci. This volume.

78. NEWSHOLME, E. A. 1977. Ann. N.Y. Acad. Sci. This volume.

79. SALTIN, B. 1973. Oxygen transport by the circulatory system during exercise in man. *In* Factors Limiting Physical Performance. J. Keul, Ed. : 235–251. Georg Thieme Verlag. Stuttgart.

80. NORDESJÖ, L.-O. 1974. The effect of quantitated training on the capacity for short and prolonged work. Acta Physiol. Scand. Suppl. 405.

81. SALTIN, B. *et al.* Unpublished observations.

INTRAMUSCULAR SUBSTRATE UTILIZATION DURING PROLONGED EXERCISE *

Birgitta Essén

Department of Clinical Physiology
Karolinska Hospital
S-104 01 Stockholm
Sweden

Analyses of respiratory exchange ratios suggest that both lipids and carbohydrates contribute to energy metabolism during prolonged muscular exercise.[1] During the last ten years several studies [2-6] have shown that the glycogen stores of the striated muscles are important substrate sources during prolonged heavy exercise whereas only a few studies [7-9] have as yet considered the importance of the contribution of local triglycerides to energy metabolism.

It is known that the human skeletal muscle contain fiber types with different metabolic characteristics.[10] The type I fibers have a higher oxidative capacity than the type II fibers, and type IIA fibers have a greater oxidative capacity than the more glycolytic type IIB fibers. At rest all fibers reveal a similar glycogen content, whereas during running and bicycle exercise different rates of glycogen depletion have been found.[5, 6, 11]

In this article attention will be paid to the storage and utilization of lipids and carbohydrates in the skeletal muscle of man as well as to factors regulating preference of substrate utilization. This information is based on data from a number of biopsy studies with analyses made not only on mixtures of different types of muscle fibers, but also on single fibers or pooled fibers of the same type.

METHODS

In the last few years detailed information concerning intramuscular substrate utilization in man during physical exercise has been obtained using the needle-biopsy technique.[12] Measurements of glycogen or triglyceride content in muscle samples show to what extent the substrate is utilized. With a recently developed technique [10] it has furthermore been possible to make quantitative analyses of substrate content in a defined type of fiber: The muscle sample is freeze-dried and individual fibers are dissected out under a dissection microscope ($40-80\times$). Parts of the single fiber are subjected to myofibrillar ATPase-staining and identified, whereas the remaining portion of the fiber is used for biochemical analyses. If needed, pooled fibers of the same type can be used for the analyses.

INTRAMUSCULAR STORE OF SUBSTRATE

Intracellular substrates in human skeletal muscle constitute a rather large amount of stored energy. Normal muscle glycogen content in man is 80–100

* This work was supported by a grant from the Swedish Medical Research Council (04X–04554).

mmoles of glucose per kg wet weight, and if we assume a total muscle mass of 25–30 kg, the muscles contain 400–500 g of glucose or 6500 kJ. The intramuscular triglyceride content in man varies greatly but is normally around 5–15 mmole/kg wet weight, which gives a total store in the muscles of 200–300 g or 10,000 kJ. At rest mean glycogen content in human muscle is similar in type I (355 mmole/kg dry weight, d.w.) and type II fibers (359 mmole/kg d.w.).[10] Triglyceride content in type I and II fibers reveal that type I fibers contain 2–3 times as much triglyceride (207 mmole/kg d.w.) as type II fibers (74 mmole/kg d.w.) (TABLE 1).

SUBSTRATE UTILIZATION

The proportion of energy derived from the intramuscular substrate stores of glycogen and triglycerides is influenced by several factors such as mode, intensity, and duration of work, involvement of different muscle groups, and recruitment pattern of fiber types, as well as diet and physical fitness. These factors will be discussed in greater detail.

TABLE 1

TRIGLYCERIDE AND GLYCOGEN CONCENTRATION IN TYPE I AND II FIBERS IN MAN MEASURED ON TYPE I AND II FIBERS DISSECTED OUT FROM FREEZE-DRIED BIOPSIES *

	Type I	Type II
Triglyceride mmole/kg dry weight	207±86	74±46
Glycogen mmole/kg dry weight	355±140	359±92

* Values are means ± standard deviations of 17 subjects and are taken from Reference 10.

Work Intensity and Duration

At work intensities higher than 90% of the maximal oxygen uptake ($\dot{V}_{O_2 max}$) glycogen is the most important substrate. At submaximal intensities (55%–85% $\dot{V}_{O_2 max}$) (FIGURE 1) glycogen concentration decreases in a curvilinear fashion with time, the most rapid decline being observed at the onset of exercise when the uptake of glucose from the blood is small.[9] A delay in energy production from oxidative phosphorylation due to insufficient oxygen supply and resulting in the formation of lactate during the first minutes of exercise might contribute to the high rate of glycolysis. At intensities of 70%–80% $\dot{V}_{O_2 max}$, nearly all glycogen in the muscle is utilized within 1–2 hours and this often coincides with exhaustion.[3] Several studies have shown that the initial glycogen concentration in the muscle before exercise correlates closely with the maximal work duration at these intensities indicating that the availability of glycogen could be a limiting factor for the ability to perform a prolonged exercise.[13, 14] After 1–2 hours of exercise at 50%–60% $\dot{V}_{O_2 max}$ or after 3 hours at 30% $\dot{V}_{O_2 max}$[6, 9]

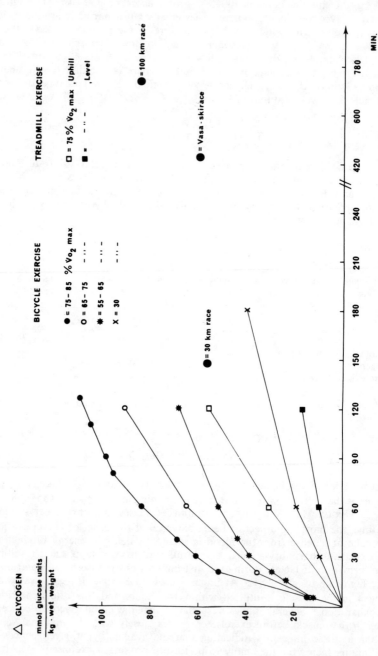

FIGURE 1. Glycogen utilization in the quadriceps femoris (vastus lateralis) at different work intensity and with different mode and duration of exercises. Values are taken from References 3–6, 8, 9, 11, 18, and 26.

a decline in glycogen concentration of only 50%–60% is observed, which suggests that at these low work intensities lipids are the most important substrate source as is also indicated by the finding of a low respiratory exchange ratio. Simultaneous measurements of the uptake of free fatty acids (FFA) by the exercising muscles and the respiratory quotient indicate that at moderate work intensities blood-borne FFA account for only about 50% of the total lipid oxidation and the rest derives from local lipid stores.[15] That intramuscular triglycerides also contribute to energy metabolism in this situation is further supported by the finding of a 25%–30% reduction in triglyceride content after 60–100 minutes at 55%–70% $\dot{V}_{O_2\,max}$[7, 9] (FIGURE 2). It is also possible that FFA can be released from adipose tissue interspersed between the muscle cells and diffuse directly to the muscle cell.

Mode of Exercise and Involvement of Muscle Groups

The involvement of the different muscle groups of the leg varies greatly with type of exercise (FIGURES 1 & 3).

During bicycle exercise the quadriceps femoris muscles are heavily involved as seen both from electromyographic recordings[16] and from the marked *glycogen* depletion in this muscle group. During exercise performed on the treadmill at 75%–80% of $\dot{V}_{O_2\,max}$ for 1–2 hours a more marked glycogen depletion occurs in the soleus and the gastrocnemius than in the vastus lateralis of the quadriceps muscles, indicating that the calf muscles are more heavily involved in running.[17, 18] However, when uphill running was performed, a 3 times greater glycogen depletion was found in the vastus lateralis indicating that this muscle is engaged more in uphill running. In subjects participating in a cross-country race over 30 km involving uphill, level, and downhill running (estimated mean intensity was 83% $\dot{V}_{O_2\,max}$) a glycogen depletion of 50%–60% was observed in the vastus lateralis.[11] During a 100-km race with a mean working time of 12 hours, during which the mean intensity was estimated to be 60%–70% $\dot{V}_{O_2\,max}$, the glycogen concentration in the vastus lateralis declined by 64%, and in the gastrocnemius there was still a large amount of glycogen at the end of the race.[26] During the Vasa ski race over a distance of 86 km with a duration of 7–8 hours, a glycogen depletion of 50%–60% has been observed in the vastus lateralis whereas the depletion in deltoideus muscle was as much as 80%–90%.[19] In running or skiing at intensities of 70%–85% $\dot{V}_{O_2\,max}$ the glycogen depletion is often smaller than in bicycle exercise at comparable intensities. Both in running and skiing the greatest rate of glycolysis in muscles is seen in the early phase of exercise. Thus in the above-mentioned 30-km race and the Vasa ski race the most dominating glycogen depletion occurred before half of the race had been covered.

The intramuscular *triglyceride* stores obviously play an essential role in prolonged submaximal running or skiing. Thus the triglyceride content in vastus lateralis decreased by 30% after a 30-km race[11] and by 37% after a 100-km race.[26] After the Vasa ski race a depletion of 50% in triglycerides was observed[8] (FIGURE 2).

The above-mentioned studies indicate that there exist a great variation in utilization of intramuscular energy stores owing to a great difference in muscle involvement in various types and intensities of work. Furthermore, caution

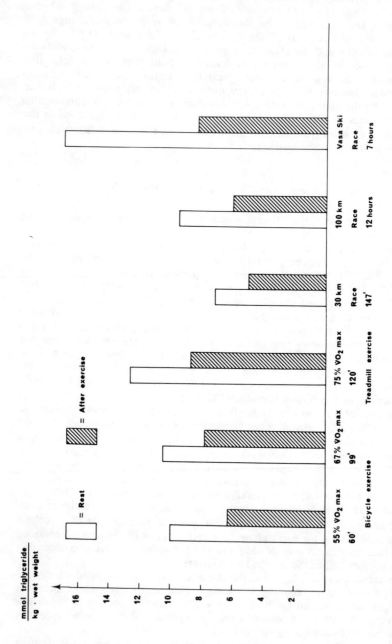

FIGURE 2. Triglyceride concentration in quadriceps femoris (vastus lateralis) at rest and after different modes of exercise. Values are from References 7–9, 11, 16, and 26.

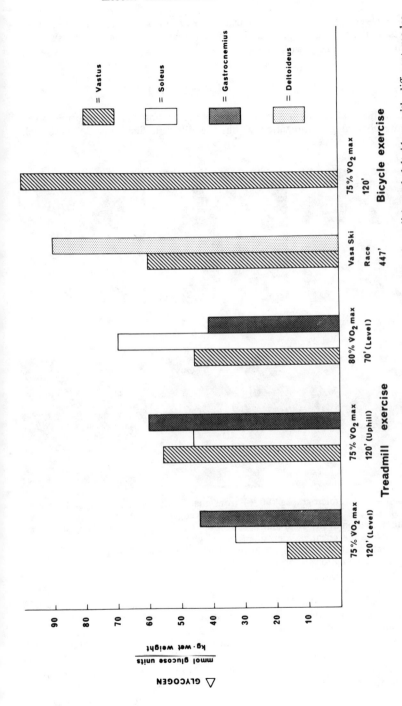

FIGURE 3. Glycogen utilization in soleus, gastrocnemius, quadriceps femoris (vastus lateralis), and deltoideus with different modes of exercise. Values are from References 8, 17, 18, and 19.

must be taken when making conclusions regarding substrate utilization from biopsies as the total amount of active muscle mass is not known and substrate utilization might change with time.

Involvement of Fiber Types

Histochemical techniques have been applied in order to get information on substrate content and utilization within the different fiber types. These tech-

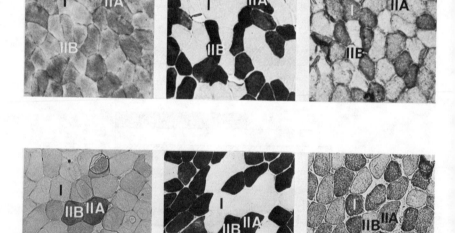

FIGURE 4. Photomicrographs (90×) from quadriceps femoris at rest and after exercise, illustrating serial sections stained for glycogen (PAS), myofibrillar ATPase after preincubation at pH 10.3, and lipid (oil red 0). (Top) At rest. (Bottom) After exercise. Note the equal staining intensity for glycogen in all fiber types at rest but the more intense staining for lipids in type I fiber. After exercise a depletion pattern can be observed only for glycogen.

niques are only semiquantitative but give valuable information about the qualitative picture in the muscle. It has been shown with PAS staining that all fiber types contain a similar glycogen content whereas staining with oil red 0 reveal that type I fibers contain a greater amount of lipid than type IIA fibers, which in turn contain more lipids than type IIB fibers (FIGURE 4). The depletion pattern of glycogen has been studied especially in relation to prolonged exercise. At intensities of 30%–85% $\dot{V}_{O_2\,max}$ the first fiber type that reveals a loss of glycogen is the type I fiber, but as exercise continues there is also a progressive depletion of glycogen occurring in type II fibers.[5] More glycolytic fibers are activated when exercise exceeds the capacity of the oxidative fibers. Usually type IIA fibers are depleted before type IIB fibers. The loss of glycogen observed in the different fiber types has suggested that these fibers have been recruited during exercise. The glycogen depletion pattern as revealed by histochemical analyses, although elucidating the recruitment pattern, cannot be taken as evidence of the extent to which the different fibers have been active since glycogen is not the only substrate for energy metabolism. Intramuscular triglyceride as well as blood-borne FFA and glucose are utilized simultaneously at most work intensities. This is specially true at low work intensity ($\approx$30% $\dot{V}_{O_2 max}$), where the contribution from lipids is greater than from carbohydrates, and even though some fibers are depleted of glycogen, they may still be utilizing lipids. The quantitative analysis available[10] might further elucidate the intramuscular substrate content and utilization during exercise in the different fiber types in man.

The recruitment of the type I and II fibers is illustrated by the following study. Five subjects performed continuous bicycle exercise at 50%–60% $V_{O_2 max}$ (mean work load 155 W) for 60 minutes. Biopsy samples were obtained from the quadriceps femoris muscle both at rest and at the end of exercise, and glycogen content was analyzed in individual type I and II fibers. The mean glycogen content at rest was similar for the two fiber types although large variations were found within each fiber type. The glycogen content at rest was 348 ± 89 mmole/kg dry weight in type I fibers and 402 ± 89 mmole/kg dry weight in type II fibers. After exercise a considerable decrease of glycogen was found in type I fibers (123 ± 166 mmole/kg d.w.), whereas a much smaller depletion of glycogen was found in type II fibers (302 ± 185 mmole/kg d.w.) (FIGURE 5), supporting the view that mainly type I fibers are involved in exercise of low intensity.[6] The same subjects then performed intermittent exercise (15 sec work, 15 sec rest) for 60 minutes at nearly twice the intensity (300 W). During continuous exercise this intensity demanded 100% $\dot{V}_{O_2 max}$. The mean total glycogen utilization after 60 minutes of intermittent exercise (300 W) was similar to that found during continuous submaximal exercise for 60 minutes at approximately half the work intensity (155 W).[9] However, after intermittent exercise the type II fibers showed a low glycogen content (129 ± 115 mmole/kg d.w.) (FIGURE 6), which indicates that, at higher work intensities and/or at onset of exercise with more intense tension development, the type II fibers are recruited.

Regulatory Factors

The rate of substrate utilization in the skeletal muscle is controlled not only by neural and hormonal mechanisms, but also by metabolic mechanisms. Changes in the ADP/ATP ratio influences the phosphorylase as well as the phosphofructokinase (PFK) activity, thus acting as an important feedback mechanism regulating the rate of glycolysis.

An interplay also exists between lipid and carbohydrate utilization. Thus in vitro studies have shown that oxidation of fatty acids elevates the concentration of citrate in the muscle,[20] which in turn causes inhibition at the PFK-step. As a result, the glucose-6-phosphate level is elevated, which inhibits the hexokinase activity, thereby decreasing the uptake of glucose from the blood. These

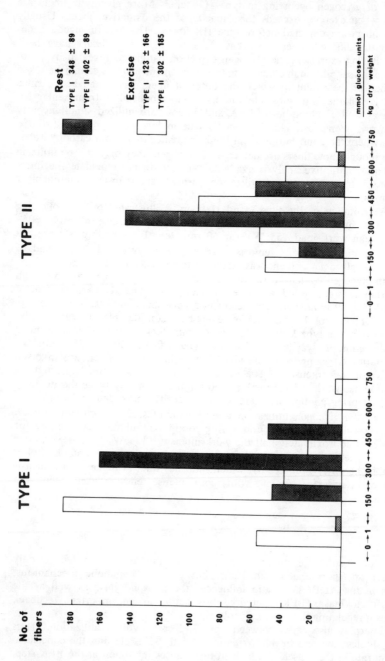

FIGURE 5. The distribution of type I and II fibers containing different amounts of glycogen at rest and after 60 min of continuous exercise at 50%–60% $\dot{V}_{O_2max}$ (155 W). Mean values from 5 subjects. From 25 to 75 type I and II fibers were dissected out from each biopsy. Values at right show mean glycogen content in type I and II fibers at rest and after exercise (± standard deviation).

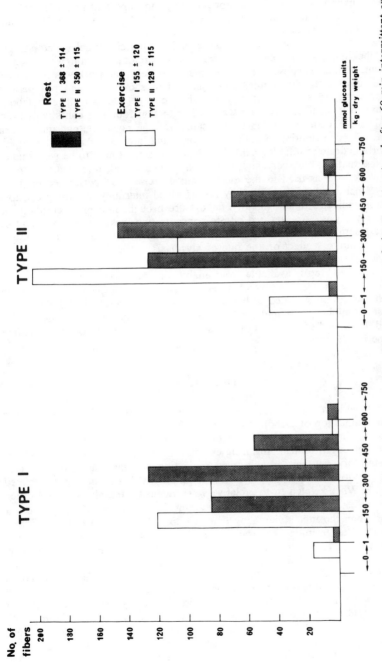

FIGURE 6. The distribution of type I and II fibers containing different amounts of glycogen at rest and after 60 min intermittent exercise (15 sec work, 15 sec rest) at 300 W. The data are mean values from 5 subjects. From 25 to 75 type I and II fibers were dissected out from each biopsy. Values at right show mean glycogen content in type I and II fibers at rest and after exercise (± standard deviation).

observations indicate that citrate probably plays an important role as a metabolite regulating substrate utilization by suppressing glycolysis when fatty acids are available for oxidation.

The preference of substrate by the exercising muscle and the factors regulating the interplay between carbohydrate and lipid utilization were studied using intermittent exercise as an experimental model. The work was performed by five subjects for 60 minutes and consisted of short work and rest periods (15 sec work, 15 sec rest) at a very high intensity (300 W). The metabolic response to intermittent exercise was similar to that found in continuous exercise (155 W) with approximately the same average power output and oxygen uptake. The contribution of both blood-borne and intramuscular stores of lipids and carbohydrate to total leg oxidative metabolism was found to be very similar in these situations.[9] A very high rate of glycolysis would have occurred if the same work load as used in the intermittent exercise were performed continuously. When work of high intensity is performed intermittently, the great lipid oxidation indicates that regulatory factors are brought into play retarding the rate of glycolysis. An elevated citrate concentration was found at the end of each rest period supporting the suggestion that high citrate concentration might have an inhibitory effect on the rate of glycolysis at the PFK level thus facilitating an enhanced lipid oxidation.[21] Further evidence that PFK activity could be an inhibited step is available from analyses of metabolites before and after the PFK-step in the glycolysis. Thus the glucose-6-phosphate concentration was shown to be elevated, whereas the sum of glyceraldehyd-3-phosphate, fructose-1,6-diphosphate, and dihydroxyacetonphosphate concentrations was decreased at the end of each rest period as compared to the end of the preceding work period (FIGURE 7).

Physical Activity

Cross-sectional studies have shown a similar glycogen utilization in relation to total combustion of carbohydrates in trained and untrained subjects performing exercise at the same relative work intensity.[3, 5] After physical training, however, glycogen utilization during exercise is decreased and lower values for the respiratory quotient are observed indicating a greater contribution from lipids to the total energy metabolism concomitantly with a significantly increased $\dot{V}_{O_2 max}$.[22] When related to the relative work intensity, the glycogen utilization in the muscle does not change after training but a glycogen-saving effect is obvious when the metabolic changes are compared at the same absolute work before and after training. The trained muscle induces changes towards a greater oxidative capacity via increased mitochondrial content[23] and increased enzymatic activity for oxidative metabolism,[24] which may account for the enhanced oxidation of lipids, which in turn evidently has a sparing effect on glycogen degradation. When substrate utilization in the muscle of trained and untrained subjects is compared in cross-sectional studies, it is of importance to remember that the local adaptation occurs only in those muscles having been trained. In runners the most suitable muscle for studies of this type is the gastrocnemius; the vastus lateralis is not a trained muscle in a subject whose training model is mostly endurance running. This might explain why many studies on the metabolic effect of physical training have failed to show any change in substrate utilization using the biopsy technique.

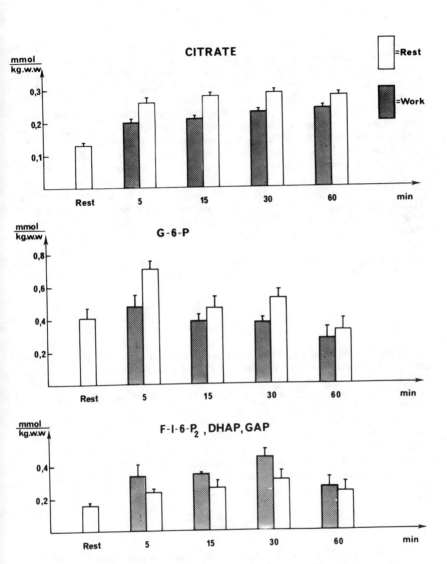

FIGURE 7. The concentrations of citrate, glucose-6-phosphate (G-6-P), and the total sum of fructose-1-6-diphosphate (F-1-6-P_2), dihydroxyacetonphosphate (DHAP), and glyceraldehyde-3-phosphate (GAP) during intermittent exercise (15 sec work, 15 sec rest) at 300 W in subjects originally at complete rest or at rest after a previous work period. The samples were obtained at rest and after 5, 15, 30, and 60 min of exercise. Values are means ± standard errors. Concentrations are expressed in mmoles per kg wet weight.

Diet

The glycogen stores in the muscle can be influenced by the composition of diet. During a resting period even great variations in the carbohydrate content of the diet will influence the glycogen concentration only to a very small extent. If, however, intense exercise precedes a period of carbohydrate-rich diet, the glycogen content is markedly increased, whereas it remains low with a carbo-hydrate-low diet.[13] This overshoot in glycogen content following a carbohydrate-rich intake is restricted to those groups of muscles having taken part in the preceding exercise. By lowering the carbohydrate content of the diet, one finds a considerable reduction in work time.[13] On the other hand it is possible to extend the capacity for prolonged heavy exercise by increasing the amount of carbohydrates in the diet. These findings support the importance of carbo-hydrate as fuel at heavier work intensities.[13, 14] The mechanisms for the increased glycogen synthesis after a carbohydrate-rich diet is not well understood. One factor that has been discussed is an increased activity of glycogen synthetase, the key enzyme in regulation of glycogen synthesis, although a significant increase has never been shown.[25] It is also not known if the overshoot in glycogen occurs selectively in one fiber type or similarly in all fiber types. This cannot be elucidated from histochemical data and has to await quantitative analyses on individual fibers.

SUMMARY

Large stores of intramuscular substrates are found in the different fiber types of human skeletal muscle, and with prolonged exercise both glycogen and tri-glyceride stores are utilized. The contribution from intramuscular glycogen stores is greatest at higher work intensities while triglyceride stores are utilized at moderate intensities.

In man all fiber types have a similar glycogen content whereas the highest lipid content is found in the more oxidative fibers. The muscle metabolism is well adapted to the supply of substrate as well as to the demand for energy. Among several regulatory mechanisms, changes in citrate concentration seems to be an important factor in the interplay between carbohydrate and lipid metabolism.

REFERENCES

1. CHRISTENSEN, E. H. & O. HANSEN. 1939. Zur methodik der respiratorischen quotient-bestimmungen in ruhe und bei arbeit. II. Untersuchungen über die verbrennungsvorgänge bei langdauernder, schwerer muskelarbeit. III. arbeits-fähigkeit und ernährung. Skand. Arch. Physiol. **81:** 137–171.
2. BERGSTRÖM, J. & E. HULTMAN. 1967. A study of the glycogen metabolism during exercise in man. Scand. J. Clin. Lab. Invest. **19:** 218–228.
3. HERMANSEN, L., E. HULTMAN & B. SALTIN. 1967. Muscle glycogen during prolonged severe exercise. Acta Physiol. Scand. **71:** 129–139.
4. SALTIN, B. & J. KARLSSON. 1971. Muscle glycogen utilization during work of different intensities. *In* Muscle Metabolism During Exercise. B. Pernow & B. Saltin, Eds. Vol. **11:** 289–299. Plenum Press. New York, N.Y.

5. GOLLNICK, P. D., R. B. ARMSTRONG, C. W. SAUBERT IV, W. L. SEMBROWICH, R. E. SHEPERD & B. SALTIN. 1973. Glycogen depletion patterns in human skeletal muscle fibres during prolonged work. Pflügers Arch. **344:** 1–12.
6. GOLLNICK, P. D., K. PIEHL & B. SALTIN. 1974. Selective depletion pattern in human muscle fibres after exercise of varying intensity and at varying pedalling rates. J. Physiol. (Lond.) **241:** 45–51.
7. FRÖBERG, S. O., L. A. CARLSON & L-G. EKELUND. 1971. Local lipid stores and exercise. In Muscle Metabolism During Exercise. B. Pernow & B. Saltin, Eds. Vol. **11:** 307–313. Plenum Press. New York, N.Y.
8. FRÖBERG, S. O. & F. MOSSFELDT. 1971. Effect of prolonged strenuous exercise on the concentration of triglycerides, phospholipids and glycogen in muscle of man. Acta Physiol. Scand. **82:** 167–171.
9. ESSÉN, B., L. HAGENFELDT & L. KAIJSER. 1977. Substrate utilization in intermittent exercise in man. J. Physiol. **265:** 489–506.
10. ESSÉN, B., E. JANSSON, J. HENRIKSSON, A. W. TAYLOR & B. SALTIN. 1975. Metabolic characteristics of fibre types in human skeletal muscle. Acta Physiol. Scand. **95:** 153–165.
11. COSTILL, D. L., P. D. GOLLNICK, E. JANSSON, B. SALTIN & E. M. STEIN. 1973. Glycogen depletion pattern in human muscle fibres during distance running. Acta Physiol. Scand. **89:** 374–383.
12. BERGSTRÖM, J. 1962. Muscle electrolytes in man. Determined by neutron activation analysis on needle biopsy specimens. A study on normal subjects, kidney patients, and patients with chronic diarrhoea. Scand. J. Clin. Invest. Suppl. **14:** 1–110.
13. BERGSTRÖM, J., L. HERMANSEN, E. HULTMAN & B. SALTIN. 1967. Diet, muscle glycogen, and physical performance. Acta Physiol. Scand. **71:** 140–150.
14. KARLSSON, J. & B. SALTIN. 1971. Diet, muscle glycogen, and endurance performance. J. Appl. Physiol. **31:** 203–206.
15. HAVEL, R. J., B. PERNOW & N. L. JONES. 1967. Uptake and release of free fatty acids and other metabolism in the legs of exercising man. J. Appl. Physiol. **23:** 90–96.
16. HENRIKSSON, J. & F. BONDE-PETERSEN. 1974. Integrated electromyography of quadriceps femoris muscle at different exercise intensities. J. Appl. Physiol. **36:** 218–220.
17. COSTILL, D. L., K. SPARKS, R. GREGOR & C. TURNER. 1971. Muscle glycogen utilization during exhaustive running. J. Appl. Physiol. **31:** 353–356.
18. COSTILL, D. L., E. JANSSON, P. D. GOLLNICK & B. SALTIN. 1974. Glycogen utilization in leg muscles of men during level and uphill running. Acta Physiol. Scand. **91:** 475–481.
19. BERGSTRÖM, J., E. HULTMAN & B. SALTIN. 1973. Muscle glycogen consumption during cross-country skiing (the Vasa Ski Race). Int. Z. Angew Physiol. **31:** 71–75.
20. RANDLE, P. J., E. A. NEWSHOLME & P. B. GARLAND. 1964. Regulation of glucose uptake by muscle. 8. Effects of fatty acid, ketone bodies and pyruvate, and of alloxan diabetes and starvation, on the uptake and metabolic fate of glucose in rat heart and diaphragm muscle. Biochem. J. **93:** 652–655.
21. PARMEGGIANI, A. & R. H. BOWMAN. 1963. Regulation of phosphofructokinase activity by citrate in normal and diabetic muscle. Biochem. Biophys. Res. Commun. **12:** 4, 268–273.
22. KARLSSON, J., L.-O. NORDESJÖ & B. SALTIN. 1974. Muscle glycogen utilization during exercise after physical training. Acta Physiol. Scand. **90:** 210–217.
23. MORGAN, T. E., L. A. COBB, F. A. SHORT, R. ROSS & D. R. GUNN. 1971. Effects of long-term exercise on human muscle mitochrondria. In Muscle Metabolism During Exercise. B. Pernow & B. Saltin, Eds. Vol. **11:** 87–96. Plenum Press. New York, N.Y.

24. HENRIKSSON, J. & J. S. REITMAN. 1976. Quantitative measures of enzyme activities in type I and II muscle fibers of man after training. Acta Physiol. Scand. **97:** 392–397.
25. HULTMAN, E., J. BERGSTRÖM & A. E. ROCH-NORDLUND. 1971. Glycogen storage in human skeletal muscle. *In* Muscle Metabolism During Exercise. B. Pernow & B. Saltin, Eds. Vol. **11:** 273–288. Plenum Press. New York, N.Y.
26. ESSÉN, B. Unpublished observations.

GLUCOSE TURNOVER DURING EXERCISE IN MAN *

John Wahren

*Department of Clinical Physiology
Karolinska Institute
Huddinge Hospital
S-141 86 Huddinge, Sweden*

Introduction

Uptake of blood glucose by contracting skeletal muscle has been recognized for almost 90 years.[1] However, following the discovery of the important role of the plasma free fatty acids as energy-yielding substrates,[2-4] glucose was generally relegated to a minor role with respect to energy metabolism in muscle. In recent years studies have been made in man of the quantitative contributions of blood glucose to the energy needs engendered by exercise, and it is now clear that blood glucose plays an important role in the supply of fuel to contracting muscle. The contribution made by blood glucose appears to be primarily determined by the duration and the intensity of the exercise performed.

Resting Muscle

The respiratory quotient (RQ) of muscle in the resting state is close to 0.7, indicating the almost total dependence of muscle on the oxidation of fatty acids.[5] Uptake of glucose accounts for less than 10% of the total oxygen consumption by muscle. The overall rate of glucose utilization by muscle is about 20 to 25 mg per minute,[5] no more than 10% to 15% of the total body glucose turnover. Since some of the glucose consumed within the muscle bed reflects glycolysis by blood cells, it is clear that muscle is relatively unimportant in glucose disposal in the resting state. Instead, the major site of glucose consumption in this state is the brain.[6]

Glucose Uptake by Exercising Forearm Muscle

The forearm is a useful experimental model for quantitative metabolic studies inasmuch as it permits the accurate measurements of both brachial artery blood flow and arterial-venous (a-v) differences in the metabolites utilized or produced by exercising forearm muscle, thus allowing quantitative determinations of the net uptake or production of muscle metabolites.[7]

In the resting state there is a small positive a-v difference for glucose across the deep forearm tissues, indicating glucose uptake.[5] At the onset of heavy, rhythmic forearm exercise this difference becomes smaller and after 1 to 2 minutes it is reversed, indicating a net release of glucose from the forearm.[8-9]

* This work was supported by the Swedish Medical Research Council (19-X-3108) and the National Institute of Health (AM-13526).

45

Since glucose-6-phosphatase is not present in muscle tissue, the mechanism behind this finding probably does not involve hydrolysis of glucose-6-phosphate. Some clues may be provided by the breakdown pattern of glycogen, in which most of the glycosyl units are converted to glucose-6-phosphate by the action of myophosphorylase. In the degradation process, debranching of the glycogen molecules involves certain formation of free glucose, corresponding to 8% to 10% of the glycogen.[10] During conditions of low-to-moderate rates of glycogenolysis, this glucose is probably phosphorylated rapidly in the hexokinase reaction, whereas during heavy exercise with rapid glycogen degradation, increased amounts of intracellular glucose will be formed. At this time the hexokinase reaction may be operating slowly or not at all, due in part to inhibition by the accumulation of glucose-6-phosphate. Under such circumstances it is

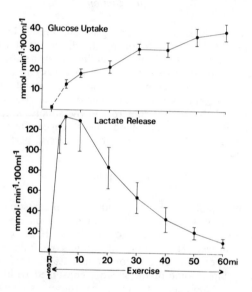

FIGURE 1. Glucose uptake and release of lactate by the forearm tissues [mean ± standard error (SE)] at rest and during prolonged forearm exercise using a hand ergometer (work load 1.5 W).

possible that the transport of glucose across the cell membrane into the cell is reversed. This transient release of glucose from muscle to blood is quantitatively insignificant, but the observation may help explain the divergent results previously reported for glucose uptake by muscle during exercise in man.

After the initial 1–2 minutes of exercise the forearm muscles show a small net uptake of glucose and a considerable release of lactate. As work continues, glucose uptake increases progressively and the release of lactate gradually subsides as illustrated in FIGURE 1.[9] Quantitative calculations show that net glucose uptake by forearm muscle may be 15 times the basal value after 10 minutes of exercise and as much as 35 times after 60 minutes.[9] The contribution of glucose to the total carbohydrate oxidation as well as to the total oxidative metabolism of forearm muscles can be estimated from the local RQ and the a-v differences for oxygen, glucose, and lactate. Such calculations show that the major part of the oxygen uptake is being used for carbohydrate oxidation after 10 minutes of exercise; lactate is released in excess of the simultaneous glucose uptake, suggesting that muscle glycogen is the dominant source of carbohydrate substrate. However, at the end of a longer period of exercise (40–60 minutes) the situation has changed: The RQ value now indicates that about half of the oxidative metabolism is carbohydrate oxidation, nearly all of which can be accounted for by glucose uptake from the blood.[9]

During the early phase of exercise, lactate output from contracting muscle is at its peak (FIGURE 1), lower rates of lactate release being seen with increasing duration of work at submaximal work loads. It used to be considered that lactate output is a sign of muscle hypoxia even during mild exercise. However, measurements of the steady-state oxidation-reduction level of mitochondrial NAD of contracting skeletal muscle have demonstrated adequate oxygenation even during lactate production.[11] This indicates that lactate production is not necessarily a result of hypoxic stimulation of anaerobic glycolysis. Instead, at mild to moderate levels of work it may reflect an imbalance between the rate of glycolysis and the rate of pyruvate utilization in the citric acid cycle. But although lactate release does not necessarily imply muscle hypoxia, it does not rule out the possibility of hypoxia during the initial phase of exercise or during very heavy work.

Glucose Uptake during Leg Exercise

Owing to the small muscle volume involved, glucose utilization during forearm exercise does not substantially challenge the blood glucose homeostasis. However, during exercise with the large muscle groups of the leg the concentration of blood glucose changes little during short-term mild to moderately heavy exercise.[12] In contrast, exercise that continues 90 minutes or more causes a significant fall in blood glucose concentration.[13-14] Genuine hypoglycemia (blood glucose below 40 mg/100 ml) is rare; it has sometimes been observed in marathon runners,[15] in patients on low carbohydrate diets,[16] and in insulin-treated diabetic patients.

In healthy individuals exercising on a bicycle ergometer at mild-to-strenuous work loads, the a-v difference for glucose and the leg blood flow both rose at all levels of working intensity.[12] Net glucose uptake by the leg increased 7-fold above the resting value after 40 minutes of light exercise and 10- and 20-fold at the heavier work intensities (FIGURE 2). Leg glucose uptake rose gradually during the entire period of exercise, in keeping with the observations from forearm exercise. For leg exercise, blood glucose oxidation accounts for a growing fraction of both the total and the carbohydrate oxidation of the leg during progressive exercise at all levels of work intensity (FIGURE 3), thereby helping to make up for the gradually diminishing stores of glycogen in the exercising muscle. Thus, although muscle glycogen is likely to be the dominant carbohydrate substrate during the initial phase of exercise, the utilization of blood glucose rises steadily with time. After 40 minutes of exercise, blood glucose can (if we assume that the glucose taken up by the leg muscles is completely oxidized) sustain as much as 75% to 90% of the carbohydrate metabolism and 30% to 35% of the total oxidative metabolism of the leg (FIGURE 3).

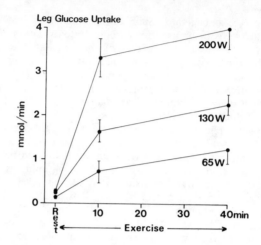

FIGURE 2. Glucose uptake by the legs during bicycle ergometer exercise at different work loads (mean ± SE).

As mild leg exercise is continued beyond 40 minutes the rate of glucose utilization increases further, reaching a peak at 90–180 minutes at which time glucose uptake may account for 35%–40% of total metabolism (FIGURE 4). Mild hypoglycemia may subsequently develop and leg uptake of glucose declines slightly.[13]

Examination of the glucose exchange across the cerebral circulation reveals that glucose remains the dominating substrate oxidized during exercise and that its rate of utilization is unchanged from the resting state.[17] Moreover, during one-leg exercise, the glucose uptake by the nonexercising leg is unchanged or slightly increased above the basal level.[18] These observations thus refute the previously advanced hypothesis that part of the increased uptake of blood

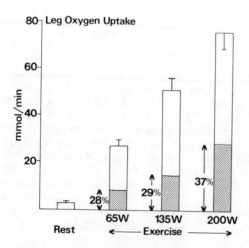

FIGURE 3. Leg oxygen uptake at rest and after 40 min of bicycle exercise at work loads of 65, 130, and 200 W. The hatched area indicates the proportion of the oxygen uptake that may be accounted for by glucose oxidation (mean ± SE).

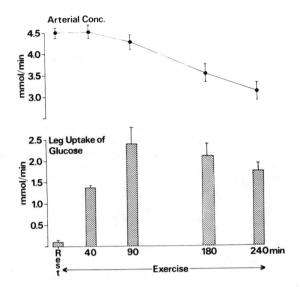

FIGURE 4. Arterial concentration and leg uptake of glucose at rest and during 4 hours of prolonged exercise (mean ± SE).

glucose to the exercising muscles is provided for by a reduced uptake to inactive muscle or to the brain.

With regard to the mechanism behind the rise in glucose uptake to muscle during exercise, it is noteworthy that exercise induces a significant fall in the plasma insulin concentration (FIGURE 5),[12, 13, 19] possibly as a consequence of increased liberation of catecholamines.[20, 21] It has been postulated that exercise-induced hypoinsulinemia serves to limit blood glucose uptake by muscle, thereby increasing its availability to the brain. However, this does not appear to be

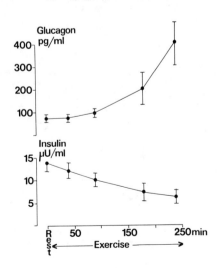

FIGURE 5. Arterial concentrations of insulin and glucagon during prolonged mild exercise (mean ± SE).

the case since glucose uptake by muscle increases during exercise in the face of falling concentrations of insulin. Furthermore, insulin-withdrawn diabetic patients also show a marked rise in muscle glucose utilization during physical exertion.[22] One can therefore conclude that glucose uptake during exercise does not depend on the ability to secrete increased quantities of insulin. It is still conceivable, however, that the presence of low concentrations of insulin' exert a permissive effect on glucose uptake by contracting muscle,[23] and it should be noted that the augmented blood flow and enlarged capillary surface area during exercise augment the total delivery of insulin to the working muscle. It has also been suggested that the contractile process results in the release by muscle of a humoral substance ("muscle activity factor") that stimulates glucose utilization by exercising muscle.[24] However, subsequent studies involving perfused muscle have failed to show such a humoral factor.[23, 25]

Hepatic Glucose Production

The stimulation of glucose utilization by muscle that characterizes exercise suggests that blood glucose homeostasis can be achieved only by an increase in glucose production. Except in very prolonged starvation, in which state the kidney produces glucose,[26] the liver is the sole site of glucose production and release into the blood stream. In the resting state the rate of hepatic glucose production is approximately 150 mg/min; 75% is produced by glycogenolysis and the remainder by gluconeogenesis from lactate, pyruvate, glycerol, and glucogenic amino acids.[7, 27]

During short-term exercise, splanchnic glucose uptake increases 2–5 times, depending on the intensity of the work performed [12] and keeps pace with the increment in glucose utilization by muscle tissue (FIGURE 6). This increased glucose production results almost entirely from augmented glycogenolysis; except for a transient rise in lactate consumption, splanchnic uptake of gluconeo-

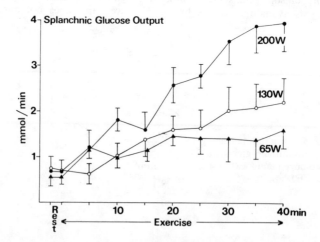

FIGURE 6. Splanchnic glucose output (mean ± SE) at rest and during bicycle exercise at work loads of 65, 130, and 200 W.

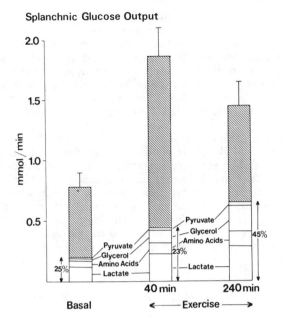

FIGURE 7. Splanchnic glucose output and uptake of glucogenic precursor substrates in the basal state and during prolonged exercise (mean ± SE).

genic precursors remains unchanged from the resting state.[12] As a consequence of the absolute rise in total glucose production, the relative contribution from gluconeogenesis falls from 25% in the resting state to 16% after 40 minutes of mild exercise and to less than 6% after the same period of severe exercise.[12] The total amount of glucose released from the liver during 40 minutes of heavy work is estimated to be 18 g, no more than 20%–25% of the total hepatic glycogen stores in the postabsorptive state.[16]

As exercise extends beyond 40 minutes, a slight imbalance between the rates of hepatic production and peripheral utilization of glucose as well as an increasing reliance on hepatic gluconeogenesis are observed. During prolonged mild exercise, splanchnic glucose output doubles in 40 minutes and thereafter remains constant for 3–4 hours (FIGURE 7).[13] The relative contribution from gluconeogenesis to overall hepatic glucose output, estimated from substrate balances across the splanchnic bed, increases from 25% in the basal state to 45% during prolonged exercise, a 3-fold rise in the absolute rate of gluconeogenesis.[13] Splanchnic uptake of alanine, lactate, and pyruvate doubles, and glycerol utilization increases 10 times. These increments in splanchnic uptake of glucose precursors are largely a result of augmented fractional extraction. Thus, fractional extraction of alanine by the splanchnic bed increases from the resting level (35%–40%) to almost 90% in prolonged exercise.[13] The overall importance of gluconeogenesis in prolonged exercise is underscored by the estimation that 50–60 g of hepatic glycogen is mobilized in 4 hours of exercise, a 75% depletion of the total liver glycogen stores.[13]

With regard to the factors responsible for the augmented glucose output during exercise, it is noteworthy that serum insulin decreases in short-term [12] as well as in prolonged exercise. Since the liver is highly sensitive to small changes in insulin,[28] one could expect such a decrease to result in stimulation of hepatic glycogenolysis and gluconeogenesis. At heavy work intensities [21, 29] and during prolonged exercise involving mild hypoglycemia,[13] increases in plasma glucagon may also contribute to hepatic glucose production. In addition, increments in growth hormone [30] and catecholamines [21] may be of importance in this context. Recent studies suggest that changes in the circulating levels of insulin, glucagon, and glucose are not the sole (or primary) determinants of hepatic glucose production in exercise. When the concentrations of insulin, glucagon, and glucose in plasma are maintained at basal levels during exercise by means of an intravenous glucose infusion this fails to influence the normal 2–3-fold increase in hepatic glucose production.[31] Furthermore, infusion of insulin and maintenance of hyperinsulinemia do not inhibit exercise-induced stimulation of hepatic glucose output.[31] Thus, factors other than the prevailing concentrations of insulin and glucagon contribute to the regulation of hepatic glucose output in exercise. Sympathetic adrenergic activity and release of catecholamines are both augmented in exercise and may be of importance for this regulation.

Glucose Administration in Connection with Exercise

All of the results discussed above were obtained in the postabsorptive, basal metabolic state. Since some form of nutrition (usually rich in carbohydrate) is often taken in connection with heavy exercise or athletics, it is of interest to determine to what extent muscle substrate utilization can be modified when extra glucose is supplied. Available data indicate that glucose administration does not significantly reduce muscle glycogen consumption during strenuous exercise.[32] In contrast, during light exercise (less than 50% of maximal oxygen uptake) glycogen utilization is diminished following glucose administration.[33]

Recently the metabolic fate of glucose ingested in connection with exercise has been examined.[34, 35] Glucose feeding is found to be accompanied by significantly elevated levels of blood glucose and insulin and failure of glucagon concentration to rise during exercise, as well as markedly augmented glucose uptake by the exercising legs. Blood-borne glucose could thus account for 50%–60% of the total oxidative fuel consumption as compared to 30%–40% in controls (FIGURE 8). Moreover, glucose ingestion was found to result in diminished splanchnic uptake of the glucogenic precursors lactate, pyruvate, glycerol, and alanine, indicating decreased hepatic gluconeogenesis. These observations thus suggest that exercise fails to overcome the inhibitory influence of glucose administration on hepatic gluconeogenesis, previously well established in resting subjects.[28]

The metabolic and hormonal responses noted during exercise were similar when glucose was administered before and during exercise. Thus, whether glucose is ingested prior to or during the course of exercise, hyperglycemia is seen in combination with reversal of exercise-induced inhibition of insulin secretion and suppression of exercise-induced stimulation of glucagon secretion. In addition, fuel utilization by muscle shifts from fat to glucose, and splanchnic uptake of gluconeogenic precursors is inhibited.[34-35]

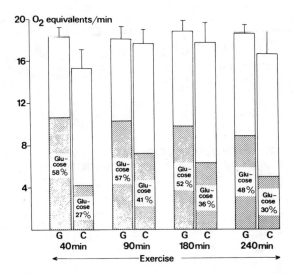

FIGURE 8. Leg oxygen uptake (total height of the bars, mean ± SE) during prolonged exercise after oral glucose ingestion (G) and in controls (C). The hatched area indicates that portion of the oxygen uptake which can be accounted for by glucose oxidation.

References

1. CHAUVEAU, M. A. & M. KAUFMANN. 1887. Expériences pour la détermination du coefficient de l'activité nutritive et respiratoire des muscles en repos et en travail. C.R. Acad. Sci. **104**: 1126–1132.

2. DOLE, V. P. 1956. A relation between non-esterified fatty acids in plasma and the metabolism of glucose. J. Clin. Invest. **35**: 150–154.

3. GORDON, R. S., JR. & A. CHERKES. 1956. Unesterified fatty acids in human blood plasma. J. Clin. Invest. **35**: 206–212.

4. LAURELL, S. 1956. Plasma free fatty acids in diabetic acidosis and starvation. Scand. J. Clin. Lab. Invest. **8**: 81–82.

5. ANDRES, R., G. CADER & K. L. ZIERLER. 1956. The quantitatively minor role of carbohydrate in oxidative metabolism by skeletal muscle in intact man in the basal state. Measurements of oxygen and glucose uptake and carbon dioxide and lactate production in the forearm. J. Clin. Invest. **35**: 671–682.

6. BONDY, P. K. & P. FELIG. 1974. Disorders of carbohydrate metabolism. In Duncan's Diseases of Metabolism. Genetics and metabolism. P. K. Bondy & L. E. Rosenberg, Eds., 7th edit. : 221–340. W. B. Saunders Company. Philadelphia, Pa.

7. WAHREN, J. 1966. Quantitative aspects of blood flow and oxygen uptake in the human forearm during rhythmic exercise. Acta Physiol. Scand. **67**(Suppl. 269): 1–93.

8. WAHREN, J. 1970. Human forearm muscle metabolism during exercise. IV. Glucose uptake at different work intensities. Scand. J. Clin. Lab. Invest. **25**: 129–135.

9. JORFELDT, L. & J. WAHREN. 1970. Human forearm muscle metabolism during exercise. V. Quantitative aspects of glucose uptake and lactate production during prolonged exercise. Scand. J. Clin. Lab. Invest. **26**: 73–81.

10. FIELD, R. A. 1966. Glycogen deposition diseases. *In* The Metabolic Basis of Inherited Diseases. : 141–177. McGraw-Hill Book Company. New York, N.Y.

11. JÖBSIS, F. F. & W. N. STAINSBY. 1968. Oxidation of NADH during contractions of circulated mammalian skeletal muscle. Resp. Physiol. **4:** 292–300.

12. WAHREN, J., P. FELIG, G. AHLBORG & L. JORFELDT. 1971. Glucose metabolism during leg exercise in man. J. Clin. Invest. **50:** 2715–2725.

13. AHLBORG, G., P. FELIG, L. HAGENFELDT, R. HENDLER & J. WAHREN. 1974. Substrate turnover during prolonged exercise in man: Splanchnic and leg metabolism of glucose, free fatty acids and amino acids. J. Clin. Invest. **53:** 1080–1090.

14. YOUNG, D. R., R. PELLIGRA, J. SHAPIRA, R. R. ADACHI & K. SKRETTINGLAND. 1967. Glucose oxidation and replacement during prolonged exercise in man. J. Appl. Physiol. **23:** 734–741.

15. LEVINE, S. A., B. GORDON & C. L. DERICK. 1924. Some changes in the chemical constituents of the blood following a marathon race. J. Amer. Med. Assoc. **82:** 1778–1779.

16. HULTMAN, E. & L. H. NILSSON. 1971. Liver glycogen in man: Effect of different diets and muscular exercise. *In* Muscle Metabolism during Exercise: Proceedings of a Karolinska Institutet Symposium held in Stockholm, Sweden, September 6–9, 1970. B. Pernow & B. Saltin, Eds. : 143–151. Plenum Press. New York, N.Y.

17. AHLBORG, G. & J. WAHREN. 1972. Brain substrate utilization during prolonged exercise. Scand. J. Clin. Lab. Invest. **29:** 397–402.

18. AHLBORG, G., L. HAGENFELDT & J. WAHREN. 1975. Substrate utilization by the inactive leg during one-leg or arm exercise. J. Appl. Physiol. **39:** 718–723.

19. HUNTER, W. M. & M. Y. SUKKAR. 1968. Changes in plasma insulin levels during muscular exercise. J. Physiol. (London) **196:** 110–112.

20. HÄGGENDAL, J., L. H. HARTLEY & B. SALTIN. 1970. Arterial noradrenaline concentration during exercise in relation to the relative work levels. Scand. J. Clin. Lab. Invest. **26:** 337–342.

21. GALBO, H., J. J. HOLST & N. J. CHRISTENSEN. 1975. Glucagon and plasma catecholamine responses to graded and prolonged exercise in man. J. Appl. Physiol. **38(1):** 70–76.

22. WAHREN, J., L. HAGENFELDT & P. FELIG. 1975. Splanchnic and leg exchange of glucose, amino acids and free fatty acids during exercise in diabetes mellitus. J. Clin. Invest. **55:** 1303–1314.

23. BERGER, M., S. HAGG & N. B. RUDERMAN. 1975. Glucose metabolism in perfused skeletal mucle: Interaction of insulin and exercise on glucose uptake. Biochem. J. **146:** 231–238.

24. GOLDSTEIN, M. S. 1961. Humoral nature of hypoglycemia in muscular exercise. Amer. J. Physiol. **200:** 67–70.

25. SZABO, A. J., R. J. MAHLER & O. ASABO. 1972. Influence of exercise upon serum factors and its secondary effect on glucose utilization by the resting muscle. Horm. Metab. Res. **4:** 139–143.

26. OWEN, O. E., P. FELIG, A. P. MORGAN, J. WAHREN & G. F. CAHILL, JR. 1969. Liver and kidney metabolism during prolonged starvation. J. Clin. Invest. **48:** 574–583.

27. FELIG, P. 1973. The glucose-alanine cycle. Metabolism **22:** 179–207.

28. FELIG, P. & J. WAHREN. 1971. Influence on endogenous insulin secretion on splanchnic glucose and amino acid metabolism in man. J. Clin. Invest. **50:** 1702–1711.

29. FELIG, P., J. WAHREN, R. HENDLER & G. AHLBORG. 1972. Plasma glucagon levels in exercising man. N. Engl. J. Med. **287:** 184–185.

30. HUNTER, W. M., C. C. FONSEKA & R. PASSMORE. 1965. The role of growth hormone in the mobilization of fuel for muscular exercise. Quart. J. Exp. Physiol. Cog. Med. Sci. **50:** 406.

31. FELIG, P., J. WAHREN & R. HENDLER. 1974. Sensitivity of hepatic glucoregulatory mechanisms in exercising man. Endocrinology 94(Suppl.): 172 (Abstr.).
32. HULTMAN, E. 1967. Studies on muscle metabolism of glycogen and active phosphate in man with special reference to exercise and diet. Scand. J. Clin. Lab. Invest. 19(Suppl. 94): 63.
33. HULTMAN, E. 1971. Muscle glycogen stores and prolonged exercise. In Frontiers of Fitness. R. J. Shephard, Ed., Charles C Thomas. Springfield, Ill.
34. AHLBORG, G. & P. FELIG. 1976. Influence of glucose ingestion on the fuel-hormone response during prolonged exercise. J. Appl. Physiol. 41: 683–688.
35. AHLBORG, G. & P. FELIG. 1977. Substrate utilization during prolonged exericse preceded by the ingestion of glucose. Amer. J. Physiol. In press.

AMINO ACID METABOLISM IN EXERCISE *

Philip Felig

Department of Internal Medicine
Yale University School of Medicine
New Haven, Connecticut 06510

The fuel requirements of exercising muscle are largely met by the oxidation of glucose and free fatty acids. Amino acids are less important with respect to overall fuel economy. On the other hand, amino acids represent the carbon skeletons for *de novo* glucose synthesis. In addition, the utilization of amino acids as glucose precursors or as an oxidizable substrate represents the dissolution of body protein stores. Thus, with respect to overall glucose hemeostasis, the maintenance of body protein reserves, and the transfer of nitrogen between muscle and liver, amino acids occupy a central role.[1] This review will examine the effects of exercise on the metabolism of amino acids in muscle and liver as gleaned from studies in human subjects employing arterial and venous catheter techniques to study substrate exchange.

Amino Acid Exchange in the Resting State

In the resting condition, a net flux of amino acids exists between muscle tissue (the major reservoir of body protein) and nonmuscular tissues, particularly the liver, the kidney, and, to a lesser extent, the brain (FIGURE 1). While virtually all amino acids with the exception of serine show a net release from muscle tissue, alanine and glutamine exceed all other amino acids in their net release from muscle.[2-4] The predominance of alanine in the amino acid output from muscle is largely accounted for by the transamination of glucose-derived pyruvate.[2, 5, 6] With respect to the source of the amino groups for the synthesis of alanine, recent data suggest that the branched chain amino acids (valine, leucine, and isoleucine) may be particularly important as nitrogen donors.[6, 7]

Complementing the outflow of amino acids from muscle tissue is a net uptake of amino acids by the liver and, to a lesser extent, by the kidney, the gastrointestinal tract, and the brain [4, 8, 9] (FIGURE 1). As in the case of muscle output, alanine predominates in the uptake of amino acids by the liver and is quantitatively the most important gluconeogenic amino acid.[8] Because of the predominance of alanine in the amino acid output from the muscles, as well as its uptake by the liver, and in view of the evidence that the carbon skeleton of alanine is largely derived from pyruvate,[2, 5] a glucose-alanine cycle involving muscle and liver has been described.[2, 10, 11] Recent studies, however, suggest that some of the carbon skeletons of alanine may be derived from other amino acids,[12, 13] thus raising the possibility that alanine transfer between muscle and liver represents not only recycling of carbon skeletons, but may represent *de novo* synthesis of glucose as well. Regardless of the extent to which the carbon

* The work from the author's laboratory described in this review was supported by grants AM 13526 and RR 125 from the National Institutes of Health.

skeletons of alanine are recycled or synthesized *de novo* from other amino acids, it is clear that alanine represents a means of conveying nitrogen groups from muscle to liver.

In addition to the utilization of amino acids by the liver, both the gastrointestinal tract and the kidney represent important sites of amino acid uptake. In this transfer of amino acids to the gut and kidney, glutamine exceeds all other amino acids in quantitative importance. In the kidney, glutamine represents an important precursor for ammonia synthesis.[14] Glutamine is also taken up by the gastrointestinal tract where it may serve as an energy-yielding substrate for transport processes.[4, 15, 16] A net uptake of amino acids is also demonstrable for brain tissue; the branched chain amino acid valine is taken up in significant quantities by the cerebrovascular bed.[9]

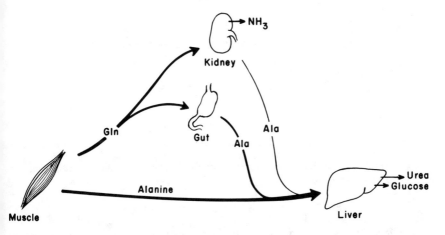

FIGURE 1. Interorgan amino acid exchange in the resting postabsorptive state.

Muscle Amino Acid Exchange During Exercise

During exercise amino acid exchange across contracting muscle undergoes both quantitative as well as qualitative changes. Whereas a variety of amino acids are released by the resting muscle, during exercise a net output is observed only in the case of alanine (FIGURE 2).[5] Thus for all other amino acids the net exchange is too small or variable to reach significant levels. With respect to alanine, the output of this amino acid increases in proportion to the severity of the exercise performed.[5] The major factor determining alanine output during exercise appears to be the availability of pyruvate. This is indicated by the direct linear relationship between plasma alanine and pyruvate levels during exercise.[5] In addition, in subjects in whom pyruvate output from muscle is limited, as in the case of McArdle's syndrome, a corresponding decline in alanine output from muscle is observed.[17]

Of particular interest is the source of the nitrogen groups for alanine synthesis in muscle during exercise. Inasmuch as no net uptake of amino acids by exercising muscle is observed during short-term exercise, it would appear that

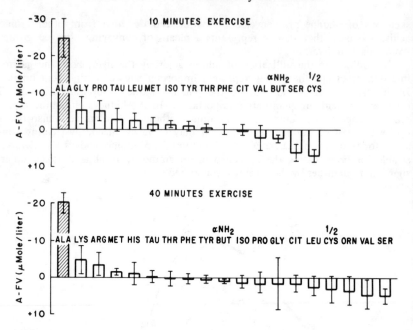

FIGURE 2. Influence of exercise on arterial-venous differences of amino acids across the leg. A consistent net output (negative A-V difference) is observed only in the case of alanine. Absolute alanine output increases 2–5-fold depending on the severity of the exercise.[11]

endogenous amino acids within muscle tissue represent the amino donors for alanine synthesis. As noted above, in the resting state the branched chain amino acids appear to be particularly important as nitrogen donors for alanine synthesis. A similar situation may exist during exercise, although direct evidence of such a relationship is not available at present. An additional source of amino groups may be derived from the purine-nucleotide cycle (the interconversion of adenosine monophosphate and inosine monophosphate).[18] The sequence of events encompassed by the purine-nucleotide cycle results in the liberation of ammonia in muscle tissue.[18] The utilization of ammonia for alanine synthesis requires the presence of glutamate dehydrogenase. This enzyme has generally been felt to be present primarily in liver tissue.[19] However, recent studies from our laboratory indicate the presence of substantial activity of glutamate dehydrogenase in mitochondria from muscle tissue.[20, 21] In fact, the activity of this enzyme is comparable to that of leucine aminotransferase activity in muscle tissue.[21] Furthermore, physiologic concentrations of leucine increase the activity of glutamate dehydrogenase in muscle tissue [20, 21] (as in the case of the liver enzyme [19]). Thus, the nitrogen for alanine synthesis in muscle tissue may be derived from catabolism of branched chain amino acids or alternatively by way of utilization of the ammonia generated in the purine-nucleotide cycle. Leucine may thus contribute to alanine synthesis during exercise both as a substrate as well as an activator of glutamate dehydrogenase [21] (FIGURE 3).

During prolonged exercise (exercise extending for 2–4 hr), output of alanine from muscle tissue continues to be observed.[22] In addition, a net uptake of the branched chain amino acids is demonstrable across the exercising leg muscle after 2–4 hours.[22] These findings thus suggest that extramuscular proteins (e.g., liver proteins) provide a source of amino groups for muscle utilization when exercise is prolonged (see below).

Amino Acid Metabolism by Liver

The uptake of alanine by the liver observed in the resting state continues at similar rates during exercise.[5] Inasmuch as an increase in muscle alanine output occurs with exercise, the failure of hepatic uptake to increase concomitantly results in an accumulation of alanine in arterial blood. Thus the characteristic change in arterial amino acid concentrations during exercise is an increase in arterial alanine while little change is noted for the remaining amino acids.[5] Since blood flow to the splanchnic bed generally declines by 30%–50% during exercise,[5, 23] the maintenance of alanine uptake at resting levels represents in part, an increase in fractional extraction of this amino acid. With more prolonged exercise (extending for 2–4 hr), alanine uptake shows a net increase above resting levels [22] (FIGURE 4). This increment in alanine uptake is due to a further rise in fractional extraction.[22] In fact, fractional extraction of alanine in very prolonged exercise reaches levels of 90%, which exceeds that observed in other circumstances of increased gluconeogenesis such as diabetes,[24] prolonged starvation,[8] or obesity.[25] This increase in fractional extraction of alanine thus provides for a greater contribution from gluconeogenesis to overall glucose production than is observed at rest. The increment in gluconeogenesis allows, in turn, for ongoing glucose output from the liver at rates that are 2–3 times the resting level, despite a progressive depletion of hepatic glycogen stores.[26] Thus, after 2–4 hours of exercise, the net contribution from gluconeogenesis to glucose output from the liver has doubled, in part as a consequence of increased alanine utilization. In addition, the augmented extraction of alanine from the liver results in a fall in arterial concentration so that peak levels of alanine in arterial blood are observed during short-term rather than long-term exercise.[22]

As noted above, during prolonged exercise branched chain amino acids are extracted from arterial blood by contracting muscle.[22] The source of these branched chain amino acids for muscle uptake is the splanchnic bed. After 2–4 hours of exercise, a net splanchnic release is demonstrable for valine, leucine, and isoleucine.[22] These findings thus suggest that breakdown of liver proteins

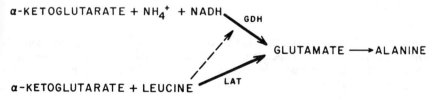

FIGURE 3. Dual role of leucine in alanine synthesis in exercise. Leucine serves as a substrate (catabolism via leucine aminotransferase) as well as a stimulus (activation of glutamate dehydrogenase) in enhancing alanine synthesis in muscle.[20, 21]

may provide additional fuel for exercising muscle in the form of branched chain amino acids.

Influence of Carbohydrate Ingestion

In subjects fed carbohydrates during the course of prolonged exercise, the patterns of fuel utilization by muscle and substrate uptake by the liver are markedly altered.[27] Glucose ingestion during prolonged exercise results in an

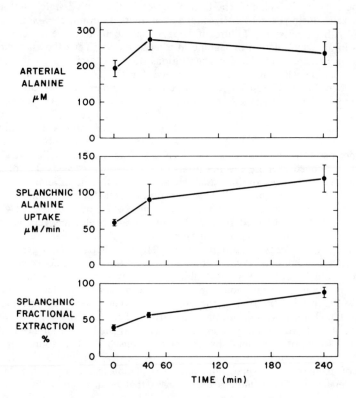

FIGURE 4. Alanine metabolism during prolonged submaximal exercise.[22] As exercise extends beyond 40 minutes, arterial concentration declines while uptake by the splanchnic bed increases.

increase in the glucose consumption by contracting muscle and a diminution in lipolysis and fatty acid utilization by such tissues. The intake of glucose also has an effect upon amino acid exchange across the liver. In contrast to the marked increase in fractional extraction of alanine observed with prolonged exercise,[22] the fractional extraction of alanine during prolonged exercise following carbohydrate intake falls by 30%.[27] Thus the effect of glucose consumption during exercise is a sparing of body fat stores with respect to fuel uptake by muscle and a sparing of gluconeogenic substrate with regard to its utilization by liver. The factors mediating this change in substrate metabolism are the increase in circulating insulin and the reduction in glucagon induced by carbohydrate ingestion.[27]

Recovery from Exercise

In contrast to the effects of carbohydrate ingestion, the effect of recovery from exercise on amino acid metabolism by liver is an exaggeration of the situation observed during exercise. Specifically, the net uptake of alanine by the splanchnic bed is increased during recovery, reflecting an augmented flow to the splanchnic bed as well as an ongoing increase in fractional extraction of this amino acid by hepatic tissues.[28] In contrast, alanine output from muscle falls rapidly following exercise.[28] The net effect is a reduction in arterial alanine levels as splanchnic uptake of this amino acid exceeds net output from muscle tissue. The consequence of this increase in gluconeogenic substrate utilization by the liver is an enhancement of glycogen repletion in liver. Thus, during recovery from exercise, gluconeogenic precursor uptake remains high while glucose output has returned to basal, resting levels.[28]

Exercise and Diabetes

The diabetic state is a situation in which the principal hormonal abnormality is a deficiency of insulin. Inasmuch as exercise is also characterized by a fall in insulin levels,[22, 23] one might anticipate that exercise might accentuate some of the metabolic abnormalities in diabetes. On the other hand, exercise results in stimulation of glucose utilization, and thus might be expected to have an ameliorative effect on diabetes.[29] In fact, the response to exercise in the diabetic suggests both an exaggeration as well as an amelioration of the diabetic syndrome.[30, 31]

In the diabetic, short-term exercise is associated with an absolute increment in alanine uptake by the splanchnic bed.[30] This rise in alanine utilization for gluconeogenesis is a consequence of augmented fractional extraction of this amino acid. A similar increase in alanine uptake is not observed in normal individuals unless exercise is extended for 2–4 hours.[5, 22] Thus the effect of exercise on diabetes is to accentuate the already increased rate of gluconeogenesis that characterizes diabetes, whereas the effect of diabetes is to accelerate the gluconeogenic response to exercise.[30, 31] In contrast to the changes in hepatic metabolism of alanine, the uptake of glucose and the output of alanine by the exercising muscle are comparable in diabetics and nondiabetic subjects during exercise.[30] The similar increment in glucose utilization thus provides strong evidence that glucose uptake during exercise is not dependent on an increase in insulin secretion.

The accelerated response of the diabetic to exercise as indicated by hepatic uptake of alanine is also demonstrable with regard to branched chain amino acid metabolism. During short-term exercise in the diabetic a net flow of branched chain amino acids (valine, leucine, and isoleucine) from liver to muscle tissue is observed.[30] A similar response, as noted above, is not demonstrable in healthy subjects until 2–4 hours of exercise have elapsed.[22] Thus the dependence on amino acids derived from liver tissue as a fuel for exercising muscle is accelerated in the diabetic as compared to nondiabetic subjects. This utilization of branched chain amino acids earlier in exercise may reflect the lesser availability of glycogen stores in the muscle of hyperglycemic, insulin-dependent diabetic patients.[32]

Summary

During exercise, release of alanine from muscle tissue is stimulated in proportion to the severity of the exercise and in proportion to the availability of glucose-derived pyruvate. The amino groups for alanine synthesis are provided by *in situ* breakdown of branched chain amino acids as well as by utilization of ammonia formed in the purine-nucleotide cycle. During short-term exercise, alanine uptake by the liver remains at resting levels, resulting in an accumulation of this amino acid in arterial blood. During prolonged exercise, alanine uptake by the liver increases so that gluconeogenesis provides a greater proportion of total glucose output from the liver. Alanine output from muscle remains stable so that concentrations of alanine in arterial blood show a decline as exercise continues for 2–4 hours. In prolonged exercise, branched chain amino acids are released from liver and taken up by muscle, thus providing an additional fuel for the contracting muscle tissue. Ingestion of carbohydrates reduces the uptake of gluconeogenic amino acids by the liver whereas recovery from exercise is characterized by an increased utilization of alanine by the liver. In diabetic subjects the response to exercise is accelerated, as reflected by an increase in the net uptake of alanine by the liver and a transfer of branched chain amino acids from liver to muscle tissue during the first 40 minutes of exercise. Thus, during exercise, alanine provides a means of transferring nitrogen and gluconeogenic carbon skeletons from muscle to liver while branched chain amino acids provide a protein-derived oxidizable fuel, which is transferred from liver to muscle.

References

1. FELIG, P. 1975. Amino acid metabolism in man. Ann. Rev. Biochem. **44:** 933–953.
2. FELIG, P., T. POZEFSKY, E. MARLISS *et al.* 1970. Alanine: Key role in gluconeogenesis. Science **167:** 1003–1004.
3. MARLISS, E. B., T. T. AOKI, T. POZEFSKY, *et al.* 1971. Muscle and splanchnic glutamine and glutamate metabolism in postabsorptive and starved man. J. Clin. Invest. **50:** 814–817.
4. FELIG, P., J. WAHREN & L. RAF. 1973. Evidence of inter-organ amino-acid transport by blood cells in humans. Proc. Nat. Acad. Sci. U.S.A. **70:** 1775–1779.
5. FELIG, P. & J. WAHREN. 1971. Amino acid metabolism in exercising man. J. Clin. Invest. **50:** 2703–2714.
6. ODESSEY, R., E. A. KHAIRALLAH & A. L. GOLDBERG. 1974. Origin and possible significance of alanine production by skeletal muscle. J. Biol. Chem. **249:** 7623–7629.
7. PALAIOLOGOS, G. & P. FELIG. 1976. Effects of ketone bodies on amino acid metabolism in isolated rat diaphragm. Biochem. J. **154:** 709–716.
8. FELIG, P., O. E. OWEN, J. WAHREN, *et al.* 1969. Amino acid metabolism during prolonged starvation. J. Clin. Invest. **48:** 584–594.

9. FELIG, P., J. WAHREN & G. AHLBORG. 1973. Uptake of individual amino acids by human brain. Proc. Soc. Exp. Biol. Med. **142:** 230–231.
10. MALLETTE, L. E., J. EXTON & R. R. PARK. 1969. Control of gluconeogenesis from amino acids in the perfused rat liver. J. Biol. Chem. **244:** 5713–5723.
11. FELIG, P. 1973. The glucose-alanine cycle. Metabolism **22:** 179–207.
12. GOLDSTEIN, L. & E. A. NEWSHOLME. 1976. The formation of alanine from amino acids in diaphragm muscle of the rat. Biochem. J. **154:** 555–558.
13. GARBER, A. J., I. E. KARL & D. M. KIPNIS. 1976. Alanine and glutamine synthesis and release from skeletal muscle. II. The precursor role of amino acids in alanine and glutanine synthesis. J. Biol. Chem. **251:** 836–843.
14. OWEN, E. E. & R. R. ROBINSON. 1963. Amino acid extraction and ammonia metabolism by the human kidney during the prolonged administration of ammonium chloride. J. Clin. Invest. **42:** 263–270.
15. WINDMUELLER, H. G. & A. E. SPAETH. 1974. Uptake and metabolism of plasma glutamine by small intestine. J. Biol. Chem. **249:** 5070.
16. FELIG, P., J. WAHREN, I. KARL, et al. 1973. Glutamine and glutamate metabolism in normal and diabetic subjects. Diabetes **22:** 573–576.
17. WAHREN, J., P. FELIG, R. J. HAVEL, et al. 1973. Amino acid metabolism in McArdle's syndrome. N. Engl. J. Med. **288:** 774–777.
18. LOWENSTEIN, J. M. 1972. Ammonia production in muscle and other tissues: The purine nucleotide cycle. Physiol. Rev. **52:** 382–414.
19. McGIVAN, J. D., N. M. BRADFORD & J. B. CHAPPELL. 1974. Biochem. J. **142:** 359–364.
20. PALAIOLOGOS, G. & P. FELIG. 1976. Kinetic studies of glutamate dehydrogenase (aminating) (EC 1.4.1.2) from rat diaphragm mitochondria. Fed. Proc. **35:** 299.
21. PALAIOLOGOS, G. & P. FELIG. 1977. Influence of L-leucine on glutamate dehydrogenase activity in isolated rat diaphragm. Submitted for publication.
22. AHLBORG, G., P. FELIG, L. HAGENFELDT & J. WAHREN. 1974. Substrate turnover during prolonged exercise in man: Splanchnic and leg metabolism of glucose, free fatty acids, and amino acids. J. Clin. Invest. **53:** 1080–1090.
23. WAHREN, J., P. FELIG, G. AHLBORG & L. JORFELDT. 1971. Glucose metabolism during leg exercise in man. J. Clin. Invest. **50:** 2715–2725.
24. WAHREN, J., P. FELIG, E. CERASI, et al. 1972. Splanchnic and peripheral glucose and amino acid metabolism in diabetes mellitus. J. Clin. Invest. **51:** 1870–1878.
25. FELIG, P., J. WAHREN, R. HENDLER & T. BRUNDIN. 1974. Splanchnic glucose and amino acid metabolism in obesity. J. Clin. Invest. **53:** 582–590.
26. HULTMAN, E., L. H. NILSSON. 1971. Liver glycogen in man: Effect of different diets and muscular exercise. In Muscle Metabolism during Exercise: Proceedings of a Karolinska Institute Symposium held in Stockholm, Sweden, September 6–9, 1970. B. Pernow & B. Saltin, Eds. : 143–151. Plenum Press. New York, N.Y.
27. AHLBORG, G. & P. FELIG. 1976. Influence of glucose ingestion on fuel-hormone response during prolonged exercise. J. Appl. Physiol. **41:** 683–688.
28. WAHREN, J., P. FELIG, R. HENDLER, et al. 1973. Glucose and amino acid metabolism during recovery after exercise. J. Appl. Physiol. **34:** 838–845.
29. MARBLE, A. 1971. Insulin in the treatment of diabetes. In Joslin's Diabetes Mellitus. Eleventh edit. A. Marble, P. White, R. F. Bradley, et al., Eds. : 287–301. Lea and Febiger. Philadelphia.
30. WAHREN, J., L. HAGENFELDT & P. FELIG. 1975. Splanchnic and leg exchange of glucose, amino acids, and free fatty acids during exercise in diabetes mellitus. J. Clin. Invest. **55:** 1303–1314.
31. FELIG, P. & J. WAHREN. 1975. Fuel homeostasis in exercise. N. Engl. J. Med. **293:** 1078–1084.
32. ROCH-NORLUND, A. E., J. BERGSTROM, H. CASTENFORS, et al. 1970. Muscle glycogen in patients with diabetes mellitus: Glycogen content before treatment and the effect of insulin. Acta Med. Scand. **187:** 445–453.

FREE FATTY ACID TURNOVER AND THE AVAILABILITY OF SUBSTRATES AS A LIMITING FACTOR IN PROLONGED EXERCISE

Philip D. Gollnick

Department of Physical Education for Men
Washington State University
Pullman, Washington 99164

From contemporary literature the misconception can easily be gotten that the question of what fuels are used during muscular exercise is new. The question, however, is not new and neither for that matter are most of the answers. A general interest in this question undoubtedly dates back to the inception of athletic or combative activity of man. Indeed, evidence exists to suggest that the Greeks and Romans were concerned with what was the best food for maximum performance. In the middle of the 19th century the renowned German physiologist von Liebig [1] stated that the protein of skeletal muscle was consumed during work and that large quantities of meat should be eaten to replenish its loss. Although this was shown to be incorrect in 1866,[2] it is surprising that now more than a century later a large percentage of modern-day coaches and athletes still espouse the belief that large quantities of meat must be consumed during periods of heavy exercise to replace the "used up protein."

The question of the relative importance of fats and carbohydrates for the working muscle has also been debated for a long time. In 1896 Chauveau [3] stated that carbohydrates were the only fuel that could be oxidized by the working muscles. This concept received support in 1916 from Fletcher and Hopkins,[4] in 1924 from Meyerhof,[5] and in 1926 from Hill.[6] However, work from the Zuntz laboratory [7-9] from 1896 to 1901 on intact man did not substantiate the Chauveau hypothesis and in fact suggested that both fats and carbohydrates could serve as fuels for muscular work. Numerous studies in the period between 1900 and 1930 [10-14] in which the respiratory exchange ratio (RER) of man and dogs was measured supported the concept that both fat and carbohydrate were oxidized by the working organism. Such total body measurements, however, could not eliminate the possibility that the contractile activity of the muscles themselves was carried out exclusively at the expense of a carbohydrate breakdown. The studies of Himwich and Rose [15] in 1927 may have been the first measurement of the arteriovenous difference for oxygen and carbon dioxide across skeletal muscle at rest and during work. In these studies fed and starved dogs were examined. It was observed that in fed dogs the respiratory quotient (RQ) of muscle was about 0.92 at rest and 0.94 during exercise. In starved dogs (5 to 15 days without food) these values were 0.80 both at rest and after exercise. These studies clearly indicated that fat was providing a major portion of the substrate for the muscle. Much later a large number of similar studies [16-20] were conducted both on man and dogs to firmly establish that both fats and carbohydrates were used as energy sources by the muscle during work. The observation of Fritz and coworkers [21] that stimulated isolated muscle took up and oxidized fatty acids was conclusive proof that skeletal muscle could use fat to support the exercise metabolism.

Likewise, studies concerning the influence of diet on the substrate oxidized during exercise are not new. Around the turn of the century Zuntz and co-workers [7-9] reported a series of studies in which the respiratory exchange ratio (RER) of individuals was measured both at rest and during exercise following dietary manipulation. These studies generally demonstrated a lower RER during work after consumption of fat diets for a number of days prior to the work. A summary of some work conducted by Frentzel and Reach [7] in the Zuntz laboratory is presented in TABLE 1. These data illustrate that a reduction in both the rest and work RER occurred after the consumption of a high fat diet for one week. These studies were subsequently confirmed by Krogh and Lindhard in 1920,[12] by Cathcart and Burnett in 1925,[11] and by Marsh and Murlin in 1928.[13] Anderson and Lusk [10] in 1917 reported a similar dietary effect on the rest and exercise RER of the dog.

The anecdotal comments from the subjects studied by Krogh and Lindhard and by Marsh and Murlin are interesting and informative. Following the fat

TABLE 1

THE INFLUENCE OF DIET ON THE RESPIRATORY EXCHANGE RATIO (RER)
OF MAN DURING WORK *

Subject	Diet	RER	Work (kcal/kg·min)
Frentzel	Fat	0.773	2.066
	Carbodyrate	0.889	1.980
Reach	Fat	0.781	2.119
	Carbohydrate	0.900	2.086

* Values are from 176 experiments. (From Frentzel & Reach.[7])

diet the subjects generally experienced a subjective feeling that the work was harder. They were not inclined to do either physical or mental work under this condition. In contrast, after 5 days on a carbohydrate diet the work seemed extremely easy. Marsh and Murlin reported that one of their subjects experienced a feeling of dizziness while working on the cycle ergometer and afterward expressed fear that he might have fallen off. These symptoms are now commonly recognized as being those of hypoglycemia.

In a now classical study of the influence of diet on work performance, Christensen and Hansen [22] followed the RER during exercise and recorded total endurance time for subjects after a mixed diet, a high fat diet, and a high carbohydrate diet. They clearly demonstrated that the RER was lower both at rest and during exercise after consumption of a high fat diet and that total work endurance time was only about 70% that of the mixed diet condition. The RER was much higher at rest after the high carbohydrate diet, and although it fell during exercise it did not go below the resting value for the mixed diet condition. Under these conditions total work endurance was about twice that of the mixed diet condition. Subsequent studies by our contemporary Scandinavian colleagues,[23-25] in which biopsy samples were taken from the leg muscles, have clearly demonstrated that the glycogen content of the muscle is radically altered by the different diets and that this is responsible for the differences in work capacity. These rather old principles are currently being rediscovered almost daily and used by athletes engaged in endurance activities.

In spite of the fact that it had been demonstrated that fats are used as fuels for exercise before the turn of the century, the mechanisms by which the energy stores of adipose tissue participated in this process remained obscure into the middle of this century. A first step in unraveling this process was the demonstration of Szent-Györgyi and Tominaga [26] in 1924 that a small amount of free fatty acid (FFA) existed in the blood plasma of man. Cohn and associates [27] thereafter established that the FFA was found in the albumin fraction of plasma. The physiological significance of the albumin-bound FFA of plasma as a transport of FFA from the adipose tissue to peripheral tissue was clearly established by Dole [28] and Gordon and Cherkes.[29] Soon thereafter it was established that although the FFA level in plasma was small the turnover was high and that this represented a major energy source for a variety of peripheral tissue.

Measurement of plasma FFA turnover rates via the infusion of albumin-bound, ^{14}C-labeled, long chain fatty acids made it possible to quantitate their role under a variety of metabolic states including exercise. These studies demonstrated that the turnover rate of plasma FFA was related to its concentration in the plasma,[30] that plasma FFA levels are sharply elevated under a variety of conditions including fasting,[28, 29] and prolonged endurance exercise,[31-39] and that under such conditions a large percentage of metabolism is supported by the oxidation of fatty acids whose origin had been the triglyceride pool of the adipose tissue.

During most conditions of prolonged exercise the concentration of glucose in the blood remains remarkably constant. However, as Wahren has pointed out,[40] working muscle does take up and oxidize blood-borne glucose. Furthermore, this can represent a significant source of energy for the muscle. The source of this blood glucose is undoubtedly the glycogen reserves of the liver. One method for estimating the importance of liver glycogen to metabolism during work is to take liver samples and analyze them for glycogen throughout the work bout. Our studies with animals using this method have revealed a significant contribution to work metabolism and also that the blood glucose remains high until the glycogen stores of the liver are nearly depleted.[41]

An estimation of the total amount of FFA and glucose available to the muscle during rest and exercise can be made from the concentrations of these substances in the blood and the blood flow through the muscle. Using existing data for blood flow through a single leg [42, 43] and the concentrations of glucose and FFA in the blood,[44] estimates such as those presented in TABLE 2 can be made of the availability of blood-borne metabolites to the muscles. These estimates demonstrate that the substrate flow through a muscle during exercise far exceeds the metabolic requirement of the exercise and probably the catabolic capacity of the metabolic pathways. This illustrates the importance of the regulatory mechanisms for limiting the overall contribution that extramuscular substrates make to the work metabolism.

Regulation of substrate entry into muscle is influenced both by intra- and extra-muscular factors. It is well established that a membrane-bound carrier system exists for the translocation of glucose from the blood into muscle.[45] This system is influenced by hormonal factors and by intracellular levels of metabolic intermediates such as ATP, AMP, glucose-6-PO$_4$, free glucose, and so forth, which operate by altering the activity of the enzyme hexokinase. During prolonged exercise insulin levels in the blood probably decline, whereas the levels of the intramuscular regulators result in an inhibition of hexokinase. The net effect is an inhibition of a massive uptake of glucose from the blood by the contracting muscle. If allowed to proceed unabated such an uptake of glucose would rapidly deplete the supply of blood glucose and that of the liver. This would have a disastrous effect on the central nervous system, which is dependent upon this as its major energy source. FFA uptake, as indicated earlier, is dependent upon its concentration in the plasma. However, although the plasma level increases during exercise, the fractional extraction rate decreases.[46] Nevertheless, the net result of the increased blood flow and the fractional extraction is an elevated FFA uptake by working muscles. No membrane carrier system for the movement of FFA into muscle has been identified and it is assumed

TABLE 2

An Estimate of the Substrate Available to One Leg from the Circulation of a Subject at Rest and during Exercise *

	Rest	Exercise †
Blood flow (liter/min)	0.45	6.00
Blood glucose (mM)	5.00	5.00
Glucose perfusion (mmoles/min)	2.25	30.00
O$_2$ equivalent of glucose flow (liter/min)	0.30	4.03
Plasma FFA (mEq/liter)	0.50	2.00
FFA perfusion (mEq/min)	0.12 ‡	6.60
O$_2$ equivalent of FFA flow (liter/min)	0.06	3.40
Total body $\dot{V}_{O_2}$ (liter/min)	0.30	2.50
Estimated Q (liter/min)	6.00	16.00
$\dot{V}_{O_2}$ of leg	0.03	1.20

* Estimates are made from data previously published.[42–44]
† Approximately 60% of $\dot{V}_{O_2}$ max.
‡ Plasma volume estimated from a hematocrit of 45%.

that the uptake occurs by a simple diffusion through the plasma membrane of the muscle.

Following the demonstration that fats are oxidized by working muscle during exercise, the question of the relative importance of plasma FFA to the exercise metabolism remained unsettled. Measurement of FFA turnover and oxidation from isotopic infusion studies led to estimates that FFA could account for 25% to 90% of the total exercise metabolism.[35, 47, 48] Pernow and Saltin [49] have studied the role of local versus blood-borne substrates with a unique one-leg exercise model. On day 1 subjects exercised first with one leg and after a 60 min rest with the other leg. After the exercise the subjects consumed a low carbohydrate diet to maintain a low muscle glycogen concentration. The experimental protocol was repeated on day 2 except that the work load was reduced so that it elicited 50% rather than 75% of the one-leg maximal oxygen uptake. In addition, nicotinic acid was administered during the 60-min rest period to block lipolysis. During the first leg exercise with reduced glycogen (day 2) the RER was lower than the day 1, indicating a greater reliance upon the oxidation of fat. Elevation in both plasma FFA and glycerol indicated enhanced lipolysis. Exercise following blockage of lipolysis was accompanied by an elevation in the RER, a small rise in plasma glycerol, a sharp drop in blood glucose, and a reduction in total work capacity. These experiments demonstrate that under conditions of reduced muscle glycogen an enhanced uptake of plasma FFA can serve as an energy source. However, FFA cannot completely substitute for the carbohydrate during moderately severe exercise. When, however, the contribution of plasma FFA is restricted, work capacity is severely inhibited.

In an additional experiment Saltin and associates [50] evaluated the relative importance of local glycogen stores as compared with blood-borne substrates during leg exercise. Subjects performed two-legged bicycle exercises one day after the glycogen content of one leg had been reduced by exercise and maintained low by a high fat-protein diet. Work loads requiring 60% and 80% of the maximal oxygen uptake were performed before and after nicotinic acid infusion. Under the first condition the RQ across the "low" glycogen leg was lower than that of the normal leg during both work loads in spite of the increased plasma FFA and the greater glucose uptake by this leg. Blood glucose remained relatively constant throughout the exercise although both legs had taken up a significant amount of glucose from the blood. Following the administration of nicotinic acid the total body RER increased as did the RQ across both working legs with the difference observed in the "normal" condition being abolished under this condition. A rapid uptake of glucose occurred during both the 60% and 80% $\dot{V}_{O_2}$ max loads, and a sharp fall in blood glucose ensued. These data demonstrated that glycogen availability does influence the metabolic characteristics of the muscle and its relative reliance upon blood-borne substrates.

With FFA uptake and oxidation being dependent upon their concentration in plasma and from the increased oxidative potential of endurance-trained skeletal muscle, it might be expected that an enhanced rate of lipolysis would accompany training. This could be envisaged as a mechanism for providing more FFA to the muscle to support the increased ability to oxidize fat. Although there are exceptions,[51] the general observation is that plasma FFA levels of trained subjects are actually lower than those of untrained individuals during exercise.[52-54] This could be related either to a depressed rate of lipolysis or to an elevated rate of uptake by the working muscle. The lower RER of trained subjects at similar relative work loads as untrained subjects supports the concept of an elevated extraction and oxidation of FFA following training. Examination of the triglyceride lipase activity of adipose tissue has failed to reveal any alteration in this enzyme.[55, 56] Shepherd and coworkers [57] have examined the adenylate cyclase and phosphodiesterase activities of fat cell ghosts from trained and untrained rats. Adenylate cyclase activity was unchanged by training whereas phosphodiesterase activity was elevated. This suggests that training blunted rather than enhanced lipolysis.

Summary

A continual hydrolysis and release of FFA from the triglycerides stores of adipose tissue occurs during prolonged moderately severe exercise. The uptake and oxidation of plasma FFA by the working skeletal muscles represents a major source of energy during such exercise. During light and moderately intense prolonged exercise, lipolysis and the release of FFA from the adipose tissue exceeds uptake by peripheral tissue and the net result is an increase in plasma FFA levels. FFA uptake appears to be related to plasma concentrations and uses no membrane transport system. As work intensity increases the release of FFA from adipose tissue declines and the relative contribution of the plasma FFA to the work metabolism declines until at high work rates there is an almost complete reliance on the intramuscular glycogen reserves. At work loads above about 65% of the individual's aerobic capacity the limiting factor for prolonged exercise appears to be the glycogen stores of the working muscle. When these stores are depleted the work either must stop or its intensity be reduced. Trained individuals have a greater capacity to oxidize fats at high work loads than do untrained subjects. This, however, is not matched by an increased capacity for lipolysis. Why intramuscular glycogen stores are required for prolonged relatively severe exercise when the amount of FFA and glucose that perfuses the skeletal muscles under such conditions is theoretically capable of supporting the exercise metabolism is unknown.

REFERENCES

1. VON LIEBIG, J. 1842. Animal Chemistry or Organic Chemistry in its Application to Physiology and Pathology. W. Gregory, translator. Taylor and Walton. London.
2. VON PETTENKOFER, M. & C. VOIT. 1866. Untersuchungen ueber dem Stoffverbrauch des normalen Menschen. Z. Biol. 2: 459–573.
3. CHAUVEAU, A. 1896. Source et nature du potentiel directment utilise dans le travail musculaire d'après les exchanges respiratoires, chez l'homme en etat d'abstinence. C.R. Acad. Sci. (Paris). 122: 1163–1221.
4. FLETCHER, W. M. & F. G. HOPKINS. 1916. The respiratory process in muscle and the nature of muscular motion. Proc. R. Soc. London (B) 89: 444–467.
5. MEYERHOF, O. 1924. Chemical Dynamics of Life Phenomena. Philadelphia, Pa.
6. HILL, A. V. 1926. Muscular Activity. Baltimore, Md.
7. FRENTZEL, J. & F. REACH. 1901. Untersuchungen zur Frage nach der Quelle der Muskelkraft. Pfluegers Arch. 83: 477–508.
8. ZUNTZ, N. 1896. Ueber die Rolle des Suckers im thierischen Stoffwechsel. Arch. Physiol. : 538–577.
9. ZUNTZ, N. 1901. Ueber die Bedeutung der Verschiedenen Nahrstoffe als Erzeuber der Muskeldraft. Pfluegers Arch. 83: 557–571.
10. ANDERSON, R. J. & G. LUSK. 1917. The interrelation between diet and body condition and the energy production during mechanical work. J. Biol. Chem. 32: 421–445.
11. CATHCART, E. P. & W. A. BURNETT. 1925. The influence of muscle work on metabolism in varying conditions of diet. Proc. Ry. Soc. London (B) 99: 405–426.
12. KROGH, A. & J. LINDHARD. 1920. The relative value of fat and carbohydrate as sources of muscular energy. Biochem. J. 14: 290–363.
13. MARSH, M. E. & J. R. MURLIN. 1928. Muscular efficiency on high carbohydrate and high fat diets. J. Nutrition 1: 105–137.
14. HEINEMAN, H. N. 1901. Experimentelle Untersuchung am Menschen ueber den Einfluss der Muskelarbeit auf den Stoffverbrach und die Bedeutung der einzelnen Nahrstoffe als Quelle der Muskelkraft. Pfluegers Arch. 83: 441–476.
15. HIMWICH, H. E. & M. I. ROSE. 1927. The respiratory quotient of exercising muscle. Amer. J. Physiol. 81: 485–486.

16. CHAPLER, C. K. & W. N. STAINSBY. 1968. Carbohydrate metabolism in contraction dog skeletal muscle in situ. Amer. J. Physiol. **215:** 995–1004.

17. CORSI, A., M. MIDRIO & A. L. GRANSTA. 1969. In situ utilization of glycogen and blood glucose by skeletal muscle during tetanus. Amer. J. Physiol. **216:** 1534–1541.

18. DIPRAMPERO, P. E., P. CERRETELLI & J. PIIPER. 1969. O_2 consumption and metabolite balance in the dog gastrocnemius at rest and during exercise. Pfluegers Arch. **309:** 38–47.

19. KARLSSON, J., S. ROSSELL & B. SALTIN. 1972. Carbohydrate and fat metabolism in contracting canine skeletal muscle. Pfluegers Arch. **331:** 57–69.

20. ANDRES, R., G. CADER & K. L. ZIERLER. 1956. The quantitative minor role of carbohydrates in the oxidative metabolism by skeletal muscle in intact man in the basal state. Measurements of oxygen and glucose uptake and carbon dioxide and lactate production in the forearm. J. Clin. Invest. **35:** 671–682.

21. FRITZ, I., D. G. DAVIS, R. H. HOLTROP & H. DUNDEE. 1958. Fatty acid oxidation by skeletal muscle during rest and activity. Amer. J. Physiol. **194:** 379–386.

22. CHRISTENSEN, E H. & O. HANSEN. 1939. Arbeitsfähiget und Ehrnährung. Skand. Arch. Physiol. **81:** 160–175.

23. BERGSTRÖM, J. & E. HULTMAN. 1966. Muscle glycogen synthesis after exercise: An enhancing factor localized to the muscle cells in man. Nature **210:** 309–310.

24. BERGSTRÖM, J., L. HERMANSEN, E. HULTMAN & B. SALTIN. 1967. Diet, muscle glycogen and physical performance. Acta Physiol. Scand. **71:** 140–150.

25. HERMANSEN, L., E. HULTMAN & B. SALTIN. 1967. Muscle glycogen and prolonged severe exercise. Acta Physiol. Scand. **7:** 129–139.

26. SZENT-GYÖRGYI, A. & T. TOMINAGA. 1924. Die quantitative Bestimmung der freien Blut fettsäuren. Biochem. Z. **146:** 226–238.

27. COHN, E. J., W. L. HUGHES, JR. & J. H. WEARE. 1947. Preparation and properties of serum and plasma protein. XIII. Crystallization of serum albumins from ethanol-water mixtures. J. Amer. Chem. Soc. **69:** 1753–1761.

28. DOLE, V. P. 1956. A relation between non-esterified fatty acids in plasma and the metabolism of glucose. J. Clin. Invest. **35:** 150–154.

29. GORDON, R. S., JR. & A. CHERKES. 1956. Unesterified fatty acid in human blood plasma. J. Clin. Invest. **35:** 206–212.

30. ARMSTRONG, D. T., R. STEELE, N. ALTSZULER, A. DUNN, J. S. BISHOP & R. C. DEBODO. 1961. Regulation of plasma free fatty acid turnover. Amer. J. Physiol. **201:** 9–15.

31. BASU, A., R. PASSMORE & J. A. STRONG. 1960. The effect of exercise on the level of nonesterified fatty acids in the blood. Quart. J. Exp. Physiol. **45:** 312–317.

32. CARLSON, L. A., S. FRÖBERG & S. PERSSON. 1965. Concentration and turnover of the free fatty acids of plasma and concentration of blood glucose during exercise in horses. Acta Physiol. Scand. **63:** 434–441.

33. FREIDBERG, S. J., P. B. SHER, M. C. BOGDONOFF & E. H. ESTS, JR. 1963. The dynamics of plasma free fatty acid metabolism during exercise. J. Lipid Res. **4:** 34–38.

34. HUNTER, W. H., C. C. RONSEKA & R. PASSMORE. 1965. Growth hormone: Important role in muscular exercise in adults. Science **150:** 1051–1053.

35. HAVEL, R. J., A. NAIMARK & C. R. BORCHGREVIN. 1963. Turnover rate and oxidation of free fatty acids of blood plasma in man during exercise: Studies during continuous infusion of palmitate-1-C^{14}. J. Clin. Invest. **42:** 1054–1063.

36. HAVEL, R. J., L. A. CARLSON, L-G. EKELUND & A. HOLMGREN. 1964. Turnover rate and oxidation of different free fatty acids in man during exercise. J. Appl. Physiol. **19:** 613–618.

37. PAUL, P. 1975. Effects of long lasting physical exercise and training on lipid

metabolism. *In* Metabolic Adaptation to Prolonged Physical Exercise. H. Howard & J. R. Poortmans, Eds. S. A. Karger, A. G. Basel, Switzerland.

38. ISSEKUTZ, B., JR., H. L. MILLER, P. PAUL & K. RODHAL. 1969. Aerobic work capacity and plasma FFA turnover. J. Appl. Physiol. **20:** 293–296.

39. MILLER, H., B. ISSEKUTZ, JR. & K. RODHAL. 1963. Effect of exercise on the oxidation of fatty acids in the dog. Amer. J. Physiol. **205:** 167–172.

40. WAHREN, J. 1977. Glucose turnover during exercise in man. Ann. N. Y. Acad. Sci. This volume.

41. ARMSTRONG, R. B., C. W. SAUBERT, IV, W. L. SEMBROWICH, R. E. SHEPHERD & P. D. GOLLNICK. 1974. Glycogen depletion in rat skeletal muscle fibers at different intensities and duration of exercise. Pfluegers Arch. **352:** 243–256.

42. SALTIN, B., K. NAZAR, D. L. COSTILL, E. STEIN, E. JANSSON, B. ESSÉN & P. D. GOLLNICK. 1976. The nature of the training response: Peripheral and central adaptations to one-legged exercise. Acta Physiol. Scand. **96:** 289–305.

43. WAHREN, J. & L. JORFELDT. 1973. Determination of leg blood flow during exercise in man: An indicator-dilution technique based on femoral venous dye infusion. Clin. Sci. Mod. Med. **45:** 135–146.

44. GOLLNICK, P. D., R. B. ARMSTRONG, C. W. SAUBERT, IV, W. L. SEMBROWICH, R. E. SHEPHERD & B. SALTIN. 1973. Glycogen depletion patterns in human skeletal muscle fibers during prolonged work. Pfluegers Arch. **344:** 1–12.

45. MORGAN, H. E., D. M. REGEN & C. R. PARK. 1964. Identification of a mobile carrier-mediated sugar transport system in muscle. J. Biol. Chem. **239:** 369–374.

46. HAVEL, R. J., B. PERNOW & N. L. JONES. 1967. Uptake and release of free fatty acids and other metabolites in the legs of exercising man. J. Appl. Physiol. **23:** 90–96.

47. CARLSON, L. A., L-G. EKLUND & L. ÖRO. 1963. Studies on blood lipids during exercise. IV. Arterial concentration of plasma free fatty acids and glycerol during and after prolonged exercise in normal men. J. Lab. Clin. Med. **61:** 724–729.

48. ISSEKUTZ, B., JR. & P. PAUL. 1966. The role of extramuscular energy sources in the metabolism of the exercising dog. Fed. Proc. **25:** 334–339.

49. PERNOW, B. & B. SALTIN. 1971. Availability of substrates and capacity for prolonged heavy exercise in man. J. Appl. Physiol. **31:** 416–422.

50. SALTIN, B., B. ESSÉN, E. JANSSON, P. D. GOLLNICK & B. PERNOW. Availability of substrates and leg metabolism during exercise in man. In Press.

51. KEUL, J., E. DOLL & G. HARALAMBIE. 1970. Freie Fettsauren, Glycerin und Triglyceride im arteriellen und femoralvenosen Blut vor und nach vierwachigen korperlichen Training. Pfluegers Arch. **316:** 194–204.

52. JOHNSON, R. H., J. L. WALTON, H. A. KREBS & R. H. WILLIAMSON. 1969. Metabolic fuels during and after severe exercise in athletes and non-athletes. Lancet **ii:** 452–455.

53. JOHNSON, R. H. & J. L. WALTON. 1972. The effect of exercise upon acetoacetate metabolism in athletes and non-athletes. Quart. J. Exp. Physiol. **57:** 73–79.

54. WINDER, W. W., K. M. BALDWIN & J. O. HOLLOSZY. 1975. Exercise induced increase in the capacity of the rat skeletal muscle to oxidize ketones. Can. J. Physiol. Pharmacol. **53:** 86–91.

55. ASKEW, E. W., G. L. DOHM, R. H. HUSTON, T. W. SNEED & R. P. DOWDY. 1973. Response of rat tissue lipases to physical training and exercise. Proc. Soc. Exp. Biol. Med. **41:** 123–129.

56. MCGARR, J. A., L. B. OSCAI & J. BORENSZATJN. 1976. Effect of exercise on hormone-sensitive lipase activity in rat adipocytes. Amer. J. Physiol. **230:** 385–388.

57. SHEPHERD, R. E., W. L. SEMBROWICH, H. E. GREEN & P. D. GOLLNICK. 1977. Effect of physical training on control mechanisms of lipolysis in rat fat cell ghosts. J. Appl. Physiol. In press.

HORMONAL REGULATION DURING PROLONGED EXERCISE *

H. Galbo, E. A. Richter, and J. Hilsted

*Institute of Medical Physiology B
University of Copenhagen
Copenhagen, Denmark*

J. J. Holst

*Department of Clinical Chemistry
Bispebjerg Hospital
Copenhagen, Denmark*

N. J. Christensen

*2nd Clinic of Internal Medicine
Kommunehospitalet
Aarhus, Denmark*

J. Henriksson

*The August Krogh Institute
University of Copenhagen
Copenhagen, Denmark*

Although both the sympathetic and parasympathetic nervous system may modulate the function of the pancreatic α- and β-cells, the role of neural mechanisms in the physiologic regulation of insulin and glucagon secretion is unclear.[1] During prolonged exercise plasma insulin concentrations decrease in man,[2-4] dog,[5] and rat[6-8] (FIGURE 1), probably due to inhibition of insulin release.[9, 10] When α-adrenergic receptors were blocked in man by phentolamine (Regitin), insulin concentrations during exercise were larger than in control experiments without drugs.[4] Also, larger plasma insulin levels were found in rats during exercise when the function of the sympathetic nervous system was inhibited by blockade of α-adrenergic receptors,[7, 8] by immunosympathectomy,[11] or by chemical sympathectomy.[47] Furthermore, in rats α-adrenergic blockade abolished the exercise-induced inhibition of insulin release.[10] In man[12, 13] as well as in rats[14] a diminished rise of plasma catecholamine levels in trained individuals during exercise is accompanied by a smaller decrease in plasma insulin levels. Available evidence thus indicates that during prolonged exercise α-adrenergic activity inhibits insulin secretion.

Plasma glucagon concentrations increase during prolonged exercise (FIGURES 1, 2 & 3). In rats the exercise-induced increase in plasma glucagon concentration has been ascribed to stimulation of α-adrenergic[7] as well as β-

* This work was supported by grants from the NOVO Research Foundation, The Danish Medical Research Council, Idrættens Forskningsråd, Den Lægevidenskabelige Forskningsfond for Storkøbenhavn, Færøerne og Grønland, and The P. Carl Petersen Foundation.

72

adrenergic [8, 11] receptors. In man, however, we found that prolonged sub-maximal running elicited a much larger glucagon response than short-term maximal running, even though plasma catecholamine concentrations were larger during maximal running (FIGURE 2). Furthermore, the plasma concentration of glucagon, which is a rapidly cleared hormone, was still elevated 30 minutes after prolonged exercise, whereas the catecholamines at that time had decreased markedly. It was concluded that in man increments in catecholamines could not account completely for the glucagon response to prolonged exercise.[2] The lack of significant influence of the autonomic nervous system on the exercise-induced secretion of glucagon in man has been confirmed in experiments in which exhaustive running was performed during α-adrenergic blockade with phentolamine (Regitin) and during parasympathetic blockade with atropine.[4] Neither did β-adrenergic blockade with propranolol (Inderal) inhibit glucagon secretion in man during prolonged exercise.[3] On the contrary, when compared with control experiments, plasma glucagon concentrations increased more rapidly during exhaustive exercise when β-adrenergic receptors were blocked

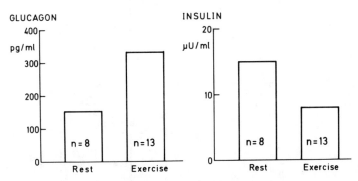

FIGURE 1. Plasma glucagon and insulin concentrations in rats at rest and after heavy exercise (1 hr of swimming with a tail weight of 4% of the body weight).

and also when lipolysis was blocked by nicotinic acid (FIGURE 3). These differences could not be explained by differences in the plasma concentrations of free fatty acids, alanine, and lactate,[3] substrates that may influence pancreatic α-cell secretion.[1] Also plasma epinephrine concentrations, which normally increase gradually throughout prolonged exercise in man,[2-4, 12] increased more rapidly during exercise after administration of propranolol or nicotinic acid (FIGURE 4). Since the intensified glucagon and epinephrine responses to exercise after administration of these drugs were closely related to increased rates of decline in plasma glucose concentrations,[3] and since glucose concentrations may modulate glucagon [1] as well as epinephrine concentrations,[15, 16] it was suggested that decreased glucose availability significantly enhances the secretion of these hormones during prolonged exercise in man.[3] In agreement with this hypothesis, maintenance of euglycemia by glucose-infusion during β-adrenergic blockade markedly reduced the glucagon and epinephrine responses to exercise in man.[17] Simultaneously norepinephrine concentrations were not changed by glucose-infusion, in accordance with the finding that the secretion of epinephrine is much more dependent on glucose concentrations than is the secretion of norepi-

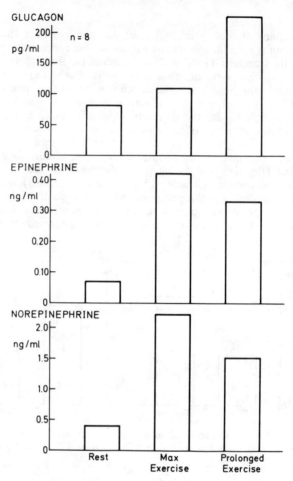

FIGURE 2. Plasma glucagon and plasma catecholamine concentrations in man at rest and after short term maximal and prolonged submaximal exercise.

nephrine.[15, 16] Glucose administration has also been shown to reduce markedly the glucagon concentrations reached during exercise in rats [7, 8] and dogs [18] as well as the epinephrine concentrations reached during exercise in dogs.[19] These findings led to the hypothesis [3] that during prolonged exercise glucose-sensitive cells in CNS and pancreas, possibly sensitized by low insulin concentrations,[1, 20] establish a hormonal response that favors glucose production and lipid mobilization. As a consequence, an enhanced hormonal response to exercise would be expected when available glycogen stores are small or hard to mobilize, and plasma glucose concentrations accordingly decline more rapidly during exercise. That this seems to be the case appears from our recent preliminary experiments. When exercise was performed after intake of a fat diet, glucose concentrations declined more rapidly than after a carbohydrate diet. Simultaneously the responses to exercise of glucagon, epinephrine, growth hormone, and cortisol were intensified. When glucose concentrations were restored by glucose infusion during continued exercise, the concentrations of glucagon and epinephrine were markedly reduced, while norepinephrine and insulin levels were principally unchanged. Also compatible with our hypothesis is the finding that the exercise-induced increase in plasma glucagon was lessened, when a glucose sparing effect was introduced by increasing plasma free fatty acids.[21] Furthermore, in trained individuals carbohydrate stores are increased,[14, 22] and the tendency to a decline of plasma glucose concentrations during exercise is less.[13, 14, 22] Consistently during exercise, plasma glucagon concentrations in man[13] and in rats[14] as well as plasma epinephrine concentrations in man[12, 13] and in rats,[47] and the urinary excretion rate of epinephrine in the rat[23] were smaller in trained than in untrained individuals.

Plasma growth hormone concentrations have previously been shown to increase during exercise in man.[12, 13, 24-26] The increase could be suppressed by glucose[24, 25] and by infusion of phentolamine (Regitin),[26] which also may suppress the growth hormone release after insulin-induced hypoglycemia. Some authors found that human growth hormone rose to a greater extent during exercise in untrained than in trained individuals,[13, 27] whereas other authors found that the degree of elevation was not affected by physical training.[12] In the rat, increased[11] as well as decreased[28] plasma growth-hormone levels after prolonged exercise have been reported.

Plasma corticosteroid concentrations, which also are promoted by glucose deprivation,[29] have been shown to increase during heavy exercise in rats[11, 30, 31] and in man.[12, 13, 32, 33, 34] When the work load exceeds a critical level of about 60% of the individual maximal oxygen uptake[13, 33] an increased rate of secre-

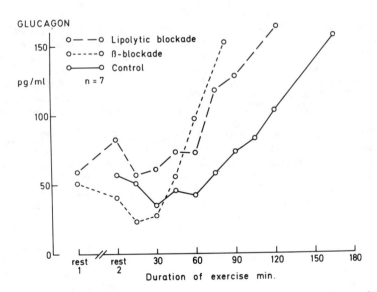

FIGURE 3. Plasma glucagon concentrations in man at rest and during prolonged exercise. When rest-1 samples had been drawn nicotinic acid (lipolytic blockade) or propranolol (β-blockade) was administered.

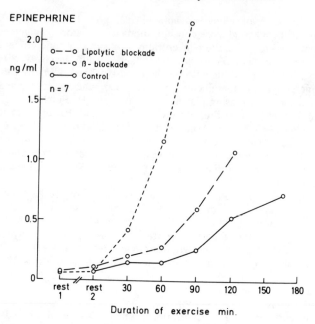

FIGURE 4. Plasma epinephrine concentrations in man at rest and during prolonged exercise. When rest-1 samples had been drawn nicotinic acid (lipolytic blockade) or propranolol (β-blockade) was administered.

tion of cortisol [34] exceeds the increased rate of removal of cortisol, which is found also during light exercise.[34] Increased [13] as well as unchanged [12] and decreased [27, 35] plasma corticosteroid concentrations have been found during exercise in trained individuals as compared with untrained individuals. Finally, since hypoglycemia may stimulate the release of thyroid-stimulating hormone (TSH),[36, 37] it should be mentioned that, in contrast to previous findings,[38, 39] serum concentrations of TSH recently have been reported to increase during exercise.[40]

The depicted pattern of hormonal changes during prolonged exercise, *i.e.,* decreased plasma concentrations of insulin and increased plasma concentrations of glucagon, catecholamines, growth hormone, thyroid-stimulating hormone, and corticosteroids ought to favor mobilization of free fatty acids and hepatic glucose production. In accordance with this, exercise-induced lipolysis has been inhibited by β-adrenergic blockade,[3, 11, 19, 26, 41] adrenomedullectomy,[31, 42] chemical sympathectomy with 6-OH-dopamine,[42] immunosympathectomy,[11] adrenalectomy,[8, 30, 31] hypophysectomy,[11, 41] and insulin-infusion,[47] whereas lipolysis was increased during exercise in diabetics [43] and after pancreatectomy.[44] However, a normal lipolytic response to exercise has also been described after β-adrenergic blockade,[8, 11] adrenomedullectomy,[11, 30, 41] and adrenalectomy with corticosteroid replacement therapy.[41] Glucagon does not seem to be indispensable for exercise-induced mobilization of free fatty acids.[3, 6, 11]

The exercise-induced hepatic glycogen depletion was not inhibited by β-adrenergic blockade,[3, 19, 41] adrenomedullectomy,[30, 31, 41, 42] chemical sympa-

thectomy with 6-OH-dopamine,[42] adrenalectomy (with [41] or without [30, 31] replacement therapy), and hypophysectomy.[41] However, in some studies of
adrenomedullectomy and adrenalectomy [30, 31] the decline of blood glucose concentrations during exercise was more marked than in control experiments.
Furthermore, the exercise-induced hepatic glycogen depletion has been diminished by chemical sympathectomy with 6-OH-dopamine in a dose [47] that was
larger than previously used,[42] and by blocking the release of catecholamines at
nerve endings with drugs in adrenal-demedullated rats.[30]

During exercise the decrease in hepatic glycogen content as well as the
increase in blood glucose concentrations were diminished in rats treated with
glucagon-antibodies (FIGURE 5). This finding suggests that glucagon may
enhance hepatic glycogen depletion during exercise.[6] Also, in antibody-treated
exercising rats, however, a decrease in hepatic glycogen concentrations was
observed (FIGURE 5). Furthermore the effect of neutralization of glucagon with
antibodies on hepatic glycogen depletion during exercise seems only to be
marked when insulin concentrations are markedly decreased.[47] Even if insulin [5, 9, 43, 44] and glucagon [5, 13] concentrations are constant, hepatic glucose
production may increase during exercise. The concentration of insulin required
for exercise to stimulate glucose uptake in the working muscles is undoubtedly
very low.[45]

As described above it seems as if the hormonal response to exercise is
blunted in trained individuals. Nevertheless, the need for blood-borne substrates
during exercise is not diminished after training.[11, 22, 44] Accordingly, we have
to propose that training causes increased sensitivity to the hormonal changes
that occur during exercise. In fact it has been shown that adipose tissue lipolysis
is more sensitive to epinephrine in trained than in untrained rats.[46]

It is evident that the regulation of fuel mobilization during exercise is multifactorial. The different hormones act in concert and may probably substitute
for each other. We do not know enough about the relative role of the different
hormones in this interplay.

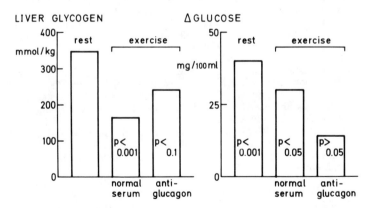

FIGURE 5. The influence of glucagon-antibody administration in rats on hepatic
glycogen depletion and change in blood glucose concentration during heavy exercise.
(Glycogen concentrations were expressed as mmoles of glucose per kg of wet tissue.
Blood glucose concentrations were measured before as well as after a 60 min period
of either rest or exercise).

The present survey does not pretend to be complete and may be biased, since it has focused on the possibility that the hormonal response to exercise (and with that the amount of mobilized fuel) is influenced by glucose-sensitive receptors. However, in this way the supply of fuels may have relation to the demand of the working muscles. Furthermore, it is in any case difficult to ignore the similarity between the hormonal response to prolonged exercise and the hormonal responses to states of glucoprivation such as fasting, hypoglycemia, and deoxyglucose administration.

References

1. GERICH, J. E., M. A. CHARLES & G. M. GRODSKY. 1976. Regulation of pancreatic insulin and glucagon secretion. Ann. Rev. Physiol. **38:** 353–388.
2. GALBO, H., J. J. HOLST & N. J. CHRISTENSEN. 1975. Glucagon and plasma catecholamine responses to graded and prolonged exercise in man. J. Appl. Physiol. **38:** 70–76.
3. GALBO, H., J. J. HOLST, N. J. CHRISTENSEN & J. HILSTED. 1976. Glucagon and plasma catecholamines during beta-receptor blockade in exercising man. J. Appl. Physiol. **40:** 855–863.
4. GALBO, H., N. J. CHRISTENSEN & J. J. HOLST. 1976. The role of the autonomic innervation in the control of glucagon and insulin responses to prolonged exercise in man. Acta Physiol. Scand. (Suppl. 440): 175.
5. VRANIC, M., R. KAWAMORI, S. PEK, N. KOVACEVIC & G. A. WRENSHALL. 1976. The essentiality of insulin and the role of glucagon in regulating glucose utilization and production during strenuous exercise in dogs. J. Clin. Invest. **57:** 245–255.
6. GALBO, H. & J. J. HOLST. 1976. The influence of glucagon on hepatic glycogen mobilization in exercising rats. Pflügers Arch. **363:** 49–53.
7. HARVEY, W. D., G. R. FALOONA & R. H. UNGER. 1974. The effect of adrenergic blockade on exercise-induced hyperglucagonemia. Endocrinology **94:** 1254–1258.
8. LUYCKX, A. S. & P. J. LEFEBVRE. 1974. Mechanisms involved in the exercise-induced increase in glucagon secretion in rats. Diabetes **23:** 81–93.
9. CONARD, V., H. BRUNNENGRABER, R. VANROUX, A. DESCHAEPDRIJVER, E. MOERMANS & J. R. M. FRANCKSON. 1969. Influence of muscular exercise on glucose regulation. *In* Biochemistry of Exercise. J. R. Poortmans, Ed. Vol. **3:** 114–115. Karger. Basel, Switzerland.
10. BRISSON, G. R., F. MALAISSE-LAGAE & W. J. MALAISSE. 1971. Effect of phentolamine upon insulin secretion during exercise. Diabetologia **7:** 223–226.
11. LUYCKX, A. S., A. DRESSE, A. CESSION-FOSSION & P. J. LEFEBVRE. 1975. Catecholamines and exercise-induced glucagon and fatty acid mobilization in the rat. Amer. J. Physiol. **229:** 376–383.
12. HARTLEY, L. H., J. W. MASON, R. P. HOGAN, L. G. JONES, T. A. KOTCHEN, E. H. MOUGEY, F. E. WHERRY, L. L. PENNINGTON & P. T. RICKETTS. 1972. Multiple hormonal responses to prolonged exercise in relation to physical training. J. Appl. Physiol. **33:** 607–610.
13. BLOOM, S. R., R. H. JOHNSON, D. M. PARK, M. J. RENNIE & W. R. SULAIMAN. 1976. Differences in the metabolic and hormonal response to exercise between racing cyclists and untrained individuals. J. Physiol. (Lond.) **258:** 1–18.
14. RICHTER, E. A., H. GALBO & J. J. HOLST. 1976. Training-induced diminution of the glucagon and insulin responses to prolonged exercise in rats. Acta Physiol. Scand. (Suppl. 440): 151.
15. CHRISTENSEN, N. J., K. G. M. M. ALBERTI & O. BRANDSBORG. 1975. Plasma catecholamines and blood substrate concentrations: Studies in insulin induced

hypoglycaemia and after adrenaline infusions. Europ. J. Clin. Invest. **5:** 415–423.

16. NIIJIMA, A. 1975. The effect of 2-deoxy-D-glucose and D-glucose on the efferent discharge rate of sympathetic nerves. J. Physiol. (Lond.) **251:** 231–243.

17. GALBO, H., N. J. CHRISTENSEN & J. J. HOLST. 1976. Glucose-induced decrease in glucagon and epinephrine responses to exercise in man. Acta Physiol. Scand. (Suppl. 440): 179.

18. BÖTTGER, I., E. M. SCHLEIN, G. R. FALOONA, J. P. KNOCHEL & R. H. UNGER. 1972. The effect of exercise on glucagon secretion. J. Clin. Endocrinol. Metab. **35:** 117–125.

19. NAZAR, K., Z. BRZEZINSKA & S. KOZLOWSKI. 1975. Sympathetic activity during prolonged physical exercise in dogs: Control of energy substrate utilization. *In* Metabolic Adaptation to Prolonged Physical Exercise. H. Howald & J. R. Poortmans, Eds. Vol. **7:** 204–210. Birkhäuser Verlag. Basel, Switzerland.

20. SZABO, O. & A. J. SZABO. 1972. Evidence for an insulin-sensitive receptor in the central nervous system. Amer. J. Physiol. **223:** 1349–1353.

21. RENNIE, M. J., W. W. WINDER & J. O. HOLLOSZY. 1976. A sparing effect of increased plasma fatty acids on muscle and liver glycogen content in the exercising rat. Biochem. J. **156:** 647–655.

22. BALDWIN, K. M., R. H. FITTS, F. W. BOOTH, W. W. WINDER & J. O. HOLLOSZY. 1975. Depletion of muscle and liver glycogen during exercise. Protective effect of training. Pflügers Arch. **354:** 203–212.

23. ÖSTMAN, I., N. O. SJÖSTRAND & G. SWEDIN. 1972. Cardiac noradrenaline turnover and urinary catecholamine excretion in trained and untrained rats during rest and exercise. Acta Physiol. Scand. **86:** 299–308.

24. GLICK, S. M. 1968. Normal and abnormal secretion of growth hormone. Ann. N.Y. Acad. Sci. **148:** 471–487.

25. HANSEN, AA.P. 1971. The effect of intravenous glucose infusion on the exercise-induced serum growth hormone rise in normals and juvenile diabetics. Scand. J. Clin. Lab. Invest. **28:** 195–205.

26. HANSEN, AA.P. 1971. The effect of adrenergic receptor blockade on the exercise-induced serum growth hormone rise in normals and juvenile diabetics. J. Clin. Endocr. **33:** 807–812.

27. MIKULAJ, L., L. KOMADEL, M. VIGAS, R. KVETNANSKY, L. STARKA & P. VENCEL. 1975. Some hormonal changes after different kinds of motor stress in trained and untrained young men. *In* Metabolic Adaptation to Prolonged Physical Exercise. H. Howald & J. R. Poortmans, Eds. Vol. **7:** 333–338. Birkhäuser Verlag. Basel, Switzerland.

28. FEDERSPIL, G., G. UDESCHINI, C. DE PALO & N. SICOLO. 1975. Role of growth hormone in lipid mobilization stimulated by prolonged muscular exercise in the rat. Horm. Metab. Res. **7:** 484–488.

29. BRODOWS, R. G., F. X. PI-SUNYER & R. G. CAMPBELL. 1973. Neural control of counter-regulatory events during glucopenia in man. J. Clin. Invest. **52:** 1841–1844.

30. MALING, H. M., D. N. STERN, P. D. ALTLAND, B. HIGHMAN & B. B. BRODIE. 1966. The physiologic role of the sympathetic nervous system in exercise. J. Pharm. Exp. Ther. **154:** 35–45.

31. STRUCK, P. J. & C. M. TIPTON. 1974. Effect of acute exercise on glycogen levels in adrenalectomized rats. Endocrinology **95:** 1385–1391.

32. FOLLENIUS, M. & G. BRANDENBERGER. 1975. Effect of muscular exercise on day-time variations of plasma cortisol and glucose. *In* Metabolic Adaptation to Prolonged Physical Exercise. H. Howald & J. R. Poortmans, Eds. Vol. **7:** 322–325. Birkhäuser Verlag. Basel, Switzerland.

33. DAVIES, C. T. M. & J. D. FEW. 1973. Effects of exercise on adrenocortical function. J. Appl. Physiol. **35:** 887–891.

34. FEW, J. D. 1974. Effect of exercise on the secretion and metabolism of cortisol in man. J. Endocrinol. **62:** 341–353.
35. FRENKL, R., L. CSALAY & G. CSÁKVÁRY. 1975. Further experimental results concerning the relationship of muscular exercise and adrenal function. Endokrinologie **66:** 285–291.
36. GUANSING, A. R., Y. LEUNG, K. AJLOUNI & T. C. HAGEN. 1975. The effect of hypoglycemia on TSH release in man. J. Clin. Endocrinol. Metab. **40:** 755–758.
37. LEUNG, Y., A. R. GUANSING, K. AJLOUNI, T. C. HAGEN, P. S. ROSENFELD & J. J. BARBORIAK. 1975. The effect of hypoglycemia on hypothalamic thyrotropin-releasing hormone (TRH) in the rat. Endocrinology **97:** 380–384.
38. TERJUNG, R. L. & C. M. TIPTON. 1971. Plasma thyroxine and thyroid-stimulating hormone levels during submaximal exercise in humans. Amer. J. Physiol. **220:** 1840–1845.
39. FEDERSPIL, G., P. FRANCHIMONT & M. T. HAZEE-HAGELSTEIN. 1976. Serum TSH and prolactin levels during prolonged muscular exercise. Horm. Metab. Res. **8:** 323–324.
40. GALBO, H., L. HUMMER, I. B. PETERSEN, N. J. CHRISTENSEN & N. BIE. 1977. Thyroid and testicular hormone responses to graded and prolonged exercise in man. Europ. J. Appl. Occupat. Physiol. **36:** 101–106.
41. GOLLNICK, P. D., R. G. SOULE, A. W. TAYLOR, C. WILLIAMS & C. D. IANUZZO. 1970. Exercise-induced glycogenolysis and lipolysis in the rat: Hormonal influence. Amer. J. Physiol. **219:** 729–733.
42. SEMBROWICH, W. L., C. D. IANUZZO, C. W. SAUBERT IV, R. E. SHEPHERD & P. D. GOLLNICK. 1974. Substrate mobilization during prolonged exercise in 6-hydroxydopamine treated rats. Pflügers Arch. **349:** 57–62.
43. WAHREN, J., L. HAGENFELDT & P. FELIG. 1975. Splanchnic and leg exchange of glucose, amino acids, and free fatty acids during exercise in diabetes mellitus. J. Clin. Invest. **55:** 1303–1314.
44. PAUL, P. 1971. Uptake and oxidation of substrates in the intact animal during exercise. Adv. Exp. Med. Biol. **11:** 225–247.
45. BERGER, M., S. HAGG & N. B. RUDERMAN. 1975. Glucose metabolism in perfused skeletal muscle. Interaction of insulin and exercise on glucose uptake. Biochem. J. **146:** 231–238.
46. ASKEW, E. W., R. L. HUSLON, C. C. PLOPPER & A. L. HECKER. 1975. Adipose tissue cellularity and lipolysis. J. Clin. Invest. **56:** 521–529.
47. GALBO, H. *et al.* Unpublished results.

THE REGULATION OF INTRACELLULAR AND EXTRACELLULAR FUEL SUPPLY DURING SUSTAINED EXERCISE

E. A. Newsholme

Department of Biochemistry
University of Oxford
Oxford, OX1 3QU
England

INTRODUCTION

Prolonged physical activity, such as that occurring in the marathon run or longer endurance races, causes a marked stimulation not only in the flux of metabolites through the energy-producing pathways in muscle, but also in the rate at which fuels are mobilized from the storage tissue of the body (i.e., liver and adipose tissue). There are at least three general problems in metabolic regulation that are posed by this increase in the rate of fuel provision and oxidation. First, how is the rate of ATP production within the muscle regulated *precisely* in relation to the rate of ATP utilization by the contractile process: this problem applies to all types of physical activity including short bursts of violent activity as well as endurance exercise. Secondly, how is the rate of mobilization of fuels from the storage tissues regulated *precisely* to the rate of fuel oxidation by the muscles: this is particularly relevant to endurance exercise in which glucose and fatty acids are mobilized from liver and adipose tissue (respectively), and yet the concentrations of these fuels in the blood (especially glucose) remain fairly constant. Thirdly, how is the rate of oxidation of endogenous carbohydrate (i.e., muscle glycogen) regulated in relation to the rate of oxidation of fatty acids by the muscle: this problem is particularly relevant to the marathon runner who, by dietary manipulation prior to the race, can raise the level of glycogen in his muscles so that oxidation of this energy reserve can play a substantial role in ATP formation during the race. These problems are discussed in detail in the following sections.

CONTROL OF CARBOHYDRATE UTILIZATION IN MUSCLE IN RELATION TO THE RATE OF ATP UTILIZATION

Importance of the Maintenance of the ATP/ADP Concentration Ratio in Muscle

It is known that ATP does not function as a store of chemical energy in the cell. Its concentration in muscle is only 5–7 μmole/g fresh muscle,[1] which would be depleted in less than a second during intense muscular activity unless it was resynthesized at a rate equal to that of utilization.[2] In combination with ADP, ATP functions as an energy transfer system in the cell: the generation of ATP from ADP during the oxidation of fuels (e.g., glucose) conserves chemical energy, which is utilized in a number of processes (e.g., muscular contrac-

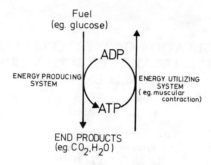

FIGURE 1. The role of the ATP/ADP couple in energy transfer in muscle. The ATP/ADP concentration ratio remains remarkably constant under very different conditions of steady-state flux. There is no store of energy in this system, so that a change in rate of utilization of ATP must cause the same change in rate of production.

tion, FIGURE 1). The ATP-ADP system couples the oxidative processes of the cell with the contractile process in such a way that the latter process is totally dependent upon the former. Thus when contractile activity is increased, the rate of fuel oxidation must also be increased. Furthermore, to avoid large transient changes in the ATP/ADP concentration ratio, the rate of fuel oxidation must be regulated *rapidly* and *precisely* according to the rate of ATP utilization by the contractile process. Indeed, this ratio of oxidation to utilization is known to remain constant under these conditions. For example, the initiation of flight in the insect, which increases the rate of ATP turnover several hundred-fold, results only in small changes in the ATP-ADP concentration ratio (TABLE 1).

The reason for this remarkable constancy of the ATP/ADP ratio may be to maintain what the author terms the "kinetic efficiency" of the energy-producing and energy-utilizing processes in the muscle. Since ATP is chemically very similar to ADP, the catalytic site of enzymes that react with these nucleotides cannot totally distinguish between them. This lack of complete discrimination manifests itself as competitive inhibition of the enzyme activity by one

TABLE 1

CONCENTRATIONS OF ADENINE NUCLEOTIDES AND INORGANIC PHOSPHATE (P_i) IN LOCUST FLIGHT MUSCLE AT REST AND AFTER FLIGHT

	Metabolite Concentration (μmole/g fresh wt)		
Metabolites	Resting Muscle	10 sec Flight	3 min Flight
ATP	5.06 ± 0.20 (13)†	4.58 ± 0.13 (19)	4.32 ± 0.10 (10)
ADP	0.43 ± 0.03 (7)	0.96 ± 0.05 (12)	1.10 ± 0.09 (10)
AMP	0.06 ± 0.01 (7)	0.12 ± 0.01 (10)	0.12 ± 0.02 (12)
P_i	9.30 ± 1.2 (9)	13.5 ± 1.2 (10)	11.9 ± 0.7 (9)
ATP/ADP	11.8	4.8	3.9

* After Rowan.[3]
† Numbers in parentheses indicate number of tests performed.

nucleotide in relation to the other. Thus, enzymes that utilize ADP as substrate are inhibited by ATP and enzymes that utilize ATP as substrate are inhibited by ADP [4] (TABLE 2). Consequently, if the intracellular ATP/ADP concentration ratio increased, the activity of enzymes catalyzing the conversion of ADP into ATP would be inhibited, whereas if the ratio decreased, the activity of enzymes catalyzing ATP utilization would be inhibited (TABLE 2). It is likely that small changes in this concentration ratio in the cell would cause only slight inhibition, but any reduction in the activity of enzymes catalysing important regulatory reactions in the cell could reduce the rate of ATP formation and/or the performance of mechanical work. In this way, the kinetic efficiency of energy transfer in the muscle would be reduced. Although a reduction in this kinetic efficiency may have little obvious effect in the everyday life of a "normal" human subject enjoying the benefits of civilization, it could seriously

TABLE 2

INHIBITION OF ATP-PRODUCING AND ATP-UTILIZING ENZYME ACTIVITIES
BY ADENINE NUCLEOTIDES

Enzyme	Substrate	Inhibitor	Type of Inhibitor
Hexokinase[5]	ATP	ADP	Competitive
3-Phosphoglycerate kinase[5]	ADP	ATP	Competitive
Pyruvate kinase[5]	ADP	ATP	Competitive
Creatine phosphokinase[5]	ATP	ADP	Competitive
Phosphoenol pyruvate carboxylase[5]	GTP	GDP	Competitive
Fatty acyl-CoA synthetase[5]	ATP	ADP	Competitive
Adenylate kinase[5]	ATP	ADP	Mixed type
Actomyosin ATPase[6]	ATP	ADP	
Adenine nucleotide translocase *[7]	ADP	ATP	

* The inward transport of ADP by heart muscle mitochondrial translocase is not specific for ADP so that an increase in the ATP concentration in the cytoplasm could reduce the activity of the translocase.

interfere in the performance of an athlete. The challenge of competition demands that the formation, transfer, and utilization of biological energy in the muscle occurs with maximum efficiency. In other words, changes in the concentration of intracellular adenine nucleotides should be minimal during changes in the rate of energy utilization in muscle.

*The Fructose-6-Phosphate–Fructose-Diphosphate Substrate Cycle:
A Mechanism for Increasing Sensitivity in Metabolic Control of Glycolysis*

The need for maintenance of kinetic efficiency of energy transfer in muscle of an athlete during competitive performance has been emphasized above. Minimal changes in the concentration of adenine nucleotides would be incurred if the rate of ATP production was regulated in relation to the rate of ATP utilization by a direct feedback control mechanism.

In the early stages of sustained exercise (10–15 min) it is likely that glucose is the major fuel for the muscle. During this period, the rate of glycolytic flux (and the citric acid cycle plus electron transport chain) must be sufficient to provide enough energy for the demands of the contractile process. Consequently, the rate of glycolysis is controlled in relation to the energy requirement of the muscle. The three nonequilibrium reactions in the early stages of glycolysis that are regulated in relation to the energy requirements of the muscle are glucose transport, hexokinase, and phosphofructokinase.[2] There is little biochemical information on the mechanism of the control of glucose transport. The activity of hexokinase is regulated by the changes in the concentration of glucose-6-phosphate, which in turn is regulated by the activity of phosphofructokinase. The latter enzyme is regulated by a feedback mechanism dependent upon the rate of ATP utilization. Phosphofructokinase is inhibited by ATP, but this inhibition is relieved by AMP, inorganic phosphate, fructose diphosphate, and NH_4^+. A small decrease in the ATP/ADP concentration ratio in the muscle causes larger increases in the concentration of AMP, NH_4^+, and inorganic phosphate, and these latter changes are largely responsible for the increase in activity of phosphofructokinase.[2, 8] Thus, the feedback system involves changes in concentrations of regulators that are dependent upon the changes in the ATP/ADP concentration ratio (FIGURE 2).

A major problem in the regulation of glycolysis in muscle is sensitivity of phosphofructokinase to the changes in concentrations of these metabolic regulators. In particular, the increase in rate of energy utilization that occurs when a resting muscle is maximally activated is large, but the changes in concentrations of the metabolic regulators (AMP, fructose diphosphate, inorganic phosphate, and NH_4^+) may not be sufficient to produce the necessary increase in activity of phosphofructokinase. (The limits imposed on changes in concentration of metabolic regulators and the sensitivity of enzyme activities to these changes have been extensively discussed elsewhere.[2, 9, 10]) In some muscles, the reaction catalyzed by phosphofructokinase is opposed by a reaction catalyzed by the enzyme, fructose-diphosphatase. There is some evidence to support the

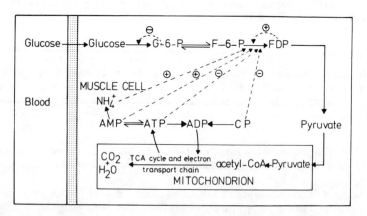

FIGURE 2. Regulation of glycolysis in muscle at the glucose transport, hexokinase, and phosphofructokinase reactions. The abbreviaitons G6P, F6P, FDP, represent glucose-6-phosphate, fructose-6-phosphate, fructose-1,6-diphosphate, respectively.

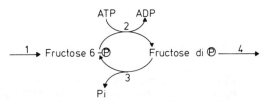

FIGURE 3. The fructose-6-phosphate–fructose-1,6-diphosphate cycle. Reaction 1 represents the flux into fructose-6-phosphate from glycogenolysis or glucose utilization or both. Reactions 2 and 3 represent phosphofructokinase and fructose-1,6-diphosphatase, respectively, and reaction 4 represents the flux into the remainder of the glycolytic pathway.

view that these two enzymes are simultaneously active in resting muscle so that fructose-6-phosphate is converted to fructose diphosphate, but this is converted back into fructose-6-phosphate through the activity of fructose-diphosphatase. This constitutes a substrate cycle between fructose-6-phosphate and fructose-diphosphate (FIGURE 3). The role of this cycle is considered to be to provide very sensitive metabolic control at this enzymatic level.[9-11]

The sensitivity in control provided by a substrate cycle is defined as follows:

$$\text{sensitivity} = 1 + \frac{\text{cycling rate}}{\text{flux}},$$

where sensitivity is defined as the ratio of the relative change in flux to the relative change in regulator concentration.[11] The ratio, cycling rate to flux, refers to the situation in the muscle under control (i.e., resting) conditions, so that, in order to provide an increased sensitivity over and above that provided by a noncycling system, the ratio must be large when the muscle is at rest. However, it has been shown that a high rate of cycling will produce a significant amount of heat [11] and the maintenance of such high cycling rates for prolonged periods could result in hyperthermia. This problem is overcome if it is assumed that high rates of cycling (and therefore a large ratio of cycling rate to flux) occur in resting muscle *only* when exercise is anticipated. Thus, it has been suggested that certain hormones (e.g., adrenaline, noradrenaline) increase the rate of cycling between fructose-6-phosphate and fructose-diphosphate in resting muscle when exercise is anticipated (or under conditions of stress).[11] A high rate of cycling under this condition would increase the sensitivity of the phosphofructokinase system to control by metabolic regulators, so that, if muscular activity followed the anticipation, the rate of ATP production could rapidly and precisely increase to meet the new demand for ATP by the contractile system.

In the absence of substrate cycling at this level, larger changes in concentrations of the feedback regulators may be required in order to regulate satisfactorily the rate of glycolytic flux. However, large changes in the concentrations of these regulators can only be obtained at the expense of large changes in the ATP/ADP concentration ratio. The latter would result in kinetic inefficiency of energy metabolism in muscle (see above). Thus, the ability to control the rate of substrate cycling under resting, anticipatory conditions would appear to be important for the athlete. It is suggested that one role of athletic training, especially interval training, is to increase the capacity of such substrate cycles,

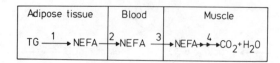

FIGURE 4. The provision of fatty acid for oxidation in muscle by lipolysis in adipose tissue. (1) The lipolytic reaction in adipose tissue. (2) The release of fatty acid by adipose tissue. (3) The uptake of fatty acid by muscle. (4) The oxidation of fatty acids in muscle.

and/or improve their response to changes in hormone levels. Consequently, large changes in flux through the ATP-producing and ATP-utilizing processes would be obtained upon initiation of exercise with only minimum changes in concentrations of metabolic regulators: kinetic efficiency would be maintained despite very high rates of ATP turnover.

THE ROLE OF THE TRIGLYCERIDE-FATTY ACID CYCLE IN THE REGULATION OF FATTY ACID MOBILIZATION FROM ADIPOSE TISSUE

The oxidation of long-chain fatty acids by muscle provides a considerable proportion of the energy required during prolonged exercise (e.g., marathon running, see below). The fatty acids are derived from the triglyceride stores in the adipose tissue. The process of lipolysis in the adipose tissue converts triglyceride into fatty acids, which are released into the bloodstream and transported to the muscle (FIGURE 4).

In adipose tissue, the process of lipolysis occurs simultaneously with that of esterification, so that triglyceride is broken down to fatty acids, which are re-activated and re-esterified to form triglyceride. Thus a substrate cycle between triglyceride and fatty acid is present in adipose tissue [2, 11] (FIGURE 5). It is suggested that one role of this substrate cycle is to provide a sensitive control mechanism for fatty acid mobilization. Thus small changes in blood levels of lipolytic and/or antilipolytic hormones and other lipolytic regulators

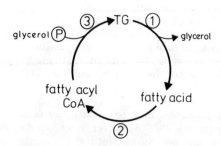

FIGURE 5. The triglyceride-fatty acid substrate cycle. Reaction (1) is catalyzed by triglyceride lipase (plus di- and monoglyceride lipases); reaction (2) by fatty acyl CoA synthetase, and reaction (3) represents the esterification process. TG represents triglyceride and glycerol ⓟ represents glycerol-1-phosphate. The simultaneous activities of enzymes catalyzing the three processes result in the substrate cycle.

(e.g., ketone bodies) may exert marked changes in the rate of fatty acid mobilization from adipose tissue. However, a direct feedback control mechanism may operate between muscle and adipose tissue in order to provide a more precise mechanism of control of fatty acid mobilization that would complement the hormonal control. If the rate of fatty acid utilization by muscle increased (because of increased contractile activity) this could result in a decrease in the concentration of fatty acids in the blood and hence that in the adipose tissue. Since the concentration of fatty acid in adipose tissue is not saturating for the esterification process,[12, 13] a decrease in concentration would reduce the rate of esterification. Hence the rate of fatty acid mobilization would increase. Furthermore, since fatty acids inhibit the activity of triglyceride lipase [14, 15] a decrease in the fatty acid concentration in adipose tissue would increase the rate of lipolysis. Consequently, an increased rate of utilization of fatty acids in muscle, causing a decrease in fatty acid concentration in adipose tissue, will lead to increased mobilization of fatty acids from adipose tissue (FIGURE 6). The opposite changes would, of course, result from a decreased rate of utilization of fatty acids in muscle.

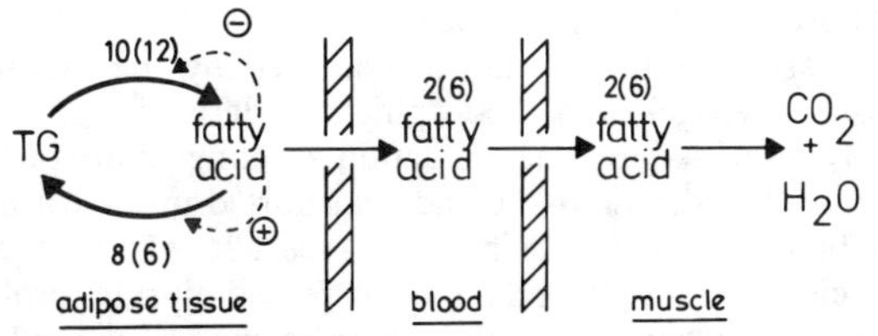

FIGURE 6. Feedback control of fatty acid mobilization from adipose tissue via the triglyceride-fatty acid cycle. The numbers represent the (hypothetical) rates of the various processes. The numbers in parenthesis indicate the changes in rates produced by an increased rate of fatty acid utilization by muscle.

It is possible that athletic training, and especially interval training, increases the capacity of the triglyceride-fatty acid substrate cycle in adipose tissue. Consequently, an increase in the cycling/flux ratio, which could be produced by changes in hormone concentrations prior to the exercise, could provide a very sensitive control mechanism so that the rate of fatty acid mobilization could be modified by small changes in the level of fatty acids.

INTERRELATIONSHIP BETWEEN FAT AND CARBOHYDRATE OXIDATION IN MUSCLE

The amounts of fuel stored in the different tissues in the average human subject are given in TABLE 3. Glycogen appears to be a major store of fuel within muscle itself and it is utilized under both aerobic and anaerobic conditions.[2] Approximately 100 g of glycogen is also stored in the liver and it is released (as glucose) from the liver into the bloodstream during muscular activity. It is well known that muscle glycogen can be increased markedly by dietary manipulations.[17] In some individuals the glycogen level in muscle can be raised to 4 g/100 g muscle. It is generally accepted amongst athletes that this elevated glycogen level in the muscle plays an important role in sustaining muscular activity during a marathon run. A simple calculation emphasizes the importance of this glycogen: If the content of glycogen in muscle is 4 g/100 g of muscle, the total glycogen in the muscles of the leg will be 600 g (assuming 1.5 kg of leg muscle); the complete oxidation of this glycogen will provide 2220 kcal of energy (assuming that oxidation of 1 g of glucose produces 3.7 kcal energy). Furthermore, the release of 100 g of glucose by the liver (from glycogen) should provide an additional 370 kcal, so that the total energy available from carbohydrate oxidation in the marathon runner is approximately 2579 kcal. If the marathon runner expends energy at the rate of 18 kcal/min, carbohydrate oxidation should provide sufficient energy for 143 minutes of marathon running, the entire duration of the run.

Unfortunately, the above calculations assume that the transfer of chemical energy from carbohydrate oxidation to the ADP-ATP energy couple (see above) and the transduction of this chemical energy into mechanical activity are 100% efficient. There is no doubt that these processes will not be 100% efficient, but it is not possible to give an accurate value for their efficiency. If the overall efficiency of these processes is 70%, carbohydrate oxidation could provide 70% of the energy required during the marathon run; if it is 50%, the carbohydrate oxidation would provide 50% of the energy.

The question arises as to the fuel that is used by the marathon runner in addition to muscle glycogen and blood glucose (derived from liver glycogen). It is undoubtedly provided by the oxidation of long-chain fatty acids, which are mobilized from the adipose tissue and transported in the form of an albumin complex in the bloodstream to the muscles (see above). It is well established that the fatty acid level in the blood is increased during prolonged exercise including the marathon run [18] and that there is increased oxidation of fat by the muscle during prolonged exercise. However, the oxidation of fatty acids by the muscle is not merely a process that supplements carbohydrate oxidation for energy production in muscle. It plays an important regulatory role, which ensures that if fatty acids are available, they will be oxidized in preference to carbohydrate so that blood glucose will be conserved for tissues that have a high or an absolute dependence on this fuel for energy provision (e.g., brain, red and white blood cells). Thus there is now considerable evidence that fatty acid

TABLE 3

FUEL RESERVES IN THE AVERAGE HUMAN SUBJECT *

Fuel	Tissue	Fuel Reserves in Average Man	
		kcal	g
Triglyceride	Adipose tissue	100,000	15,000
Glycogen	Liver	200	70
	Muscle	400	120
Glucose	Body fluids	40	20
Protein	Muscle	25,000	6,000

* After Cahill & Owen.[16]

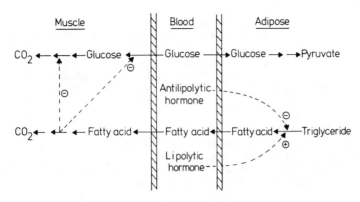

FIGURE 7. Mechanism of regulation of the blood glucose level via the glucose-fatty acid cycle. The mechanisms of regulation of glucose utilization in muscle by fatty acid oxidation are given in FIGURE 8. Examples of lipolytic hormones include adrenaline, noradrenaline, glucagon, and growth hormone. The most potent antilipolytic hormone is insulin. Since the author considers that changes in the blood glucose level do not play an important role in the regulation of fatty acid release due to changes in rate of esterification, this regulatory link has been omitted (c.f. Reference 2, page 227).

oxidation in muscle decreases glucose utilization by this tissue.* In the early stages of the exercise, liver glycogen may be degraded more readily than adipose tissue triglyceride, so that glucose will be more important than fatty acids. Nonetheless, after the first few minutes of a period of sustained exercise, fatty acids will be used to a progressively greater extent and that, perhaps after 20 minutes, they may be the major *blood-borne* fuel for the muscle. However, the fuel requirement of the marathon run appears to be considerably greater than can be supplied by the oxidation of fatty acids alone, hence the importance of the elevation of muscle glycogen to the marathon runner. (At the present time it is unclear whether mobilization, transport, or uptake is the factor limiting the rate of oxidation of fatty acid in the muscle.) The author suggests that, for the major period of the marathon run, the energy requirement of the athlete is provided by oxidation of both endogenous glycogen and exogenous fatty acid (perhaps in the ratio 70/30, see above). The importance of fatty acid oxidation is that it will restrict the utilization of glycogen to that required to supplement the energy *not* provided by fatty acid oxidation. If fatty acid oxidation did not restrict glycogen utilization (via control of glycolysis, FIGURE 7), the glycogen reserves of the muscle would be utilized more rapidly, so that they would become exhausted before completion of the race. If this occurred, only the blood-borne fuels could be used (i.e., fatty acids and glucose). However, as indicated above, the rate of fatty acid oxidation alone cannot provide energy

---

* Experiments with isolated muscle preparations (perfused rat heart, isolated rat diaphragm, and isolated rat leg muscles) demonstrate that fatty acid oxidation inhibits glucose utilization by specific biochemical mechanisms [19-21] (FIGURE 7). An increase in the blood fatty acid level, produced physiologically or artifically in animals or man, decreases the overall rate of glucose utilization *in vivo*.[2]

at the rate required for the marathon-runnning activity (i.e., 18 kcal/min): it may be only able to provide approximately 30% of the energy requirement. Although fatty acid oxidation can inhibit glucose utilization, this inhibitory effect is removed if the energy demand by the muscle exceeds that that can be provided by fatty acid oxidation. The regulation of glucose utilization by fatty acid oxidation is achieved, in part, by the inhibitory effect of citrate on the enzyme phosphofructokinase [2, 19] (FIGURE 8). However, it is well established that an increase in the concentration of any (or all) of the deinhibitors of phosphofructokinase (e.g., AMP, NH_4^+, inorganic phosphate, and fructose diphosphate, FIGURE 2) will reduce citrate inhibition of the enzyme and hence increase the rate of glycolysis and glucose utilization.[2, 19, 22]

Thus if the rate of fatty acid provision to muscle provides just sufficient fatty acid oxidation for the energy requirements of the working muscle, a

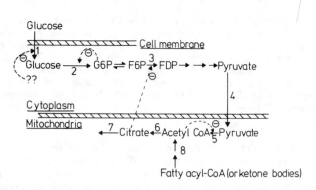

FIGURE 8. Mechanism of control of glycolysis by fatty acid oxidation in muscle. The reactions are as follows: (1) membrane transport of glucose; (2) hexokinase; (3) phosphofructokinase; (4) pyruvate transport into the mitochondrion; (5) pyruvate dehydrogenase; (6) citrate synthase; (7) further reactions of the citric acid cycle; (8) β-oxidation system (or pathway of ketone body utilization). The dotted lines indicate allosteric regulatory mechanism by which some nonequilibrium reactions of glycolysis are controlled via the rate of fatty acid (and/or ketone body) oxidation in muscle. The allosteric factor regulating glucose transport is unknown.

further increase in work by that muscle would reduce the ATP/ADP concentration ratio, increase the concentrations of AMP, inorganic phosphate, and NH_4^+ (and possibly fructose-diphosphate), and hence increase the flux through glycolysis. This would occur despite the inhibitory effects of fatty acid oxidation, since citrate inhibition of phosphofructokinase is relieved by increases in the concentration of AMP etc. (see above). Thus if an increased energy demand by muscle could not be met by increased fat mobilization, an increase in the rate of glucose utilization would have to occur. In the absence of muscle or liver glycogen, which will represent the condition of an athlete towards the end of a marathon run, utilization of blood glucose would cause a reduction in the level of blood glucose. In particular, the glucose concentration in the local environment of the muscle may fall considerably. This could result in fatigue. A decrease in the local concentration of glucose in the muscle might impair nervous function and hence this could give rise to physiological exhaustion.

Alternatively, the reduction in glucose concentration would lower the rate of glycolysis (because of depletion of substrate) and, in the absence of any other alternative fuel to supplement fatty acid oxidation, the rate of energy formation in the muscles would be decreased. The muscle could respond only by reducing energy utilization, i.e., causing a reduction in mechanical activity, which is known as physiological exhaustion (although the biochemical details of the mechanism of exhaustion are unknown). Hence the elevated level of glycogen in the muscles of marathon runners provides a fuel that, if it can be utilized to supplement fatty acid oxidation throughout the entire period of the marathon run, would enable the high caloric expenditure of this activity to be maintained throughout the run without inducing physiological exhaustion. It should be clear that a combination of adequate fuel supply and efficient and sensitive metabolic regulation (in order to ensure that the correct proportions of fat and carbohydrate are used in relation to the energy demands of the muscle) is required for a satisfactory performance from a marathon runner.

References

1. BEIS, I. & E. A. NEWSHOLME. 1975. Biochem. J. **152:** 23–32.
2. NEWSHOLME, E. A. & C. START. 1973. Regulation in Metabolism. Wiley & Sons. London.
3. ROWAN, A. 1975. D.Phil. thesis. Oxford University.
4. WATTS, D. C. 1971. *In* Biochemical Evolution and The Origin of Life. E. Schoffeniels, Ed. : 150–173. North Holland. Amsterdam.
5. BARMAN, T. E. 1969. Enzyme Handbook. Vols. I and II. Springer-Verlag. Berlin.
6. MARUYAMA, K. & J. W. S. PRINGLE. 1967. Arch. Biochem. Biophys. **120:** 225–228.
7. BEIS, I. & E. A. NEWSHOLME. 1976. J. Mol. Cell. Cardiology. **8:** 863–876.
8. SUGDEN, P. H. & E. A. NEWSHOLME. 1975. Biochem. J. **150:** 113–122.
9. CRABTREE, B. & E. A. NEWSHOLME. 1975. *In* Insect Muscle. P. N. R. Usherwood, Ed. : 405–500. Academic Press. London.
10. NEWSHOLME, E. A. & B. CRABTREE. 1973. Symp. Soc. Exp. Biol. **26:** 429–460.
11. NEWSHOLME, E. A. & B. CRABTREE. 1976. Biochem. Soc. Symp. **41:** 61–110.
12. BALLY, P. R., G. F. CAHILL, B. LEBOUEF & A. E. RENOLD. 1960. J. Biol. Chem. **235:** 333–336.
13. KERPEL, S., E. SHAFRIR & B. SHAPIRO. 1961. Biochem. Biophys. Acta **227:** 608–617.
14. RODBELL, M. 1965. Ann. N.Y. Acad. Sci. **131:** 302–314.
15. BURNS, T. W., P. E. LANGLEY & G. A. ROBINSON. 1975. Metabolism **24:** 265–276.
16. CAHILL, G. F. & O. E. OWEN. 1965. *In* Carbohydrate Metabolism and its Disorders. F. Dickens, P. J. Randle & W. J. Whelan, Eds. Vol. **1:** 497–522. Academic Press. New York, N.Y.
17. BERGSTRÖM, J. L., E. HERMANSEN, E. HULTMAN & B. SALTIN. 1967. Acta Physiol. Scan. **71:** 140–150.
18. GOLLNICK, P. D. 1977. Ann. N.Y. Acad. Sci. This volume.
19. NEWSHOLME, E. A. & P. J. RANDLE. 1964. Biochem. J. **93:** 641–651.
20. CUENDET, G. S., E. G. LOTEN & A. E. RENOLD. 1975. European Association for Study of Diabetes Meeting. Munich 1975. Abstract No. 42.
21. RUNDERMAN, N. B. Personal communication.
22. NEWSHOLME, E. A. 1970. *In* Essays in Cell Metabolism. W. Bartley, H. L. Kornberg & J. R. Quayle, Eds. : 189–223. Wiley-Interscience. London.

DISCUSSION

Bengt Saltin, *Moderator*

University of Copenhagen
Copenhagen, Denmark

P. MILVY (*Mt. Sinai School of Medicine, New York, N.Y.*): Dr. Saltin, you talked of endurance training, which trains the cardiovascular system as well as the skeletal muscles. Could you comment on endurance of weight lifters or discus throwers? Do you find a similar muscle fiber distribution in these athletes?

B. SALTIN: In strength-trained athletes there may be no special fiber composition or there may be found a predominance of type II or fast-twitching fibers, as would be expected. However, in these athletes there is not a high activity of mitochondrial enzymes or a high degree of capillarization. If anything, the reverse is true. That is, there is a dilution of mitochondria in these athletes, with mitochondrial enzyme activities about one half of what is seen with normal subjects.

B. CERRETELLI (*SUNY at Buffalo, Buffalo, N.Y.*): You showed that the IIB (FT$_b$) fibers increased their oxidative activity with training; yet this seems in a way a contradiction to the fact that they are fast fibers, built for anaerobic activity. Does this mean that the functional usage of the fibers changes with training, that is, the percentage contribution of anaerobic and aerobic metabolism that they use?

B. SALTIN: I think that the changes that we see in capillarization and oxidative potential of fibers, especially the type IIA (FT$_a$) and type IIB (FT$_b$) fibers, are important and have significance for performance during running of one, two, or three hours. At workloads of 60% to 70% of $\dot{V}_{O_2 \, max}$, type I (ST) fibers are preferentially used. As these fibers become depleted of glycogen, there is an increased use of type IIA (FT$_a$) and finally type IIB (FT$_b$) fibers, so success in the later stages of prolonged running is to a large degree dependent upon whether or not those fibers, recruited at the end, can perform aerobically.

QUESTION: I would like to ask if Dr. Essén has any data on the composition of the lipid fraction that she extracts from the freeze-dried muscle?

B. ESSÉN (*Karolinska Institutet, Stockholm, Sweden*): The method that we are using measures triglycerides. I must say that we also measure monoglycerides with this techniques, although it has been shown that the concentration of monoglycerides in muscles is very low. We have no information on the fatty acid composition of these fats, although we have made some preliminary attempts.

K. W. ELLINGWOOD (*University of Florida, Gainesville, Fla.*): I would like to ask Dr. Wahren if he had measured insulin levels in his experiments?

J. WAHREN (*Karolinska Institutet, Stockholm, Sweden*): The general finding in our experiments and others is that the blood insulin concentration falls during exercise from a basal level of say 10 to 15 $\mu U/ml$ to about one half of that during exercise. At the same time, glucagon concentration rises, particularly during heavy and prolonged exercise. In the prolonged exercise glucagon levels rose from 100 pg/ml to about 400–500 pg/ml. I believe that the glucagon levels may be important in stimulating hepatic glucogenesis during prolonged exercise. In our glucose ingestion studies we saw that the insulin levels rose quite markedly, although the rise was blunted by the exercise. That is, the rise was not as much as it otherwise would be had the subjects been at rest.

A. KUNIN (*University of Vermont, Burlington, Vt.*): I am interested in the effect of glucose ingestion or some other sugar precursor such as maple syrup, sucrose, or candy during long distance running. Does this correspond to the intravenous glucose administration that you gave your exercising subjects?

J. WAHREN: I think that our data shows that glucose ingestion, both before and during exercise, is readily absorbed from the gut and transported from the liver to the exercising muscles. The contribution this made was considerable, and it would seem to provide a grounds for facilitating further work. In this situation there was a relative hyperglycemia all through the work period, so that the blood sugar was higher as compared to the control subjects who received no glucose. Our glucose was given by oral ingestion of a 60% glucose solution. In spite of the fact that this was a highly concentrated glucose solution, it appears as if it was readily absorbed.

D. RUDIKOFF (*Queens College, Flushing, N.Y.*): Is it possible to increase the glycogen content of the liver in a way analogous to carbohydrate loading of muscle?

J. WAHREN: From data that derives from studies of Dr. Hultman and others in Stockholm a similar pattern seems possible. If the liver glycogen is depleted prior to exercise and then a carbohydrate-rich diet is provided, the liver glycogen will rise and reach higher levels than before. So the "overshoot" phenomenon does seem to also exist in the liver. It may also be said that it appears as if the carbohydrate content of the liver rather closely follows the intake of sugar; i.e., 12 hours without a carbohydrate intake will markedly deprive the liver of its glycogen content. This is true also at rest.

E. J. COLT (*St. Luke's Hospital, New York, N.Y.*): What are the relative contributions of muscle glycogen and blood glucose, from liver glycogenolysis and gluconeogenesis, to carbohydrate utilization during exercise?

J. WAHREN: While I have focused essentially on blood glucose, the contribution of muscle glycogen is of great importance, particularly during the initial phase of exercise when blood glucose will contribute very little. As exercise continues, the contribution of blood glucose increases as the muscle glycogen stores decline. After 40 minutes of exercise, under the conditions I have discussed, blood glucose can account for 30% to 40% of the total turnover of fuel. In the legs, at this same time, indications are that blood glucose accounts for between 75% and 90% of the carbohydrate utilization.

D. S. KRONFELD (*University of Pennsylvania, Philadelphia, Pa.*): We have done some diet studies on racing huskies who do a marathon distance in 90 minutes, three days in a row. A carbohydrate-loading diet tends to give them problems. We have compared three types of diets: a primarily carbohydrate diet, a diet about equal in carbohydrate and fat, and a diet with almost no carbohydrate. We believe that a very low-carbohydrate diet facilitates fat mobilization and our studies show that this results in increased performance. Based on these dog studies, we feel that a prolonged low-carbohydrate diet may prove beneficial for human distance running, although we have not seen any studies where people were trained for long periods of time on a low-carbohydrate diet.

P. D. GOLLNICK (*Washington State University, Pullman, Wash.*): I think that is a very interesting comment. However, I think your dog study shows two things; it demonstrates a marked species difference, and also recalls that Eskimos can survive quite well and also exercise on high-fat diets. As far as the studies of the prolonged feeding of man of high-fat diets, it is a question of what you mean by prolonged. Krogh and Lidnhard kept subjects on high-fat diets for 2 to 3 weeks and they found that it was exceedingly difficult for these subjects to sustain that diet as they experienced nausea and diarrhea.

A. GILLESPIE (*Ohio State University, Columbus, Ohio*): Can the success of Lasse Viren in the 1976 Olympics be explained in terms of glycogen depletion and free fatty acid metabolism? Can the three events he entered be explained by the selective recruitment of different fiber types in these different events?

P. D. GOLLNICK: That is a very difficult question to answer because I know of no data on this subject, especially his fiber type. It seems to me that these three events, the 5,000 m, 10,000 m, and marathon are not so very different in that they are all endurance events, although the 5,000 m may be more of an exception to this.

K. M. BALDWIN (*University of California, Irvine, Calif.*): Your data, Dr. Galbo, shows that insulin levels go down during exercise of progressive duration. Dr. Wahren has shown very convincingly that glucose uptake by the muscle is enhanced under similar conditions. Would you speculate that this response of glucose uptake is occurring independently of insulin?

H. GALBO (*University of Copenhagen, Copenhagen, Denmark*): I will speculate that, yes. Very convincing experiments using isolated perfused muscle have shown that insulin must be present to allow for increased glucose uptake in muscle during exercise. But perhaps insulin acts only permissively, and only low insulin concentrations must be present to provide full stimulus for glucose uptake during exercise.

J. WAHREN: I agree with Dr. Galbo that we can't draw certain conclusions regarding the need of insulin for glucose uptake during exercise. Although the insulin level falls to a great extent during exercise, perhaps the increased blood flow through the exercising tissues as well as the concomitant increase in capillary surface area together provide for more insulin being offered to the tissues during exercise compared to the resting state. Thus the local "insulinization," if I may use such a term, is perhaps as great during exercise as it is during rest even though the arterial level of insulin falls.

H. GALBO: I do not agree with Dr. Wahren's interpretation because it has been shown in rats, and perhaps in humans, that insulin secretion is decreased during exercise. This means that the turnover of insulin is inhibited during exercise.

E. A. NEWSHOLME (*University of Oxford, Oxford, England*): Is there any evidence that administration of factors other than oral glucose, such as the amino acids leucine or arginine, which will stimulate insulin release, will cause a decrease in exercise performance?

H. GALBO: We increased insulin levels through administration of an alpha-adrenergic blocker and found that this treatment diminished the exercise performance. This performance decrement was not due to the elevated insulin levels. To my knowledge increased insulin levels through the procedure you have described has not been done.

W. R. DRUCKER (*University of Virginia, Charlottesville, Va.*): Studies in the field of shock have demonstrated an increased uptake of glucose in the face of a diminished insulin concentration. The interpretation of this effect is that there is a decreased energy content in the muscles as evidenced by a reduced ATP content through changes in intracellular pH. I wonder if you are aware of similar data on exercising muscles that would explain this enhanced glucose uptake accompanied by a reduced energy content in the muscle.

H. GALBO: As I understand your question, I can say that when we blocked lipolysis with nicotinic acid or with beta-adrenergic blockade, we saw from muscle biopsies and other measures that glucose uptake was enhanced. From this data I suppose that an inhibited local glycogen breakdown allows an increased uptake of glucose from the blood. I believe that we shall hear more about this problem.

R. ALTEVEER (*Hahnemann Medical College, Philadelphia, Pa.*): From the data presented in this symposium many substrate changes occur during exercise. However, I believe that to properly understand substrate utilization it is necessary to perform labeling experiments to see whether you get radio-labeled carbon dioxide out. Do we agree that this simple labeling approach is the way to understand substrate utilization?

E. A. NEWSHOLME: I totally disagree with that comment, and let me illustrate this with an example. We know that there is no net biochemical pathway in higher animals for the conversion of fat into carbohydrate. Yet if you take a ^{14}C-labeled fatty acid and feed it to a tissue, particularly liver or kidney, you can get 60% of that label appearing in glucose. This is due either to enzyme-catalyzed biochemical exchange or because the metabolism is complicated. Therefore, if you give a labeled substrate and find that you get no labeled carbon dioxide, this is no real indication that it is not being oxidized. It may be an indication that the pathway is more complicated than the textbooks tell us.

R. ALTEVEER: Obviously I was not referring to interconversions. But to get energy out of muscle in the final analysis it must come out as CO_2, or I suppose ketone bodies. In other words to determine how much energy is derived from glucose, for example, then we must look for labeled glucose going to labeled CO_2.

E. A. NEWSHOLME: Again, I disagree. The labeled glucose may not yield labeled carbon dioxide because the label has been exchanged with glycogen or protein or triglyceride.

J. WAHREN: I would like to take an intermediate position because there are, in fact, a number of good isotope experiments indicating that free fatty acids are oxidized as we have heard in this symposium and that glucose is being taken up and oxidized in approximately the manner I have described. In addition, labeled alanine experiments indicate that alanine contributes to hepatic gluconeogenesis. I therefore feel that despite the exchange effect, many of these label experiments provide good support for the results that we have heard. I would also like to address a question to Dr. Newsholme. We have found that in our 4-hour exercised subjects, that despite a progressively rising arterial concentration of free fatty acids that could produce as much as 60% of the total metabolism, there was a continued large uptake of glucose. I wonder if you would like to comment on this in regard to your statement that free fatty acids may inhibit glucose uptake in muscle? I wonder whether this relates more to the heart muscle than it does to skeletal muscle.

E. A. NEWSHOLME: The question would be what would happen to an exercising muscle, which is undoubtably using fuel, if you reduced the availability of fat? Would that muscle take up the same amount or more of carbohydrate? I would suggest, without having done the experiment, that it would in fact take up more glucose if you reduced the rate of fat oxidation. There is a balance between the two: an increase in fat oxidation does not inhibit total glucose utilization; it is just inhibited in relation to what it would be if you had no fat oxidation. You are balancing the two energy systems. The evidence for this has been based on heart and diaphragm muscle simply because these were preparations that could be used. But I understand that very recent evidence indicates that this also happens in rat skeletal muscle.

D. THOMASHOW (*Harlem Hospital Center, New York, N.Y.*): Cholestyramine is a drug used in treating familial hyperlipidemia. In addition to binding bile acids in the gut, this drug also increases the fractional catabolism of low-density liproproteins. Are you aware of any studies where this drug has been used in exercise studies?

E. A. NEWSHOLME: You have raised an interesting point, and that is how important are plasma triglycerides, whether chylomicrons or low-density lipo-proteins, as a fuel for exercising muscle. It is known that triglycerides can be used by the isolated heart, but in terms of skeletal muscle, I think our data is still very poor. I think that this is a very important point because the plasma concentration of triglycerides is usually much higher than that of fatty acids.

G. SHEEHAN (*Riverview Hospital, Red Bank, N.J.*): As a number of us here are athletes than physiologists, we need to translate the information we have heard into something to help our running performance. My understanding from this symposium is that carbohydrate loading is not so important since we can take and utilize sugar during the race. Therefore, my question is: what is the ideal way to supply and regulate carbohydrates to the working muscles?

E. A. NEWSHOLME: One of the limitations is that the carbohydrate stores of the liver are relatively small, and that dietary manipulation used to elevate muscle glycogen concentrations do not seem to be as effective in raising liver carbohydrate stores. I am concerned that carbohydrates taken in during a run may have an osmotic effect, and withdraw water from the body, reducing extracellular fluid volume. Further, the mere presence of glucose in the gut can have an insulinogenic effect, causing insulin release and hence a reduction in free fatty acid mobilization. From earlier comments about the subjective beneficial effect of sugar ingestion it may be a quantitative problem how much glucose you take and in what form it is taken.

A. KUNIN: I think that if one keeps one's fluids up throughout the race, and does not get too dehydrated, that the ingestion of carbohydrate in some form will supply more glucose to the exercising muscle.

K. ELLINGWOOD: Since many athletes train both morning and afternoon, and it seems to me that the morning workout will have the effect of reducing muscle glycogen stores so that during the afternoon training session there is a greater reliance on fat as a fuel. I think if an athlete has a diet high in proteins and fats following the morning training session, that this will enhance the metabolic ability to utilize fat and that this may be a useful adaptive response in allowing them to switch to fat as a fuel more effectively.

E. A. NEWSHOLME: Your point is that in terms of training, you are training under a situation where very little blood-borne fuel other than fatty acids is available. You, therefore, have a training regimen that will first of all metabolize glycogen stores and then switch on an improved system to mobilize and oxidize fatty acids. I would still like to believe, that after an initial 10 to 20 minutes, you are utilizing both fat and carbohydrate. I would still argue, that despite the fast race pace, that both fuels must be used simultaneously to provide degree of cohesion of control between the two fuels to ensure fuel stability.

PHYSIOLOGICAL DEFENSES AGAINST HYPERTHERMIA OF EXERCISE *

Ethan R. Nadel, C. Bruce Wenger, Michael F. Roberts,
Jan A. J. Stolwijk, and Enzo Cafarelli

*John B. Pierce Foundation Laboratory
Department of Epidemiology and Public Health
Yale University School of Medicine
New Haven, Connecticut 06519*

During intensive exercise such as marathon running, heat is produced in the contracting muscles at rates in excess of 1100 W, on the order of 15 to 18 times of the basal metabolic rate. Practically all of this heat is rapidly transferred from the muscles to the blood and carried to the body core in the venous return. A heat production of this magnitude is sufficient to raise the body core temperature of an average-sized individual by $1°$ C every 5 minutes if no temperature regulatory mechanisms were activated. Since a marathon runner is able to sustain this level of exercise for 2 to 3 hours [1] with body core temperature maintained at a relatively constant level between 39 and $41°$ C,[2, 3] it is evident that the temperature regulatory system must be highly efficient. It is well established that in the presence of a thermal load, thermal receptors in specialized sites within the hypothalamus sense the increased body temperature and in response direct an integrated reflex whereby the excess heat is transferred via increased cutaneous circulation to the skin surface, where it can be dissipated by physical means, primarily the evaporation of sweat. In this case the great amount of heat produced during running is balanced by the heat dissipated to the environment and the new steady state of internal body temperature is maintained until some new perturbation is introduced. In the following paragraphs we will describe studies that were intended to elucidate the characteristics and sensitivity of the temperature regulatory system in humans during exercise. Since the rate of heat storage (and hence the new steady state of internal body temperature) is primarily determined by the rapidity of the temperature regulatory response, most of our studies were conducted during the 20 to 30 minute initial transient of exercise.

Energy Transfers

Figure 1 is a schematic diagram that illustrates the pathways for energy transfer from body core to skin to environment. There are several modes of transfer, dependent upon both the physiological response and the physical characteristics of the environment. The rate of transfer of energy from core to skin is the product of the average core-to-skin temperature gradient and the transfer coefficient, or the overall skin conductance. The overall conductance of heat is the sum of a fixed conductance (according to the thickness of the subcutaneous

---

* This work was supported in part by National Institutes of Health Grants ES–00354, ES–00123, and HL–17732.

fat layer) by passive conduction and a variable conductance by the convective transfer from core to skin in the circulation. During conditions of low vascular resistance in the skin, the flow of blood to the skin can be more than twenty times greater than during maximal skin vasoconstriction, and the rate of transfer of heat from core to skin per unit of temperature difference is accordingly greater. Thus, the ability to increase skin blood flow in the face of a thermal load is a primary defense against hyperthermia. It should be remembered, however, that the net transfer of energy is the product of the conductance and the core-to-skin temperature difference. Even when the skin blood flow is high, the heat flux may be relatively limited if the core-to-skin thermal gradient is small.

The delivery of body heat to the skin surface would be of little value if the heat were not able to be readily dissipated to the environment. As can be seen

$$h_{sk} (T_{in} - \bar{T}_{sk}) = h_e (P_{sk} - \phi P_a) + h_{r+c} (\bar{T}_{sk} - T_a)$$

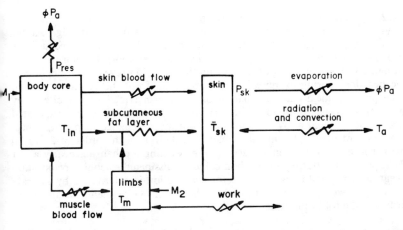

FIGURE 1. A schematic representation of the avenues for thermal exchanges from the human body to the environment. The equation above the model describes the energy balance in heat transfer and temperature terms.

from FIGURE 1, there are several avenues for the transfer of body heat to the environment. Energy exchanges from skin to environment by radiation and convection are the product of the combined transfer coefficient and the skin-to-environment temperature gradient. Although the radiative heat transfer coefficient is independent of air velocity, the convective heat transfer coefficient is variable and increases with air velocity according to the equation

$$h_c = 8.60 v^{0.531},$$

where h_c is the convective heat transfer coefficient in $W \cdot m^{-2} \cdot {}^\circ C^{-1}$, and v is the air velocity in $m \cdot s^{-1}$. This equation was derived by Nishi and Gagge [4] for freely moving subjects using the naphthalene sublimation technique. Since running at marathon race speeds produces a high effective air velocity, the convective heat transfer coefficient is increased by a factor of 6 to 7, and the heat loss due to convection accordingly is greater. Convective losses are minimized, however, on a warm day when the skin-to-ambient temperature gradient is small.

Energy exchanges by radiation may be large in some circumstances but are usually not. Lee [5] found that the incident solar radiation in the desert varied between 100 and 250 W·m^{-2}, with the minimum exposure during the middle of the day when the sun is at its zenith. Maximum heat gain conditions were toward the midafternoon when air and ground temperatures were higher. Normally on warm days, the thermal load from solar radiation is considerably lower than in the desert and is usually more than equalized by the convective loss, especially when the latter is elevated due to the high air velocity accompanying running.

Another avenue for energy loss to the environment is from the respiratory tract via evaporation. Increased evaporative water loss accompanies the increased minute ventilation during exercise and can be accurately estimated (up to 75% of maximal aerobic power) according to the following equation: [6]

$$E_{res} = 0.0023 \ M(44 - P_a),$$

where E_{res} is the respiratory evaporative heat loss in W·m^{-2}; M, the metabolic rate in W·m^{-2}; and P_a, the ambient water vapor pressure in mmHg. Above 75% of maximal aerobic power this equation is no longer valid because the ratio of minute ventilation to oxygen uptake increases above the normal value of around 23 liters per liter of O_2. Solving this equation reveals that about 5% of the heat loss during exercise is via evaporation from the respiratory tract.

The primary means for dissipation of the thermal load of exercise is by evaporation of sweat from the skin surface. Each gram of water evaporated carries about 0.6 kcal away from the skin during the change in phase. Since, in conditions of maximal demand humans can deliver on the order of 20 to 30 grams per minute to the skin surface via the sweating mechanism, nearly all of the heat production during a marathon could be dissipated solely by evaporation of sweat in ideal conditions. The rate of evaporation is determined by the rate of sweating as well as by certain physical characteristics of the environment, as described in the following equation: [7]

$$E_{sk} = h_e \ (P_{sk} - P_a) \ A_W/A_D,$$

where E_{sk} is the skin evaporative heat loss in W·m^{-2}; h_e, the evaporative heat transfer coefficient in W·m^{-2}·mmHg^{-1} equal to h_c (2.2° C·mmHg^{-1}) at atmospheric pressure with h_c being the convective heat transfer coefficient; P_{sk} is the water vapor pressure at skin temperature in mmHg; P_a, the ambient water vapor pressure in mmHg; A_W, the wetted area of skin in m^2; and A_D, the DuBois body surface area in m^2.

The critical role of sweating rate in the transfer of heat from skin to environment is seen in the above equation in the factor P_{sk}. For the most part, increases in sweating rate cause an increase in P_{sk}, widening the skin-to-ambient humidity gradient and thereby increasing evaporative rate in given conditions.

In the following paragraphs we will discuss the physiological factors that determine heat transfer to the skin by their control of the rate of skin blood flow and those factors that affect the evaporative heat transfer from skin to environment by their control of the rate of sweat secretion. We will also consider factors which modify the control mechanisms, thereby affecting the overall heat transfer.

Control of Skin Blood Flow

Three healthy subjects exercised on a modified Monark cycle ergometer for 30 min at 30%, 50%, and 70% of maximal aerobic power ($\dot{V}_{O_2 \, max}$) in ambient temperatures of 15°, 25°, and 35° C, with ambient water vapor pressure less than 18 mmHg. The cycle ergometer had been modified to allow the subject to sit in a contour chair behind the pedals and thereby free his arms from any activity during exercise.[8] Exercise was employed to vary internal temperatures during an experiment.[9] Different ambient temperatures were used to vary mean skin temperature independently of internal temperature. Internal temperature was continuously measured in the esophagus (T_{es}) and eight skin temperatures were monitored once per minute, with a weighted average ($\overline{T}_{sk}$) based upon the product of regional area and local relative thermal sensitivities.[10] Forearm

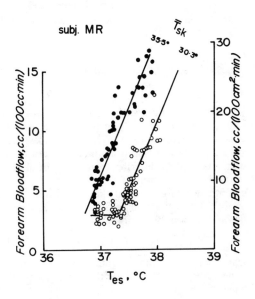

FIGURE 2. Forearm blood flow as a function of esophageal and mean skin temperatures during exercise at 15° and 35° C. The data taken at 25° C were omitted for clarity. These data are representative of those for each subject. (After Wenger et al.[12])

blood flow was measured twice per minute by venous occlusion plethysmography.[11] Since forearm muscle blood flow is not significantly increased during body heating,[12] increases in forearm blood flow were taken as representing increases in skin circulation. The forearm was maintained at a constant temperature (around 35° C) in all of these experiments, thereby eliminating the possibility of local arm temperature changes modifying the total response characteristic.

Two important findings were evident from the data from these experiments. Forearm skin blood flow (BF) was linearly related to T_{es} at any level of $\overline{T}_{sk}$. The effect of modifying $\overline{T}_{sk}$ was to shift the T_{es} threshold for vasodilation without changing the slope of the $BF:T_{es}$ relationship. This effect is shown in FIGURE 2. Increasing $\overline{T}_{sk}$ lowered the T_{es} threshold for vasodilation and shifted the $BF:T_{es}$ relation accordingly. Thus, T_{es} and $\overline{T}_{sk}$ combine additively in the determination of BF.

The second finding was that there was no significant effect of exercise intensity on the relation between BF and T_{es}, once values taken during the first minute of exercise, the adjustment phase, were discarded. We have seen transient changes in forearm blood flow at the onset of exercise that were not related to temperature changes. We consider these as emotional or compensatory adjustments which are short-lived and uncommon in experienced subjects. Thus, we were able to fit the data from the three subjects to a linear additive model, as follows:

$$BF = 8.01(T_{es}) + 0.85 \ (\overline{T}_{sk}) - 321,$$

where BF is the forearm blood flow in $ml \cdot 100 \ ml^{-1} \cdot min^{-1}$. This model had an average multiple linear correlation coefficient of 0.87 for the three subjects. In fact, we were able to improve the average multiple correlation coefficient to 0.90 by adding a term that accounted for the effect of exercise intensity. However, since the coefficient of this term varied considerably between subjects, and since the improvement was negligible, we felt the simpler model had greater physiological and predictive value.

Control of Sweating Rate

In experiments that had a similar design, we investigated the control of both local sweating rate (using resistance hygrometry to measure chest sweating rate [13]) and whole body evaporative rate (using the Potter platform scale to continuously measure rate of weight loss during exercise [14]). We found that sweating rate was well accounted for by the same type of linear additive model that was used to describe the control of skin blood flow. Further, the ratio of the proportional control constants for T_{es} and $\overline{T}_{sk}$ were similar for the control of both sweating rate and skin blood flow; i.e., a given change in T_{es} produced about 9 times the change of response as did the same change in $\overline{T}_{sk}$. The best fit for the model describing the control of whole body evaporative rate was

$$E_{sk} = [197(T_{es}) + 23(\overline{T}_{sk}) - 8012] \ \exp \ (0.1 \ \overline{T}_{sk} - 3.4),$$

where E_{sk} = evaporative rate from the skin in $W \cdot m^{-2}$. The exponential factor is necessary to account for the direct local effect of skin temperature on sweat gland function.

Because of the similarity in the control equations for both skin blood flow and sweating rate, we have represented both effector systems as being responsive to a common central nervous system drive for heat dissipation. The negative feedback control systems are described by the conceptual model in FIGURE 3. In this model internal and mean skin temperatures are the primary feedback elements to the integrator within the central nervous system (we know, from many animal studies, that the integrator is located within the hypothalamus [15]). Two important implications are drawn from this model. The first is that the central drive for heat dissipation is common to both effector systems and is the consequence of the addition of internal and skin temperature inputs. Secondly, any modifications that are induced in the control system must occur either within the central nervous system, by alteration of the reference, or at the periphery, at the level of the effector. In the latter case the modification should be multiplicative with the central drive in the determination of the response. Thus, by examination of the relationship between the thermal inputs and response outputs before and following interventions such as physical training, one can determine the magnitude of the change in the controlling system and the site of occurrence.

Modifications in the Control Systems

There are a number of ways in which the linear relationship between the sweating rate and central drive can be modified. In the presence of a given central drive, an increase in skin wettedness suppresses the sweating rate.[16] Increasing the evaporative power of the environment provides for the removal of water standing on the skin surface and reverses this suppression. The evaporative power of the environment is related to both the evaporative heat transfer coefficient and the ambient water vapor pressure. An increase in air velocity, such as one encounters during running, enhances evaporation and actually potentiates the sweating rate at a given central drive. Conversely, increased

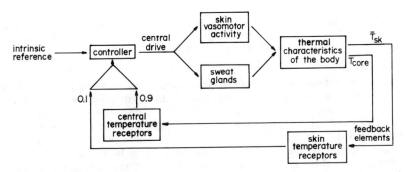

FIGURE 3. A conceptual model describing the negative feedback control of skin blood flow and sweating rate.

ambient humidity reduces the evaporative power and suppresses the sweating rate at a given central drive. The end result of a decrease in sweating rate is decreased evaporative cooling and a higher internal body temperature.

The effect of the evaporative power of the environment upon sweating rate is illustrated in FIGURE 4. Increasing the air velocity around the exercising subject increased the gain of the relation between sweating rate and internal temperature. In the mathematical model, this is described as a multiplicative effect, having its influence at the periphery. At an air velocity of 2.2 m·s⁻¹, approximately half of what a runner would encounter during a 5-minute mile on a still day, it is evident that the required evaporation would be achieved at a lower internal temperature. If a runner required an evaporative rate of 15 g·min⁻¹ to achieve a steady state, he or she could do so at an internal temperature of 38.2° C if the body were exposed to a high air velocity, but would reach the steady state at 39.2° C if the air velocity were minimal. Any barrier between the skin and the environment reduces the air velocity at the level of the skin surface and therefore reduces the evaporative capacity of the microenvironment.

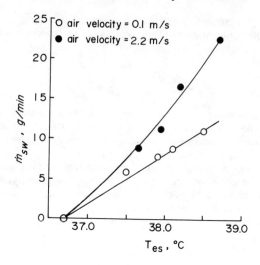

FIGURE 4. The relation between whole body sweating rate ($\dot{m}_{sw}$) and esophageal temperature (T_{es}) at two air velocities. $\overline{T}_{sk}$ was around 34° C. (From Nadel and Stolwijk.[16] By permission of the American Physiological Society.)

According to our observations this suppresses the actual sweating rate at a given central drive, causing higher body temperatures than would otherwise occur.

A different method for enhancing sweating at a given level of central drive is associated with physical training and/or heat acclimatization. It is well established that both physically fit [17, 18] and heat-acclimatized individuals [19] maintain a lower internal temperature when challenged by a heat and exercise test. Studies such as these show that the responsiveness of the sweating mechanism is improved by repeated exposures to internal thermal loads (exercise) or external thermal loads (ambient heat).

We showed recently [20] that physical training and heat acclimation produce increased sweating at a given central drive by somewhat different mechanisms. Physical training results in an increased sensitivity of the sweating response per unit change in central drive. The average increase in gain was 67% for six subjects. There was also a small decrease in the internal temperature threshold for sweating. Heat acclimation increased the sweating rate at a given central drive by lowering the internal temperature threshold for sweating without a change in gain. The reduction in sweating threshold averaged 0.3° C for the six subjects.

It has been shown that mild dehydration, or hypohydration, results in a steady-state internal temperature that is higher than that in normally hydrated conditions during exercise.[21, 22] To maintain a steady-state internal temperature, the rate of heat dissipation must balance the rate of heat production. It follows that the elevation in internal temperature in hypohydrated conditions is the consequence of either an increase in the internal temperature threshold for sweating or, more likely, a reduction in the sensitivity of the sweating response. In the latter case, the increment in sweating rate is lower per unit of internal temperature increase, and the sweating rate required for the steady state is achieved at a higher central drive.

A schematic representation of the peripheral influences on the relation between sweating rate and central sweating drive is shown in FIGURE 5. Factors such as physical training or increased air velocity increase the sensitivity of the control mechanism and allow the steady state to be reached at a lower central sweating drive. Conversely, factors such as hypohydration (or, presumably, increased plasma osmolarity) or increased skin wettedness reduce the sensitivity of the control mechanism and result in the steady state being reached at a higher central drive.

We have recently shown [23] that the skin blood flow alterations with physical training and heat acclimation are relatively similar to the alterations in sweating rate, except that there was no consistent change in the slope of the skin blood flow-to-internal temperature relation with acclimation. Improved sweating responsiveness may provide physically fit individuals with a small cardiovascular advantage in that the skin blood flow demand is slightly lower at a given central drive during exercise. However, the primary changes with training and heat acclimation appear to be a reduction in response thresholds, thereby providing a lower operating temperature during the steady state. The primary advantage of a lower temperature during exercise is that the individual has a greater margin of safety between operating and limiting temperatures. The major cardiovascular advantages that accompany physical training and heat acclimation probably are not the result of changes in the temperature regulatory mechanisms per se, but probably are more closely tied into improved abilities to maintain an adequate circulating blood volume.

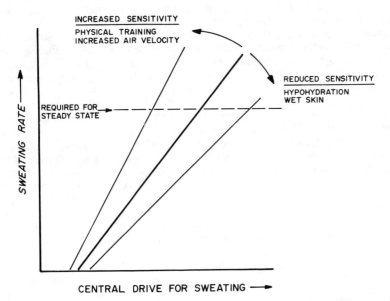

FIGURE 5. A hypothetical representation of the mechanism by which certain peripheral influences modify the linear relation between the sweating rate and central sweating drive.

Maintenance of Central Circulation

One of the primary problems encountered during exercise in warm conditions is that the individual is incapable of rapidly dissipating the metabolic and solar radiative thermal loads and the internal body temperature climbs to very high levels. The progressive hyperthermia is accentuated if the ambient humidity is high, for the reasons described in previous sections. Because both skin blood flow and skin venous volume increase with the rise in internal temperature, the body is presented with the problem of providing adequate circulation to both the skin and muscle vasculature. Further compounding the circulatory problem in these conditions, Harrison *et al.*[24] have confirmed that there is a decrease in circulating plasma volume that amounts to more than 15% during 50 minutes of moderate exercise. Maintenance of cardiac filling pressure would appear to be difficult in the face of these compromises. Indeed, it is well known that heat-induced syncope is the consequence of an impairment in cardiac filling pressure, which itself results from a combination of several occurrences, such as reduction in venomotor tone and reduction in circulating blood volume.

About ten years ago Rowell *et al.*[25] made perhaps the only systematic study of central circulatory responses of unacclimatized men to exercise in a hot environment. Rowell *et al.*[26] have also shown that there was a decrease of 20% in splanchnic blood flow during exercise in the heat and speculated that the redistribution of blood flow from splanchnic to skin beds might be sufficient to eliminate the need for an increase in cardiac output over that during exercise in cooler conditions. They validated this hypothesis for conditions of low and moderate exercise in the heat. However, during heavy exercise in the heat ($T_a = 43°$ C), cardiac output was about 2 liters per minute lower than in a 26°C environment over the 15 minutes of exercise. Thus, when the oxygen demand was low, the reductions in splanchnic circulation were sufficient to compensate for the increases in skin circulation and reduced circulating blood volume. However, during heavy exercise in the heat, the stroke volume and cardiac output were reduced and muscle demands were presumably met by increased oxygen extraction during these bouts.

In experiments designed to extend these observations, we have recently found that during 20 minutes of moderate exercise the body is able to maintain cardiac output in a 36° C environment despite a very high skin blood flow and a considerable decrease in circulating plasma volume. FIGURE 6 illustrates the circulatory responses as a function of internal (esophageal) temperature during these bouts. Each plotted point is the average of data from two identical experiments, with the exception of the changes in plasma volume, which were from a single experiment. Cardiac output was estimated at 4–5 minute intervals by a modified CO_2 rebreathing technique.[27] The change in plasma volume was estimated from the change in hemoglobin concentration in serial samples of venous blood taken from a butterfly catheter placed in a superficial cubital vein. Other techniques have been described in previous sections.

We found that there was a linear decrease in plasma volume as internal temperature increased. This reduction in plasma volume was independent of the mean skin temperature. The loss of fluid from the intravascular space is probably related to increased osmotic pressure in the extravascular space, this due to mobilization of substrate and outward movement of protein, and is also related to some extent to increased capillary filtration due to reductions in precapillary resistance and increased dehydration due to sweat losses. During moderate exercise, cardiac output was independent of internal temperature. In the heat, reductions in cardiac filling pressure, which would be the result of reduced circulating blood volume and reduced venous tone, resulted in a lower

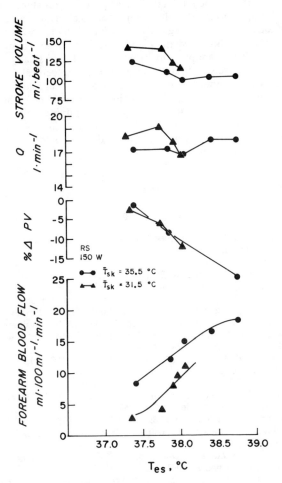

FIGURE 6. Circulatory responses to exercise in a cool and in a warm environment as a function of internal (esophageal) temperature. Each function includes averaged data from duplicate runs in each condition. Data are from a representative subject.

stroke volume; however, increased heart rate provided for the maintenance of cardiac output. Despite the fact that skin blood flow was considerably higher in the heat, cardiac output was sufficient to meet the demands from both skin and muscle at the moderate exercise intensity.

We are presently completing studies that examine the interaction between the circulatory, osmotic, and temperature regulatory systems at different levels of exercise and in different thermal environments. Studies such as these can be used to develop and refine models that have predictive as well as physiological validity. These models then provide stimulation for further experimentation and can reveal where the limiting factors to prolonged exercise reside.

In conclusion, the trained athlete has acquired a resistance to excessive hyperthermia during exercise [20] and an improved tolerance to a combined heat and exercise exposure.[18] Physiological adaptations include lower internal temperature thresholds for both sweating and vasodilation and a more sensitive sweating response. These adaptations provide for a lower steady-state internal temperature during exercise. Maintenance of a lower central drive for heat dissipation allows the runner to resist the decrease in cardiac filling pressure that would develop from greater reductions in plasma volume. There may also be improvements in venomotor tone with physical training, but this is yet unclear. Adaptations in temperature regulatory mechanisms occur along with those in other organ systems during training and provide for optimal performance in conditions of great demand.

References

1. COSTILL, D. L. & E. L. FOX. 1969. Energetics of marathon running. Med. Sci. Sports. 1: 81–86.
2. ADAMS, W. C., R. H. FOX, A. J. FRY & I. C. MACDONALD. 1975. Thermoregulation during marathon running in cool, moderate and hot environments. J. Appl. Physiol. 38: 1030–1037.
3. MARON, M. B., J. A. WAGNER & S. M. HORVATH. 1977. Thermoregulatory responses during competitive marathon running. J. Appl. Physiol. In press.
4. NISHI, Y. & A. P. GAGGE. 1970. Direct evaluation of convective heat transfer coefficient by naphthalene sublimation. J. Appl. Physiol. 29: 830–838.
5. LEE, D. H. K. 1972. Large mammals in the desert. In Physiological Adaptations, Desert and Mountain. M. K. Yousef, S. M. Horvath & R. W. Bullard, Eds.: 109–125. Academic Press. New York, N.Y.
6. MITCHELL, J. W., E. R. NADEL & J. A. J. STOLWIJK. 1972. Respiratory weight losses during exercise. J. Appl. Physiol. 32: 474–476.
7. GAGGE, A. P. 1972. Partitional calorimetry in the desert. In Physiological Adaptations, Desert and Mountain. M. K. Yousef, S. M. Horvath & R. W. Bullard, Eds.: 23–51. Academic Press, New York.
8. BIGLAND-RITCHIE, B., H. GRAICHEN & J. J. WOODS. 1973. A variable-speed motorized bicycle ergometer for positive and negative work exercise. J. Appl. Physiol. 35: 739–740.
9. SALTIN, B. & L. HERMANSEN. 1966. Esophageal, rectal and muscle temperature during exercise. J. Appl. Physiol. 21: 1757–1762.
10. NADEL, E. R., J. W. MITCHELL & J. A. J. STOLWIJK. 1973. Differential thermal sensitivity in the human skin. Pflügers Arch. Ges. Physiol. 340: 71–76.
11. WENGER, C. B., M. F. ROBERTS, J. A. J. STOLWIJK & E. R. NADEL. 1975. Forearm blood flow during body temperature transients produced by leg exercise. J. Appl. Physiol. 38: 58–63.
12. RODDIE, I. C., J. T. SHEPHERD & R. F. WHELAN. 1956. Evidence from venous oxygen saturation measurements that the increase in forearm blood flow during body heating is confined to the skin. J. Physiol. (London) 134: 444–450.
13. NADEL, E. R., R. W. BULLARD & J. A. J. STOLWIJK. 1971. Importance of skin temperature in the regulation of sweating. J. Appl. Physiol. 31: 80–87.
14. NADEL, E. R., J. W. MITCHELL & J. A. J. STOLWIJK. 1971. Control of local and total sweating during exercise transients. Int. J. Biometeor. 15: 201–206.

15. HARDY, J. D. 1960. Physiology of temperature regulation. Physiol. Rev. **41:** 521–606.

16. NADEL, E. R. & J. A. J. STOLWIJK. 1973. Effect of skin wettedness on sweat gland response. J. Appl. Physiol. **53:** 689–694.

17. PIWONKA, R. W. & S. ROBINSON. 1967. Acclimatization of highly trained men to work in severe heat. J. Appl. Physiol. **22:** 9–12.

18. GISOLFI, C. & S. ROBINSON. 1969. Relations between physical training, acclimatization and heat tolerance. J. Appl. Physiol. **26:** 530–534.

19. WYNDHAM, C. H. 1967. Effect of acclimatization on the sweat rate/rectal temperature relationship. J. Appl. Physiol. **22:** 27–30.

20. NADEL, E. R., K. B. PANDOLF, M. F. ROBERTS & J. A. J. STOLWIJK. 1974. Mechanisms of thermal acclimation to exercise and heat. J. Appl. Physiol. **37:** 515–520.

21. GREENLEAF, J. E. & B. L. CASTLE. 1971. Exercise temperature regulation in man during hypohydration and hyperhydration. J. Appl. Physiol. **30:** 847–853.

22. NIELSEN, B., G. HANSEN, S. O. JORGENSEN & E. NIELSEN. 1971. Thermoregulation in exercising man during dehydration and hyperhydration with water and saline. Int. J. Biometeorol. **15:** 195–200.

23. ROBERTS, M. F., C. B. WENGER, J. A. J. STOLWIJK & E. R. NADEL. 1977. Skin blood flow and sweating rate changes following exercise training and heat acclimation. J. Appl. Physiol. In press.

24. HARRISON, M. H., R. J. EDWARDS & D. R. LEITCH. 1975. Effect of exercise and thermal stress on plasma volume. J. Appl. Physiol. **39:** 925–931.

25. ROWELL, L. B., H. J. MARX, R. A. BRUCE, R. D. CONN & F. KUSUMI. 1966. Reductions in cardiac output, central blood volume and stroke volume with thermal stress in normal men during exercise. J. Clin. Invest. **45:** 1801–1816.

26. ROWELL, L. B., G. L. BRENGELMANN, J. R. BLACKMON, R. D. TWISS & F. KUSUMI. 1968. Splanchnic blood flow and metabolism in heat-stressed man. J. Appl. Physiol. **24:** 475–484.

27. FARHI, L. E., M. S. NESARJAH, A. J. OLSZOWKA, L. METILDI & A. K. ELLIS. 1975. Measurement of pulmonary blood flow by a rebreathing technique. Fed. Proc. **34:** 451.

INFLUENCE OF EXERCISE MODE AND SELECTED AMBIENT CONDITIONS ON SKIN TEMPERATURE *

William C. Adams

Human Performance Laboratory
Physical Education Department
University of California, Davis
Davis, California 95616

INTRODUCTION

Gisolfi and Copping [1] have noted the increasing popularity of distance running among men and women over a wide age range and that, while runners can train during the coolest hours of the day, competition is often scheduled at times when environmental heat stress is significant. Because of the necessity of dissipating high rates of metabolic heat production over a prolonged period, marathon runners are particularly susceptible to heat injury problems, a fact leading to a recent position statement by the American College of Sports Medicine. [2]

While international class marathon runners sustain a metabolic heat production exceeding 650 W/m^2 for approximately 2¼ hours, [3] thermoregulation is not generally a limiting factor in cool and moderate temperatures unless there is considerable solar radiation. [4, 5] Utilizing the partitional heat balance procedure set forth by Kerslake, [6] the limiting relative humidity and mean radiant temperature (MRT) for a lone marathon runner at a speed of 255 m/min have been detailed. [7] However, there is insufficient data to apply this method of identifying multiple combinations of limiting environmental conditions for runners of varied ability and thermoregulatory capacity. Thus, it would seem worthwhile to quantify more precisely metabolic heat production and ambient environmental combinations likely to limit performance, and particularly those that might endanger the participants' health.

Central to this approach, as pointed out by Fox, [8] is the significant intervening role of mean skin temperature ($\overline{T}_s$) in affecting the marathon runner's heat exchange between body core and the ambient environment. Nielsen [9] demonstrated that $\overline{T}_s$ is a linear function of dry bulb temperature (T_{db}) over a range from 5° to 35° C when a subject exercised indoors on a bicycle ergometer. Pugh [10] noted a similar relationship in a subject running outdoors with the T_{db} ranging from 5° to 25° C. In fact, while the heat transfer laws are fundamentally rather simple, [6] the effect of ambient conditions other than T_{db}, notably relative humidity (RH), airflow, and solar radiation on the $\overline{T}_s, T_{db}$ relationship has not been studied systematically in exercising man.

The paucity of T_s data on runners outdoors is, in the opinion of Pugh, [11] primarily due to the technical difficulties in measurement of T_s in a moving

* This study was supported in part by U.S. Air Force Grant F-44620-72-C-0011 to the Human Physiology Department, Medical School, University of California, Davis.

athlete who is sweating profusely. In an attempt to circumvent this problem, Clark, Mullan, and Pugh,[12] using AGA infrared thermovision and a rapid responding thermocouple probe, have observed that the latter can be used for estimating T_s during running, provided measurements are initiated immediately on stopping and allowance is made for the rise of temperature during the measurement. Their observations, however, were made on a single subject running at 268 m/min, and then only in cool and moderate temperatures.

The primary purpose of the present investigation was to ascertain the effects of airflow and solar radiation on the $\overline{T}_s$, T_{db} relationship during running in cool (C), moderate (M), and warm (W) temperatures. Similar relationships during outdoor bicycle riding were also studied. A secondary purpose was to examine further the validity of utilizing recovery $\overline{T}_s$ measurements for estimating $\overline{T}_s$ during running over a wide range of T_{db}, with and without airflow. Finally, pertinent observations relating to limiting environmental conditions for optimal marathon performance were examined.

TABLE 1

PHYSICAL CHARACTERISTICS OF SUBJECTS

Subject No.	Age (yr)	Ht (cm)	Wt (kg)	BSA * (m²)	Body Fat (%)†	$\dot{V}_{O_2max}$ (ml/ kg·min)	Best 5-km Time (min : sec)	Exercise Mode
1	21.3	176.7	65.9	1.80	3.63	75.97	14:37	Run & Bike
2	21.0	187.0	71.9	1.95	4.16	76.31	14:33	Run
3	21.7	176.4	59.9	1.72	3.80	76.11	14:32	Run

* BSA, body surface area.
† Percent of body weight as fat calculated from the formula of Brozek et al.[13]

MATERIALS AND METHODS

Subjects. Three highly trained college middle-distance runners, whose physical characteristics are given in TABLE 1, served as subjects. Whole body density was determined by immersion, with body fat estimated by the formula of Brozek et al.[13] Treadmill maximal oxygen uptake ($\dot{V}_{O_2 max}$) was assessed by procedures described elsewhere.[14]

Experimental Design. Subject 1 completed 28 experimental protocols, including running 11.1 km or riding a bicycle 24 km continuously for periods ranging from 37–45 min. Twelve running experiments were done indoors on a motor driven treadmill at two speeds in C (19°–21° C), M (24°–5° C), and W (29°–31.5° C) T_{db}, with airflow equivalent to the runner's speed, or in "still" air. Twelve running experiments at two speeds equivalent to those indoors with airflow, were completed outdoors on a flat, smooth macadamized surface in C, M, and W T_{db}, with clear sky solar radiation, or after sunset. Bicycle rides were done in M and W T_{db}, both with solar radiation and after sunset, at a speed requiring metabolic energy expenditure at the same percent of $\dot{V}_{O_2\,max}$ as the slow run speed outdoors ($\dot{V}_{O_2\,max}$ for bicycle riding was assumed to be 7.5% less than measured running $\dot{V}_{O_2\,max}$).[15] Subjects 2 and 3 completed a total of 16 of the 24 running protocols.

Experimental Routine. Subjects reported to the laboratory at least 3 hours after their previous meal. Running attire consisted of rubber-sole training shoes, cotton socks and briefs, and nylon shorts. During bicycle experiments, subject 1 wore cotton briefs and standard racing cycling shorts and shoes. Subjects were weighed before and after exercise, both nude and in their athletic attire, the latter to determine the amount of unevaporated sweat trapped in clothing during exercise. A rectal probe was inserted by the subject to a depth of 12 cm anterior to the external anal sphincter. The rectal probe lead, along with seven skin thermistor leads (Yellow Springs Instrument, YSI, No. 408) had been severed, and the ends of each soldered to a subminiature connector, the total weight of the "harness" being 180 g (FIGURE 1). One end led to the thermistor plug and the other to the rectal probe or skin thermistors. The skin thermistors were seated with epoxy on a No. 20 copper wire framework attached to 3.2-mm-thick lucite rings, 3.81-cm outside diameter, which were attached to the subject by surgical tape formed into flat doughnuts (FIGURE 2).

The subjects ran outdoors at two speeds (254 and 293 m/min), chosen to elicit approximately 65% and 80% of treadmill $\dot{V}_{O_2\,max}$, respectively. Maintenance of a near constant and relatively exact rate of speed was insured via observation of elapsed time at previously measured checkpoints along the course. When the runner was confronted with airflow equivalent to running speed being generated by a 0.5 HP fan, treadmill speeds indoors were the same as those outdoors. When running indoors without airflow, speed was increased 3.9% and 4.1% to account for the reduced $\dot{V}_{O_2}$ necessary for overcoming air resistance at the slow and fast speeds, respectively.[16] Fluid was imbibed only during the course of an adjunct experimental protocol, a run at 293 m/min with airflow for 21.1 km. Dry bulb, wet bulb (T_{wb}), and globe (T_g) temperatures and wind velocity were measured at 5–10 minute intervals outdoors at the starting point. Dry and wet bulb temperatures were also monitored at similar intervals indoors.

Measurement Techniques

Treadmill Runs. Skin temperature at seven sites (FIGURE 3) and rectal temperature were monitored sequentially on a YSI telethermometer (Model 44TA) at approximate 4-second intervals each minute for 7–10 minutes before exercise, during runs, and for 3 minutes after exercise. Expired air measurement and sampling methods, described previously,[14] were used to determine respiratory metabolism for 1¼ minutes at three equally spaced intervals during the run. Samples were analyzed within several minutes for CO_2 and O_2, respectively, on Beckman LB-2 and E-2 analyzers, in tandem. Expired air volumes were corrected to STPD, and respiratory metabolism values calculated according to procedures outlined by Consolazio, Johnson, and Pecora.[17] Heart rate was determined from an electrocardiogram recorded during the first 10 seconds of each sampling period.

Outdoor Runs. Pre-exercise T_s and T_{re} were monitored for 7 to 10 minutes as indoors before treadmill runs. Within 1 minute prior to initiating running, the subject's harness connector was uncoupled from its mate leading to the thermistor jacks of the telethermometer. Upon completion of the run, the harness connector was recoupled, and within 5–10 seconds after the run, T_s and T_{re} were monitored sequentially at approximate 3-second intervals for 2½–3 minutes as in recovery following treadmill runs. Although half of the outdoor runs were done in clear-sky solar radiation, all pre- and postrun T_s measurements were taken in the shade with minimal airflow. In 20 experiments, pre- and postrun, near steady-state $\bar{T}_s$ telethermometer values were compared to those obtained by a Barnes infrared radiometer at sites closely adjacent to

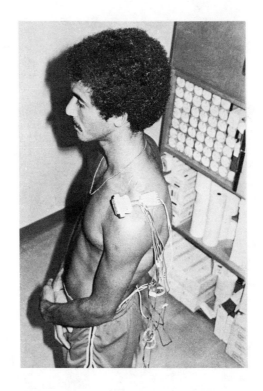

FIGURE 1. The thermistor lead harness, including sub-miniature connector and electrocardiogram leads.

the thermistor sites. The prerun $\bar{T}_s$ obtained by telethermometer readings was approximately 1 °C lower than $\bar{T}_s$ measured by radiometer, whereas there was no significant difference between the two techniques in measurements taken from 3–4 minutes postrun.

Verification of virtually similar $\dot{V}_{O_2}$ values for running outdoors and for running at the same speed on the treadmill indoors with airflow equivalent to running speed, was done on one occasion with subject 1. A standard ¼-ton pickup truck was equipped to measure respiratory metabolism, with a wooden frame mounted on the truck bed to support the expired air collection tubing. The subject ran near the cab window at approximately 1 m distance from the right side, breathing through a low-resistance Daniel's valve mounted on a

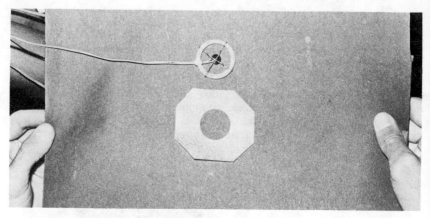

FIGURE 2. The plastic ring skin thermistor applicator, with surgical tape doughnut.

plastic headpiece. Maintenance of a near constant and relatively exact rate of speed was insured via observation of checkpoints along the course. The course was a flat, smooth macadamized surface, 3.2 km in length. The first 1.2 km of the run was utilized as a warmup period, after which expired air, previously exhausted to the atmosphere through a Parkinson-Cowan gasometer (Type

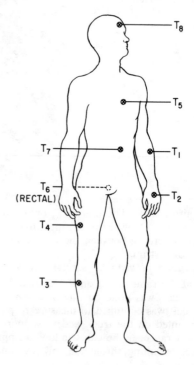

FIGURE 3. Thermistor placement sites.

CD-4) was directed into a Douglas bag for the remainder of the run. The subject rested briefly before repeating the run in the opposite direction. If pulmonary ventilation volumes for runs in opposite directions at a given speed were not within 12½%, the run was repeated (in the direction with the wind, if any) and the values for three runs averaged. Samples were taken from the Douglas bag into small rubber butyl bags and transported to the laboratory for gas analysis, as described previously, which was completed within 20 minutes after sampling.

Bicycle Riding. The same respiratory metabolism procedures described earlier were used to assess $\dot{V}_{O_2}$ for subject 1, an experienced occasional touring cyclist, at two bicycling speeds judged to yield values slightly below and above that of the slow running speed. Using Pugh's curve [18] and measured $\dot{V}_{O_2}$ values at speeds of 31.4 and 34.2 km/hr, a riding speed of 31.8 km/hr was found to require $\dot{V}_{O_2}$ at the same percent of estimated bicycle $\dot{V}_{O_2\,max}$ (62.7%) as that for measured running $\dot{V}_{O_2\,max}$, i.e., an absolute value of 7.5% less than that for running. The subject rode at his preferred pedaling rate, 79 rev/min, on a racing style bicycle, weighing 10.8 kg, with 68.6 cm wheel diameter, 2.38 cm tire cross section, and with tire pressure of 6.33 kg/cm². The subject assumed a modified racing position with both hands placed on the top rung of the dropped racing handle bars. A smooth, level macadamized out-and-back course of 8.04 km was used. The subject rode against the wind (if any) once and with the wind (if any) twice, totalling 24.0 km in approximately 45 minutes. Skin temperature and T_{re} were measured before and after riding, using the same procedures described earlier for outdoor running.

Thermal Exchange Analysis. Skin temperature values for the first 75 seconds of recovery from 25 test runs completed by all subjects in a wide variety of ambient conditions were used to determine how much the arithmetic mean differed from the weighted formula procedure of Hardy and DuBois.[19] Except for the postexercise bicycle comparisons, which differed from 0.3°–0.5° C, the arithmetic mean was found to agree within 0.25° C of the weighted mean. Because of ease of computation and what was felt to be an acceptable deviation from the weighted $\overline{T}_s$, the simple arithmetic $\overline{T}_s$ was used in all subsequent analyses.

Partitional heat exchange analyses for subject 1 were completed for the following conditions: (1) fast speed runs in M and W T_{db}, indoors with airflow and outdoors after sunset; (2) fast speed runs in C, M, and W T_{db}, indoors without airflow, and outdoors in direct solar radiation; (3) slow speed runs in W T_{db}, indoors without airflow, and outdoors in direct solar radiation; and (4) bicycle riding in W T_{db} with direct solar radiation. Procedures for calculating partitional heat exchange analyses were the same as those utilized by Adams and colleagues,[7] except that respiratory weight and heat loss were estimated according to formulas advanced by Mitchell and associates.[20]

Statistical Analysis. Visual inspection of end-run $\overline{T}_s$ data for subject 1 indicated no appreciable difference due to running speed at a given T_{db} for indoor runs with airflow. Hence, data from these runs were pooled to develop a regression analysis of $\overline{T}_s$ on T_{db}, the r being 0.95. Subsequently, a linear regression for all of subject 1's outdoor runs after sunset, was calculated and found not to be significantly different from the regression line for indoor runs with airflow.[21] The statistical analysis utilized includes testing whether parallel lines through the respective means can be regarded as an acceptable fit, and if so, whether they can be regarded as coincident, i.e., as a single line. Several other $\overline{T}_s$, T_{db} regression line comparisons were also made with this procedure. In each case, the 0.05 level of significance was applied.

RESULTS

Since T_s observations were made each minute during indoor treadmill runs, it was possible to analyze variation in $\overline{T}_s$ response with time. A comparison of time-course variation between subjects for the slow run (254 m/min), with airflow, is depicted in FIGURE 4. The mean T_{db} during subject 1's run was 21.0° C, while that for subject 2 was 21.4° C. Other intersubject comparisons revealed little difference in absolute $\overline{T}_s$, or in the trend of response.

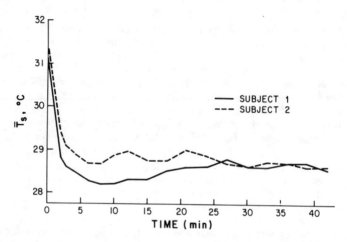

FIGURE 4. Intersubject variation in mean skin temperature response during a treadmill run with airflow.

An example of $\overline{T}_s$ response for subject 1 during treadmill running at the slow speed in C and M T_{db} with airflow equivalent to the runner's speed, is depicted in FIGURE 5. Also shown is the $\overline{T}_s$ response during runs at both speeds in W T_{db}. There is a drop of approximately 2° C from the prerun control $\overline{T}_s$ within the first 5 minutes in all runs, with only minor fluctuations thereafter. Absolute differences in $\overline{T}_s$ can be attributed primarily to T_{db} variation in the three conditions. Clearly, there is no substantial difference in the pattern of response attributable to speed of running, the 0.5° C higher $\overline{T}_s$ values for the slower run in W conditions being due largely to an equivalently higher T_{db}. There was also no appreciable difference in the pattern or magnitude of $\overline{T}_s$ response noted for the slow and fast runs in either the C or M conditions.

The time-course variation for the indoor runs without airflow followed an entirely different pattern than those with airflow. While there was a drop in $\overline{T}_s$ from the prerun control valve during the first 5 minutes for runs at both speeds, as shown in FIGURE 6 for the C T_{db} condition, it amounted to only 0.5° to

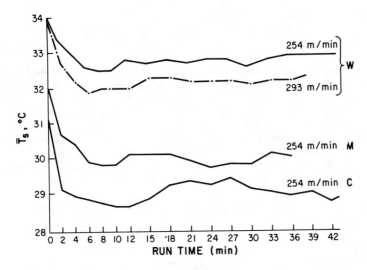

FIGURE 5. Mean skin temperature during treadmill running in cool, moderate and warm temperatures with airflow.

1.0° C. Thereafter, there was a gradual upward trend to values equal to or greater than the prerun control $\overline{T}_s$. It is also evident that the increase is greater in the faster run, which was also the case, but to a slightly lesser extent, in the M and W conditions.

Comparison of the $\overline{T}_s$ response during the fast run with airflow to that without airflow in W T_{db} is shown in FIGURE 7. Also depicted is the T_{rc} re-

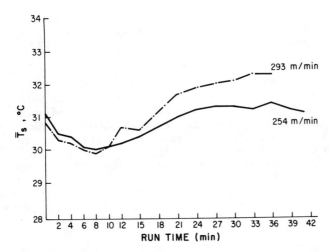

FIGURE 6. Mean skin temperature during treadmill running at two speeds in cool temperature without airflow.

sponse for these runs. It is evident that T_{re} rises almost steadily throughout the run without airflow, whereas that for the run with airflow equivalent to the runner's speed is over 0.5° C lower during the last half of the run and shows a tendency to plateau in the last 5 minutes.

In the present study, it was observed that a linear extrapolation back to time zero of the mean of the first three T_s measurements taken at each site over the course of the first 75 seconds of recovery following treadmill runs rarely differed by more than ±0.2° C from measured $\overline{T}_s$ during the last minute of running. An example of this comparison for subject 1's runs with airflow is shown in FIGURE 8. Although $\overline{T}_s$ seems to rise slightly more rapidly following the faster runs, no systematic effect of running speed or T_{db} on the accuracy of the procedure is evidenced. Similar results were observed in analyses of postrun extrapolation and end-run $\overline{T}_s$ comparisons for subjects 2 and 3.

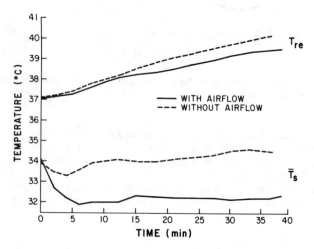

FIGURE 7. Mean skin and rectal temperatures during "fast" treadmill runs in warm temperature, with and without airflow.

Extrapolated end-run $\overline{T}_s$ values for outdoor postsunset runs of subject 1 were compared statistically to the $\overline{T}_s$ values obtained in the last minute of indoor runs with airflow. No significant difference was noted; thus, the data were combined and a regression line calculated (FIGURE 9). Also shown in FIGURE 9 are subject 1's $\overline{T}_s$ values obtained in the last minute of indoor runs without airflow and extrapolated end-exercise $\overline{T}_s$ values for outdoor runs in clear-sky solar radiation and for bicycle rides in clear sky solar radiation and after sunset.

When the end-run $\overline{T}_s$, T_{db} data for the outdoor-postsunset and the indoor-with-airflow runs of subjects 2 and 3 were compared to the regression line from subject 1's runs in the same conditions, no significant difference was found. Visual comparison of end-run $\overline{T}_s$ data for subjects 2 and 3 with that of subject 1 for the outdoor runs with clear-sky solar radiation and indoor runs without airflow revealed no substantial differences. Hence, data for all subjects were pooled to yield the regression equations shown in TABLE 2. Statistical analysis

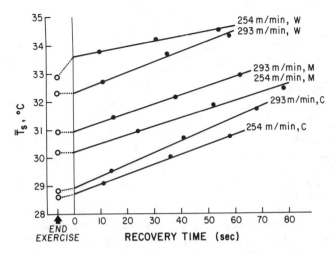

FIGURE 8. Linear extrapolation estimate of end-run mean skin temperature from recovery measurements following treadmill runs with airflow.

revealed that each of the last three regression lines differed significantly from the line calculated from the indoor-with-airflow and outdoor-postsunset data.

Relative humidity (RH) during subject 1's runs varied from 33% to 73% in the outdoor runs, being highest in the early morning and after sunset and lowest in the afternoon. Since the indoor conditions were manipulated via the laboratory's general air-conditioning and heating system, which was largely dependent on an outdoor air source, RH was highest during runs in C T_{db} and lowest during those in W T_{db}. Linear regression analysis of end-run $\bar{T}_s$ on RH for all subject 1's indoor and outdoor runs yielded an r of −0.66, while that obtained for the 12 indoor-with-airflow and outdoor-postsunset runs alone was −0.89. However, this relationship is clearly T_{db}-dependent, as when a partial

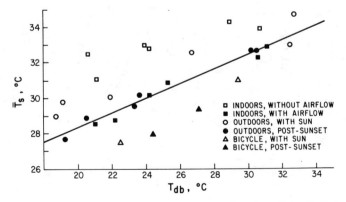

FIGURE 9. End-exercise mean skin temperature as a function of dry bulb temperature for subject 1.

TABLE 2

REGRESSION EQUATIONS OF END-EXERCISE $\overline{T}_s$ ON T_{db}

Condition	No. of Data Pts	r	Regression Equation
Indoors with airflow & outdoors postsunset	22	0.975	$y = 20.27 + 0.40x$
Indoors without airflow	9	0.863	$y = 26.45 + 0.26x$
Outdoors, clear-sky radiation	9	0.946	$y = 22.77 + 0.35x$
Outdoors, bicycle	4	0.975	$y = 14.20 + 0.58x$

correlation analysis holding T_{db} constant was calculated, the r between RH and $\overline{T}_s$ was reduced to -0.10.

Linear regression analysis of the end-run $\overline{T}_s$ and sweat rate (SR) relationship for subject 1 is depicted in FIGURE 10. It is readily apparent that SR is higher for a given $\overline{T}_s$ at the faster running speed, although the relationship is not as clear at $\overline{T}_s < 30°$ C.

The end-run T_{re} for subject 1 reflected the relative strain imposed by the various combinations of exercise intensity and indoor and outdoor ambient conditions. At the slower speed (62.7% of $\dot{V}_{O_2\,max}$) T_{re} ranged from 38.4° C in the C condition with airflow, to 39.2° C in the W conditions indoors without airflow and outdoors with solar radiation. At the faster speed (77.9% of $\dot{V}_{O_2\,max}$), end-run T_{re} ranged from 38.9° C in C and M T_{db} up to 39.5° C in the W T_{db} indoors with airflow and outdoors after sunset. End-run T_{re} for the fast runs indoors without airflow and outdoors with solar radiation ranged from 39.3° C in the C T_{db} to 40.2° C in the W T_{db}. Other data relative to thermoregulation for subject 1 during the more stressful protocols are summarized in TABLE 3.

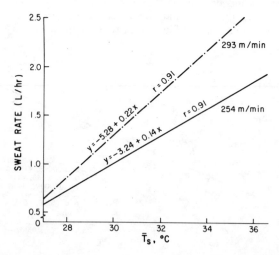

FIGURE 10. Regression lines of sweat rate on mean skin temeprature at two running speeds, including all indoor and outdoor runs.

TABLE 3

ANALYSIS OF HEAT STRESS IMPOSED BY RUNNING AT TWO SPEEDS, INDOORS AND OUTDOORS IN MODERATE AND WARM TEMPERATURES*

Run	Time of Run (min)	T_{db} (°C)	T_g (°C)	End-Run $\overline{T}_s$ (°C)	End-Run T_{re} (°C)	SR (liter/hr)	Body Heat Storage (W/m²)	Tissue Conductance (W/m² per °C) $T_{re} - \overline{T}_s$
Slow, without airflow	42.0	30.7	30.1	33.9	39.2	1.74	90.7	101.3
Slow, in sun	43.1	32.4	41.0	32.9	38.8	1.66	72.4	85.9
Fast, with airflow	38.0	25.3	25.0	30.9	38.7	1.25	96.1	74.4
Fast, with airflow	72.1	24.8	24.5	30.8	38.9	1.33	49.0	74.9
Fast, with airflow	38.0	30.6	30.1	32.3	39.5	1.72	111.6	85.9
Fast, postsunset	37.6	30.2	28.9	32.8	39.7	1.86	109.1	89.8
Fast, without airflow	36.5	28.9	28.3	34.3	40.2	2.20	158.3	123.5
Fast, in sun	37.1	32.7	45.7	34.7	40.3	2.19	184.2	119.2

* T_{db}, dry-bulb temperature; T_g, globe temperature; $\overline{T}_s$, mean skin temperature; T_{re}, rectal temperature; SR, sweat rate.

Discussion

Utilizing an AGA infrared thermovision device and a rapid-responding thermocouple probe, Clark, Mullan, and Pugh [12] have shown that the latter can be used for estimating $\overline{T}_s$ during running in C and M T_{db}, provided observations are initiated immediately and allowance is made for the approximate $1°$ C temperature rise per minute during the first 2 minutes of recovery. One objective of the present study was to examine further the validity of estimating $\overline{T}_s$ during running via measurements taken in the first 2 minutes of recovery, and particularly over a wide range of T_{db}. In the present study, linear extrapolation of the mean of the first three recovery $\overline{T}_s$ measurements at each site back to time zero rarely deviated more than $±0.2°$ C from the measured $\overline{T}_s$ during the last minute of indoor runs with airflow equivalent to running speed (FIGURE 8). Similarly close approximations were also observed following indoor runs without airflow, although the rate of $\overline{T}_s$ increase during the first 75 seconds was about one-half that of runs with airflow. Thus, since close approximations were obtained with all S_s in both runs with and without airflow, the technique would seem to have acceptable validity for predicting $\overline{T}_s$ during running in a variety of outdoor conditions.

Pugh [11] found that the $\overline{T}_s$ of athletes running outdoors in M T_{db} fell to a steady value within 20 minutes after initiating exercise, averaging several degrees below the normal values of appropriately clothed persons at rest. In the present investigation there was an initial fall in $\overline{T}_s$ from the prerun control in the first 5 minutes for all indoor runs, but with that for runs with airflow being two to three times greater than that for runs without airflow. The initial drop reflects the reflex vasoconstriction of peripheral blood vessels at the onset of strenuous exercise. [15] In the runs without airflow, convective and evaporative heat transfer were significantly reduced and $\overline{T}_s$ gradually rose as increased metabolic heat was transported to the periphery, an explanation substantiated by higher end-run $\overline{T}_s$ for the fast runs. On the other hand, the greater initial drop of $\overline{T}_s$ in the runs with airflow remained essentially steady throughout. This reflects the adequate environmental cooling capacity via convection and evaporation within the range of ambient conditions studied.

One of the major findings in the present study was the virtually identical agreement of the last-minute $\overline{T}_s$, T_{db} relationship for indoor runs with airflow equivalent to the runner's speed with that for the extrapolated end-run $\overline{T}_s$, T_{db} relationships obtained for the outdoor runs after sunset. This permitted an enlarged data pool for statistical analysis of the effects of ambient environmental variables other than T_{db} on $\overline{T}_s$.

By inspection of FIGURE 9 and TABLE 2, it can be seen that clear-sky solar radiation, with MRT ranging from $37.0°$ to $56.9°$ C in a T_{db} range from $18.7°$ to $32.7°$ C, exerts a potentiating influence on $\overline{T}_s$, amounting to approximately $1.5°$ C above that for outdoor runs after sunset and indoor runs with airflow. This agrees rather closely with Pugh's observations in Mexico City, in which it was noted that clear-sky solar radiation raised $\overline{T}_s$ between $1°$ to $2°$ C in M T_{db}. [11] Considerably larger increases were observed in subjects standing still, the difference being attributed to the high rate of evaporative and convective cooling during running. Adams and colleagues [7] noted an enhanced $\overline{T}_s$ of about $1°$ C in a single runner competing in a marathon in partly cloudy skies when compared to $\overline{T}_s$ observed during indoor runs with airflow. Increased sweat rate, in association with the greater $\overline{T}_s$, was noted for the outdoor marathon run. While a higher $\overline{T}_s$ reduces the radiation gain to the body, as well as increasing the potential for heat loss via convection and evaporation, the total reduction generally amounted to only a small fraction of the total radiation heat gain effected in clear-sky solar radiation compared to that during postsunset runs within the T_{db} range studied. Furthermore, the increased SR from the enhanced $\overline{T}_s$ effected by clear-sky solar radiation (FIGURES 9 & 10) would facilitate a secondary rise in T_{re} from increased dehydration above 3%–4% of body weight, which is typical in prolonged runs.[1, 5, 7, 22, 23]

In M conditions ($T_{db} = 20°$ to $23°$ C), Pugh[11] observed $\overline{T}_s$ of $27°$–$28°$ C for an international caliber athlete running on a treadmill at 10 mph with airflow equivalent to running speed. At similar T_{db} with no airflow, $\overline{T}_s$ was between $30°$–$31.5°$ C. Very similar $\overline{T}_s$ values were observed in the present study in this T_{db} range. However, the increased airflow velocity when subject 1 rode a bicycle at 533 m/min, as opposed to running at 254 m/min (at nearly equivalent metabolic rates), resulted in a significantly reduced $\overline{T}_s$ for a given T_{db} in postsunset conditions. Furthermore, the potentiated $\overline{T}_s$ increase effected by clear-sky solar radiation over postsunset rides at equivalent T_{db} was reduced, probably due primarily to increased convective heat loss. As the SR, $\overline{T}_s$ relationship for the bicycle rides was very nearly equivalent to that for the slow runs, the lower $\overline{T}_s$ at a given T_{db} during bicycling lowered the SR. Thus, bicyclists, riding at speeds necessitating metabolic heat production equivalent proportionally to their $\dot{V}_{O_2\,max}$ as that for runners, have considerable advantage in the maintenance of thermoregulation in W conditions that runners could not tolerate for prolonged periods (e.g., 2¼ hours).

Pugh[11] noted that RH had little effect on the steady-state $\overline{T}_s$ within the T_{db} range observed during running outdoors. Although RH was significantly related to $\overline{T}_s$ in the present study during runs indoors with airflow and postsunset runs outdoors, this was shown by partial correlation analysis to be largely due to the close relationship of RH to T_{db}, the latter being related to $\overline{T}_s$ even more closely than RH. It should be noted, however, that with the minimal cooling potential via convection and evaporation afforded in the indoor "still" air runs, $\overline{T}_s$ was significantly elevated for a given T_{db} compared to runs with airflow. Thus, in outdoor runs with very high RH (e.g., >85%) and W or hot T_{db} (where convective heat loss is minimized, or becomes a gain), one could expect elevated $\overline{T}_s$ higher than for runs at equivalent T_{db} in low RH, in which $\overline{T}_s$ would be reduced via greater evaporation of sweat produced.

Although the present study was not designed to identify precisely the limiting environmental conditions at the two running speeds used, it is instructive to examine the data obtained from this perspective. For example, the end-run T_{re} for subject 1 was 38.4 at the slower speed and 39.0 at the faster speed in the C T_{db} indoors with airflow. There was less than $0.2°$ C rise in T_{re} during the last 7 minutes of these runs, and they closely approximate the steady-state values as a function of percent $\dot{V}_{O_2\,max}$ observed by Saltin and Hermansen[24] for healthy partially trained subjects at 62.7% and 77.8%, respectively. Clearly, this subject was operating within the prescriptive zone of temperature regulation as described by Lind[25] at both workloads in these conditions.

In the most stressful environmental conditions imposed in the present study, viz., indoors without airflow at $30.7°$ C T_{db} and outdoors at $32.4°$ C T_{db} and $41.0°$ C T_g, subject 1 completed the slow speed runs with a T_{re} of $39.2°$ and $38.8°$ C, respectively. During the indoor run, T_{re} reached $38.4°$ C within 20 minutes and climbed steadily, an additional 0.85° C, in the following 24 minutes. If the same rate of increase had persisted in these conditions with minimal convective and evaporative heat loss, hyperthermic T_{re} ($>40.5°$ C) would have been reached in less than 1½ hours. Sweat rate during this run was submaximal for the subject, but sufficient to cause a significant secondary T_{re} elevation within 1¼ hour without fluid supplementation.[22, 26] Cutaneous blood flow, as indicated by calculated tissue conductance,[27] was about 80% of the maximum observed for subject 1 and storage was also submaximum, although rising with continually increasing T_{re}. Thus, it is unlikely that subject 1 could have completed the full marathon distance at 254 m/min in these conditions, primarily because of the steady metabolic heat accumulation from relatively ineffective evaporative heat loss. On the other hand, it seems possible that he might have been able to complete the full marathon distance outdoors at the slower speed in the existent W T_{db} and clear-sky solar radiation. In these conditions, T_{re}, the rate of body heat storage, tissue conductance, and SR were not as high as for the indoor run. Partitional heat exchange revealed minimal convective heat exchange, but at the low RH (26%), virtually all of the sweat

TABLE 4

COMPARISON OF END-RUN METABOLIC AND THERMOREGULATORY RESPONSES
TO A TREADMILL RUN OF 11.1 km AND 21.1 km AT 293 m/min

Length of Run (km)	Heart Rate (beats/ min)	$\dot{V}_E$ (liter/ min BTPS)	Respiratory Quotient	$\dot{V}_{O_2}$ (liter/ min)	SR (liter/ hr)	$\bar{T}_s$ (°C)	T_{re} (°C)
11.1	170	110.4	0.86	3.713	1.25	30.9	38.7
21.1	172	124.8	0.88	3.751	1.33	30.8	38.9

produced was evaporated, amounting to 675 W/m². Thus, metabolic heat production, 587 W/m², and radiation heat gain, 124 W/m², were effectively counterbalanced. Of course, adequate fluid replacement would be necessary to complete the full marathon distance.

Although subject 1 had no previous competitive running experience in races longer than 13 km, the fast speed (293 m/min) used in the present study appears to be a realistic marathon pace for him in optimal environmental conditions. His steady-state $\dot{V}_{O_2}$ at this running speed was 59.1 ml/min·kg, or 77.9% of $\dot{V}_{O_2 max}$, which is only slightly higher than the mean value for a group of national class marathon runners studied by Costill and Fox.[3] This contention is also supported by a run at that speed indoors with airflow at a T_{db} of 24.8° C over a half-marathon distance, 21.1 km. A comparison of pertinent data between this run and the 11.1 km run in the same conditions is shown in TABLE 4. It is readily apparent that, except for $\dot{V}_E$, very little difference exists between end-run values for each test. Clearly, the subject was running in a near steady-state, with very little change in HR, $\dot{V}_{O_2}$, and RQ. Furthermore, SR was submaximal, body heat storage remained nearly constant, and tissue conductance was virtually identical. Although the subject was permitted water *ad libitum* for the 21.1 km run only, he imbibed just 79 ml. His weight loss of 1.892 kg represented 2.90% of total body weight, which if continued at the same rate for the full marathon distance would have caused a significant secondary rise in T_{re}, but almost certainly not above 1° C.[7]

Inspection of the data in TABLE 3 suggests that the indoor-with-airflow and outdoor-postsunset runs in W T_{db} (30.2° to 30.6° C) might also have been continued at the same pace for the marathon distance, although T_{re}, SR, storage, and tissue conductance were significantly higher than for the half-marathon run. Furthermore, the end-run $\overline{T}_s$ of 32.3° and 32.8° C are considerably above the 28.5° C value advanced by Pugh as the upper limit for optimal marathon competition.[10]

From the data presented in FIGURE 7 and TABLE 3, there can be no question that the environmental conditions imposed in the W T_{db} fast run indoors without airflow and outdoors with clear-sky radiation are beyond subject 1's ability to maintain steady-state thermoregulation over the full marathon distance. During the fast indoor run in these conditions, T_{re} rose at an almost steady rate of 0.085° C/min, which, if maintained, would have resulted in the T_{re} exceeding 41° C shortly after 45 minutes. Although SR and tissue conductance were maximum, the ineffective evaporation effected by this still-air environment resulted in a steadily increasing heat storage, which soon would have reached maximum. Dehydration, per se, was not a significant problem, as less than 2.5% of body weight was lost during the run. Heart rate was 187 beats/min; $\dot{V}_E$, 146.1 ℓ/min (BTPS); and the RQ, 0.93, during the last minute of the run, which reflects an increased cardiorespiratory stress due largely to an excessive demand placed on the cardiovascular system by the combined cutaneous and muscular requirements.[7] The $\overline{T}_s$, T_{re}, SR, and tissue conductance for the fast outdoor run in W T_{db} with clear-sky solar radiation closely approximate those in the previously described limiting indoor still-air run in W T_{db}. Body heat storage for the outdoor run was somewhat higher, reflecting a slightly greater heat stress. Again, the subject would clearly have been forced to stop within a few minutes if he sought to maintain the same pace. Radiation heat gain to the body for this run was calculated to be 132.2 W/m², equivalent to nearly 20% of metabolic heat production, a result closely approximating outdoor observations on runners in clear-sky conditions at Mexico City by Pugh.[11]

In summary, it has been demonstrated that extrapolation of T_s measurements taken in the first 75 seconds of recovery back to time zero agree closely with T_s measured during the last minute of treadmill running at T_{db} values ranging from 20° to 31° C. It was also shown that the end-run $\overline{T}_s$, T_{db} relationship for indoor treadmill running with airflow equivalent to the runner's speed was not significantly different from that for outdoor running after sunset, whereas that for indoor runs in still-air and outdoors in clear-sky solar radiation were. The importance of forced convection on the $\overline{T}_s$, T_{db} relationship was further demonstrated by a significantly lower $\overline{T}_s$ when bicycling outdoors at a metabolic rate nearly equivalent to running outdoors at a similar T_{db}. Finally, although the present study was not specially designed to identify limiting environmental conditions during prolonged running, the data clearly illustrate the severe thermal stress imposed by high solar radiation levels when attempting to maintain normal competitive speed.

ACKNOWLEDGMENTS

The technical assistance of Mr. Richard Fadling, Electronics Technician, and the laboratory assistance afforded by Messrs. Dave Biles, Geoff Adams, and Keith Adams is gratefully acknowledged. Mr. Fadling constructed the lucite ring thermistor applicators, while Mr. John Seabury fabricated the thermistor lead, subminiature connector harness. Dr. Aaron Goldman (Mathematics Department, University of Nevada, Las Vegas) suggested the statistical procedures utilized. Drs. Edmund Bernauer and Rudolph Dressendorfer (Physical Education Department, University of California, Davis) and Dr. Carl Gisolfi (Department of Physiology and Biophysics, The University of Iowa, Iowa City) graciously agreed to review the manuscript and offered numerous helpful suggestions. Finally, especial appreciation is expressed to the subjects, Angel Martinez, Peter Sweeney, and Matt Yeo, who performed obligingly and admirably.

REFERENCES

1. Gisolfi, C. V. & J. R. Copping. 1974. Thermal effects of prolonged treadmill exercise in the heat. Med. Sci. Sports 6: 108–113.
2. American College of Sports Medicine Position Statement. 1975. Prevention of heat injuries during running. Med. Sci. Sports 7(1): vii–viii.
3. Costill, D. L. & E. L. Fox. 1969. Energetics of marathon running. Med. Sci. Sports 1: 81–86.
4. Costill, D. L. 1972. Physiology of marathon running. J. Amer. Med. Assoc. 221: 1024–1029.
5. Pugh, L. G. C. E., J. L. Corbett & R. H. Johnson. 1967. Rectal temperatures, weight losses, and sweat rates in marathon running. J. Appl. Physiol. 23: 347–352.
6. Kerslake, D. McK. 1972. The Stress of Hot Environments. University Press. Cambridge, England.
7. Adams, W. C., R. H. Fox, A. J. Fry & I. C. MacDonald. 1975. Thermoregulation during marathon running in cool, moderate and hot environments. J. Appl. Physiol. 38: 1030–1037.
8. Fox, R. H. 1960. Heat stress in athletics. Ergonomics. 3: 307–313.
9. Nielsen, M. 1938. Die regulation der korpertemperatur bei muskelarbeit. Scand. Arch. F. Physiol. 79: 193–230.
10. Pugh, L. G. C. E. 1971. Temperature regulation in athletes. Nat. Inst. Med. Res. Scientific Report for 1969–1970 (London) : 69.
11. Pugh, L. G. C. E. 1970. Mean skin temperature and sweat rates of runners in Mexico. Nat. Inst. Med. Res. Scientific Report for 1968–1969 (London) : 57–58.
12. Clark, R. P., B. J. Mullan & L. G. C. E. Pugh. 1974. Colour thermography in running. J. Physiol. 239: 81P–82P.
13. Brozek, J., F. Grande, J. T. Anderson & A. Keys. 1963. Densitometric analysis of body composition: Revision of some quantitative assumptions. Ann. N.Y. Acad. Sci. 110: 113–140.
14. Dill, D. B. & W. C. Adams. 1971. Maximal oxygen uptake at sea level and at 3,090-m altitude in high school champion runners. J. Appl. Physiol. 30: 854–859.
15. Åstrand, P.-O. & K. Rodahl. 1970. Textbook of Work Physiology. McGraw-Hill Company, New York, N.Y.
16. Pugh, L. G. C. E. 1970. Oxygen intake in track and treadmill running with observations on the effect of air resistance. J. Physiol. 207: 823–835.

17. CONSOLAZIO, C. F., R. E. JOHNSON & L. J. PECORA. 1963. Physiological Measurements of Metabolic Functions in Man. McGraw-Hill Company. New York, N.Y.
18. PUGH, L. G. C. E. 1974. The relation of oxygen intake and speed in competition cycling and comparative observations on the bicycle ergometer. J. Physiol. 241: 795–808.
19. HARDY, J. D. & E. F. DuBois. 1938. The technique of measuring radiation and convection. J. Nutr. 15: 461–475.
20. MITCHELL, J. W., E. R. NADEL & J. A. J. STOLWIJK. 1972. Respiratory weight losses during exercise. J. Appl. Physiol. 32: 474–476.
21. BROWNLEE, K. A. 1968. Statistical Theory and Methodology in Science and Engineering. John Wiley and Sons, Inc. New York, N.Y.
22. COSTILL, D. L., W. F. KAMMER & A. FISHER. 1970. Fluid ingestion during distance running. Arch. Environ. Health. 21: 520–525.
23. WYNDHAM, C. H. & N. B. STRYDOM. 1969. The danger of an inadequate water intake during marathon running. S. African Med. J. 43: 893–896.
24. SALTIN, B. & L. HERMANSEN. 1966. Esophageal, rectal and muscle temperature during exercise. J. Appl. Physiol. 21: 1757–1762.
25. LIND, A. R. 1963. A physiological criterion for setting thermal environmental limits for everyday work. J. Appl. Physiol. 18: 51–56.
26. GREENLEAF, J. E. & B. L. CASTLE. 1971. Exercise temperature regulation in man during hypohydration and hyperhydration. J. Appl. Physiol. 30: 847–853.
27. ROBINSON, S., F. R. MEYER, J. L. NEWTON, C. H. TS'AO & L. O. HOLGERSEN. 1965. Relations between sweating, cutaneous blood flow, and body temperatures in work. J. Applied Physiol. 20: 575–582.

HEAT STROKE AND HYPERTHERMIA IN MARATHON RUNNERS

C. H. Wyndham

Chamber of Mines Research Laboratories
Marshalltown, Transvaal
South Africa

University of the Witwatersrand
Johannesburg, South Africa

Introduction

Sir Adolphe Abrahams in his article on "Athletics" in the 1950 edition of the *British Encyclopaedia of Medical Practice* states:

> I am of the opinion that in healthy subjects the only serious potential risk to life from violent exercise is heat stroke—a danger well exhibited by examples I have seen of alarming collapse and, on one occasion, death. The correct precaution would be to prohibit the race in circumstances in which an occurrence might be expected—a moisture laden atmosphere, a following wind and the early afternoon of a day with a shade temperature of 85° F (29.5° C) or higher.

Sir Adolphe could not have expressed his warning about heat stroke in clearer terms, but, in spite of his warning, sports administrators still continue to arrange marathon running and cycling events in climatic conditions that are dangerous because of the risks of heat stroke.

Prevention is better than cure, but for prevention to be effective there must be a good understanding of both the circumstances that lead to the condition and its pathophysiology.

Heat Exchange

Studies in my laboratory [1-4] have demonstrated convincingly that $\dot{V}_{O_2}$ is highly correlated with gross body mass during both walking and running. In a study [4] of six males varying in weight from 63 to 102 kg, correlation coefficients of between $r = 0.85$ and $r = 0.99$ were found for walking at 3.2, 4.8, and 8.0 km/hr, and running at 8.0, 9.7, 11.3, and 12.9 km/hr (FIGURES 1 & 2). A similar, statistically significant correlation of $r = 0.71$ between $\dot{V}_{O_2}$ and body mass was found for six marathon runners when running at 18 km/hr, the speed needed to complete a standard marathon in reasonable time. The physical characteristics and $\dot{V}_{O_2 max}$ values of these six runners are given in TABLE 1 and are compared with those of two sub-4-minute milers and 80 fit young Army trainees. All of these studies were carried out in Johannesburg, which is at an altitude of 1,763 m above sea level.

The $\dot{V}_{O_2}$ values of the six marathon runners when running at 18 km/hr are given in TABLE 2, together with the percentages of $\dot{V}_{O_2 max}$, the blood lactates, and the heart rates at rest and after 30 minutes of running. The $\dot{V}_{O_2}$ varied from 2.6 l/min in the 50 kg to 3.5 l/min in the 72-kg man. All of the percent-

128

TABLE 1

PHYSICAL AND PHYSIOLOGICAL CHARACTERISTICS OF ENDURANCE ATHLETES

Subjects	Age (years)	Height (cm)	Weight (kg)	$\dot{V}_{O_2max}$ (liters/min)	$\dot{V}_{O_2max}$ (ml/min·kg)
Marathon runners					
Mou.	22	175.6	61.05	3.87	63.39
Mo.	21	182.2	63.65	3.67	57.66
H.	18	164.9	51.05	3.42	66.99
P.	20	176.5	68.90	4.28	62.15
Me.	20	183.5	71.55	4.40	61.50
S.	34	177.8	65.45	4.09	62.49
Mean	22.5	176.7	63.61	3.95	62.36
Sub-4-minute milers					
Z.	19	174.4	62.00	4.32	69.68
L.	24	183.4	65.35	4.13	63.19
Army recruits					
80 men	17–19	174.4	66.30	3.15	47.21

ages of $\dot{V}_{O_2\,max}$ used while running at 18 km/hr were in excess of 75%. One would expect, therefore, that some of these runners would be in anaerobic metabolism. Judged by the blood lactate levels after 30 minutes of running, this proved to be the case. Blood lactate levels in excess of 60 mg/100 ml were found in those runners using 85%–90% of $\dot{V}_{O_2\,max}$. Their heart rates were also in excess of 180 beats/min.

TABLE 2

LACTATE RESPONSE OF MARATHON RUNNERS AFTER 30 MINUTES AT 18 km/hr *

Subjects	Speed (km/hr)	Lactate (mg/100 ml)	$\dot{V}_{O_2}$ (liters/min)	$\dot{V}_{O_2}$ as % of maximum	Heart Rate (beats/min)
Mou.	Rest	10.86	—	—	—
	18	71.85	3.54	91.4	180
Mo.	Rest	9.90	—	—	—
	18	13.12	2.98	80.5	156
H.	Rest	9.34	—	—	—
	18	17.27	2.58	75.4	162
P.	Rest	13.72	—	—	—
	18	68.25	3.66	85.5	182
Me.	Rest	13.31	—	—	—
	18	18.29	3.42	77.7	178
S.	Rest	7.67	—	—	—
	18	27.37	3.38	82.7	189

* 10 miles per hour.

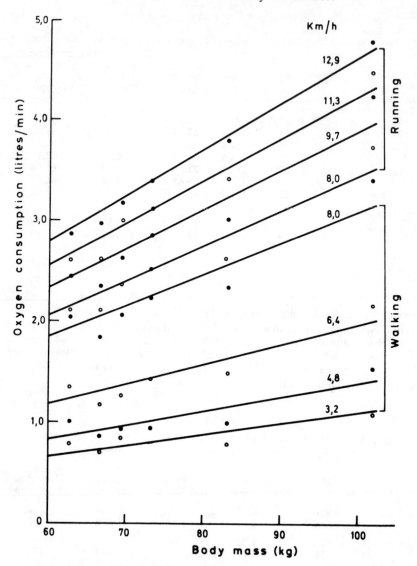

FIGURE 1. Oxygen consumption in relation to body mass and walking or running speed for six males.

The high levels of $\dot{V}_{O_2}$ recorded in these men when running at 18 km/hr would be associated with high rates of heat production. These would cause their body temperatures to rise to heat stroke levels if the human body did not have a superbly efficient mechanism for ridding itself of waste heat—the evaporation of sweat. If we consider only the heat produced by aerobic metabolism, a 60-kg runner would produce 900 kcal (3,780 kJ) per hour, and if he had no means of getting rid of waste heat his body temperature would rise to about 45° C after 30 minutes of running at 18 km/hr. All of the heat produced could, however, be dissipated by sweating 1,500 ml/hr of water and evaporating it.

Do marathon runners sweat sufficiently for these high rates of evaporation from their body surfaces? Observations by my laboratory [5] on 30 marathon runners in a 30-km race on a cool day (the dry bulb temperature rose from 9° C at 8:00 AM to 17° C at noon and relative humidity fell from 90% to 30%) showed that there is a significant correlation ($r = 0.90$) between sweat rates and body masses, irrespective of the places in which the runners finished the race (FIGURE 3). From the regression line in FIGURE 3 one can estimate that a 60-kg runner would sweat at a rate of 1,250 ml/hr. Similar high rates of

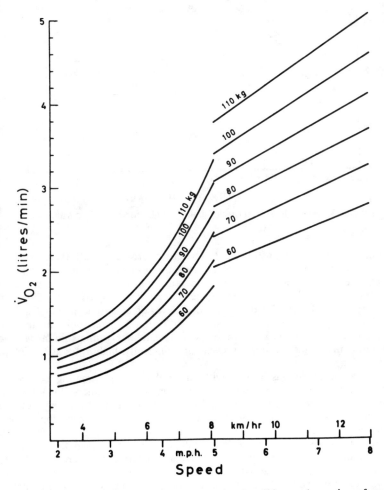

FIGURE 2. Oxygen intake at different speeds of walking and running of men of different weights.

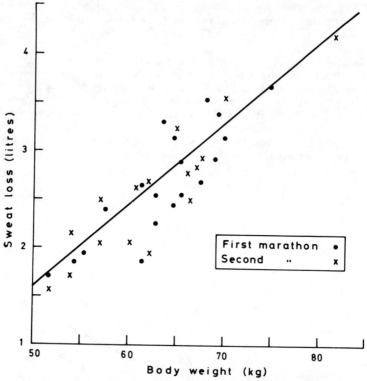

FIGURE 3. Sweat loss in terms of body weight for marathon runners.

sweating were shown by Costill et al.[6] Therefore, provided the humidity of the air is sufficiently low to allow all of the sweat to evaporate, marathon runners probably are able to sweat fast enough to remain in thermal balance with the high rates of aerobic heat production. The runners who might get into difficulty in this regard are those who develop a high level of anaerobic metabolism. A few examples of such runners were shown in TABLE 2. Anaerobic metabolism adds materially to the production of waste heat, and runners in anaerobic metabolism might not be able to sweat at sufficiently high rates to maintain thermal balance.

There are problems associated with the high rates of sweating needed to maintain thermal balance in marathon running. If the runners do not drink at a sufficient rate to replace the water losses from sweating, they may develop severe dehydration. Dehydration materially affects the ability of the human body to regulate body temperature. This is well shown in studies from my laboratory.[5] Those runners who drank sufficient water to keep their level of dehydration below 3% of body mass had rectal temperatures of around 38.5° C at the end of the 30-km race, which is normal (FIGURE 4). However, in those men who did not drink sufficient water to keep below this safe level of dehydration, there was a significant positive correlation between the rectal temperature and the extent of dehydration. From the regression line fitted to these data one can predict that runners who develop more than 5% dehydration would be likely to finish the race with rectal temperatures around 41° C. Interestingly enough, this prediction agrees well with Pugh's observation [7] on a marathon runner: On a warm day in the United Kingdom he sweated at a rate of 1,800 ml/hr and developed a rectal temperature of 41.1° C in association with 6.7% dehydration.

Hyperthermia

Body temperature is invariably raised above 38° C during a marathon run,[5, 6] and, if the runner is dehydrated, the rectal temperature may rise above 40° C. This poses the problem of whether body temperatures raised to such levels for prolonged periods of at least 2 hours in a standard marathon can cause damage to cells in vital organs. Evidence of damage to vital organs is revealed either in elevated serum enzyme levels or in deranged function of an organ.

McKechnie *et al.*[8] made a detailed study of ECG changes, serum enzymes, and blood potassium in 20 marathon runners immediately after a race and, in some, a fortnight later. They did not find any evidence of myocardial damage in the ECG. The mean values of the serum enzymes GOT, GPT, and LDH were all elevated above normal (TABLE 3). Abnormal values were found in 8, 13, and 8 of the 20 runners for GOT, GPT, and LDH, respectively. In two runners GOT was above 100 units, in one of the two GPT was above 100 units, and in both LDH was above 700 units. Serum aldolase was raised above

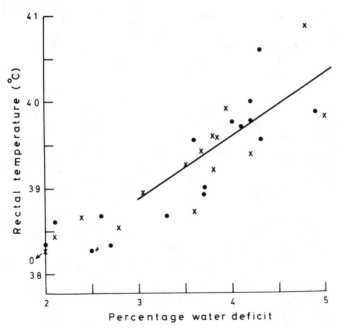

FIGURE 4. Rectal temperature in relation to percentage water deficit for marathon runners.

normal in all 20 runners and was still above normal in four of the six runners who returned for further study two weeks later. Serum potassium levels were raised in all 20 runners. Rose et al.[9] measured total LDH, total CPK, and LDH isoenzymes in six men after a standard marathon. Significant increases were found in total LDH and total CPK and in the LDH isoenzymes −3, −4, and −5 but not in the isoenzymes −1 and −2, the fractions found in cardiac muscle and the kidney.

No measurements were made of rectal temperature or of blood lactate and pH by McKechnie et al. or Rose et al. Hence we have no evidence of whether hyperthermia or metabolic acidosis played any part in the cell damage that was revealed by the raised serum enzyme levels. In an attempt to determine whether prolonged hyperthermia, without metabolic acidosis, causes cell damage, my laboratory[10] exercised 15 physically conditioned and heat-acclimatized men for 4 hours at a $\dot{V}_{O_2}$ of 1.32 l/min in hot and humid conditions. This heat stress and exercise condition caused their rectal temperatures to rise to 39°–40° C for most of the period of the experiment. The rate of exercise was chosen to give a $\dot{V}_{O_2}$ of well below 50% of the men's $\dot{V}_{O_2 max}$ values in order to ensure that they would not be in anaerobic metabolism and develop metabolic acidosis.

TABLE 3

SERUM ENZYMES IN HEAT STROKE VICTIMS, MARATHON RUNNERS, AND NORMALS

| | 44 Normal Men | 20 Marathon Runners | 40 Heat Stroke Victims | | |
| | | | Time after Heat Stroke | | |
			0 hr	48 hr	96 hr
GOT	36	60	518	1007	210
GPT	24	50	112	843	349
LDH	308	436	2058	3283	656

Control studies were made at the same work rate and for the same period in cool conditions and resulted in rectal temperature rising to a mean of 37.5° C. The serum enzymes GOT, GPT, LDH, and CPK, were significantly higher when the men's rectal temperatures were raised to 39°–40° C than at 37.5° C. The increase in serum enzyme levels in the men with hyperthermia of this order were, however, neither as consistent nor as high as those reported by Kew et al.[11] in heat stroke cases (TABLE 3), nor did the increase persist after the exercise ceased.

It seems reasonable to conclude on the available evidence that "physiological" levels of hyperthermia, i.e., rectal temperatures of below 41° C result in only mild and transient damage to cells in the human body. However, as shown in the earlier section, marathon runners commonly run at above 75% of $\dot{V}_{O_2 max}$ and some develop marked metabolic acidosis as indicated by elevated blood lactate values. The combination of mild hyperthermia and metabolic acidosis would be expected to result in more severe cell damage than hyperthermia alone, and it is probably this combination of insults to the cell that caused such high serum enzyme values in two of the runners studied by McKechnie et al. These were the two men with GOT and GPT values of over 100 units and LDH values of over 700 units. None of these runners apparently had any signs and symptoms of damage to vital organs but, in my view, it is merely a greater degree and extent of damage to vital organs that leads to the syndrome of nephropathy described by Dancaster *et al.* (1969) in two runners in a Comrades Marathon, an 80-km race between Durban and Pietermaritzburg in Natal, South Africa. Both of these cases had severe, transient renal damage and will be described in detail in the section on heat stroke.

The question may well be asked what criteria should be used to distinguish the case with hyperthermia and evidence of cell damage, as shown by elevated serum enzymes and/or deranged function of a vital organ, from a case of genuine heat stroke. Two criteria are useful in this regard. One is that there should be definite evidence of cerebral involvement for the diagnosis of heat stroke to be made. This may, on the one hand, be cerebral depression with collapse into unconsciousness with stupor or coma or cerebral stimulation with great irritability, attacks on helpers, and, finally, convulsions or fits. The other criterion is that the serum enzyme levels should be markedly elevated above normal and should continue to rise for the first 48 hours after the collapse. Difficulties arise when the collapse into unconsciousness is of short duration or the evidence of cerebral stimulation is relatively mild, such as mere irritability of the subject. It is in these cases that serial measurements of serum enzymes are of great help in arriving at a correct diagnosis.

Heat Stroke

A number of heat stroke cases have been reported as a result of prolonged, intense physical exercise in warm and hot humid weather. There was the case of the British marathon runner at the Empire Games in Canada in 1955. A fatal case of heat stroke occurred during the Tour de France in 1959[12] in a cyclist who had drugged himself with amphetamines. There were three nonfatal cases in the Danish cyclists in the hot humid weather during the Olympic Games in Rome in 1960.[13]

Heat stroke should be suspected if a marathon is run on a warm day and a runner develops some of the following premonitory symptoms and signs. He may become irritable and aggressive and may even assault anyone who tries to remonstrate with him or help him; or he may display emotional instability with hysterical weeping; or he may be apathetic and fail to respond to questioning. In this phase the subject may be disorientated in time and space. He may run the wrong way around the track and be unaware of the time of the day. He may develop an unsteady gait and a glassy stare. Finally he may collapse and become unconscious or he may have a convulsive seizure. His skin may be hot and dry or he may sweat profusely. His pulse may be rapid and feeble or it may be full and bounding.

If a marathon runner has any of these premonitory symptoms and signs and collapses, heat stroke should be suspected and an immediate rectal temperature measurement should be made. If the temperature is over 41° C, and especially if above 45° C, heat stroke should be diagnosed and emergency treatment started. The first priority is to cool the man until the rectal temperature falls to 38° C. If there is a delay in the diagnosis and the man arrives in hospital after 2 or more hours without being cooled with a rectal temperature of, say, 45° C the chances of a fatal outcome are about 7:10.[14] The best way of cooling the man is to spray water over his body and blow air over it with a strong fan.[15] Generally these resources are not available and in that case water should be thrown over the man's body and the body kept wet. Spectators should be asked to fan the man with a large piece of cardboard. The man should not be placed in a bath of ice-water as advocated by some heat physiologists. This method of treating heat stroke is dangerous because it is very difficult to control the extent of fall in rectal temperature and circulatory shock may occur, with fatal results, during the rewarming phase.

Prompt cooling of suspected heat stroke cases is the most effective way of preventing damage to vital organs. It is important to take a sample of blood from such cases as soon as possible and again at 48 and 96 hours after the collapse for the measurement of certain serum enzymes such as GOT, GPT, LDH, and CPK. TABLE 3 contains levels of these serum enzymes in samples of men at rest, after marathon running, and with heat stroke. The heat stroke values are at the time of admission to hospital and at 48 and 96 hours after admission. In definite cases of heat stroke all of these serum enzymes are markedly elevated on admission to hospital, continue to rise for the first 48 hours, and then fall but still remain above normal limits after 96 hours according to Kew et al.[11] The extent of elevation of serum enzyme levels and the length of time they are elevated are useful indicators of the amount of damage to vital organs, such as the kidney, and also are an aid to prognosis.[11]

The first priority in the treatment of a suspected case of heat stroke is cooling the patient until the rectal temperature reaches 38° C. However, this may take an hour or more and during this period it is important to take steps to prevent damage to vital organs by two of the common complications of heat stroke: These are circulatory collapse and metabolic acidosis. When these complications occur the cell is subject to three simultaneous insults. They are cell anoxia due to poor local circulation, a low pH, and hyperthermia, which increases cell metabolism. Circulatory shock is best treated by intravenous fluids, which must be given sufficiently rapidly to restore the blood pressure as soon as possibly to avoid the renal vascular shut-down that accompanies circulatory shock. Severe metabolic acidosis occurs in some cases of heat stroke. Wyndham et al.[14] reported a case with a pH of 7.280, a p_{CO_2} of 18 mmHg, a base excess of -14.5 mEq/l and standard bicarbonate of 14.4 mEq/l. Cases with severe metabolic acidosis improve dramatically when treated with intravenous bicarbonate solutions. Up to 30 g of bicarbonate is sometimes required to restore acid/base balance.

Where prompt cooling of a suspected case of heat stroke is not carried out damage may occur to certain target organs. These are the kidney,[16] the heart,[17] the liver,[18] and the brain.[14] Kidney damage with acute renal failure is a common complication of heat stroke in circumstances where men exercise vigorously in warm or hot conditions such as army recruits undergoing hard physical exercise in warm weather or miners working physically in hot and humid mines.[16, 19, 20] Scheir et al.[21] coined the apt phrase of "nephropathy associated with heat stress and exercise" for this syndrome. Most of the patients with this condition who survive the acute stage make a complete recovery, but Kew et al.[22] found that four of their forty cases of heat stroke developed chronic interstitial nephritis.

Relatively few cases of this syndrome have been reported in marathon runners. A notable exception is the occurrence of two cases during a Comrades Marathon (80 km) reported by Dancaster et al.[23] One case was a runner of

38 years of age who suffered a severe collapse during the race. He was in a stupor for some while after the collapse and passed loose stools and vomited during this phase. He passed no urine for *48 hours* after the collapse and he had a blood pressure of 200/130 and a BUN of 186 mg/100 ml. He gradually improved on intravenous therapy and conservative treatment over the next 2 weeks, and his blood pressure, BUN, and renal function returned to normal. The other case felt very ill and was dizzy after the race. He also had an episode of diarrhea. He passed only 400 ml of urine in the next four days and during this period his blood pressure rose to 160/90 and his BUN to 176 mg/100 ml. His serum GOT was 135 units; GPT, 180 units; and LDH, 1,500 units. On intravenous therapy he developed a massive diuresis of 4,000 ml on the fifth day and went on to recover completely.

It is comforting to know that if heat stroke is suspected, if the diagnosis is made sufficiently early, and if proper treatment is instituted (particularly immediate body cooling), then the chances of a fatal outcome are very low. The key issue is that the sports medical officer and track officials should be on the lookout for the occurrence of heat stroke if a marathon is run on a warm and humid day. The sports medical officer should be armed with a rectal thermometer and should not hesitate to make a rectal temperature measurement if a runner behaves abnormally and particularly if he collapses.

Recommendations [24]

(1) Running and cycling marathons should not be run in warm and humid weather. If the climatic condition over the period in which the race would be run exceeds 25° C wet bulb — globe temperature in the week prior to the race the runners are at risk from heat stroke and officials should be warned to look out for abnormal behavior on the part of the runners. If wet bulb — globe temperature exceeds 28° C the race should be called off.

(2) Adequate amounts of water should be available at least at 20-minute intervals and competitors should be warned of the dangers of dehydration and be encouraged to drink at least a cupful of water (300 ml) at these intervals.

(3) In the event of a runner behaving abnormally and collapsing, a rectal temperature measurement should be made, and if it is above 41° C, the runner should be treated for heat stroke. He should be cooled immediately, and if there are clinical signs and symptoms of stock and/or metabolic acidosis, appropriate treatment should be started during the period of cooling.

(4) A sample of blood should be taken as soon as possible and sent to a clinical pathology laboratory for estimation of the serum enzymes GOT, GPT, LDH, and CPK.

(5) If the diagnosis of heat stroke is confirmed by the serum enzyme measurements, then the runner should be admitted to hospital and a careful watch kept on renal function.

References

1. WYNDHAM, C. H. & A. J. A. HEYNS. 1969. Determinants of oxygen consumption and maximum oxygen intake of Bantu and Causasian males. Intern Z. Angew Physiol. **27:** 51–75.

2. WYNDHAM, C. H., N. B. STRYDOM, C. H. VAN GRAAN, A. J. VAN RENSBURG, C. G. ROGERS, J. S. GRAYSON & W. H. VAN DER WALT. 1971. Walk or jog for health. 1. The energy costs of walking and running at different speeds. S. Afr. Med. J. 45: 50–53.

3. WYNDHAM, C. H., W. H. VAN DER WALT, A. J. VAN RENSBURG & C. G. ROGERS. 1971. The influence of body weight on energy expenditure during walking on a road and a treadmill. Intern. Z. Angew Physiol. 29: 285–292.

4. VAN DER WALT, W. H. & C. H. WYNDHAM. 1973. An equation for the prediction of the energy expenditure of walking and running. J. Appl. Physiol. 34(3): 559–563.

5. WYNDHAM, C. H. & N. B. STRYDOM. 1969. The danger of an inadequate water intake during marathon running. S. Afr. Med. J. 43: 893–896.

6. COSTILL, D .L., W. F. KAMMER & A. FISHER. 1970. Fluid ingestion during distance running. Arch. Environ. Health 21: 520–525.

7. PUGH, L. G. C. E. 1967. Rectal temperatures, weight losses and sweat rates in marathon running. J. Appl. Physiol. 23(3): 347–352.

8. MCKECHNIE, J. K., W. P. LEARY, O. M. JOUBERT. 1967. Some electrocardiographic and biochemical changes in marathon runners. S. Afr. Med. J. 41: 722–725.

9. ROSE, L. I., J. E. BROUSSER & K. H. COOPER. 1970. Serum enzymes after marathon running. J. Appl. Physiol. 29(3): 355–357.

10. WYNDHAM, C. H., M. C. KEW, R. KOK, I. BERSOHN & N. B. STRYDOM. 1974. Serum enzyme changes in unacclimatised and acclimatised men under severe heat stress. J. Apl. Physiol. 37(5): 695–698.

11. KEW, M. C., I. BERSOHN & H. C. SEFTEL. 1971. The diagnostic and prognostic significance of serum enzyme changes in heat stroke. Trans. R. Soc. Trop. Med. Hyg. 65: 325–330.

12. BERNHEIM, I. T. & J. N. COX. 1960. Coup de chaleur et intoxication amphetamine chez un sportiff. Schweiz Med. Wochenscher. 90: 322–331.

13. SHIBOLET, S., M. C. LANCESTER & Y. DANOU. 1976. Heat stroke: A review. Aviat. Space Environ. Med. 47(3): 280–301.

14. WYNDHAM, C. H. 1966. A survey of research initiated by the Chamber of Mines into the clinical aspects of heat stroke. Proc. Mine Med. Officers Assoc. 46: 68–80.

15. WYNDHAM, C. H., N. B. STRYDOM, M. H. COOKE, J. F. MORRISON, J. S. MATITZ, P. W. FLEMING & J. S. WARD. 1959. Methods of cooling subjects with hyperpyrexia. J. Appl. Physiol. 14: 771–776.

16. KEW, M. C., C. ABRAHAMS & N. W. LEVIN. 1967. The effects of heat stroke on the function and structure of the kidney. Quart. J. Med. 36: 277–300.

17. KEW, M. C., R. B. K. TUCKER & I. BERSOHN. 1969. The heart in heat stroke. Amer. Heart J. 77: 324–335.

18. KEW, M. C., I. BERSOHN & H. C. SEFTEL. 1970. Liver damage in heat stroke. Amer. J. Med. 49: 192–202.

19. SHIBOLET, S., R. COLL & T. GILAT. 1967. Heat stroke: Its clinical picture and mechanisms in thirty-six cases. Quart. J. Med. 36: 524–548.

20. VERTEL, R. M. & T. P. KNOCHEL. 1967. Acute renal failure due to heat injury. Amer. J. Med. 43: 435–451.

21. SCHIER, R. W., J. HONO & H. I. KELLER. 1967. Nephropathy associated with heat stress and exercise. Ann. Intern. Med. 67: 350–376.

22. KEW, M. C., C. ABRAHAMS & H. C. SEFTEL. 1970. Chronic interstitial nephritis as a consequence of heat stroke. Quart. J. Med. 39: 189–199.

23. DANCASTER, C. P., W. C. DUCKWORTH & C. J. ROPER. 1969. Nepropathy in marathon runners. S. Afr. Med. J. 43: 758–760.

24. WYNDHAM, C. H. & N. B. STRYDOM. 1972. Physical exercise in high temperature. In Sportmedizen. W. Hollman, Ed. : 131–150. Springer-Verlag. Berlin.

WORK-HEAT TOLERANCE OF DISTANCE RUNNERS *

C. V. Gisolfi, N. C. Wilson, and B. Claxton

Stress Physiology Laboratory
University of Iowa
Iowa City, Iowa 52242

Introduction

The only serious threat to the physical well-being of a marathon runner is the possibility of his suffering a fatal thermal injury, namely, a heat stroke. This is such a serious problem that the American College of Sports Medicine has recently issued a position statement setting forth guidelines to be followed in conducting distance races in the heat.[1] Thus, it is appropriate for us to be concerned about the thermal tolerance of distance runners. This paper deals with three questions: How much heat tolerance does the distance runner derive from training in a cool environment? What is the thermal tolerance of marathoners for running at competitive speeds in the heat? By what practical means can the tolerance of these highly trained athletes be improved?

Heat Tolerance Derived from Training in a Cool Environment

Most environmental physiologists acknowledge the fact that physical training in a cool environment does improve the ability of a subject to sustain work in the heat.[2-13] The question is how much thermal tolerance can be derived from this physical training relative to that produced by heat acclimatization? This question remains unanswered because previous studies have (a) sometimes lacked adequate controls, (b) employed training programs varying markedly in duration and intensity, and (c) lacked an adequate standard work-heat stress to assess the improvement in thermal tolerance derived from training. Relative to the last point, acclimatization to hot dry conditions [50/27 C dry bulb/wet bulb (db/wb)] does not necessarily insure acclimatization to hot wet conditions (36/34 C db/wb).[14-18] Likewise, acclimatization to mild work (25% max $\dot{V}_{O_2}$) in the heat does not insure acclimatization to moderate (50% max $\dot{V}_{O_2}$) or severe (75% max $\dot{V}_{O_2}$) work in the heat. Thus, when we speak of the beneficial effects of training in a cool environment it is appropriate to ask, to what conditions is this trained individual more tolerant? If the standard heat stress is too severe, the beneficial effects of training could be easily obscured. If the stress is too mild, the full benefit will not be observed. The conditions to which the trained subject is more tolerant will vary with the duration and intensity of the training program.[2-13]

The controversy over the thermal benefits derived from training began in 1965 when Piwonka *et al.*[11] showed that, in winter, competitive distance runners

* This work was supported by Contract N00014–75–C–0597 from the Office of Naval Research.

performed as fully acclimatized men when subjected to moderate work ($\dot{V}_{O_2}$ 1.5 l/min) in dry heat (40/23.5 C db/wb). In 1966, Strydom et al.[19] using a mild ($\dot{V}_{O_2}$ 0.9 l/min) physical conditioning program for 12 days found no evidence of heat acclimatization in their subjects. The stress test employed in these experiments consisted of mild work in wet heat (36.1/33.9 C db/wb). Using moderate work ($\dot{V}_{O_2}$ 1.4 l/min) in dry heat (50/28 C db/wb) as their stress test, Shvartz et al.[12] also found no evidence of heat acclimatization after training. Their subjects performed hard work ($\dot{V}_{O_2}$ 1.9 l/min) during their daily training sessions, but for only 6 days. In a subsequent study by the South African group [13] using moderate work ($\dot{V}_{O_2}$ 1.5 l/min) as the conditioning stimulus and a less severe thermal stress to evaluate the effects of training (33.9/32.2 C db/wb), they found reductions in rectal temperature and heart rate for the first 2 hr of their standard 4-hr test, but thereafter rectal temperature and heart rate rose to preacclimatization levels; sweat rate did not change significantly. Gisolfi and Robinson [8] demonstrated that intense interval training 1 hr/day for 6 weeks was a more effective system of preparing men for work in the heat than prolonged mild exercise, however, their subjects were still not fully acclimatized for moderate work ($\dot{V}_{O_2}$ 1.5 l/min) in dry heat (50/27 C db/wb). In a more controlled study, using the ratio of terminal rectal temperature to performance time as an index of acclimatization, Gisolfi [7] showed that 8 weeks of interval training in a cool environment produced 50% of the total adjustment made by acclimatization to mild work ($\dot{V}_{O_2}$ 1.0 l/min) in dry heat (50/27 C db/wb).

FIGURE 1 is taken from the data of Piwonka et al.[11] showing the rectal temperature changes in highly trained distance runners and untrained subjects walking 5.6 km/hr up a 5.6% grade on the treadmill in the heat (40/23.5 C db/wb) and in a cool environment (20–25 C db). All subjects wore 8-oz khaki twill pants and shirt and army service shoes. Metabolic rate (MR) of the runners and untrained men were 240 and 261 kcal/m²·hr, respectively. Average rectal temperatures of the runners leveled off at 37.9 C in the cool room and 38.2 C in the heat, whereas those of the untrained men continued to rise throughout the walks reaching values of 38.3 C in the cool room and 39.5 C in the heat. Heart rate in the heat reached a steady state averaging 118 beats/min in the runners compared with an average of 173 beats/min at the end of work in the untrained men. Mean skin temperatures were approximately the same in both groups. Sweat rate was less in the runners than in the untrained men, but it was 2.4 times greater per degree rise of rectal temperature for the runners indicating the greater sensitivity of their sweating response to thermal stimuli. The superior tolerance of the runners was attributed to their lower heat production relative to surface area and to their more effective cardiovascular system resulting in higher tissue heat conductance. The improved cardiovascular stability and "preacclimatized state" of these men was a product of their daily training sessions, which produced marked elevations in central temperatures and stimulated the thermoregulatory responses of sweating and cutaneous blood flow.[20-22]

This study was criticized because the untrained men were working at higher metabolic rates and percentages of aerobic capacity and therefore would be expected to have higher core temperatures.[23-25] It was also criticized for the short (85 min) duration of exposure to the heat stress. Hausman et al.[26] and Wyndham et al.[27] have shown an inverse relationship between maximal oxygen uptake and the rise in body temperature under standard heat stress conditions; however, the improvement in thermal tolerance associated with heat acclimatization is not associated with an increase in max $\dot{V}_{O_2}$.[28]

FIGURE 2 shows the heart rates, rectal temperatures, and sweat rates of four distance runners and a group of six college students with the same max $\dot{V}_{O_2}$ during mild work in dry heat. The college students had completed 8 weeks of interval training. Both groups walked at 5.6 km/hr on a level treadmill (MR 160 kcal/m²·hr for both groups) and had similar mean body weight/

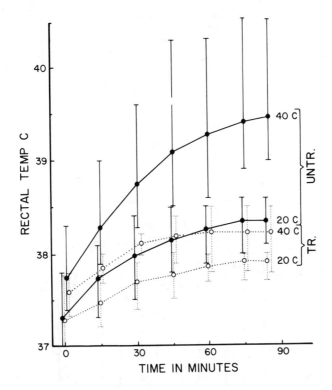

FIGURE 1. Average rectal temperatures of seven untrained men (solid lines, untr.) and five runners (dashed lines, tr.) during moderate work in the heat and in a cool environment. Vertical lines represent the range in each group. (After Piwonka *et al.*[11])

surface area ratios (38.3 and 38.5 kg/m² for the runners and trained students, respectively). The runners maintained significantly lower heart rates throughout the exposure and completed the walk with a significantly lower rectal temperature than the trained students. This difference in thermal tolerance can not be attributed to differences in sweat rate, although the runners may have had a quicker onset of sweating and/or a more efficient distribution of sweat over the body surface.[29, 30] The lower heart rates of the runners compared with the students indicates a more stable cardiovascular system suggesting a more ade-

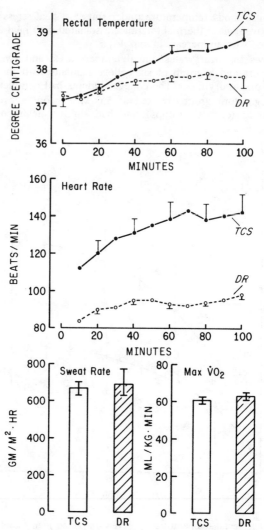

FIGURE 2. Rectal temperatures, heart rates, sweat rates, and max $\dot{V}_{O_2}$ values of six trained college students (TCS) and four distance runners (DR) during treadmill exercise in dry heat [50/27 C db/wb (dry bulb/wet bulb), wind velocity 36 m/min]. Values are means ± standard error (SE).

quate flow of blood through visceral organs [31] and a more efficient flow of heat from the core to the skin. The reason for the more stable cardiovascular condition of the runners is once again attributed to the training program of these athletes. Maximal oxygen uptake is achieved relatively quickly with intense training and would account for the similar aerobic capacities of these two groups; however, the intensive training of the runners at high energy expenditures (70%–80% max $\dot{V}_{O_2}$) for 1 to 2 hr a day for several years no doubt has produced in these men a more efficient cardiovascular system than the 8 weeks of interval training produced in the previously untrained college students. It is important to note in this regard that Lind and Bass [32] showed that the optimal exposure time for heat acclimatization was 100 min of continuous work (MR 160 kcal/m²·hr) in the heat (49/26·C db/wb). Whereas the runners often train this long at high metabolic rates and sustain high elevations in core temperatures, the students could not maintain high central temperatures for similar periods of time. The differences between these two groups would probably have been even greater had the exposure been continued for several hours.

FIGURE 3 shows the mean rectal temperatures, heart rates, metabolic rates,

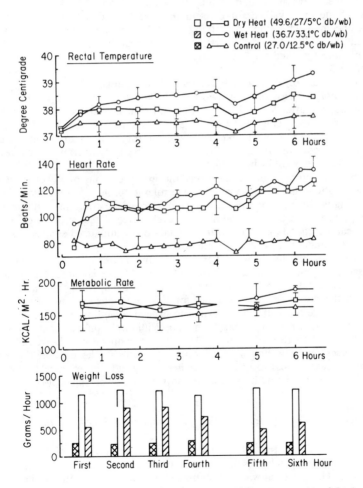

FIGURE 3. Rectal temperatures, heart rates, metabolic rates, and weight losses of four distance runners during mild treadmill exercise in dry heat, wet heat, and in a cool environment. Wind velocity was constant at 36 m/min. Mean max $\dot{V}_{O_2}$ of these men was 62.1 ml/kg·min. Values are means ± SE.

and weight losses of four distance runners walking 5.6 km/hr on a level tread-mill in dry heat, wet heat, and in a cool environment. The experiments were performed 4 to 5 weeks apart and consisted of 4 hr of continuous walking, 30 minutes for lunch in the test environment, and then 2 to 3 hr more of walking. The men drank water ad libitum, but were constantly informed of their weight loss from hour to hour and thus were successful in maintaining fluid balance. Each man in this study was running 40 to 50 miles/week through-out the experimental period and had not been exposed to heat since the preced-ing summer. A typical workout will illustrate their training regime. During the month of February with an average ambient temperature of 40 F, two of these men ran approximately 7 miles over roads and parks in 40 min. Their rectal temperatures at the end of this run were 39.8 and 39.4 C.

All of the men walked for 6 hr in the neutral and hot dry environments except one man who stopped walking after 5.5 hr in dry heat with a rectal temperature of 39.0 C and a heart rate of 136 beats/min. On the other hand, another subject walked for 7 hr in dry heat and finished with a rectal tempera-ture of 38.3 C and a heart rate of 132 beats/min. The latter subject stopped primarily because of soreness in his ankle and knee joints.

In the hot wet environment, two men walked for 6 hr while the other two subjects stopped after 5 hr. Three of the men stopped with rectal temperatures and heart rates averaging 39.3 C and 132 beats/min, respectively. The fourth subject, who was the same man who walked for 7 hr in dry heat, stopped because of discomfort from hemorrhoids. His rectal temperature was 38.2 C and his heart rate was 124 beats/min.

These data support the observations and interpretations of Piwonka et al.[11] and clearly show that distance runners can tolerate prolonged mild work in dry heat during winter months without severe physiological strain and without prior heat exposure. The average equilibrium level of rectal temperature of 38.0 C in dry heat is in good agreement with the data on acclimatized subjects of other investigators under similar climatic conditions.[33]

In wet heat, the men had higher rectal temperatures and heart rates. This increased stress is associated in part with a slight but significant increase in metabolic rate and, more importantly, to fatigue of the sweating mechanism.[34-38] Although the mechanisms responsible for this latter phenomenon are unclear, there is evidence suggesting it is related to excessive wetting of the skin.[37, 39, 40] Compared with the data of Strydom and Williams[13] on acclimatized Bantu laborers, two of these runners had similar rectal temperatures, heart rates, and weight losses over the first 4 hr of work. In general, the men in this study showed increased stress to work in wet heat; they did, however, walk continu-ously for at least 4 hr with minimal or no signs of severe physiological strain.

Thermal Tolerance for Running at Competitive Speeds in the Heat

Are these highly trained distance runners also tolerant of work in the heat at energy expenditures characteristic of endurance competition (75% max $\dot{V}_{O_2}$)? This question was first addressed by Adams et al.[2] in a rather heroic series of experiments on himself. He performed treadmill exercise at 15.3 km/hr in 10, 22, and 35 C (dry bulb) environments before and after heat acclimatization. Before acclimatization he attempted a maximal duration run in the heat and was forced to stop after 102 minutes with a rectal temperature of 40.2 C. After acclimatization, he was able to run for 135.3 minutes in this environment and stopped with a rectal temperature of 40.7 C. These elevations in core temperature were associated with reductions in both evaporative cooling and heat conductance. Although he demonstrated considerable work-heat tolerance from his training in a temperate climate, after heat acclimatization he maintained lower rectal and mean skin temperatures during his runs in the 22 and 35.4 C environments. This improvement was associated with an increase in sweat rate and an expanded blood volume (suggested by decreased hematocrit and plasma protein concentration). These data support those of Piwonka and Robinson,[41] which showed that highly trained distance runners can be further acclimatized when exposed to more stressful work-heat conditions. The data also indicated that the subject was running with a lower "set point" after the first 40–50 minutes in both the 22 and 35.4 C environments after acclimatization. Baum *et al.*[42] have also provided evidence for a lower set point in distance runners compared with control subjects based on a lower sweating threshold at rest.

Training in Sweat Clothing

Since marathon runners are not fully acclimatized for running at competitive speeds in the heat as a result of their training in a temperate environment, then how might they achieve a greater heat tolerance without the aid of climatic chambers, which are usually available only to researchers? Many distance runners train in sweat suits during early Spring to acclimatize for competition in warmer weather, however, the thermal benefits derived from training in extra clothing are controversial.[10, 43, 44] What are the benefits of distance training in sweat clothing in a cool environment?

FIGURE 4 shows the thermoregulatory responses of a marathoner who attempted to run 16 km/hr (70% max $\dot{V}_{O_2}$) for 2 hr on a level treadmill in dry heat (35/21 C db/wb, wind velocity 213 m/min) before and after 8 consecutive days of training in a cool room (23/16 C db/wb) dressed in a warm-up suit and after 6 days of running in the heat. This subject was a seasoned distance runner preparing for the Drake Marathon (which he completed in 2:32:53) at the time he participated in these experiments. For the 3-week period prior to the experimental period he was running approximately 50 miles/week, 20% of which was run on the treadmill. Training in sweat clothing consisted of running on the treadmill at speeds of 12.8 to 16 km/hr for 80 to 120 minutes in a cool temperature-controlled environment. The sweat suit was constructed of 100% stretch nylon and the jacket was zippered to the neck during experiments. Skin (chest, forearm, lateral calf) and rectal temperatures were recorded continuously during the training sessions (FIGURE 5) and during the runs in the heat (FIGURE 6). Water was consumed ad libitum during all runs. The experiments in the heat consisted of running 12.8 to 16 km/hr for 30 to 120 minutes at dry bulb temperatures ranging from 38 to 43 C. Prior to the runs in the test environment (35/21 C db/wb), the subject consumed one liter of water 1.5 hours before exercise to offset the effects of voluntary dehydration. Also shown in FIGURE 6 is a control experiment in a cool (22/15 C db/wb) environment. The max $\dot{V}_{O_2}$ of this subject before and after running in sweats and after running in the heat were 4.66, 4.57, and 4.61 l/min, respectively.

During his initial exposure to the test environment, the subject was forced to stop exercise after 60 minutes with a rectal temperature of 40.6 C and a heart rate of 174 beats/min. After training in sweat clothing for 8 days, he ran for 90 minutes and stopped with a rectal temperature of 39.5 C and a heart rate of 176 beats/min. Sweat rate increased 13.6% in g/m²·hr and 63.6% when expressed in g/m²·hr per degree C rise in rectal temperature

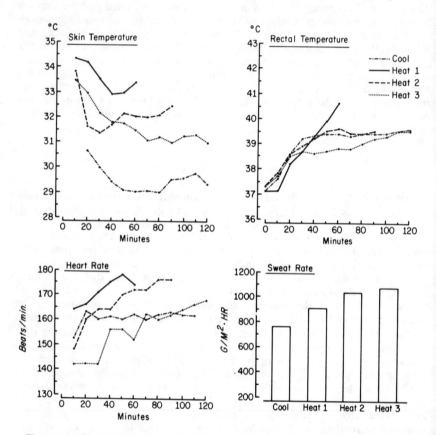

FIGURE 4. Rectal and mean skin temperatures, heart rates, and sweat rates of a marathoner during treadmill exercise in the heat (35/21 C db/wb, wind velocity 213 m/min). Runs were performed in a cool environment, before (Heat 1) and after (Heat 2) training in sweat clothing, and after training in the heat (Heat 3).

above 37 C. Mean skin and terminal rectal temperatures averaged over all running days were 33 and 39.5 C, respectively (FIGURE 5). Running without sweats in the cool room, he had a mean skin temperature averaging 29.7 C. The subject stopped running because of gastrointestinal distress, not from hyperpyrexia. Following the runs in the heat, he completed the 2-hr run with a final rectal temperature of 39.5 C and a heart rate of 168 beats/min. There was little further increase in sweat rate compared with the previous exposure,

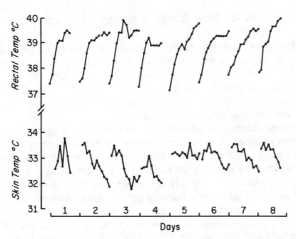

FIGURE 5. Rectal and mean skin temperatures of the marathoner in FIGURE 4 during his 8 days of training in sweat clothing. The ambient temperature was 23° C.

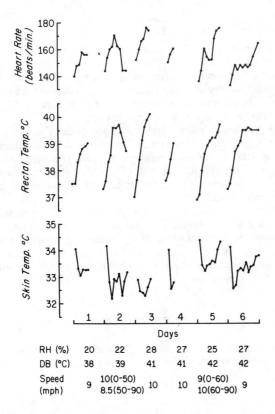

	Days					
	1	2	3	4	5	6
RH (%)	20	22	28	27	25	27
DB (°C)	38	39	41	41	42	42
Speed (mph)	9	10(0-50) 8.5(50-90)	10	10	9(0-60) 10(60-90)	9

FIGURE 6. Rectal and mean skin temperatures and heart rates of the marathoner in FIGURE 4 during his 6 days of training in the heat. Ambient temperature was gradually increased. Running speed was reduced as necessary to keep the subject exercising as long as possible in a given environment.

147

but mean skin temperatures and heart rates were lower suggesting improved evaporative cooling and a more stable cardiovascular system. Rectal temperature between 40 and 70 minutes of running were substantially lower after the runs in the heat compared with the previous exposure as well as the run in the cool room. This supports the observation of Adams et al.[2] and likewise suggests a lower set point after acclimatization.

The improved thermal tolerance after training in sweat clothing is attributed to the elevation in mean skin temperature during the training sessions. This was concluded because terminal rectal temperature during these sessions did not exceed values observed in this man running at the same speed and for the same duration without sweat clothing. Had this subject been allowed to train more than 8 days and at higher metabolic rates in sweat clothing, perhaps even a more marked improvement in thermal tolerance would have been observed. Likewise, the improvement we have observed in this man after 6 days of running at variable speeds and durations in the heat should not be considered the maximal thermal tolerance attainable by him.

Summary

Physical training in a cool environment by subjects not previously trained improves their work-heat tolerance, but can not replace heat acclimatization to the standard heat stress conditions employed by a variety of investigators. This is attributed to the inability of these subjects to sustain prolonged work at high metabolic rates. Thus, they are not maintaining high core body temperatures long enough to bring about an adaptive change to heat.

On the other hand, the intense and prolonged (years) training of long distance runners in a temperate environment at high metabolic rates has acclimatized them for at least 4 hours of mild work (MR 160 kcal/$m^2 \cdot$hr) in both hot dry (50/27 C db/wb) and hot wet (36.7/33.1 C db/wb) environments, but not for work at high energy expenditures (MR 540 kcal/$m^2 \cdot$hr) in a less severe thermal stress (35/21 C db/wb).

These highly trained athletes can improve their work-heat tolerance at high metabolic rates in a warm climate by training at competitive speeds in a cool environment dressed in sweat clothing or by training at near competitive speeds in the heat. In either of these situations the athlete is cautioned to consume water at frequent intervals to offset the dehydration associated with excessive sweating under these conditions.

Acknowledgment

The authors wish to thank Dr. Sid Robinson for his critical comments on the manuscript and the subjects who participated in these most difficult experiments.

References

1. AMERICAN COLLEGE OF SPORTS MEDICINE. Position statement. 1975. Prevention of heat injuries during distance running. Med. Sci. Sports 7(1): VII.

2. ADAMS, W. C., R. H. FOX, A. J. FRY & I. C. MACDONALD. 1975. Thermoregulation during marathon running in cool, moderate, and hot environments. J. Appl. Physiol. **38:** 1030–1037

3. ALLAN, J. R. 1965. The effects of physical training in a temperate and hot climate on the physiological responses to heat stress. Ergonomics **8:** 445–453.

4. BASS, D. E., C. R. KLEEMAN, M. QUINN, A. HENSCHEL & A. H. HEGNAUER. 1959. Mechanisms of acclimatization to heat in man. Medicine **34:** 323–380.

5. BEAN, W. B. & L. W. EICHNA. 1943. Performance in relation to environmental temperature: Reactions of normal young men to simulated desert environment. Fed. Proc. **22:** 144–158.

6. DUNCAN, S. K. O. 1964. The effects of an artificial acclimatization technique on performance in a hot climate. Ergonomics **7:** 365.

7. GISOLFI, C. V. 1973. Work-heat tolerance derived from interval training. J. Appl. Physiol. **35:** 349–354.

8. GISOLFI, C. V. & S. ROBINSON. 1969. Relation between physical training, acclimatization, and heat tolerance. J. Appl. Physiol. **26:** 530–534.

9. LOFSTEDT, B. 1966. Human Heat Tolerance. : 44. Berlingska Bocktrycheriet. Lund, Sweden.

10. MARCUS, P. 1972. Heat acclimatization by exercise-induced elevation of body temperature. J. Appl. Physiol. **33:** 283–288.

11. PIWONKA, R. W., S. ROBINSON, V. L. GAY & R. S. MANALIS. 1965. Preacclimatization of men to heat by training. J. Appl. Physiol. **20:** 379–384.

12. SHVARTZ, E., E. SAAR, N. MEYRSTEIN & B. BENOR. 1973. A comparison of three methods of acclimatization to dry heat. J. Appl. Physiol. **34:** 214–219.

13. STRYDOM, N. B. & C. G. WILLIAMS. 1969. Effects of physical conditioning on state of heat acclimatization of Bantu laborers. J. Appl. Physiol. **27:** 262–265.

14. EICHNA, L. W., W. B. BEANS, W. F. ASHE & N. NELSON. 1945. Performance in relation to environmental temperature: reactions of normal men to hot, humid (simulated jungle) environment. Johns Hopkins Hosp. Bull. **76:** 25.

15. FOX, R. H., R. GOLDSMITH, I. F. G. HAMPTON & T. J. HUNT. 1967. Heat acclimatization by controlled hyperthermia in hot-dry and hot-wet climates. J. Appl. Physiol. **22:** 39–46.

16. SHVARTZ, E. & D. BENOR. 1971. Heat acclimatization by the prevention of evaporative cooling. Aerospace Med. **42:** 879–882.

17. SHVARTZ, E., D. BENOR & E. SAAR. 1972. Acclimatization to severe dry heat by brief exposures to humid heat. Ergonomics. **15:** 563–572.

18. WYNDHAM, C. H., N. B. STRYDOM, A. MUNRO, R. K. MACPHRSON, B. METZ, G. SCAFF & J. SCHIEBER. 1964. Heat reactions of Caucasians in temperate, in hot, dry, and in hot, humid climates. J. Appl. Physiol. **19:** 607–612.

19. STRYDOM, N. B., C. H. WYNDHAM, C. G. WILLIAMS, F. F. MORRISON, G. A. C. BREDDELL, A. J. S. BENADE & M. VON RAHDEN. 1966. Acclimatization to humid heat and the role of physical conditioning. J. Appl. Physiol. **21:** 636–632.

20. GISOLFI, C. V. & S. ROBINSON. 1970. Central and peripheral stimuli regulating sweating during intermittent work in men. J. Appl. Physiol. **29:** 761–768.

21. ROBINSON, S., F. R. MEYER, J. L. NEWTON, C. H. TS'AO & L. O. HOLGERSEN. 1965. Relations between sweating, cutaneous blood flow, and body temperature in work. J. Appl. Physiol. **20:** 575–582.

22. SALTIN, B., A. P. GAGGE & J. A. J. STOLWIJK. 1970. Body temperatures and sweating during thermal transients caused by exercise. J. Appl. Physiol. **28:** 318–327.

23. ASTRAND, I. 1960. Aerobic work capacity in men and women with special reference to age. Acta Physiol. Scand. **49**(Suppl. 169): 67.

24. SALTIN, B. & L. HERMANSEN. 1965. Esophageal, rectal, and muscle temperature during exercise. J. Appl. Physiol. **21:** 1757–1762.

25. NIELSEN, M. 1938. Die Regulation der Korpertemperatur bei Muskelarbeit. Skandinav. Arch. Physiol. **79:** 193.

26. HAUSMAN, A., D. BELAWEY & J. PATIGNY. 1969. Selection criteria for rescue workers operating in hot atmospheres. Rev. Inst. Hyg. Mines **21:** 36–47.

27. WYNDHAM, C. H., N. B. STRYDOM, C. G. WILLIAMS & A. HEYNS. 1967. An examination of certain individual factors affecting the tolerance of mine workers. J. S. African Inst. Mining Met. **68:** 79–91.

28. WYNDHAM, C. H., N. B. STRYDOM, A. J. VON RENSBURG, A. J. S. BENADE & A. J. HEYNS. 1970. Relation between max V_{O_2} and body temperature in hot humid air conditions. J. Appl. Physiol. **29:** 45–60.

29. HOFLER, W. 1968. Changes in regional distribution of sweating during acclimatization to heat. J. Appl. Physiol. **25:** 503–506.

30. NADEL, E. R., K. B. PANDOLF, M. F. ROBERTS & J. A. J. STOLWIJK. 1974. Mechnisms of thermal acclimation to exercise and heat. J. Appl. Physiol. **37:** 515–520.

31. ROWELL, L. B. 1974. Human cardiovascular adjustments to exercise and thermal stress. Physiol. Rev. **54:** 75–159.

32. LIND, A. R. & D. E. BASS. 1963. Optimal exposure time for development of acclimatization to heat. Fed. Proc. **22:** 704–708.

33. ROBINSON, S., E. S. TURRELL & S. D. GERKING. 1945. Physiologically equivalent conditions of air temperature and humidity. Amer. J. Physiol. **143:** 21–32.

34. ROBINSON, S. & S. D. GERKING. 1947. Thermal balance of men working in severe heat. Amer. J. Physiol. **149:** 476–488.

35. BROWN, W. K. & F. SARGENT. 1965. Hidromeiosis. Arch. Environ. Health. **11:** 442–453.

36. HERTIG, B. A., M. L. RIEDESEL & H. S. BELDING. 1961. Sweating in hot baths. J. Appl. Physiol. **16:** 647–651.

37. NADEL, E. R. & J. A. J. STOLWIJK. 1973. Effects of skin wettedness on sweat gland response. J. Appl. Physiol. **35:** 689–694.

38. KERSLAKE, D. McK. 1972. The Stress of Hot Environments. Cambridge University Press. Cambridge, England.

39. BREBNER, D. F. & D. McK. KERSLAKE. 1964. The time course of the decline in sweating produced by wetting the skin. J. Physiol. (Lond.) **175:** 295–302.

40. COLLINS, K. J. & J. S. WEINER. 1962. Observations on arm-bag suppression of sweating and its relationship to thermal sweat-gland fatigue. J. Physiol. (Lond.) **161:** 538–556.

41. PIWONKA, R. W. & S. ROBINSON. 1967. Acclimatization of highly trained men to work in severe heat. J. Appl. Physiol. **22:** 9–12.

42. BAUM, E., K. BRUCK & H. P. SCHWENNICKE. 1976. Adaptive modifications in the thermoregulatory system of long-distance runners. J. Appl. Physiol. **40:** 404–410.

43. ALLAN, J. R., J. P. CROWDY & M. F. HAISMAN. 1965. The use of a vapour barrier suit for the practical induction of artificial acclimatization to heat. I. Winter experiment. Army Personnel Res. Estab. Rep. **4:** 65.

44. ALLAN, J. R. & M. F. HAISMAN. 1966. Modification of the physiological responses to heat stress by physical training with and without extra clothing. Army Operational Res. Estab. Rep. **11:** 64.

RENAL FUNCTION DURING PROLONGED EXERCISE

Jan Castenfors

Karolinska Institutet
Stockholm, Sweden

Introduction

For a long time it has been known that intensive exercise influences renal function. In 1878 Leube [1] reported proteinuria following strenous exercise among soldiers whose early morning urine was free of protein. In 1910 Barach [2] studied the urine of marathon runners and found protein, hyaline and granular casts, and also red blood cells. Over the past few years the mechanism and significance of the renal involvement during exercise has been extensively studied. [3-6]

The purpose of the present report is to give a comprehensive survey of renal function during exercise with emphasis on prolonged heavy exercise. In order to elucidate the effect of such exercise on renal function, this work has been subdivided into renal hemodynamics, concentration mechanisms, electrolyte excretion, and proteinuria. For data we used our results from an investigation of renal function in normal subjects during an 85-km ski race. [7, 8] Renal hemo-dynamic changes, however, could be studied only during short periods of heavy exercise under laboratory conditions, and therefore in this case data from our results in healthy volunteers are also presented. [9, 10]

Renal Hemodynamics

During rest in the supine position, renal blood flow is about 1.2 l/min or 20% of the cardiac output. Renal plasma flow (RPF) is 700 ml/min, about 15% of which is filtered through the glomeruli—the glomerular filtration rate (GFR). During exercise, the need for increased blood flow through the exercising muscles necessitates a decrease in blood flow in the splanchnic and renal circulations. This decrease in RPF and renal blood flow (RBF) is proportional to the severity of exercise (FIGURE 1). Nevertheless, renal autoregulation tries to preserve GFR, which is less markedly decreased. Thus, with increasing renal vasoconstriction, a greater part of the diminishing RPF is filtered. This relative increase in filtration is usually expressed as an increased filtration fraction (FF), which is increased from 15% to about 25% during short heavy exercise under laboratory conditions (FIGURE 2).

During prolonged heavy exercise it has been impossible to study RBF in man, and only semiquantitative evaluations of GFR (by endogenous creatinine clearance) are available. During an 85-km ski race [7] there was a mean decrease in creatinine clearance of about 30% (FIGURE 3), which agrees with other reports on prolonged exercise. [6] Urine flow also showed a decrease of about 30%, and there was a significant correlation between the decrease in urine flow and the creatinine clearance, suggesting that the decrease in urine flow was mainly due to a decrease in GFR. Even during short heavy exercise, inulin

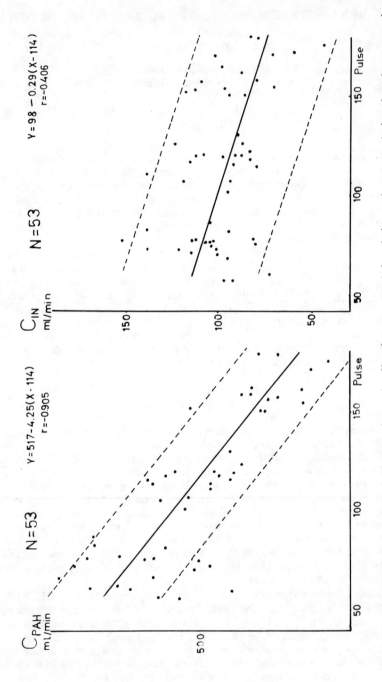

FIGURE 1. Renal plasma flow (C_{PAH}) and the glomerular filtration rate (C_{IN}) in relation to heart rate during short heavy exercise in the supine position. (After Castenfors.[3])

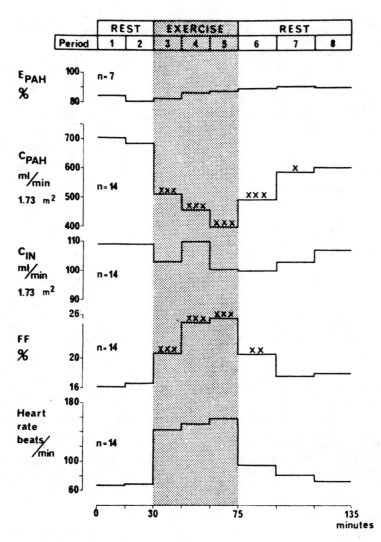

FIGURE 2. Effect of supine exercise in normal subjects on renal hemodynamics. Mean values of PAH extraction (E_{PAH}), C_{PAH}, C, FF, and heart rate are shown. x denotes a statistically significant difference compared with period 2. (From Castenfors.[10] By permission of *Acta Physiologica Scandinavica*.)

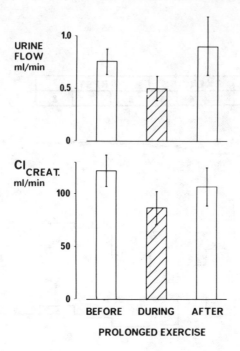

FIGURE 3. Urine flow and the glomerular filtration rate. Effect of prolonged heavy exercise on urine flow and endogenous creatinine clearance. Mean values ± standard deviations (SD). (After Castenfors *et al.*[7])

clearance (which is a more reliable measure of GFR than creatinine clearance) was not decreased more than about 30%.[3] If it is assumed that the FF was 25%, then there was approximately a 50% decrease of RPF and RBF during the ski race.

Urinary Water Excretion

Water excretion in the urine is mainly regulated by antidiuretic hormone (ADH), which is influenced by osmoreceptors in the brain and also by a volume-sensitive mechanism. During exercise, both an increase in osmolarity and a decrease in plasma volume are stimuli for the release of ADH. During short heavy exercise in well-hydrated subjects [10] with an "unphysiologically" high urine flow (10–20 ml/min), a decrease in free water clearance (C_{H_2O}) has been demonstrated, suggesting an ADH effect. The decrease in urine flow was mainly related to the decrease in C_{H_2O}.

During prolonged heavy exercise, however, with a more physiological urine flow rate (less than 1 ml/min), no significant changes in C_{H_2O} or urine/plasma creatinine ratio were found (FIGURE 4).[7] The latter is a sensitive indicator of water conservation during low urine flow rates. In some studies, a decline in urinary concentrating ability during heavy exercise has been reported.[5, 6, 11] This paradoxical absence of water retention in spite of a probable increased ADH release is difficult to explain. It may be related to a relatively smaller amount of free water available in relation to the changes in osmolar clearance during severe exercise.

Urinary Electrolyte Excretion

Physical exercise induces a significant decrease in the urinary excretion of several electrolytes, especially sodium, whereas potassium excretion increases.[3, 6]

A decrease in urinary sodium excretion during heavy exercise of short duration occurs within 15 min.[10] This is mainly related to an increase in tubular reabsorption, as the tubular rejection fraction is significantly decreased. In this situation the rather slowly acting aldosterone mechanism cannot be responsible for the sodium retention, which probably is related to poorly understood renal hemodynamic mechanisms. During prolonged heavy exercise (the ski race), there was a similar decrease in the tubular rejection fraction (FIGURE 5). This increased tubular reabsorption of sodium is, however, probably due in part to an increased aldosterone secretion, as an increased plasma renin activity was demonstrated at the end of exercise.[8] During a ski race of similar duration, an increase in both plasma renin activity and plasma aldosterone concentration has been shown.[12] The increased potassium excretion may be partly due to increased aldosterone secretion, but is probably in addition influenced by other factors such as H^+ excretion and hematuria.

Exercise Proteinuria

Proteinuria is almost invariably found during heavy and prolonged exercise. There is also an increased incidence of granular and hyaline casts and also blood cells in the urine after heavy exercise, and the name "athletic pseudonephritis" has been proposed for this phenomenon.[13]

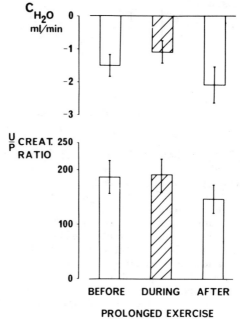

FIGURE 4. Urinary water excretion. Effect of prolonged exercise on free water clearance (C_{H_2O}) and urine/plasma creatinine ratio (U/P creat.). Mean values $\pm$ SD are given. (After Castenfors et al.[7])

In contact sports such as boxing or football, renal trauma has been suggested as a cause for these urinary findings. Regardless of the type of sport activity (contact or noncontact) similar findings in the urine have been reported.[14] Football players demonstrate the highest incidence of hematuria, which may indeed be related to renal trauma. Long distance runners, on the other hand, show the highest incidence of protein in the urine, suggesting that the proteinuria is related to other renal mechanisms.

The cause of the increased urinary protein excretion is not definitely known; it may be due to increased glomerular permeability, decreased tubular reabsorption, or a combination of both mechanisms. During prolonged heavy exercise (the ski race) there was a statistically significant increase in total protein and albumin excretion (FIGURE 6). In most subjects electrophoresis showed a predominance of albumin, and this was confirmed with a gel filtration technique.

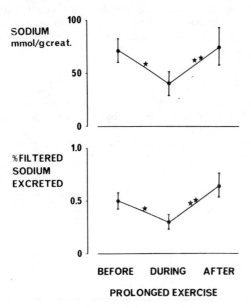

FIGURE 5. Urinary sodium excretion. Effect of prolonged heavy exercise on urinary sodium excretion and the tubular rejection fraction. Mean values ± SD are given. Stars denote statistically significant differences between the periods. (After Castenfors et al.[7])

The excretion of the low-molecular-weight protein ribonuclease was not changed during exercise. This protein can be expected to be relatively easily filtered by glomeruli and therefore more dependent on tubular reabsorption for its conservation. This suggests that tubular factors are of minor importance as a cause of exercise proteinuria.

Albumin has a molecular weight of 69,000, which is just above the "limiting pore radius" of the glomerular membrane.[15] An increased glomerular permeability would therefore favor the predominant increase of albumin, which is usually demonstrated in urine during exercise.

Several factors probably contribute to the increased glomerular permeability. Increased body temperature during exercise may be a factor, as fever produces albuminuria.[16] Another probably important factor is the renal vasoconstriction during exercise, which is characterized by an increased filtration fraction. This

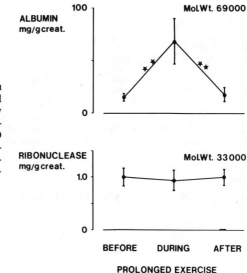

FIGURE 6. Urinary excretion of proteins. Effect of prolonged heavy exercise on the urinary excretion of albumin and ribonuclease. Mean values ± SD are given. Stars denote statistically significant differences between the periods. (After Castenfors et al.[7])

suggests a relatively more marked constriction of the efferent glomerular arterioli, resulting in an increased filtration pressure and stasis in the glomerular capillaries (FIGURE 7). This favors an increased filtration of protein through the glomerular membrane, to some extent possibly as a result of a stretch pore phenomenon. This phenomenon may also explain the increased incidence of hyaline casts and erythocytes in the urine. The urinary protein excretion is probably proportional to the severity of exercise in the individual subject, but

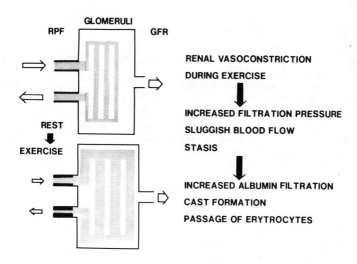

FIGURE 7. Effect of exercise on the glomerular circulation—Hypothetical scheme.

in a group of normal subjects the most important factors determining the amount of protein excreted are probably minor biological differences (genetic or acquired) in the "limiting pore radius" of the glomerular membrane.[7] Indeed, exercise has been used to demonstrate minor subclinical changes in glomerular permability in diabetic patients.[17]

Hemoglobinuria and Myoglobinuria

March hemoglobinuria and exercise myoglobinuria are rare,[18] and the pathogenesis of these conditions is not completely elucidated. March hemoglobinuria usually appears in the urine 1–3 hr after exercise performed in the upright position, and some results [19] indicate that running on a hard surface is of importance in producing this syndrome, suggesting that mechanical trauma to the erythrocyte as it passes through the foot may be a pathogenetic factor.

Exercise myoglobinuria, which appears in the urine 24–48 hr after exercise, has been attributed to a break down of muscle fibers from excessive exercise resulting in an increased myoglobin plasma concentration.[18] Myoglobin (MW 17,000) is relatively easily filtered by the glomeruli, and the increased excretion in the urine is not a sign of renal impairment.

Duration and Magnitude of the Renal Changes

After short heavy exercise, most renal parameters including proteinuria were normalized within 1 hr after the end of the exercise. After prolonged heavy exercise (the 85-km ski race) renal function parameters were normalized within about 10 hr. The small magnitude of exercise proteinuria is illustrated by the fact that in only 3 of the 15 subjects the proteinuria after prolonged severe exercise reached a level that could be detected by usual clinical tests (Albustix).

General Conclusions

During severe exercise, renal blood flow decreases to allow maximal redistribution of cardiac output to the exercising muscles. The glomerular filtration rate is relatively well maintained, resulting in an increased filtration fraction, an important mechanism in producing exercise proteinuria. Urinary water excretion is relatively little influenced during prolonged exercise. Urinary sodium excretion, however, decreases partly due to increased aldosterone secretion. The renal changes are of a transient nature and disappear rapidly after exercise. There is no indication of renal parenchymal damage during heavy prolonged exercise; almost all changes can be attributed to renal vasoconstriction during exercise.

References

1. LUEBE, W. 1878. Über auscheidung von eisweiss im harn des gesunden Menschen. Wirchows Arch. **72:** 145–157.
2. BARACH, J. H. 1910. Physiological and pathological effects of severe exercise

(the Marathon race) on the circulatory and renal system. Arch. Intern. Med. **5:** 382–405.

3. CASTENFORS, J. 1967. Renal function during exercise. With special reference to exercise proteinuria and the release of renin. Acta Physiol. Scand. **70** (Suppl. 293) : 1–44.

4. RAUCH, P. J. & I. D. WILSON. 1968. *In* Exercise Physiology. H. B. Falls, Ed. : 130–139. Academic Press. New York. N.Y.

5. KACHADORIAN, W. A. & R. E. JOHNSSON. 1970. Renal responses to various rates of exercise. J. Appl. Physiol. **28**(6): 748–752.

6. REFSUM, H. E. & S. B. STRÖMME. 1975. Relationship between urine flow, glomerular filtration and urine solute concentration during prolonged heavy exercise. Scand. J. Clin. Lab. Invest. **35:** 775–780.

7. CASTENFORS, J., F. MOSSFELDT & M. PISCATOR. 1967. Effect of prolonged heavy exercise on renal function and urinary protein excretion. Acta Physiol. Scand. **70:** 194–206.

8. BOZOVIC, L., J. CASTENFORS & M. PISCATOR. 1967. Effect of prolonged heavy exercise on urinary protein excretion and plasma renin activity. Acta Physiol. Scand. **70:** 143–146.

9. CASTENFORS, J. & M. PISCATOR. 1967. Renal hemodynamics, urine flow and urinary protein excretion during exercise in supine position at different loads. Acta Med. Scand. Suppl. **472:** 231–244.

10. CASTENFORS, J. 1967. Renal clearances and urinary sodium and potassium excretion during supine exercise in normal subjects. Acta Physiol. Scand. **70:** 207–214.

11. RAISZ, L. G., W. Y. W. AU & R. L. SCHEER. 1959. Studies of the renal concentration mechanism. III. Effect of heavy exercise. J. Clin. Invest. **39:** 8–13.

12. SUNDFJORD, J. A., S. B. STRÖMME & A. AAKVAAG. 1975. Plasma aldosteron (PA), plasma renin activity (PRA) and cortison (PF) during exercise. *In* Metabolic Adaptation to Prolonged Physical Exercise. E. H. Howald, J. R. Poortman & R. Birkhäuser, Eds. : 308–314. Verlag. Basel.

13. GARDNER, K. D. 1956. Athletic pseudonephritis—Alteration of urinary sediment by athletic competition. J. Amer. Med. Assoc. **161:** 1613–1617.

14. ALYEA, E. P., M. H. PARISH & N. C. DURHAM. 1958. Renal response to exercise —Urinary findings. J. Amer. Med. Assoc. **167:** 807–813.

15. ARTURSSON, G. & G. WALLENIUS. 1964. The clearance of dextran of different molecular sizes in normal humans. Scand. J. Clin. Lab. Invest. **1:** 81–86.

16. SCHULTZE, H. E. & J. F. HEREMANS. 1966. The urinary proteins. *In* Molecular Biology of Human Proteins : 670–731. Elsevier Publishing Co. New York, N.Y.

17. MOGENSEN, C. E. & E. VITTINGHUS. 1975. Urinary albumin excretion during exercise in juvenile diabetes. A provocation test for early abnormalities. Scand. J. Clin. Lab. Invest. **35:** 295–300.

18. STAHL, C. W. 1957. March hemoglobinuria. Report of five cases in students at Ohio State University. J. Amer. Med. Assoc. **164:** 1458–1460.

19. BUCKLE, R. M. 1965. Exertional (march) hemoglobinurea. Reduction of hemolytic episodes by use of Sorbo-Rubber insoles in shoes. Lancet **i:** 1136–1138.

SWEATING: ITS COMPOSITION AND EFFECTS ON BODY FLUIDS *

D. L. Costill

Human Performance Laboratory
Ball State University
Muncie, Indiana 47306

The marathoner's capacity to dissipate metabolically produced heat depends for the most part on his or her ability to form and vaporize sweat. The previous papers have effectively detailed the role of sweating in maintaining a thermal equilibrium during the runner's high rate of energy expenditure. As demonstrated in FIGURE 1, the magnitude of sweat production is proportional to the rate of energy expenditure (i.e., running speed).[1] It is apparent that during competition in a warm environment the marathoner may evoke sweat losses in excess of 6 liters (~2.8 liters/hr). Despite the runner's efforts to take fluids during the race, sweat loss may result in an 8% reduction in body weight and a 13%–14% loss of body water.

It is well established that a decrease in body weight of more than 2% by exercise-induced sweating places severe demands on both the cardiovascular and thermal regulatory systems.[2, 3] In light of the extreme levels of dehydration incurred during marathon competition, it is difficult to understand how these athletes are able to sustain such high rates of oxygen transport (>57 ml·kg⁻¹· min⁻¹) and heat transfer (0.24 kcal·m⁻²·min⁻¹) during the final stage of a race conducted under warm conditions.

In addition to the body water losses generated during marathon running, a myriad of nutrients are known to exist in sweat.[4] Although many investigators have examined the constituents in human sweat, little information is available to describe the mineral content of sweat during the prolonged severe stress of marathon running. The obvious questions therefore are, "what is the magnitude of the mineral losses in the marathoner's sweat?" and, "how do these losses affect body fluids and exercise performance?"

Thus, the intent of the following discussion will be to detail the composition of sweat and to describe the alterations in body fluid compartments during prolonged exercise. More specifically, attention will be given to the changes in water and electrolyte contents of muscles and plasma during exercise of long duration.

Sweat Composition

A variety of methods have been used to collect samples of sweat for chemical analyses, but most have limited sampling to a small area of the body. Recent studies by Vellar[4] have clearly shown that the isolation and trapping of sweat

---

* Portions of the research presented in this paper were supported by grants from the National Institutes of Health (AM 17083–02) and Ball State University Faculty Research Committee.

160

in either a capsule or plastic bag does not represent the composition of free flowing human sweat. A body washdown method, however, permits relative accuracy ($\pm1\%$) in determining the total ion losses in sweat during prolonged exercise and/or heat exposure.[4]

The ionic concentration of sweat may vary markedly between individuals and is strongly affected by the rate of sweating and the subject's state of heat acclimatization. In general, however, the Na^+, K^+, Cl^-, and Mg^{++} concentrations in sweat are similar to those listed in TABLE 1. When compared to electrolyte

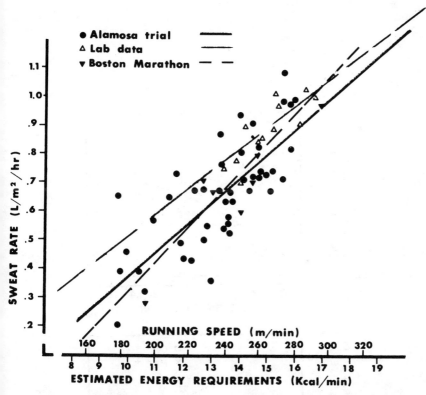

FIGURE 1. Relationship between running speed (energy expenditure) and sweating rate during treadmill (2 hrs) and marathon running.

concentrations in cellular and extracellular fluids, it is apparent that sweat is hypotonic and that the principal ions lost are those from the extracellular compartments, namely, Na^+ and Cl^-.

It should be noted, however, that the concentration of ions in sweat is influenced by a number of factors, such as sweat rate. As illustrated in FIGURES 2a and 2b, with an increasing sweating rate the concentration of Na^+ and Cl^- in sweat tends to increase, Ca^{++} concentration decreases, while K^+ and Mg^{++} concentrations remain unchanged. Thus, at the high rates of sweating reported

TABLE 1

ELECTROLYTE CONCENTRATIONS AND OSMOLALITY IN SWEAT, MUSCLE AND PLASMA

	Electrolytes (meq/liter)				Osmolarity (mOsmol/ liter)
	Na$^+$	Cl$^-$	K$^+$	Mg^{++}	
Sweat	40–60	30–50	4–5	1.5–5	80–185
Plasma	140	101	4	1.5	302
Muscle	9	6	162	31	302

* After Costill et al.[5]

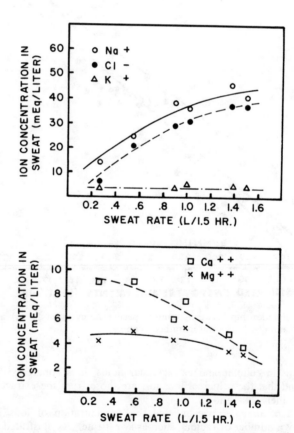

FIGURE 2. Relationship between sweat rate and the concentration of (top) Na$^+$, Cl$^-$, and K$^+$ and (bottom) Ca^{++} and Mg^{++}.

during marathon running, it is anticipated that sweat will contain relatively high levels of Na^+ and Cl^- but little K^+, Ca^{++}, and Mg^{++}.

During a recent investigation,[6] we observed that a 4.11-liter sweat loss (5.8% reduction in body weight) resulted in Na^+, K^+, Cl^-, and Mg^{++} losses of 155, 16, 137, and 13 meq, respectively. Based on estimates of the subject's body mineral contents, we have estimated that this sweat loss produced deficits in body Na^+ and Cl^- of roughly 5% to 7%. At the same time, total body K^+ and Mg^{++}, two ions principally confined to the intracellular space, decreased the estimated body content less than 1.2%. Urine electrolyte losses during these periods are usually small as a result of a diminished urine formation and increased renal Na^+ reabsorption.[7] Thus, it is apparent that during a marathon race the only ionic deficits of major concern are those of the extracellular compartments (i.e., Na^+ and Cl^-).

Water and Electrolytes in Body Fluids during Prolonged Exercise

In an effort to examine the changes in water and electrolyte contents of extracellular and intracellular compartments during and following large sweat losses, two methods have been used: First, distribution in muscle biopsy samples was determined by the chloride method previously described by Bergström.[8] The second method used to determine the changes in water and electrolytes from extracellular and intracellular spaces is based on calculations of the total loss of chloride in urine and sweat, and assumes proportionate losses of Cl^- from both the vascular and interstitial fluids.[6]

Traditionally, studies of the change in body water compartments during prolonged exercise have been limited to measurements of constituents in plasma. Attempts to measure the distribution of water and ions between intracellular and extracellular spaces during muscular activity have been invalidated by the movement of proteins and isotope markers (e.g., ^{125}I, ^{131}I-albumin, T-1824) between the various compartments.

Since the mid-1960s studies have been conducted using an isolated leg muscle preparation in the cat [9-11] and the muscle biopsy procedure [6, 8] in humans to determine the changes in water and electrolytes in muscle tissue during exercise. If we assume that the changes in plasma water and electrolytes during exertion are representative of interstitial fluids, then it is possible to describe the influence of acute exercise and subsequent dehydration on various body fluid compartments.

At the onset of exercise, there is a marked flux of water out of plasma into the active musculature. This reduction in plasma volume constitutes a decrement of roughly 13% at exercise levels generally observed during marathon competition.[12] This transcapillary fluid movement into the active tissues has been shown to occur as a result of tissue hyperosmolality.[10] The efflux of metabolic products and ions (K^+) from the active muscle fibers are therefore responsible for a decrease in plasma volume and an exercise hyperemia.

FIGURE 3 illustrates the effects of prolonged exercise and thermal dehydration (sauna exposure) on changes in plasma volume and osmolality. As previously mentioned, there is a significant decline in plasma volume at the onset of exercise. The interesting point is the fact that despite a 2.8-kg reduction in body weight during the final 110 minutes of exercise, plasma volume remained relatively constant. This is unlike the steady decline in plasma volume observed

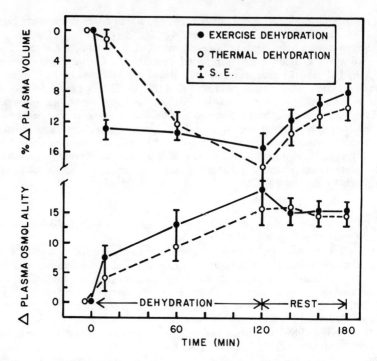

FIGURE 3. Changes in plasma volume and osmolality during exercise and thermal (sauna) dehydration. The subjects were dehydrated 4% at the end of both the exercise and heat exposures.[12]

during a similar dehydration incurred under resting heat-stress conditions. At present there is minimal data available to explain these differences in the cardio-vascular dynamics of exercise and thermal dehydration. It seems reasonable to assume, however, that the mechanisms that are responsible for the trans-capillary movement of water at the beginning of exercise (i.e., tissue hyper-osmolality) may serve to maintain plasma volume throughout prolonged severe bouts of exercise. This is supported by the fact that plasma osmolality increases throughout the exercise-dehydration, thereby exerting a strong drive to shift water from the extravascular toward the vascular compartment.

This would suggest that the body water lost during prolonged exercise is derived from interstitial and/or intracellular spaces. In an effort to determine the distribution of water between plasma and muscle during exercise, we sampled active (gastrocnemius) and inactive (deltoid) muscles and venous blood during 2 hours of treadmill running. As illustrated in FIGURE 4, muscle water (H_2O_m) increased roughly 8% in the active tissue during the early minutes of exercise. At the same time, plasma water declined by about the same proportion, while the less active muscles remained unchanged. Despite a 3.2% reduction in body weight (−2.33 kg), the additional loss from plasma amounted to less than 150 ml, with perhaps a 500 ml decrease in the active and inactive H_2O_m.

How then can we explain the loss of water in sweat without showing some marked changes in either the extracellular or intracellular volumes? If we assume that changes in plasma volume are representative of alterations in interstitial fluids, then an additional 580 g of the 2.5 kg weight loss can be accounted for. Other factors that may contribute to at least part of the exercise-sweat weight loss include the water released during the breakdown of glycogen (~370 ml), water from oxidation (~460 ml), and metabolic weight loss (~160 grams). It is, therefore, possible to account for 2.22 kg of the 2.33-kg weight loss incurred during the exercise. This remaining difference (0.11 kg) may simply be attributed to water drawn from the gut. In any event, it is reasonable to assume that the distribution of water lost via sweating may reflect osmotic pressures that are produced during the excretion of a hypotonic sweat.

What affect does exercise and sweating have on the ions in body fluids? At the onset of exercise, the exercising muscle shows a small but significant decrease in K^+ content that is paralleled by a rise in plasma K^+ (FIGURE 5). This response is similar to that in previous reports that suggest that in the early minutes of muscular activity there is an efflux of K^+ from the cell.[13] Progressive exercise-dehydration seems to have little effect on the plasma K^+ content, while K^+ appeared to re-enter the active muscles. The K^+ in the deltoid muscle, on the other hand, did not change at any time during exercise, but decreased roughly 5% after 30 minutes of recovery. However, because of individual variability, this decline was not statistically significant ($p > 0.05$).

Exercising muscle appears to slowly increase its Mg^{++} content, which is paralleled by a gradual decline in plasma Mg^{++}. Although we can only speculate, it is possible that these Mg^{++} shifts into contracting muscle are a function of increased metabolic need. Unfortunately, these data do not permit a definitive analysis of the mechanisms responsible for this change or its physiological significance.

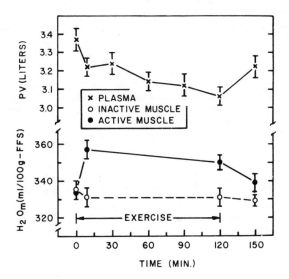

FIGURE 4. Changes in plasma volume and the water content of inactive (deltoid) and active (vastus lateralis) muscles during 2 hours of exercise.

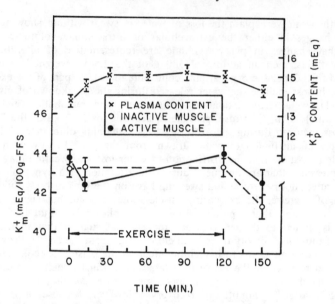

FIGURE 5. Changes in the K⁺ content of plasma (K^+_p), exercising muscles (vastus lateralis), and inactive muscles (deltoid) during exercise and recovery.

Apparently the ionic and water shifts that occur at the onset of exercise seem to have little effect on the resting membrane potential (RMP). At the end of the 2 hours of running, however, the calculated RMP [14] showed a 6 mV increase in the working muscle, but returned to the pre-exercise value (90 mV) after 30 minutes of recovery. The RMP of the inactive muscle was unaffected by either exercise or dehydration. The Cl⁻ method used in calculating the intramuscular and extramuscular water content assumes that the RMP remains constant and that 95% of the Cl⁻ in the biopsy specimen is extracellular. In light of these RMP estimates, it seems that these assumptions may not be valid during prolonged exercise, thereby falsely describing the distribution of muscle water between the extracellular and intracellular compartments.

In any event, it appears that there are marked differences between active and inactive muscles with regard to their water and ionic contents during both short-term and prolonged exercise. After 30 minutes of recovery, however, these constituents are redistributed so that both tissues have similar water and electrolyte contents. Therefore, muscle tissue sampled from a single site can be used to estimate the effects of dehydration on muscle water and electrolytes, provided the subject has been inactive for 30 minutes. These observations also suggest that attempts to calculate the distribution of muscle water and ions during exercise by the chloride method are probably invalidated because of a shift in the membrane potential.

Body Fluids Following Dehydration

Thus far we have concerned ourselves with the effects of acute exercise and sweating on body water and electrolytes. The previous discussion has shown that sweat losses may have markedly different effects on the distribution of body fluids when measured at rest and during exercise. For that reason, it seems appropriate that some attention be given to the effects of dehydration on water and ionic contents of extracellular and intracellular compartments in the hours following exercise and/or heat stress.

Since the major ions lost in sweat and urine were those of the extracellular compartment, it is not surprising to observe a disproportionately larger loss of water from plasma and interstitial spaces than from the intracellular compartment. While plasma and interstitial water decline approximately 2.5% for each percent of dehydration, the intracellular water decreased only 1.1% for each percent of dehydration.[6] The absolute loss of water from these compartments, however, was found to be quite evenly distributed between the extracellular and intracellular spaces. It is interesting to note that at all stages of dehydration, plasma water accounts for 10%–11% of the total body water loss. Except at low levels of dehydration (<2.0%), intracellular fluids contribute roughly half of the water lost from the body.

Now let us consider the water and electrolyte contents of the muscle biopsy specimens (TABLE 2). In keeping with the previous calculations of the change in intracellular water, muscle water declines steadily with progressive levels of dehydration. The change from 341 to 318 ml per 100 g FFS (fat-free solid weight) constitutes a 6.8% decrease in muscle water, which is similar to the change in intracellular water (-6.5%) determined by the loss of Cl^- in urine and sweat. The values reported in TABLE 3 for muscle Na^+, K^+, and Cl^- content were not statistically significant at any stage of dehydration. Only muscle Mg^{++} content showed a significant change, decreasing 12% following the final stage of dehydration (-5.8%).

Since these values (TABLE 2) are computed on the basis of the fat-free solid weight of the tissue, they do not reflect the concentration of the ions in muscle water. Based on the Cl^- method,[8] however, we have calculated the Na^+, K^+, and Mg^{++} concentrations in intramuscular water. As a result of the decline in muscle water, the ions present in the tissue samples were concentrated. Thus, intramuscular K^+ (K^+_i) increased significantly but Mg^{++}_i and Na^+_i remained unchanged.

Based on the preceding data and the equation by Hodgkin and Horowicz,[14] it is possible to estimate what effects dehydration might have on the muscle's resting membrane potential. Before dehydration the RMP averaged -91.4

TABLE 2

MUSCLE WATER, ELECTROLYTES, AND GLYCOGEN CONTENT BEFORE AND AFTER
VARIED DEGREES OF DEHYDRATION *

	Concentrations in Muscle Tissue per 100 g fat-free solids					
Dehydration	H_2O (ml)	Na^+ (meq)	K^+ (meq)	Cl^- (meq)	Mg^{++} (meq)	Glycogen (mmoles/kg)
0	341	9.9	46.3	6.1	9.0	115
-2.2%	329	10.4	47.4	6.6	8.3	76
-4.1%	324	11.1	47.0	8.3	8.1	61
-5.8%	318	9.6	47.8	6.2	7.9	48

* After Costill et al.[6]

mV, which is similar to previously reported values in the leg muscles of man.[15, 16] Since the concentrations of intracellular and extracellular K^+ and Na^+ increased somewhat proportionately with dehydration, the RMP remained relatively constant. Although such methods of computing the RMP must be viewed cautiously, these calculations suggest that the altered RMP observed during prolonged exercise is normalized after 30 minutes of recovery, despite severe levels of dehydration.

Thus, this series of observations demonstrate that body water lost following acute dehydration is attributed to relatively larger water losses from extracellular rather than intracellular compartments. Despite large sweat losses, the muscle K^+ content remained unchanged but increased in concentration as a result of the loss of water from the muscle tissue. However, one should not overlook the facts that these measurements were made following 30 minutes of rest and that muscle samples were obtained only from a heavily exercised muscle. Thus, shortly after exercise and/or heat-induced dehydration, there is a shift of fluids from the intracellular to the extracellular space, with some redistribution of selected ions.

Repeated Days Of Heavy Sweating

The preceding discussion of acute changes in body fluids during exercise and heavy sweating are relevant to the conditions experienced during and immediately after marathon running. In preparation for the marathon, most runners exercise for 1 to 3 hours each day, thereby experiencing large daily sweat losses. For that reason, it seems appropriate that some attention be given to the effects of training and repeated days of heavy sweating on body fluid balance.

It has been suggested that individuals who perform heavy exercise and sweat profusely on repeated days may incur deficits of selected ions, principally K^+.[17, 18] Despite many accusations, no direct evidence of tissue hypokalemia has been provided to substantiate these claims.

In an attempt to gain some insight into this problem, studies were conducted during five successive days of dehydration.[5] Although the subjects were permitted to eat and drink ad libitum, the total water, K^+, Na^+, Cl^-, and caloric intakes were closely monitored. Likewise, the daily excretion of water and ions in sweat and urine were accurately measured. These body water and electrolyte exchange data revealed that repeated days of exercise dehydration induced a renal conservation of Na^+ with a small decline in urine K^+. As a result, the subjects tended to store Na^+ (392 meq/5 days), while body K^+ remained in positive balance during the 5 days of these observations. The relatively large gains in Na^+ were accomplished by a proportionate increase in extracellular water. This is well documented by the expansion of plasma volume illustrated in FIGURE 6. It is interesting to note that a period of 48 to 72 hours was required for the elimination of this "excess" water and extracellular ion.

The mechanism apparently responsible for the conservation of Na^+ in response to successive days of dehydration is an increase in mineral corticoid function.[7] Exposure to heat, exercise, and/or dehydration results in arterial hypovolemia and relative renal ischemia. Both factors are known to be responsible for increased aldosterone production and renal sodium reabsorption.[19, 20] This point is documented by changes in plasma renin and aldosterone concentrations following a single bout (1 hr) of exercise (FIGURE 7). Despite *ad libitum* water intake, plasma aldosterone remains elevated for nearly 12 hours following such exercise.[7]

Thus, despite the sweat and urinary losses incurred during dehydration, it is reasonable to assume that marathoners probably maintain a positive Na^+, K^+, and Cl^- balance via dietary intake and renal conservation of these ions, provided food and drink are consumed *ad libitum*. Knochel *et al.*,[17] however, have observed that six men undergoing intensive physical training in a hot climate developed a mean K^+ deficit of 349 meq in the first 4 days of exercise. This deficit, estimated from measurements of ^{42}K, occurred despite a daily K^+ intake

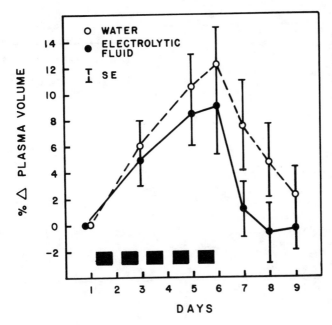

FIGURE 6. Percentage change in plasma volume during 5 days of repeated dehydration (-3% per day). During one series the subjects were only permitted to drink water, while in the second treatment thirst was satisfied by *ad libitum* ingestion of an electrolyte drink.

of 100 meq/day. Unfortunately, the balance of K^+ intake and excretion (sweat, urine, and feces) was not adequately monitored to validate the ^{42}K calculations. If, in fact, heavy sweating and exercise on repeated days can induce these large body K^+ deficits, then such changes should be detectable in muscle biopsy specimens.

For that reason, we recently conducted an investigation to determine the effects of low dietary K^+ and repeated days of heavy exercise on muscle water and electrolytes. Eight men ran sufficiently on 4 successive days to achieve a mean body weight loss of 3.1 kg (4.2% of body weight). This protocol was followed under two dietary regimens. One diet sequence provided 25 meq of

K^+ daily (low K^+ diet), while the second contained 80 meq of K^+ per day (high K^+ diet). Both diets included 180 meq of Na^+/day with an average daily caloric content of 2880 kcal.

In response to the four days of exercise-dehydration, urine production decreased from a control value of approximately 1300 ml/24 hours to a low of 600 ml/24 hours during the low K^+ dietary sequence. Although urine volume was depressed in both experimental treatments, the low K^+ diet elicited a significantly greater reduction than did the high K^+ diet. At the same time, there was a marked reduction in urine Na^+ excretion, which also seemed to be more pronounced during the low K^+ experiment. As a matter of fact, some individuals excreted less than 10 meq of Na^+ in a 24-hour period. These patterns of reduced

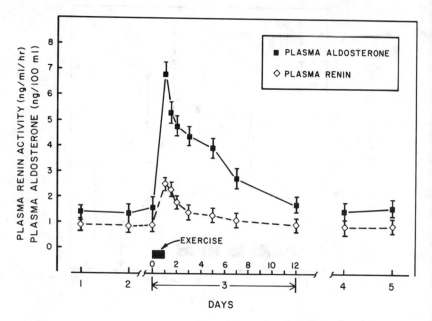

FIGURE 7. Alerations in plasma renin activity and aldosterone concentration as a result of a single 60-minute exercise bout.[7]

renal water and Na^+ excretion are similar to our earlier observations and suggest that dietary K^+ may influence renal Na^+–water conservation during repeated days of heavy exercise.[5]

Of greater interest was the rate of body K^+ lost in urine and sweat during the exercise and dietary regimens. As can be observed in FIGURE 8, there was substantially less K^+ excreted in urine during the low K^+ diet than when the men consumed the 80 meq of K^+ daily. Changes in dietary K^+ intake had no effect on sweat K^+ content.

If this lower renal K^+ excretion were a function of the reduced urine volume, then we would expect to see a decreased K^+ excretion in both dietary treatments and no change in the concentration of K^+ in urine. FIGURE 9 shows that urine

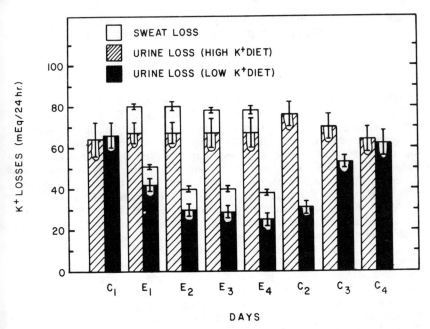

FIGURE 8. Sweat and urine K$^+$ losses during control (C) and repeated days of exercise (E). Hashed vertical bars represent values obtained during the high K$^+$ diet. Solid bars denote values during the low K$^+$ diet.

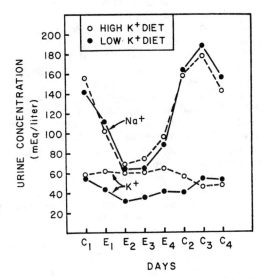

FIGURE 9. Urine Na$^+$ and K$^+$ concentrations before (C$_1$), during (E$_1$–E$_4$) and after (C$_2$–C$_4$) repeated days of exercise dehydration.

K$^+$ concentration decreased significantly during the low K$^+$ intake, but remained relatively constant during the high K$^+$ treatment. Thus, with a reduced K$^+$ intake and repeated days of dehydration, there is a selective reduction in renal K$^+$ excretion. The mechanism responsible for this apparent K$^+$ conservation is not easily explained, but may simply reflect the lower K$^+$ entry into plasma following the low K$^+$ diet.

Thus, given the dietary intake and losses (urine and sweat) of Na$^+$ and K$^+$, it is possible to approximate the average daily change in body content. Despite heavy sweating and relatively normal urine K$^+$ excretion, the subjects were able to remain in positive K$^+$ balance with an intake of 80 meq per day. When the diet contained only 25 meq of K$^+$ per day, however, the subjects incurred a body K$^+$ deficit of about 17 meq/day (-68 meq/4 days). If we assume that these men had total body K$^+$ contents of 3450 meq (42 meq/kg), then the deficits incurred in this study were roughly 2% of the body K$^+$ stores.

Muscle biopsy samples obtained at rest on the first, third, and fifth days of the experiments revealed an increase in muscle water content (H_2O_m) during both dietary conditions. In keeping with the plasma volume and Na$^+$ balance data, H_2O_m increased significantly more during the low K$^+$ diet than with the high K$^+$ intake. At the same time there was a small increase in muscle K$^+$ content and no change in plasma K$^+$. These data are compatible with the dietary K$^+$ balance data, which showed little or no change in body K$^+$ content. In any event, there is no evidence to support the concept that heavy exercise on repeated days will threaten the muscle and plasma K$^+$ stores even when the dietary K$^+$ intake is extremely low.

Conclusion

In summary, these studies demonstrate the body's capacity to minimize electrolyte losses during acute and repeated bouts of exercise and dehydration. Although there are marked shifts in water and selected ions in the exercising muscle, only during prolonged exertion is the ratio of intramuscular to extramuscular K$^+$ significantly altered, suggesting that some modifications of the muscle cell membrane may occur. Muscle tissue not engaged in the exercise seems unaffected by the sweat lost during prolonged activity but relinquishes intracellular water shortly after work is terminated. Blood, muscle, sweat, and urine measurements before and following varied levels of dehydration demonstrate that body water lost during exercise in the heat is accomplished at the expense of larger water losses from extracellular than from intracellular compartments. Moreover, the loss of ions in sweat and urine had little effect on the K$^+$ content of either plasma or muscle.

With repeated days of dehydration and heavy exercise, plasma volume increased in proportion to an increase in body Na$^+$ storage. At this point some mention should be made concerning the effect of this increased plasma water on the concentration of blood constituents. Since red blood cells and hemoglobin are confined to the vascular space, both may decrease significantly as a function of the hemodilution induced by repeated days of exercise and dehydration. This may in part explain the apparent anemia reported by sports physicians among athletes undergoing intensive training. It is also possible that such hemodilution may produce low concentrations of plasma K$^+$, which might be falsely interpreted as suggestive of a hypokalemic state. In any event, some caution should be used in the clinical interpretation of plasma concentrations of various constituents among endurance-trained athletes.

In general, it seems that the large sweat losses incurred during training and marathon competition are adequately tolerated by the runner, with concomitant adjustments in the water and electrolyte distribution of the runner's body fluid compartments. Despite the sizeable excretion of ions in sweat, the runner's large caloric intake and renal conservation of Na^+ minimize the threat of chronic dehydration and/or electrolyte deficiencies.

References

1. COSTILL, D. L., W. F. KAMMER & A. FISHER. 1970. Fluid ingestion during distance running. Arch. Environ. Health. **21:** 520–525.
2. KOZLOWSKI, C. & B. SALTIN. 1964. Effect of sweat loss on body fluids. J. Appl. Physiol. **19:** 1119–1124.
3. SALTIN, B. 1964. Circulatory responses to submaximal and maximal exercise after thermal dehydration. J. Appl. Physiol. **19:** 1125–1132.
4. VELLAR, O. D. 1968. Studies on sweat losses of nutrients. I. Iron content of whole body sweat and its association with other sweat constituents, serum iron levels, hematological indices, body surface area and sweat rate. Scand. J. Clin. Lab. Invest. **21:** 157–167.
5. COSTILL, D. L., R. COTÉ, E. MILLER, T. MILLER & S. WYNDER. 1975. Water and electrolyte replacement during repeated days of work in the heat. Aviat. Space Environ. Med. **45**(6): 795–800, 1975.
6. COSTILL, D. L., R. COTÉ & W. FINK. 1976. Muscle water and electrolytes following varied levels of dehydration in man. J. Appl. Physiol. **40**(1): 6–11.
7. COSTILL, D. L., G. BRANAM, W. FINK & R. NELSON. 1977. Exercise induced sodium conservation: Changes in plasma renin and aldosterone. Med. Sci. Sports. **8:** 209–213.
8. BERGSTRÖM, J. 1962. Muscle electrolytes in man. Determination by neutron activation analysis on needle biopsy specimens. A study on normal subjects, kidney patients, and patients with chronic diarrhea. Scand. J. Clin. Lab. Invest. **18:** 16–20.
9. KJELLMER, I. 1964. The effect of exercise on the vascular bed of skeletal muscle. Acta Physiol. Scand. **62:** 18–30.
10. LUNDVALL, J. 1972. Tissue hyperosmolality as a mediator of vasodilatation and transcapillary fluid flux in exercising skeletal muscle. Acta Physiol. Scand. (Suppl. 379): 1–142.
11. MELLANDER, S, B JOHANSSON, S. GRAY, O. JONSSON, J. LUNDVALL & B. LJUNG. 1967. The effects of hyperosmolarity on intact and isolated vascular smooth muscle. Possible role in exercise hyperemia. Angiologica **4:** 310–322.
12. COSTILL, D. L. & W. J. FINK. 1974. Plasma volume changes following exercise and thermal dehydration. J. Appl. Physiol. **37:** 521–525.
13. MILLER, H. C. & D. C. DARROW. 1941. Relation of serum and muscle electrolytes, particularly potassium to voluntary exercise. Amer. J. Physiol. **132:** 801–807.
14. HODGKIN, A. L. & P. HOROWICZ. 1959. The influence of potassium and chloride ions on the membrane potential of single muscle fibers. J. Physiol. (Lond.) **148:** 127–160.
15. HODGKIN, A. L. & P. HOROWICZ. 1959. The influence of potassium and Resting membrane potential difference of skeletal muscle in normal subjects and severely ill patients. J. Clin. Invest. **50:** 49–59.
16. JOHNS, R. J. 1960. Microelectrode studies of muscle membrane potential in man. Neuro. Disorders **38:** 704–713.

17. KNOCHEL, J. P., L. N. DOTIN & R. J. HAMBURGER. 1972. Pathophysiology of intense physical conditioning in a hot climate. I. Mechanisms of potassium depletion. J. Clin. Invest. **51:** 242–255.
18. SCHAMADAN, J. L. & W. D. SNIVELY, JR. 1967. Potassium depletion as a possible cause for heat stroke. Ind. Med. Surg. **36:** 785–788.
19. HARTROFT, P. M. & S. HARTROFT. 1961. Regulation of aldosterone secretion. Brit. Med. J. **1:** 1171–1179.
20. BARTTER, F. C. & D. S. GANN. 1960. On the hemodynamic regulation of the secretion of aldosterone. Circulation **21:** 1016–1021.

POTASSIUM DEFICIENCY DURING TRAINING IN
THE HEAT

James P. Knochel

Renal Section
Veterans Administration Hospital
Dallas, Texas 75216

Department of Internal Medicine
University of Texas
Southwestern Medical School
Dallas, Texas 75235

Approximately one-half of the young men who sustain acute heat stroke or severe heat exhaustion during training programs in hot weather demonstrate hypokalemia during the acute phase of their illness.[1] Hypokalemia under such conditions does not necessarily indicate potassium deficiency. When exposed to heat normal subjects hyperventilate. The resulting respiratory alkalosis induces transfer of potassium ions into the liver and skeletal muscle cells and consequently may cause hypokalemia.[2] In contrast, it has been observed that some patients who have sustained acute heat stroke during intense physical exertion display modest hypokalemia *even in the presence of severe lactic acidosis.*[1] As opposed to effects of acute alkalosis, acute metabolic acidosis would be expected to produce acute hyperkalemia. Therefore, the findings in this group of patients would suggest that potassium deficiency might have existed before the onset of heat stroke.

Studying the effects of brief, modest exercise under conditions of experimental heat stress, other investigators have shown evidence that modest potassium deficiency may occur after a period of several days.[3,4] Independently, others have observed polyuria and hyposthenuria, both unresponsive to posterior pituitary extract [5] and the finding of vacuolar nephropathy in a group of military recruits with acute heat stroke who had a history of polyuria and polydispsia before they became ill.[6] These findings could have resulted from potassium deficiency.

In our own experience and that of others with military recruits and football players,[1,7,8] acute heat stroke that occurs during or after intense physical activity has been associated with muscle necrosis (rhabdomyolysis). Potassium deficiency is now recognized as a cause of rhabdomyolysis.[9,10]

Because of the foregoing evidence, a study was designed to examine the effects of intense conditioning in hot as well as cool climates in young men undergoing basic military training.

Methods

Detailed methods of procedure have previously been published.[11,12] Briefly, six healthy volunteers were studied during the first five weeks of basic training in hot weather. For comparison, 16 additional subjects were studied during cooler weather. Dietary intake was constant and consumed entirely by each

175

subject. Potassium intake was 106 meq/day. Sodium intake was constant but variable for each group and ranged between 150 and 350 meq/day. In all subjects, the training program was stereotyped. The studies were conducted on the same day each week for 5 consecutive weeks. Besides routine measurements of electrolytes in plasma, special studies included weekly measurements of total exchangeable potassium (^{42}K), secretion and excretion of aldosterone, plasma renin activity, total body water, and extracellular fluid volume. The latter two measurements were derived from either body density or tritium dilution and radiosulfate dilution, respectively. Renal function was assessed serially by measuring plasma creatinine concentration, endogenous creatinine clearance, and inulin clearance. Electrolyte losses in sweat were assessed from aqueous eluates of clothing. For the latter purpose, all clothing worn during the study had been rinsed in distilled water, dried and issued to the volunteers on the morning of the study. Their clothing was collected in plastic bags the following morning and eluted with distilled water.

In order to properly interpret the value for total body potassium, each subject underwent estimations of lean body mass each week volumetrically by water displacement in a total body volumeter.[13]

Results

Average values for total exchangeable potassium in the six subjects training in hot weather are shown in TABLE 1. In this table are shown serial values for exchangeable ^{42}K for all subjects training in the heat. [Their maximum deficits occurred on either the 4th, 11th, or 18th day.] The average maximum

TABLE 1

AVERAGE VALUES FOR TOTAL EXCHANGEABLE POTASSIUM IN SIX SUBJECTS
TRAINING IN HOT WEATHER *

Day of Training	^{42}K (meq)	LBM † (kg)	^{42}K/LBM (meq/kg)	K Sweat ‡ (meq/ 24 hr)	Urine K (meq/ 24 hr)	Urine Na (meq/ 24 hr)
Control §	3252	62.5	52.2	28	56	201
	±449	±8.3	±4.7	±14	±14	±112
4	2903	63.5	45.0	37	64	191
	±418	±7.4	±3.7	±12	±14	±65
11	2789	65.7	42.5	24	56	254
	±440	±6.8	±5.2	±16	±12	±125
18	2996	66.2	45.3	23	72	231
	±311	±6.2	±3.2	±15	±9	±117
25	3235	67.5	47.8	23	74	197
	±481	±5.9	±4.0	±16	±10	±139
32	3450	66.4	52.1	21	50	131
	±380	±6.2	±4.1	±15	±4	±69

* All values are means ± standard deviations (SD).
† Lean body mass.
‡ Does not include K lost in dripped sweat or that adhering to body surface.
§ Sixteen subjects training in cooler weather served as controls.

TABLE 2

RANGE AND AVERAGE VALUES FOR ALDOSTERONE EXCRETORY AND SECRETORY RATES
FOR SIX SUBJECTS TRAINING IN HOT WEATHER *

Day	Aldosterone		Plasma Renin Activity † (μg/dl/3 hr)	Total Body Water (liters)
	Excretion (μg/24 hr)	Secretion (μg/24 hr)		
Control ‡	19.8	172	399	45.8
	±9.9	±121	±210	±6.1
4	13.2	117	408	47.2
	±5.2	±81	±160	±5.5
11	20.1	108	305	48.1
	±6.7	±84	±157	±4.9
18	21.2	99	458	48.5
	±7.9	±67	±330	±4.6
25	14.8	159	514	49.3
	±7.9	±109	±362	±4.4
32	13.8	161	549	48.6
	±6.5	±98	±293	±4.6

* All data are expressed as means ± SD.
† Sample collected before arising.
‡ Sixteen subjects training in cooler weather served as controls.

deficit for these six subjects was 517 meq. The late rise of total body potassium was probably the result of cooler weather and diminished losses of potassium by sweating. Recovery of potassium from clothing eluates showed that a substantial amount of potassium was lost by sweating. The measured values in the clothing eluates minimize the actual losses because of unrecovered sweat from the body surface and that lost by dripping. Although frank hypokalemia did not occur, serum potassium values were in the lower range of normal. Total daily potassium excretion into the urine averaged 67 meq/day on the day when potassium deficiency was at its height for each subject. Sodium excretion into the urine was approximately 50% of intake.

TABLE 2 shows the range and average values for aldosterone excretory and secretory rates. In terms of sodium intake these values were considerably higher than those usually observed in non-heat-stressed subjects. Plasma renin activity was measured in the morning before arising and again at noon in order to determine the effects of upright posture. To our surprise, it was common to find some morning values exceptionally elevated and especially so when considered in terms of sodium intake. In many of the subjects, the corresponding value obtained at noon was often less than that observed in the morning.

Total body water estimated from body density rose in each subject. Lean body mass also rose indicating that the decline of exchangeable ^{42}K was not catabolic in origin. By the end of the training period, total body water had risen substantially in all subjects.

In the trainees studied during hot weather, endogenous creatinine clearance showed a slight fall during the first week. Thereafter, it rose so that the final value exceeded that considered to be normal for subjects of this age. Because of this observation, glomerular filtration rates were estimated by inulin clearance and extracellular fluid volumes by radiosulfate dilution in the remainder of the subjects undergoing training in cooler weather. Both of these were observed to rise significantly by the 28th day of training (TABLE 3).

Discussion

These studies show that significant potassium depletion may occur in healthy young men undergoing intensive training in hot weather. This occurs despite provision of adequate nutrition and normal potassium intake. To incur an average potassium deficit of 517 meq after approximately two weeks of training would require a net daily loss of approximately 40 meq. Men training under such conditions have been shown to produce up to 12 liters of sweat per day.[14] Since the average potassium concentration in sweat is 9 meq/l,[15] losses in sweat alone could exceed the normal dietary intake. If the kidney could conserve potassium under such conditions, the net deficit would be small. However, it

TABLE 3

GLOMERULAR FILTRATION RATES AND FLUID VOLUMES FOR SIX SUBJECTS TRAINING IN HOT WEATHER

	Creatinine Clearance (ml/min/ 1.7 m²)	Inulin Clearance (ml/min/ 1.72 m²)	Total Body Water (liters)	Extra-cellular Volume (liters)
Control *	114	101	46.6	14.7
	±10	±7	±2.6	±0.7
Day 28	131	123	49.7	16.8
	±6	±6	±1.9	±0.5
p	< 0.001	< 0.001	< 0.001	< 0.001

* Sixteen subjects training in cooler weather served as controls.

was noted in these subjects that when potassium deficiency was maximum, average daily excretion of potassium into the urine ranged between 41 to 79 meq and averaged 67 meq/day. Such losses would generally be considered inappropriately high in other situations wherein potassium deficiency was incurred by extrarenal means. For example, in potassium deficiency induced by diarrhea, it is unusual to observe potassium excretion into the urine in quantities greater than 20 meq/day.[16] That the rate of excretion in these subjects was higher suggests excessive mineralocorticoid activity. Indeed, as suggested by Conn several years ago,[17] heat acclimatization in many respects resembles mineralocorticoid escape. In the latter situation, combined administration of a mineralocorticoid such as desoxycorticosterone or aldosterone, in conjunction with sodium chloride, will cause wasting of potassium into the urine. However, if aldosterone or desoxycorticosterone was administered in the same dosage but in the absence of sodium chloride, potassium wasting into the urine does not occur. In subjects training in hot weather, sodium excretion was apparently sufficient to prevent potassium conservation. Aldosterone secretion rates were abnormally elevated in terms of sodium intake. Consequently, it would appear that potassium was lost into the urine under the influence of aldosterone-mediated sodium exchange for potassium at the renal tubular site. Abetting this process was development of an expanded extracellular fluid volume and an increase of glomerular filtration rate. Potassium deficiency did not occur in any subjects studied during cooler weather. In contrast, the latter men showed an increase of total body potassium in proportion to the rise in lean body mass as one would anticipate as a result of physical conditioning. The most important difference among the subjects training in hot and those training in cooler weather was the difference in sweat potassium losses. Subjects training in cool weather did not sweat significantly and they did not become potassium deficient.

What might the possible consequences of potassium deficiency under such conditions be? In our subsequent studies, it was shown that rhabdomyolysis can be readily induced in the potassium deficient dog by exercise.[10] There are at least two mechanisms whereby rhabdomyolysis could occur in the potassium-deficient animal or man. The first is ischemia of skeletal muscle during exercise. In health, muscle contraction is associated with release of potassium ions into the interstitial fluid of the muscle. At this site, increased potassium concentration causes vasodilitation, which in turn initiates the increased muscle blood flow during exercise. The normal increase of muscle blood flow during exercise subserves at least three major functions. First it allows delivery of fuel to energize contraction. Second, it facilitates delivery of heated blood away from the muscle to prevent local overheating. Third, it facilitates delivery of chemical metabolites out of working muscle. At least for a period of time, the potassium deficient animal can perform muscular work at an intensity equal to normal. However, during this exercise, in contrast to normal, the deficient animal shows virtually no increase in muscle blood flow. Based upon these observations, muscle ischemia during exercise must be considered a cause of rhabdomyolysis.[10, 18]

In other studies [19] we have shown that, when sufficiently severe, potassium deficiency leads to a subnormal resting transmembrane potential of skeletal muscle cells, abnormal accumulation of salt and water in the cells, and eventually a release of creatine phosphokinase from the muscle irrespective of exercise.

Another important consequence of muscle potassium deficiency is defective storage and synthesis of glycogen.[20] During hard, sustained muscular work, provision of oxygen is inadequate to permit complete oxidation of glucose to CO_2 and water. Therefore, under such conditions, the most important chemical fuel providing replenishment of ATP for muscle contraction is glycogen.

Many investigators have clearly shown a requirement of potassium ions for glycogen synthesis.[21] In the dog, muscle glycogen virtually disappears after potassium deficiency.[20] The same probably happens in man.[22]

Another important aspect of glycogen metabolism in skeletal muscle is that referred to as supercompensation.[23] In this process, a single bout of exhaustive muscular exercise sufficient to deplete muscle glycogen will be followed by an increased rate of glycogen synthesis and storage. By the third or fourth day after such exercise, muscle glycogen content may reach values three to four times that which had existed previously. In recent studies on the dog, we have shown that not only does muscle glycogen content fall to almost unmeasureable values in potassium deficiency, but exercise no longer is followed by an increase in resting muscle glycogen content.[23] In these studies, potassium deficiency of only 10% or 15% of the total body content was sufficient to produce this abnormality. Loss of glycogen from skeletal muscle as the result of potassium deficiency establishes a situation somewhat analogus to that of McArdle's syndrome. In this disease, muscle phosphorylase is absent or deficient.[24] Therefore, muscle glycogen cannot be utilized during exercise. In the event of strenuous exercise, muscle necrosis and myoglobinuria may occur. Thus by analogy at least, potassium deficiency induces a sort of acquired McArdle's syndrome in which glycogen is unavailable as a fuel.

If healthy young men become potassium deficient as a result of strenuous training in hot climates, it would seem likely that their muscle performance could become limited and further that a potential for rhabdomyolysis may materialize.

Logical criticism has been assigned to the suggestion made earlier [25] that potassium deficiency may somehow be related to heat stroke as it occurs in military recruits or football players training in hot climates.[26] Quite obviously, young healthy men who develop heat stroke on the first day of their training who have no previous history of illness and no reason why potassium deficiency should exist are not likely to have developed heat stroke on the basis of potassium deficiency. Nevertheless, it may yet play a role in those who develop heat exhaustion or heat stroke after a week or two of training. It seems quite possible that potassium deficiency could have an adverse effect on skeletal muscle performance and perhaps on cardiovascular performance as well.[27] It may also impair sweat production.[28]

The final issue concerns whether or not potassium supplementation should be provided during training in hot weather. Certainly, providing extra potassium in the diet by ingesting foods with a large potassium content would appear to be ideal. However, providing 40 meq of potassium each day in such foods could be quite expensive. On the other hand, I would consider it potentially dangerous to ingest those types of chemical potassium supplements that are readily soluble and rapidly absorbed by the gut. Thus, the usual hyperkalemia of exercise could be exaggerated sufficiently to pose a hazard of cardiotoxicity.[29, 30] Perhaps some of the newer preparations [31] that provide slow absorption of potassium over a period of many hours would not only be more safe but also more economical.

References

1. KNOCHEL, J. P. 1974. Environmental heat illness. Arch. Int. Med. **133:** 841–854.
2. IAMPIETRO, P. R. 1963. Heat-induced tetany. Fed. Proc. **22:** 884–886.
3. STREETEN, D. D. P., J. W. CONN, L. H. LOUIS, S. S. FAJANS, H. S. SELTZER, R. D. JOHNSON, R. D. GITTLER & A. H. DUBE. 1960. Secondary aldosteronism: Metabolic and adrenocortical responses of normal men to high environmental temperatures. Metab. (Clin. Exp.). **9:** 1071.
4. GORDON, R. S. JR. & H. L. ANDRES. 1966. Potassium depletion under heat stress. Fed. Proc. **25:** 1372.
5. LADELL, W. S. S., J. C. WATERLOW & M. F. HUDSON. 1944. Desert climate, physiological and clinical observations. Lancet **ii:** 491–508.
6. SOBEL, S., *et al.* 1963. Renal mechanisms in heat stroke. Clin. Res. (Abstr) **11:** 252.
7. KNOCHEL, J. P., *et al.* 1961. The renal, cardiovascular, hematologic and serum electrolyte abnormalities of heat stroke. Amer. J. Med. **30:** 299–309.

8. VERTEL, R. M. & J. P. KNOCHEL. 1967. Acute renal failure due to heat injury: An analysis of ten cases associated with a high incidence of myoglobinuria. Amer. J. Med. **43:** 435–451.

9. GROSS, E. G., J. D. DEXTER & R. G. ROTH. 1966. Hypokalemic myopathy with myoglobinuria associated with licorice ingestion. N. Engl. J. Med. **274:** 602–606.

10. KNOCHEL, J. P. & E. M. SCHLEIN. 1972. On the mechanism or rhabdomyolysis in potassium depletion. J. Clin. Invest. **51:** 1750–1759.

11. KNOCHEL, J. P., L. N. DOTIN & R. J. HAMBURGER. 1972. Pathophysiology of intense physical condition in a hot climate. I. Mechanisms of potassium depletion. J. Clin. Invest. **51:** 242–255.

12. KNOCHEL, J. P., L. N. DOTIN & R. J. HAMBURGER. 1974. Heat stress, exercise, and muscle injury: Effects on urate metabolism and renal function. Ann. Int. Med. **81:** 321–328.

13. ALLEN, T. H. 1963. Measurement of human body fat: A quantitative method suited for use by aviation medical officers. Aerospace Med. **34:** 907–912.

14. ROBINSON, S. & A. H. ROBINSON. 1954. Chemical composition of sweat. Physiol. Rev. **34:** 202–206.

15. SCHWARTZ, I. L. & J. H. THAYSEN. 1956. Excretion of sodium and potassium in human sweat. J. Clin. Invest. **35:** 114–120.

16. HUTH, E. J., R. D. SQUIRES & J. R. ELKINTON. 1959. Experimental potassium depletion in normal human subjects. II. Renal and hormonal factors in the development of extracellular alkalosis during depletion. J. Clin. Invest. **38:** 1149–1156.

17. CONN, J. W. 1963. Aldosteronism in man. Some clinical and climatological aspects. J. Amer. Med. Assoc. **183:** 775–790.

18. KNOCHEL, J. P. 1972. Exertional rhabdomyolysis (Editorial). N. Engl. J. Med. **287:** 927–929.

19. BILBREY, G. L., N. W. CARTER & J. P. KNOCHEL. 1973. Skeletal muscle resting membrane potential in potassium deficiency. J. Clin. Invest. **52:** 3011–3018.

20. BLACHLEY, J., J. P. KNOCHEL & J. LONG. 1974. Impaired muscle glycogen synthesis and prevention of muscle glycogen supercompensation by potassium deficiency (Abstr.). Clin. Res. **22(3):** 517A.

21. GARDNER, L. I., N. B. TALBOT, C. D. COOK, H. BERMAN & C. URIBE. 1950. The effect of potassium deficiency on carbohydrate metabolism. J. Lab. Clin. Med. **35:** 592–602.

22. BERGSTROM, J. & E. HULTMAN. 1965. The effect of thiazides, chlorthalidone and furosemide on muscle electrolytes and muscle glycogen in normal subjects. Acta. Med. Scand. **180:** 363–376.

23. BERGSTROM, J. & E. HULTMAN. 1966. Muscle glyocgen synthesis after exercise. An enhancing factor localized to the muscle cells in man. Nature (Lond.) **210:** 309–310.

24. MCARDLE, B. 1951. Myopathy due to a defect in muscle glycogen breakdown. Clin. Sci. **10:** 13–33.

25. KNOCHEL, J. P. & R. M. VERTEL. 1967. Salt loading as a possible factor in the production of potassium depletion, rhabdomyolysis, and heat injury. Lancet **i:** 659–665.

26. SHIBOLET, S., M. C. LANCASTER & V. DANON. 1976. Heat stroke: A review. Clin. Med. **47(3):** 280–301.

27. KNOCHEL, J. P., F. D. FOLEY, JR. & H. L. WALKER. 1970. Effect of potassium (K) depletion on cardiac output and lactate response to exercise in the dog. Clin. Res. **18:** 92.

28. MASSRY, S. G. & J. W. COBURN. 1962, 1972. Clinical Disorders of Fluid and Electrolyte Metabolism, 2nd Edit. Chap. 31, Clinical physiology of heat exposure : 1089–1115. McGraw-Hill Book Company. New York, N.Y.

29. ROSE, K. D., J. A. URSICK & R. D. MACA. 1972. Exercise and serum potassium flux: Myocardial metabolic implications. *In* Myocardiology. E. Bajusz & G. Rona, Eds. : 673–683. University Park Press. Baltimore, Md.
30. KNOCHEL, J. P. 1975. Dog days and siriasis. How to kill a football player (Editorial). J. Amer. Med. Assoc. **233:** 513–515.
31. ISHAY, D. B. & K. ENGELMAN. 1973. Bioavailability of potassium from a slow-release tablet. Clin. Pharm. Therapeut. **14:** 250–258.

DISCUSSION

David L. Costill, *Moderator*

Ball State University
Muncie, Indiana 47306

D. L. COSTILL: There is no single factor that poses a greater threat to the marathoner's health and performance than does hyperthermia. In addition to the demands placed on the cardiovascular system to transport nutrients to the running musculature, the circulatory system must transfer metabolically produced heat from the active tissues to the body surface where it is to be dissipated to the environment via the evaporation of sweat. Any factor that tends to overload the cardiovascular system or reduce the sweat evaporation can drastically impair the marathoner's performance and risk overheating. A second result of the evaporative body water loss is the excretion of ions in sweat. It has been suggested that large electrolyte losses in sweat may induce muscle cramping, upset body water balance, and impair muscular function. Thus the body's efforts to maintain a thermal equilibrium may result in large losses of essential body water and electrolytes, thereby placing even greater restraints on the marathoner's capacity to endure the 26 miles of competition. The papers in this section have offered an opportunity to view the interaction between body temperature regulation and body fluid balance. The following discussion will reveal the complex physiologic systems that are forced to function at near maximal capacities to support the runner's performance and to minimize the danger of heat injury.

A. CRAIG (*University of Rochester, Rochester, N.Y.*): Dr. Nadel, your studies of exercise and the rise in body temperature suggest a centrally controlled mechanism. Is that the control variable? And if so, what is the comparator?

E. R. NADEL (*Yale University, New Haven, Ct.*): We feel that it is probably the hypothalamic temperature that is the important variable in evaluating the nervous input and sending out the appropriate regulatory outflow, in this case sending out the messages for the heat dissipation responses. There have been a number of studies where the small area of the brainstem, the hypothalamus, has been heated and cooled and a very small total caloric input is added or subtracted from the brain, and yet one can get a fairly large response, out of proportion to the heat input thermoregulatory response. For that reason we are fairly confident from neurophysiological studies with animals that the comparator and the integrator is in the hypothalamus. In our studies all we can do is take the best measure that we can of internal temperature, esophageal temperature, and use it as the primary piece of input information to the brain. Skin temperature is also important, but this, as we mentioned, is only about 10% as important as the internal temperature. There may be temperature receptors in muscles or the spinal cord, but we have no way of separating these in humans.

D. E. CASTRO (*SUNY at Binghampton, Binghampton, N.Y.*): I realize this question is rather general and perhaps a little speculative, but in your studies of the body's capability to resist overheating, have you noticed any evidence of the ability to selectively control the mechanisms of sweating versus peripheral blood flow? For example, at a very high temperature, say in a very hot race, peripheral blood flow might be not too valuable in cooling the body as compared to sweating. Is it possible for the body to emphasize one more than the other?

E. R. NADEL: The skin blood flow is of course important to get the heat from the core to the skin. In other words the heat is carried in the blood according to the specific heat and flow rate of the blood to the skin. From this standpoint, this is the most important vehicle for carrying heat from core to skin. If you didn't have that vehicle then you would effectively trap all the heat within the body core, and the sweating that you do would just be cooling the shell. In terms of selective information being transmitted to the sweat glands and to the skin basal motor outflow areas, I think the two must be closely linked.

E. COLT (St. Luke's Hospital, New York, N.Y.): Dr. Wyndham, you may recall that in the summer of this year there was a report in the Annals of Internal Medicine describing the runner who collapsed in the 1973 Boston Marathon, apparently from hyperthemia. He remained in a coma for about 50 days and then died, at the end of which time an autopsy revealed that he had a massive myocardial infarction with normal coronary arteries. Is myocardial infarction seen as a part of the syndrome of hyperthermia? Do you think that this man's death was in fact myocardial infarction as a primary event or secondary to hyperthermia?

C. H. WYNDHAM (Marshalltown, South Africa): I can only report the experience of the group working in the General Hospital in Johannesburg, which has seen more heat stroke cases than anyone in the world. They certainly have not recorded this in their reports of myocardial infarction. Most of the hyperthermic cases, however, are young men in their twenties. They are not individuals in the age group that you are talking about. I think this is one difficulty in relating the Johannesburg data to this particular case. One thing I think that I would like to stress is the need for sports administrators and sports medical officers associated with marathon running to carry rectal thermometers with them. We had a similar sort of experience to the one you mentioned. One of our best runners in South Africa went to the Athens marathon about 4 or 5 years ago. This was a particularly hot and humid day and his coach forgot to take any fluids for him to drink during the race. As a result, the runner ran the entire marathon without taking any fluids. He ran to 20 miles where he became totally disoriented. For 6 months this fellow behaved in a most irrational fashion. We couldn't find any EEG changes that characterize heat stroke, but we were convinced that he had experienced heat stroke. Even today some of his close associates feel that he is not mentally as normal as he was before.

A. S. KUNIN (University of Vermont, Burlington, Vt.): I wonder if any of these studies were done on white athletes. I think it might be very interesting to see how they did in terms of heat regulation and sweating. Those of us who followed the track events at the Montreal Olympic Games remember the Black athletes who won in the shorter and sprint events.

C. H. WYNDHAM: Yes, these we reported here have been done on white athletes. We have data on Black athletes, but they are not applicable to this paper. Certainly our studies in comparing Black and white athletes in heated climates raise an interesting point. Unfortunately, our subject population is often composed of medical students whom I regard as not characteristic of the general population. Nevertheless, when we make comparisons with these individuals, one finds that the Black has a higher degree of acclimatization than the white. But when you put them both through a very vigorous acclimatization procedure, they show similar capacities for heat tolerance.

J. P. KNOCHEL (*Southwestern Medical School, Dallas, Texas*): I would like to comment on the question about myocardial infarction. I reported a case in 1961 in the *American Journal of Medicine* of a young soldier who had a transmural infarct with perfectly normal coronary arteries. I've seen two since. Just a month or two ago there was one reported in the *American Heart Journal*, again normal coronary arteries. I would like to ask a question of Dr. Wyndham. When you exposed people to just generated hyperthermia, was there any change in their CPK, independent of LDH?

C. H. WYNDHAM: We didn't have a CPK on the case I mentioned, because we went through a period of changing the method during our studies. Some methodological problems developed, but we have some recent information that shows that plasma CPKs are elevated in the men with hyperthermia.

A. CLAREMONT (*University of Wisconsin, Madison, Wisc.*): This is just a comment on the papers by Drs. Gisolfi and Wyndham. We have recently tested a nationally ranked runner who has run a 2-hour 15-minute marathon. He has had the problem of heat syncope during previous marathons, which was very puzzling in light of his outstanding performance. He weighs only 47 kilograms. In the experiment, he ran for us at 10 miles an hour for 82 minutes, which was the termination point. In that time he reduced his body weight by over 5%. In other words, he sweat at approximately 1.2–1.3 liters per hour. At that time he had a core temperature of 39.3° C, which is quite acceptable and tolerable. However, if we extrapolate that over another hour with the same sweating rate, he would acquire a 7% deficit from dehydration and a core temperature sufficient to bring about the symptoms. Thus, it should be emphasized that I'm really trying to push that frequent fluid feedings beyond satiation are essential for maximal endurance performance.

S. J. MANN (*Montefiore Hospital, Bronx, N.Y.*): Dr. Gisolfi, in the experiments that you were just relating, in view of the effect on body temperature from the percent dehydration, was the water consumption of the subjects measured?

C. V. GISOLFI: Yes. He was a seasoned subject and had been through experiments in the laboratory for several years. In a previous project we studied the consumption of fluid during 2-hour runs on the treadmill with six subjects. These men were reluctant to consume both cool and warm fluids at the beginning of the experiments. Later in the study, however, they looked forward to the experiments where they were able to drink. In some of the other experiments they had to run two hours without consuming anything. In essence, what I'm saying is that they learned how to drink.

S. J. MANN: Since the runner's shirt covers over 30% of the body surface, how will his/her dress affect the runner on cloudy-versus-sunny, humid-versus-dry, or windy-versus-calm days? Are there guidelines that should be followed?

C. V. GISOLFI (*University of Iowa, Iowa City, Iowa*): I think that is exactly what Dr. Adams is trying to answer with his studies. I think the data that he presented here today provide some of the first solid answers.

J. DEMPSEY (*University of Wisconsin, Madison, Wisc.*): You report a large drop in skin temperature in the acclimatized man. Is there a difference in the skin blood flow during prolonged exercise in the long distance athlete?

C. V. GISOLFI: There does not seem to be much of a difference in the sweat rate yet these men do have lower skin temperatures, and as pointed out by Dr. Nadel and a variety of other people there is a quicker onset of sweating in the trained athlete and in the acclimatized individual. This may be a result of a more even distribution of sweat over the body surface. In a paper by Hoffer in 1968, he showed that there was more sweating on the limbs of an acclimatized individual than an unacclimatized person, and that there was more effective evaporative cooling as a result. I suspect that the decrease in heart rate and the improved cardiovascular stability in these subjects is related to cutaneous blood flow. In a study by Robinson in 1965, trained athletes were found to have higher heat conductance values. They were profusing the skin with more blood.

D. THOMASHOW (*Harlem Hospital Center, New York, N.Y.*): Dr. Castenfors, you said that the change of sodium excretion occurred fairly early in exercise. If that's the case, then I imagine you're postulating that the renal sodium conservation was not secondary to autonomic changes? Do you know of any xenon washout studies either in athletes or in transplanted kidney patients who have been exercised to see if the same effect occurs?

J. CASTENFORS (*Karolinska Institutet, Stockholm, Sweden*): No, some people have suggested that there is some nervous regulation of renal tubular absorption.

E. J. ZAMBRASKI (*Rutgers University, New Brunswick, N.J.*): Studies at the University of Iowa have shown that there is a direct neural control over sodium reabsorption in the proximal tubule independent of hemodynamic changes. The same increase in sympathetic nerve activity that produces a renal vasoconstriction probably increases sodium reabsorption to partially explain the antidiuresis seen in exercise.

T. D. NOAKES (*University of Capetown, Capetown, South Africa*): Dr. Castenfors, you mentioned that the renal involvement during exercise is transient, which is borne out by the low incidence of renal problems in the standard marathon. In South Africa, one of our most popular ultramarathon races is over 56 miles. The incidence of acute renal failure after that race in runners is quite alarming. There have been eight cases of acute renal failure; that means patients who required regular dialysis. This does not include a large proportion of cases who responded rapidly to conservative treatment. It is possible that these symptoms are related to hyperthermia and/or dehydration. Unfortunately these runners are only identified 24 or 48 hours after the race. At that time it is very difficult to relate their problem to either hyperthermia or dehydration.

D. S. KRONFELD (*University of Pennsylvania, Philadelphia, Pa.*): I've had quite a lot of experience with canoe racing in Australia. We found two things most bothersome. One was hyperventilation in the heat. The other one has to do with a decrease in plasma volume. In 80° F and 112° F environments we have observed plasma shifts of water of up to 2 liters. In the heat, this seems to make it difficult for the athletes to recover. We found mean blood pressures down to 60 mmHg with a tendency to faint 15 to 20 minutes after exercise. I wondered whether Dr. Costill saw this response in marathon runners.

D. L. COSTILL: The transcapillary movement of plasma water is common to all exercise and is somewhat proportional to the exercise intensity. In this regard, I would like to know if you sampled blood from a forearm vein in these canoeists?

D. S. KRONFELD: Yes, we did.

D. L. COSTILL: This poses some problem for interpretation. The transcapillary movement of water that you're attempting to measure is the result of movement out of the plasma into active muscle tissue. This uptake of water is dependent, in part, on the hyperosmolarity of the tissue. In canoeists, I would expect that the forearm lactate levels are extremely high at the end of exercise. Thus, the fluid shifts may be extremely large across the arm, but not necessarily representative of the total plasma water loss. When exercising at 70%–80% of one's aerobic capacity, the marathoner usually shows a plasma water loss of 8%–16% because of this transcapillary shift. This would amount to no more than a 600 ml decrease in plasma volume, certainly less than your observations.

P. G. HANSON (*University of Wisconsin, Madison, Wisc.*): Some of our patients engage in regular exercise and also take diuretics. Dr. Knochel, do you think that this could pose a problem or do we need to take greater care in checking potassium? Is the sodium-potassium ratio an accurate assessment?

J. P. KNOCHEL (*Southwestern Medical School, Dallas, Texas*): Serum potassium concentration does not reflect intracellular potassium losses. A 600 meq body deficit of potassium may only be associated with a 0.4 meq/liter drop in the serum.

R. L. WESTERMAN (*Kalamazoo, Mich.*): The untrained individual who is suddenly exposed to heat and exercise may get into some difficulties. There may be a very different situation in the individual who is training regularly. There may be a readjustment of any potassium deficiencies that might have existed. I do not believe that anybody has really done good work to show what time course may exist for body potassium under these conditions.

COMMENT: I have been impressed with how often hypokalemia is associated with patients in renal failure. In a number of individuals we have found the presence of myoglobinuria and believe that the renal failure was directly related not only to those things that you showed but also to the presence of myoglobinuria. I wondered if you might speak to that thought in relation to myoglobinuria, renal hypokalemia, and the production of renal failure in some of the long distance runners.

J. P. KNOCHEL: Recently we had a patient who had run 5 miles and collapsed. This person was an occasional runner and he had been taking diuretics trying to induce some weight loss. When he collapsed his body temperature was 108° F, and he required dialysis for 2 weeks. This man, on the day he was admitted, had frank myoglobinuria and had a serum uric acid of 44 mg%. His BUN at the time of admission was only 17. So this man had a massive amount of muscle necrosis, which rapidly was converted to uric acid. I think people who are running, are not hydrated, and have injured muscles are prime candidates to develop acute renal failure. Obviously, if they are potassium deficient this would increase the jeopardy.

A. S. KUNIN: I think you try to put too many things into one box. If a patient who has hypokalemia also has polyuria, they won't run into trouble with a concentration of their urine. However, the individual that you're talking about sounds like there was massive dehydration and massive muscle necrosis, and I think sometimes it gets a little bit too complicated to explain in complete detail.

J. P. KNOCHEL: I think that the emphasis I placed on a large volume of urine, the nephrogenic diabetes insipidus, has been a very rare occurrence in these men. Most people with this have urines that are very concentrated, very acid.

A. S. KUNIN: Then it's not due to the potassium loss, it's due to the dehydration.

D. L. COSTILL: Dr. Knochel, I had read your paper and wondered how you were ever able to produce such extremely large potassium deficits when we know that sweat only contains 4–5 meq/liter. A marathon runner training 20 miles per day probably doesn't lose more than 4 or 5 liters of sweat. That means they are losing 20 to 25 meq of potassium per day. We have tried to induce deficits in these athletes, but fail to see more than a 1% decline in total body potassium in 4–5 days of training. Even in individuals who ingested only 25 meq of potassium per day, we failed to show more than a 70 meq potassium deficit after 4 days of exercise-dehydration (−4% dehydration per day). Thus I fail to be convinced that heavy sweating and exercise on repeated days offers a major threat to the training endurance athlete, especially when they are permitted to eat *ad libitum*.

J. P. KNOCHEL: The subjects in our studies consumed a very salty diet, like everybody in the military.

D. L. COSTILL: Yes, I know. Most people do not realize how much sodium they injest each day. We observed that subjects who were allowed to eat *ad libitum* consumed nearly twice the value reported in the clinical physiology textbooks.

CENTRAL CIRCULATORY FUNCTION DURING PROLONGED EXERCISE

L. Howard Hartley *

Department of Medicine
Harvard Medical School
Beth Israel Hospital
Boston, Massachusetts 02215

Dynamic muscular exercise induces predictable changes of the central circulation. With the onset of exercise, the heart rate increases from resting levels to a value that changes very little between 5 and 10 minutes of work. If exercise continues for a long period of time, the heart rate continues to rise. In FIGURE 1 the initial changes are indicated between the filled circles at rest and 10 minutes of exercise. The gradual drift of heart rate with prolonged exercise is indicated between the second filled symbol at 10 minutes and the third at 1 hour. The extent to which the heart rate will rise during prolonged work depends upon the intensity and the duration of exercise. At an intensity of about 70%–80% of maximal the heart rate quickens about 30 beats per minute or about 15%–20%.[1, 2] At lower intensities, the changes in heart rate are less, and after physical conditioning the increase in heart rate with prolonged work is less.[3]

The mechanical efficiency of man decreases with the passage of time. The usual increase in oxygen uptake during prolonged work is between 5% and 10% of the value at 10 minutes. This greater oxygen uptake is probably due to increased fat consumption during the prolonged work. The extent of the increase in oxygen uptake is not sufficient to explain completely the changes in heart rate that are observed during prolonged exercise.[2]

Body temperature also increases during prolonged work. Ekelund and Holmgren found a 1.6° C rise during 50 minutes of work.[1] Jose reported that the intrinsic heart rate is increased by 7 beats per minute per 1° C rise.[4] Hence the effect of temperature can explain only a small part of the heart rate rise during prolonged exercise.

Cardiac output measured by either the Fick method or dye dilution method does not change during prolonged exercise.[1, 2] Hence the stroke volume is changing reciprocally with the heart rate. Whether the changes in stroke volume are caused by the changes in heart rate or are causing the increase in heart rate is not certain. However, some evidence does suggest that the stroke volume may be reduced primarily.

The right ventricular diastolic pressure was 2.7 mmHg in the patients who had exercised for 10 minutes at a heart rate of 148 beats per minute in the study of Ekelund.[1] At 50 minutes, when the heart rate had reached 171 beats per minute, the filling pressure was 0. Corresponding values for diastolic pressure in the pulmonary artery indicated that at 10 minutes the pressure was 12.5 mmHg and fell to 9.5 after 50 minutes of work. These figures indicate that the filling pressures of both the right and left ventricles fall with the passage of time.

* Recipient of National Heart Institute Career Development Award Number KO HL 32645.

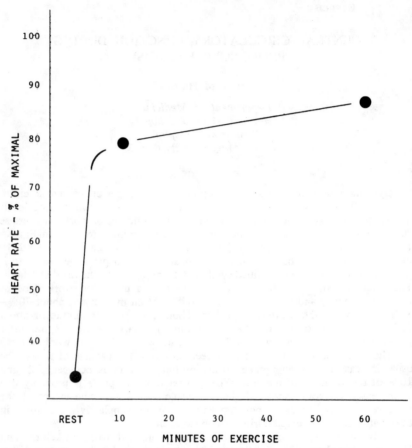

FIGURE 1. The adjustments of heart rate during prolonged heavy work.

Radiographic heart volumes are reduced at the time that the fall in ventricular filling pressures is occurring.

The reason for a decrease in filling pressure of the heart is not entirely clear. Plasma volume is reduced between 10 and 50 minutes of exercise,[1] but the reduction is small and not sufficient to explain the fall in stroke volume. The reduction in flow to the splanchnic and renal beds during prolonged exercise is even more pronounced than is the case during short-term work.[6] Presumably the increased volume of the venous bed is partly induced by augmentation of skin blood flow and partly by mechanisms that have not been clearly defined. Peripheral distribution of the intravascular volume seems to be the most likely explanation for the fall in venous return that occurs with prolonged work.

Ekelund observed that the radiographic heart volume increased in some of his subjects near exhaustion.[5] Although this suggests a change of either myocardial performance or compliance, the observation would be more impressive if intracardiac pressures rose simultaneously. Animal studies have indicated that myocardial performance can be altered by prolonged severe exercise.[7] In TABLE 1 the reduction in performance of isolated trabecular muscles from the left ventricles of rats is demonstrated.[7] The sedentary controls did not run, the trained controls ran downhill, and the exhausted rats ran uphill until they were exhausted. The control groups were not significantly different from each other, and the exhausted group had a lower peak developed tension and a lower velocity of contraction for any combination of preloads or afterloads. Electron microscopy of the rat myocardium after exhaustive exercise has been reported to show abnormalities of cellular structure.[8]

The mean arterial pressure has been found to be reduced over the 10-minute values if exercise persists to an hour.[1, 2] The extent of the reduction is variable, but the decrement is about 10 mmHg. Since the cardiac output does not change, this must represent a decrease in systemic vascular resistance. The mechanism of such a change is not completely understood, but dilation of the vessels to the skin is at least part of the explanation. The fall in resistance could contribute to the heart rate increase during exercise through carotid sinus stimulation. Splanchnic and renal vascular beds have reduced flows during exercise and are further reduced during prolonged work.[6] Blood flow to the exercising muscles during prolonged work has not been adequately studied.

The heart rate increment during prolonged work appears to be mediated by the autonomic nervous system. In FIGURE 2, the results of atropine administration on the heart rate response to work and of determination of circulating norepinephrine levels are demonstrated. On the abscissa are minutes of exercise at 70% to 80% of maximal work intensity. On the ordinate of the upper panel are the increases in heart rate that were induced by atropine administration intravenously.[9] On the ordinate of the lower panel are the values of plasma norepinephrine in micrograms per liter.[10] From 10 minutes to 1 hour the parasympathetic nervous system is almost completely withdrawn and the sympathetic nervous activity increases. These autonomic adjustments are probably the mechanism by which the heart rate increases during work.

Physiological responses very similar to the changes occurring during prolonged work can be induced during shorter exercise. If a mild work load (40% of maximal) is performed before and after a heavier work load (80% of maximal), the heart rate will be higher. TABLE 2 summarizes the results of such an experiment.[10] The heart rate is increased after the heavy work load compared to before. Some important differences, however, between this shorter exercise and prolonged exercise do occur. After the heavier work load there is no change in arterial pressure, oxygen uptake, or body temperature. The

TABLE 1

THE EFFECTS OF EXHAUSTIVE EXERCISE ON LEFT VENTRICULAR TRABECULAR MUSCLE PERFORMANCE IN THE RAT

	Peak Developed Tension (grams/mm²)	Velocity of Contraction (L_0/sec)
Sedentary controls ($n=8$)	2.5 ± 0.3	2.06 ± 0.1
Trained controls ($n=7$)	2.3 ± 0.2	2.38 ± 0.08
Exhausted ($n=11$)	1.1 ± 0.2	1.38 ± 0.18

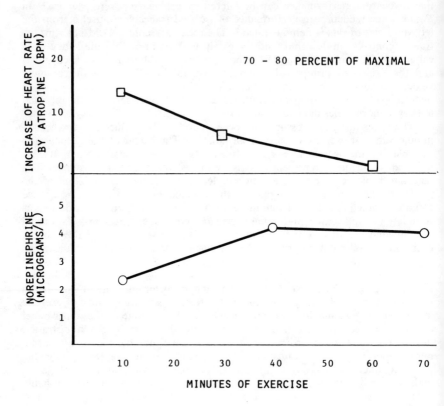

FIGURE 2. Autonomic nervous system activity during prolonged heavy work as judged by atropine blockade and plasma norepinephrine levels.

TABLE 2

THE CARDIOVASCULAR RESPONSE TO MILD EXERCISE BEFORE AND 10 MINUTES AFTER A HEAVY WORK LOAD *

	40% Maximal Work before 80% Load	after 80% Load 40% Maximal Work
Oxygen uptake (liters/min)	1.44	1.47
Heart rate (beats/min)	103.0	119.0
Cardiac output (liters/min)	13.0	12.9
Stroke volume (ml)	124.0	104.0
Arterial pressure (mmHg)	115.0	116.0

* Average values of 6 tests.

noraderenaline levels are not increased, but the administration of atropine completely ablated the effects of the previous work suggesting that withdrawal of parasympathetic tone was necessary for the effect. Although the exact relationship between this experimental protocol and prolonged work cannot be stated for certain, it does seem to indicate that it is possible to generate the heart rate changes without the presence of a fall in systemic vascular resistance, an increase in oxygen uptake, or a rise in body temperature.

The contribution of these cardiovascular changes in causing fatigue is not clear. Saltin performed experiments in which exercise testing was performed before and after a long bout of heavy, exhaustive exercise.[2] At 90 minutes after the exercise had finished, the submaximal heart rate was still elevated by 16 beats per minute. The maximal oxygen uptake was an average of 0.07 liters less (not significant in 15 subjects), the maximal work time was reduced by an average of 2.6 minutes, and the maximal blood lactate was reduced by 4.5 mmoles per liter. These findings suggest that the oxygen transporting characteristics of the individual are not impaired and that tissue and peripheral factors rather than central factors are probably responsible for the onset of fatigue.

In conclusion, the heart rate continues to rise during prolonged work above the initial 10-minute value. The increase in heart rate is mediated by parasympathetic nervous activity withdrawal and sympathetic activation. Part of the increment is caused by the increases in oxygen uptake and body temperature. The reduction in stroke volume is associated with decreased venous return to the heart, and this may be one of the mechanisms for the heart rate increase. Myocardial performance may be adversely affected by prolonged exercise; however, the evidence for such impairment is convincing only in experimental animals. Systemic vascular resistance is decreased, and this decrement contributes to the heart rate increase as well. The effects of heavy work on subsequent mild work indicates that an increase in heart rate can be induced without a fall in systemic vascular resistance. The central circulatory changes that occur with prolonged work do not seem to alter the oxygen-delivering capabilities of the cardiovascular system. The mechanism for fatigue probably resides in the muscle cells.

References

1. EKELUND, L. G. & A. HOLMGREN. 1964. Circulatory and respiratory adaptation during long-term, non-steady state exercise in the sitting position. Acta Physiol. Scand. **62**: 240–255.
2. SALTIN, B. 1964. Aerobic work capacity and circulation at exercise in man. Acta Physiol. Scand. **62** (Suppl. 230).
3. EKBLOM, B. 1970. Effect of training on circulation during prolonged severe exercise. Acta Physiol. Scand. **78**: 145–150.
4. JOSE, A. D., F. STITT & D. COLLISON. 1970. The effects of exercise and changes in body temperature on the intrinsic heart rate in man. Amer. Heart J. **79**: 488–497.
5. EKELUND, L., A. HOLMGREN & C. OVENFORS. 1967. Heart volume during prolonged exercise in the supine and sitting position. Acta Physiol. Scand. **70**: 88–98.
6. ROWELL, L. 1974. Human cardiovascular adjustments to exercise and thermal stress. Physiol. Rev. **54**: 75–159.
7. MAHER, J., A. GOODMAN, R. FRANCESCONI, W. BOWERS, L. HARTLEY & E. ANGLAKOS. 1972. Responses of rat myocardium to exhaustive exercise. Amer. J. Physiol. **222**: 207–212.

8. KING, D. & P. GOLLNICK. 1970. Ultrastructure of rat heart and liver after exhaustive exercise. Amer. J. Physiol. **218:** 1150–1155.
9. HARTLEY, L., B. PERNOW, H. HAGGENDAL, J. LACOUR, J. DELATTRE & B. SALTIN. 1970. Central circulation during submaximal work preceded by heavy exercise. J. Appl. Physiol. **29:** 818–823.
10. HARTLEY, L., J. MASON, R. HOGAN, L. JONES, T. KOTCHEN, E. MOUGEY, F. WHERRY, L. PENNINGTON & P. RICKETTS. 1972. Multiple hormonal responses to prolonged exercise in relation to physical training. J. Appl. Physiol. **33:** 607–610.

REGULATION OF SKIN CIRCULATION DURING PROLONGED EXERCISE *

John M. Johnson

University of Texas Health Science Center
San Antonio, Texas 78284

INTRODUCTION

Major demands on the circulation attending prolonged exercise are maintenance of blood flow to working skeletal muscle, dissipation of heat arising from the increased metabolic activity of skeletal muscle and maintenance of arterial blood pressure. The cardiovascular system is often unable to meet these competing demands in such events as the marathon. Cardiac output is constant or little changed during prolonged steady-state exercise.[1, 2] Even when exercise is performed in hot environments, cardiac output is not increased over levels achieved at the same level of work in a cool environment.[3, 4] Also, there are only small further reductions in visceral blood flow after the first few minutes of exercise.[5, 6] If blood flow to active skeletal muscle is maintained during prolonged exercise, skin blood flow and the regulation of internal temperature must suffer. Manifestations of this limitation have been observed [7-10] where rectal temperatures as high as 41° C were measured after distance races.

Skin thus represents the principle site of competition between thermal and nonthermal demands on blood flow distribution during exercise. Were the skin circulation regulated solely by body temperature, blood flow to skin would rise to high levels with the elevation in internal temperature accompanying exercise. In the face of a constant cardiac output, active muscle blood flow and/or arterial blood pressure would fall markedly in such a setting. However, if skin blood flow did not rise during exercise, internal temperature would quickly reach levels of extreme hyperthermia.

Few studies have dealt directly with the competitive nature of regulation of the cutaneous circulation during prolonged exercise. Thus, studies have dealt with the responses of the cutaneous circulation to heating at rest [11, 12] or with the responses during exercise [13-15] but have not considered the similarities or differences between the two settings.

The focus here, therefore, is on the control of skin blood flow during exercise. The objective is to show how competing demands for cardiac output limit skin blood flow. Emphasis is placed on how such control differs from that observed at rest. Specific problems attacked here include (a) whether skin blood low is lower during exercise than at the same level of internal temperature at rest, (b) the response of skin blood flow to prolonged work, (c) whether the reflex response of skin blood flow to rising skin temperature is influenced by exercise, and (d) the response of skin blood flow to the combination of heat stress and exercise when work in the heat is prolonged.

* This work was supported by National Heart and Lung Institute Grants HL–09773 and HL–16910.

195

Methods employed in this study have been reported in detail elsewhere. Since there is currently no method for the measurement of total skin blood flow, alterations in the vasomotor state of skin were assessed from changes in skin blood flow of the forearm. The neurogenic control of forearm skin blood flow reflects that over most of the body surface.[16] Further, the increase in forearm blood flow reflects the pattern and extent of increments in total skin blood flow during whole body direct heating at rest.[17, 18] Briefly, changes in skin blood flow were assessed by measuring changes in forearm blood flow. Since forearm muscle blood flow does not rise during whole-body direct heating,[19] indirect heating,[20, 21] local heating of the forearm,[22] or leg exercise,[13, 23] elevations in forearm blood flow are confined to skin. Forearm blood flow was measured by venous occlusion plethysmography with a mercury-in-silastic circumference gauge.[24] Internal temperature was measured as esophageal temperature with a thermocouple at the level of the left atrium. Skin temperature was measured as the electrical average of ten thermocouples placed at representative sites over the body surface. Whole-body skin temperature was controlled in some studies by dressing the subject in a water-perfused suit and passing hot or cold water through the suit tubing.[25, 26] Exercise was performed at a constant level on a bicycle ergometer. Workloads were chosen to represent moderate levels of exercise.

Response of Skin Blood Flow to Rising Internal Temperature

A first step in the study of the cutaneous circulation during exercise was to find whether its regulation was indeed modified by upright exercise. A number of studies have noted an initial forearm or hand vasoconstriction with the onset of leg exercise, which was succeeded by a steady vasodilation as exercise continued.[13-15, 27] Zelis et al.[15] found the initial forearm vasoconstriction to include both skin and muscle and to vary with the level of work. It was not clear from these studies whether the cutaneous vasoconstriction was of only a transient nature or, alternatively, whether the skin remained vasoconstricted relative to the level of internal temperature.

Thus the critical question was, is this response different than what would have been observed at rest at the same level of internal temperature? To force internal temperature to rise at rest, it was necessary to conduct studies at an elevated skin temperature (controlled by water-perfused suits). Therefore, all of these studies were performed at the same elevated skin temperature. A temperature of 38° C was chosen as a level that would yield an elevation of approximately 1°–1.5° C in internal temperature at rest, and had been observed in exercise in hot, natural environments.[28] Thus the relationship of forearm blood flow to internal temperature was observed in four settings: supine rest, supine exercise, upright rest, and upright exercise.[29]

FIGURES 1 and 2 show representative results from this study. Note that in FIGURE 1 the elevations in forearm blood flow and in internal temperature are considerably less in the upright than in the supine posture. These findings are consistent with earlier findings that the skin is vasoconstricted by orthostasis,[30, 31] and that this vasoconstriction is sustained in the face of a competing thermoregulatory drive for vasodilation.[32, 33] FIGURE 2 compares the responses to upright and supine exercise. Note that the postural effects mentioned above persist. FIGURE 3 relates forearm blood flow to esophageal temperature in each of the

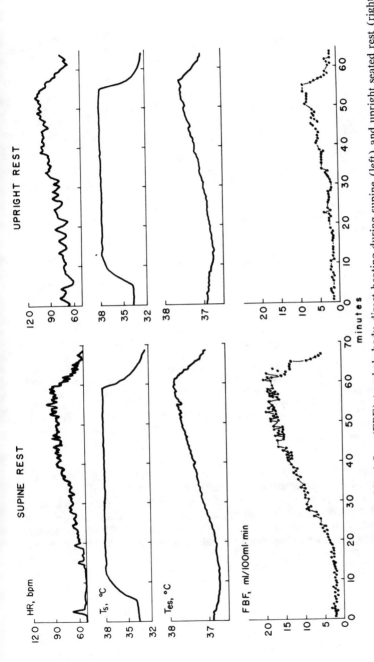

FIGURE 1. Response of forearm blood flow (FBF) to whole-body direct heating during supine (left) and upright seated rest (right) in one subject. Whole-body skin temperature (T_s) was held at 38° C in each case. Note that during upright rest, esophageal temperature (T_{es}) rose more slowly, indicating a relatively vasoconstricted skin. This point is borne out by the low levels of FBF achieved in the upright posture. Responses in heart rate (HR) are also shown. (From Johnson et al.[20] By permission of the American Physiological Society.)

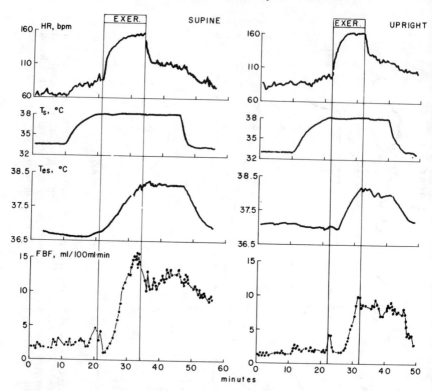

FIGURE 2. Responses of FBF, T_{es}, and HR to upright (right) and supine (left) exercise at a T_s of 38° C in one subject. Symbols and abbreviations are as in FIGURE 1. The periods of exercise are denoted by the vertical lines. Work load was 750 kpm/min (125 W) in each case. Note the more marked rise in FBF during supine (as compared to upright) exercise. (From Johnson et al.[29] By permission of the American Physiological Society.)

four conditions. There are several points to be made from these data. First, at a given level of internal temperature, forearm blood flow is lower in the upright position than in the supine posture either at rest or during exercise. Second, in either the upright or the supine posture, at a given level of internal temperature forearm blood flow was lower during exercise than at rest. Third, the forearm vasoconstriction relative to internal temperature is greatest when upright posture and exercise are combined.

These results offer direct confirmation that skin remains relatively vasoconstricted during exercise. Although there is some elevation in skin blood flow as exercise continues and internal temperature rises, this elevation is much less than that observed at rest. Thus skin is on the efferent arm of vasoconstrictor reflexes associated with exercise per se, as are the splanchnic,[6, 34] renal,[5, 35] and resting skeletal muscle[13-15, 23] circulations. This augmented vasoconstrictor drive to skin yields an attenuated response to thermoregulatory reflexes arising from elevations in internal temperature. Such an attenuated response must exist at high levels of work, as maximum oxygen intake can be reached in a hot environment.[36] However, sufficient heat stress can reduce maximal oxygen consumption,[37] indicating that a large fraction of the cardiac output can be directed to skin in that setting.

Response of Skin Blood Flow to Prolonged Exercise in Normal Environments

Given the responses noted in the preceding section, one would predict similar restrictions on skin blood flow during upright exercise in a cool or neutral environment. An additional vasoconstricting drive would arise from the lower levels of skin temperature in that setting, as opposed to the elevated skin temperatures used in the study mentioned above. Several studies [1, 2, 38] noted progressive cardiovascular adjustments and responses to prolonged exercise. These include steadily falling central venous pressure, stroke volume, and mean arterial pressure, with a steadily rising heart rate and little or no change in cardiac output. Possible mechanisms for these changes have been recently reviewed.[17] Briefly, one explanation for these findings (the so-called cardiovascular drift)

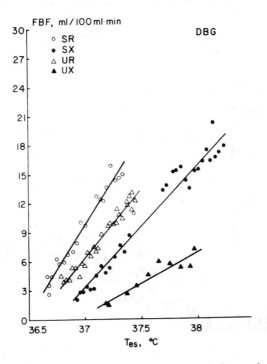

FIGURE 3. Composite of responses in FBF to rising T_{es} during supine rest (SR), supine exercise (SX), upright rest (UR), and upright exericse (UX) in one subject. Skin temperature was 38° C in all cases. Data from each experiment were fitted with a regression line, as shown. Note that at a given level of T_{es}, FBF is reduced by upright posture both at rest and during exercise and that FBF is reduced by exercise in either posture. Abbreviations as in FIGURE 1. (From Johnson et al.[29] By permission of the American Physiological Society.)

is that prolonged heavy work results in myocardial fatigue.[2, 38] Such a notion is supported to some extent by the finding of increased duration of systole attending prolonged exercise.[1] An alternative explanation offered by Rowell [17] points out that some or all of these changes might be accounted for by a steady peripheral displacement of blood volume. Such a displacement would reduce filling pressures and stroke volume. Heart rate increases would compensate for the reduction in stroke volume, maintaining cardiac output. A logical site for such a peripheral displacement of blood volume is the cutaneous vascular bed. Raising local compliance or pressure in cutaneous veins would raise this volume. Cutaneous venous pressure would passively rise in response to a similar increase in skin blood flow.

Consistent with this explanation, we observed a progressive increase in forearm skin blood flow during one hour of continuous exercise.[23] The workload was 600 kpm/min (100 W) for one subject and 750 kpm/min (125 W) for the other four subjects. FIGURE 4 shows results from one of these experiments.

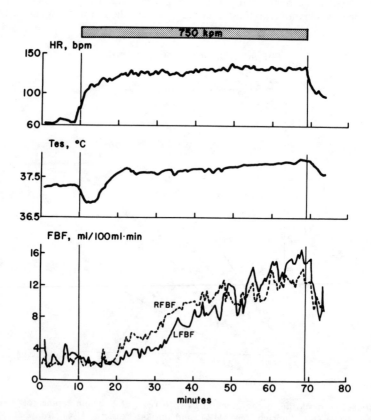

FIGURE 4. Responses of FBF, T_{es}, and HR to one hour of exercise (750 kpm/min; 125 W) in a neutral environment (ambient temperature 24° C). LFBF is left forearm blood flow and RFBF is right forearm blood flow. Other abbreviations as in FIGURE 1. (From Johnson & Rowell.[23] By permission of the American Physiological Society.)

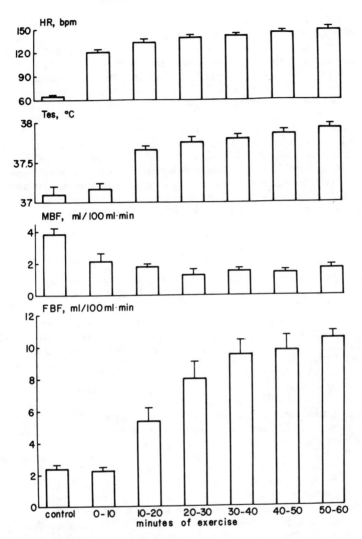

FIGURE 5. Composite responses of HR, T_{es}, forearm muscle blood flow (MBF), and FBF during rest and one hour of exercise from all subjects studied. Each bar shows the mean and standard error of the response for each parameter for each 10-min period. MBF was measured from the clearance of a depot of [^{125}I]-antipyrine injected 1 cm into the brachioradiolis muscle. Other abbreviations as in FIGURE 1. (From Johnson & Rowell.[23] By permission of the American Physiological Society.)

Thus we see a progressive rise in forearm blood flow, beginning at about 10 minutes of exercise and continuing throughout the remainder of the work period. FIGURE 5 shows the responses of the entire group, averaged over each 10-minute interval of exercise. Although skin blood flow progressively rose, and may indeed account for other circulatory changes attending prolonged exercise, the final levels achieved were still less than what would be expected at a comparable level of internal temperature in a resting individual.

The problems associated with the combination of an elevated internal temperature and a relatively low skin blood flow become increasingly severe with the level of work or environmental temperature. Rectal temperature is maintained at essentially the same level for a given workload over a wide variation in environmental temperatures,[39] indicating skin blood flow must be increased with environmental temperature. This increment in skin blood flow is apparently met by further redistribution of flow from the viscera,[40, 41] as cardiac output is not increased.[3, 4] However, as environmental conditions become more extreme, internal temperature is no longer stable and visceral blood flow reaches potentially ischemic levels.[42] Similarly, high levels of heat production can stress the ability of the cardiovascular system both to meet thermoregulatory needs and to deliver oxygen to skeletal muscle. Clearly, the combination of high levels of exercise and heat stress tax the cardiovascular system to severe limits.

Influence of Skin Temperature during Exercise

The foregoing studies show that competition between body temperature regulation and exercise per se for the control of skin blood flow yields a vasoconstriction relative to the level of body temperature and a vasodilation relative to drives from upright posture and exercise. One notable difference between studies at high and neutral levels of skin temperature was that skin blood flow increased from the beginning when exercise was performed at a high level of skin temperature (FIGURE 2) but failed to increase for the first 10 minutes of exercise in the study performed at a low skin temperature (FIGURE 4). This observation indicates that skin temperature plays an important role in the responses to rising internal temperature during exercise. However, observations on resting man assign only a minor role to skin temperature.[11, 12] On the other hand, Rowell et al.[25] noted a marked rise in cardiac output in response to a rise in whole-body skin temperature during exercise.

Is the reflex response to an elevation in skin temperature altered during exercise? Also, to what extent can the above elevation in cardiac output be ascribed to direct (nonreflex) effects of heating the skin? To answer these questions, whole-body skin temperature was rapidly raised during exercise, as well as at rest. Forearm blood flow was measured in both arms. One arm was left exposed to ambient conditions, or controlled at 32° C, thus reflecting reflex vasomotor adjustments. The other arm was warmed according to the whole-body skin temperature protocol, thus reflecting responses to combined direct and reflex effects of raising skin temperature.

FIGURE 6 shows an example of one such study. At 10 minutes, exercise was initiated at 525 kpm/min (88 W) and at a skin temperature of 32° C. At 30 minutes, skin temperature was rapidly elevated toward 38° C. Esophageal temperature (T_{es}) fell transiently, and during this period of rising skin temperature and reduced or unchanged esophageal temperature forearm blood flow rose markedly in both arms. Forearm blood flow (FBF) showed only a small further rise while skin temperature was held at 38° C and internal temperature rose above preheating levels. This was usually the case. FIGURE 7 shows the relation between FBF and T_{es} during the same protocol in another subject. In this case the workload was 750 kpm/min (125 W). Again, there was a prompt elevation in forearm blood flow in both arms with the elevation in skin temperature with no change in esophageal temperature. This corresponds to the vertical portion of the data in FIGURE 7. Here, as in most subjects the level of forearm blood flow leveled off, despite a marked further rise in esophageal temperature. Of the six subjects studied with this protocol, four showed this "leveling off" phe-

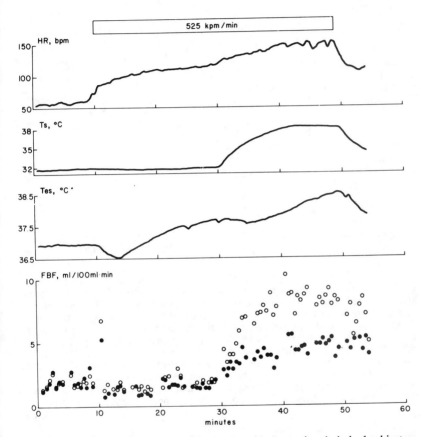

FIGURE 6. FRB, T_{es}, and HR responses to a rapid change in whole body skin temperature (T_s) during upright exercise (525 kpm/min; 88 W). The left forearm (open symbols) was warmed along with the rest of the body and the right forearm (closed symbols) was kept at 32° C throughout. At 10 min, exercise began and continued until 50 min. Between 30 and 40 min, T_s and the local temperature of the left forearm were raised to 38° C. Note the marked rise in FBF to each arm during the period of depressed T_{es} between 30 and 38 min. Abbreviations as in FIGURE 1.

nomenon. Application of the same protocol to resting men revealed little or no elevation in forearm blood flow with rising skin temperature in the arm held at a neutral temperature, and only a modest elevation in the blood flow to the arm heated with the rest of the body. As in previous studies most of the increase in FBF was due to rising internal temperature during whole-body direct heating

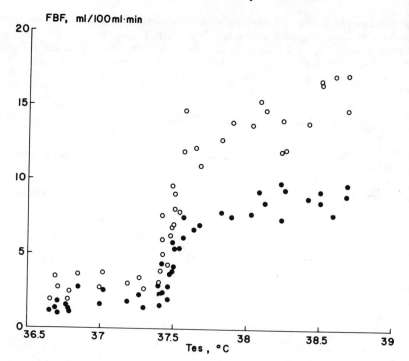

FIGURE 7. FBF vs T_{es} from a protocol like that shown in FIGURE 6. The open symbols represent FBF from the arm heated according to the whole-body T_s protocol and the closed symbols represent FBF from the arm kept cool. The horizontal portion of the data (in the lower left hand portion of the plot) are from the period of rising T_{es} and essentially constant FBF during the first few minutes of exercise at low T_s. The vertical portion of the data show the response during the period of rapidly rising T_s (imposed by water perfused suits) with unchanging T_{es}. The horizontal portion of the data in the upper right of the figure represent the final 10 min of exercise at a T_s of 38° C. Data from the left (warmed arm, open symbols) indicate the response to combined effects of rising T_s, T_{es}, and local temperature while data from the arm kept cool indicate reflex responses only. Abbreviations as in FIGURE 1.

at rest;[11, 12, 29] thus the roles of skin and internal temperatures appear to be somewhat reversed between rest and exercise. That is, during whole-body direct heating at rest, there is only a minor contribution by skin temperature and a major contribution by internal temperature to cutaneous vasodilation. During exercise, there appears to be a major effect of skin temperature. TABLE 1 shows the results of multiple linear regression analysis of data from these protocols. These coefficients show the rise in forearm blood flow per ° C rise in internal temperature and skin temperature, respectively. Data are given for both the cool arm and the arm warmed with the rest of the body, both at rest and during exercise. Note the increase in the response to skin temperature and the decrease in the response to internal temperature during exercise as opposed to rest. These coefficients probably do not apply to all levels of exercise. It is also likely that the level of internal temperature is a major determinant of the response to rising skin temperature. For example, one might hypothesize that the combined vaso-constrictor drives from low skin temperature, upright posture, and exercise would be sufficient to mask effects of vasodilator drive from increased internal temperature. When skin temperature is suddenly raised, however, much of this previously suppressed vasodilator drive is allowed to act, and skin blood flow rises markedly. Although this explanation is consistent with these observations, other models of control could also explain the data. The point here is that it is currently unclear how the various drives for skin blood flow interact, and that linear additive models for control of the cutaneous circulation by skin and internal temperatures are presumptive. Nevertheless, two points are evident from this analysis. First, the reflex vasomotor responses in skin to elevations in skin and/or internal temperature are markedly altered during exercise (as compared to rest). Second, the elevation in cardiac output with whole-body

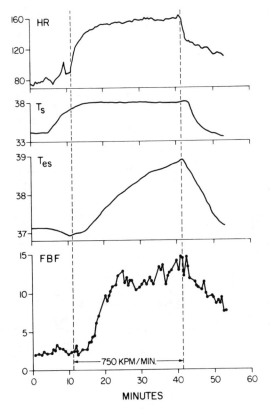

FIGURE 8. FBF, T_{es}, and HR responses to prolonged (30 min) exercise at high T_s (38° C). At 5 min T_s was elevated and when it had reached 38° C the subject began to exercise (125 W or 750 kpm/min). Note the rapid rise in FBF until 25 min (when T_{es} had reached approximately 38° C) after which there was little or no fur-ther rise in FBF, despite a marked further elevation in T_{es}. Abbreviations as in FIGURE 1.

direct heating at rest [26] or during exercise [25] includes a significant component due to the direct local effects of elevating skin temperature.

Taken together, the results from the three experiments discussed so far indicate the effect of skin temperature is essentially to inhibit or permit reflex vasomotor responses in skin to internal temperature. Thus, with exercise at a cool skin temperature, internal temperature rises appreciably, but is not accompanied by a similar response in skin blood flow (FIGURES 4 & 5). Removal of

TABLE 1

RESULTS OF REGRESSION ANALYSIS FOR FBF RESPONSE TO CHANGE IN T_s AND T_{es} AT REST AND DURING EXERCISE *

Subject	Arm Treatment	Regression Coefficients	
		α (FBF/T_{es})	β (FBF/T_s)
DG (rest)	C	9.78	NS
	W	10.15	0.80
DG (825 kpm/min; 135 W)	C	3.77	1.28
	W	3.89	2.53
RK (rest)	C	10.19	0.12
	W	7.93	1.03
RK (600 kpm/min; 100 W)	C	3.69	1.44
	W	5.16	2.54
GN (rest)	C	17.45	0.17
	W	24.35	0.48
GN (750 kpm/min; 125 W)	C	1.13	1.05
	W	2.08	1.76
DW (rest)	C	14.78	NS
	W	10.09	1.49
DW (750 kpm/min; 125 W)	C	NS	2.74
	W	NS	2.53
SF (750 kpm/min; 125 W)	C	1.62	0.72
	W	3.15	1.36
JJ (525 kpm/min; 88 W)	C	NS	0.42
	W	NS	1.02

* See FIGURE 6 for specific protocol. Subjects are listed according to whether the study was done at rest or during exercise. Work loads are given in parenthesis. Regression coefficients for the arm kept cool (C) and for the arm warmed according to the whole-body T_s protocol (W) show the rise in FBF per degree rise in T_{es} (α) and the rise in FBF per degree rise in T_s (β). NS indicates the value was not significantly different from 0. Units for α and β are ml/100 ml·min·°C.

this inhibition due to low skin temperature (by elevating skin temperature) before (FIGURES 2 & 3) or during exercise (FIGURES 6 & 7) allows much of the effect of the elevation in internal temperature to become manifest. Parenthetically, skin blood flow is reflexly controlled by two distinct arms of the sympathetic nervous system.[16, 43] It is consistent with these results and the findings of others [11, 12, 43, 44] that the vasoconstrictor arm is responsive to changes in skin temperature, while the vasodilator arm is responsive to changes in internal temperature. As vasoconstrictor outflow to skin is also increased by upright posture and exercise, it seems likely that such augmented vasoconstrictor outflow would restrict responses to rising vasodilator outflow. Thus, during the first few minutes of upright exercise at a cool skin temperature, internal temperature could rise by a significant amount without a corresponding rise in skin blood flow. This is what we observed. Withdrawal of a significant portion of the vasoconstrictor outflow due to rising skin temperature would allow the effects of previously overridden vasodilator outflow to become manifest. The findings in the foregoing experiment are consistent with such a scheme of control for skin blood flow.

Responses to Prolonged Exercise at High Skin Temperature

Whatever the involvement of the two arms of the sympathetic nervous system in the control of skin blood flow, the "leveling off" phenomenon was unexpected. Heat stress at even higher levels of skin and internal temperatures reveal no comparable phenomenon at rest.[12, 19] To insure that such an observation was not in some way dependent on the specific protocol, we elevated skin temperature to 38° C just prior to the initiation of 30 minutes of exercise.[45] FIGURE 8 shows the results of one such study. This protocol is identical to that in the first series of experiments reported here, except that the duration of exercise was extended to 30 minutes. As seen in the experiment shown in FIGURE 8, forearm blood flow rose with internal temperature in a linear fashion. However, at an esophageal temperature of approximately 38° C, forearm blood flow leveled off. Thus skin blood flow responds to rising internal temperature during exercise only over a limited range of internal temperature.

Although not all subjects revealed the "leveling off" phenomenon as dramatically as in this case, most did. Further, no subject showed more than a modest rise in forearm blood flow above an esophageal temperature of 38° C, despite further large increments in internal temperature. Such a phenomenon shows that the ability of the cardiovascular system to meet extreme challenges to temperature regulation during exercise is severely limited. Only when skin temperature is raised, as in this experiment, is cardiac output known to rise when heat stress is added to exercise.[25] Even in that case the elevation in cardiac output is limited. Redistribution of blood flow from nonactive regions is also limited, leaving only active muscle as a possible source of blood flow to skin. Therefore, given that the supply of blood is limited, skin blood flow must have a limitation of its response during exercise. This is borne out by the observation, here, of the apparent upper limit to forearm skin blood flow. Such an upper limit would contribute to the hyperthermia of exercise in natural environments such as the marathon.

DISCUSSION

The experiments reported here show skin blood flow to be responsive to more than thermoregulatory drives. During exercise skin is vasoconstricted at any given level of internal temperature (relative to supine rest). Both posture and exercise per se contribute to the vasoconstrictor drive, while high internal temperature and skin temperature contribute to competing drives for vasodilation. Thus, at a given level of internal temperature, skin blood flow is less during exercise than at rest. These observations offer direct corroboration of a low skin blood flow in exercise predicted [17] on the basis of (a) no increase in cardiac output, (b) limited redistribution capacity from the viscera, and (c) the ability to sometimes (but not always) achieve maximal oxygen consumption during exercise in the heat. The only situation wherein cardiac output is increased by heat stress during exercise occurs when the skin over the entire body surface is heated to high levels, as by water perfused suits. Even in this extreme situation, the elevation in skin blood flow (i.e., cardiac output) is limited. Thus, the elevation in cardiac output of only 2–2.5 liters/min observed previously,[25] and the constancy of forearm blood flow above an internal temperature of approximately 38° C were both observed to accompany a rapid elevation in skin temperature during exercise.

What are the consequences of such a competitive scheme of control for skin blood flow? First, the ability of the body to lose heat is compromised during exercise. Although sweat rate may be extremely high, convective transfer of heat to the surface is determined by skin blood flow. Second, compensatory vasoconstriction of splanchnic and renal vascular beds becomes extreme during the combination of heat stress and exercise. Rowell et al.[42] observed hepatic venous oxygen contents as low as 0.5 ml O_2/100 ml blood during heavy exercise in a hot environment. They also observed an outpouring of hepatic glucose that is often the sign of hepatic ischemia. Renal function is also subject to compromise, as indicated by findings of protein, red blood cells and myoglobin in urine following exercise in the heat.[46, 47] Clearly, as duration or humidity or level of exercise or ambient conditions become more extreme, the probability of heat stroke increases markedly. Comprehensive treatments of heat stroke [48–50] show the incidence of heat deaths and disorders to be greatest when exercise, cardiovascular disease, and hot, humid environments are combined.

A third consequence of vasomotor adjustments in skin is the redistribution of blood volume to cutaneous veins. As cutaneous blood flow rises, blood volume in cutaneous veins must also passively increase. Cutaneous venomotor activity has only been studied for short durations of exercise.[14, 51, 52] There is a marked cutaneous venoconstriction at the initiation of exercise. As internal temperature rises, cutaneous venous compliance returns toward resting levels. If local skin temperature or whole body skin temperature is elevated, cutaneous venoconstrictor responses to exercise are abolished. At any level of cutaneous venous compliance, cutaneous blood volume will passively rise as veins are distended by rising skin blood flow. A high cutaneous blood volume is efficacious for heat elimination, i.e., linear velocity of blood is low, allowing time for heat transfer.

However, a high cutaneous blood volume poses a problem for the central cardiovascular adjustments to exercise. As cutaneous blood volume rises, blood volume in other areas falls accordingly. Central blood volume and probably splanchnic blood volume fall, as does right atrial pressure.[25] The consequent fall in cardiac filling pressures leads to a reduction in stroke volume.[1, 25] Compensatory increments in heart rate maintain cardiac output in a neutral environment,[1, 2] but may fail to do so in hot ambient conditions.[4] Ironically, the mechanism that tends to slow the accumulation of blood in cutaneous veins is vasoconstriction (i.e., lowering the rate of filling) rather than venoconstriction (lowering the ultimate volume).

With respect to the marathon, the relevance of these observations of cutaneous vasomotor and venomotor adjustments to prolonged work or to work in the heat is as follows. First, work rates are generally quite high[53] and internal temperature often rises to high levels. Marathons are often conducted when ambient conditions (i.e., temperature and humidity) are elevated. Pugh et al.[8] and Wyndahm et al.[9] found the rectal temperature of marathon winners to be about 41° C in mild environmental conditions. Heat stroke, injury, or death have occurred following marathon running, or cycling, with rectal temperatures as high as 43° C.[45] Pathology of renal and splanchnic regions associated with excessive body temperatures following competitive events are common.[48-50, 54] As sweat rates are usually high, these high levels of internal temperature are due to relatively low levels of skin blood flow. Finally, measurements of air temperature do not consider the radiant heat loads to which the competitor is subjected. On a clear day, solar radiation can be a major source of heat. Simulation of solar radiant heating can yield skin temperatures of 37°–41° C in exposed areas at rest.[55-57] However, equivalent data from exercise are unavailable.

Thus skin blood flow participates in reflexes other than those involved in temperature regulation. The temperature we maintain in conditions other than supine rest is largely the resultant of competing vasodilator and vasoconstrictor drives to skin. When drives for vasoconstriction are great, as the result of upright posture, exercise, or disease, temperature regulation can fall victim to blood pressure regulation and/or to adjustments to exercise. When heat stress becomes severe then even blood pressure regulation can fail, with pathologic consequences for renal and splanchnic tissues. The common findings of anuria and nausea are therefore not surprising. As the marathon represents possibly the greatest stress to which man voluntarily taxes his cardiovascular system, problems arising from competition for control of skin blood flow are a natural consequence.

ACKNOWLEDGMENTS

The author is grateful for helpful suggestions from Dr. Loring B. Rowell and Dr. Ethan R. Nadel.

REFERENCES

1. EKLUND, L. G. 1972. Circulatory and respiratory adaptation during prolonged exercise. Acta Physiol. Scand. **70** (Suppl. 292).
2. SALTIN, B. & J. STENBERG. 1964. Circulatory response to prolonged severe exercise. J Appl. Physiol. **19:** 833–838.
3. WILLIAMS, C. G., G. A. G. BREDELL, C. H. WYNDHAM, N. B STRYDOM, J. F. MORRISON, J. PETER, P. W. FLEMING & J S. WARD. 1962. Circulatory and metabolic reactions to work in the heat. J. Appl. Physiol. **17:** 625–638.
4. ROWELL, L. B., H. J. MARX, R. A. BRUCE, R. D. CONN & F. KUSUMI. 1966. Reductions in cardiac output, central blood volume, and stroke volume with thermal stress in normal men during exercise. J. Clin. Invest. **45:** 1801–1816.
5. GRIMBY, G. 1965. Renal clearances during prolonged supine exercise at different loads. J. Appl. Physiol. **20:** 1294–1298.
6. ROWELL, L. B., K. K. KRANING II, T. O. EVANS, J. W. KENNEDY, J. R. BLACKMON, & F. KUSUMI. 1966. Splanchnic removal of lactate and pyruvate during prolonged exercise in man. J. Appl. Physiol. **21:** 1773–1783.

7. ROBINSON, S. 1949. Physiological Adjustments to Heat. L. H. Newburgh, Ed. : 193–231. W. B. Saunders Company. Philadelphia, Pa.

8. PUGH, L. G. C. E., J. L. CORBETT & R. H. JOHNSON. 1967. Rectal temperatures, weight losses, and sweat rates in marathon running. J. Appl. Physiol. **23:** 347–352.

9. WYNDHAM, C. H. & N. B. STRYDOM. 1969. The danger of inadequate water intake during marathon running. S. Afr. Med. J. **43:** 893–896.

10. COSTILL, D. L., W. F. KAMMER & A. FISHER. 1970. Fluid ingestion during distance running. Arch. Environ. Health **21:** 520–525.

11. WYSS, C. R., G. L. BRENGELMANN, J. M. JOHNSON, L. B. ROWELL & M. NIEDERBERGER. 1974. Control of skin blood flow, sweating, and heart rate: role of skin vs. core temperature. J. Appl. Physiol. **36:** 726–733.

12. WYSS, C. R., G. L. BRENGELMANN, J. M. JOHNSON, L. B. ROWELL & D. SILVERSTEIN. 1975. Altered control of skin blood flow at high skin and core temperatures. J. Appl. Physiol. **38:** 839–845.

13. BLAIR, D. A., W. E. GLOVER & I. C. RODDIE. 1961. Vasomotor responses in the human arm during leg exercise. Circ. Res. **9:** 264–274.

14. BEVEGARD, B. S. & J. T. SHEPHERD. 1966. Reaction in man of resistance and capacity vessels in forearm and hand to leg exercise. J. Appl. Physiol. **21:** 123–132.

15. ZELIS, R., D .T. MASON & E. BRAUNWALD. 1967. Partition of blood flow to the cutaneous and muscular beds of the forearm at rest and during leg exercise in normal subjects and in patients with heart failure. Circ. Res. **24:** 799–806.

16. FOX, R. H. & O. G. EDHOLM. 1963. Nervous control of the cutaneous circulation. Brit. Med. Bull. **19:** 110–114.

17. ROWELL, L. B. 1974. Human cardiovascular adjustments to exercise and thermal stress. Physiol. Rev. **54:** 75–159.

18. KOROXENIDIS, G. T. & J. T. SHEPHERD. 1961. Cardiovascular response to acute heat stress. J. Appl. Physiol. **16:** 869–872.

19. DETRY, J.-M. R., G. L. BRENGELMANN, L. B. ROWELL & C. WYSS. 1972. Skin and muscle components of forearm blood flow in directly heated resting man. J. Appl. Physiol. **32:** 506–511.

20. EDHOLM, O. G., R. H. FOX & R. K. MACPHERSON. 1956. The effect of body heating on the circulation in skin and muscle. J. Physiol. (London) **134:** 612–619.

21. RODDIE, I. C., J. T. SHEPHERD & R. F. WHELAN. 1956. Evidence from venous oxygen saturation measurements that the increase in forearm blood flow during body heating is confined to the skin. J. Physiol. (London) **134:** 444–450.

22. JOHNSON, J. M., G. L. BRENGELMANN & L. B. ROWELL. 1976. Interaction between local and reflex influences on human forearm skin blood flow. J. Appl. Physiol. **41:** 826–831.

23. JOHNSON, J. M. & L. B. ROWELL. 1975. Forearm skin and muscle vascular responses to prolonged leg exercise in man. J. Appl. Physiol. **39:** 920–924.

24. WHITNEY, R. J. 1953. The measurement of volume changes in human limbs. J. Physiol. (London) **121:** 1–27.

25. ROWELL, L. B., J. A. MURRAY, G. L. BRENGELMANN & K. K. KRANING II. 1969. Human cardiovascular adjustments to rapid changes in skin temperature during exercise. Circ. Res. **24:** 711–724.

26. ROWELL, L. B., G. L. BRENGELMANN & J. A. MURRAY. 1969. Cardiovascular responses to sustained high skin temperature in resting man. J. Appl. Physiol. **27:** 673–680.

27. CHRISTENSEN, E. H., M. NIELSEN & B. HANNISDAHL. 1942. Investigations of the circulation in the skin at the beginning of muscular work. Acta Physiol. Scand. **4:** 162–170.

28. ROWELL, L. B., K. K. KRANING II, J. W. KENNEDY & T. O. EVANS. 1967. Central circulatory responses to work in dry heat before and after acclimatization. J. Appl. Physiol. **22:** 509–518.

29. JOHNSON, J. M., L. B. ROWELL & G. L. BRENGELMANN. 1974. Modification of the skin blood flow-body temperature relationship by upright exercise. J. Appl. Physiol. **37:** 880–886.

30. BEISER, G. D., R. ZELIS, S. E. EPSTEIN, D. T. MASON & E. BRAUNWALD. 1970. The role of skin and muscle resistance vessels in reflexes mediated by the baroreceptor system. J. Clin. Invest. **49:** 225–231.

31. ROWELL, L. B., C. R. WYSS & G. L. BRENGELMANN. 1973. Sustained human skin and muscle vasoconstriction with reduced baroreceptor activity. J. Appl. Physiol. **34:** 639–643.

32. CROSSLEY, R. J., A. D. M. GREENFIELD, G. C. PLASSARAS & D. STEPHENS. 1966. The interrelation of thermoregulatory and baroreceptor reflexes in the control of blood vessels in the human forearm. J. Physiol. (London) **183:** 628–636.

33. JOHNSON, J. M., M. NIEDERBERGER, L. B. ROWELL, M. M. EISMAN & G. L. BRENGELMANN. 1973. Competition between cutaneous vasodilator and vasoconstrictor reflexes in man. J. Appl. Physiol. **35:** 798–803.

34. ROWELL, L. B., J. R. BLACKMON & R. A. BRUCE. 1966. Indocyanine green clearance and estimated hepatic blood flow during mild to maximal exercise in upright man. J. Clin. Invest. **43:** 1677–1690.

35. CHAPMAN, C. B., A. HENSCHEL, J. MINCKLER, A. FORSGREN & A. KEYS. 1948. The effect of exercise on renal plasma flow in normal male subjects. J. Clin. Invest. **27:** 639–644.

36. ROWELL, L. B., G. L. BRENGELMANN, J. A. MURRAY, K. K. KRANING II & F. KUSUMI. 1969. Human metabolic responses to hyperthermia during mild to maximal exercise. J. Appl. Physiol. **26:** 395–402.

37. PIRNAY, F., R. DEROANNE & J. M. PETIT. 1970. Maximal oxygen consumption in a hot environment. J. Appl. Physiol. **28:** 642–645.

38. HARTLEY, L. H. & B. SALTIN. 1968. Reduction of stroke volume and increase in heart rate after a previous heavier submaximal workload. Scand. J. Clin. Lab. Invest. **22:** 217–223.

39. NIELSEN, M. 1938. Die Regulation der Korpertemperatur bei Muskelarbeit. Skand. Arch. Physiol. **79:** 193–230.

40. ROWELL, L. B., J. R. BLACKMON, R. H. MARTIN, J. A. MAZZARELLA & R. A. BRUCE. 1965. Hepatic clearance of indocyanine green in man under thermal and exercise stress. J. Appl. Physiol. **20:** 384–394.

41. RADIGAN, L. R. & S. ROBINSON. 1949. Effects of environmental heat stress and exercise on renal blood flow and filtration rate. J. Appl. Physiol. **2:** 185–191.

42. ROWELL, L. B., G. L. BRENGELMANN, J. R. BLACKMON, R. D. TWISS & F. KUSUMI. 1968. Splanchnic blood flow and metabolism in heat-stressed man. J. Appl. Physiol. **24:** 475–484.

43. EDHOLM, O. G., R. H. FOX & R. K. MACPHERSON. 1957. Vasomotor control of the cutaneous blood vessels in the human forearm. J. Physiol. (London) **139:** 455–465.

44. RODDIE, I. C., J. T. SHEPHERD & R. F. WHELAN. 1957. The vasomotor nerve supply to the skin and muscle of the human forearm. Clin. Sci. **16:** 67–74.

45. BRENGELMANN, G. L., J. M. JOHNSON, L. B. ROWELL, L. HERMANSEN & H. D. PATTON. 1976. Upper limit to skin blood flow in exercising man. Fed. Proc. **35:** 482.

46. SCHRIER, R. W., H. S. HENDERSON & C. C. TISHER. 1967. Nephropathy associated with heat stress and exercise. Ann. Int. Med. **67:** 356–376.

47. SMITH, R. F. 1968. Exertional rhabdomyolysis in naval officer candidates. Arch. Int. Med. **121:** 313–319.

48. LEITHEAD, C. S. & A. R. LIND. 1964. Heat Stress and Heat Disorders. Davis. Philadelphia, Pa.

49. ELLIS, F. P. 1972. Mortality from heat illness and heat-aggravated illness in the United States. Environ. Res. **5:** 1–58.

50. SHIBOLET, S., M. C. LANCASTER & Y. DANON. 1976. Heat stroke: A review. Aviat. Space Environ. Med. **47:** 280–301.

51. ROWELL, L. B., G. L. BRENGELMANN, J. M. R. DETRY & C. WYSS. 1971. Venomotor responses to rapid changes in skin temperature in exercising man. J. Appl. Physiol. **30:** 64–71.
52. ZITNIK, R. S., E. AMBROSIONI & J. T. SHEPHERD. 1971. Effect of temperature on cutaneous venomotor reflexes in man. J. Appl. Physiol. **31:** 507–512.
53. COSTILL, D. L. & E. L. FOX. 1969. Energetics of marathon running. Med. Sci. Sports. **1:** 81–96.
54. WYNDHAM, C. H. 1973. The physiology of exercise under heat stress. Ann. Rev. Physiol. **35:** 193–220.
55. STOLWIJK, J. A. J. & J. D. HARDY. 1965. Skin and subcutaneous temperature changes during exposure to intense thermal radiation. J. Appl. Physiol. **20:** 1006–1013.
56. NADEL, E. R., R. W. BULLARD & J. A. J. STOLWIJK. 1971. Importance of skin temperature in the regulation of sweating. J. Appl. Physiol. **31:** 80–87.
57. HARDY, J. D. 1963. Thermal effects of solar radiation in man. Solar Effects on Building Design, No. **1007:** 19–30.

MYOCARDIAL BLOOD FLOW AND OXYGEN CONSUMPTION DURING EXERCISE

Charles R. Jorgensen, Frederick L. Gobel,
Henry L. Taylor, and Yang Wang

*Department of Medicine
and
Laboratory of Physiological Hygiene
University of Minnesota Medical School
Minneapolis, Minnesota 55455*

Our concepts of what variables determine myocardial oxygen consumption $(M\dot{V}_{O_2})$ have evolved considerably over the last six to seven decades. Perhaps the earliest significant investigation of this problem was published in 1912 showing that oxygen use in an isovolumetrically contracting preparation was proportional to the product of pulse rate and left ventricular pulse pressure.[1] For many years stroke work, the product of stroke volume and arterial pressure, was considered the primary factor, although it was recognized early that pressure work is more expensive than volume work and that pressure changes reflect changes in ventricular wall tension only if ventricular volume is not altered.[2] Very comprehensive approaches have thought in terms of contractile element work,[3] an entity based on the three component model of muscle and requiring several difficult measurements and some assumptions in its calculation. Our current understanding is relatively complete and is the result of the work of many investigators, primarily with *in vitro* preparations. A number of factors have been identified as determinants of myocardial oxygen consumption [4-7] (TABLE 1), but the major factors are: (a) the heart rate; (b) internal work, the stress or tension in the wall of the ventricle; (c) the contractile state of the heart; and (d) external work.

The heart rate is listed first because it provides the summing factor for most of the other variables listed, which are determined on a per beat basis.[8] Furthermore, in experiments comparing severe exercise and pacing to the same heart rate, it was suggested that the tachycardia alone was responsible for about one-third the increment in coronary blood flow that normally occurs during strenuous exercise.[9]

The second factor, internal or pressure-generation work, accounts for about 50% of the oxygen consumption of the heart doing external work at a high level.[7] The expression given for the wall stress is the familiar law of Laplace and indicates that the stress is a function of intraventricular pressure, intraventricular radius (volume), and ventricular wall thickness. Although this equation is for a sphere and the left ventricle is not spherical, it should be noted that expressions for more appropriate shapes (the prolate spheroid or the ellipsoid of revolution) have exactly the same form with the radius replaced by the semiminor axis and the one-half replaced by a dimensionless multiplier, which is a function of the semimajor and semiminor axes.[10] The term "tension" has been used interchangeably with the term "stress" in the literature on cardiac mechanics,[10] but the two terms do have different physical meanings and there would appear to be merit in distinguishing between them in physiology also.

Stress is the force per unit cross-sectional area of a material,[10] and thus has units of dynes/cm². Tension is a force that produces an extension [10] and thus has units of dynes, although for hollow structures it has been defined as the force per unit length of circumference [11] and thus has units of dynes/cm and is equal to wall stress times wall thickness. A third equation has been used to calculate total force in dynes across the cross-sectional area of the heart muscle at the equator [11] or against the entire surface area of the inner wall of the ventricle.[12] The distinction between these variables is pertinent in discussing $M\dot{V}_{O_2}$ in that the oxygen consumption when measured per 100 g left ventricular myocardium is related to the stress.[13] Of interest in this regard are hypertrophied and dilated hearts. It has been suggested that a rise in stroke energy expenditure is causally related to myocardial hypertrophy.[14] With hypertrophy, wall thickness is increased so that the wall stress,[12, 15] and likewise the energy expenditure per unit mass of contractile tissue per beat,[14, 16, 17] are

TABLE 1

DETERMINANTS OF OXYGEN CONSUMPTION OF THE HEART
(9–64 ml per 100 g left ventricle per minute)

Major Determinants
1. Heart rate
2. Internal work, intramyocardial stress or tension
$$\sigma = PR/2h$$
$$T = PR/2$$
$$TF = \pi PR^2$$
3. Contractile state
4. External work, load $\times$ shortening
$$SW = P \times SV$$

Others
5. Basal cardiac metabolism (nonbeating, nondepolarized)
6. Depolarization
7. Activation and relaxation
8. ? Maintenance of the active state

restored to or toward normal. In contrast to wall stress, wall tension and total force would be increased in pressure-overloaded or dilated hearts, and it is not clear which of the latter two expressions would best relate to total left ventricular blood flow.

Although we use the term "contractility" extensively in cardiac physiology, it remains a difficult concept to define and a hard variable to measure.[10] Nevertheless, there has been a considerable amount of work indicating that changes in inotropic state are associated with substantial changes in $M\dot{V}_{O_2}$, and with what measurement techniques are available it has been suggested that the contractile state may account for up to 35% of $M\dot{V}_{O_2}$ along with such other variables as basal cardiac metabolism.[7]

In contrast to the thinking in the early years of this century, external work is not the dominant factor determining $M\dot{V}_{O_2}$ but might account for only about 15%.[7]

Basal cardiac metabolism has been listed as a minor determinant even though it is recognized that measurements of the oxygen consumption of the arrested heart are as high as 20%–25% of measurements of the $M\dot{V}_{O_2}$ in intact subjects at rest.[18] However, presumably this "basal" metabolism remains constant with increased cardiac activity while the other variables mentioned will increase markedly.[18]

At this point it is worth remembering several features of cardiac physiology. The heart is an aerobic organ with little capacity to function anaerobically or to incur an oxygen debt. Furthermore, the oxygen saturation of coronary venous blood is very low as the heart is extracting from the blood most of the oxygen available. Therefore any increase in the heart's demands for oxygen must be met primarily by increasing myocardial blood flow (MBF), so that among the various possible mechanisms for the regulation of blood flow in different regional circulations, it would appear that for the coronary circulation the metabolic theory is dominant.[19] Thus, measurements of myocardial blood flow closely parallel measurements of myocardial oxygen consumption although the normal human heart does have some capacity to increase the latter by increasing oxygen extraction by as much as 50%.[20-22] This is more of a factor in species such as the dog where there is a greater increase in hematocrit with exercise.[23]

A discussion of myocardial blood flow and oxygen consumption during exercise then comes down to a consideration of what changes occur in the primary determinants of myocardial oxygen consumption during exercise. This varies somewhat with such factors as age, type of exercise being performed (dynamic or static), the muscle groups involved, the body position, the state of physical training, and the presence or absence of disease. For purposes of simplicity we will consider primarily upright, dynamic, leg exercise in healthy, young individuals and will emphasize maximal performances of well-trained persons. Data from animals will also be reviewed where pertinent to certain issues.

The heart rate might be expected to increase by 2½–4 times resting values at maximal exercise.[20, 24] This immediately suggests that marked increases in MBF will occur.

To estimate the changes in left ventricular wall stress we have to consider the changes in systemic arterial pressure and ventricular volume. Acute changes in wall thickness would have to be small and inversely proportional to changes in ventricular volume since total left ventricular mass would not change acutely.

Unfortunately most of the available data on arterial pressure during exercise was measured in the brachial or femoral arteries and hence over-estimates the pressure load on the heart as measured in the aorta because of the well-known phenomenon of peripheral amplification of the systolic blood pressure.[24] A recent study in our laboratory showed a linear relationship between aortic and brachial artery pressure with the aortic pressure being equal to 37 mmHg plus two-thirds of brachial artery pressure ($r = 0.83$).[25] In general the greatest increase in aortic systolic pressure from rest to maximal exercise was about 50%. It should be noted that these pressures were measured in the usual way with a catheter having both end and side holes being directed against the flow axis and therefore stagnation or impact pressure was being measured. Measurements made with the catheter tip pointing downstream so that static or distending pressure is being measured reveal that the aortic systolic pressure rises only slightly with increasing levels of exertion.[26]

The changes that occur in left ventricular volume with exercise have been debated for many years but a fairly clear picture is available at present. Direct measurements of left ventricular diameter or volume [27-30] in animals indicate that the increase in stroke volume that occurs with mild work is accomplished by ejecting to a lower end systolic volume with end diastolic volume remaining the same. With maximal exercise there is in addition an increase in end diastolic volume, which might be estimated to be 15% as the heart utilizes the Frank-Starling mechanism to increase stroke volume. Studies in man in the upright position are limited to determinations of overall transverse diameter or volume of the heart determined from chest roentgenograms. These indicate that with the onset of upright exercise the overall heart volume initially increases about 10% then decreases somewhat towards resting size with increasing levels of submaximal exercise,[31] and the transverse diameter decreases slightly from rest to mild exercise.[32] Thus, what data is available for humans is compatible with the animal data.

Since stroke volume is increasing by as much as 150% [30, 33] to 200% [34, 35] while the systolic ejection period is decreasing by 50%,[20] the rate of ejection increases markedly during exercise. At maximal exertion such measures of contractility $(dP/dt)/P$ and isolength velocity have increased to 250% and 220% of control, respectively.[30]

The changes in external cardiac work during exercise are implicit in the changes in arterial pressure and stroke volume mentioned above.

Thus, with the exception of left ventricular end diastolic volume, all the major determinants of myocardial oxygen consumption change markedly with graded exercise, some of the variables linearly and some nonlinearly. Remembering the tight coupling between myocardial metabolic demand and myocardial blood flow we find it obvious that striking increases in coronary flow must occur during exercise. This sort of survey provides one with a qualitative answer, but to know the actual magnitude of the response and its relation to the degree of exercise requires actual measurement. Studies done during graded exercise in animals reveal increases in coronary blood flow of between 3 and 6 times resting values at heavy exercise.[9, 23, 36-40] In recent years there has been increasing interest in the transmural distribution of myocardial blood flow, and it has been shown that at rest endocardial flow exceeds epicardial flow by a ratio of between 1.1 and 1.3 to 1. With graded exercise there is a progressive decrease in this ratio so that at maximal exertion endocardial and epicardial flow are equal.[39, 40]

Most of the data in the literature on myocardial flow in man is for mild levels of exercise in the supine position. Many of the determinants of $M\dot{V}_{O_2}$ are difficult or impractical to measure in exercising man. Therefore several years ago we set out to determine if simpler measurements could give us some idea of energy demands of the heart over a wide range of exercise intensity. Data were obtained at two or three levels of exertion in ten normal young male volunteers. MBF was measured by the nitrous oxide saturation method, which yields flow in units of ml per 100 g left ventricle per minute in lieu of obtaining the absolute flow for the whole heart. Heart rate was obtained from the electrocardiogram and phasic blood pressure was measured with a catheter in the ascending aorta. Various hemodynamic variables were correlated with myocardial blood flow and oxygen consumption by regression techniques. It was found that the product of heart rate (HR) and systolic blood pressure (BP) considered as a single variable correlated best with myocardial oxygen consumption, the correlation coefficient being quite high at 0.90.[20] (FIGURE 1).

This quantity is similar to what was termed the index of cardiac effort [41] but may more simply be called the rate-pressure product (RPP).

When one includes in the product the systolic ejection period to obtain the tension-time index (TTI) [better termed pressure-time per minute (PTM)] or the triple product, the correlation actually becomes poorer, although the difference is not statistically significant. Similar measurements were carried out in a separate group of subjects after giving the beta-adrenergic blocking agent pro-

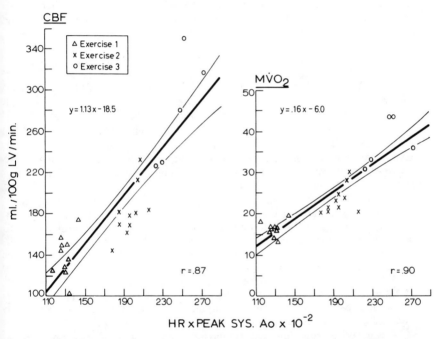

FIGURE 1. Relationship of coronary blood flow (CBF) (left) or myocardial oxygen consumption ($M\dot{V}_{O_2}$) (right) and the rate-pressure prduct (HR × PEAK SYS. Ao × 10^{-2}). The regression line is the heavy straight line, and the lighter curved lines indicate the 95% confidence zones for the slope of the regression line; r=correlation coefficient.

pranolol in doses that decreased myocardial contractility and significantly lengthened the ejection period. The correlation coefficients between myocardial flow or oxygen consumption and the TTI became much worse, in contrast to the persistently good correlations with the RPP.[21] We feel that the deficiencies of any index including the systolic ejection period have been clearly demonstrated.

In contrast, the heart rate alone is almost as good an index of $M\dot{V}_{O_2}$ as the RPP ($r = 0.88$),[20] suggesting at first that including the blood pressure is unnecessary. This is deceptive, however, as it occurs because for this simple dynamic exercise the heart rate and blood pressure are strongly correlated ($r = 0.73$). We have recently reanalyzed the data by performing a three-variable rather than two-variable linear regression, considering the heart rate and blood pressure as separate variables rather than combined into a product. This yields the regression equation

$$M\dot{V}_{O_2} = 0.24 \text{ HR} + 0.16 \text{ BP} - 29.9, \quad r = 0.89.$$

Since the ranges of the two variables were similar (HR 99–173, mean 134 beats/min, BP 111–160 mmHg, mean 133 mmHg), the fact that the coefficients were sizable on both the heart rate and blood pressure terms indicates both variables were important determinants of the $M\dot{V}_{O_2}$. When one considers interventions where BP does not rise pari passu with HR, the necessity of including BP in the index becomes even more evident. In a third group of subjects studied in our laboratory, myocardial oxygen consumption was measured during static work alone or static plus dynamic exercise. The isometric exercise was chosen since it induces a more marked change in blood pressure than dynamic exercise. Again the RPP correlated best with $M\dot{V}_{O_2}$ and the TTI was a much poorer index.[22] Others have compared the responses to supine leg exercise and atrial pacing at rest supine. The slope of the regression of $M\dot{V}_{O_2}$ on HR was much lower during pacing than exercise, but the relationship between $M\dot{V}_{O_2}$ and the RPP fell along the same regression line as during exercise.[42] Myocardial oxygen consumption on a per beat basis increases with exercise and decreases with pacing,[20] hence the importance of including some variable influencing $M\dot{V}_{O_2}$/beat in an index.

We conclude that the rate-pressure product is a good index of myocardial metabolic needs, and that even though ventricular volume,[43] contractility, and external cardiac work do determine the absolute value of myocardial oxygen consumption, actually measuring them appears to be of lesser importance in studying relative values during exercise. The usefulness of this index for clinical purposes has been pointed out.[44, 45]

Although our work has all been done using centrally measured blood pressure, there is a direct relationship between aortic and brachial artery pressure,[25] so use of a peripheral pressure measurement will still yield a valid RPP but with a slightly different slope of the regression line with $M\dot{V}_{O_2}$.[22, 46]

The measurements done before and after propranolol administration raise one further point. After giving propranolol the repeat exercise load was altered to achieve the same heart rate, 129 beats/minute, as before propranolol and nearly twice the external work load was required, 112 versus 63 watts. Nevertheless, the systemic blood pressure was the same so that the RPP was the same, 150 before propranolol and 154 after. Correspondingly the myocardial oxygen consumption was the same, 20.8 versus 22.1 ml per 100 g left ventricle per minute, but this was achieved by a significantly lower myocardial blood flow and a significantly higher coronary arteriovenous difference.[21] These data emphasize that the stress on the heart is not necessarily proportional to the degree of exertion and that there is a separation of the metabolic load for the body as a whole induced by a given intervention from the concomitant metabolic demands of the heart (FIGURE 2). Since physical training produces a significantly lower heart rate at any given level of submaximal exercise,[24] it is apparent that the oxygen demands of the heart would likewise be lower.

We have left then to consider the magnitude of myocardial blood flow at maximal exertion in the normal person and, in particular, in the championship level endurance athlete. At rest at a heart rate of 75 beats per minute and an aortic systolic blood pressure of 120 mmHg, MBF is 85 ml per 100 g left ventricle per minute.[20] For a heart rate of 190 beats/minute and aortic systolic blood pressure of 170 mmHg at maximal exercise for both untrained subjects and athletes,[20, 25, 33, 47] the MBF can be calculated from the regression equation to be 345 ml per 100 g left ventricle per minute, an increase of four times. However, the endurance athlete has the capacity to generate a much higher stroke volume, values up to 200 ml/beat being reported,[47] achieved by a significantly increased heart volume [24, 47–49] and an increase in contractility brought

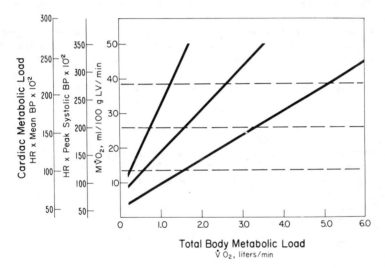

FIGURE 2. Illustration of the variable relationship between total body metabolic load ($\dot{V}_{O_2}$) and the cardiac metabolic load, expressed as either myocardial oxygen consumption ($M\dot{V}_{O_2}$) or its hemodynamic correlate, the rate-pressure product. The dashed lines represent the upper limits of myocardial oxygen supply that might be seen in patients with varying severities of coronary artery disease.

about by changes in the intrinsic physiology and biochemistry of cardiac muscle.[50] With the increase in end-diastolic volume there will be hypertrophy to keep wall stress constant,[12, 15] and even though only modest changes in wall thickness are demonstrable in the athlete,[48, 49] left ventricular mass may be 50% greater than normal.[48] Therefore our regression equation will underestimate the level of MBF at maximal exertion in the endurance athlete, even though there is some evidence indicating hearts of trained subjects are more efficient in converting chemical energy to external work,[50] and it seems reasonable to suggest that an athlete working near or at maximal will have a MBF per unit mass 4–5 times the normal resting value and an even greater increase in total left ventricular flow. This corresponds to the magnitude of increase documented in animals alluded to earlier. This is within the capability of the human coronary circulation as it has been demonstrated in man that the MBF can go from 80 ml per 100 g left ventricle per minute at rest to 400 ml per 100 g left ventricle per minute during pharmacologically induced maximal coronary vasodilatation with dipyridamole.[51]

Coronary flows of this magnitude are probably reached and sustained during competition in distance running and other racing activities. The heart rate increases rapidly during the initial stages of a race and reaches approximately 180 beats per minute within half a minute.[52] Estimates[53] and actual measurements[54] of cardiorespiratory responses during competitive marathon running show levels of total body oxygen consumption between 68% and 100% of maximal at various stages of the race with heart rate, stroke volume, and cardiac output being maintained at greater than 90% maximal. This would imply that myocardial blood flow and oxygen consumption are also near maximal throughout the race.

The question might be suggested: Is MBF a limiting factor to physical performance in the absence of disease? It appears to be established that the limitation to maximal total body oxygen consumption is not pulmonary or the metabolic capacity of the muscles, but cardiac—the maximal cardiac output and oxygen extraction, or the capacity to develop pressure against a particular total peripheral resistance.[55] Subjects exercised to maximal capacity while breathing hypoxic gas mixtures develop the same heart rates and blood pressure suggesting coronary flow is not limiting since it must actually be increased given the decreased oxygen content of the blood.[56] Similarly during exhaustive exercise the heart rate, aortic pressure, and cardiac output are continuing to rise while there is shift of blood flow from the endocardial to the epicardial layers of the myocardium suggesting this redistribution is not a limiting factor.[40] Since the capillary density of the hearts of trained animals increases, one would not expect limitations in flow at the microscopic level to be a limiting factor to the athlete's maximal capacity.[57] It appears the limitation must lie in the mechanics or pumping ability of the heart,[55, 57, 58] as well as the maximal attainable heart rate.

References

1. ROHDE, E. 1912. Über den Einfluss der mechanischem Bedingungen auf die Tätigkeit und den Sauerstoffverbrach der Warmblüterherzens. Arch. Exp. Path. Pharm. **68**: 401–434.
2. EVANS, C. L. & V. MATSUOKA. 1915. The effect of various mechanical conditions on the gaseous metabolism and efficiency of the mammalian heart. J. Physiol. London **49**: 378–405.
3. BRITMAN, N. A. & H. J. LEVINE. 1964. Contractile element work: A major determinant of myocardial oxygen consumption. J. Clin. Invest. **43**: 1397–1408.
4. BRAUNWALD, E. 1971. Control of myocardial oxygen consumption. Physiologic and clinical consideration. Amer. J. Cardiol. **27**: 416–432.
5. SONNENBLICK, E. H. & C. L. SKELTON. 1971. Myocardial energetics: Basic principles and clinical implications. New Eng. J. Med. **285**: 668–675.
6. ROSS, J., JR. 1972. Factors regulating the oxygen consumption of the heart. *In* Changing Concepts in Cardiovascular Disease. H. I. Russek & B. L. Zohman, Eds. : 20–31. The Williams and Wilkins Co. Baltimore, Md.
7. BURNS, J. W. & J. W. COVELL. 1972. Myocardial oxygen consumption during isotonic and isovolumic contractions in the intact heart. Amer. J. Physiol. **223**: 1491–1497.

8. ANTIC, R., L. J. HIRSCH, L. M. KATZ, E. BOYD & A. BRAUER. 1965. The factors controlling myocardial oxygen consumption per stroke and per minute. Acta Cardiol. **20:** 309–323.
9. VATNER, S. F., C. B. HIGGINS, D. FRANKLIN & E. BRAUNWALD. 1972. Role of tachycardia in mediating the coronary hemodynamic response to severe exercise. J. Appl. Physiol. **32:** 380–385.
10. MIRSKY, I., D. N. GHISTA & H. SANDLER, Eds. 1974. Cardiac Mechanics: Physiological, Clinical and Mathematical Considerations. John Wiley and Sons, Inc., New York, N.Y.
11. BADEER, H. S. 1963. Contractile tension in the myocardium. Amer. Heart J. **66:** 432–434.
12. HOOD, W. P., JR., C. E. RACKLEY & E. L. ROLETT. 1968. Wall stress in the normal and hypertrophied human left ventricle. Amer. J. Cardiol. **22:** 550–558.
13. BADEER, H. 1960. Effect of heart size on the oxygen uptake of the myocardium. Amer. Heart J. **60:** 948–954.
14. BADEER, H. S. 1972. Development of cardiomegaly. Cardiology **57:** 247–261.
15. GROSSMAN, W., D. JONES & L. P. McLAURIN. 1975. Wall stress and patterns of hypertrophy in the human left ventricle. J. Clin. Invest. **56:** 56–64.
16. BADEER, H. S. 1971. Myocardial blood flow and oxygen uptake in clinical and experimental cardiomegaly. Amer. Heart J. **82:** 105–119.
17. MALIK, A. B., A. TOMIO, H. O'KANE & A. S. GEHA. 1973. Cardiac function, coronary flow, and oxygen consumption in stable left ventricular hypertrophy. Amer. J. Physiol. **225:** 186–191.
18. McKEEVER, W. P., D. E. GREGG & P. C. CANNEY. 1958. Oxygen uptake of the nonworking left ventricle. Circ. Res. **6:** 612–623.
19. RUBIO, R. & R. M. BERNE. 1975. Regulation of coronary blood flow. Prog. Cardiovasc. Dis. **18:** 105–122.
20. KITAMURA, K., C. R. JORGENSEN, F. L. GOBEL, H. L. TAYLOR & Y. WANG. 1972. Hemodynamic correlates of myocardial oxygen consumption during upright exercise. J. Appl. Physiol. **32:** 516–522.
21. JORGENSEN, C. R., K. WANG, Y. WANG, F. L. GOBEL, R. R. NELSON & H. L. TAYLOR. 1973. Effect of propranolol on myocardial oxygen consumption and its hemodynamic correlates during upright exercise. Circulation **48:** 1173–1182.
22. NELSON, R. R., F. L. GOBEL, C. R. JORGENSEN, K. WANG, Y. WANG & H. L. TAYLOR. 1974. Hemodynamic predictors of myocardial oxygen consumption during static and dynamic exercise. Circulation **50:** 1179–1189.
23. KHOURI, E. M., D. E. GREGG & L. R. RAYFORD. 1965. Effect of exercise on cardiac output, left coronary flow and myocardial metabolism in the unanesthetized dog. Circ. Res. **17:** 427–437.
24. ÅSTRAND, P.-O. & K. RODAHL. 1970. Textbook of Work Physiology. McGraw-Hill Book Company. New York, N.Y.
25. GALICHIA, J., J. DANIEL, C. JORGENSEN & F. GOBEL. 1976. The effect of age on central to peripheral amplification of the arterial pulse during upright exercise. (Abstr.) Amer. J. Cardiol. **37:** 137.
26. MARX, H. J., L. B. ROWELL, R. D. CONN, R. A. BRUCE & F. KUSUMI. 1967. Maintenance of aortic pressure and total peripheral resistance during exercise in heat. J. Appl. Physiol. **22:** 519–525.
27. WILDENTHAL, K. & J. H. MITCHELL. 1969. Dimensional analysis of the left ventricle in unanesthetized dogs. J. Appl. Physiol. **27:** 115–119.
28. ERICKSON, H. H., V. S. BISHOP, M. B. KARDON & L. D. HORWITZ. 1971. Left ventricular internal diameter and cardiac function during exercise. J. Appl. Physiol. **31:** 473–478.
29. HORWITZ, L. D., J. M. ATKINS & S. J. LESHIN. 1972. Role of the Frank-Starling mechanism in exercise. Circ. Res. **31:** 868–875.
30. VATNER, S. F., D. FRANKLIN, C. B. HIGGINS, T. PATRICK & E. BRAUNWALD.

1972. Left ventricular response to severe exertion in untethered dogs. J. Clin. Invest. **51:** 3052–3060.

31. HOLMGREN, A. & C. O. OVENFORS. 1960. Heart volume at rest and during muscular work in the supine and in the sitting position. Acta Med. Scand. **167:** 267–277.

32. PHILLIPS, W. J., H. B. HIGGINBOTHAM, H. FRERKING & R. PAINE. 1966. Evaluation of myocardial state by synchronized radiography and exercise. N. Engl. J. Med. **274:** 826–829.

33. EKBLOM, B., P.-O. ÅSTRAND, B. SALTIN, J. STENBERG & B. WALLSTRÖM. 1968. Effect of training on circulatory response to exercise. J. Appl. Physiol. **24:** 518–528.

34. MITCHELL, J. H., B. J. SPROULE & C. B. CHAPMAN. 1958. The physiological meaning of the maximal oxygen intake test. J. Clin. Invest. **37:** 528–547.

35. ÅSTRAND, P.-O., T. E. CUDDY, B. SALTIN & J. STENBERG. 1964. Cardiac output during submaximal and maximal work. J. Appl. Physiol. **19:** 268–274.

36. ESSEX, H. E., J. F. HERRICK, E. J. BALDES & F. C. MANN. 1939. Influence of exercise on blood pressure, pulse rate, and coronary blood flow of the dog. Amer. J. Physiol. **125:** 614–623.

37. VAN CITTERS, R. L. & D. I. FRANKLIN. 1969. Cardiovascular performance of Alaska sled dogs during exercise. Circ. Res. **24:** 33–42.

38. VATNER, S. F., C. B. HIGGINS, S. WHITE, D. PATRICK, D. FRANKLIN & D. P. McKOWN. 1971. The peripheral response to severe exercise in untethered dogs before and after complete heart block. J. Clin. Invest. **50:** 1950–1960.

39. BALL, R. M., R. J. BACHE, F. R. COBB & J. C. GREENFIELD, JR. 1975. Regional myocardial blood flow during graded treadmill exercise in the dog. J. Clin. Invest. **55:** 43–49.

40. SANDERS, T. M., F. C. WHITE & C. M. BLOOR. 1975. Myocardial blood flow distribution in the conscious pig during steady state and exhaustive exercise. Fed. Proc. **34:** 414.

41. KATZ, L. N. & H. FEINBERG. 1958. The relation of cardiac effort to myocardial oxygen consumption and coronary flow. Circ. Res. **6:** 656–669.

42. HOLMBERG, S. & E. VARNAUSKAS. 1971. Coronary circulation during pacing-induced tachycardia. Acta. Medica Scand. **190:** 481–490.

43. SIMAAN, J. 1974. Left ventricular volume as a determinant of myocardial oxygen consumption. Cardiovasc. Res. **8:** 534–540.

44. GOLDSTEIN, R. E. & S. E. EPSTEIN. 1973. The use of indirect indices of myocardial oxygen consumption in evaluating angina pectoris. Chest **63:** 302–306.

45. AMSTERDAM, E. A., J. L. HUGHES, III, A. N. DEMARIA, R. ZELIS & D. T. MASON. 1974. Indirect assessment of myocardial oxygen consumption in the evaluation of mechanisms and therapy of angina pectoris. Amer. J. Cardiol. **33:** 737–743.

46. FERGUSON, R. J., P. GAUTHIER, P. CÔTÉ & M. G. BOURASSA. 1975. Coronary hemodynamics during upright exercise in patients with angina pectoris. (Abstr.) Circulation **52**(Suppl. II): 115.

47. EKBLOM, B. & L. HERMNSEN. 1968. Cardiac output in athletes. J. Appl. Physiol. **25:** 619–625.

48. MORGANROTH, J., B. J. MARON, W. L. HENRY & S. E. EPSTEIN. 1975. Comparative left ventricular dimension in trained athletes. Ann. Int. Med. **82:** 521–524.

49. ROESKE, W. F., R. A. O'ROURKE, A. KLEIN, G. LEOPOLD & J. S. KARLINER. 1976. Noninvasive evaluation of ventricular hypertropy in professional athletes. Circulation **53:** 286–292.

50. SCHEUER, J., S. PENPARGKUL & A. K. BHAN. 1974. Experimental observations on the effects of physical training upon intrinsic cardiac physiology and biochemistry. Amer. J. Cardiol. **33:** 744–751.

51. TAUCHERT, M., K. KOCHSIEK, H. W. HEISS, B. E. STRAUER, D. KETTLER, H. D. REPLOH, G. RAU & H. J. BRETSCHNEIDER. 1972. Measurement of coronary blood flow in man by the argon method. *In* Myocardial Blood Flow in Man.

Methods and Significance in Coronary Disease. A. Maseri, Ed. : 139–144. Minerva Medica. Torino, Italy.

52. McArdle, W. D., G. F. Foglia & A. V. Patti. 1967. Telemetered cardiac response to selected running events. J. Appl. Physiol. **23:** 566–570.

53. Fox, E. L. & D. L. Costill. 1972. Estimated cardiorespiratory responses during marathon running. Arch. Environ. Health **24:** 316–324.

54. Maron, M. B., S. M. Horvath, J. E. Wilkerson & J. A. Gliner. 1976. Oxygen uptake measurements during competitive marathon running. J. Appl. Physiol. **40:** 836–838.

55. Rowell, L. B. 1974. Human cardiovascular adjustments to exercise and thermal stress. Physiol. Rev. **54:** 75–159.

56. Lamb, L. E., R. J. Kelly, W. L. Smith, A. D. LeBlanc & P. C. Johnson. 1969. Limiting factors in the capacity to achieve maximum cardiac work. Aerospace Med. **40:** 1291–1296.

57. Leon, A. S. 1972. Comparative cardiovascular adaptation to exercise in animals and man and its relevance to coronary heart disease. Adv. Exp. Med. Biol. **22:** 143–174.

58. Epstein, S. E., B. F. Robinson, R. L. Kahler & E. Braunwald. 1966. The mechanism normally limiting the maximal cardiac output (Abstr.). Clin. Res. **14:** 245.

THE INTERPLAY BETWEEN PERIPHERAL AND CENTRAL FACTORS IN THE ADAPTIVE RESPONSE TO EXERCISE AND TRAINING

Bengt Saltin

August Krogh Institute
Copenhagen University
Copenhagen, Denmark

One of the classical questions within the field of exercise physiology is whether there is a central or a peripheral limitation to a person's maximal oxygen uptake. Although many fascinating experimental models have been used to solve the problem, no final solution has as yet become commonly accepted. In the search for the limiting factor, training studies have also been performed. Clausen and colleagues [1,2] have used a model where they have trained the legs or the arms and tested the arms and legs separately. They concluded that if a large enough muscle mass is involved in the training (i.e., legs), the capacity of the heart is enhanced and the work capacity of the untrained extremities (arms) is also improved. These results thus point at a central limitation. In recent experiments where only one leg was trained results were obtained partly at variance with their conclusion.[3] In this paper the one-leg training results will be briefly mentioned. In addition a further analysis of the data will be presented as well as some results from a one-leg training study in progress.[4] The main focus of the presentation will be on maximal exercise, but as quite interesting findings were obtained for the one-legged submaximal heart rate response, some of these data will also be elaborated upon.

SUBJECTS AND PROTOCOL

In the first study 13 young healthy students participated. Eight of them trained only one leg, five times a week for 4 weeks. The other five subjects trained first one of the legs and then the other at each session. The training was of the endurance type and lasted for 30–45 minutes per leg and training session. Approximately 3000 kJ were performed per week by each leg. Each subject performed submaximal and maximal one-legged exercise with each leg before and after the training, and as well, did ordinary two-legged exercise. Heart rate, oxygen uptake, and blood lactate were measured, and the activity of succinate dehydrogenase was assayed using muscle samples from each leg.

In our second study seven healthy men participated. They all had one leg injured playing soccer. Within 2–3 days after the injury the healthy leg was exercised. Heart rate, oxygen uptake, and blood lactate were measured. From each leg a biopsy was taken, which was used for the analysis of muscle fiber composition, capillary density, and the activity of succinate dehydrogenase. While the injured leg was in a cast for 4–6 weeks, the other leg was kept on a training schedule of one-legged exercise for two to three 30-minute sessions a week at 600 kpm/min (100 W). The exercise intensity was intended to be comparable to normal activity level for the leg. After the cast was removed,

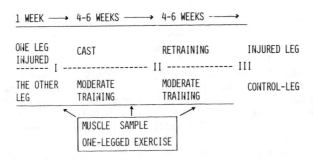

FIGURE 1. A summary of the protocol for study II.

as soon as the subject could pedal with his injured leg (usually 2–3 days), biopsies and one-legged exercise tests were repeated. After another 6–8 weeks when the two legs were comparable in size and work capacity, these measurements were done a third time. A schematic schedule of protocol for the experiments is found in FIGURE 1.

RESULTS

Study I. A One-Leg Training Model

An increase in the oxidative potential of the muscle tissue was only found in the trained leg (FIGURE 2). The one-legged maximal oxygen uptake was also significantly enlarged only in the trained leg (FIGURE 2). Before the training period, the maximal oxygen uptake of one leg amounted to 80%–81% of the

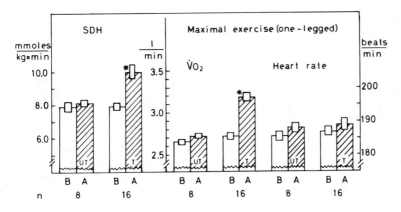

FIGURE 2. The activity of succinate dehydrogenase of the thigh muscles of the untrained (UT) and the trained (T) legs before (B) and after (A) the training period. Included in the graph are also the oxygen uptake and the heart rate at maximal exercise. The open bars at the top of each bar represent the standard error (SE) and a star denotes a significant difference ($p < 0.001$). (After Saltin *et al.*[3])

two-leg maximal oxygen uptake, and after training, the untrained leg was 73%–75% whereas the trained leg reached 85% of the two-leg maximal oxygen uptake.

Maximal heart rate in one-legged exercise was 10–12 beats lower that in the two-legged maximal exercise, and no significant changes were observed with the training period. In the submaximal exercise (100 W) with one leg, heart rate averaged 160 beats/min when the leg was untrained (FIGURE 3). When performing the same exercise with the leg still untrained after the training period, the heart rate was 156 beats/min. This should be compared with the leg which became trained where a drop in heart rate of 14 beats/min was noticed. Also the blood lactate concentration was only significantly reduced after the training when the submaximal exercise was performed with the trained limb (FIGURE 3).

As pointed out earlier, eight of the subjects trained only one limb, whereas five subjects trained first one limb and then the other in each training session.

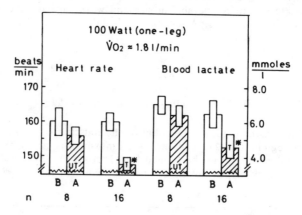

FIGURE 3. Heart rate response and blood lactate concentration at submaximal exercise in the same group of subjects as in FIGURE 2. (After Saltin *et al.*[3])

As the amount of training was identical for each leg, one could say that there is a situation where one group of subjects had twice as much cardiac training (II) as the other group (I), the local training of the trained leg being very similar in both groups.

When a comparison is made for the two-legged maximal oxygen uptake before and after training, both groups increased by 0.3 liters/min (8%–9%). The response to one-legged exercise performed with the trained leg was also surprisingly similar in the two groups (TABLE 1). The increase in one-legged maximal oxygen uptake, the reduction in submaximal heart rate, and the blood lactate concentration were significantly changed as an effect of the training, but between groups no difference could be established. Not even a trend could be detected for a more marked improvement in the group with twice as much training.

Thus these results indicate that an improved central cardiovascular performance could not be elicited unless the exercising extremity was trained. Further,

TABLE 1

SUMMARY OF THE CHANGES FOUND IN SUBJECTS PERFORMING ONE-LEGGED EXERCISE
AFTER TRAINING ONE (I) OR BOTH (II) LEGS *

	Group	Before Training	After Training	Difference
V_{O_2max} (liters/min)	I	2.59	3.10	+0.51
	II	2.83	3.25	+0.43
Heart rate (beats/min)†	I	161	152	−9
	II	160	146	−14
Blood lactate (mmole/liter)†	I	7.1	4.4	−2.6
	II	6.1	4.7	−1.4

* After Saltin et al.[3] When both legs were trained they were exercised separately.
† During a 100-W work rate.

it appears that for an endurance training response the peripheral adaptation is at least as important as any central factor.

Study II. Healthy Leg versus Injured Leg Model

In a one-legged submaximal bicycle exercise, the control (healthy) leg did not vary much in either heart rate or blood lactate response at the three test occasions (FIGURE 4). The injured leg closely followed the activity level; i.e., submaximal heart rate was the highest after the period of inactivity, and so was the blood lactate concentration (FIGURE 4).

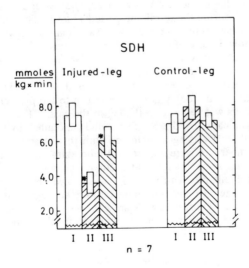

FIGURE 4. Succinate dehydrogenase activity for the injured and the control leg of seven subjects in study II. Star denotes p <0.001 and the open bar at the top of a bar represents the SE. (After Ingemann-Hansen.[4])

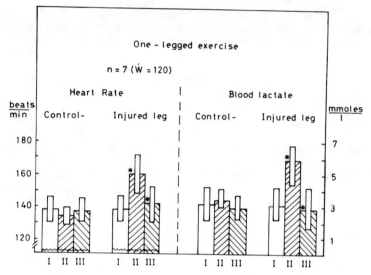

FIGURE 5. Heart rate and blood lactate at a work load of 120 W ($\dot{V}_{O_2}$ 1.2 liters/min) for the seven subjects of study II. (After Ingemann-Hansen.[4])

In this study not only were measurements of the activity of succinate de-hydrogenase performed as a marker for the oxidative potential of the muscle, but also muscle fiber typing and determination of capillary density were in-cluded. All three variables varied with the activity level of the extremity. The SDH activity of the leg in the cast was reduced by 50% and returned to almost the preinjured level during the retraining period (FIGURE 5). In the control leg no significant changes were observed. The two main groups of muscle fiber types did not change in any of the legs or in any phase of the study. Between the subgroups of the fast-twitching fibers (FT) an interesting observation was made. In the inactivated leg a reduction in the FT_a fibers occurred and the number of FT_b fibers was concomitantly increased (p < 0.05). With the re-training a "normalization" took place, i.e., a return to the preinjury distribution. The size of the fibers was reduced in the leg in the cast. This reduction in fiber size was only significant for the ST fibers and amounted to about 15%. A reversal to control level was again obtained with the retraining. In the control leg no changes in fiber size were apparent. Preliminary analysis of the capillary density indicates that some changes did occur in the casted leg. The reduction in the number of capillaries with inactivity was, however, not greater than the reduction in fiber size. In the retraining period the degree of capillarization followed the fiber size. Thus, no significant changes in diffusion conditions may have been the result of the changes in activity levels for the limbs.

DISCUSSION

The striking observation in these studies is the very close relationship be-tween the local adaptation to the training and the cardiovascular performance. This appears to be true for submaximal as well as for maximal exercise intensities as manifested by the lower submaximal heart rate response and the larger maximal oxygen uptake when exercising with the trained limb. What is less apparent is the mechanism brought into play to explain the regulation.

Heart Rate Regulation

Cardio-acceleration can be elicited both by cortical influence on the vaso-motor center and by afferent inflow of impulses from exercising muscles. The immediate interpretation could be that with such a marked local muscle adaptation as resulted from the training, the lowered submaximal response is the result of a less pronounced peripheral drive. What cannot be ruled out, however, is that the hypotrophy of the muscle fibers brings about more centrally activated motor units when exercising submaximally with the more inactive leg. EMG recordings from the thigh do not support the idea of a greater motor unit involvement as the integrated EMG activity is, if anything, less when a given tension is produced with the least trained leg. However, the interpretation of the EMG is difficult and probably can not be used to rule out the possibility that there is a difference in cortical influence on the vasomotor center and the spinal motor neuron.

In view of the strong support for a peripheral control system to exist for the heart rate response in exercise, the following may be said based on the present findings.

Since the same absolute work load is used in the submaximal exercise when exercising with the trained and untrained limbs, the mechano-receptor output should then be similar, and ruled out as the explanation for the elevated heart rate observed when the most inactive leg is exercising. Mitchell and coworkers [5] have ample evidence for the importance of the nerve endings of the muscle in mediating the impulse traffic responsible for the cardiovascular control. It is further demonstrated that chemical stimuli such as elevated K^+ and osmolarity affect these nerve endings.[6] In view of these findings the results of the present studies could be explained by a more pronounced peripheral drive as lactate concentrations in the muscle tissue and the release of lactate (and thus the osmolarity) were higher in the exercising muscles of the inactive leg (FIGURE 6).

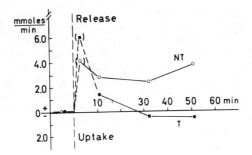

FIGURE 6. Lactate flux in the untrained (NT) and the trained (T) leg when performing ordinary two-legged exercise 1 hour of exercise at 70% of maximal oxygen uptake. The values within parentheses at 3 min are based on the arterio-venous difference for lactate of that time and leg blood flow determinations at 10 min. (After Saltin et al.[3])

A problem with osmolarity being the stimulus for the peripheral drive is that as time passes while exercising, lactate production may gradually become lowered and the difference between the legs diminished. It is of note, however, that during a one-hour exercise period at 70% of maximal oxygen uptake (two-leg), the difference between the trained and the untrained leg in lactate release did persist (FIGURE 6). Thus, the present data may give a base for proposing a metabolic factor to be the stimulus for the peripheral drive. In addition, the possibility exists that with each depolarization of the muscle cell the flux of K^+ out of the activated fibers also affects the small nerve endings in the muscle.

The Factor Limiting Maximal Oxygen Uptake

Both Gleser[7] and Davies and Sargeant[8, 9] came to the conclusion that the periphery limited maximal oxygen uptake in one-legged exercise. They based this conclusion on somewhat different grounds.

Gleser[7] argues that neither before nor after the one-legged training did cardiac output reach maximum in one-legged as compared to two-legged exercise. However, the difference between the one-legged and two-legged maximal cardiac output after training was very small. In fact, some of the subjects had the same cardiac output or higher in the one-legged maximal work. Moreover, after training, the stroke volume was the highest during the one-legged exercise. Thus, from the data provided by Gleser, it appears more difficult to completely exclude the central circulation from being the limiting factor also in one-legged exercise. The argument of Davies and Sargeant[8] was based on the fact that they were unable to demonstrate an enhancement of maximal oxygen uptake in one-legged exercise breathing a high oxygen mixture (45% O_2 in N_2) whereas a 10% increase in $\dot{V}_{O_2\,max}$ was seen in the two-legged exercise, which is quite surprising.

It is thus questionable whether any of the above-cited studies provide enough information for a definite conclusion whether or not the periphery or the central circulation limit oxygen uptake in one-legged and two-legged exercise.

In the present study, tests of the nontrained leg showed a minor increase in $\dot{V}_{O_2\,max}$, especially among those who performed the endurance training. In addition, all subjects in our study demonstrated an improvement in the two-legged $\dot{V}_{O_2\,max}$, producing a small change in the ratio between the one-legged and two-legged $\dot{V}_{O_2\,max}$ before and after training. The conclusion from this can be that the one-legged training caused some improvement of the central circulation, which could be transferred to nontrained muscles. This is in agreement with the findings of Clausen et al.,[1, 2] who did see enhancement as a result of leg training of the work capacity and oxygen uptake of the nontrained arms. The improvement after training was related to the capacity of the central circulation to further increase systemic arterial pressure, thereby increasing perfusion pressure and blood flow to the arms. Whether their findings should be taken as proof that cardiac factors are also critical in exercise that utilizes a smaller percent of the total muscle mass cannot be settled. Among the local factors studied in the present work, most interest is focused on the role of the oxidative capacity of the muscle and the capillarization for the enhancement of maximal oxygen uptake. Henriksson[10] argues that as the oxidative enzymes decline much more rapidly than the maximal oxygen uptake during detraining, the oxidative potential of the muscle is not a determinant for the maximal aerobic power. He may be right, but the present data do indicate that oxygen extraction is more complete in the trained leg. This could have been explained by a greater capillary density, but, as shown in the study of the injured sportsmen, diffusing conditions may not change significantly over the studied period. Based on the very close coupling between activity level of the limb, its SDH activity, and maximal oxygen uptake found in every phase of the present two experiments, it is tempting to ascribe a crucial role to the oxidative potential of the muscle.

SUMMARY

(1) Local adaptation of skeletal muscles (fibers) only occurs in the extremity involved in the training.

(2) Work performance and maximal oxygen uptake were significantly increased only in the trained leg, and the "transfer" to the untrained leg was very small.

(3) The classical sign of a training effect with a lowered submaximal heart rate response could only be elicited when exercising the trained leg. Lactate concentration and release of lactate were also lower when the trained leg performed the exercise.

(4) The present results suggest that the local adaptation of skeletal muscle to training is of primary importance for enhancing work capacity and oxygen uptake.

(5) The results also indicate that there may exist a peripheral factor in the regulation of the heart rate response during exercise. Moreover, the data favor the hypothesis of a chemical receptor playing a role in such a peripheral control system.

REFERENCES

1. CLAUSEN, J. P., K. KLAUSEN, B. RASMUSSEN & J. TRAP-JENSEN. 1973. Central and peripheral circulatory changes after training of the arms or the legs. Amer. J. Physiol. **225:** 675–682.
2. CLAUSEN, J. P. 1976. Circulatory adjustments to dynamic exercise and effect of physical training in normal subjects and in patients with coronary artery disease. Progr. in C.-V. Disease. XVIII: 459–495.
3. SALTIN, B., K. NAZAR, D. L. COSTILL, E. STEIN, E. JANSSON, B. ESSÉN & P. D. GOLLNICK. 1976. The nature of the training response; Peripheral and central adaptations to one-legged exercise. Acta Physiol. Scand. **96:** 289–305.
4. INGEMANN-HANSEN, T., J. HALKJAER-KRISTENSEN & B. SALTIN. 1977. Adaptations to one-legged exercise during immobilization and training. Abstract. Intern. Congress in Paris.
5. MITCHELL, J. H. et al. 1977. Ibid.
6. WILDENTHAL, K., D. S. MIERZWIAK, N. S. SKINNER, JR. & J. H. MITCHELL. 1968. Potassium-induced cardiovascular and ventilatory reflexes from the dog hindlimb. Amer. J. Physiol. **215:** 542–548.
7. GLESER, M. A. 1973. Effects of hypoxia and physical training on hemodynamic adjustments to one-legged exercise. J. Appl. Physiol. **34:** 655–659.
8. DAVIES, C. T. M. & A. J. SARGEANT. 1974. Physiological responses to one- and two-legged exercise breathing air and 45% oxygen. J. Appl. Physiol. **36:** 142–148.
9. DAVIES, C. T. M. & A. J. SARGEANT. 1975. Effects of training on the physiological responses to one- and two-legged work. J. Appl. Physiol. **38:** 377–381.
10. HENRIKSSON, J. 1977. Human skeletal muscle adaptation to physical activity. Thesis. Karolinska Institutet, Stockholm, Sweden.

POSSIBLE ROLE OF MUSCLE RECEPTORS IN THE CARDIOVASCULAR RESPONSE TO EXERCISE *

Jere H. Mitchell, William C. Reardon,
D. Ian McCloskey,† and Kern Wildenthal

*The Pauline and Adolph Weinberger Laboratory
for Cardiopulmonary Research
Department of Internal Medicine
University of Texas Health Science Center
Southwestern Medical School
Dallas, Texas 75235*

The mechanisms that are responsible for bringing about the cardiovascular changes that occur during muscular exercise remain incompletely understood. It would seem that a neurogenic mechanism is responsible since the onset of the changes in heart rate, arterial pressure, and contractile state of the left ventricle is so rapid.

Over the years, two general theories of neurogenic control of the cardiovascular responses to exercise have evolved (FIGURE 1). An early suggestion that one or both of two distinct mechanisms might exist was published by Johansson in 1894.[1] One postulate holds that the cardiovascular responses are due to a direct action of central command in the motor cortex on the medullary cardiovascular center (central control); the other holds that the responses are reflexly elicited by afferent neural activity from receptors in the skeletal muscles or joints on the medullary cardiovascular center (peripheral control). Obviously, these two theories are not mutually exclusive.

The hypothesis that the cardiovascular responses during exercise are due to a direct action of higher motor centers on the cardiovascular center (central irradiation) was elaborated most clearly by Krogh and Lindhard.[2, 3] Asmussen, Christensen, and Nielsen[4] thought they had found support for this hypothesis when they showed that the cardiac output response during dynamic leg exercise was related to the intensity of the work, even when circulation to the legs was blocked and the oxygen consumption was halved. Ochwadt et al.[5] and Asmussen et al.[6] found that heart rate and blood pressure responses were greater at a given work load when muscular strength was reduced by partial curarization. Thus, the cardiovascular response was related to the greater motor command needed to achieve a given level of muscular work when the subject was weaker. This finding suggested that central irradiation was involved. Freyschuss demonstrated an increase in blood pressure and heart rate in subjects whose muscles were unable to respond to command signals to perform handgrips.[7] The muscular groups involved in handgripping were paralyzed by injection of succinylcholine into the brachial artery. Significant cardiovascular responses developed

---

* This work was supported by a grant from the National Heart and Lung Institute (HL 06296), by Pauline and Adolph Weinberger, and by the Southwestern Medical Foundation.

† Currently at the School of Physiology & Pharmacology, University of New South Wales, Sydney, Australia.

232

in response to intended isometric handgrips, although the changes were less than with handgrips in the absence of succinylcholine.

Goodwin, McCloskey, and Mitchell investigated the cardiovascular response of human subjects to isometric exercise in experiments where the central motor command required to achieve a given tension was varied.[8] High-frequency vibration of a muscle excites the primary afferent nerves of muscle spindles. If the primary afferents are activated in a contracting muscle, they reflexly cause an involuntary increase in motor activation of the muscle, so that less central command is required to maintain the same tension. On the other hand, if the spindle afferents are activated in the antagonists of a contracting muscle, they cause reflex inhibition of the contracting muscle, so that a greater central command is required and the subject perceives that the conscious effort has increased. When the same muscle tension was achieved with less central command during isometric exercise, the resultant hypertension and tachycardia decreased; and when the same tension was achieved with more central com-

CARDIOVASCULAR CONTROL
DURING EXERCISE

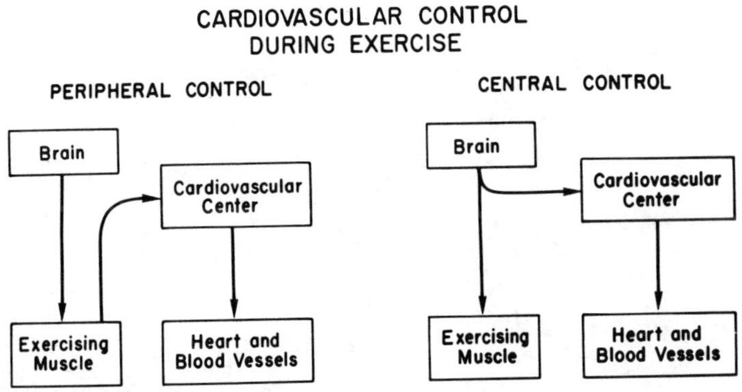

FIGURE 1. Diagrammatic representation of two postulated mechanisms for cardiovascular control during exercise.

mand, the resultant hypertension and tachycardia increased. It was concluded, therefore, that there is radiation of cardiovascular control centers by the descending central command during voluntary isometric contraction in man.

The hypothesis that the cardiovascular responses during exercise are due to a reflex originating in contracting skeletal muscle received its first major experimental support in the work of Alam and Smirk.[9, 10] They demonstrated an increase in blood pressure and in heart rate while the leg was performing predominantly isometric exercise during local circulatory occlusion. After exercise stopped the responses remained until the vascular occlusion was removed. They concluded that receptors located in the skeletal muscles were activated by some byproduct of the contraction and stimulated a reflex increase in blood pressure and heart rate. Similar conclusions were reached by Staunton, Taylor, and Donald.[11]

More recent work by Hollander and his co-workers has also suggested the existence of a muscle-heart reflex.[12, 13] In their studies in conscious man, exercise induced by direct electrical stimulation of the skeletal muscle caused an increase in heart rate that was identical in its time course and magnitude to one obtained during voluntary contraction of the same muscle.

In this paper we will be concerned only with the peripheral control or skeletal-muscle–cardiovascular-reflex theory. For this concept to be viable, the neural pathway for the reflex must be present. Studies have shown that a pressor response can be elicited when the central cut end of a muscle nerve is stimulated.[14–16] To define this reflex further a study was performed in anesthetized dogs to elicit cardiovascular changes by stimulating the central cut end of a nerve from skeletal muscle.[16] The experimental preparation for this study is shown in FIGURE 2. Measurements were made of aortic pressure, left ventricular pressure, aortic flow, and heart rate. In some of the studies heart rate, aortic

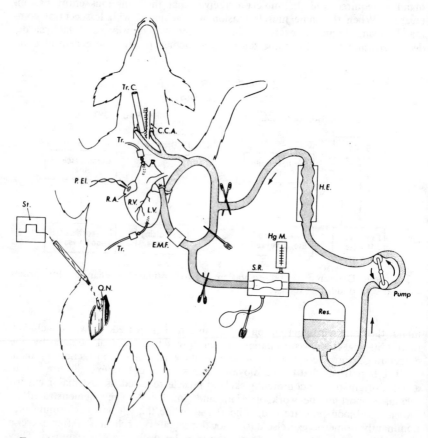

FIGURE 2. Preparation for stimulation of afferent fibers from skeletal muscle during measurement of cardiovascular variables: (Tr.C) tracheal cannula; (C.C.A.) common carotid artery; (R.A.) right atrium; (R.V.) right ventricle; (L.V.) left ventricle; (E.M.F.) electromagnetic flowmeter transducer; (S.R.) Starling resistance; (Hg M.) mercury manometer; (Res.) blood reservoir; (Pump) rotor pump; (H.E.) heat exchanger; (P.El.) pacing electrode; (Tr.) pressure transducer; (St.) Grass stimulator; (Q.N.) quadriceps nerve. (From Mitchell *et al.*[16] By permission of *Circulation Research*.)

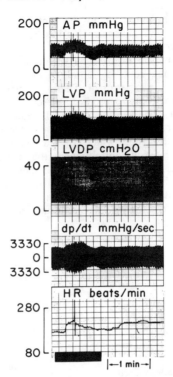

FIGURE 3. Pressor response to stimulation of afferent fibers of the quadriceps nerve: (AP) aortic pressure; (LVP) left ventricular pressure; (LVDP) left ventricular diastolic pressure; (dp/dt) rate of left ventricular pressure development; and (HR) heart rate. Stimulation of the quadriceps nerve at 25 times threshold for the flexion response is indicated by the black bar. (From Mitchell *et al.*[16] By permission of *Circulation Research*.)

pressure, and aortic flow were controlled; in others these factors were allowed to vary by disconnecting the Grass stimulator and excluding the Starling resistance, blood reservoir, and rotor pump from the extracorporeal circuit. In the controlled studies the heart was paced at a rate well above the spontaneous rate, while the aortic pressure and aortic flow were maintained constant by setting the Starling resistance and rotor pump, respectively. The quadriceps nerve was dissected free for several centimeters from its cut peripheral end and mounted on a pair of electrodes. Small-sized, high-threshold afferent fibers were activated by stimulations at 5 to 25 times the threshold for the flexion reflex.

An example of the response observed when the small-sized, high-threshold afferent fibers from muscle were stimulated is shown in FIGURE 3. There was an increase in aortic pressure, left ventricular pressure, maximal rate of left ventricular pressure development, and heart rate, and a decrease in left ventricular end-diastolic pressure.

When aortic pressure, aortic flow, and heart rate were held constant during stimulation of the central and of the quadriceps nerve, there was still an increase in the maximal rate of left ventricular pressure development and no change in end-diastolic pressure. Thus, stimulation of these afferent fibers caused an increase in the contractile state of the left ventricle. The administration of propranolol abolished the changes in heart rate and contractile state of the left ventricle. This demonstrates the importance of the cardiac beta-adrenergic receptors in the response observed in this anesthetized dog preparation.

It was next necessary to show that contraction of skeletal muscle by stimulating neural input below the central motor command could cause appropriate cardiovascular changes. This has been accomplished in several studies.[17-20] In our experiments a laminectomy was performed on anesthetized cats and the spinal cord was exposed by an incision through the dura.[18, 20] Both dorsal and ventral spinal roots L_5, L_6 and S_2 downward were always cut, leaving L_7 and S_1 for use in the experiment. The experimental preparation used for stimulation of the ventral roots to produce exercise in one hind limb of the cat is shown in FIGURE 4. The ventral roots of L_7 and S_1 were cut close to their exit from the spinal cord and placed over a pair of electrodes. Electrical stimulation of the spinal ventral roots, which contain predominantly motor fibers to skeletal muscle, was used to elicit contractions in the muscles of one hind limb. The corresponding dorsal roots, which carry the sensory input from the muscle to the brain, were left intact. Periods of simulated exercise of 30 to 45 seconds were given. Measurements were made of heart rate, arterial pressure, left ventricular pressure, and the rate of left ventricular pressure development.

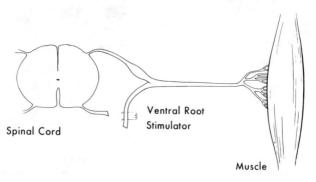

Spinal Cord

Ventral Root Stimulator

Muscle

FIGURE 4. Preparation for simulated exercise. Muscles in a hindlimb were caused to contract by stimulating the peripheral cut ends of the ventral roots of spinal segments L_7 and S_1. Afferent nerves from the contracting muscles entered the spinal cord in the dorsal roots of these segments; other dorsal roots supplying the hindlimb were cut.

The response to simulated exercise is shown in FIGURE 5. At the arrow muscular contraction was induced by stimulation of the ventral root. During induced exercise there was an increase in heart rate, arterial pressure, left ventricle systolic pressure, and the maximal rate of left ventricle pressure development. After the cessation of exercise all these factors returned to control values. Vascular occlusion applied before the conclusion of muscular contraction could maintain the pressor response.[18] In this respect the findings in cats are similar to those of Alam and Smirk [9, 10] and others [11] in man.

As shown in FIGURE 4 it would also be possible to section the dorsal roots receiving afferents from the exercising muscle. After such sectioning the increase in heart rate, arterial pressure, left ventricular systolic pressure, and left ventricular rate of pressure development were all abolished. This means that the changes induced by simulated exercise were not mediated by release into the circulation of active compounds, but rather was caused by a local phenome-

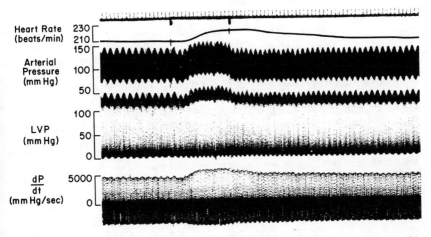

Heart Rate (beats/min)
Arterial Pressure (mm Hg)
LVP (mm Hg)
$\frac{dP}{dt}$ (mm Hg/sec)

FIGURE 5. Response to induced exercise: (LVP) left ventricular pressure; (dp/dt) rate of left ventricular pressure development. Time marks are at intervals of 1 second. Exercise was induced between bars. (From Mitchell *et al.*[20] By permission of the *American Journal of Physiology*.)

non in the contracting muscle, which produced changes in afferent or sensory input into the cardiovascular center. The responses maintained by vascular occlusion after a contraction are also abolished when the dorsal roots are sectioned.[18]

The type of sensory or afferent fibers coming from skeletal muscle are shown in TABLE 1. All these fibers run into the dorsal roots. Types Ia and Ib are myelinated with a diameter of 12 to 20 μm and a conduction velocity of 70 to 120 meters/sec. The Ia fiber originates in the primary ending of the muscle spindle and the Ib fiber in the Golgi tendon organ. The type II fiber is myelinated with a diameter of 4 to 12 μm and a conduction velocity of 15 to 70 meters/sec. This fiber innervates the secondary ending of the muscle spindle. The type III fiber is myelinated with a diameter less than 4 μm and a conduction

TABLE 1

CLASSIFICATION OF SENSORY (AFFERENT) FIBERS FROM SKELETAL MUSCLES

Type	Diameter	Velocity (meters/sec)	Receptor
Ia	12–20 μm, myelinated	70–120	Muscle spindle, primary ending
Ib	12–20 μm, myelinated	70–120	Golgi tendon organ
II	4–12 μm, myelinated	15–70	Muscle spindle, secondary ending
III	<4 μm, myelinated	12–24	Pressure-pain receptors
IV	Unmyelinated	0.5–2	Pain: unknown

velocity of 12 to 24 meters/sec. This fiber originates in so-called pressure-pain receptors, among others. The type IV fiber is unmyelinated with a conduction velocity of 0.5 to 2 meters/sec and principally originates in free nerve endings. Some of these free nerve endings mediate sensations of pain; however, whether or not they play any other physiological role is unknown.

Studies were performed to identify the type of afferent fiber that was responsible for the cardiovascular changes that were observed during induced exercise. Direct current anodal block of the dorsal roots receiving afferents from the exercising muscle was used to block preferentially large myelinated fibers.[18] This should include types Ia and b, II, and even the large type III fibers. The technique is demonstrated in FIGURE 6. A test stimulator was placed on the sciatic nerve. Test stimuli were delivered here by a second isolated stimulator. This elicited a compound action potential that was picked up from a sampling slip of dorsal root beyond the anodal blocking electrode. The compound action potential was displayed on an oscilloscope and photographed. Test stimuli were applied and anodal block was used until the sampled compound action potential showed that the large myelinated afferents had been blocked. After this procedure was carried out, the test stimuli were turned off and the ventral roots were again stimulated to produce contraction of the muscles of the hind limb.

The results of experiments performed before and after anodal block are shown in FIGURE 7. In the upper panel is shown blood pressure during the control study when no anodal block was being applied. The sample compound action potential is shown on the right. When the ventral root was stimulated causing contraction of the muscles of the hind limb there was an increase in both systolic and diastolic blood pressure. In the middle panel the anodal block was applied. The sampled action potential on the right shows that the large myelinated fibers have been blocked. During stimulation of the ventral roots there is still an increase in arterial blood pressure. In the lower panel the anodal block was turned off and exercise again produced by ventral root stimulation with the usual response. In this and all similar experiments, when the large

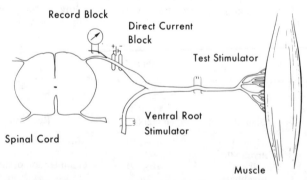

FIGURE 6. Preparation for exercise during anodal block with direct current. Direct current could be passed between two electrodes placed under the intact dorsal roots. The degree of block achieved was gauged by stimulating the sciatic nerve high in the back of the thigh with the test stimulator, and monitoring the changes produced by the block in the compound action potential recorded from a slip of the dorsal root after it had passed the blocking region.

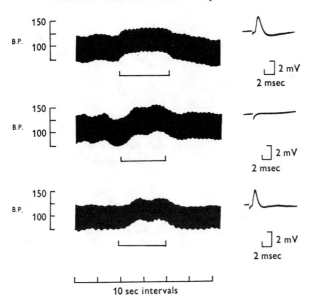

FIGURE 7. Blood pressure response to induced exercise during anodal block. Records of arterial blood pressure (B.P.) and the compound action potential are shown from three periods of exercise: (upper panel) control period of exercise before anodal block; (middle panel) period of exercise after anodal block just sufficient to block the A-wave of the compound atrium potential; (lower panel) control period of exercise after removal of the block. (From McCloskey & Mitchell.[18] By permission of the *Journal of Physiology*, London.)

myelinated fiber types I, II, and large type III were blocked there was no effect on the response of blood pressure during induced exercise.

Local anesthetic block of the dorsal roots receiving afferents from the exercising muscle was used to block preferentially small myelinated type III fibers and unmyelinated type IV fibers.[18] The technique is demonstrated in FIGURE 8. Test stimuli again were used to elicit the compound action potential, which was picked up from a sampling slip of dorsal root beyond the local anesthetic block in the spinal cord. Test stimuli were applied and then 0.125% lidocaine was applied to the dorsal root.

Bouts of exercise were performed both before and during the local anesthetic block and results are shown in FIGURE 9. In the upper panel exercise was performed before applying lidocaine and an increase in blood pressure occurred. In the middle panel during stimulation of the ventral root after lidocaine there is no change in arterial blood pressure even though the sampled action potential on the right shows no change. In the bottom panel after the anesthetic block has disappeared there is again an increase in arterial blood pressure during exercise of the hind limb muscles. Thus the exercise response disappeared but the compound action potential caused by type I, type II, and large type III fibers was still present. Therefore, one must assume that when the small type III and type IV fibers are blocked, the response disappears.

In summary these studies show that a peripheral control or skeletal-muscle–

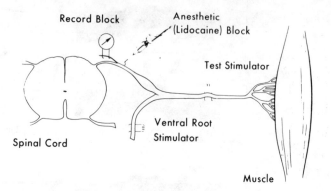

FIGURE 8. Preparation for exercise during anesthetic block. Lidocaine (0.125%) could be applied to the dorsal roots to produce a local anesthetic block. The degree of block achieved was monitored as described in FIGURE 7.

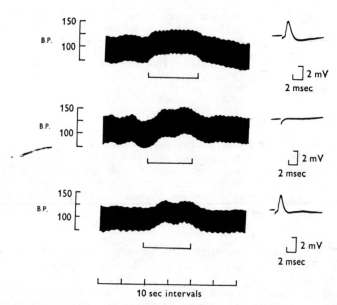

FIGURE 9. Blood pressure response to induced exercise during anesthetic block. Records of arterial blood pressure (B.P.) and the compound action potential are shown from three periods of exercise: (upper panel) control period of exercise before anesthetic block; (middle panel) period of exercise several minutes after application of lidocaine to the dorsal roots; (lower panel) control period of exercise after the lidocaine had been washed away. (From McCloskey & Mitchell.[18] By permission of the *Journal of Physiology*, London.)

circulation reflex does exist and that the afferent fibers of this reflex are small type III or type IV fibers. These fibers principally originate in free nerve endings.

There are two major questions that remain concerning this skeletal-muscle–circulation reflex. First, what are the factors that activate the receptors involved in this reflex physiologically during contraction? Work from our laboratory has suggested possible roles for increases in interstitial potassium and in hyperosmolarity in activating the receptors,[21, 22] but their physiological importance remains uncertain. Second, how important is the peripheral control mechanism in the conscious exercising animals in comparison to central command? Final answers to these questions require more experimental work.

References

1. JOHANSSON, J. E. 1894. Ueber die Einwirkung der Muskelthätligkeit auf die Athmung und die Herzthätigkeit. Scand. Arch. Physiol. **5:** 20–66.
2. KROGH, A. & J. LINDHARD. 1913/14. The regulation of respiration and circulation during the initial stages of muscular work. J. Physiol. (London) **47:** 112–136.
3. KROGH, A. & J. LINDHARD. 1917. A comparison between voluntary and electrically induced muscular work in man. J. Physiol. (London) **51:** 182–201.
4. ASMUSSEN, E., E. H. CHRISTENSEN & M. NIELSEN. 1940. Kreislaufgrösse und cortikal-motorische Innervation. Skand. Arch. Physiol. **83:** 181–187.
5. OCHWADT, B., E. BÜCHERL, H. KREUZER & H. H. LOESCHCKE. 1959. Beeinflussung der Atemsteigerung bei Muskelarbeit durch partiellen neuromuskulären Block (Tubocurarin). Pflügers Arch. **269:** 613–621.
6. ASMUSSEN, E., S. H. JOHANSEN, M. JORGENSEN & M. NIELSEN. 1965. On the nervous factors controlling respiration and circulation during exercise; experiments with curarization. Acta Physiol. Scand. **63:** 343–350.
7. FREYSCHUSS, U. 1970. Cardiovascular adjustment to somatomotor activation. Acta Physiol. Scand. Suppl. **342:** 1–63.
8. GOODWIN, G. M., D. I. McCLOSKEY & J. H. MITCHELL. 1972. Cardiovascular and respiratory responses to changes in central command during isometric exercise at constant muscle tension. J. Physiol. (London) **266:** 173–190.
9. ALAM, M. & F. H. SMIRK. 1937. Observations in man upon a blood pressure raising reflex arising from the voluntary muscles. J. Physiol. **89:** 372–383.
10. ALAM, M. & F. H. SMIRK. 1938. Observations in man upon a pulse-accelerating reflex from the voluntary muscles of the legs. J. Physiol. **92:** 167–177.
11. STAUNTON, H. P., S. H. TAYLOR & K. W. DONALD. 1964. The effect of vascular occlusion on the pressor response to static muscular work. Clin. Sci. **27:** 283–292.
12. PETRO, J. K., A. P. HOLLANDER & L. N. BOUMAN. 1970. Instantaneous cardiac acceleration in man induced by a voluntary muscular contraction. J. Appl. Physiol. **29:** 794–798.
13. HOLLANDER, A. P. & L. N. BOUMAN. 1975. Cardiac acceleration in man elicited by a muscle-heart reflex. J. Appl. Physiol. **38:** 272–281.
14. LAPORTE, Y., P. BESSOU & S. BOUISSET. 1960. Action reflexe des differents types de fibres afferentes d'origin musculaire sur la pression sanguine. Arch. Ital. Biol. **98:** 206–228.
15. SKOGLUND, C. R. 1960. Vasomotor reflexes from muscle. Acta Physiol. Scand. **50:** 311–327.
16. MITCHELL, J. H., D. S. MIERZWIAK, K. WILDENTHAL & W. D. WILLIS, JR. 1968. Effect on left ventricular performance of stimulation of an afferent nerve from muscle. Circ. Res. **22:** 507–518.

17. COOTE, J. H., S. M. HILTON & J. F. PEREZ-GONZALES. 1971. The reflex nature of the pressor response to muscular exercise. J. Physiol. (London) **215:** 789–804.
18. McCLOSKEY, D. I. & J. H. MITCHELL. 1972. Reflex cardiovascular and respiratory responses originating in exercising muscle. J. Physiol. (London) **224:** 173–186.
19. FISHER, M. L. & D. O. NUTTER. 1974. Cardiovascular reflex adjustments to static muscular contractions in the canine hindlimb. Amer. J. Physiol. **226:** 648–655.
20. MITCHELL, J. H., W. C. REARDON & D. I. McCLOSKEY. In press. Reflex effects on circulation and respiration from contracting skeletal muscle. Amer. J. Physiol.
21. WILDENTHAL, K., D. S. MIERZWIAK, N. S. SKINNER, JR. & J. H. MITCHELL. 1968. Potassium-induced cardiovascular and ventilatory reflexes from the dog hindlimb. Amer. J. Physiol. **215:** 542–548.
22. WILDENTHAL, K., D. S. MIERZWIAK & J. H. MITCHELL. 1969. Acute effects of increased serum osmolality on left ventricular performance. Amer. J. Physiol. **216:** 898–904.

PULMONARY ADAPTATION TO EXERCISE: EFFECTS OF EXERCISE TYPE AND DURATION, CHRONIC HYPOXIA AND PHYSICAL TRAINING*

J. A. Dempsey, N. Gledhill, W. G. Reddan,
H. V. Forster, P. G. Hanson, and A. D. Claremont

Pulmonary Physiology Laboratory
Department of Preventive Medicine
University of Wisconsin
Madison, Wisconsin 53706

A precise, efficient response of the pulmonary system to the increased energy demands imposed by rhythmic muscular work is well recognized as a necessary first line of defense in ensuring adequate systemic oxygen transport. We shall describe some critical aspects of this response in short-term muscular work and then examine how this response might be altered—both acutely by varying types of exercise and chronically by physical training and hypoxic environments.

Short-term exercise in healthy man at sea level may be used as the criterion response for purposes of comparison with other states. Some essential features of this pulmonary response are shown in TABLE 1. Note that arterial oxygen tension (P_{O_2}) is maintained near resting levels even to exhaustion and that arterial P_{CO_2} is maintained through moderate exercise levels and only falls as hyperventilation responds to the metabolic acidosis of heavy work. The efficiency with which this blood gas and acid-base homeostasis is achieved is remarkable, as evidenced by the absence of dyspneic sensations until exhaustive work levels are approached and the fact that the pulmonary vasculature is capable of receiving the entire cardiac output with minimal changes in right- or left-sided pressures and no accumulation of pulmonary extravascular water. The only significant sign of any "inefficiency" in pulmonary gas transport during exercise is the progressive widening of the alveolar to arterial P_{O_2} difference $[(A - a)D_{O_2}]$ (see below).

Several key mechanisms or characteristics underlie this homeostatic pulmonary response to short-term exercise. To name a few: (1) the complex combination of primary and feedback input to medullary neurons (see FIGURE 5 for details) ensures an isocapnic hyperpnea and high alveolar P_{O_2}; (2) a portion of this feedback system, i.e., that from respiratory muscle and lung stretch receptors to brain and spinal motor neurons, dictates a combination of breathing frequency and tidal volume that ensures a near ideal "minimum work" generation by the chest wall; and (3) the large reserve capabilities of the lung are such that the metabolic capacity of respiratory muscles, the mechanical limits of the lungs, airways, and parenchyma for gas flow and volume expansion, and the expansion capabilities of the pulmonary capillary network are barely taxed in exhaustive short-term work.

* This work was supported by the National Heart, Lung and Blood Institute Grant 17540 and Career Development Award 00149, by the Wisconsin Heart Association and by the University of Wisconsin Graduate School.

243

Pulmonary gas transport or the magnitude of the alveolar to arterial P_{O_2} difference [$(A - a)D_{O_2}$] is critically dependent upon ventilation ($\dot{V}_A$) to perfusion ($\dot{Q}$) relationships—both the overall $\dot{V}_A:\dot{Q}$ for the lung and the relative distributions of $\dot{V}_A$ and $\dot{Q}$ throughout the lung. Gledhill et al.[1] have studied the effects of exercise in health on the steady-state elimination of inert gases,[2] a technique that—unlike conventional radioactive tracer methods—permits the quantitation of $\dot{V}_A:\dot{Q}$ distribution throughout the lung. An example of these findings during mild exercise (TABLE 2) reveals the following pertinent conclusions: (1) Overall, $\dot{V}_A$ increases more than $\dot{Q}$ during exercise, resulting in a higher overall $\dot{V}_A:\dot{Q}$ with increasing exercise intensity (e.g., $\dot{V}_A:\dot{Q} \gtrless 5$ in maximum work). Hence, during exercise, the low $\dot{V}_A:\dot{Q}$ compartments are eliminated from participation in gas exchange—an adjustment that is critical to avoiding arterial hypoxemia and CO_2 retention in the face of increased metabolic demand and declining mixed venous P_{O_2} and rising P_{CO_2}. (2) Unexpectedly, $\dot{V}_A:\dot{Q}$ dispersion or distribution did not become more uniform during

TABLE 1

ARTERIAL BLOOD GAS HOMEOSTASIS: HEALTHY MAN IN SHORT-TERM WORK
(4–8 MINUTES) AT SEA LEVEL

	$\dot{V}_{O_2 max}$ %	Arterial Blood P_{O_2} (mmHg)	P_{CO_2}	pH	[HCO_3^-] (meq/ℓ)	Alveolar to Arterial P_{O_2} (mmHg)
Rest	—	90	40	7.40	25	10
Light work	20–30	88	42	7.38	25	12
Moderate work	40–60	90	40	7.38	23	15
Heavy work	65–85	90	35	7.34	19	18
Maximum work	100	93	30	7.29	14	25

exercise. In view of the more uniform topographical (or interregional) distribution of $\dot{V}_A$ or $\dot{Q}$ found during exercise using radioactive tracers,[3] our findings point to an exercise-induced intraregional inhomogeneity in $\dot{V}_A:\dot{Q}$ distribution. (3) The quantitation of $\dot{V}_A:\dot{Q}$ distribution permits calculation of end-capillary blood gases and hence a partitioning of factors causing the observed $(A - a)D_{O_2}$. Note that the increased $(A - a)D_{O_2}$ during exercise is attributable mostly to the contribution from an anatomical shunt of mixed venous blood (~1% of cardiac output).

We will now examine a variety of conditions which may alter the pulmonary response to exercise. The effects of short-term work in varying *body postures and during tethered crawl swimming* were tested in healthy subjects (FIGURES 1 & 2). We postulated an improved pulmonary gas exchange secondary to a more homogeneous topographical $\dot{V}_A:\dot{Q}$ distribution with supination and immersion. At rest, $(A - a)D_{O_2}$ was narrowed and DL_{CO} significantly higher in the supine posture, but during exercise and particularly heavy exercise no clear effects of posture or immersion were evidenced other than small differences in ventilatory response at moderate workloads. These data confirm the idea ex-

TABLE 2

PULMONARY VENTILATION TO PERFUSION RATIO ($\dot{V}_A:\dot{Q}$) DURING EXERCISE:
RESULTS OF MULTIPLE INERT GAS ANALYSIS

	Rest ($\dot{V}_{O_2}=0.27$ liters/min)	Mild Work ($\dot{V}_{O_2}=1.1$ liters/min)
Mixed-venous blood gas values (mmHg)		
P_{O_2}	39	31
P_{CO_2}	45	52
$\dot{V}_A$ *and* $\dot{Q}$ *(liters/min)*		
$\dot{V}_A$	5.4	25.6
$\dot{Q}$	5.8	11.7
$\dot{V}_A:\dot{Q}$		
Mean	0.93	2.3
Dispersion *	±0.34	±0.46
Range	0.49–2.1	0.93–6.6
P_{O_2} *(mmHg)*		
Alveolar	100 ⎫ 7 †	108 ⎫ 9 †
End pulmonary capillary	93 ⎭ ⎫ 3 ‡	99 ⎭ ⎫ 8 ‡
Arterial	90 ⎭	91 ⎭
Alveolar to arterial difference, $(A-a)D_{O_2}$	10	17

* Log of standard deviation (SD).
† Portion of the $(A-a)D_{O_2}$ due to $\dot{V}_A:\dot{Q}$ inhomogeneity.
‡ Portion of the $(A-a)D_{O_2}$ due to anatomical shunt. We assume that limitations
to alveolar capillary diffusion contribute nothing to the $(A-a)D_{O_2}$.

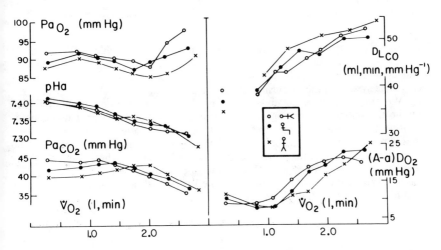

FIGURE 1. Effects of posture on pulmonary response to short-term (4–6 min)
workloads ($n=6$). Exercise diffusion capacity (DL_{CO}) was measured with the single-
breath method at rest and steady-state method during exercise. Postural effects were
negligible in moderate to heavy work.

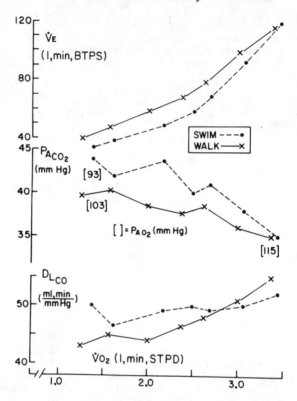

FIGURE 2. Effects of tethered swimming (4–5 min per load) on ventilation and DL_{CO} (steady-state method) in trained swimmers ($n=9$). Swimming effects were limited to a relative underventilation and mild CO_2 retention in moderate work.

pressed above that intraregional rather than only topographical differences in $\dot{V}_A:\dot{Q}$ distribution determine alveolar to arterial gas exchange during exercise and demonstrate that it is difficult to improve upon an already near-ideal gas exchange system in the exercising healthy upright man.

We emphasize that steady-state exercise in laboratory conditions may not mimic the pulmonary response to the unsteady states encountered under competitive conditions. For example, the sprint crawl is often preceded by 20 or more minutes of volitional hyperventilation, with the swimmer beginning the race at high lung volume, which he maintains while apneic throughout the 20+ seconds of a 50-yard sprint. Note below the changes in alveolar (end-tidal) gases obtained immediately before and the first breath after practice time trials in a highly trained sprinter (mean of four trials).

	Quiet Rest	50-yd. Sprint (21.0 sec)	
		Before	After
Alveolar P_{CO_2} (mmHg)	41	23	68
Alveolar P_{O_2} (mmHg)	96	124	47

The pulmonary response to *prolonged heavy exercise* at constant workload (60%–75% of maximum $\dot{V}_{O_2}$) in the fit but not highly trained individual is most notably characterized by a progressive, time-dependent tachypneic hyperventilation and hypocapnia (FIGURE 3). This "ventilatory drift" is analogous to the well-known progressive tachycardia or "cardiovascular drift" in prolonged work and is accompanied by gradually rising intravascular temperatures and a

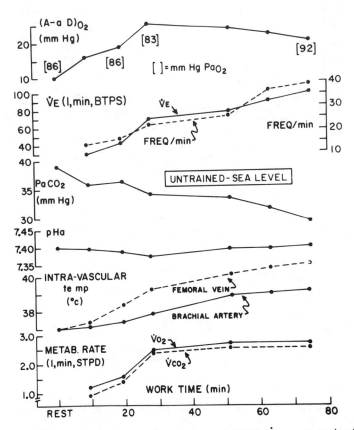

FIGURE 3. Pulmonary response to long-term work (66% $\dot{V}_{O_2max}$ at sea level in fit but untrained subjects ($n=6$, $\dot{V}_{O_2max}=50\pm2$ ml/kg). All blood gases were corrected to observed vascular temperatures. During the prolonged heavy work phase increases in $\dot{V}_E$, breathing frequency, and heart rate (148 to 175) were 40%, 70%, and 18%, respectively.

near-perfect regulation of arterial [H+]. In the sea-level native after 2–5 weeks sojourn at high altitudes, this ventilatory drift is similar in nature to that seen at sea level but is markedly accentuated (FIGURE 4). Alveolar to arterial O_2 transport is well maintained during prolonged work, i.e., at sea level and even at 3100 m arterial P_{O_2} remains at or above resting levels and $(A-a)D_{O_2}$ narrows slightly with exercise duration. There are, of course, limits to even the healthy lung's capability for alveolar-capillary diffusion and blood gas homeostasis, as may be noted at 4300 m where arterial hypoxemia worsens with intensity and duration of work despite the extreme levels of hyperventilation.

The potential *mediators of "hyperventilatory drift"* in prolonged exercise are outlined in FIGURE 5. They are viewed as overriding stimuli—superimposed on the basic system of primary and feedback stimuli which operate in combina-

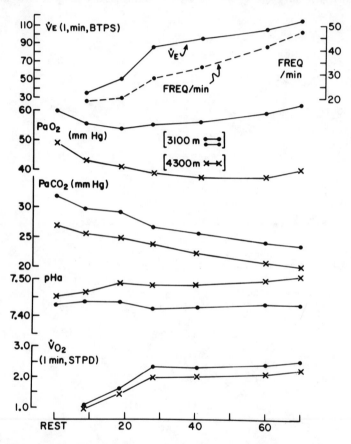

FIGURE 4. Pulmonary response to long-term work (70% $\dot{V}_{O_2max}$) after 10 days to 3 weeks at high altitudes in the same subjects as in FIGURE 3 ($\dot{V}_{O_2max}$ at 3100 m = 45 ±2 ml/kg). Vascular temperature changes were similar to those at sea level (FIGURE 3). At 3100 m during the prolonged heavy work phase, increases in $\dot{V}_E$, breathing frequency, and heart rate (157 to 179) were 35%, 67%, and 15%, respectively.

tion to ensure a fairly precise eucapnic hyperpnea in short-term moderate work. While we are as yet unable to determine precisely which of these overriding stimuli are responsible for ventilatory drift, the evidence to date points to three possibilities: (1) The *[H+] stimulus,* although a dominant factor in the hyperventilation of short-term heavy exercise, must play a small or negligible role in prolonged work—simply because a metabolic acidosis is not incurred in arterial

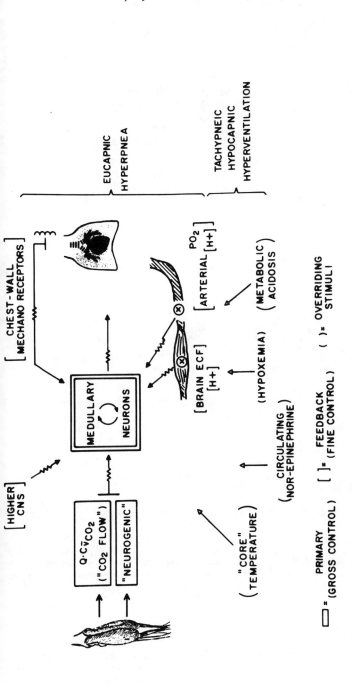

FIGURE 5. Schema for regulation of exercise hyperpnea and hyperventilation. Eucapnic hyperpnea is maintained (in short-term work) by a precise combination of 1 or 2 "primary" drives originating in working muscle [4] with both chemical and mechanical feedback or "error" control. During prolonged heavy work in normoxia or hypoxia a number of stimuli override this basic control system resulting in a progressive tachypneic, hypocapnic hyperventilation.

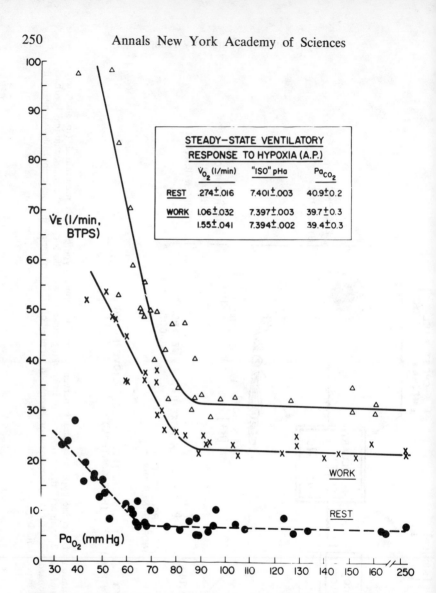

FIGURE 6. Mild exercise (treadmill walking) combined with hypoxemia causes a multiplicative effect on steady-state ventilatory response. Each point represents 15 min of breathing a hypoxic, normoxic, or hyperoxic gas with continuous adjustment of inspired CO_2 so as to maintain a steady arterial P_{CO_2}.

blood (FIGURES 3 & 4). We do not, however, know if [H⁺] homeostasis at the level of intracranial chemoreceptors is similarly maintained. (2) A *thermal drive* to ventilation has been documented in man under conditions of increased ambient and core temperature [5, 6] and may be important during prolonged work as evidenced by the absence of hyperventilation when skin temperature was cooled sufficiently to prevent most of the rise in core temperature.[7] However,

TABLE 3

EFFECTS OF EXERCISE, HYPOXIA, AND THEIR COMBINATION ON
CATECHOLAMINE EXCRETION (27 EXPERIMENTS IN 3 SUBJECTS)

	Rest Hypoxia	Work Normoxia Light	Work Normoxia Moderate	Work + Hypoxia Light	Work + Hypoxia Moderate
V_{O_2} (liter/min)	0.27	1.1	1.6	1.1	1.6
Pa_{O_2} (mmHg)	56	100	110	55	56
Epinephrine + norepine-phrine urinary excretion (% of resting control values)*	168%	100%	182%	200%	467%

* Each experimental condition consisted of 20 min of exercise and/or hypoxia. Urine catecholamine excretion was obtained from samples collected 5 min after each of these conditions and compared to control samples obtained in the resting normoxia state at 20-min intervals over the 60 min preceding each condition and at 30–40 min following each condition of hypoxia and/or exercise. These control excretion values averaged 0.024 μg/min (range 0.020 to 0.031).

we emphasize the preliminary nature of these data and the fact that the site or mode of action of this proposed thermal drive remains unknown. (3) *Circulating norepinephrine* acting via carotid body chemoreceptors may be a key mediator of hyperventilatory response—particularly in hypoxic exercise. Supportive, circumstantial evidence is shown from the work of Jackson *et al.* in our laboratory: (a) hypoxemia and even mild exercise produce multiplicative effects on ventilation (FIGURE 6); (b) these same conditions in combination have an interactive effect on norepinephrine excretion (TABLE 3); and (c) infused norepinephrine, like mild exercise, potentiates the ventilatory response to hypoxia (FIGURE 7). We suspect, because of the substantial magnitude of

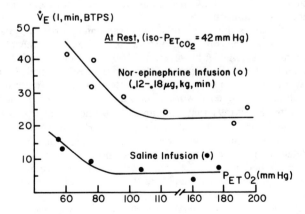

FIGURE 7. Norepinephrine intravenous infusion causes a multiplicative effect on steady-state ventilatory response to hypoxia at rest. Each point represents 25 min of isocapnic hypoxia, or normoxia plus saline (control), or norepinephrine infusion

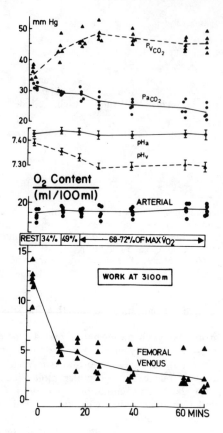

FIGURE 8. Arterial and femoral venous O_2 content and acid-base status during prolonged work at 3100 m ($n=6$). Note venous O_2 contents falling to < 2 ml/100 ml, as $C(a\text{-}v)_{O_2}$ widens with duration of heavy work. Arterial and femoral venous pH remain constant throughout the prolonged heavy work phase.

the hyperventilatory drift, that its mediation would require a combination of these stimuli acting simultaneously.

Of what *significance* is this substantial hyperventilatory drift *to systemic O_2 transport and tissue metabolism?* During exercise at sea level the effects on arterial O_2 content are negligible; however, at 3100 m, hyperventilation is essential to maintaining arterial O_2 content (Ca_{O_2}) near resting levels [7] and this adaptation may be critical in view of the very low levels of femoral venous C_{O_2} and P_{O_2} achieved in long-term work (FIGURE 8). On the other hand, additional data suggests (FIGURE 9) that, so long as blood flow is high and H^+ concentration reasonably well regulated, end-capillary P_{O_2} in working skeletal muscle must reach extremely low levels ($\sim <5$ mmHg) before significant changes are detected in the energy state of the muscle. In other words, O_2 content in arterial blood presented to the working muscle becomes a rather minor consideration if the "critical" capillary P_{O_2} is so low that a near maximum femoral arterio-venous O_2 content difference may be achieved for maintaining high levels of steady-state energy metabolism during prolonged work.

We think, then, that protection of [H^+] homeostasis rather than O_2 transport may present a much more crucial role for hyperventilation in prolonged work. Note the constancy of both arterial and femoral venous pH during the prolonged phase of heavy work (FIGURE 8). The importance of [H⁺] homeostasis to muscle metabolism in exercising man is poorly understood, but a sufficient amount of data from *in situ* and *in vitro* preparations are available which clearly demonstrate a tight coupling of pH with some ATP-linked cellular processes [9] and show the level of ECF [H⁺] to be a critical determinant of skeletal muscle metabolic rate, lactate production and uptake, and contractile strength.[10, 11] Unfortunately, hypocapnia during exercise does not serve [H⁺] homeostasis in all of the body's ECF, and the poorly buffered brain ECF is a notable exception. The result is a vasoconstrictive response of cerebral arterioles to local alkalosis, which is initiated during exercise around 30 mmHg Pa_{CO_2} (FIGURE 10) and is maintained during prolonged work.[7] The concomitant reductions in cerebral O_2 transport and cerebral capillary P_{O_2} produced no detectable effects on cerebral oxidative metabolism—although this analysis of cerebral arterio-venous differences would not be sensitive to more subtle metabolic changes, such as reduced brain neuro-transmitter turnover, which are known to occur with even mild levels of cerebral hypoxia.[12]

Hence, hypocapnia during prolonged work has both positive and negative implications for tissue metabolism. Quantitation of the true net effects of these observations awaits delineation of [H⁺] effects at the cellular level.

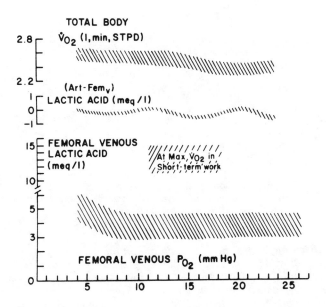

FIGURE 9. Changes in femoral venous and arterial–femoral-venous lactate and $\dot{V}_{O_2}$ as femoral venous P_{O_2} falls with time during prolonged work. Combined data from six subjects working for 70 min at 65%–72% $\dot{V}_{O_2max}$ at sea level and high altitude. As judged from the ratios of mixed to femoral arterio-venous O_2 content differences,[8] blood flow to the legs was high and constant throughout prolonged work. Also noted (in the lower panel) is the plasma lactic acid concentration and femoral venous P_{O_2} achieved in 2–4 min of maximum work at sea level. It appears that hypoxemia, per se, in working muscle capillaries must be extremely severe (< 5–10 mmHg) before evidence of tissue anoxia is evident.

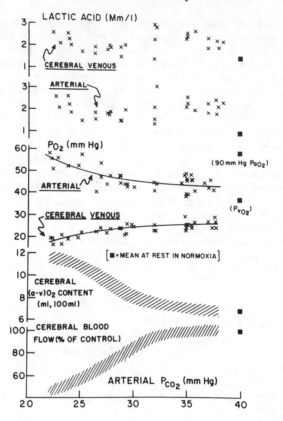

FIGURE 10. Changes in relative cerebral blood flow (CBF), arterial and cerebral venous C_{O_2}, P_{O_2}, and lactic acid, with varying levels of steady-state hypocapnia during moderate supine exercise ($n=5$, $P_{I_{O_2}}=105$ mmHg). CBF fell with Pa_{CO_2} below ~30 mmHg Pa_{CO_2}. Hyperventilation increased arterial P_{O_2} but cerebral venous P_{O_2} fell to <20 mmHg bcause of reduced CBF. Arterial–cerebral–venous lactate (or glucose) differences were not affected by these reductions in CBF.

The effects of various chronic conditions on the pulmonary response to work are most readily demonstrated in disease states; and mild exercise stress is sometimes helpful as a fairly sensitive tool for diagnosis of gas exchange abnormalities.[13] The cases shown in FIGURE 11 represent inadequate ventilatory response to work for a variety of reasons and include two otherwise healthy persons who, for unexplained reasons, show mild and severe CO_2 retention during exercise.

Negative effects on the pulmonary response to work are, then, numerous and often demonstrable at even the earliest stages in the pathogenesis of lung disease, but it has been much more difficult to document factors that might exert a positive chronic influence on lung functions. For example, it seems logical to postulate—and many have—that biological adaptation to chronic physical training would include the lungs and/or associated ventilatory control systems. Certainly there is strong evidence to link metabolic rate and gas exchange surface area or lung volume as an explanation for differences among species,[14] between wild and domestic animals within a species [15] and for the observed increase in lung surface area in genetically or pharmacologically induced chronic elevations in metabolic rate.[16, 17] We have looked carefully for this adaptation at various stages of training in endurance athletes—crewmen, swimmers, and trackmen—and have failed to confirm this hypothesis.[18] The only consistent finding of ourselves and others is that training causes a reduced V_E at any given V_{O_2} in moderate to heavy work, and this is usually explained by a reduced metabolic acidosis and/or V_{CO_2} with training.[13] We have also examined what we believed to be ideal conditions for producing pulmonary adaptations, i.e., sedentary, healthy sea-level natives training 2–3 hours daily in a hypoxic environment at 3100 m altitude (FIGURES 12A & 12B; TABLE 4). We saw substantial increases in maximum V_{O_2} and reductions in heart rate and plasma lactate during submaximal work, but failed to detect training effects on exercise diffusion capacity (DL_{CO}) and $(A - a)D_{O_2}$ or on the ventilatory response to either exercise or imposed chemical stimuli at rest. The results pertain to data obtained in these subjects both during their 8 weeks of training at 3100 m and after returning to sea level. Similarly, we found no significant differences, in these respects, between athletic and sedentary adult natives of 3100 m.

One interpretation of these data is that the healthy "untrained" pulmonary system is already endowed with a reserve, which *by itself* is capable of attaining olympian-sized work capacities. Accordingly, the well-documented stress—

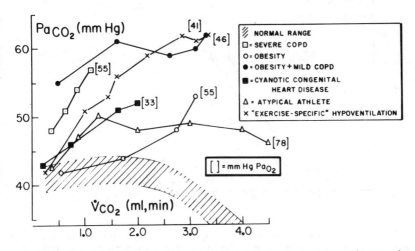

FIGURE 11. Atypical CO_2 retention during short-term steady-state work, secondary mainly to: (1) a ventilatory pump that is incapable of producing the required flow rates (chronic obstructed lung disease); (2) restricted diaphragmatic response (obesity); (3) combination of (1) and (2); and (4) a high ventilatory response, but right-to-left shunt of mixed venous blood (cyanotic congenital heart disease). The moderate and severe hypoventilation and CO_2 retention in the healthy untrained subject ($\times$) and endurance athlete (crewman) were associated with very low breathing frequencies during exercise and severely depressed ventilatory response to CO_2 and hypoxia at rest.

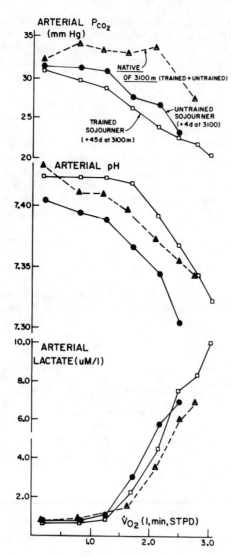

FIGURE 12A. Acid-base status during short-term exercise at 3100 m in sojourners before and after training ($n=5$) and a mixed group of trained and untrained natives to 3100 m ($n=14$) (see also TABLE 4). Training at 3100 m had no significant effects on these responses, but the native of 3100 m maintained isocapnic hyperpnea until heavy work loads were reached.

adaptation phenomena elicited by daily physical training in heart, skeletal muscle, and the sympatho-adrenal system—does not occur in the pulmonary system simply because it is really not "stressed" often enough near its capabilities. That is not to say that the healthy lung in both young and adult animals and man is incapable of adaptation to truly chronic stress. Significant functional and morphologic change has been shown following pneumonectomy [19] and most consistently in hypobaric hypoxia.[15, 20, 21] Further, the healthy human native or long-term resident (of ≤3 years) at high altitudes shows a near-ideal adaptation to moderate exercise in his hypoxic environment. That is, he does not exhibit tachypneic hyperventilation as does the short-term sojourner and yet

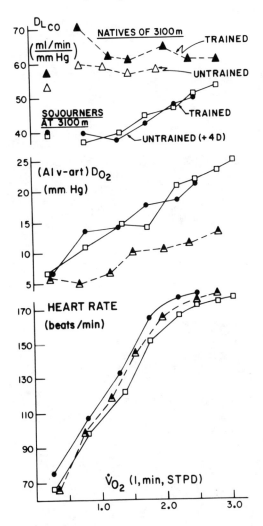

FIGURE 12B. Pulmonary O$_2$ transport and diffusing capacity (DL_{CO}) during short-term exercise at 3100 m. DL_{CO} was measured by the single-breath technique at rest and steady-state technique during exercise. Training in the sojourners produced no consistent effects and there were no significant differences between trained and untrained natives of 3100 m. Note, however, the extremely high DL_{CO} and narrowed alveolar to arterial P_{O_2} [$(A-a)D_{O_2}$] in the natives.

maintains arterial O$_2$ content near resting levels because of a narrowed $(A-a)D_{O_2}$ and extremely high alveolar-capillary diffusion and pulmonary capillary blood volume (FIGURES 12A & 12B).[22]

Finally, it is important to emphasize that physical training may conceivably elicit adaptive changes in the pulmonary system under very specific conditions that, to date, have not received sufficient scrutiny. For example, the stage of lung maturation (during growth) or degeneration (with the aging process) may be an important determinant of training effectiveness, although the available data in either young animals[23] or diseased adult lung[24] show no consistent effects of training on pulmonary gas exchange. More promising are findings that the diaphragm, like other skeletal muscle, may show adaptation of fiber type and oxidative capacity to training in young and older animals[25] and that

TABLE 4

CHARACTERISTICS, $\dot{V}_{O_2 max}$, AND VENTILATORY RESPONSE TO CHEMICAL STIMULI IN SEDENTARY (CONTROL) AND TRAINING SOJOURNERS AT 3100 M AND IN NATIVES OF 3100 M

	Sea-Level Natives Sojourning at 3100 m						Natives of 3100 m * (1–3 generations at 3100 m)
	Trainees			Controls			
		3100 m			3100 m		
	250 m	4th Day	45th Day	250 m	4th Day	45th Day	
Age (yr)	22.3 (1.8)†						19.8 (1.3)
Height (cm)	176.4 (2.1)			179.5 (1.7)			176.8 (1.9)
Weight (kg)	69.0 (3.0)	68.9 (3.0)	67.3 (2.5)	76.3 (1.8)	75.2 (1.5)	75.5 (1.8)	69.2 (2.3)
Hemoglobin (g)	14.8 (0.17)	15.4 (0.18)	15.4 (0.67)	15.0 (0.2)	14.6 (0.2)	15.7 (0.2)	16.6 (0.3)
TLC (liters)	6.01 (0.07)			6.31 (0.07)			6.08 (0.19)
$\dot{V}_{O_2 max}$ (ml/kg)	41.3 (0.44)	36.4 (1.9)	44.6 (2.3)	45.2 (2.6)	40.0 (2.7)	40.4 (2.6)	40.0 (1.3)
Resting CO_2 response $(\Delta\dot{V}_E/\Delta P_{A CO_2})$	3.2 (0.8)	3.5 (0.6)	4.9 (1.2)	2.7 (0.5)	3.8 (0.4)	5.6 (0.8)	2.6 (0.3)
Resting isocapnic hypoxic response $[\Delta\dot{V}_E(\text{liter/min})$ from $P_{A O_2}$ 250 to 40 mmHg]	29 (5)	46 (8)	47 (5)	27 (7)	44 (16)	44 (8)	23 (2)

* All these characteristics, except $\dot{V}_{O_2 max}$, were not significantly different in the athletic and nonathletic natives and hence values are pooled for both groups. Mean $\dot{V}_{O_2 max}$ was 44 ml/kg in the athletic native and 35 ml/kg in the nonathletic native.
† Standard deviation.

humans can improve the capacity for sustaining high levels of voluntary ventilation through daily "endurance" training of respiratory and accessory muscles.[26] We have recently examined ventilatory response to prolonged heavy work under laboratory and field conditions in highly trained, competitive distance runners.

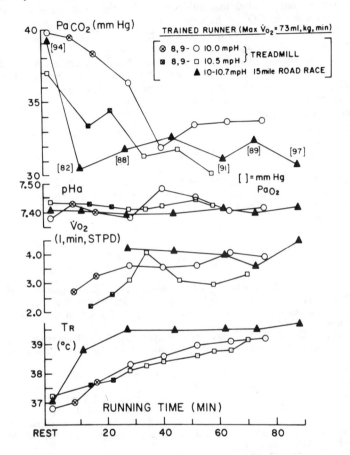

FIGURE 13. Changes in arterial blood gases and acid-base status during prolonged heavy work (70%–75% $\dot{V}_{O_2max}$) in a trained endurance runner. All values corrected to body temperature. Data obtained during exercise (twice under laboratory conditions and once during a 16-mile road race). Hyperventilation and hypocapnia were significant in all three instances, but tended to subside somewhat with duration of exercise.

Preliminary results in six runners (FIGURE 13) show that they do experience significant hypocapnia in prolonged work accompanied by maintained or alkaline arterial H+ concentrations and rising core temperatures. However, relative to his untrained contemporaries, the runner's hyperventilation and tachypnea were not as severe nor progressive with exercise duration, and occasionally the level of hyperventilation actually lessened with time of running. It has been suggested that the endurance athlete may possess an inherent "insensitivity" to chemical stimuli and that responses to chemical stimuli at rest are predictive of the ventilatory response to work.[27-29] Our data are consistent in part with this idea because we have found that subjects at the high and low extremes of ventilatory response to CO_2 or hypoxia also hyperventilate and hypoventilate, respectively, during exercise in normoxia or hypoxia [30, 31] (FIGURES 11 & 12). However, we have also found that the resting ventilatory response to chemical stimuli in a wide variety of endurance athletes is highly heterogeneous and not unlike that of the normal, nonathletic population. Hence, we believe that any modification in the athlete's ventilatory response to prolonged work is most likely attributable to lower levels of ventilatory stimuli, such as core temperature or circulating norepinephrine.

Acknowledgments

We wish to acknowledge the technical assistance of Jean Vaughn, Monique Wanner, and Naomi Wells and the collaboration of James Thoden, Edward Vidruk, John Thomson, Frank Cerny, Louis Chosy, and G. A. doPico in many of these studies.

References

1. GLEDHILL, N., A. B. FROESE & J. A. DEMPSEY. 1977. Ventilation to perfusion distribution during exercise and health. *In* Muscular Exercise and the Lung. J. A. Dempsey & C. E. Reed, Eds. : 325–343. University of Wisconsin Press. Madison, Wisconsin.
2. WAGNER, P. D., H. A. SALTZMAN & J. B. WEST. 1974. Measurement of continuous distribution of ventilation-perfusion ratios: Theory. J. Appl. Physiol. **36:** 588–599.
3. BAKE, B., J. BJORN & J. WIDIMSKY. 1968. The effect of sitting and graded exercise on the distribution of pulmonary blood flow in healthy subjects studied with the ^{133}xenon technique. Scand. J. Clin. Lab. Invest. **22:** 99–106.
4. WASSERMAN, K., B. WHIPP, R. CASABURI, W. BEAVER & H. BROWN. 1977. CO_2 flow to the lungs and ventilatory control. *In* Muscular Exercise and the Lung. J. A. Dempsey and C. E. Reed, Eds. : 103–136. University of Wisconsin Press, Madison, Wisc.
5. CUNNINGHAM, D. & J. O'RIORDON. 1957. The effect of a rise in the temperature of the body on the respiratory response to CO_2 at rest. Quart. J. Exper. Physiol. **42:** 329–336.
6. MACDOUGALL, J. D., W. G. REDDAN, C. R. LAYTON & J. A. DEMPSEY. 1974. Effects of metabolic hyperthermia on performance during heavy prolonged exercise. J. Appl. Physiol. **36:** 538–544.
7. DEMPSEY, J., J. THOMSON, S. C. ALEXANDER, H. V. FORSTER & L. CHOSY. 1975. Respiratory influences on acid-base status and their effects on O_2 transport during prolonged muscular work. *In* Metabolic Adaptation to Prolonged Physical Exercise. H. Howald & J. R. Poortmans, Eds. Birkhäuser Verlag. Basel, Switzerland.
8. DEMPSEY, J., J. M. THOMSON, H. FORSTER, F. CERNEY & L. CHOSY. 1975. HbO_2 dissociation in man during prolonged work in chronic hypoxia. J. Appl. Physiol. **38:** 1022–1029.

9. DANFORTH, W. H. 1965. Activation of glycolytic pathway in muscle. *In* Control of Energy Metabolism. B. Chase & R. Estabrook, Eds. : 287–294. Academic Press. New York, N.Y.

10. HARKEN, A. H. 1976. Hydrogen ion concentration and oxygen uptake in an isolated canine hindlimb. J. Appl. Physiol. **40:** 1–5.

11. FITZGERALD, R. S., F. GARFINKEL, E. SILKEGELD & S. LOSAUFOFF. 1971. Factors in the interpretation of mouth occlusion pressure during measurements of chemosensitivity. Chest **70**(Suppl): 145–148.

12. DAVIS, J., N. CARLSSON, V. MACMILLAN & B. K. SIESJO. 1973. Brain tryptophon hydroxylation: Dependence on arterial oxygen tension. Science **182:** 72–74.

13. JONES, N. L. 1976. Use of exercise in testing respiratory control mechanisms. Chest **70**(Suppl): 169–172.

14. TENNEY, S. M. & J. E. REMMERS. 1963. Comparative quantitative morphology of the mammalian lung: Diffusing area. Nature **197:** 54–56.

15. WEIBEL, E. R. 1973. Morphological basis of alveolar-capillary gas exchange. Physiol. Rev. **53:** 419–495.

16. GEELHAAR, A. & E. R. WEIBEL. 1976. Morphometric estimation of pulmonary diffusion capacity. III. The effect of increased O_2 consumption in Japanese waltzing mice. Resp. Physiol. **11:** 354–366.

17. BURRI, P. H., P. GEHRI, K. MÜLLER & E. R. WEIBEL. 1976. Adaptation of the growing lung to increased $\dot{V}_{O_2}$. I. IDPN as inducer of hyperactivity. Resp. Physiol. **28:** 129–140.

18. REUSCHLEIN, P. L., W. G. REDDAN, J. F. BURPEE, J. B. L. GEE & J. RANKIN. 1968. The effect of physical training on the pulmonary diffusing capacity during submaximal work. J. Appl. Physiol. **24:** 152–153.

19. BRODY, J. S. & W. J. BUBAIN. 1973. Hormonal influence on postpneumonectomy lung growth in the rat. Resp. Physiol. **19:** 344–355.

20. BARTLETT, D. & J. E. REMMERS. 1971. Effects of high altitude exposure on the lungs of young rats. Resp. Physiol. **13:** 116–125.

21. CERNY, F. C., J. DEMPSEY & W. G. REDDAN. 1973. Pulmonary gas exchange in nonnative residents of 3100 m. J. Clin. Invest. **52:** 12.

22. DEMPSEY, J. A. 1975. Determinants of acquired changes in pulmonary gas exchange in man via chronic hypoxic exposure. *In* Progress in Resp. Research. H. Herzog, Ed. Vol. **9:** 180–186. S . Karger. Basel, Switzerland.

23. BARTLETT, D. 1970. Postnatal growth of the mammalian lung: Influence of exercise and thyroid activity. Resp. Physiol. **9:** 50–57.

24. PAEZ, P., E. PHILLIPSON, M. MOSANGKAY & B. SPROULE. 1967. The physiological basis of training patients with emphysema. Amer. Rev. Resp. Dis. **95:** 944–953.

25. LIEBERMAN, D., L. MAXWELL & J. FAULKNER. 1972. Adaptation of guinea pig diaphragm muscle to aging and endurance training. Amer. J. Physiol. **222:** 556–560.

26. LEITH, D. E. & M. BRADLEY. 1976. Ventilatory muscle strength and endurance training. J. Appl. Physiol. **41:** 508–516.

27. BYRNE-QUINN, E., J. V. WEIL, I. SODAL, G. FILLEY & R. GROVER. 1971. Ventilatory control in the athlete. J. Appl. Physiol. **30:** 91–95.

28. REBUCK, A. S. & J. READ. 1971. Pattern of ventilatory response to CO_2 during recovery from asthma. Clin. Sci. **31:** 14–20.

29. REBUCK, A. S., N. L. JONES & E. J. M. CAMPBELL. 1972. Ventilatory response to exercise and to CO_2 rebreathing in normal subjects. Clin. Sci. **43:** 861–867.

30. DEMPSEY, J. A., W. REDDAN, J. RANKIN & B. BALKE. 1966. Alveolar-arterial gas exchange during muscular work in obesity. J. Appl. Physiol. **21**(6): 1807–1814.

31. DEMPSEY, J. A. 1976. CO_2 response: Stimulus definition and limitations. Chest **70**(Suppl): 114–118.

THE HEMODYNAMIC AND METABOLIC ALTERATIONS ASSOCIATED WITH ACUTE HEAT STRESS INJURY IN MARATHON RUNNERS *

Thomas F. O'Donnell, Jr.

Departments of Surgery and Medicine
Tufts University School of Medicine
Tufts-New England Medical Center Hospital
Boston, Massachusetts 02111

Newton-Wellesley Hospital
Newton, Massachusetts 02162

Naval Hospital
Beaufort, South Carolina 29902

INTRODUCTION

One of the key mechanisms in the body's defense against heat stress is the maintenance of a hyperdynamic circulatory response until the heat load is dissipated. As a result of a release of sympathetic vasomotor tone, cutaneous blood flow rises three or fourfold in order to facilitate external heat loss. Cardiac output increases 50% to 75% during heat stress, paralleling the elevated peripheral blood flow. In resting man, when skin temperature is kept constant but elevated, the increase in cardiac output is accounted for by elevated cutaneous flow.[1] Muscle blood flow is not enhanced appreciably. If exercise is superimposed on the heat gain from environmental sources, the endogenous heat load of 65 to 85 kcal/hr from basal metabolism may escalate to 400–600 kcal/hr. Not only does the working muscle mass compound the total heat gain, but also it requires increased blood flow to supply oxygen and energy substrates. Thus, the circulatory stress of a man exercising in hot and humid conditions differs from that encountered by a resting subject in similar environmental situations. Metabolic needs may compete with thermoregulatory demands.

The circulatory system of the marathon runner demonstrates certain adaptive responses to exercise that are characterized by lowered heart rate and increased stroke volume index. In effect, cardiac contractility is enhanced and may prove of benefit during periods of heat stress. In this manner, the conditioned athlete's cardiovascular response to heat stress probably differs from that of the nonconditioned but equally youthful subject.[2] Because of the close relationship of the hemodynamic response to the metabolic response, biochemical changes during heat stress may also be different in these two groups. It is the purpose of this study to examine the hemodynamic and metabolic responses of eight marathon runners treated for heat stress injury during the 1976 Boston Athletic Association (BAA) Marathon. Dry bulb temperatures at that event were in the 90s (32°–38° C) and humidity was greater than 60%—conditions well recognized as conducive to the development of heat stress. Of the 2,000 participants, approximately 16 were treated at various hospitals for heat stress illnesses. The data on eight marathon runners will be compared to similar observations obtained on 15 young nonconditioned Marines previously reported by this author.[3]

---

* Opinions expressed in this article are those of the author and do not reflect those of the Navy or Marine Corps at large.

METHODS AND MATERIALS

Eight participants in the 1976 BAA marathon were studied. All patients exhibited some form of heat stress injury, and all were brought immediately to the Newton-Wellesley Hospital by police ambulance. Our participants' heat stress injury occurred at a distance of between 13.75 and 19.5 miles of the marathon route. Upon arrival at the hospital, rectal temperature, heart rate, and blood pressure were obtained. The eight patients were triaged into two groups by clinical criteria: heat stroke or heat exhaustion.[4] Those subjects with heat stroke were cooled to 101° F (38.3° C) by packing in ice and vigorous massage, and received an infusion of Ringer's lactate.[5] By contrast, those participants with heat exhaustion received an infusion of Ringer's lactate alone with volume replacement assessed by urine output and postural signs. Venous blood samples were drawn for electrolytes, blood urea nitrogen, and creatinine, as determined by standard laboratory measures.[6] All patients were questioned as to their previous residence and training regimen when fully alert.

RESULTS

Environmental Data. TABLE 1 presents the dry bulb temperatures at various distances along the marathon route at a time when humidity was approximately 62%, and wind velocity varied between 4 to 8 knots.

Clinical Data. None of the patients were world class runners, and only two were "official" marathon entries. Seven of the eight patients resided in the north, where they had undergone their premarathon training. The mean age of the participants was 28 years (range: 17 through 38 years) and all were males. Six of the eight subjects demonstrated mental confusion on initial examination. None were anhidrotic, although the three patients with elevated rectal temperatures had flushed skin.

Circulatory Data. TABLE 2 demonstrates the admission hemodynamic and temperature data for the eight patients. Three patients were hypotensive. No patient had a pulse pressure greater than 40 mmHg. Of note were the strikingly low heart rates, despite increased rectal temperatures in several of these patients. One patient was extremely bradycardic (patient No. 6) with a heart rate of

TABLE 1

ENVIRONMENTAL DATA ALONG THE COURSE OF THE 1976 BOSTON MARATHON

Distance (Miles)	Dry Bulb Temperature * (° C)
0	37.2
6.8	33.3
10.5	31.1
13.8 †	32.2
17.8 †	30.2

* Relative humidity was 62% for all temperatures.

† Interval between which patients demonstrated acute heat stress syndrome.

TABLE 2

HEMODYNAMIC DATA

Subject Number	Rectal Temperature (° C)	Mean Arterial Pressure (mmHg)	Pulse Pressure (mmHg)	Heart Rate (beats/min)
1	40.5	67	20	62
2	38.4	84	36	96
3	38.3	93	40	68
4	39.0	84	34	60
5	39.2	103	40	70
6	40.0	68	25	48
7	38.0	111	34	74
8	40.6	68	25	58

48 beats/min. Electrocardiograms were performed in five patients and all showed some minor abnormalities (atrial premature beat in one; S-T segment elevation, three; sinus bradycardia, two; voltage criteria for LVH, three; and first degree heart block, two.)

Metabolic Data. Six and five patients, respectively, had serum sodium and chlorides at the upper range of normal, while four patients showed elevated

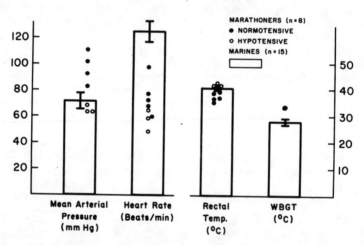

FIGURE 1. This figure compares hemodynamic and environmental data from 15 Marine recruits to the 8 marathoners. Although mean arterial pressure and rectal temperature are comparable in the two groups, heart rate is markedly decreased in the marathoners. The environmental conditions, indicated by the wet bulb globe temperature (WBGT), were more severe for the marathoners than for the group of Marines.

serum potassium levels. By contrast, carbon dioxide combining power was normal in all patients. Three patients had elevation of their blood urea nitrogen, one patient to 30 mg/100 ml. Plasma hemoglobin levels were increased in two patients to 12.4 and 22 mg%, respectively.

DISCUSSION

This study demonstrates that the responses of eight marathon runners to heat stress differs in many respects from those of the less conditioned subject.

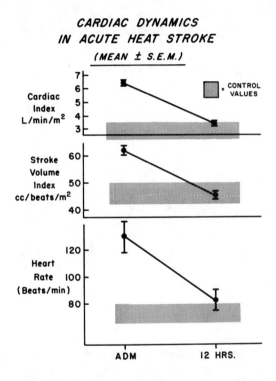

FIGURE 2. This figure demonstrates cardiac dynamics on admission with acute heat stroke (left side of panel) and twelve hours following treatment (right side of panel). Cardiac index, stroke volume index, and heart rate are all elevated on admission. The increase in cardiac index results from both an elevated heart rate and an enhanced stroke volume index.

These differences are best appreciated by comparing our eight marathon runners to a group of 15 Marine recruits subjected to heat stress previously studied by this author.[3] As will be appreciated in FIGURE 1, environmental conditions during the marathon were more severe than those experienced by the Marine recruits. That not more than sixteen participants developed heat stress injuries during the 1976 BAA marathon despite the hot and humid condition may be related to the constant cooling of the runners by water hoses along the route. Since seven of the eight marathoners resided and trained in the North prior to the race, lack of acclimatization played an important role in the development of heat stress injury. A similar prevalence of Northerners was observed in our study of 15 Marine recruits with heat stress injury. Because of the sudden change from a cool environmental condition to a hot and humid condition, the well-described endocrinologic, renal, and circulatory adaptations had not had time to develop.[7] Other major risk factors, such as fatigue and dehydration, may also have played a role in the development of heat stress injury in the marathoners. Lack of physical conditioning and obesity obviously were absent in the marathon runners but were present in several of the Marine recruits.

Although two of the clinical manifestations of heat stress injury, confusion and weakness, were similar to those shown by the nonconditioned Marines, the

TABLE 3

BIOCHEMICAL DATA

Subject Number	Potassium (meq/liter)	Sodium (meq/liter)	Chloride (meq/liter)	Carbon Dioxide (meq/liter)	Blood Urea Nitrogen (mg/ 100 ml)
Normal range	135–145	3.5–5.2	90–110	20–30	8–20
1	145	4.2	—	—	17
2	144	3.8	111	24.0	19
3	141	4.6	106	27.5	32
4	145	4.0	110	26.0	18
5	145	5.2	107	24.5	14
6	145	5.1	105	27.5	21
7	139	5.4	105	26.0	17
8	143	5.2	108	27.5	21

three marathoners with heat stroke differed in one major respect—they were sweating despite a markedly increased rectal temperature. This nonanhidrotic form of heat stroke has been described with prolonged exercise in highly acclimatized Israeli soldiers[8] and in Army recruits.[9] Exercise-induced heat stroke may differ from that observed in the elderly population, which occurs generally at rest. Austin and Berry[10] noted 100% of their cases were anhidrotic. By contrast, in the young athlete the endogenous heat load overwhelms the heat dissipating mechanisms before "sweat fatigue" may ensue. Of further interest was the cerebral symptom of confusion observed in the other five marathoners who did not have elevated rectal temperatures and were suffering from heat exhaustion. Rectal temperature, therefore, assumes an important differential finding in the clinical diagnosis of the various heat stress disorders.[7]

The hemodynamic responses of the eight marathon runners are compared to the 15 Marine recruits in FIGURE 1. Rectal temperature and mean arterial pressure are relatively comparable. Heart rate, however, is inappropriately low in seven of the eight marathoners, particularly in the three hypotensive subjects with heat stroke. Many authors [11-13] have observed the close relationship between a central and peripheral circulatory response in heat stress. The marked increase in cutaneous flow acts like an arteriovenous shunt so that cardiac output is increased 3–4-fold.[14] When exercise is combined with exposure to hot and humid conditions even greater stress is placed on circulatory homeostasis. Muscle blood flow is increased because of metabolic demands, but in turn muscle work results in a 7–10-fold increase in endogenous heat production. Deep muscle temperatures may rise to 41.1° C (106° F), so that the temperature of the blood draining from the muscle beds and the liver may be significantly higher than rectal temperature. Most investigators feel that the central circulatory response is determined by the resistances of the various regional vascular beds. Thus, in the exercising heat-stressed individual, splanchnic blood flow must decrease to compensate for the combination of increased skin and muscle blood flow. The limitations on venous return in the exercising heat-stressed individual alters the central response. Cardiac output and stroke volume are less than in the resting heat-stressed subject.[15]

Controversy exists as to whether the central response, that is, increased cardiac output, results predominantly from an increased heart rate or from a concomitant increase in stroke volume. Koroxenides [1] felt that cardiac output was increased principally as a result of an elevated heart rate, but Burch and Hyman [16] observed that the 4-fold increase in cardiac output was accompanied by a 3-fold elevation in stroke volume. FIGURE 2 demonstrates the results of cardiodynamic studies in eight Marine recruits with acute heat stroke studied by this author.[17] It will be noted that the markedly increased cardiac index resulted from both an elevated heart rate and an increased stroke volume index. It can be appreciated from this data that the limiting factor in the circulatory response to heat stress is the ability of the heart to meet the demands required by peripheral blood flow. Either cardiac failure or lack of selective shunting of blood within the splanchnic region may result in circulatory decompensation. On the other hand, the direct toxic effect of heat on thermally labile enzymes may also lead to decreased myocardial contractility as we have observed in one Marine recruit.[17] As has been demonstrated by the experimental work of Gold [13] and of Daily and Harrison,[12] circulatory failure results in high mortality in heat stress injuries.

The cardiovascular response of the right marathoners to heat stress was unique. Mean arterial pressure and urine output were maintained at normal or near normal levels. In view of the low heart rate and the clinical evidence of vasodilatation, stroke volume index was apparently increased to maintain cardiac output. This would be consistent with previous circulatory studies in conditioned athletes where an increased stroke volume index was the main circulatory adaptation to repetitive exercise.[2] Further adaptive changes in the circulatory response may be related to selective regional shunting such as in the splanchnic or muscle beds.[19]

Whether enhanced vagal tone was the basis for the bradycardia observed in the marathoners is unknown. The electrocardiographic findings, however, in several of the marathoners (increased P-R interval and first degree heart block) make increased parasympathetic activity a possibility. Whatever the cause of the bradycardia, it is in striking contrast to the tachycardia of the nonconditioned Marines.

The metabolic data demonstrated in TABLE 2 is in agreement with our previous findings and those of Schreier.[20] The marginal elevations in sodium are probably related to the hypotonic sweat loss, which was significant by the 15th mile of the marathon. Serum potassium levels, however, differ from those observed in the Marine recruits. Actual hyperkalemia was observed in four marathoners. The elevated potassium may be related to changes in muscle membrane permeability secondary to prolonged exercise.[5] Such a hypothesis is strengthened by the finding of myoglobinemia in previous studies of exercising man.[21] The slight elevation in blood urea nitrogen is consistent with dehydration and with alterations in renal dynamics as described by Schreier and others.[20, 22]

SUMMARY

Studies of clinical, metabolic, and hemodynamic responses to heat stress in eight marathon runners have demonstrated several important differences from those observed in nonconditioned subjects. Three marathoners manifested a nonanhidrotic form of heat stroke, a phenomenon not observed in our Marine recruits. Five patients with heat exhaustion evidenced signs of severe mental confusion despite apparently adequate hemodynamic function. Heart rate was significantly lower in all eight marathoners in comparison to the 15 Marine recruits. This latter observation suggests that either selective regional shunting of blood or increased stroke volume index occurs in marathoners subject to heat stress.

ACKNOWLEDGMENTS

The author wishes to express his gratitude for the help of the surgical, medical, resident, and nursing staffs of the Newton-Wellesley Hospital in caring expertly for these patients.

REFERENCES

1. KOROXENIDIS, G. T., J. T. SHEPHERD & R. J. MARSHALL. 1961. Cardiovascular response to acute heat stress. J. Appl. Physiol. 16(5): 869–872.
2. GRIMBY, G. & B. SALTIN. 1971. Physiological effects of physical training in different ages. Scand. J. Rehab. Med. 3: 6–14.
3. O'DONNELL, T. F. 1975. Acute Heat Stroke. J. Amer. Med. Assoc. 234: 824–828.
4. EDITORIAL. 1968. Heat Stroke. Lancet ii: 31–32.
5. O'DONNELL, T. F. 1971. Medical problems of recruit training: A research approach. U. S. Navy Med. 586: 28–34.
6. BERGMEYER, H. U. 1965. Methods of enzymatic analysis. Academic Press. New York, N.Y.
7. KNOCHEL, J. P. 1974. Environmental heat illness. Arch. Intern. Med. 133: 841–862.
8. GILAT, T., S. SHIBOLET & E. SHOHAR. 1963. Mechanism of heat stroke. J. Trop. Med. Hyg. 66: 204–212.
9. KNOCHEL, J. P., W. R. BEISEL, E. G. HERNDON, E. S. GERARD & K. G. BARRY. 1961. The renal, cardiovascular, hematologic, and serum electrolyte abnormalities of heat stroke. Amer. J. Med. 30: 299–309.
10. AUSTIN, M. G., J. W. BERRY. 1956. Observations on 100 cases of heat stroke. J. Amer. Med. Assoc. 161: 1525–1529.

11. WILSON, G. 1940. The cardiopathology of heat stroke. J. Amer. Med. Assoc. **114:** 557–558.
12. DAILY, W. M. & T. R. HARRISON. 1948. A study of the mechanism and treatment of experimental heat pyrexia. Amer. J. Med. Sci. **215:** 42–55.
13. GOLD, J. 1960. Development of heat pyrexia. J. Amer. Med. Assoc. **173:** 1175–1182.
14. DETRY, J-M. R., G. L. BRENGELMANN, L. B. ROWELL & C. WYSS. 1972. Skin and muscle components of forearm blood flow in directly heated resting man. J. Appl. Physiol. **32**(4)**:** 506–511.
15. ROWELL, L. B., J. A. MURRAY, G. L. BRENGELMANN & K. K. KRANING. 1969. Human cariovascular adjustments to rapid changes in skin temperature during exercise. Circ. Res. **24:** 711–724.
16. BURCH, G. E. & A. HYMAN. 1977. Influence of a hot and humid envoironment upon cardiac output and work in normal man and in patients with chronic congestive heart failure at rest. Amre. Heart J. **53:** 665–675.
17. O'DONNELL, T. F. & G. H. A. CLOWES. 1972. The circulatory abnormalities of heat stroke. N. Engl. J. Med **287:** 734–737.
18. MOORE, F. T., S. A. MARABLE & E. OGDEN. 1966. Contractility of the heart in abnormal temperatures. Ann. Thor. Surg. **2**(3)**:** 446–450.
19. ROWELL, L. B., G. L. BRENGELMANN, J. R. BLACKMON & J. A. MURRAY. 1970. Redistribution of blood flow during sustained high skin temperature in resting man. J. Appl. Physiol. **28:** 415–420.
20. SCHREIR, R. W., J. HANO, H. I. KELLER, R. M. FINKEL, P. F. GILLILAND, W. J. CIRKSENA & P. E. TESCHAN. 1970. Renal, metabolic, and circulatory response to heat and exercise. J. Int. Med. **73:** 213–223.
21. GREENBERG, J. & L. ARNENSON. 1967. Exertional rabnomyolysis with myoglobinuria in a large group of military recruits. Neurology **17:** 216–222.
22. KEW, M. C., C. ABRAHAMS, N. W. LEVIN, et al. 1967. The effects of heat stroke on the function and structure of the kidney. Quart. J. Med. **35:** 277–300.

DISCUSSION

Loring B. Rowell, *Moderator*

University of Washington
Seattle, Washington 98195

L. B. ROWELL: Dr. Hartley, is there any direct or indirect evidence, other than what you cited from Ekelund's work, that there is any impairment of cardiac function in man during prolonged exercise?

L. H. HARTLEY (*Harvard University, Boston, Mass.*): I think the evidence in man is very slim. The strongest evidence is from animal experiments, but we are not sure that the changes are like those reported for man. I think the changes in heart volume reported for man are difficult to interpret because they were not associated with changes in right ventricular pressure. I do not think that there is convincing evidence that myocardial function is decreased in man.

J. WAHREN (*Karolinska Institute, Huddinge, Sweden*): Dr. Hartley pointed out that oxygen uptake increases some 5% to 10% during prolonged work. He suggested that this is due to a shift in substrate utilization from carbohydrates to free fatty acids. I would like to point out that during prolonged exercise there is a gradual increase in the oxygen uptake of the liver from approximately 50 ml per minute at the onset of exercise to some 100 to 150 ml per minute during the later phase of the exercise period. This reflects the synthetic work of the liver in that gluconeogenesis increases. This hepatic synthesis proceeds with a respiratory quotient (RQ) that is close to zero because oxygen is consumed in the process without carbon dioxide release. Thus, part of the increase in total oxygen uptake during prolonged work could be caused by increased hepatic oxygen uptake. Accordingly, the RQ value for the body as a whole should be interpreted very cautiously.

A. CRAIG (*University of Rochester, Rochester, N.Y.*): Dr. Johnson, in your experiments you were measuring total forearm blood flow. How representative is that of skin blood flow over the entire body surface?

J. M. JOHNSON (*University of Texas, San Antonio, Texas*): I wish we had a definitive answer to your question. I can say that the neurogenic control of forearm blood flow is similar to that seen over most of the body surface. That is, the forearm has both a vasoconstrictor system and an active vasodilator system. The areas known to lack this dual control are the apical regions, the hands and the feet, so that the forearm might not reflect the changes in these regions. Incidentally, it is now well documented that increases in forearm blood flow during heating are confined to skin; blood flow to underlying muscle does not increase. With regard to the range of blood flow, the only evidence we have that changes in forearm skin blood flow reflect the changes in most of the body skin is based upon very indirect calculations. Measurements of increased cardiac output and changes in blood flow to major vascular beds (e.g., splanchnic, renal, muscle) during heating provide estimates of the increase in total skin blood flow. These agree with estimates of total skin blood flow obtained by extrapolating the changes in forearm blood flow to the total body surface area.

L. B. ROWELL: Just to expand what Dr. Johnson said, the work of Blair and his colleagues in England would suggest that patterns of changing forearm skin

270

blood flow follow closely the changes seen in all regions (except hand and feet) of the four limbs.

A. LAVERE: Dr. Jorgensen, would you describe the coronary sinus catheter? How deeply was it inserted into the sinus to make sure that only sinus blood was sampled? Would you comment on the safety of this procedure during exercise?

C. R. JORGENSEN (*University of Minnesota, Minneapolis, Minn.*): The catheter was a No. 6 or No. 7 *Goodell Rubin,* standard coronary sinus catheter. We generally tried to put it within a few centimeters of the left heart border as seen fluoroscopically, which meant it was 6 to 8 cm into the coronary sinus. We checked the oxygen saturation of withdrawn blood to make sure the catheter was in the coronary sinus, and then after we got the subjects up onto the bicycle we again checked the oxygen saturation to be sure the catheter had not been displaced. By using indocyanine green dye we showed that blood samples would become contaminated with right atrial blood only if the catheter was just barely into the sinus orifice, or in by only 1 or 2 cm. We feel we obtained good samples of cardiac venous blood. As for safety, I repeat, that subjects were not performing maximal exercise because we had to have a fairly long period of steady-state exercise in order to accomplish the measurements. Exercise required somewhere around 55% or 60% of maximal oxygen uptake. We had no problems or complications with this procedure. We were careful to place the catheter in an area where it was still mobile, not wedged into a vein.

J. G. HAYDEN (*Lahey Clinic Foundation, Boston, Mass.*): Could you also elaborate on your measurement of arterial pressure? You indicated that you measure central aortic blood pressure rather than peripherally measured arterial pressures because systolic pressures would not be accurate. Could you elaborate somewhat on this and indicate exactly how this discrepancy or this inaccuracy would be introduced by utilizing brachial or radial artery pressure?

C. R. JORGENSEN: Well, I do not think it would be right to say that it is inaccurate to use brachial artery pressure since it is still linearly related to aortic pressure and to myocardial oxygen consumption. If one used brachial artery pressure the rate-pressure product would still be a good predictor of myocardial oxygen consumption; the slope of that regression line would simply be a little different from that obtained using aortic pressure. Others have obtained data similar to ours using peripheral pressures and have shown that peripheral measurements still correlate well. I think brachial artery pressures, direct or indirect (cuff), provide reasonable estimates.

L. B. ROWELL: As to how the discrepancy between aortic and peripheral systolic pressures occurs, peripheral arteries can be regarded as compliant tubes connected to the aorta. As pressure waves move down peripheral vessels, pulse wave amplitude and systolic pressure increase due to wave reflection and resonance characteristics of the vessels. Thus, use of peripherally measured systolic pressure could lead to overestimates of true myocardial O_2 consumption.

E. ELDRED (*Massachusetts General Hospital, Boston, Mass.*): Dr. Saltin, when your subjects exercised with the untrained leg I believe you did not observe the bradycardia associated with training.

B. SALTIN (*University of Copenhagen, Cophagen, Denmark*): That is correct.

E. ELDRED: It is known that the lactate can be a limiting factor in exercise. You showed that lactate levels in the trained leg were lower than in the control leg. Since the lactate produced in working muscle can be removed by nonexercising muscles, is it possible that the lactate going to the control leg could be a training factor by the fact that there is an increase in lactate level in that leg?

B. SALTIN: I think it is a possibility, yes.

J. G. HAYDEN: I suggest that because in similar studies we found a very significant training-induced bradycardia when the control leg was exercised as well.

J. A. DEMPSEY (*University of Wisconsin, Madison, Wisc.*): Over the last 15 years Tipton and others have shown in rats and in other animals that a training effect occurs with the isolated heart preparation upon stimulation. How do you think this fits with your suggestion that this is purely a local effect?

B. SALTIN: The surprising thing in our results is the finding of no significant increase in maximal oxygen uptake or the reduction in submaximal heart rate when exercise was performed with the control or the untrained leg. But we did see some changes, and I cannot say whether they were of the magnitude associated with these intrinsic changes in the heart. I am definitely not excluding the possibility that central changes take place.

L. B. ROWELL: Were you to condition a small fraction of the total muscle mass, say a forearm, would you expect any central or cardiac effect? In other words, is it possible that training with one leg is not a sufficient stimulus to actually effect a central change at the heart?

B. SALTIN: This question, as you know, is not easily answered. What I can say is that maximal one-legged exercise can utilize about 80% of maximal oxygen uptake. We found no significant increase in that percentage after training the one leg. Thus we are clearly not taxing or using the maximal capacity of the central circulation in one-legged exercise.

J. A. DEMPSEY: I would like to address a two-part question to Dr. Saltin. First, you have been using the needle biopsy technique to obtain muscle samples for the analysis of SDH (succinate dehydrogenase) activity. Does the time interval between insertion of the needle into the muscle and when it is frozen a few seconds later affect this enzyme activity? Second, you and your associates have examined the high energy phosphates in such muscle samples. What effect does this delay in freezing have on these compounds? I pose this second question because of data that have shown for brain and heart that a delay of a few milliseconds in freezing can cause problems in accurately assessing the *in vivo* concentration of these compounds.

B. SALTIN: Let me start by saying that we have been using SDH activity only as a marker for changes in aerobic capacity that occur in response to any experimental treatment. I am not suggesting that it is the only Krebs cycle enzyme that is important or rate-limiting. Your question was whether the time delay in extraction and freezing of a needle biopsy sample will affect this enzyme activity. Actually the time delay may in fact be less than occurs when animals are sacrificed and the muscle sample is dissected out. The latter may require a delay of one-half minute or more. We have compared the enzyme activity of dog muscle that was rapidly frozen *in situ* with samples whose freezing was delayed to simulate the time required to remove and freeze a needle biopsy sample. There were no differences in enzyme activity associated with the two methods of sampling.

Now for the second part of your question. Of course the turnover of high energy phosphates is extremely fast, milliseconds. But the interesting thing is that if one compares a piece of skeletal muscle left at room temperature for several minutes with a piece frozen immediately (within 5 or 10 seconds) the only difference is increased lactate and a decreased glycogen in the former. Even the decrease in glycogen is fairly small. Under these conditions ATP and CP (creatine phosphate) levels remain rather constant until lactate concentration approaches 20 or 25 mmole/kg. Only then do the ATP and CP levels drop. This suggests that the high glycolytic capacity of skeletal muscle keeps ATP and CP levels high even after the biopsy sample has been taken. In contrast, the tissues that you mentioned, heart and brain, have low glycolytic capacities; thus, one would expect marked changes in the high energy phosphate levels with any delay in freezing these tissues.

L. B. ROWELL: Dr. Mitchell, when you stimulated the unmyelinated C fibers you saw a rise in pressure of about 20 to 30 mmHg, which is about the full change in blood pressure that you saw with exercise, whereas the changes in ventilation were in the order of only 15% to 25% during stimulation. One would expect to see increases of 20-fold with severe exercise. This suggests to me that the primary importance of these afferent fibers is their effect on blood pressure and that their input to the respiratory centers is really almost insignificant. Would you agree?

J. H. MITCHELL (*University of Texas, Dallas, Texas*): I would agree with that. I think that both the respiratory and the cardiovascular centers receive input from the higher centers and also from the periphery, and that there is an interplay between these two. I also think that the responses of heart rate and blood pressure are quite different. For example, as you know, when one keeps an extremity occluded after exercise, elevated blood pressure is maintained. It is as if the reflex is able to keep pressure elevated but not heart rate, which in recent work was seen to return to control values. So there are probably different control mechanisms for blood pressure and for heart rate. And I think that there is also a difference in the control mechanism for ventilation and the circulation, but I still think there is an interplay of these two.

L. B. ROWELL: You mentioned increases in muscle interstitial potassium concentration and osmolarity as possible stimuli affecting these unmyelinated afferent fibers. Would you favor potassium over osmolarity? The basis of my question is that you would expect altered osmolarity to exert more or less of a transient effect. However, if you consider the amount of potassium that could be generated by skeletal muscle action potentials, it appears that an augmented potassium concentration could be sustained around the C fibers, as proposed by Hnik, for example.

J. H. MITCHELL: Right. I think that we do not really know. If one measures venous potassium from an exercising limb, that may increase by only 1 meq/liter. There are now some recent studies wherein interstitial potassium concentration was determined using potassium electrodes; muscle potassium levels were reported to reach as high as 15 to 20 meq/liter during contractions (Hnik). What we are planning to do next is to reproduce the interstitial potassium changes that occur in exercising muscle by injecting potassium. The object is to see whether potassium levels and ventilatory and circulatory responses are related.

QUESTION: These small fibers carry pain. Will inducing pain in the muscle have the same effect as exercise?

J. H. MITCHELL: Our animals did not feel pain but your point is a good one. These fibers seem to be the ones that we always said were there to signal claudication. The major question is whether these fibers play any physiological role when they are activated without the perception of pain. Unfortunately I cannot answer it at the moment. In some studies, particularly on humans who have been walking, the changes in heart rate and blood pressure that attend claudication in the legs occur before the patients report pain. Also, when these fibers are activated by arterial occlusion of an exercised limb, the subject may experience pain, but in those who experience no pain, the blood pressure responses are the same as in those who had pain.

L. B. ROWELL: And if you deliberately try to generate pain by occluding limbs in a nonexercising subject the pressor response that results is rather small compared to the pressor response that Dr. Mitchell has described, i.e., the one that attends exercise and ischemia of the exercising or exercised limb.

K. M. BALDWIN (*University of California, Irvine, Calif.*): Have you considered stimulating different types of motor units in the muscles to see if different muscle fiber types might elicit different responses?

J. H. MITCHELL: It would be very interesting to look at the response from pure white muscle compared to pure red muscle. It is something we want to do. It is a good point.

J. G. HAYDEN: Dr. Dempsey, in your discussion of the gradual increase in ventilation, which I gather you define by the fall in arterial P_{CO_2}, in the presence of constant pH, you dismiss metabolic acidosis rather quickly. I don't understand the reasons for this. It seems to me that the whole thing could be explained by a metabolic acidosis induced by tissue hypoxia, resultant lactic acidosis, and a secondary hyperventilation that is a compensatory mechanism to maintain pH. Would not this explain your findings?

J. A. DEMPSEY: Yes it could. I think that the hyperventilation in short-term, very heavy exercise is probably induced by metabolic acidosis as a primary drive. But in prolonged, less severe exercise we have a problem because arterial pH does not fall. In other words, the regulation is perfect. If you want to postulate that bicarbonate concentration is itself a drive, and I do not know of any evidence for that even in the brain, then fine. I will accept that as a potential explanation for the long-term changes in ventilation. But when pH stays normal or slightly alkaline, I find it difficult to accept this idea. But I also have a difficult time explaining why the pH regulation is so near-perfect in prolonged work.

J. D. SINCLAIR (*University of Auckland, Auckland, New Zealand*): I would like to ask two question. First, you seem to have emphasized the rise in temperature as a stimulus to increased ventilation during prolonged exercise. I wonder why in shorter term exercise a rise of body temperature seems not to be associated with hyperventilation. My second question is were you using Dr. Peter Wagner's multiple inert gas technique? Anyone associated with physiology for the last 20 years has, I think, assumed that ventilation was more evenly related to blood flow during exercise than at rest. You show the opposite. I wonder whether you think Wagner's technique is in fact reliable enough to accept that observation, and if so what you have in mind to explain it?

J. A. DEMPSEY: First, temperature is not thought to be a drive in short-term work simply because it just does not change enough.

L. B. ROWELL: What if you force a rapid temperature change? It still does not appear to affect ventilation.

J. A. DEMPSEY: Do you mean preheating a man before exercise begins?

L. B. ROWELL: No, I mean that if one suddenly raises body temperature during exercise by rapidly raising skin temperature, the subject does not hyperventilate.

J. A. DEMPSEY: Well, I would not approach the problem that way. The question was what is the importance of rising body temperature during prolonged work; does it explain hyperventilation? Rather than trying to answer that question by artificially increasing body temperature more. I would try to remove any thermal drive. When we actually did that during prolonged exercise, ventilation decreased. But in short-term work, this maneuver did not change ventilation. In answer to the second question about inert gas analysis, I think that there are real problems with this technique that are not yet resolved. This is particularly true in certain disease states with severe ventilation/perfusion ratio abnormalities. However, the evidence also shows that this technique is valid and consistent when it is applied to a normal person in whom ventilation/perfusion ratio distributions are uniform. That is a brief statement about a long story with which Dr. Wagner and others are currently dealing. I think I can explain why the differences between radioisotope studies and inert gas analysis occur. With radioisotope studies, we are looking at the lung in one plane, topographically. This tells us nothing about intraregional differences in ventilation/perfusion ratios. We now know that there are many facters contributing to intraregional differences in ventilation/perfusion ratio distributions. For example, just the cardiac effect on mixing in the gas phase is extremely important to gas exchange. In essence, what we are saying here is that during exercise there is still significant heterogeneity in intraregional ventilation/perfusion ratio distribution. It is not much greater than at rest, but it is not any less. So, in short, I do not see where our assessment of "functional" ventilation/perfusion ratio distribution is incompatible with the topographical ventilation/perfusion ratio distribution obtained from radioisotope studies.

T. S. SCANLON (*Naval Regional Medical Center, San Diego, Calif*): If you do not believe that there is a metabolic acidosis, what maintains the pH constant? If you take a patient, place him on a ventilator and drop his P_{CO_2}, his pH will rise.

J. A. DEMPSEY: Yes, but that is because with an acute decrease in P_{CO_2} his bicarbonate has not fallen significantly. Bicarbonate has fallen slightly in prolonged work, but acidosis does not occur. I have no problem with that. Bicarbonate has fallen, CO_2 has fallen, pH is constant. When pH stays constant under these conditions, then one presumes that there must be feedback regulation involving hydrogen ions somewhere. I would like to believe that hydrogen ion concentration is involved, but I have two problems with this. First, the gradual rise in ventilation during prolonged work is substantial. Ventilation increases approximately 35% to 40% and respiratory frequency about 65% to 70%. Second, to explain these changes via hydrogen ion drive alone, one would need a substantial and progressive arterial acidosis. We saw none. If anything, a mild alkalosis occurred during prolonged work. So we postulate that some substantial "non-hydrogen ion drive" to ventilation must be involved and that rising body temperature could be the stimulus.

QUESTION: Dr. O'Donnell, you demonstrated very elegantly that supply may not meet circulatory demands during heat stroke. Yesterday Dr. Knochel mentioned the occurrence of myocardial infarction during heat stroke, and in particular the case of a Boston Marathoner who died in 1973, presumably having suffered from heat stroke. At autopsy the victim was found to have suffered a myocardial infarction. I think another member of the audience mentioned that he had seen myocardial infarction in a couple of recruits and that all of these people had normal coronary arteries. Would you care to comment on this?

T. F. O'DONNELL (*Tufts-New England Medical Center, Boston, Mass.*): Yes. I agree with Jim Knochel that myocardial infarction does occur with heat stroke. One has only to turn to the elegant pathological studies carried out by

Malamud in the 1940s to document this. He showed subendocardial infarcts in many patients who suffered heat stroke injuries. They were young Army recruits (about 150 men in all) who presumably did not have any previous cardiac disease and whose coronary arteries were free of atheroma.

COMMENT: I believe that what you are describing is subendocardial infarction. I believe the Boston Marathoner had a massive infarction of the entire wall of the heart.

T. F. O'DONNELL: Well, I personally have not seen an acute myocardial infarction in a young heat stroke victim, but Jim Knochel has treated such a case. One would just have to extrapolate a bit further from Dr. Jorgensen's data on maximal coronary blood flow to suggest that this certainly could happen. A point must be reached where the demands for oxygenated blood and nutrient substrate by the heart cannot be met so that myocardial damage must occur. I must hasten to say that the serum enzyme elevations alone described by Dr. Wyndham do not provide a firm basis for the diagnosis of heat stroke. It is a clinical diagnosis. My experience in treating about 35 patients with heat stroke is that the marked elevations that Dr. Wyndham demonstrated are unusual and may be related to associated exercise. It is usually seen in patients with concomitant exertional rhabdomyolysis and not with heat stroke *per se*.

J. G. HAYDEN: Did you measure either blood gases or muscle enzymes in any of these patients, either the marine recruits or the marathoners? Also, in your opinion is there any relationship between the heat exhaustion that you described in these individuals and the genetically determined so-called malignant hyperpyrexia that one sees in certain strains of pigs and also in some human subjects under anesthesia? In the latter there seems to be a breakdown within the muscle sarcoplasmic reticulum. A severe metabolic acidosis and muscle-induced hyperpyrexia develops. There is some indication, I gather, of a genetic or at least an individual predilection toward heat exhaustion. Is any analogy between these two conditions a legitimate speculation?

T. F. O'DONNELL: To answer your first question: Yes, we have measured arterial blood gases. Most of the patients have a metabolic acidosis with respiratory compensation. Usually their pH levels are about 7.48–7.52 with a decreased P_{CO_2}. Only when they develop a low flow state do we see metabolic acidosis. Secondly, we have also measured muscle enzymes in these patients and they generally have only marginal elevations, nothing like those shown yesterday. We have observed marked enzyme increases only in patients who have exertional rhabdomyolysis. I have studied about 45 of these latter patients while with the Marine Corps. Marked elevations in muscle enzymes in young patients who have been treated rather promptly after sustaining heat injury are unusual. Your third question about whether there is a genetic predisposition toward heat exhaustion is a good one. In those patients who had heat stroke and were not medically discharged from the Marine Corps, one of them developed heat stress injury several months later in Viet Nam. Thus, one might speculate that there may be an individual, perhaps genetic, predisposition in this disease.

C. H. WYNDHAM (*Marshalltown, South Africa*): You seem to be a little vague on this question of your diagnosis of heat stroke. I would like to know more details. What are the mental aberrations that these individuals show? Second, how soon after the occurrence of heat injury do you measure rectal temperature? Thirdly, I would like to know what serum enzyme levels you measured?

T. F. O'DONNELL: In answer to your first question: The diagnosis of heat stroke is a clinical one, as defined in a *Lancet* editorial, and consists of the triad of: (1) hyperpyrexia, (2) mental changes, (3) dry hot skin—the last is not invariable. As for mental aberrations, the patient may go anywhere from a semicomatose combative state to frank coma. As for rectal temperatures, our Marine patients' rectal temperature ranged from 109° to the lowest in our series of 106 ° F. As far as the marathoners', theirs were slightly lower (106 ° F). In respect to the serum enzymes, as I stated earlier, and Jim Knochel has previously commented on, they were somewhat lower than the ones that you reported. Individual data on our Marines were reported in the *Journal of the American Medical Association.**

* O'DONNELL, T. F. 1975. Acute heat stroke. J. Amer. Med. Assoc. **234:** 824–828.

OVERVIEW

Michael L. Pollock *

*Institute for Aerobics Research
Dallas, Texas 75230*

Many factors such as energy output (maximal and submaximal), biomechanics, body composition, nutritional status, and psychological factors have been associated with success in distance running.[1-4] It has been the desire of both the researcher and the coach to be able to predict with high reliability the best performer in a competitive race. Investigations determining the characteristics of world caliber distance runners have included only small samples of elite runners and/or have dealt with a limited number of test variables, and therefore have not resulted in reliable predictions.[1, 4, 5, 6] Costill *et al.*[2, 7, 8] have looked at a greater variety of test variables to predict endurance performance. Variables such as maximum oxygen uptake ($\dot{V}_{O_2\,max}$), rate of $\dot{V}_{O_2}$ expenditure, body composition, and muscle fiber typing have been shown to predict top performers within groups with a wide range of ability, but these predictions are limited when groups are homogeneous.[2, 7, 8]

The purpose of this study was to investigate a large sample of elite runners with a more comprehensive test battery than had been previously used. To accomplish an investigation of this magnitude required the cooperation of many athletes and investigators. It was not difficult to establish the research team. The researchers were eager to participate in what appeared to be a unique opportunity and experience. The initial organizing committee included: Michael L. Pollock, Kenneth H. Cooper, and William Walker, Institute for Aerobics Research; David Costill, Ball State University; Peter Cavanagh, Pennsylvania State University; William Morgan, University of Wisconsin; and Kenny Moore, Olympic marathoner and staff writer for *Sports Illustrated*. Other investigators in this project are listed within their respective manuscripts found in this section.

As mentioned, it was relatively easy to establish a research team for this investigation, but it was difficult to recruit a large amount of elite runners who would be available for extensive testing over a 3- to 4-day period. Also, the image of researchers was poor with many of our outstanding athletes. Fortunately, Kenny Moore thought the project had important implications for runners and felt that he could convince many elite runners of the merits of the study. In an initial letter to them he stated that:

> The experiences of top U.S. distance runners with physiological research in many cases have not been happy. Those of you who were on the last Pan-Am team or the Munich Olympic team will recall that on both occasions blood was taken from athletes under the pretense that it was part of the routine physical examination necessary to be admitted to the team. In fact (we learned too late), it was part of someone's private study, the results of which have yet to be made known to those who participated. (In 1971, it was only the last man in line,

* Present address: Department of Medicine, Mt. Sinai Medical School, Milwaukee, Wisc.

Liquori, who flatly refused to surrender his blood, was admitted to Colombia anyway, and so demonstrated to the rest of us how we had been taken.)

The result of such abuses has been the growth of a very healthy suspicion of all doctors wielding needles. The purpose of this letter is to allay that suspicion with regard to the proposed study at the Dallas Aerobic Center this fall.

He went on to say that the project would provide them valuable information about themselves and also be an important learning experience. It was in this spirit that the project was formulated and the athletes agreed to participate. Twenty of 24 elite distance runners who were contacted volunteered to participate in the study. Fifteen of the 20 volunteers came to the Institute for Aerobics Research, Dallas, Texas, during January 2–5, 1975. Five others came at a later date. All testing was completed by April 1, 1975. Because of logistical problems, the biomechanics and muscle biopsy information was not collected on the five runners who were tested at the later time.

For comparative purposes, eight good runners were also evaluated; five of them being members of a local university track team. All of these men were actively engaged in endurance training and competition, but were not considered elite.

On another occasion a sample of ten young, lean sedentary men were tested on a limited number of variables. The variables included noninvasive analysis of cardiac function, and determination of maximal working capacity and body composition.

The performance and training characteristics of the 20 elite runners are shown in TABLE 1. The group included 12 middle to long distance runners (M-LD), primarily 3- to 6-milers, and eight marathon runners who had won or placed high in national and/or international competition in the two years prior to testing. Seventeen of the elite runners were American, one was Kenyan, and two were Irish. Altogether, the group included 17 runners who were members of either a Pan American or Olympic team, and/or who had earned a National Collegiate Athletic Association (NCAA) or American Amateur Athletic Union (AAU) title. One runner (Prefontaine) held ten different American distance records.

In response to a questionnaire concerning their training the year prior to testing, it was found that the group as a whole trained 85 miles per week. When they were dichotomized by best running distance, the M-LD runners averaged 75.4 miles per week while the marathoners averaged 100.7. Although there was some overlap in training methods, the M-LD runners used more high intensity interval training.

The good runners were all highly trained, but had significantly slower performance times than the elite distance runners. Their miles trained per week was also significantly lower than the elite group (average 60 mi/week).

Prior to coming to Dallas for testing, the runners were sent a general description of the project and testing protocols. Each investigator informed the subjects of the potential risk involved concerning each particular test. They were also informed that their individual results would be held confidential and not be published without their permission. Only one runner wished to remain anonymous.

The testing was conducted over a 3½-day period. TABLE 2 shows the testing schedule and instructions for training and dietary control prior to the administration of each test. Muscle biopsy procedures were performed in the afternoon of day 1 and prior to any training. Of the questionnaires, only the written

TABLE 1

PERFORMANCE AND TRAINING CHARACTERISTICS OF ELITE RUNNERS

Subject	Best Distance Performance*	Olympic-Pan Am Competitor	NCAA or AAU Competition	Best Performance (min:sec)					Training (miles/week)
				440 yd	1 mi	3 mi	6 mi	Marathon	
Brown	M-LD	Yes	First	:52.0	4:04.5	13:27.4	27:51.0	—	70
Castaneda	M-LD	Yes	Second	:52.4	3:58.5	13:10.5	27:22.4	147:30	100
Crawford	M-LD	Yes	—	:48.8	3:57.7	13:13.4	29:58.0	176:00	45
Cusak	Marathon	Yes	First	:54.0	4:00.4	13:10.0	27:40.0	133:39	120
Galloway	Marathon	Yes	Second	:53.3	4:11.0	13:17.0	27:21.0	139:37	110
Geis	M-LD	Yes	First	—	3:58.0	12:55.8	—	—	70
Johnson	M-LD	No	First	:49.6	3:58.6	13:18.6	27:52.8	—	70
Kardong	M-LD	Yes	Third	—	4:01.9	12:57.6	28:00.6	138:06	100
Kennedy	Marathon	No	Third	:51.0	4:22.0	14:45.0	30:03.0	139:58	90
Manley	M-LD	Yes	First	:52.1	4:01.4	13:22.2	29:30.0	149:29	75
Moore	Marathon	Yes	First	:52.0	4:03.7	13:16.0	27:47.4	131:36	65
Ndoo	M-LD	Yes	First	:53.0	4:08.0	13:26.0	28:07.8	142:15	90
Pate	Marathon	No	—	:56.0	4:17.0	14:11.0	29:15.0	135:30	70
Prefontaine	M-LD	Yes	First	:51.6	3:54.6	12:51.8	26:51.8	—	90
Rose	M-LD	Yes	First	:51.6	3:58.4	13:14.0	—	—	90
Shorter	Marathon	Yes	First	:54.6	4:02.5	12:52.0	27:09.0	130:30	70
Tuttle	M-LD	No	First	:53.7	4:08.9	13:20.2	27:40.0	137:00	120
Wayne	Marathon	No	—	—	4:07.4	13:58.0	28:56.0	136:16	100
Williams	Marathon	No	—	:55.3	4:12.4	13:47.3	28:54.1	135:18	110
11 †	M-LD	Yes	Second	:52.0	3:57.8	13:23.4	27:30.0	—	89

* M-LD, middle-long distance runner.
† Subject's name kept anonymous.

psychological tests were administered under controlled conditions. Medical history and previous training record forms were filled out at the subjects' leisure.

Blood was drawn from all subjects the morning of day 2. The noninvasive measures of cardiac function, and body composition and pulmonary function tests were administered on the morning of days 2 or 3. Other tests were scheduled systematically so that each participant had plenty of time to get from station to station. Treadmill filming and determination of submaximal and maximal working capacity tests were administered on alternate days.

The 6-mile run results were to be used as a criterion measure for predicting the performance level of the runners, but because of various problems incurred in the administration of this test, it was excluded from the final analysis. The 6-mile race was held on the afternoon of the fourth day at a local stadium,

TABLE 2

GENERAL ITINERARY FOR TESTING RUNNERS

Day	Test	Test Condition
1	Muscle biopsy	No training
	Questionnaires,	Begin 14-hour fast
	medical, phychological, and	
	previous training record	
2, 3	Blood drawing	14-hour fast
	Body composition	14-hour fast
	Noninvasive cardiac function	14-hour fast
	Pulmonary function	14-hour fast
	Psychological interview	
	Treadmill, submaximal and maximal	3-hour fast
	working capacity	
	Treadmill, filming	
	Physical examination	3-hour fast
4	6-mile race	

which had an all-weather track. The day was clear with the temperature brisk (12° C), humidity 45%, and the wind gusting up to 25 mph. The exact distance of this event was the first choice of most of the runners in the study. The race itself was excellent with Gary Tuttle winning in 28:00 minutes, but the fact that many of the participants did not run made it of little value for research purposes. Prefontaine cancelled because of an important race scheduled for the following weekend; Castanda had severe blisters on his feet and could not run; Geis was having chondromalacia of the knee and did not want to race; Kennedy was recovering from a hip injury and could not run hard on the turns; and, the five runners who came at a later time obviously did not attend the race. Therefore only 11 of 20 actually started the race and two of these men did not finish.

The authors wish to thank Quinton Instruments (Seattle, Wash.) for their financial support of this project, and members of the Aerobics Activity Center for housing the athletes during their stay in Dallas. Appreciation also goes to the United States Track Coaches Association for their support in the planning of this investigation. Special appreciation goes to the athletes who participated in this project in the hope of adding scientific information to the literature that would ultimately help both the coach and the athlete.

References

1. ÅSTRAND, P. O. & K. RODALE, Eds. 1970. Textbook of Work Physiology. 1st edit. McGraw-Hill Book Company. New York, N.Y.
2. COSTILL, D. L. 1972. Physiology of marathon running. J. Amer. Med. Assoc. **221:** 1024–1029.
3. DANIELS, J. 1974. Physiological characteristics of champion male athletes. Res. Quart. **45:** 342–348.
4. MORGAN, W. P. & D. L. COSTILL. 1972. Psychological characteristics of the marathon runner. J. Sports Med. Phys. Fit. **12:** 42–46.
5. SALTIN, B. & P. O. ÅSTRAND. 1967. Maximal oxygen uptake in athletes. J. Appl. Physiol. **23:** 353–358.
6. WYNDHAM, C. H., N. B. STRYDOM, A. J. VAN RENSBURG & A. J. S. BENADE. 1969. Physiological requirements for world-class performances in endurance running. S. Afr. Med. J. **43:** 996–1002.
7. COSTILL, D. L., H. THOMASON & E. ROBERTS. 1973. Fractional utilization of the aerobic capacity during distance running. Med. Sci. Sports **5:** 248–252.
8. COSTILL, D. L., J. DANIELS, W. EVANS, W. FINK, G. KRAHENBUHL & B. SALTIN. 1976. Skeletal muscle enzymes and fiber composition in male and female track athletes. J. Appl. Physiol. **40:** 149–154.

MEDICAL EXAMINATION AND ELECTROCARDIOGRAPHIC ANALYSIS OF ELITE DISTANCE RUNNERS

L. W. Gibbons, K. H. Cooper, R. P. Martin, and M. L. Pollock

Institute for Aerobics Research
Dallas, Texas 75230

Much has been written about the electrocardiograms (ECG) of athletes. Abnormalities simulating organic heart disease often occur in apparently healthy, young, highly conditioned individuals who would seem to have excellent cardiovascular function, and be unlikely to have significant cardiovascular abnormalities.[1-5] Some of these ECG abnormalities are physiologically reasonable and explainable as a result of the training process (bradycardia, increased precordial R wave voltage, increased PR interval); others are more difficult to explain physiologically.

This current study is particularly enlightening for the following reasons: The individuals studied, all world class middle-long distance or marathon run-

TABLE 1

WORLD CLASS DISTANCE RUNNERS ($n=20$)

Variable	Mean	Range
Age, yr	26.2 (21.7) *	21–32
Height, cm	177.0 (180.6)	167.1–184.2
Weight, kg	63.1 (63.2)	53.6–69.9
$\dot{V}_{O_2max}$, ml/kg·min	76.9 (54.2)	71.3–84.4

* Control group values in parentheses.

ners, represent one of the most highly conditioned groups of athletes ever studied (mean maximal oxygen uptake = 76.9 ml/kg·min; range 71 to 84) (TABLE 1). Secondly, electrocardiograms were monitored during and immediately following maximal exercise. Most of the electrocardiographic studies on athletes have examined only resting ECGs [6-9] or have only looked at ECGs taken a few minutes following vigorous exercise.[2, 5, 10, 11] Thirdly, the scope of the cardiovascular evaluation of these athletes was extremely broad and included complete medical history and physical examination, chest X ray, resting ECG, maximum stress ECG, echocardiography, phonocardiography, and vectorcardiography (VCG). The results of echocardiography, vectorcardiography, and phonocardiography are reported by Underwood and Swade.[12]

METHODS

Twenty world class distance runners volunteered for participation in this study. All subjects completed a detailed medical history questionnaire, and were then interviewed concerning that history by a physician. This was followed by a thorough medical examination. A standard chest X ray, PA and lateral, was

283

made and a standard 12-lead resting electrocardiogram was recorded in supine and standing positions. Lead V_5 was also recorded following 30 seconds of hyperventilation. The resting ECG was followed by submaximal and maximal treadmill tests.

A description of the submaximal treadmill test is reported elsewhere.[13] Following an appropriate rest (10 minutes) a maximal treadmill test was performed to exhaustion. The maximal treadmill test used was a protocol designed by Åstrand,[14] and modified by Pollock et al.[15] It was a continuous multistage run test performed to voluntary exhaustion. The treadmill speed was 11 mph. Elevation was started at 0% and was raised 2½% every 2 minutes. The test was monitored continuously by a standard, multilead exercise cable system and a single channel ECG recorder (Model 1500B, Hewlett-Packard, Paramus, N.J.). A modified V_4 lead (electrode placed half way between V_4 and V_5) was monitored during exercise; leads I, II, III, AVR, AVL, AVF, and V_4 immediately following and at 1, 3, and 5 minutes of recovery. For the purpose of this study, V_4 will represent the modified V_4 placement. After the immediate ECG tracing was completed in the standing position, the subject was asked to sit for the rest of the recovery period. Blood pressure was determined at rest and at 1, 3, and 5 minutes of recovery. Only the results of the maximal treadmill test will be reported here; metabolic data from the submaximal and maximal tests are reported by Pollock.[13]

Ten control subjects with similar body build to the elite runners, who were not competitive athletes, were given resting and stress electrocardiograms in an identical fashion except that the treadmill speed was slowed (6.5 to 7.5 mph) to compensate for their lack of training. The submaximal test was not performed by the control group.

Resting and stress electrocardiograms were interpreted independently by three physicians. A consensus was arrived at by discussion if differences in interpretation were present. Resting ECGs were evaluated according to standard criteria outlined by Marriot.[16] In evaluating the exercise ECGs, ST depression was considered abnormal if magnitude of depression reached 1 mm, measured from the $Q - Q$ baseline, for at least 0.08 seconds.

RESULTS

History and Physical Examination

Aside from the various musculoskeletal problems one would expect to encounter in a group of runners training an average of 86 miles per week, the subjects related very few serious medical problems in their medical histories. A few runners have had infectious mononucleosis, one reported a kidney stone, and one had experienced recurrent chest pain at rest; otherwise detailed histories were strikingly negative.

On examination, pulse rates (mean 47 beats/min) and blood pressures (mean 117/74, right arm, sitting) were low as expected. Precordial cardiac impulses were not unusually prominent and were notable only in one instance. Six runners had systolic murmurs, Grade I or Grade II. All murmurs were thought to be functional by the examiners. Very few third and fourth heart sounds were audible and no clicks were heard. Examination of other systems was in general unremarkable. Despite the common history of numerous past

LARGE P WAVES

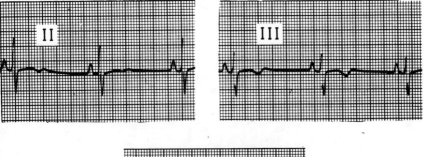

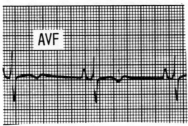

FIGURE 1. Short strips of the resting ECG recordings from leads II, III, and AVF of one of the elite marathon runners. Note the large amplitude (>3 mm) and peaked nature of the P waves.

SECOND DEGREE AV BLOCK

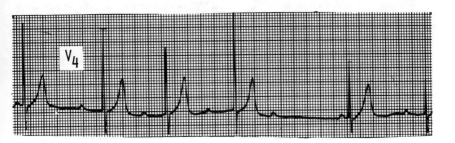

FIGURE 2. A continuous rhythm strip (lead V_4) from the resting ECG of an elite middle distance runner. Note the Wenckebach type of second degree AV block.

musculoskeletal difficulties, only two individuals had significant musculoskeletal problems at the time of examination. One runner had chondromalacia and one had significant unilateral hip pain of uncertain etiology.

Resting ECG

Four of the 20 runners had abnormally tall P waves (>2.5 mm) in inferior leads (example in FIGURE 1). In each case a large orthostatic component was present, but the changes from supine to standing were not unidirectional. In

RESTING ST ELEVATION - A

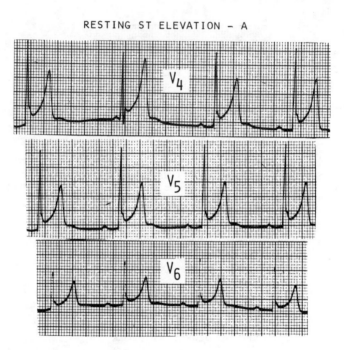

FIGURE 3. Short strips of leads V_4, V_5, and V_6 from the resting ECG of an elite long distance runner. Note the significant upsloping ST elevation (early repolarization).

two the P waves were much larger on standing, in two the opposite was true. Three controls also showed significant orthostatic variation in P wave size but in no instance was amplitude above 2 mm.

Some type of AV block was present in three runners. In addition to one routine first degree block there were two cases of second degree block (example in FIGURE 2). One runner showed classic second degree block with Wenckebach. One had a variable PR interval as long as 0.40 sec with some dropped beats. In all cases the block disappeared at low levels of exercise. No instances of AV block were seen in controls.

A crista pattern (incomplete right bundle branch block) was present in

QRS VOLTAGE - B

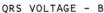

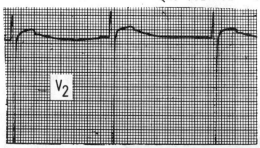

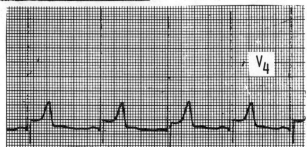

FIGURE 4. Leads V₂ and V₄ from the resting ECG of an elite middle distance runner. Note first the 3 mm of horizontal ST elevation, and second the large-amplitude QRS voltage in both leads (>40 mm).

QRS VOLTAGE - A

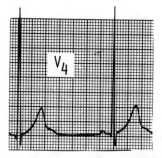

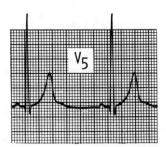

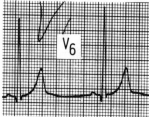

FIGURE 5. Leads of V₄, V₅, and V₆ from the resting ECG of an elite long distance runner. The QRS amplitude in V₄ is nearly 45 mm.

anterior precordial leads in six athletes and in one control. This has been commonly reported in numerous studies on athletes.[1]

Striking ST elevation (early repolarization), usually in anterior precordial leads, was present in all but six of the world class runners (examples in FIGURES 3 & 4). Often, segments were completely horizontal and significantly elevated (as much as 4 mm). Conversely, ST elevation was seen in only one of the controls. In all cases the elevation disappeared with exercise and was still absent when all leads were scanned immediately following exercise.

Not surprisingly, precordial R wave voltages were large in the elite runners. Mean R wave amplitude in V_4 was 34 mm (18–54 mm range) (example in FIGURE 5). In terms of standard criteria (R or S wave in precordial lead >25 mm; in standard or limb lead >20 mm)[16] all 20 tracings had abnormally high voltage. None of the supine tracings exhibited other ST or T abnormalities commonly associated with LVH, however. Large R wave voltage was not uncommon among the lean controls; 40% of controls had "abnormal" voltage in standard or precordial leads. However, mean R voltage in V_4 was only 24 mm, significantly lower than mean V_4 R wave voltage in the elite group.

Orthostatic inversion of T waves in inferior leads was seen in five runners. It is interesting to note that three of these individuals were in the group that showed significant ST depression with exercise (also in inferior leads). There was no associated orthostatic ST depression in any of the runners and no significant ST or T wave changes with hyperventilation. Among controls, there was no ST depression or T inversion with standing or hyperventilation, though some orthostatic T flattening did occur.

Despite large left precordial voltages for the runners, most axes were near vertical. Mean QRS axis was +80°. Mean axis in controls was similar (75.5°). One runner, however, had left axis deviation, and VCG confirmed left axis deviation and left anterior hemiblock.[12]

Maximal Exercise ECG

The most unexpected finding in this group of superbly conditioned distance runners occurred immediately following exercise. Five of 20 runners showed significant ST depression (0.08 sec duration, 1 mm depression) after maximal exercise (examples in FIGURES 6–8). Only lead V_4 was monitored during exercise; no changes were seen during exercise nor during recovery in this lead. ST depression was seen only in inferior leads (II, III, AVF). In two instances, changes were present immediately on stopping and became less evident during recovery. In two instances changes were evident throughout the recovery period. In one case abnormalities were present only at 5 minutes of recovery.

DISCUSSION

It is not surprising to find that a group of world class distance runners has had few significant medical problems, and exhibits virtually no abnormalities on physical examination. Excellent past and present health would seem to be a prerequisite to withstanding the great physiologic stresses of competitive distance running. It is interesting to note the frequency of Grade I or Grade II systolic murmurs in the group (30%). These murmurs were characteristic of murmurs of flow rather than abnormal anatomy. Ejection time was not prolonged [12] and auscultation was not carried out during or following exercise to evaluate its effects on the murmurs. Stroke volume was larger in the athletes than in controls, which would increase aortic root flow; however, echocardiography showed aortic root diameter in systole to also be significantly larger in the athletes.[12]

The purpose of this paper is not to catalogue the unusual features of electrocardiograms of athletes. This has been done previously with larger groups.[1, 2, 10]

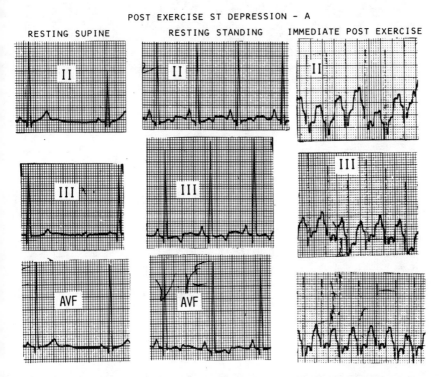

POST EXERCISE ST DEPRESSION - A

RESTING SUPINE   RESTING STANDING   IMMEDIATE POST EXERCISE

FIGURE 6. Leads II, III, and AVF from the resting supine, resting standing, and immediate postexercise ECG of one elite long distance runner. Note the orthostatic T wave inversion in these leads and the postexercise ST segment depression. Orthostatic T wave inversion was seen in three of the five runners who had postexercise ST depression.

It is interesting to note, however, that the same kinds of resting ECG abnormalities are present in this group of elite distance runners. This fact underscores the importance of looking beneath apparent ECG abnormalities in otherwise normal, healthy individuals before becoming overly concerned with ECG changes or overly cautious in allowing strenuous activity. The electrocardiogram cannot be interpreted in a vacuum.

The large QRS voltages seen in highly trained athletes have been thought to reflect various degrees of ventricular dilatation and/or hypertrophy. It would

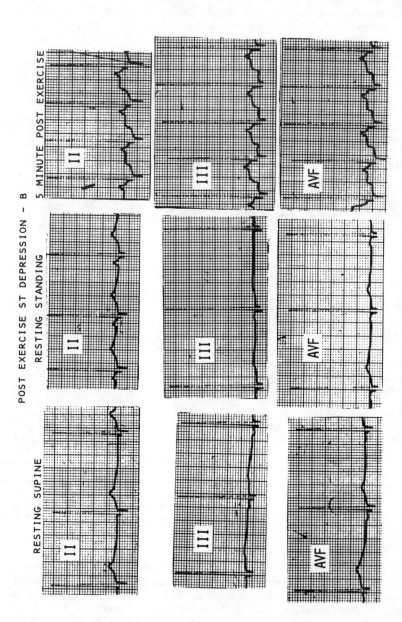

FIGURE 7. Leads II, III, and AVF from the resting, supine, resting standing, and 5-minute postexercise ECG of an elite middle distance runner. Note the significant postexercise ST depression, this time without associated orthostatic T wave inversion.

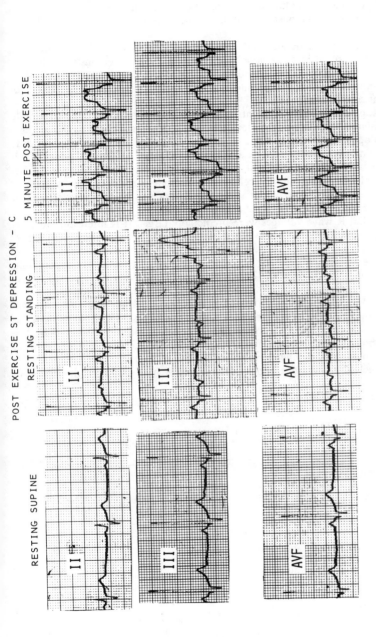

FIGURE 8. Leads II, III, and AVF from resting supine, resting standing, and 5-minute postexercise ECG of another elite middle distance runner. Orthostatic T wave inversion with postexercise ST depression.

not seem surprising then, in this group, to expect some increase in atrial voltage and atrial size, a possible explanation for the tall P waves seen in 20% of the group. Vectorcardiographic measurements did show that seven of 20 athletes (and no controls) demonstrated at least one criterion for right atrial hypertrophy.[12]

The benign nature of second degree AV block in athletes, probably due to a physiologic increase in vagal tone with training, is well demonstrated by two cases from this study. Understanding the cardiovascular demands of a sub-2-hour-20-minute marathon (26 miles) helps greatly to ease one's suspicions of significant cardiovascular disease.

The appearance of ST segments in some of these runners is quite striking to the uninitiated. But again, ST elevation (early repolarization) has been regularly catalogued in studies of athletes' ECGs.[1] Similar ST changes are known to occur commonly in young black individuals, whether athlete or nonathlete.[17] Some writers have suggested that the high incidence of this finding in studies done on athletes might simply be due to the high percent of blacks in those athlete groups.[1] Only one of our study population was black, however, and he was not one of the 80% with significant ST elevation.

Precordial R wave voltages were predictably large. It is interesting to compare electrocardiographic criteria with other parameters commonly used to assess heart size. On chest X rays none of the runners was thought to have an enlarged heart; in two subjects, the heart was judged to be at the upper limits of normal size. And in one, the question of right ventricular fullness was raised. Using vectorcardiography, only six runners had abnormal QRS voltage (greater than 2.0 mV), but the correlation with voltage measured on scalar tracings was quite good ($r = 0.63$). The five runners with the largest QRS voltage on VCG were the same five runners who had the largest V_4 voltage on routine electrocardiography. Eight of the highest ten voltages on VCG were found in eight of the ten runners showing highest voltages on ECG (TABLE 2).

With echocardiography, three of the runners had slightly high values for

TABLE 2

WORLD CLASS DISTANCE RUNNERS:
ECG VOLTAGE VERSUS VCG VOLTAGE

	ECG Voltage		VCG Voltage
Runner No.	R Wave Height V_4 (mm)	Runner No.	QRS Voltage H Plane (mV)
1	54	1	3.20
2	44	4	2.60
3	41	2	2.40
4	40	3	2.25
5	40	5	2.20
6	37	8	2.06
7	36	12	1.75
8	35	6	1.73
9	35	10	1.55
10	34	18	1.50

TABLE 3

WORLD CLASS DISTANCE RUNNERS:
ECG VOLTAGE COMPARED WITH LEFT VENTRICULAR INTERNAL DIAMETER (DIASTOLE)
AND WALL THICKNESS (DIASTOLE)

Runner No.	LV Int. Diameter (mm)	Runner No.	LV Wall Thickness (mm)
2	56.0	1	11.6
1	56.0	9	11.4
7	56.0	17	11.4
11	56.0	8	10.4
18	55.4	16	10.2
8	53.0	20	10.2
3	52.2	6	10.0
5	51.8	13	10.0
10	51.4	14	10.0
4	50.8	6	9.8

left ventricular wall thickness: 11.6, 11.4, and 11.4 mm (upper limits of normal = 11 mm). Only one of these subjects, however, was included in the top eight ECG or VCG voltage measures. In general, the relationship between echocardiographic measurements of wall thickness and ECG — VCG measurements of voltage was poor. There was much better association between the ECG — VCG data with echocardiographic-derived measures of left ventricular internal diameter in diastole (LVIDD). The ten runners with largest measures of LVIDD included all five runners with the largest VCG — ECG voltages, and eight of the top ten with the largest VCG — ECG voltage measurements (TABLE 3). Hence large voltage on ECG or VCG seems to correlate much better with dilitation than with hypertrophy of myocardial muscle in this population. Still, however, measurements of dilatation were surprisingly normal. Four subjects had an LVIDD of 56 mm, the upper limit of normal, and none were above that.[12]

Raskoff, Goldman, and Cohn [3] found only 70% of their marathon runners met ECG voltage criteria for left ventricular hypertrophy (LVH), and only 12% had a larger than normal LV internal diameter in diastole (LVIDD). Five runners (20%) had an abnormal LV wall thickness and high voltage on scalar ECG did not correlate well with LV wall thickness or with LVIDD. These authors concluded that LVH was indeed present but was "slight" and that the echocardiographic measurements were simply less sensitive in picking up that degree of LVH. Roeske, O'Rourke, and Klein found a much higher percentage of professional basketball players to have measurements suggestive of true LVH: 11 of 42 athletes (25%) met stringent Estes [19] criteria for LVH on ECG.[1] Only ten subjects had satisfactory echocardiograms, but 40% of these had abnormal LVIDD and 60% had abnormal LV wall thickness.

In our study, impressive voltage on ECG is not supported by data from physical examination, chest X ray, nor echocardiographic measures of wall thickness or chamber size in suggesting significant cardiac enlargement. Indeed, these runners' hearts are larger than controls', but few of these noninvasive measures of heart size are clearly outside normal limits. With the amount of intense cardiovascular training, the exceptional functional capacity, the impressive values for maximum oxygen uptake and the large voltages on scalar ECG, what is striking to the observer is the *normality*, not the abnormality, of these measurements.

Certainly, some of the increase in precordial R wave voltage is due to the slender build of the runner and not solely due to cardiac changes. R wave height was abnormal in four of the lean, healthy, nonathletic controls; one control subject had an R wave in V_4 of 44 mm. This subject had borderline elevation of QRS voltage (2.0 mV) in the H plane on VCG.

Vertical QRS axes despite large QRS voltages would seem to be more a function of youth and slender body build than of conditioning since the axes of lean, nonconditioned controls did not differ significantly from those of the runners.

The most interesting aspect of this study is the occurrence of significant ST depression in five of 20 elite distance runners (25%). ST depression immediately following exercise has been previously reported in distance runners but only rarely [10, 11, 20] and generally in populations that included runners in their 40s or 50s—where coronary heart disease (CHD) would seem more plausible. Hunt [5] reported that eight of 20 teenage swimmers had up to 0.2 mV ST depression on ECGs taken serially 3 to 30 minutes following "all out" sprints of 110 yards. Two of the ECGs were reported to be still abnormal after 30 minutes. Six of the eight abnormal ECGs were classified as showing "false" ST depression; two as showing "true" ST depression. Roeske, O'Rourke, and Klein [3] and Raskoff, Goldman, and Cohn [4] found no ST depression in the athletes whom they tested on the treadmill; however, Roeske did a submaximal test only, and Raskoff monitored only the V_5 lead.

It is interesting to speculate on possible reasons for the high incidence of ST depression in this population—one of the most highly conditioned groups of individuals ever studied as a group. None of these five runners with ST depression had any known cardiovascular disease, nor any symptoms suggestive of disease, nor any significant abnormality on cardiovascular examination, or any significant abnormality on chest X ray. Nonetheless, one possibility is that the ST changes are truly manifestations of coronary ischemia. The age, the lack of other significant risk factors, and the superb functional capacity of this population make this highly unlikely, of course. Without accompanying angiographic data or long-term follow-up one cannot be unequivocally certain, however. It is well known that in some individuals with significant coronary disease, impressive athletic performance is still possible,[21] however, probably not this quality of performance.

It is known that left ventricular hypertrophy may cause ST depression in the absence of significant coronary disease.[22] This might be considered a possible cause of the abnormalities; however, mean R wave voltage was lower in those with ST depression than in the remainder of the group. Also, echocardiographic measurements of left ventricular wall thickness were not significantly different in those with ST depression; thus hypertrophy does not appear to help in the explanation of the ST abnormalities.

With the magnitude of cardiovascular work of which these runners are capable, and the correspondingly high myocardial oxygen demands, one might speculate that an abnormal subendocardial oxygen supply/demand state could arise even with no significant coronary atherosclerosis. Conceivably, at the peak output required by a maximum exercise test in these superbly conditioned runners, the oxygen demand might become too great for delivery even through normal coronaries. This type of physiologic ischemia could conceivably result in abnormal ST depression in a population whose coronary arteries were perhaps slightly congenitally smaller than their fellow runners.

Another possibility is that the ST segment changes are due to vasoregulatory abnormalities. Many of the characteristics of our elite runners make this an attractive explanation. It has been reported that excessive autonomic tone may cause "false positive" ST depression in young, healthy individuals with few coronary risk factors and without typical ischemic symptoms.[23] This vasoregulatory abnormality is usually attributed to excess sympathetic tone but presumably might also occur with excessive vagal tone. Orthostatic ST and T wave changes are commonly associated with the ST abnormalities seen during or following exercise in this syndrome. Hunt[5] reported a high incidence (9/19) of T wave lability in his healthy teenage swimmers who showed a high prevalence of postexercise ST depression. Froelicher *et al.*[24] reported positional T wave changes in six of 11 young, apparently healthy subjects with normal resting ECG, abnormal stress ECG, and normal coronary angiography—presumably the identical situation to that in our elite runners.[13] Orthostatic T wave changes in Froelicher's study were less common in those with angiographically demonstrable coronary disease though they did occur. The fact that ST changes in our study were seen in inferior leads also seems to fit this vasoregulatory explanation. These were the same leads in which orthostatic T changes occurred prior to exercise in three of the five subjects in question. Exercise-induced ST changes due to ischemia, hypertrophy, or abnormal supply/demand relationships might be expected to more likely occur in lateral precordial leads rather than solely in inferior leads, at least in some of the five cases.

Other explanations for the ST depression seen in this highly conditioned group are possible (transient coronary spasm, for example), though none seem especially attractive. Doing detailed invasive studies to provide more definitive answers is difficult to approve in this healthy, asymptomatic population. Yet, paradoxically, the fact that these individuals do appear to demonstrate such superb cardiovascular health makes these electrocardiographic abnormalities associated with exercise all the more intriguing and tempting for further study.

REFERENCES

1. LICHTMAN, J., R. A. O'ROURKE, A. KLEIN & J. S. KARLINER. 1973. Electrocardiogram of the athlete. Arch. Intern. Med. **132:** 763–770.
2. NAKAMOTO, K. 1969. Electrocardiograms of 25 marathon runners before and after 100 meter dash. Japan. Circ. J. **33:** 105–128.
3. RASKOFF, W. J., S. GOLDMAN & K. COHN. 1976. The "athletic heart." J. Amer. Med. Assoc. **236:** 158–162.
4. ROESKE, W. R., R. A. O'ROURKE & A. KLEIN. 1976. Noninvasive evaluation of ventricular hypertrophy in professional athletes. Circulation **53(2):** 286–292.
5. HUNT, E. A. 1963. Electrocardiographic study of 20 champion swimmers before and after 110-yard sprint swimming competition. Canad. Med. Assoc. J. **88:** 1251–1253.
6. VANGANSE, W., L. VERSEE, W. EYLENBOSCH & K. VUYLSTEEK. 1970. The electrocardiogram of athletes. Brit. Heart. J. **32:** 160–164.
7. VENERANDO, A. & V. RULLI. 1964. Frequency morphology and meaning of the

ECG anomalies found in Olympic marathon runners and walkers. J. Sports Med. and Phys. Fitness. **3:** 135–141.

8. ROSE, K. D. 1969. Relationship of cardiac problems to athletic participation. J. Amer. Med. Assoc. **208**(12): 2319–2324.

9. NEVINS, M. A., A. LEVY & L. J. LYON. 1974. When a pro athlete's heart mimics heart disease. Phys. Sports. Med. (Jan. 1974): 27–30.

10. BECKNER, G. L. & T. WILSON. 1954. Cardiovascular adaptions to prolonged physical effort. Circulation **9:** 835–846.

11. SMITH, W. G., K. J. CULLEN & I. O. THORBURN. 1964. Electrocardiograms of marathon runners in 1962 commonwealth games. Brit. Heart J. **26:** 469–476.

12. UNDERWOOD, R. & J. SCHWADE. 1977. Noninvasive analysis of cardiac function of elite distance runners—Echocardiography, vectorcardiography and cardiac intervals. Ann. N.Y. Acad. Sci. This volume.

13. POLLOCK, M. 1977. Submaximal and maximal working capacity of elite distance runners. Part I: Cardiorespiratory fitness. Ann. N.Y. Acad. Sci. This volume.

14. ÅSTRAND, P. O. & K. RODAHL, Eds. 1970. Textbook of Work Physiology. McGraw-Hill Book Company. New York, N.Y.

15. POLLOCK, M., R. BOHANNON, K. COOPER, J. AYRES, A. WARD, S. WHITE & A. C. LINNERUD. 1976. A comparative analysis of four protocols for maximal treadmill stress testing. Amer. Heart J. **92**(1): 39–46.

16. MARRIOT, H. J. 1972. Practical Electrocardiography. 5th ed. Williams and Wilkins Co. Baltimore, Md.

17. THOMAS, J., E. HARRIS & G. LASSITER. 1960. Observations on the T wave and ST segment changes in the precordial electrocardiogram of 320 young negro adults. Amer. J. Cardiol. **5:** 468–472.

18. SENTER, R. J. 1969. Analysis of Data. Scott Foresman and Co. Cincinnati, Ohio.

19. ROMHILT, D. W. & E. H. ESTES, JR. 1968. A point score system for the ECG diagnosis of left ventricular hypertrophy. Amer. Heart J. **75:** 752.

20. GRIMBY, G. & B. SALTIN. 1966. Physiological analysis of physically well-trained middle-aged and old athletes. Acta Med. Scand. **179:** 512–526.

21. KAVANAUGH, T. 1977. Marathon running of select coronary men. Ann. N.Y. Acad. Sci. This volume.

22. WONG, H. O. 1969. Impaired maximum exercise performance with hypertensive cardiovascular disease. Circulation **39:** 633–638.

23. FRIESINGER, G. C., R. O. BIERN, I. LIKAR & R. E. MASON. 1972. Exercise electrocardiography and vasoregulatory abnormalities. Amer. J. Cardiol. **30:** 733–740.

24. FROELICHER, V. F., F. G. YANOWITZ, A. J. THOMPSON & M. C. LANCASTER. 1973. The correlation of coronary angiography and the electrocardiographic response to maximal treadmill testing in 76 asymptomatic men. Circulation **38:** 597–604.

NONINVASIVE ANALYSIS OF CARDIAC FUNCTION OF ELITE DISTANCE RUNNERS—ECHOCARDIOGRAPHY, VECTORCARDIOGRAPHY, AND CARDIAC INTERVALS

Ronald H. Underwood and Jack L. Schwade

Dallas Diagnostic Association
Medical City Dallas Hospital
Dallas, Texas 75230

INTRODUCTION

A number of variables have been described pertaining to the phenomenon of the "athlete's heart." Electrocardiographic, vectorcardiographic, radiographic, and recently echocardiographic variables have been analyzed, and conflicting reports have been generated suggesting that the athlete's heart may be diseased or that it may exhibit superior function.[1-5] We had the opportunity to perform noninvasive cardiac evaluation of a group of world class distance runners during active training. We assessed them for evidence of chamber hypertrophy and dilatation, and we also looked for evidence of diminished or increased cardiac function by a variety of parameters.

MATERIAL AND METHODS

Twenty world class athletes were studied during active training; all were distance runners. Two control populations were also studied. One consisted of a group of eight university distance runners; the other was a group of ten age- and weight-matched lean nonathletes from a local university. Details of the populations studied are presented elsewhere.[6] All studies were done in the early morning after an overnight fast, with the subjects in the supine position. Vector-cardiograms were recorded using the Frank lead reference system[7] on an Instant Vectorcardiogram—1B (Instruments for Cardiac Research, Syracuse, N.Y.). Still vectorcardiographic loops were taken in the frontal, left saggital, and transverse planes with appropriate magnification to identify all components of the P, QRS, and T loops. The loops were interrupted at 2.5-msec intervals. Vectorcardiograms thus obtained were evaluated for direction and magnitude of the initial, maximal, and terminal QRS vectors; rotation of the P, QRS, and T loops; direction and magnitude of the maximum atrial vectors; presence and direction of ST vector; and mean QRS and QRS-T angles.

Phonocardiograms were recorded using a Kent Cambridge Type 01077 recorder (Cambridge Instrument Company, Inc., Ossining, N.Y.). A Kent Cambridge Pulse 53642 transducer was used for recording carotid pulse tracings and apex cardiograms. Heart sounds were recorded with the transducer in the second right, second left, and fourth left intercostal spaces adjacent to the sternum, and at the apex as defined by the point of maximum impulse.

Recordings were made on Kodak Linagraph Type 1895 light-sensitive paper at a paper speed of 100 mm/sec. Calculations of heart rate, PQ interval, QRS interval, QS_2, isovolumic contraction time (ICT), isovolumic relaxation time

(IRT), left ventricular ejection time (LVET), left ventricular ejection time index (LVETI), pre-ejection period (PEP), pre-ejection period index (PEPI), and the ratio of PEP/LVET were done on each subject.

Echocardiograms were obtained with a Smith Kline Instruments Model 0–14 transducer and a modified Ekoline 20A ultrasonic unit (Smith Kline Instrument Company, Philadelphia, Pa.) interfaced with Kent Cambridge Type 01077 direct writing recorder at a paper speed of 100 mm/sec on Kodak Linagraph Type 1895 light-sensitive paper. Using the T-scan technique, the posterobasal left ventricular wall and interventricular septum were visualized. Correct transducer position was determined by directing part of the ultrasonic beam off the posterior mitral leaflet. Measurements of left ventricular wall thickness in systole (WTS) were made at the point of maximum excursion; wall thickness in diastole (WTD) was measured at the peak of the R wave of the simultaneously recorded electrocardiogram. Septal thickness was measured just before atrial systole inferior to the distal margins of the mitral leaflets. Measurements of left ventricular internal diameter in diastole (LVIDD) and in systole (LVIDS) were made and calculation of end diastole volume (EDV), end systolic volume (ESV), stroke volume (SV), and ejection fraction (EF) were made using the method of Pombo, Troy, and Russell.[8] D-E and E-F slopes, aortic root diameter in diastole (AoRDD) and in systole (AoRDS, and left atrial diameter in diastole (LADD) and in systole (LADS) were measured.[9] Posterior wall excursion and velocity were determined, and the mean rate of circumferential fiber shortening was calculated according to the method of Cooper, O'Rourke, Karliner et al.[10] Left ventricular mass was calculated using the method of Troy, Pombo, and Rackley.[11]

The analysis of variance was used to determine differences between groups. The significance among the various treatments was found using either Duncan's multiple range test or the dummy coding in analysis of variance models.[12]

RESULTS

Vectorcardiography

The direction of the mean atrial vector in the frontal plane was between +30 and +90 degrees in 16 of 20 of the elite or world class runners (80%), and was directed abnormally rightward in four (20%). The direction of the mean atrial vector in the good runners was normal in 7 of 8 (88%); it was abnormally directed rightward in one runner. The direction of the mean atrial vector in the control group was normal in all cases. The maximum atrial voltage directed anteriorly was less than 0.10 mV in all of the good runners and the control group, and in all but one of the world class athletes in whom there was abnormal anterior displacement. The maximum atrial voltage measured posteriorly was less than 0.10 mV in all subjects. The maximum atrial voltage measured inferiorly was less than 0.18 mV in 18 of 20 world class runners (95%), in seven of eight good runners (88%), and in all of the control group. Two world class runners and one good runner had increased forces in the inferior vector measuring greater than 0.18 mV; the direction of the mean atrial vector was greater than +69° in these subjects, but was not abnormally directed. The loops in the frontal plane were narrow in these subjects. The four world class runners who demonstrated abnormal rightward direction of the mean atrial vector in the frontal plane all had normal magnitude of vectors directed anteriorly and inferiorly. In no instance did the time of atrial activation exceed 50 msec in any of the three groups. In the world class runners the QRS rotation in the frontal plane was clockwise or figure of eight with major rotation clockwise in 18 of 20 (90%) and counterclockwise in two (10%). In the good runners, rotation in the frontal plane was clockwise or figure of eight with the major portion clockwise in all subjects. In the control group, rotation in the frontal plane was clockwise or figure of eight with major direction of the loop clockwise in 9 of 10 subjects (90%) and counterclockwise in one subject. The rotation in the transverse plane was counterclockwise or figure of eight with the major direction counterclockwise in all three groups. In the saggital plane the rotation was counterclockwise or figure of eight with major portion of the loop counterclockwise in all three groups (TABLE 1).

Direction of the initial QRS loop was to the right and anterior in all subjects and was superiorly directed in all but one of the world class athletes and all but one of the good athletes. The initial QRS vector was directed inferiorly. The duration of the QRS loop was less than 85 msec in all subjects.

Mean QRS axis was between 0 and +90 degrees in all subjects except one of the world class runners who had left axis deviation and left anterior hemiblock. Two of the world class runners, none of the good runners, and two of the control group showed abnormal anterior displacement of the 35-msec vector. One of the world class and one of the good runners had discordant QRS-T vectors. The maximum deflection QRS measured less than 2.0 mV in 14 of 20 (70%) of the world class runners. In 6 of 20 (30%) of the world class runners voltage criteria for left ventricular hypertrophy was present.[13] In one of the good athletes and in one of the control group, QRS voltage exceeded 2.0 mV. None of the subjects manifesting increased QRS voltage had discordant QRS-T angles, abnormal ST vectors, or open T loops.

Thirteen of 20 (65%) of the world class runners had nonspecific ST vectors. Eleven of these were directed leftward, anteriorly, and inferiorly; one leftward, anteriorly, and superiorly; and one rightward, anteriorly, and inferiorly. Four of eight (50%) of the good runners had nonspecific ST vectors. All were directed leftward, anteriorly, and inferiorly. Seven of 10 (70%) control had nonspecific ST vectors. Six of seven were directed leftward, anteriorly, and inferiorly; one was directed leftward, posteriorly, and inferiorly.

Phonocardiography

The PQ time was normal in 17 of 20 (85%) of the elite or world class runners; three subjects had first degree AV block. None of the good runners or control subjects had abnormal PQ times. The QRS interval was normal in 18 of 20 (90%) of the world class runners; two had lengthening of the QRS interval of 100 and 104 msec. One good runner had a QRS interval of 100 msec. The QRS interval was normal in all control subjects. Determinations of QS_2, isovolumic contraction time, left ventricular ejection time, pre-ejection period, and ratio of PEP/LVET did not differ significantly among the groups. The isovolumic relaxation time was not statistically different between the world class (128 ± 18.2 msec) and the good runners (119.8 ± 9.7 msec). Both groups of athletes had significantly longer IRT than the control (103.0 ± 13.8 msec) group ($p < 0.003$). The resting heart rate was significantly slower in

TABLE 1

VECTORCARDIOGRAPHIC CHARACTERISTICS *

Athlete	Mean Atrial Vector FP	Maximum Atrial Voltage Ant	Post	Inf	Atrial Time (msec)	Rotation QRS Loop FP	TP	SP	QRS-T Angle FP	Mean QRS Vector FP	ST Vector R-L	A-P	S-I	Initial QRS Loop-Direction R-L	A-P	S-I	QRS Voltage (mV) Left	Post	Ant	Duration QRS Loop (msec)
							Elite Distance Runners													
DB	30°	0.06	0.10	0.0	32.5	CW	CCW	CCW	18°	38°	0	0	0	R	A	S	1.55	0.88	0.32	52.5
DB	77°	0.10	0.04	0.20	35.0	8	CCW	CCW	5°	43°	L	A	I	R	A	S	2.25	1.25	0.45	52.5
TC	84°	0.05	0.04	0.21	40.0	CW	CCW	CCW	14°	33°	0	0	0	R	A	S	1.73	0.14	1.65	55.0
JC	43°	0.08	0.04	0.08	32.5	CW	CCW	CCW	53°	63°	L	A	I	R	A	S	1.25	1.65	0.70	52.5
NC	53°	0.02	0.02	0.10	30.0	8	CCW	CCW	10°	73°	R	A	I	R	A	S	1.48	0.40	0.59	57.5
JG	82°	0.06	0.03	0.10	40.0	CCW	CCW	CCW	4°	48°	L	A	I	R	A	S	1.75	0.25	0.78	52.5
PG	88°	0.05	0.0	0.10	37.5	CW	CCW	CCW	77°	55°	0	0	0	R	A	S	1.60	0.60	0.35	52.5
JJ	105°	0.05	0.0	0.12	50.0	CW	CCW	8	20°	62°	0	A	I	R	A	S	1.30	0.90	0.75	67.5
DK	79°	0.03	0.03	0.08	47.5	CW	CCW	CCW	7°	19°	L	A	S	R	A	I	1.14	0.27	0.23	62.5
DK	64°	0.03	0.0	0.05	27.5	CW	CCW	CCW	20°	56°	L	A	0	R	A	S	0.73	0.64	0.24	57.5
MM	67°	0.07	0.0	0.06	35.0	CW	CCW	CCW	10°	34°	L	0	I	R	A	S	2.20	0.23	0.50	60.0
KM	54°	0.06	0.0	0.10	42.5	CW	CCW	CCW	21°	40°	0	A	0	R	A	S	2.40	0.50	0.55	60.0
PN	48°	0.08	0.0	0.10	35.0	CW	CCW	CCW	30°	50°	L	A	I	R	A	S	2.60	1.30	0.50	45.0
RP	88°	0.05	0.0	0.16	45.0	8	CCW	8	20°	59°	0	A	0	R	A	S	1.50	0.60	0.50	52.5
SP	165°	0.05	0.0	0.08	45.0	8	CCW	CCW	8°	7°	L	A	I	R	A	S	2.06	0.88	0.25	55.0
NR	75°	0.06	0.0	0.10	42.5	8	CCW	8	9°	58°	L	A	I	R	A	S	1.30	0.58	0.23	85.0
FS	91°	0.08	0.04	0.11	35.0	CCW	CCW	8	28°	-28°	L	A	I	R	A	S	1.12	0.60	0.30	55.0
GT	91°	0.05	0.04	0.12	50.0	CW	CCW	CCW	18°	39°	L	A	0	R	A	I	1.48	0.73	0.42	52.5
RW	54°	0.16	0.05	0.10	37.5	8	CCW	CCW	64°	54°	L	A	0	R	A	S	1.35	0.42	1.22	60.0
DW	75°		0.0	0.16	37.5			8	3°	14°	L	A	S	R	A	S	3.20	0.40	0.40	65.0

Good Runners

DB	109°	0.05	0.0	0.09	50.0	CW	CCW	CCW	30°	59°	O	O	O	R	A	S	1.18	0.27	0.40	35.0
BC	73°	0.03	0.0	0.03	—	CW	CCW	CCW	5°	18°	O	A	O	R	A	S	1.05	0.73	0.25	52.5
RF	37°	0.05	0.0	0.07	32.5	∞	CCW	CCW	9°	46°	O	O	O	R	A	I	1.48	0.12	0.32	62.5
PK	79°	0.05	0.0	0.08	32.0	CW	CCW	CCW	9°	58°	O	O	O	R	A	S	1.05	0.92	0.40	57.5
FN	54°	0.09	0.06	0.16	52.0	CW	CCW	CCW	33°	54°	L	A	I	R	A	S	1.50	1.15	0.09	60.0
RP	54°	0.10	0.03	0.10	42.5	CW	CCW	CCW	7°	46°	L	A	I	R	A	S	1.75	0.75	0.35	80.0
HP	69°	0.08	0.06	0.20	45.0	∞	∞	∞	10°	38°	O	O	O	R	A	S	1.80	0.40	0.35	64.0
PP	61°	0.06	0.03	0.12	32.5	CW	CCW	∞	4°	28°	L	A	I	R	A	S	2.07	0.34	0.20	55.0

Nonathletic Controls

JB	39°	0.04	0.0	0.08	37.5	CW	CCW	CCW	5°	47°	O	O	I	R	A	S	1.30	0.60	0.35	60.0
MB	77°	0.05	0.0	0.10	32.5	∞	∞	∞	2°	56°	L	P	O	R	A	S	1.37	0.0	0.32	60.0
RG	64°	0.04	0.0	0.08	32.5	∞	CCW	CCW	9°	38°	O	O	I	R	A	S	2.00	0.30	0.60	60.0
LJ	90°	0.05	0.0	0.15	35.0	CW	CCW	CCW	5°	52°	L	A	O	R	A	S	0.95	0.55	0.75	60.0
BL	67°	0.04	0.02	0.16	35.0	CCW	∞	∞	38°	68°	O	O	I	R	A	S	1.32	0.62	0.33	52.5
TM	21°	0.03	0.0	0.04	47.5	∞	CCW	CCW	9°	36°	L	A	O	R	A	I	1.34	0.30	0.52	60.0
BM	67°	0.05	0.0	0.08	50.0	CW	CCW	CCW	7°	58°	L	A	I	R	A	I	0.42	0.76	0.17	62.5
TM	83°	0.05	0.03	0.11	37.5	CW	CCW	CCW	3°	56°	L	A	I	R	A	S	1.00	0.43	0.35	42.5
SR	63°	0.05	0.0	0.16	40.0	CW	CCW	CCW	8°	58°	L	A	I	R	A	S	1.03	0.72	0.40	72.0
RR	48°	0.05	0.02	0.07	35.0	CW	CCW	CCW	3°	58°	L	A	I	R	A	S	0.73	0.60	0.27	55.0

* Abbreviations: FP, frontal plane; TP, transverse plane; SP, saggital plane; Ant or A, anterior; Post or P, posterior; Inf or I, inferior; S, superior; CW, clockwise; CCW, counter clockwise.

the world class (46.6 ± 4.6 beats/min) and good (47.6 ± 5.3 beats/min) runners compared to the control (57.1 ± 8.4 beats/min) group (p < 0.007). For the phonocardiographic data, see TABLE 2.

Echocardiography

Measurements of septal thickness, left ventricular wall thickness at end-diastole and end-systole, posterior wall excursion and velocity, ejection fraction, mean velocity of circumferential fiber shortening, D-E slope and E-F slope were not statistically significantly different among the three groups studied (TABLE 3). There was no difference in the left ventricular internal diameter in diastole between the world class (50.9 ± 4.0 mm) and the good (50.0 ± 3.8 mm) runners; both groups of athletes had internal dimensions significantly greater than the control (46.2 ± 4.7 mm) group (p < 0.025). The left ventricular internal

TABLE 2

PHONOCARDIOGRAPHIC CHARACTERISTICS

Variable	Elite Runners	Good Runners	Control	p Values
Heart rate, beats/min	46.6±4.6 * (40.0–56.0)†	47.6±5.3 (41.0–56.0)	57.1±8.4 (43.0–75.0)	<0.0005
R–R interval, msec	1288.5±134.9 (1080.0–1512.0)	1269.8±131.2 (1072.0–1440.0)	1072.4–155.3 (800.0–1392.0)	NS
P–Q interval msec	171.4±31.8 (120.0–240.0)	188.1±89.7 (140.0–408.0)	137.2±26.7 (96.0–160.0)	NS
QRS duration, msec	68.1±19.3 (40.0–104.0)	66.3±25.0 (40.0–100.0)	63.8±16.7 (44.0–88.0)	NS
QS₂, msec	434.4±26.6 (366.0–480.0)	438.0±20.7 (408.0–480.0)	421.6±24.7 (392.0–460.0)	NS
Isovolyumetric construction time (ICT), msec	63.2±20.5 (32.0–96.0)	61.4±28.0 (20.0–95.2)	59.5±24.8 (20.0–88.0)	NS
Isovolumetric relaxaton time(IRT), msec	128.0±18.2 (96.0–160.0)	119.8±9.7 (100.0–132.0)	103.0±13.8 (80.0–120.0)	<0.0003
Left ventricular ejection time (LVET), msec	333.8±18.4 (300.0–360.0)	326.5±24.1 (300.0–360.0)	325.6±15.6 (300.0–356.0)	NS
Left ventricular ejection time index (LVETI), msec	414.2±18.1 (378.2–477.0)	407.4±21.6 (378.8–435.0)	424.3±20.9 (396.9–455.5)	NS
Pre-ejection period (PEP), msec	100.8±17.0 (60.0–136.0)	111.5±16.2 (80.0–132.0)	94.0±28.7 (44.0–120.0)	NS
Pre-ejection period index (PEPI), msec	119.6±16.6 (78.4–154.8)	130.6±17.5 (98.0–152.3)	116.9±28.3 (66.4–150.0)	NS
PEP/LVET	0.3±0.04 (0.2–0.4)	0.35±0.08 (0.2–0.5)	0.27±0.09 (0.1–0.4)	NS

* Mean±standard deviation.
† Range.

TABLE 3

ECHOCARDIOGRAPHIC CHARACTERISTICS

Variable	Elite Runners	Good Runners	Control	p Values
Septal thickness(ST), mm	11.3±1.9* (9.2–16.0)†	10.1±0.9 (8.4–11.0)	10.0±1.85 (7.8–14.0)	NS
Wall thickness, diastole (WTD), mm	9.8±1.0 (7.4–11.6)	9.5±0.6 (8.8–10.2)	8.7±2.4 (5.0–13.0)	NS
Wall thickness, systole (WTS), mm	15.2±2.0 (10.0–18.8)	14.2±2.1 (12.6–18.2)	14.5±2.2 (12.7–19.8)	NS
Posterior wall excursion (PWE), mm	12.7±2.9 (8.0–18.0)	10.8±2.1 (8.2–14.6)	12.2±3.5 (6.0–17.4)	NS
Posterior wall velocity (PWV), mm/msec	51.4±11.4 (35.4–76.8)	52.5±14.5 (32.6–75.8)	50.5±6.3 (38.6–58.8)	NS
Left ventricular internal diam, diastole (LVIDD), mm	51.0±3.8 (42.3–56.2)	49.7±3.8 (44.0–56.2)	46.7±3.9 (40.2–52.8)	<0.02
Left ventricular internal diam, systole (LVIDS), mm	34.2±4.4 (20.0–39.6)	34.1±3.3 (30.2–39.8)	31.7±2.8 (27.0–37.4)	NS
End-diastolic volume (EDV), ml	141.2±30.0 (79.0–185.8)	139.9±29.8 (89.2–185.8)	108.6±28.2 (68.0–155.9)	<0.02
End-systolic volume (EDV), ml	44.1±14.2 (12.7–65.0)	42.3±12.6 (28.8–66.0)	33.6±9.0 (20.6–53.0)	NS
Stroke volume (SV), ml	96.4±21.2 (66.0–133.1)	88.5±25.9 (52.9–119.8)	74.4–24 (38.6–102.9)	<0.05
Ejection Fraction (EF), (%)	67±7 (53–84)	67±9 (53–79)	68±7 (57–79)	NS
Left ventricular output (LVO), ml	4495.8±1376.4 (2850.0–8079.2)	4184.2±1168.4 (2454.6–5553.8)	4270.7±1648.7 (2161.0–6997.0)	NS
Excursion, anterior mitral valve, mm	21.4±3.7 (15.7–29.8)	18.0±4.0 (11.3–24.3)	21.6±4.3 (15.0–28.8)	NS
D–E slope, mm/sec	373.1±83.1 (231.0–505.2)	298.2±63.2 (219.5–397.0)	344.4±90.0 (194.8–495.8)	NS
E–F slope, mm/sec	177.7±45.6 (80.3–258.0)	152.9±40.2 (100.0–202.8)	171.9±43.4 (84.8–248.8)	NS
Aortic root diam, diastole (AoRDD), mm	28.7–3.0 (23.2–36)	27.3±2.1 (24.0–30.4)	27.3±3.4 (23.0–32.8)	NS
Aortic root diam, systole (AoRDS), mm	32.1±3.0 (26.8–37.2)	31.5±2.4 (27.8–36.2)	28.9±3.5 (22.8–34.4)	<0.03
Left atrial diam, diastole (LADD), mm	24.9±4.2 (16.0–32.6)	23.8±2.5 (21.0–27.0)	17.5±4.3 (12.6–26.2)	=0.0003
Left atrial diam, systole (LADS), mm	33.5±4.7 (23.3–42.2)	31.3±3.3 (27.5–37.0)	27.3±4.6 (20.6–34.8)	=0.005
Heart rate, beats/min	48.3±6.9 (38.0–60.7)	47.9±7.1 (38.6–61.3)	57.1±7.3 (47.0–68.0)	=0.007

TABLE 3—*Continued*

ECHOCARDIOGRAPHIC CHARACTERISTICS

Variable	Elite Runners	Good Runners	Control	p Values
Left ventricular mass (LVM), g	189.0±34.9 (137.8–273.2)	172.2±24.1 (130.4–194.1)	134.6±29.5 (76.8–179.8)	=0.006
Right ventricular internal diam, diastole (RVIDD), mm	18.6±4.6 (12.0–26.0)	18.0±5.0 (13.0–25.0)	11.7±3.0 (7.0–16.0)	<0.002
Mean velocity, circumferential fiber shortening (V_{cf}), circ/sec	0.73±0.13 (0.47–0.99)	0.70±0.19 (0.43–0.02)	0.72±0.1 (0.55–0.88)	NS

* Mean±standard deviation.
† Range.

diameter in systole was not significantly different between the three groups, although both groups of runners had slightly larger measurements. End diastolic volume was significantly different between both groups of runners and the control group ($p < 0.02$). There was no significant difference between the world class runners and the good runners. End-diastolic volume in the world class runners averaged 140.5 ± 31.7 ml (range: 65 to 186 ml), 130.9 ± 29.8 ml (range: 89 to 186 ml) in the good runners, and 103.0 ± 36.9 ml (range: 38 to 156 ml) in the control group. There was a statistically significant difference in the stroke volume between the world class (96.4 ± 21.2 ml) runners and the control (74.4 ± 24.0 ml) group ($p < 0.05$). There was no significant difference between the world class runners and the good (88.5 ± 25.9 ml) runners. There was no difference in the RVIDD between the world class (18.6 ± 4.6 mm) and the good (18.0 ± 5.0 mm) athletes. Both groups of runners had right ventricular internal dimensions significantly greater than the control (11.7 ± 3.1 mm) group ($p < 0.002$). Aortic root diameter in diastole was not statistically different among the three groups. There was a statistically significant difference in the aortic root diameter in systole between the world class (32.1 ± 3.0 mm) and the control (28.9 ± 3.5 mm) group ($p < 0.03$). There was no significant difference between the world class and the good (31.5 ± 2.4 mm) runners. The left atrial diameter during ventricular diastole was significantly greater in the world class (25.0 ± 4.2 mm) and good (23.8 ± 2.5 mm) runners than in the control (17.5 ± 4.3 mm) groups ($p < 0.0003$). The left atrial diameter during ventricular systole was significantly greater in the world class (33.5 ± 4.7 mm) athletes as compared to the control (27.3 ± 4.6 mm) group ($p < 0.005$). There was no significant difference between the world class and the good (31.3 ± 3.3 mm) runners. Two of the world class runners, one of the control group, and none of the good runners had septal thicknesses in excess of 12 mm. Both of the world class runners who exhibited this abnormality had ratios of septal thickness to wall thickness in diastole in excess of 1.5. The control subject did not. Both the world class athletes (189.8 ± 34.9 g) and the good athletes (172.3 ± 24.1 g) had significantly larger left ventricular mass determinations than the control (134.6 ± 29.4 g) group ($p < 0.0006$).

DISCUSSION

Vectorcardiography

Normal mean atrial vectors are directed inferiorly and leftward. Right atrial vectors are oriented anteriorly, and left atrial vectors are oriented posteriorly, reflecting their anatomic location in the body. Right atrial hypertrophy is manifest by an increase in the anteriorly directed vectors, and the magnitude usually exceeds the normal upper limit of 0.1 mV in the transverse plane, 0.18 mV in the sagittal plane, and 0.20 mV in the frontal plane. Additionally, the loop in the frontal plane often is narrow. The direction of the P vector is typically normal, between $+15°$ and $+90°$, although the vector tends to be vertical in position, closer to $+90°$.[13] One world class runner had abnormal anterior displacement of the P vector. Of the 20 world class runners, 7 (35%) demonstrated at least one criterion for right atrial hypertrophy. However, none of the athletes with abnormal direction of the mean atrial vector had voltage criteria for hypertrophy. One good runner had voltage criteria for right atrial hypertrophy (0.20 mV in the frontal plane) with a normal mean atrial vector. None of the control subjects had any criteria for right atrial hypertrophy. A P loop that is large and more or less vertical in its direction is related to the finding of "P pulmonale" in the scalar electrocardiogram. The fact that the time of atrial activation was normal in all subjects explains the narrowness of the P wave in the conventional electrocardiograms;[13] only with an increase in the time of atrial activation will the P wave become abnormally wide.

Rotation of the QRS loop was normal in all planes in all subjects, as was direction of the initial QRS vector. Time of ventricular activation was normal (≤ 85 msec) in all subjects. Roeske, O'Rourke, Klein *et al.*[4] reported that half of their athletes had 50% or more of the QRS vector anterior in the transverse plane, comparing their work to that of Arstila and Koivikko[2] who reported a similar finding in eight (17%) of 46 endurance athletes. With this criterion as evidence for right ventricular hypertrophy, four (20%) world class runners, two (25%) good runners, and three (30%) control subjects manifest this disorder. Using the more stringent criteria of Chou, Helm, and Kaplan,[13] two (10%) world class runners, two (25%) good runners, and two (20%) control subjects had 70% or more of the transverse loop located anteriorly. No subject had greater than 20% of the area of the QRS loop located in the right inferior quadrant in the frontal plane. The ST vector in Type B right ventricular hypertrophy is oriented posteriorly, to the right, and superiorly.[13] No subject studied had this direction of the ST vector. Thus, vectorcardiographic criteria for right ventricular hypertrophy were not significantly different in the three groups studied.

Left ventricular hypertrophy was suggested by voltage criteria in six (30%) of 20 world class runners, in one (13%) of eight good runners, and in one (10%) of ten control subjects. These data are consistent with that reported by Beckner and Winsor[1] (33%) and by Roeske, O'Rourke, Klein, *et al.*[4] who reported similar findings. None of the subjects with increased QRS voltage had signs of myocardial ischemia such as discordant QRS-T angles, abnormal ST vectors, or open T loops.

Nonspecific ST vectors were common in all groups. In left ventricular hypertrophy the spatial ST vector is opposite to the $QRS_s\hat{E}$ loop and its magnitude is often increased.[13] The J point (point of termination of the QRS$_8$Ê loop) is located to the right, anterior, and superior to the point of origin. No subject examined had this abnormal location of the J point. One of the world class runners and one of the good runners had discordant QRS-T vectors. Neither of these athletes had voltage criteria for left ventricular hypertrophy.

Mean QRS axis was normal and was between 0 and +90° in all subjects except one world class runner in whom left axis deviation due to left anterior hemiblock was present. Rosenbaum [14] states that left anterior hemiblock almost invariably indicates left ventricular disease. Coronary artery disease alone or in complication with hypertension, Chagasic myocarditis, cardiomyopathy, and aortic valvular disease are among the known clinical causes of left anterior hemiblock, none of which were clinically present in our subject. Left anterior hemiblock occurring in the absence of other clinical abnormalities in a young person may be a sequel of myocarditis or it may be due to a congenital anomaly of the conduction system.[15] Whatever the cause of the left anterior hemiblock in our subject, it produces no other measurable deficit in his cardiovascular system, either at rest or with the stress of world class competition.

Phonocardiography

Inasmuch as all of the individuals studied were asymptomatic and had no evidence of clinical heart disease, it is not surprising that systolic time intervals were normal. The possibility that chronic volume overload, similar to the situation encountered in the patient with valvular insufficiency [3] might be present in endurance athletes is not borne out by the systolic time intervals in the present study. The only variables that were significantly different among the groups studied were the isovolumic relaxation time and the heart rate. The isovolumic relaxation time is the period in diastole that begins with aortic valve closure and ends with mitral valve opening. This interval is shortened by conditions in which the left atrial pressure is elevated, such as mitral stenosis, and is lengthened by systemic vascular hypertension.[16] The principle reason for the longer isovolumic relaxation time in the athletes studied is probably related to the fact that the left atrial pressure diminishes with increase in the R-R interval.[17] Heart rate in the runners is significantly slower than in the control group; this allows a longer diastolic filling period with consequent lower left atrial pressure and resultant lengthening of the isovolumic relaxation time.

Echocardiography

Left ventricular end-diastolic diameter was increased in both groups of runners compared to the control group. End-systolic diameters were slightly greater in the runners than in the control subjects (TABLE 3), but the difference was not statistically significant. In contrast to the study of Raskoff et al.[5] who reported three of 25 (12%) local amateur long distance runners with left ventricular end-diastolic diameter greater than 56 mm, none of our subjects had evidence of left ventricular dilatation, although four world class and one good runner measured 56 mm, the upper limit of normal. They also reported four subjects (16%) with ejection fractions greater than 80%; only one world class runner in our study had this finding, and there was no difference in the average ejection fraction among the groups. Left ventricular end-diastolic volume was increased in the runners. Our data are similar to that reported by Roeske et al.[4] in that average left and right ventricular end-diastolic dimensions were significantly greater in the athletes than in the control population, and in that neither ventricle seemed to predominate. In spite of increased right ventricular dimensions and vectorcardiographic evidence of right ventricular hypertrophy in a few subjects, septal motion in systole and diastole was normal,[18] lending credence to the hypothesis that the hypertrophy is "physiologic." Left atrial dimensions in systole and diastole were increased in the runners. Both world class runners and good runners had significantly greater left atrial diameter in diastole ($p < 0.0003$); in systole the difference was significant only between the world class runners and the control group ($p < 0.005$). Reasons for the increase in left atrial dimensions are not apparent in the present study. It is probable that the increase is due to increased flow during training. An alternate possibility is that the left ventricular hypertrophy is not entirely "physiologic" and that the left atrium dilates partly in response to the increased left ventricular mass that the runners in our study demonstrate. Both groups of runners had left ventricular masses that were significantly greater than the control group ($p < 0.0006$). Stroke volume was significantly greater in the world class runners than in the control group ($p < 0.05$); there was no statistical difference between world class runners and good runners or between good runners and controls, although the good runners had larger stroke volumes than the controls. The resting heart rate was significantly slower in the athletes than in the control group, and there was no difference in the resting left ventricular output between the groups. The finding of larger resting stroke volumes in the athletes is similar to the data of Morganroth et al.[3] who found statistically significant differences in stroke volume of their swimmers and runners compared with wrestlers and normal subjects. Similarly Roeske et al.[4] found increased resting stroke volume in their study of professional basketball players. There was no difference in the ejection fraction between the three groups; average ejection fractions in all three groups were remarkably similar and all were normal. There was also no difference in mean velocity of circumferential fiber shortening (V_{cf}) between the groups and no subject had a V_{cf} greater than 1.02 circumferences per second. Thus there was little evidence of superior or supranormal cardiac function in the basal state. In contrast to Morganroth et al.[3] who found no differences in aortic root transverse diameters, we found a slight but statistically significant difference in aortic root diameter in systole. There was no difference in the aortic root diameters measured in diastole in both groups of runners. Whether the apparently increased compliance of the aortic root seen in the runners is due to the effect of training or whether this represents different genetic endowment is not answered by the present study, but it is a question that should be relatively easy to answer by doing sequential studies in athletes in and out of training. Left ventricular free wall thickness was normal in all subjects. Mean septal thickness was normal in all groups. Two of the world class runners had septal thicknesses in excess of 12 mm, which is accepted as the upper limit of normal.[9] Septal thickness was 16.0 and 15.6 mm in these athletes, and the ratio of septal to left ventricular free wall thickness was greater than 1.5:1 in both. One of the control subjects had a septal thickness of 14.0 mm, but his septal/free wall ratio was normal. No abnormal systolic anterior motion of the mitral valve was present in any subject, and despite one criterion for asymmetrical septal hypertrophy[19] it is unlikely that any of our subjects have hypertrophic obstructive cardiomyopathy. The problem of assessing patients for possible asymmetric septal hypertrophy has been discussed by Shah [20] who urges caution in assigning this diagnosis on the basis of limited criteria. Roeske *et al.*[4] reported septal/posterior wall thickness ratios greater than 1.3 in four of ten athletes and five of ten control subjects, and they also urged caution in the interpretation of apparently abnormal echocardiographic data in young, tall, normal males.

SUMMARY AND CONCLUSIONS

There is suggestive evidence of right atrial hypertrophy in 35% of the elite or world class runners, three of whom had voltage criteria. Left ventricular hypertrophy was suggested by voltage criteria in 30% of the world class runners, in one of the good runners, and in one of the control subjects. Nonspecific ST vectors were common in all groups. One of the world class runners demonstrated left anterior hemiblock. Systolic time intervals were normal in all groups. The isovolumic relaxation time was lengthened in the runners compared to the control subjects and this was probably due to thet lower heart rate in the athletes. Left ventricular internal diameter during diastole and end diastolic volumes were larger in the athletes than in the control population. Stroke volumes were larger, but there was no difference in the ejection fraction, posterior wall excursion, posterior wall velocity, or mean velocity of circumferential fiber shortening. Left atrial dimensions were increased in the runners. Aortic root diameters measured in systole were significantly larger in the world class runners. Measurements of the interventricular septum were normal except for two of the world class runners who had septal thicknesses above normal. Both of these runners had an abnormal ratio of septal thickness to left ventricular free wall thickness. There were no other findings to suggest hypertrophic obstructive cardiomyopathy. Left ventricular free wall thickness was normal. Left ventricular mass was significantly greater in the runners. Although the athletes as a group clearly had larger hearts, they tended to cluster towards the upper limit of normal and few demonstrated pathologically abnormal measurements.

REFERENCES

1. BECKNER, G. L. & T. WINSOR. 1954. Cardiovascular adaptations to prolonged physical effort. Circulation **9:** 835–846.
2. ARSTILA, M. & L. KOIVIKKO. 1964. Electrocardiographic and vectorcardiographic signs of left and right ventricular hypertrophy in endurance athletes. J. Sports Med. Fitness **14:** 166.
3. MORGANROTH, J., B. J. MARON, W. L. HENRY & S. E. EPSTEIN. 1975. Comparative left ventricular dimensions in trained athletes. Ann. Intern. Med. **82:** 521–524.
4. ROESKE, W. R., R. A. O'ROURKE, A. KLEIN, G. LEOPOLD & J. S. KARLINER. 1976. Noninvasive evaluation of ventricular hypertrophy in profesional athletes. Circulation **52**(2): 286–292.
5. ROSKOFF, W. J., S. GOLDMAN & K. COHN. 1976. The "Athletic Heart". J. Amer. Med. Assoc. **236**(2): 158–162.
6. POLLOCK, M. L. 1977. Characteristics of elite class distance runners: Overview. Ann. N. Y. Acad. Sci. This volume.

7. FRANK, E. 1956. An accurate, clinically practical system for spatial vectorcardiography. Circulation **13:** 737–749.
8. FEIGENBAUM, H., R. L. POPP, S. B. WOLFE, B .L. TROY, J. F. POMBO, C. L. HAINE & H. T. DODGE. 1972. Ultrasound measurements of the left ventricle. Arch. Intern. Med. **129:** 461–467.
9. FEIGENBAUM, H. 1972. Echocardiography. Lea & Febiger. Philadelphia, Pa.
10. COOPER, R. H., R. A. O'ROURKE, J. S. KARLINER, K. L. PETERSON & G. R. LEOPOLD. 1972. Comparison of ultrasound and cineangiographic measurements of the mean rate of circumferential fiber shortening in man. Circulation **46:** 914–923.
11. TROY, B. L., J. POMBO & C. E. RACKLEY. 1972. Measurement of left ventricular wall thickness and mass by echocardiography. Circulation **45:** 602–611.
12. HARVEY, W. R. 1960. Least squares analysis of variance with unequal subclass numbers. Agricultural Research Services 20–8.
13. CHOU, T-C, R. A. HELM & S. KAPLAN. 1974. Clinical Vectorcardiography. 2nd edit. Grune & Stratton. New York, N.Y.
14. ROSENBAUM, M. B., M. V. ELIZARI & J. O. LAZZARI. 1970. The Hemiblocks. Tampa Tracings. Oldsmar, Florida.
15. SUMMER, R. G., J. H. PHILLIPS, W. J. JACOBY, JR. & D. H. TUCKER. 1967. Forme fruste of endocardial cushion defect. Amer. J. Med. Sci. **254:** 266–283.
16. LEO, T. & H. HULTGREN. 1959. Phonocardiographic characteristics of tight mitral stenosis. Medicine **38:** 85–101.
17. TAVEL, M. E. 1974. Clinical phonocardiography and external pulse recording. 2nd edit. Year Book Medical Publishers, Inc. Chicago, Ill.
18. POPP, R. L., S. B. WOLFE, T. HIRATA & H. FEIGENBAUM. 1969. Estimation of right and left ventricular size by ultrasound. A study of the echoes from the interventricular septum. Amer. J. Cardiol. **24:** 523–530.
19. HENRY, W. L., C. E. CLARK & S. E. EPSTEIN. 1973. Asymmetric septal hypertrophy: Echocardiographic identification of the pathognomonic anatomic abnormality of IHSS. Circulation **47:** 225–233.
20. SHAH, P. M. 1975. IHSS—HOCM—MSS—ASH? Circulation **51:** 577–580.

SUBMAXIMAL AND MAXIMAL WORKING CAPACITY OF ELITE DISTANCE RUNNERS.
PART I: CARDIORESPIRATORY ASPECTS*

M. L. Pollock †

Institute for Aerobics Research
Dallas, Texas 75230

Maximal oxygen uptake ($\dot{V}_{O_2 max}$) has been described as an important characteristic of endurance athletes.[1-4] Early investigations by Robinson, Edwards, and Dill,[1] and Saltin and Åstrand[2] reported $\dot{V}_{O_2 max}$ values above 80 ml/kg·min for distance runners and cross-country skiers. Saltin and Åstrand[2] further documented a differentiation in $\dot{V}_{O_2 max}$ in a variety of athletic types.

A more recent study showed that although $\dot{V}_{O_2 max}$ differentiated well in endurance athletes of diverse abilities, there was a limitation of using $\dot{V}_{O_2 max}$ to predict distance running performance of good runners.[5] Costill *et al.*[6] and Costill, Thomason, and Roberts[5] found that the fractional utilization of $\dot{V}_{O_2}$ at a standard running speed to be an important measure in predicting performance capacity in good distance runners. Running efficiency from the standpoint of energy expenditure may also be an important factor in differentiating distance runners.[7-9]

It has been suggested that differences may exist in some metabolic variables between elite marathon runners (26.2 miles or 42 km) and other elite types of middle-long distance runners (1–6 miles or 1,500–10,000 m).[9, 10] As metabolic and efficiency differences may prove more predictive in differentiating among elite runners, it was the purpose of this investigation to study the submaximal and maximal metabolic characteristics of a large sample of elite runners to observe if specific differentiation into the types of runner could be made.

Methods

The subjects for this investigation included 20 elite distance runners (ER), eight good distance runners (GR), and ten untrained lean college students (UL). The ERs were further divided in accordance with their best performance capabilities. The two groups included eight marathon runners and 11 middle-long distance runners (M-LD). One runner (Kardong) was too difficult to classify and was not used in this phase of the data analysis. The performance and training characteristics for the running groups are described in an earlier paper of this volume.[11] The basic physical characteristics for the groups are shown in TABLE 1. None of the UL subjects had been in regular training for at least 2 years prior to testing, and none had participated in distance running events on a regular basis.

The subjects reported to the laboratory after a minimum of a 3-hour fast. Resting values for heart rate (HR), systolic and diastolic blood pressure (SBP

* This work was supported by Quinton Instruments, Seattle, Wash.
† Present address: Department of Medicine, Mount Sinai Medical Center, 950 N. 12th St. P.O. Box 342, Milwaukee, Wisc. 53201.

and DBP), and a standard 12-lead electrocardiogram (ECG) were determined prior to submaximal and maximal treadmill testing. Resting HR, SBP, and DBP were determined in the supine, sitting, and standing positions, but only the sitting values will be discussed in this paper. The maximal treadmill test used was a protocol designed by Åstrand [4] and modified by Pollock et al.[12] It was a continuous, multistage run test, which was performed to voluntary exhaustion. The speed of the run was held constant at 11.0 mph (5 m/sec). The treadmill grade was set initially at 0% and subsequently elevated 2.5% every 2 minutes until termination of the test. The submaximal test, which preceded the maximal test by approximately 10 minutes, was a continuous 11-minute run performance at 0% grade. The speed was set at 10 mph (4.5 m/sec) for the first 7 minutes and subsequently increased to 12 mph (5.5 m/sec) for the last 4 minutes.

It should be noted that the UL group did not have the capability to attempt the submaximal and maximal tests as described above. Thus they were not administered the submaximal test, and the maximal test was modified to accommodate their ability to run. The speed of the treadmill was adjusted to exhaust each subject in 7 to 10 minutes; this time period is considered adequate for maximal physiological adjustments to occur.[4, 13] The treadmill speed for the UL group ranged between 6.5 and 7.5 mph (3–3.5 m/sec). The grade change sequence was the same as described for the ER and GR groups.

Electrocardiogram and HR were monitored continuously on both tests by a standard, multilead exercise cable system and a single-channel ECG recorder (Model 1500B, Hewlett-Packard, Paramus, N.J.), and cardiotachometer (Model 611, Quinton Instruments, Seattle, Wash.). A modified V_4 lead (electrode was placed halfway between V_4 and V_5) was monitored during exercise; leads I, II, III, AVR, AVL, AVF, and V_4 were recorded immediately following and during 1 and 3 minutes of recovery from the submaximal test and 1, 3, and 5 minutes from the maximal test. For the purpose of this study V_4 refers to the modified position described above. Heart rate was recorded at 30-second intervals during exercise and recovery. Blood pressure was determined by the ausculation technique with the pressure cuff attached to the left arm. The measurement was determined while the subjects were at rest and during recovery. The time sequence for monitoring blood pressure during recovery was the same as described for ECG determination. Since accurate BP determinations are difficult to obtain during treadmill running, this measurement was omitted from the exercise phase of the tests. Upon completion of both the submaximal and maximal tests the subjects were seated as quickly as possible for their respective recovery periods.

During the submaximal test, expired air samples were collected during minutes 4–5, 5–6, 6–7, 8–9, 9–10, and 10–11 in 150-liter meteorological balloons. Aliquots were analyzed for O_2 and CO_2 content on Beckman OM-11 polarographic O_2 and LB-2 infrared CO_2 gas analyzers. Calibration gases and analyzers were checked by a modified Lloyd Haldane gas analyzer. Pulmonary ventilation (V_E) was determined by means of a gas meter (Model CD-4, Instrumentation Associates, Inc., New York, N.Y.) and calibrated by a tissot gasometer (150 L, W. E. Collins, Co., Braintree, Mass.) The smallest inside diameter of the system was 3.18 cm. The metabolic techniques and procedures outlined by Consolazio, Johnson, and Pecora [14] were followed.

For determination of blood lactic acid, 2 to 3 ml of blood were drawn from the antecubital vein 3 minutes after both the submaximal and maximal treadmill

TABLE 1

PHYSICAL CHARACTERISTICS AND RESTING CARDIOVASCULAR VARIABLES OF ELITE DISTANCE RUNNERS, GOOD RUNNERS, AND UNTRAINED MEN

Subject	Age (yr)	Height (cm)	Weight (kg)	RHR * (beats/min)	SBP * (mmHg)	DBP * (mmHg)	HV * (ml)	Hv/Weight (ml/kg)
Elite M–LD Runners †								
Brown	22	187	74.1	47	118	86	1019	13.8
Castaneda	23	178	62.8	49	120	78	1082	17.2
Crawford	27	172	58.0	46	112	80	1043	18.0
Geis	21	179	66.3	42	112	78	1240	18.7
Johnson	25	175	62.1	48	130	82	860	13.8
Manley	32	178	69.4	57	120	90	1113	16.0
Ndoo	28	169	53.6	55	106	86	1186	22.1
Prefontaine	23	170	66.3	42	122	80	1399	21.1
Rose	23	176	59.2	51	110	73	766	12.9
Tuttle	27	177	60.9	51	138	70	1142	18.8
11 ‡	27	170	60.9	39	—	—	1106	18.2
Mean	25.4	175.9	63.1	47.9	119	80	1087	17.3
(±SD) §	(3.2)	(5.1)	(5.3)	(5.3)	(9.7)	(6.1)	(172)	(2.97)
Elite Marathon Runners								
Cusak	23	175	64.2	40	120	80	1148	17.9
Galloway	29	181	65.0	43	104	70	921	14.2
Kennedy	27	167	55.8	46	110	80	817	14.6

Moore	31	184	64.2	43	118	82	1229	19.1
Pate	28	178	57.0	54	114	74	766	13.4
Shorter	27	178	61.3	46	112	70	732	11.9
Wayne	25	172	61.3	46	108	70	755	12.3
Williams	29	177	66.1	42	108	72	1136	17.2
Mean	27.4	176.8	62.1	45.0	112	75	938	15.1
(±SD)	(2.5)	(5.4)	(3.7)	(4.5)	(5.4)	(5.1)	(203)	(2.7)
Unclassified Kardong	26	192	69.9	55	120	84	1108	15.6
Total elite runners Mean	26.2	177.1	63.1	47.1	116	78	1028	16.4
(±SD)	(2.95)	(6.0)	(4.8)	(5.3)	(8.5)	(6.2)	(191)	(2.92)
Good runners (n=8) Mean	21.3	181.1	67.5	52.4	124	81	998	14.9
(±SD)	(2.55)	(3.9)	(3.8)	(6.5)	(9.3)	(7.2)	(191)	(2.28)
Untrained lean men (n=10) Mean	20.7	180.5	63.2	65.0	114	75	—	—
(±SD)	(3.13)	(6.4)	(5.5)	(9.7)	(9.0)	(7.9)	—	—

* RHR, resting heart rate; SBP, systolic blood pressure; DBP, diastolic blood pressure; HV, heart volume.
† M–LD, middle-long distance.
‡ Name held anonymous.
§ Standard deviation.

tests. The enzymatic method described by Henry *et al.*[15] was used in the analysis of lactic acid.

Heart volume (HV) was determined from a posteroanterior and lateral chest roentgenograms taken in the standard position. The method and calculations are described by Barnhard *et al.*[16]

Standard descriptive statistics were used to analyze data by groups: ER, GR, and UL, and ER subgroups M-LD and marathon.[17, 18] The analysis of variance was used to determine differences between groups. The significance among the various treatments was found from using the Duncan Multiple Range Test. A p value equal to or less than 0.05 was accepted as significant.

Results

The physical characteristics and resting values for HR, SBP, DBP, and HV are listed in TABLE 1. The data show the age of the ER to be significantly older than the GR and UL groups. No difference in age was found between the latter two groups. The age difference between groups was a result of the GR and UL men being recruited mainly from universities. There were no significant differences among groups in height, and the ER group was significantly lower in body weight than the GR. Other body composition measures of these groups are discussed by Pollock *et al.*[19] The data show that all three groups are considered lean and relatively similar in their external physical make-up.

The resting HR for the ER group was significantly lower when compared to the other two groups, while the GRs were significantly lower than the UL group. All resting BP values were nonsignificant among groups, except for SBP between ER and GR. The HV values were considered large for both running groups and were nonsignificant if compared to each other. No heart volume data were collected on the UL group.

There were no significant differences found in the variables shown in TABLE 1 among the ERs when dichotomized into marathon and M-LD groups. The values for HV tended to be larger for the M-LD group ($p < 0.10$), but as shown in TABLE 1 a large variation existed among runners.

Maximal treadmill performance and cardiorespiratory function results are shown in TABLE 2. The ERs were significantly higher in $\dot{V}_{O_2 max}$ than both the GR and UL groups, and the GRs significantly higher than the UL subjects. Maximal treadmill performance time (TMT) was significantly longer for the ER group when compared to the GRs. As mentioned earlier, the UL group was not capable of performing at the same running speeds as the ER or GR groups; therefore, comparison of TMT was not attempted.

The maximal treadmill run data showed two significant differences between the M-LD and marathon groups. The M-LD runners were significantly higher in $\dot{V}_{O_2 max}$ (4.7 ml/kg·min) and their TMT was 25 seconds longer.

The $\dot{V}_{O_2}$ response during the submaximal test for the ER and GR groups are shown in FIGURE 1. The data for minutes 4–7 show the ERs to be more efficient than the GRs at the 10-mph speed (4.5 m/sec) when expressed as actual values. The results expressed in percent of $\dot{V}_{O_2 max}$ showed the ERs to be significantly lower both at the 10-mph and 12-mph speeds. In fact, the run was considered near maximum for several of the GRs. Heart rate and $\dot{V}_E$

values for this test showed the same difference between groups. Serum lactic acid levels measured after the submaximal test were also significantly different between groups: 31 versus 69 mg% for the ER and GR groups, respectively. Thus, the submaximal running test clearly differentiated the running ability of the ER and GR groups.

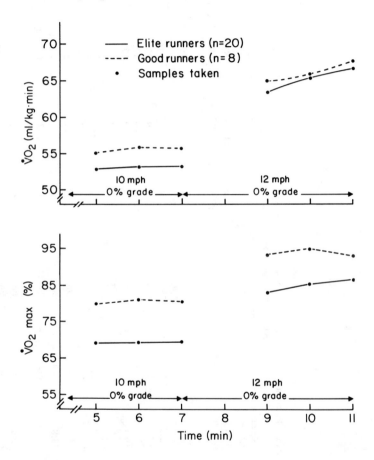

FIGURE 1. Oxygen intake ($\dot{V}_{O_2}$) expressed in absolute (ml/kg·min) values (top) and relative to $\dot{V}_{O_2max}$ (%, bottom) for elite and good distance runners. Although this was a continuous 11-min run, metabolic measures were only determined at minutes 4–5, 5–6, 6–7, 8–9, 9–10, and 10–11.

The submaximal run data for the M-LD and marathon groups are shown in FIGURE 2. The data showed that the marathon group was significantly lower in $\dot{V}_{O_2}$ (ml/kg·min) for every minute at both running speeds. The values for percent $\dot{V}_{O_2}$ and serum lactic acid were not significantly different between groups. Serum lactic acid levels were 31 mg% for both elite running groups.

TABLE 2

MAXIMAL TREADMILL PERFORMANCE AND CARDIORESPIRATORY FUNCTION OF ELITE DISTANCE RUNNERS, GOOD RUNNERS, AND UNTRAINED MEN

Subject	TMT * (min:sec)	$\dot{V}_{O_2}$ * (ml/ kg·min)	$\dot{V}_E$ * (liters/min)	HR * (beats/min)	Respiratory Exchange Ratio	Lactate (mg%)	SBP * (mmHg)	DBP * (mmHg)
Elite M–LD Runners †								
Brown	7:30	77.9	167	195	1.08	116	192	80
Castaneda	7:00	76.8	196	196	1.07	112	190	82
Crawford	7:00	75.5	156	191	1.10	117	170	70
Geis	8:00	79.9	170	186	1.12	119	200	70
Johnson	8:30	79.9	167	206	1.11	140	172	78
Manley	7:15	76.1	176	198	1.12	119	170	80
Ndoo	7:15	80.8	176	194	1.07	108	165	80
Prefontaine	8:30	84.4	195	210	1.11	122	200	80
Rose	8:00	79.0	152	198	1.16	128	198	95
Tuttle	8:15	82.7	161	214	1.13	127	182	80
11 ‡	6:30	74.0	148	198	1.04	72	210	85
Mean	7:36	78.8	169.5	198.7	1.10	116.4	186.3	80.0
(±SD)	(0:35)	(3.2)	(15.8)	(8.2)	(0.03)	(17.1)	(15.3)	(6.8)
Elite Marathon Runners								
Cusak	6:45	79.0	160	204	1.04	64	208	80
Galloway	7:15	73.0	164	196	1.16	139	188	85

	TMT*	$\dot{V}O_2$	$\dot{V}_E$	HR	R		SBP	DBP
Kennedy	7:30	72.4	154	195	1.14	130	170	85
Moore	7:30	74.2	174	192	1.10	119	192	72
Pate	7:00	76.9	166	204	1.06	116	180	70
Shorter	7:15	71.3	151	195	1.10	95	180	78
Wayne	7:15	72.9	155	192	1.10	117	200	80
Williams	7:00	73.3	186	188	1.10	97	185	68
Mean	7:11	74.1	163.4	195.8	1.10	117.6	187.9	77.3
(±SD)	(0:15)	(2.6)	(11.6)	(5.7)	(0.04)	(15.4)	(12.1)	(6.6)
Unclassified								
Kardong	8:45	77.4	189	198	1.10	123	200	80
Total elite runners								
Mean	7:30	76.9	168	198	1.10	114	188	79
(±SD)	(0:36)	(3.6)	(14.6)	(7.1)	(0.03)	(19.3)	(13.6)	(6.5)
Good runners (n=8)								
Mean	5:30	69.2	169	195	1.05	109	193	83
(±SD)	(1:01)	(3.7)	(10.7)	(8.1)	(0.03)	(23.1)	(23.9)	(8.1)
Untrained lean men (n=10)								
Mean	—	54.2	132	197	1.11	—	165	70
(±SD)	—	(6.6)	(14.8)	(8.9)	(0.03)	—	(21.8)	(12.7)

* TMT, maximal treadmill test time, till exhuastion; $\dot{V}O_2$, oxygen uptake $\dot{V}_E$, pulmonary ventilation; HR, heart rate; SBP, systolic blood pressure; DBP, diastolic blood pressure.
† M–LD, middle-long distance.
‡ Name held anonymous.

Discussion

The lower resting heart rates (RHR) found among the runners has been shown previously [4, 20, 21] and is attributed to a greater efficiency of heart function at rest.[4, 22-24] The increased efficiency of heart function at rest was found by Underwood and Schwade [25] who reported that the stroke volume was signifi-

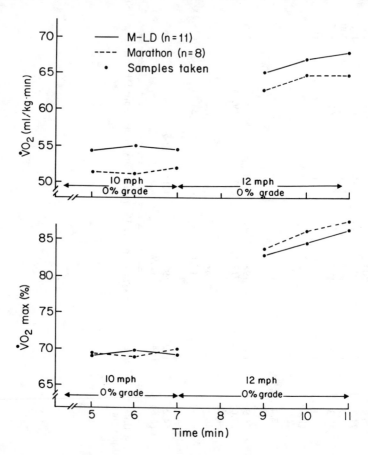

FIGURE 2. Oxygen intake ($\dot{V}_{O_2}$) expressed in absolute (ml/kg·min) values (top) and relative to $\dot{V}_{O_2max}$ (%, bottom) for elite middle-long distance (M–LD) and marathon runners. Although this was a continuous 11-min run, metabolic measures were only determined at minutes 4–5, 5–6, 6–7, 8–9, 9–10, and 10–11.

cantly larger at rest (95, 85, and 72 ml for the ER, GR, and UL groups, respectively) for both running groups if compared to the UL group.

Although the RHR were in agreement with previous reports,[4, 20, 21] the high maximum heart rates (HR_{max}) found in the running groups was surprising. Most studies have shown young trained runners to have HR_{max} values of approximately 180 to 195 beats/min.[2, 4, 5, 21, 24, 26-30] The average HR_{max} values in this study were 5 to 10 beats/min higher. In fact, five runners had values over 200 beats/min. Why the runners in this study had generally higher HR_{max} values than previously reported is not known at this time. Since the testing protocol utilized in this study was similar to other studies,[5, 27, 28] protocol differences were not considered a factor in the observed difference in HR_{max}.

The results showed a significantly greater range in the difference between RHR and HR_{max} in the ER and GRs if compared to the UL group, and ERs if compared to the GRs. This difference represents a 4.2-fold increase in HR for the ERs, a 3.7-fold increase for the GRs, and a 3.0-fold increase for the UL group. The larger stroke volume at rest and greater range of increase in RHR to HR_{max} for the runners would reflect a significantly greater cardiac reserve for the running groups.[4]

Larger heart volumes (HV) of endurance athletes has been shown many times.[22-24, 31, 32] Roskamm[24] in a comparison of different types of athletes showed long distance skiers and cyclists to have the largest HV measures, and weight lifters, gymnasts, and sedentary controls the lowest. The HV for the runners in this study are comparable to those reported for other endurance athletes,[23, 32] although Medved[32] reported values up to 1700 ml for a few well-trained athletes (a water polo player and a cyclist). However, when the HV of the ERs was reported relative to body weight, the ERs in this study have higher values. The question as to the relative significance of a large HV to physiological function and performance is still in question. Although the average value was quite high for the runners in this investigation, a wide range of volumes was observed and only moderate-($p < 0.05$)-to-low correlations were found between HV and $\dot{V}_{O_2 max}$ and TMT ($r = 0.59$ and 0.15, respectively).

Whether the large HV found in the runners in this study can be attributed to genetic factors or to years of rigorous training is not known. In a review of the question of cardiac hypertrophy in marathon runners, Van Liere[31] could find no longitudinal data on endurance athletes to enable him to answer this question. Since HV does not appear to change much during endurance training of sedentary persons,[4, 24, 33, 34] the genetic factor appears a more plausible explanation at this time. The higher relative value for HV for ERs can be partially attributed to their body type and low body weight and fat. The latter variables are partially attributable to their training habits. The question of cardiac hypertrophy in the ERs is discussed in detail by Gibbons et al.[35] and Underwood and Schwade[25] and thus will not be discussed here.

The high $\dot{V}_{O_2 max}$ values of the ERs are comparable to other studies.[2, 4, 26, 36] It was interesting to note the range in values (71.3 to 84.4 ml/kg·min) found among the ER group. The lowest value was found in Olympic marathon champion (1972, Munich, Germany) Shorter. The $\dot{V}_{O_2 max}$ of 71.3 ml/kg·min was comparable to the 71.2 value determined on him in October 1972. The highest $\dot{V}_{O_2 max}$, and one of the highest values reported for a runner, was that of Prefontaine, an outstanding M-LD runner.

The lower $\dot{V}_{O_2 max}$ for an outstanding marathoner is in agreement with Costill et al.[6] who found that elite marathoner Clayton had a $\dot{V}_{O_2 max}$ of 69.7 ml/kg·min. It appears that although a high $\dot{V}_{O_2 max}$ (>70 ml/kg·min) is a requisite for distance running success, it is not a high predictor of success among ERs.[5] Although there was a significant difference in the $\dot{V}_{O_2 max}$ (78.8 vs 74.1 ml/kg·min) of ERs when divided into M-LD and marathon groups, the correlation between $\dot{V}_{O_2 max}$ and treadmill performance time was only moderate ($r = 0.58$). As mentioned in the Overview section [11] not enough of the ERs competed in the 6-mile race, which was conducted on the fourth day of the experiment, to warrant a correlational analysis. However, Costill et al.[5] has found a high correlation between $\dot{V}_{O_2 max}$ and success in running 10 miles in a cross-section of runners, but a low correlation in an elite group.

It was interesting to note the small but significant metabolic and performance differences between the M-LD and marathon groups. The ML-D runners had a higher $\dot{V}_{O_2 max}$ (+4.7 ml/kg·min) and longer TMT (+25 sec) than the marathon group, but marathon runners were significantly more efficient on the submaximal run test. Part of the differences between ER groups may be accounted for by the quantity and quality of training accomplished prior to testing. As shown in the Overview section,[11] the training characteristics of the two groups were different. The marathon runners trained approximately 25 miles/week more than the M-LD group, but the M-LD runners did more high intensity interval training. How much effect the differences in training characteristics of the ERs had is only speculative but it is felt that high intensity interval training might be more advantageous for the M-LD group on the TMT.

Several investigators have noted that top marathoners appear to be more efficient at a standard running speed than other distance runners.[7-9, 37] The results from this investigation, which represents data from a large sample of ERs, supports this notion. Although the magnitude of difference in efficiency was only 4.5% at the 12 mph (5.5 m/sec) running speed, it would be of considerable importance over the marathon distance (26.2 miles or 42 km). It should be noted that although Shorter was shown to be the lowest of the ER group in $\dot{V}_{O_2 max}$, he was the most efficient on the submaximal treadmill run test. His average $\dot{V}_{O_2}$ of 57 ml/kg·min at the 12 mph speed was similar to the 59 ml/kg·min found for Clayton.[6] Both of these elite marathon runners are capable of working at a larger fraction of their $\dot{V}_{O_2 max}$ (>85%) during competition than most marathon runners who approximate 75% to 80%.[6, 9]

In summary, twenty elite runners (ER), eight good runners (GR), and ten untrained lean young men (UL) were evaluated on selected resting, submaximal and maximal tests of working capacity and cardiovascular-respiratory function. The results showed superior characteristics of ERs compared to GRs and UL young men in resting heart rate, $\dot{V}_{O_2 max}$, and submaximal and maximal working capacity. When ERs were divided into marathon and middle-long distance (M-LD) running groups, the M-LD group was significantly higher than the marathon group in $\dot{V}_{O_2 max}$ and treadmill performance time, while the marathon group had significantly lower submaximal $\dot{V}_{O_2}$ values (ml/kg·min) than the M-LD group. These findings further substantiate the superior ability of ERs, and show subtle, but significant differences between elite marathon and M-LD runners. Although certain trends do exist in the data for ERs, some overlapping of values found among many of the runners make interpretation complex. Possibly future multivariate analysis, taking into account a greater diversity of variables, will elicit more definitive results and enable the prediction of running success in elite runners.

Addendum

As shown in TABLES 1 and 2 Kardong was listed as unclassified. At the time of testing he was considered by most as a M-LD runner, but because he had recently shown marathon running ability (2:18:06), it was decided to put him in the unclassified category. From the time of the test (January 75) to the 1976 (May) U.S. Olympic marathon trials, Kardong slowly increased his mileage and began to think of himself as a potential marathoner. Most of the change in training and attitude occurred after January 1976 (personal communication). Subsequent history has shown him to qualify third in the 1976 U.S. Olympic trials (2:13:54) and place fourth in the Olympic marathon in Montreal (2:11:15). Because of the long time span between the testing and his later marathon accomplishments, it would be difficult and possibly misleading to derive inference from his initial testing data. Even so, it is interesting to note his submaximal treadmill run data followed the average of the marathon group, thus showing his potential as a marathon runner.

Acknowledgments

Appreciation goes to J. Ayres, A. Ward, and J. Sass for their help in data collection, and to S. White for data analysis. Further appreciation goes to Dr. R. Burns, Methodist Hospital, Dallas, Texas, for the determination of heart volume.

References

1. ROBINSON, S., H. T. EDWARDS & D. B. DILL. 1937. New records in human power. Science 85: 409–410.
2. SALTIN, B. & P. O. ÅSTRAND. 1967. Maximal oxygen uptake in athletes. J. Appl. Physiol. 23: 353–358.
3. WYNDHAM, C. H., N. B. STRYDOM, A. Y. VAN RENSBURG & A. J. S. BENADE. 1969. Physiological requirements for world-class performances in endurance running. S. Afr. Med. J. 43: 996–1002.
4. ÅSTRAND, P. O. & K. RODALE, Eds. 1970. Textbook of Work Physiology. 1st edit. McGraw-Hill Book Co., New York, N.Y.
5. COSTILL, D. L., H. THOMASON & E. ROBERTS. 1973. Fractional utilization of the aerobic capacity during distance running. Med. Sci. Sports 5: 248–252.
6. COSTILL, D. L., G. BRANAM, D. EDDY & K. SPARKS. 1971. Determinants of marathon running success. Int. Z. Angew. Physiol. 29: 249–254.
7. PUGH, L. G. C., J .L. CORBETT & R. H. JOHNSON. 1967. Rectal temperatures, weight losses, and sweat rates in marathon running. J. Appl. Physiol. 23: 347–352.
8. COSTILL, D. L. & E. WINROW. 1970. A comparison of two middle-aged ultra-marathon runners. Res. Quart. 41: 135–139.
9. COSTILL, D. L. 1972. Physiology of marathon running. J. Amer. Med. Assoc. 221: 1024–1029.
10. DANIELS, J. 1974. Physiological characteristics of champion male athletes. Res. Quart. 45: 342–348.
11. POLLOCK, M. L. 1977. Characteristics of elite class distance runners: Overview. Ann. N.Y. Acad. Sci. This volume.
12. POLLOCK, M. L., R. L. BOHANNON, K. H. COOPER, J. J. AYRES, A. WARD, S. R. WHITE & A. C. LINNERUD. 1976. A comparative analysis of four protocols for maximal treadmill stress testing. Amer. Heart J. 92: 39–46.
13. TAYLOR, H L., Y. WANG, L. ROWELL & G. BLOMQVIST. 1963. The standardization and interpretation of submaximal and maximal tests of working capacity. Pediatrics 32: 703–715.
14. CONSOLAZIO, F., R. JOHNSON & L. PECORA. 1963. Physiological Measurements of Metabolic Methods in Man. 1st edit. McGraw-Hill Book Co., New York, N.Y.

15. HENRY, R. J., D. C. Cannon & J. W. WINKELMAN, EDS. 1974. Clinical Chemistry Principles and Techniques. Harper and Row Company. New York, N.Y.
16. BARNHARD, H. J., J. A. PIERCE, J. W. JOYCE & J. H. BATES. 1960. Roentgenographic determination of total lung capacity. Amer. J. Med. 28: 54–60.
17. EDWARDS, A. 1956. Statistical Methods for the Behavioral Sciences. Rinehart Press. New York, N.Y.
18. CROXTON, F. 1953. Elementary Statistics with Application in Medicine and the Biological Sciences. Dover Publications. New York, N.Y.
19. POLLOCK, M. L., A. JACKSON, J. AYRES, A. WARD, A. C. LINNERUD & L. R. GETTMAN. 1977. Body composition of elite class distance runners. Ann. N.Y. Acad. Sci. This volume.
20. DILL, D. B., S. ROBINSON & J. C. ROSS. 1967. A longitudinal study of 16 champion runners. J. Sports Med. Phys. Fitness 7: 1–27.
21. POLLOCK, M. L. 1973. The quantification of endurance training programs. In Exercise and Sport Sciences Reviews, J. Wilmore, Ed. Academic Press. New York, N.Y.
22. HERXHEIMER, H. 1931. Size of heart in participants in olympic games in Amsterdam. Klin. Woch. Berlin 8: 402–405
23. BEVEGÅRD, B. S. & J. T. SHEPHARD. 1967. Regulation of the circulation during exercise in man. Physiol. Rev. 47: 178–213.
24. ROSKAMM, H. 1967. Optimum patterns of exercise for healthy adults. Canad. Med. Assoc. J. 96: 895–899.
25. UNDERWOOD, R. H. & J. L. SCHADE. 1977. Non-invasive analysis of cardiac function of elite distance runners—Echocardiography, vectorcardiography, and cardiac intervals. Ann. N.Y. Acad. Sci. This volume.
26. EKBLOM, B. & L. HERMANSEN. 1968. Cardiac output in athletes. J. Appl. Physiol. 25: 619–625.
27. DANIELS, J. & N. OLDRIDGE. 1970. The effects of alternate exposure to altitude and sea level on world-class middle-distance runners. Med. Sci. Sports. 2: 107–112.
28. COSTILL, D. L. & E. WINROW. 1970. Maximal oxygen intake among marathon runners. Arch. Phys. Med. Rehab. 51: 317–320.
29. LEITCH A. G. & L. CLANCY. 1976. Maximal exercise studies in Scottish athletes. Brit. J. Sports Med. 10: 62–66.
30. KOESLAG, J. H. & A. W. SLOAN. 1976. Maximal heart rate and maximal oxygen consumption of long-distance runners and other athletes. J. Sports Med. 16: 17–21.
31. VAN LIERE, E. J. 1971. The question of cardiac hypertrophy in marathon runners 11: 246–251.
32. MEDVED, R. J. & V. I. MEDVED. 1976. To which limit values has the athlete's heart enlarged? J. Sports Med. 16: 138–143.
33. SALTIN, B., G. BLOMQVIST, J. H. MITCHELL, R. L. JOHNSON, K. WILDENTHAL, C. B. CHAPMAN. 1968. Response to exercise after bed rest and after training. Circulation 37 and 38: Suppl. VII.
34. EKBLOM, B. 1970. Effect of physical training on circulation during prolonged severe exercise. Acta. Physiol. Scand. 78: 145–158.
35. GIBBONS, L. W., K. H. COOPER, R. P. MARTIN & M. L. POLLOCK. 1977. Medical examination and electrocardiography of elite runners. Ann. N.Y. Acad. Sci. This volume.
36. ÅSTRAND, P .O. 1955. New records in human power Nature 176: 922–923.
37. DILL, D. B. 1965. Marathoner DeMar: Physiological studies. J. Nat. Cancer Inst. 35: 185–191.

SUBMAXIMAL AND MAXIMAL WORKING CAPACITY OF ELITE DISTANCE RUNNERS. PART II. MUSCLE FIBER COMPOSITION AND ENZYME ACTIVITIES *

W. J. Fink, D. L. Costill, and M. L. Pollock

Human Performance Laboratory
Ball State University
Muncie, Indiana 47306

Institute for Aerobic Research
Dallas, Texas 75230

Recent use of histochemical and biochemical methods have provided some insight into the characteristics and function of skeletal muscle in trained and untrained men and women.[1, 2] However, little information is available to describe the fiber composition and metabolic potential in high-caliber endurance runners. The present study afforded an opportunity to examine the muscle fiber composition and selected oxidative and glycolytic enzymes of champion distance runners.

METHODS

Fourteen elite distance runners, 18 good middle distance runners, and 19 untrained men were used as subjects in this study. Selected individual characteristics of these men have been reported earlier.[3] Muscle samples were obtained from the lateral head of the gastrocnemius by a needle biopsy procedure.[4] The decision to sample this muscle was based on previous research,[5] which demonstrated that during endurance running the muscles of the lower leg (gastrocnemius and soleus) are metabolically more active than those of the thigh. The muscle specimen was divided into two parts. One portion was mounted in OCT (Ames) and frozen in isopentane cooled with liquid nitrogen for histochemical analysis. The remaining piece of the sample was quickly frozen in liquid nitrogen and later weighed for enzyme determination.

The muscle samples frozen for histochemical analysis were sectioned (10 μm thick) in a cryostat at $-20°$ C and stained for myosin adenosine triphoschatase (ATPase) and alpha-glycerophosphate dehydrogenase. These and other histochemical methods employed in this study have been described earlier.[3, 6] Quantitative measurements of muscle enzymes were performed for phosphorylase (total activity), lactic dehydrogenase (LDH), succinic acid dehydrogenase (SDH), and malic acid dehydrogenase (MDH). These procedures followed the general principles described by Lowry.[7] In addition, the LDH isoenzymes in the muscle samples were determined by a heat labile method described by Wróblewski and Gregory.[18]

* This work was supported by grants from the National Institutes of Health (AM 17083–02), the Ball State University Faculty Research Committee, and Quinton Instruments.

323

RESULTS AND DISCUSSION

Muscle Fiber Composition

On the average, the elite distance runners possess significantly more ST fibers than either the untrained men or the good middle distance runners. Although previous reports have noted a large percentage ST fibers in the skeletal muscles of distance runners, the values reported here for Galloway, Pate, and Tuttle are the highest observed in the human gastrocnemius.[6] It should be noted that three elite runners (Brown, Johnson, and Kardong) having the lowest percentage ST fibers have all achieved the greatest success in the shorter events (3000 m steeplechase and 5000 m). This is in keeping with our recent observations on middle distance (800–5000 m) runners, whose fiber composition ranged from 40.5% to 69.4% ST.[6]

It has previously been suggested that the percent ST fibers may be a factor governing success in distance running.[2, 6] However, this factor alone does not discriminate between the abilities of these elite runners. When the data from the good and elite distance runners were combined in the analyses, we observed a significant relationship between the percent ST fibers and the runners' best 6-mile performance ($r = -0.62$).

The cross-sectional areas of the muscle fibers varied markedly among the participants. Since this may in part be the result of varied degrees of fiber shortening at the time the samples were mounted, some caution should be used in comparing fiber areas between individuals. On the average, however, the elite runners' ST fibers were 29% larger than the FT fibers ($p < 0.05$). No differences were found between the two fiber types in the good middle distance runners or the untrained men (TABLE 1). Both fiber types were larger in the runners than those observed in the untrained men. Saltin[8] has proposed that training for endurance and strength may result in selective hypertrophy of the ST and FT fibers, respectively. Since middle distance running places metabolic demands on both ST and FT fibers, it is not surprising that their cross-sectional areas are roughly the same size. This is in contrast to the large ST fibers of the elite distance runners. Several of these men (e.g., Castaneda, Moore, Tuttle) have fiber areas that are greater than those previously reported for weight-lifters and shot-putters having more than twice the body mass of these runners.[6]

As a result of the relatively larger ST fiber, 82.9% of the cross-sectional area of the elite runners' muscle was composed of ST fibers. If it is true that ST fibers are responsible for developing a large fraction of the tension needed during distance running, the elite runners would be at a decided advantage in having more ST fibers accessible to perform this task.

Muscle Enzyme Activities

Muscular adaptations to exercise are characterized by an enhanced capacity to produce ATP.[9, 10] This can, in part, be attributed to quantitative increases in selected glycolytic and Krebs Cycle enzymes. Comparative studies have shown a positive relationship between the ability of a muscle to perform prolonged exercise and the activity of its respiratory enzymes.[11, 12] In the present study, muscle SDH activity was measured because it is generally considered representative of total mitochondrial protein and oxidative capacity of the muscle.[13]

On the average, muscle SDH activity of the elite and good runners was 3.4-fold and 2.8-fold greater, respectively, than that measured in the untrained men (TABLE 1). The levels of SDH activity in the muscle of the elite runners (21.6 μmoles/g·min) was significantly greater (p < 0.05) than that of the middle distance runners (17.7 μmoles/g·min). It is probable that this differ-

TABLE 1

MUSCLE ENZYME ACTIVITIES AND FIBER COMPOSITION

		Fiber Area (μm^2)		% Area	Enzyme Activity (μmoles/g·min)		
	% ST	FT	ST	ST	LDH	Phosp.	SDH
Elite distance runners							
Brown	69	5683	4941	72	670	9.6	16.9
Castaneda	79	15141	5739	91	775	7.3	19.3
Galloway	96	6315	3180	98	640	11.4	19.8
Geis	79	4848	3744	83	876	8.5	15.8
Johnson	60	5427	5052	62	764	12.2	24.4
Kardong	50	8685	7140	55	620	9.5	31.9
Manley	83	6946	4495	88	636	8.3	24.4
Moore	83	10865	7429	88	767	6.9	20.7
Ndoo	78	9472	5810	85	768	4.1	18.6
Pate	92	6794	5085	94	1000	7.2	26.4
Prefontaine	27	8027	10624	72	811	9.6	22.2
Shorter	80	9101	8458	81	673	4.2	16.7
Tuttle	98	10293	11516	98	718	6.9	26.4
Wayne	82	9190	7578	85	723	6.5	18.5
Mean	79.0	8342	6485	82.9	746	8.0	21.6
(SE)	(3.5)	(724)	(657)	(3.1)	(28)	(0.6)	(1.2)
Good middle distance runners							
Mean	61.8*	6378*	6284	62.1*	788	8.9	17.7*
(SE)	(2.9)	(400)	(420)	(2.6)	(37)	(0.7)	(1.0)
Untrained men							
Mean	57.7*	5460*	4947*	60.0*	843*	8.6	6.4*
(SE)	(2.5)	(552)	(496)	(2.7)	(33)	(0.8)	(0.6)

* Significant difference (p < 0.05) between identified mean and mean for elite distance runners.

ence is associated with variations in training duration and/or intensity. Since in humans ST fibers tend to show greater oxidative capacity, as measured by an intense NADH$_2$-tetrazolium reductase stain, it seems logical that runners having the highest percent ST fibers might also develop the greatest SDH activity.[14] The present data do not support this concept, however, since there was little relationship between percent ST fibers and SDH activity ($r = 0.22$). Certainly training can enhance the oxidative capacity of the FT fibers, which probably explains the fact that the highest SDH activity (31.9 μmoles/g·min) was found in the subject having the smallest percent ST fibers (50%).

Values for malic acid dehydrogenase activity were roughly twice as great in the elite runners (435 μmoles/g·min) as in the untrained men (237 μmoles/g·min). On the other hand, there was no difference between the MDH activities of elite and middle distance runners (467 μmoles/g·min). These values are similar to those recently observed in trained and untrained cyclists (unpublished).

In terms of glycolytic enzyme activities, there was no significant difference between the muscle phosphorylase activities of the trained and untrained men. The effects of endurance training on glycolytic enzymes appear uncertain. Holloszy et al.[16] have been unable to discern any change in either phosphorylase or LDH activities in rat gastrocnemius muscle following endurance treadmill training. Baldwin et al.[9] observed reductions in glycolytic enzyme activities in rat muscle composed of fast twitch red fibers following training. In contrast, they found significant increases in the glycolytic potential of the slow twitch intermediate soleus muscle. In studies by Eriksson et al.[17] young men required to cycle exhaustively 3 times per week for more than 20 min at each session showed an 85% increase in phosphofructokinase (PFK) activity after 6 weeks of training. The authors suggest that increased biosynthesis of some glycolytic enzymes (e.g., PFK) may necessitate exercise of greater intensity than that used in training studies with small animals. If we assume that phosphorylase activity parallels the changes in phosphofructokinase, we can conclude that the endurance training methods employed by the runners in the present study failed to enhance the glycolytic capacity of the running musculature.

In an earlier paper [6] we reported a strong relationship ($r = -0.70$) between the LDH activity and the percentage of the muscle area composed of ST fibers (% area ST). Although the means presented in TABLE 1 concur with this finding, the individual data for the elite runners show little relationship between percent area ST and LDH activity ($r = -0.25$). Since LDH does not function as a rate-limiting enzyme in glycolysis, these individual variations in LDH activity are probably more academic than physiologically important.

The thermal labile method for determining LDH isoenzyme activities demonstrated that the endurance trained runners have substantially more heart form of LDH (LDH$_H$) than muscle type (LDH$_M$). The muscle of untrained men, on the other hand, was found to have a predominance of LDH$_M$ activity. These findings support recent data by Sjödin [15] that suggest that endurance training produced an increase in relative activity of the heart specific isoenzyme.

SUMMARY

The present study confirms earlier observations that the musculature of elite distance runners is characterized by a high predominance of ST fibers. Although the percent ST fibers effectively discriminates between good and elite distance runners, fiber composition alone is a poor predictor of distance running success within the group of elite runners. Muscle enzyme measurements suggest that the 11 to 20 miles (17.7 to 32.2 km) of daily training performed by the elite runners produced a significantly greater increase in muscle SDH activity than was observed in the good distance runners, who were running 7 to 11 miles (11.3 to 17.7 km) per day. Although such endurance training enhances the oxidative capacity of the muscle, it apparently has little influence on the enzymes of glycogenolysis.

REFERENCES

1. COSTILL, D. L., P. D. GOLLNICK, E. D. JANSSON, B. SALTIN & E. M. STEIN. 1973. Glycogen depletion patterns in human muscle fibers during distance running. Acta Physiol. Scand. **89:** 374–383.
2. GOLLNICK, P. D., R. B. ARMSTRONG, C. W. SAUBERT IV, K. PIEHL & B. SALTIN. 1972. Enzyme activity and fiber composition in skeletal muscle of untrained and trained men. J. Appl. Physiol. **33:** 312–319.
3. COSTILL, D. L., W. J. FINK & M. L. POLLOCK. 1976. Muscle fiber composition and enzyme activities of elite distance runners. Med. Sci. Sports. **8:** 96–100.
4. BERGSTRÖM, J. 1962. Muscle electrolytes in man. Scand. J. Clin. Lab. Invest. **68.**
4. BERGSTRÖM, J. 1962 Muscle electrolytes in man. Scand. J. Clin. Lab. Invest. **68.**
5. COSTILL, D. L., E. JANSSON, P. D. GOLLNICK & B. SALTIN. 1974. Glycogen utilization in leg muscles of men during level and uphill running. Acta Physiol. Scand. **91:** 475–481.
6. COSTILL, D. L., J. DANIELS, W. EVANS, W. FINK, G. KRAHENBUHL & B. SALTIN. 1976. Skeletal muscle enzymes and fiber composition in male and female track athletes. J. Appl. Physiol. **40:** 149–154.
7. LOWRY, O. H. & J. V. PASSONNEAU. 1972. A Flexible System of Enzymatic Analysis. Academic Press. New York.
8. SALTIN, B. 1973. Metabolic fundamentals in exercise. Med. Sci. Sports **5:** 137–146.
9. BALDWIN, K. M., W. W. WINDER, R. L. TERJUNG & J. O. HOLLOSZY. 1973. Glycolytic enzymes in different types of skeletal muscle: adaptation to exercise. Amer. J. Physiol. **225:** 962–966.
10. HOLLOSZY, J. O. 1967. Biochemical adaptations in muscle. J. Biol. Chem. **242:** 2278–2282.
11. LAWRIE, R. A. 1953. The activity of the cytochrome system in muscle and its relation to myoglobin. Biochem. J. **55:** 298–305.
12. PAUL, M. H. & E. SPERLING. 1952. Cyclophorase system XXIII. Correlation of cyclophorase activity and mitochondrial density in striated muscle. Proc. Soc. Exp. Biol. Med. **79:** 352–354.
13. HOLLOSZY, J. O., L. B. OSCAI, I. J. DON & P. A. MOLÉ. 1970. Mitochondrial citric acid cycle and related enzymes: Adaptative response to exercise. Biochem. Biophys. Res. Commun. **40:** 1368–1373.
14. DUBOWITZ, V. & M. H. BROOKE. 1973. Muscle Biopsy: A Modern Approach. : 51–61. W. B. Saunders Co. Philadelphia, Pa.
15. SJÖDIN, B. In press. Effect of physical training on LDH activity and LDH isoenzyme pattern in human skeletal muscle. Proceedings of the International Congress of Physical Activity Sciences.
16. HOLLOSZY, J. O., L. B. OSCAI, P. A. MOLÉ & I. J. DON. 1971. Biochemical adaptations to endurance exercise in skeletal muscle. Muscle Metabolism during Exercise. B. Pernow & B. Saltin, Eds.) Plenum Press, New York, N.Y.
17. ERIKSSON, B. O., P. D. GOLLNICK & B. SALTIN. 1972. Muscle metabolism and enzyme activities after training in boys 11–13 years old. Acta Physiol. Scand. **87:** 231–239.
18. WRÓBLEWSKI, F. & K. F. GREGORY. 1961. Lactic acid dehydrogenase isoenzymes. Ann. N.Y. Acad. Sci. **94:** 912–932.

A BIOMECHANICAL COMPARISON OF ELITE AND GOOD DISTANCE RUNNERS

Peter R. Cavanagh, Michael L. Pollock, and Jean Landa

Biomechanics Laboratory
Pennsylvania State University
University Park, Pennsylvania 16802

Institute for Aerobics Research
Dallas, Texas 75230

INTRODUCTION

This paper reports the results of the biomechanical phase of a multidisciplinary study of elite distance runners.[1] There are some intriguing differences between this aspect of the study and several of the physiological and medical aspects. A variable such as muscle fiber composition or maximal oxygen uptake gives us information that overwhelmingly reflects the genotype of the individual.[2] The biomechanical measurements, however, are essentially quantitative expressions of running style and this factor is basically a learned response to a given set of anthropometric and physiological constraints. It is important to mention at the outset that the term "skilled runner," which is often found in the literature, is generally used to classify athletes on the basis of average running velocity over a certain distance. It is by no means axiomatic that athletes classified as skilled according to the criterion of running velocity exhibit the best form or style. Indeed the criteria for good style that are applied by coaches still rest on somewhat of an empirical base, since sport scientists have not yet produced an adequate theoretical model to allow the effects of parameter variation to be studied. The major objective of the present study is to make a comparison between groups of elite and good distance runners on variables such as stride length and rate, lower limb kinematics, swing phase kinetics, and center of gravity motion. The sample sizes are large enough to apply statistical methods to determine if significant differences exist. The two groups were significantly different ($p < 0.02$) in oxygen uptake during a standardized submaximal treadmill run at 4.47 m/sec (10 mph). (The means for the good and elite groups were 55.6 and 52.6 ml·kg⁻¹·min⁻¹, respectively.) This raises the possibility that these differences may be due in part to biomechanical differences between the good and elite athletes.

REVIEW OF LITERATURE

Early insight into the mechanics of running was provided by Fenn[3,4] and Elftman[5] who produced work of outstanding quality, which was to remain unequalled for more than 30 years. Much of the literature following these landmark papers is cited in two recent reviews.[6,7] Despite a considerable volume of studies on the mechanics of running, much of the work has been concerned with sprinting or with distance runners running at maximum velocities. Few investigations have made comparisons between runners of international caliber and varsity athletes, and most of the samples used were relatively small.

Hubbard [8] in an early study hypothesized that "trained runners" would use ballistic movements more effectively than untrained runners. He also made further suggestions concerning foot posture during contact and support, which were not adequately documented. Fenn [4] indicated that the single "outstanding" sprinter in his sample had a higher knee lift than the other athletes, a contention supported by Saito *et al.* [9] in studies of one untrained and three trained sprinters. Miura *et al.* [10] have proposed that "good" distance runners can be characterized by: small vertical oscillations of the center of gravity, complete hip extension during the support phase, greater knee flexion immediately following foot strike, greater knee flexion during swing phase, and the maintenance of hip extension after takeoff.

Considerable attention has been given to the combinations of stride length and stride rate exhibited at various velocities. [6] In a longitudinal study Nelson and Gregor [11] found that varsity distance runners tended to decrease their stride length at a given velocity over a period of 4 years. Dillman [6] summarized other literature with the statement that at a given speed poorer runners will tend to have higher stride rates. Complementing the scientific literature there is a considerable amount of "authoritative opinion," exemplified by Bowerman, [12] in which successful track coaches give their own personal opinions on important determinants of running style.

In summary there is not a large literature base that defines differences between distance athletes of different caliber.

METHODS OF DATA COLLECTION

A total of 22 distance runners were filmed at 100 frames/second from the front and from one side while they ran on a level treadmill at four steady speeds between 4.96 and 6.44 meters/second (11.1 and 14.4 mph). Only the results from the slowest speed and from the camera recording movements in the sagittal plane are reported here. This speed would represent a marathon time of 2:21:43 or a mile in 5:24.

The elite sample consisted of five middle–long distance runners (mean 3-mile time 13:10.2) and nine marathon distance runners (mean marathon time 2:15:52) while of the good runners five were classified as middle–long distance (mean 3-mile time 15:16.7) and three as marathon distance (mean marathon time 2:34:40).

Prior to the filming session small contrasting markers were placed on the various segment endpoints, on the shoe and over bony landmarks (FIGURE 1). A total of 12 anthropometric measurements were also taken for use in predictive equations for the determination of lower limb segment weights, moments of inertia and center of gravity locations. [13, 14] The estimated plane of movement of the right side of the body was calibrated by filming an object of known dimensions. The subjects ran for ten minutes at a speed of 4.47 m/sec (10 mph) before filming began. The speeds were then presented in ascending order with approximately ten strides being filmed at each condition.

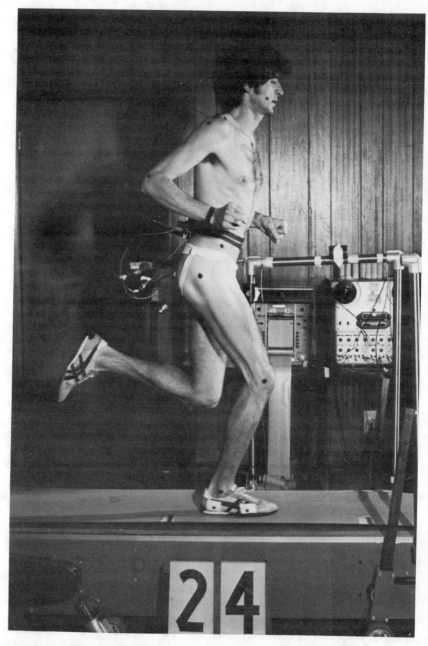

FIGURE 1. Subject running on the treadmill showing a similar field of view to that of the movie camera. Subject is wearing an accelerometer at the waist. Results of these studies are not reported here.

METHODS OF DATA ANALYSIS

The coordinates of the projection of the body markers on a sagittal plane for one complete running cycle (right foot-strike to next right foot-strike) were obtained from a Bendix digitizing system and were subsequently processed by a digital computer with plotting facilities. To enable comparisons to be made between runners with slightly differing cycle times, the data were subjected to time dilation by linear interpolation so that each complete running cycle was represented by 98 equally spaced data points. Time information was obtained from light markers placed on the film edge by LEDs driven by a crystal-controlled oscillator.

To obtain information concerning the vertical movement of the center of gravity from data of only one side of the body it was considered inaccurate to use approximations of hidden data points. An assumption of left-right symmetry was therefore made and a complete set of coordinates for the left (hidden) side were generated by making the right side coordinates relative to the head marker and specifying these as the relative coordinates of the left side one-half a running cycle later. Considerable motion of the hip marker was detected and this was corrected on the data from each frame of film by constraining the trunk segment to remain the same length throughout the running cycle. The new location of the hip marker was therefore at a fixed distance from the head marker along the line joining hip and head markers. Dempster's [15] coefficients were used to ascribe relative masses to the 11 body segments used in the analysis. To determine net muscular torques at the hip and knee joints during the swing phase the methods described in a previous investigation of walking [16] were used. The equations of motion for the thigh and a combined shank and foot segment were derived from the free body diagram shown in FIGURE 2. Clauser's [13] equations were used to obtain estimates of segment weight and center of gravity locations and Drillis and Contini's [14] coefficients of 0.25 and 0.303 were used for the radii of gyration of the thigh and combined shank and foot segments, respectively.

RESULTS

Stride Rate and Stride Length

Stride length was defined as the distance between successive ground contacts of the right and left feet, and stride rate as the total number of right and left foot-ground contacts per minute. Relative stride length was calculated as the ratio of stride length to trochanter height. Since the speed of the treadmill was known, stride length and stride rate could be calculated by estimating from film the time taken for approximately 10 strides.

The mean values and standard deviations for these stride parameters are given in TABLE 1. As a group the good runners took both longer strides and longer relative strides than the elite runners, resulting in mean stride frequencies that differed by over 9 strides per minute. The level of significance of these differences ($p = 0.064$) was however greater than the α level established for this study ($\alpha \leq 0.05$).

TABLE 1 also shows values for times of swing, flight, and support. These data were obtained from the single cycle of running for which coordinates were obtained. These differences were not significant at the 0.05 level.

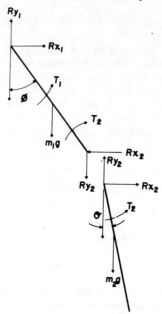

FIGURE 2. Free body diagrams for the thigh (above) and for a combined shank and foot segment. The net torque due to muscular activity at the hip (T_1) and knee (T_2) are shown in the positive direction at the proximal end of the limb (i.e., positive torque tends to flex the hip and extend the knee).

TABLE 1

A COMPARISON OF STRIDE PARAMETERS BETWEEN ELITE AND GOOD RUNNERS *

	Stride Length (meters)	Relative Stride Length †	Stride Rate (steps/ min)	Swing Time (msec)	Flight Time (msec)	Support Time
Elite	1.56	165%	191.0	431	120	205
$n=14$	(0.17)		(10.74)	(31.3)	(14.0)	(11.6)
Good	1.64	172%	182.0	458	130	201
$n=8$	(0.16)		(8.80)	(31.2)	(16.7)	(5.4)

* None of the means are significantly different at the 0.05 level. Values in parentheses represent the standard deviation.
† Relative stride length $=100 \times$ (stride length/trochanter height).

The range of stride lengths led to a variation of over 42 strides per minute in the whole sample at the same running speeds. The range of leg lengths was also considerable, however, and an important difference between groups existed in the stride-length–leg-length relationships. The correlation between these two variables was 0.67 for the elite group but −0.10 for the good runners. These results indicate that regardless of leg length, the good runners tended to take long strides while the elite athletes took shorter strides, which were better related to their leg lengths.

The longitudinal study of Nelson and Gregor [11] has indicated that at the same velocity good college distance runners tended to shorten their strides over a four year period during which their performance improved. The work of Högberg [7] has also shown that in a single subject oxygen intake increased at over twice the rate at stride lengths above the optimum value than at stride lengths below this value. It would therefore appear safer to understride than overstride and it seems likely that the good group in the present study were doing the latter. The results presented here suggest that those of Miura [10] *et al.* were biased by the fact that their trained runners were running faster than the untrained runners leading to the erroneous conclusion that the longer stride lengths were advantageous.

Angular Kinematics

The mean patterns of hip and knee joint motions are shown in the thigh-knee diagrams of FIGURE 3. The conventions used for angles and an analysis of the use of angle-angle diagrams are given by Cavanagh and Grieve.[18] These diagrams show that there is a remarkable similarity between good and elite runners with only slight differences during the swing phase distinguishing the two groups.

It is apparent that considerable hip extension occurred before foot-strike and that knee flexion had also begun before contact with the ground was made. Following foot-strike, 25 degrees of knee flexion occurred while the thigh was maintained at the same orientation of about 30 degrees to the vertical. It is interesting to note that the knee was never fully extended throughout the running cycle and at the end of the support phase knee extension was almost the same as the value at foot-strike. Toe-off occurred at this point of maximum knee extension and during the early part of the swing phase, the knee flexed while hip flexion did not begin immediately. Maximum knee flexion during swing was approximately 120 degrees and occurred as the thigh was some 25 degrees in front of the vertical. The latter part of the swing phase was characterized by knee extension about a static and then slightly extending hip.

These mean curves have been redrawn in FIGURE 4, together with bands representing ±1 standard deviation and the total range encountered. The variances are, in general, smaller during support than during swing. However, it should be noted that two variances are shown on each diagram—one for knee and one for thigh angle—and the angle with smallest time derivative tends to dominate the visual representation shown. Particularly notable is the large range of knee flexion during swing exhibited by the elite runners. This was due to two athletes, one middle-long distance and one marathon distance, who almost touched their buttock with the heel during swing phase.

To emphasize the similarities between the groups in the coordinated patterns of hip and knee motion, four postures stated by previous investigators [9], [10], [19] to distinguish runners of different ability have been shown in FIGURE 5. These include maximum knee flexion during support and swing, maximum hip flexion during swing and the position of the limb at foot-strike. No significant differences exist between groups in the joint angles at these points in the cycle reinforcing the similarity expressed in the thigh-knee diagrams.

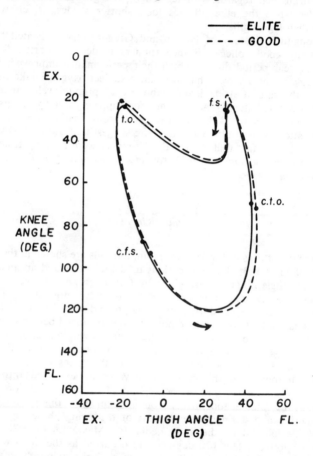

FIGURE 3. Mean thigh-knee diagrams for the good and elite groups. One complete running cycle is shown starting at foot-strike (f.s.) on the right side, proceeding through right toe-off (t.o.) and contralateral foot-strike and toe-off (c.f.s. and c.t.o., respectively).

When motion at the ankle joint is considered, the mechanism of the longer stride of the good runners becomes apparent. The ankle-knee diagrams shown in FIGURE 6 reveal the similarities during early and middle support that existed in the thigh-knee diagrams. However, in the final phases of plantar thrust the groups separate clearly with the good runners plantar flexing, on average, 10

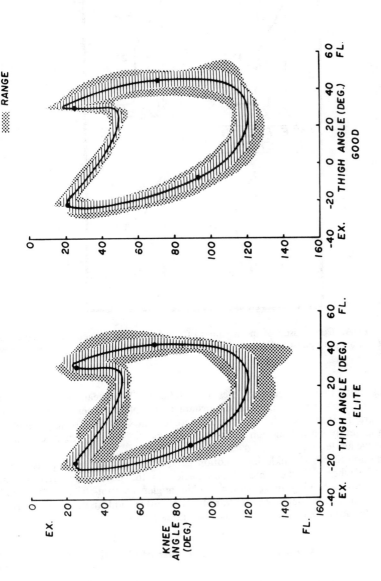

FIGURE 4. The same mean thigh-knee diagrams shown in FIGURE 3 (solid lines) but with ±1 standard deviation (horizontal shading) and range (dot shading). The solid circles indicate the cycle landmarks identified in FIGURE 3.

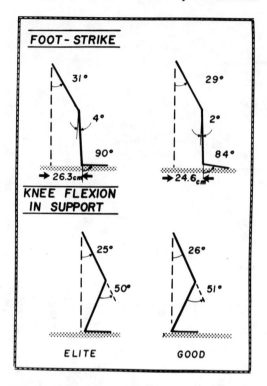

FIGURE 5A. Comparison of mean values of good and elite runners in two postures during the support phase; at foot-strike (above) and at the point of maximum knee flexion.

degrees more than the elite athletes ($p \leq 0.002$). The mean posture of the lower limb for the two groups at the instant of toe-off has been reproduced in the diagram. It is interesting that the differences in stride length are achieved with apparently similar motion at the hip and knee joints and a marked difference at the ankle joint.

The differences in ankle joint motion persist through the swing phase until foot-strike when a higher rate of dorsiflexion in the good runners results in both groups achieving more similar ankle angles at foot-strike. The good runners exhibit considerably more variability in ankle joint angles than the elite runners (FIGURE 7) in both plantar flexion and dorsiflexion.

Vertical Motion of the Center of Gravity

The subjects were in general asymmetric in the motion of their centers of gravity, casting some doubt on the assumption of symmetry of limb motion used in the calculations. Since the head and trunk together weight the location of the center of gravity by over 55%, it is the motion of these segments that still indicate an asymmetric gait despite the assumptions made. The schematic diagram in FIGURE 8 indicates the method of analysis. The mean rise in the center of gravity per stride was taken as the average of the rise from both right and left legs. An index of asymmetry was obtained by dividing the mean rise by the range of vertical excursion—leading to a value of 1.0 for perfect symmetry and a value less than 1.0 for an asymmetric pattern.

Present results confirmed the observations of Fenn that most of the flight phase was spent in descent, since take-off occurred just before the peak of vertical oscillation was reached. A comparison of the two groups revealed that the good athletes had slightly, but not statistically significantly, greater amplitude of vertical oscillation (mean values 8.0 cm and 7.6 cm for good and elite groups, respectively). When power output against gravity is calculated (per kilogram of body weight), the two groups have virtually identical mean values (2.37 watt·kg⁻¹ and 2.36 watt·kg⁻¹). This is due to the elite group exhibiting a 5% greater stride rate and a 5% smaller vertical oscillation than the good runners. The total range of values for mean oscillation in the present study was only 3.1 cm (6.2 to 9.3 cm).

The two groups were significantly different, however, in their indices of asymmetry ($p < 0.05$). The elite athletes tended to be more symmetrical than

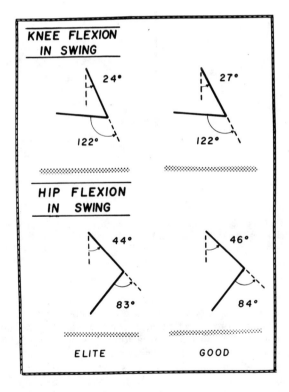

FIGURE 5B. Similar comparison of two postures during the swing phase; the point of maximum knee flexion (above) and maximum hip flexion (below). None of the differences are significant. ($\alpha \leq 0.05$).

the good runners (mean values were 0.73 and 0.8 for the index of asymmetry in the good and elite groups, respectively).

Net Torques Due to Muscular Activity

The calculated values for the torques during the swing phase due to muscular activity at the hip and knee joints revealed closely similar mean patterns between the two groups of runners (FIGURES 9–12). The phasing of applied

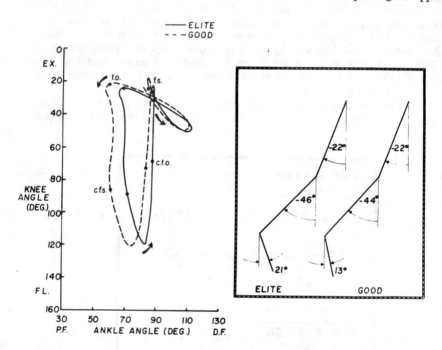

FIGURE 6. Mean ankle-knee diagrams for the good and elite groups. Diagrams begin at foot-strike on the right side (f.s.) and describe one complete running cycle through toe-off (t.o.), contralateral foot-strike (c.f.s.), and contralateral toe-off (c.t.o.).

torques is rather similar to that discussed in the literature.[5, 20, 21] At toe-off there is a torque tending to flex the hip while at the knee some runners exhibit a net flexor torque and some a net extensor torque. This is generally followed in the first third of the swing phase by a torque tending to extend the knee joint (FIGURE 11), after which there appears to be a phase of little or zero torque at the knee, which some investigators have termed a ballistic phase.[21]

In late swing the dominant action at each joint reverses being flexor at the knee joint to retard the rapidly extending leg, and flexor at the hip joint. None of the differences in peak torque values after toe-off were significantly different between groups.

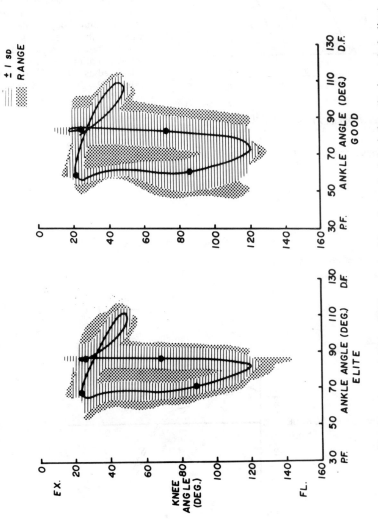

FIGURE 7. The same mean ankle-knee diagrams shown in FIGURE 6 with ±1 standard deviation (horizontal shading) and the range (dot shading). The solid circles represent the same cycle landmarks shown in FIGURE 6.

VERTICAL OSCILLATION
AND
ASYMMETRY

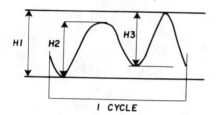

I CYCLE

FIGURE 8. A schematic diagram of the vertical movement of the total body center of gravity with respect to an external reference frame. Mean vertical motion per stride was calculated as $(H2+H3)/2$. The value $(H2+H3)/2H1$ was used as an index of asymmetry.

$$\text{MEAN OSCILLATION} = \frac{(H2+H3)}{2}$$

$$\text{ASYMMETRY} = \frac{(H2+H3)}{2 \times HI}$$

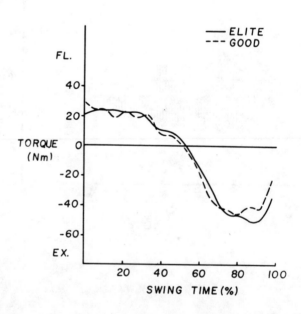

FIGURE 9. Mean net torque at the hip joint due to muscular activity for the two groups during the swing phase. A positive torque tends to flex the hip.

It should be pointed out that while the phases of activity were similar to those previously reported, there is a surprising variation in the magnitude of peak torques reported by various investigators. Plagenhoef,[20] for example, cites values in excess of 800 Nm for peak hip flexor torque at toe-off, and Dillman[21] reports values of 270 Nm for knee-extensor torque at toe-off. Whereas the

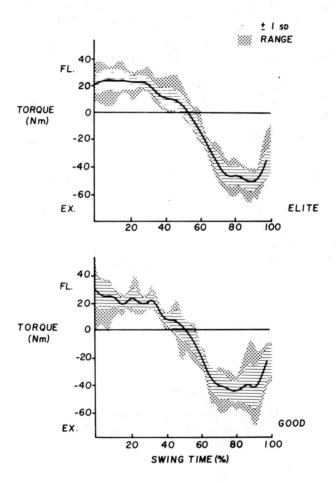

FIGURE 10. The same data as shown in FIGURE 9 with the addition of ±1 standard deviation and the range.

subjects in these two studies were running faster than those in the present study, the instantaneous values cited would appear to be close to or above the maximal steady isometric torques that these joints are capable of producing.[22] While it is known that eccentric muscle activity can generate values higher than isometric values,[23] it would seem unlikely that running requires such a maximal activation of the lower limb muscle mass during the swing phase.

SUMMARY AND DISCUSSION

It is apparent that only minor differences have been located between the two groups of athletes in the present study. These have centered principally around the longer strides being taken by the good athletes and concomitant changes in variables associated with this increased stride length. The good athletes also tended to be more asymmetrical than the elite athletes in their vertical motion.

There are several limitations to the present study that must be considered in the interpretation of the results. Firstly, the subjects were filmed during treadmill running, and as Dillman [6] has pointed out, there is by no means a consensus of opinion regarding the similarities or differences between treadmill and overground running. The problem is further complicated by the fact that there were differences within the present group of subjects in familiarity with running on the treadmill. Some athletes had previous experience and were at ease with the procedure while others were experiencing treadmill running for the first time. This may have affected the patterns of motion recorded. Also, only motion in the sagittal plane has been considered in this report and a more complete analysis would consider motion in all three planes.

The basic question still remains: Is efficient running a function of good style, a function of subcellular biochemistry, or some weighting of both, and what other factors are important? It is unfortunately not possible to give a definitive answer from this study. However, the lack of major significant differences in the biomechanical variables between the two groups leads one to believe that both the good and elite groups of athletes contain a similar range of running

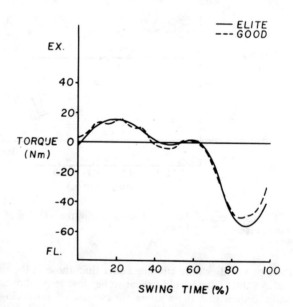

FIGURE 11. Mean net torque at the knee joint due to muscular activity in the swing phase for both groups. A positive torque tends to extend the knee.

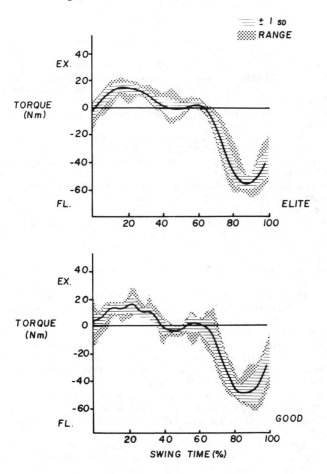

FIGURE 12. The same data as shown in FIGURE 11 with the addition of ±1 standard deviation and the range.

styles. The possibility must therefore be proposed that some of the elite runners have form or style that is worse than runners classified as good in the present study. The technique of multiple regression analysis appears to be promising for the identification of which of the many variables studied in all aspects of this present multidisciplinary project are important for efficient running.

The comparative approach used so far will not, by itself, identify aspects that make up good form in distance running. It is hoped that future work with this present data base will lay the ground work for such a statement. It is also likely that factors that currently elude precise measurement are important for efficient running. Notable amongst these are storage and recovery of elastic energy following heel contact mentioned by Fenn[4] and confirmed experimentally to be important more recently by Cavagna[24] and Asmussen.[25]

REFERENCES

1. POLLOCK, M. L. 1977. Characteristics of elite class distance runners: Overview. Ann. N.Y. Acad. Sci. This volume.
2. KOMI, P. V., J. T. VIITASALO, M. HAVU, A. THORSTENSSON & J. KARLSSON. 1976. Physiological and structural performance capacity: Effect of heredity. In Biomechanics. Vol. 5A. P. V. Komi, Ed. : 118–123. University Park Press. Baltimore, Md.
3. FENN, W. O. 1930. Frictional and kinetic factors in the work of sprint running. Amer. J. Physiol. **92:** 583–611.
4. FENN, W. O. 1930. Work against gravity and work due to velocity changes in running. Amer. J. Physiol. **93**(2)**:** 433–462.
5. ELFTMAN, H. 1939. Forces and energy changes in the leg during walking. Amer. J. Physiol. **125:** 339–352.
6. DILLMAN, C. J. 1975. Kinematic analyses of running. In Exercise and Sport Sciences Reviews. Vol. 3. J. H. Wilmore, Ed. : 193–218. Academic Press, Inc. New York, N.Y.
7. JAMES, S. L. & C. E. BRUBAKER. 1973. Biomechanical and neuromuscular aspects of running. In Exercise and Sport Sciences Reviews. Vol. 1. J. H. Wilmore, Ed. : 189–216. Academic Press, Inc. New York, N.Y.
8. HUBBARD, A. W. 1939. An experimental analysis of running and of certain fundamental differences between trained and untrained runners. Res. Quart. **20:** 28–38.
9. SAITO, M., T. HOSHIKAWA, M. MIYASHITA & H. MATSUI. 1972. An analysis of motion patterns of the hip, the knee and the ankle joint in relation to running speed. In Review of Our Researches, 1970–1973. H. Matsui, Ed. : 70–72. Dept. of Physical Education, University of Nagoya. Nagoya, Japan.
10. MIURA, M., K. KOBAYASHI, M. MIYASHITA, H. MATSUI & H. SODEYAMA. 1973. Experimental studies on biomechanics on long distance runners. In Review of Our Researches, 1970–1973. H. Matsui, Ed. : 46–56. Dept. of Physical Education, University of Nagoya. Nagoya, Japan.
11. NELSON, R. C. & R. J. GREGOR. 1976. Biomechanics of distance running: A longitudinal study. Res. Quart. **47**(3)**:** 417–428.
12. BOWERMAN, B. & G. S. BROWN. 1971. The secrets of speed. Sports Illustrated **35**(5)**:** 22–29.
13. CLAUSER, C. E., J. T McCONVILLE & J W. YOUNG. 1969. Weight, Volume, and Center of Mass of Segments of the Human Body. Report number AMRL–TR–69–70. Aerospace Medical Research Laboratory. Wright-Patterson Air Force Base, Ohio.
14. DRILLIS, R. & R. CONTINI. 1966. Body Segment Parameters. Technical Report No. 1166.03. Newk York University, School of Engineering and Science. University Heights, N.Y.
15. DEMPSTER, W. T. 1955. Space Requirements of the Seated Operator. WADC Technical Report 55–159. Wright Air Development Center. Wright-Patterson Air Force Base, Ohio.
16. CAVANAGH, P. R. & R. J. GREGOR. 1975. Knee joint torque during the swing phase of normal treadmill walking. J. Biomech. **8:** 337–344.
17. HÖGBERG, P. 1952. How do stride length and stride frequency influence the energy-output during running? Arbeitsphysiologie, **14:** 437–441.
18. CAVANAGH, P. R. & D. W. GRIEVE. 1973. The graphical display of angular movement of the body. Brit. J. Sports Med. **7**(1,2)**:** 129–133.
19. DESHON, D. E. & R. C. NELSON. 1964. A cinematographical analysis of sprint running. Res. Quart. **35**(4)**:** 451–455.
20. PLAGENHOEF, S. 1968. A kinetic analysis of running. Track & Field Quart. Rev. : 56–63.
21. DILLMAN, C. J. 1971. A kinetic analysis of the recovery leg during sprint run-

ning. *In* Biomechanics: Proceedings of C.I.C. Symposium. J. Cooper, Ed. : 137–165. Athletic Institute. Chicago, Ill.

22. CLARKE, H. H. 1966. Muscular Strength and Endurance in Man. Prentice-Hall Inc. Englewood Cliffs, N.J.

23. ASMUSSEN, E., O. HANSEN & O. LAMMERT. 1965. The relation between isometric and dynamic muscle strength in man. Communications from the Testing and Observation Institute of the Danish National Association for Infantile Paralysis. No. 20.

24. CAVAGNA, G. A., B. DUSMAN & R. MARGARIA. 1968. Positive work done by a previously stretched muscle. J. Apl. Physiol. 24(1): 21–32.

25. ASMUSSEN, E. & F. BONDE-PETERSON. 1974. Apparent efficiency and storage of elastic energy in human muscles during exercise. Acta Physiol. Scand. 92: 537–545.

BLOOD CHEMISTRY AND LIPID PROFILES OF ELITE DISTANCE RUNNERS*

Randolph P. Martin, William L. Haskell, and Peter D. Wood

Stanford Heart Disease Prevention Program
Stanford University School of Medicine
Stanford, California 94305

INTRODUCTION

The hematological, chemical, and lipoprotein profiles of 20 elite distance runners, eight good runners, and selected age-matched nonrunning controls were determined with the following three questions serving as a basis for analysis of the results. First, were there any particular hematological or chemical values that could explain the superior performance capacity of the elite or good runners? Secondly, could any of their laboratory values be considered "abnormal" when compared to nonrunning age-matched controls, a theme reminiscent of the electrocardiographic and cardiovascular physical finding often recorded [1] in endurance athletes? And thirdly, does the high level of endurance-type training exhibited by these runners offer some protection from the development of coronary heart disease? The last question was particularly intriguing because of the frequent speculation that lack of physical activity is associated with an increased incidence of coronary artery disease clinical manifestations. Since elevations in plasma cholesterol, especially when it occurs in certain of the lipoprotein fractions, has been associated closely with an increased risk of premature coronary artery disease, and since several recent publications [2, 3] have demonstrated a favorable influence of physical activity on the distribution of cholesterol among the lipoproteins, it was of particular interest to focus attention on the lipoprotein profiles exhibited by the elite runners who have exercised at high levels daily for at least several years and therefore should be deriving maximum "protective effect" from their leisure time exertional activities.

MATERIALS AND METHODS

Subjects

The age, training, and performance characteristics of the 20 elite runners and the eight good runners have been described previously in this symposium.[4] The age-matched controls for analysis of the hematological and chemical profiles were 95 males ages 21–34 (mean 28.6 years) who had undergone hematological and chemical testing as part of their physical examination procedure at the Cooper Clinic in Dallas, Texas. The age-matched controls for cholesterol, triglycerides, and lipoprotein quantification were 72 men, 26 to 30 years of age,

* This work was supported in part by Contract NIH–2161–L and grant HL 14174 from the National Heart, Lung and Blood Institute, National Institutes of Health.

who were randomly selected from participants in a prevalence survey of Stanford University employees conducted during 1973–75.

Analytical Methods

Both runners and controls were asked to fast overnight for 12 to 14 hours (nothing by mouth except water) prior to the clinic visit during which time a blood sample was obtained. Also, all participants were requested not to exercise vigorously during this fasting period so that the values obtained from the blood analysis would reflect the chronic status of the runners and not be the result of a recent bout of exercise. Adherence to the requirements for fasting and abstinence from recent exercise was checked by interview at the time of blood drawing. Venous blood samples were obtained in the morning using vacutainer tubes with the subjects in a recumbent position. Hematological and chemical analysis on the 28 runners and their 95 age-matched controls was performed at the commercial laboratory routinely used by the Institute for Aerobics Research and the Cooper Clinic (Ford Clinical Laboratory, Denton, Texas). The total cholesterol and triglyceride values for the 28 runners and 72 controls were performed at the Stanford University Medical Center lipid laboratory using the AutoAnalyzer II method according to the cooperative Lipid Research Clinics protocol.[5] Plasma was prepared from the blood drawn in two 15-ml EDTA vacutainers within two hours and was kept at 4° C. Plasma total cholesterol and plasma triglyceride concentrations were determined on the AutoAnalyzer II using a zeolite-treated isopropanol extract. The instrument remained standardized according to the Lipid Research Clinic criteria during all analysis.[5] Determination of the plasma concentrations of cholesterol and high density, low density, and very low density lipoproteins (HDL, LDL, and VLDL) in the runners and controls was done using a combined ultracentrifugal and heparin-manganese precipitation method.[5] HDL accuracy was constantly monitored using a plasma of known HDL cholesterol concentration, supplied by the Lipid Standardization Laboratory, Center for Disease Control in Atlanta, Georgia.

RESULTS

Hematology

The hematological results (means and standard deviations) for the elite runners, good runners, and controls are provided in TABLE 1. Also included are the normal ranges used by the laboratory for each variable. There were no significant differences in the hemoglobin concentrations among the three groups. However, as can be seen in TABLE 1 and FIGURE 1, the hematocrit was significantly lower for the runners and their average value fell at the lower limits of this laboratory's normal range. There was no significant difference between the red or white blood cell concentration of the elite runners and the good runners and the mean values for both running groups fell in the lower portion of this laboratory's normal range.

TABLE 1

SELECTED HEMATOLOGY MEASUREMENTS *

Variable	Elite Runners ($n=20$)	Good Runners ($n=8$)	Nonrunners ($n=95$)	Normal Values †
Hemoglobin (g)	15.5±0.9	15.6±0.70	15.8±1.11	14–18
Hematocrit (%)	43.8±2.5 ‡	43.6±1.7 ‡	47.2±3.27	42–52
RBC (10^6)	5.11±0.35	5.19±0.29	—	4.6–6.2
WBC (10^3)	5.60±0.97	5.65±0.69	—	4.8–10.8
MCV (μm^3)	85.9±2.9	84.3±3.2	—	80–94
MCH (pg^3)	30.4±1.1	30.0±0.9	—	27–31
MCHC (%)	35.6±0.8	35.9±0.4	—	32–36

* Mean ± standard deviation.

† RBC, red blood cells; WBC, white blood cells; MCV, mean cellular volume; MCH, mean cellular hemoglobin; MCHC, mean cellular hemoglobin capacity.

‡ Normal range used by Ford Laboratory, Denton, Texas.

§ Difference from nonrunners p ≤0.05.

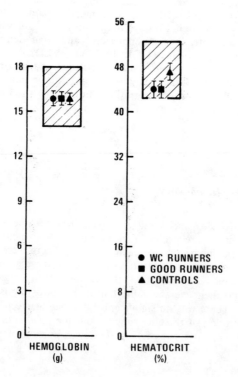

FIGURE 1. Hemoglobin and hematocrit values for elite (world class) runners, good runners, and nonrunning controls. Mean values ± standard error (SE) are given.

● WC RUNNERS
■ GOOD RUNNERS
▲ CONTROLS

HEMOGLOBIN (g)

HEMATOCRIT (%)

TABLE 2

BLOOD CHEMISTRIES

Variable †	Elite Runners (n=20)	Good Runners (n=8)	Nonrunners (n=95)	Normal Range ‡
SGOT (μmole/ml)	35.8±8.2 §	27.9±3.3	24.3±16.1	7–40
LDH (μmole/ml)	230±33.3 §	204±19.2 §	169±29.2	100–225
Alka. phos. (μmole/ml)	63.9±18.4	63.9±14.9	57.4±16.7	30–85
Total Bilirubin (mg%)	1.075±0.43 §	1.175±0.36 §	0.744±0.341	0.15–1.00
Uric Acid (mg%)	5.8±0.59	6.45±0.49	6.55±1.14	2.5–8.0
Total Protein (g%)	7.25±0.35	7.15±0.28	7.36±0.49	6.0–8.0
Albumin (g%)	4.87±0.35	5.04±0.20	4.67±0.30	3.5–5.0
Creatinine (mg%)	0.935±0.067	0.925±0.067	1.124±0.141	0.7–1.4
Bun (mg%)	18.0±3.49	21.3±4.00 §	16.3±3.64	10–20
Calcium (mg%)	10.1±0.40	10.5±0.29	9.7±0.48	8.5–10.5
Glucose (mg%)	97.8±7.1	96.5±8.9	101.6±9.9	65–110

* Mean ± standard deviation.
† SGOT, serum glutamic oxaloacetic transaminase; LDH, lactic dehydrogenase; Alk. phos., alkaline phosphatase; BUN, blood urea nitrogen.
‡ Normal range used by Ford Laboratory, Denton, Texas.
§ Difference from nonrunners: $p \leq 0.05$.

Blood Chemistry

The biochemical results and their normal ranges are provided in TABLE 2 and FIGURES 2–5. Significant elevations of the enzymes serum glutamic oxalo-acetic transaminase (SGOT) and lactate dehydrogenase (LDH) were found in the runners with the elite runners having a significantly higher SGOT and LDH than the good runners. The SGOT level for the elite runners was at the upper limits of this laboratory's normal, and the LDH value was elevated above the upper limits of normal (FIGURE 2). The alkaline phosphatase (alka. phos.) for the three groups was not significantly different and fell well within the laboratory's normal range. Total bilirubin was significantly higher in both groups of runners than the controls but did not show significant variations between the elite runners and the good runners. No attempt was made to fractionate the bilirubin. Other liver function studies such as total protein and albumin while falling in the higher levels of the laboratory normal, were not significantly different between the two running groups and the control group (FIGURE 3). The fasting blood sugar levels for the runners and the controls exhibited no significant differences and fell well within the laboratory's normal range (FIGURE 4). The creatinine values for the runners were lower than those of the controls but not significantly so. The blood urea nitrogen (BUN) was significantly higher in the good runners as compared to controls while the slight elevation in the elite runners was not significant. Serum calcium levels were slightly higher for the runners than for the controls but these differences were not significant.

Lipids and Lipoproteins

TABLE 3 contains the cholesterol and triglyceride results for the runners and the control group. Plasma triglycerides were significantly lower for both groups of runners versus the controls, but no difference existed between the two running groups. The elite runners had a slightly lower cholesterol value than either the good runners or the controls, but none of these differences were significant. However, elite runners did have a significantly lower LDL cholesterol fraction when compared to the controls. Also, the LDL cholesterol fraction of the elite runners was significantly lower than the LDL cholesterol fraction of the good runners, while the inverse was true for HDL cholesterol: it was slightly higher in the elite runners than in the good runners.

DISCUSSION

As can be seen in FIGURE 1, there were no significant differences in the hemoglobin concentration among the three groups. The hematocrit concentration for the runners was significantly lower than the controls and fell at the lower limits of the laboratory's normal range. This finding is similar to previous reports on endurance runners. In fact, the hematocrit values obtained for the elite and good runners were identical to those obtained by Brotherhood and colleagues in England on 40 male distance runners of similar age.[6] He, as have others, found a significant increase in total blood volume and postulated this as the reason for the low hematocrit in endurance athletes. Although we did not measure red blood cell breakdown products, such as haptoglobin, Brother-

TABLE 3

PLASMA CHOLESTEROL AND TRIGLYCERIDE VALUES *

Variable †	Elite Runners ($n=20$)	Good Runners ($n=8$)	Nonrunners ($n=72$)
Total Cholesterol (ml/100 ml)	175±26.3 ‡	185±35.5	189±36.4
HDL Cholesterol (ml/100 ml)	56±12.1 ‡	52±10.9	49±10.5
LDL Cholesterol (ml/100 ml)	108±24.5 ‡	121±29.5	124±35.6
VLDL Cholesterol (ml/100 ml)	11±5.2 ‡	12±11.8	15±7.5
Total Triglycerides (ml/100 ml)	74±25.2 ‡	73±39.7	92±37.3
HDL/LDL	0.56 *	0.45	0.39
HDL/Total Cholesterol	0.32	0.28	0.26

* Mean ± standard deviation.
† HDL, high density lipoprotein; LDL, low density lipoprotein; VLDL, very low density lipoprotein.
‡ Difference from nonrunners: $p \leq 0.05$

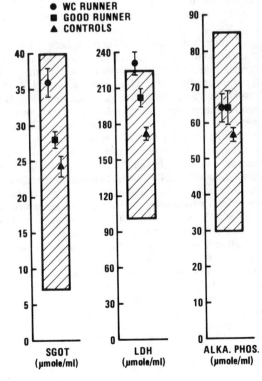

FIGURE 2. Serum glutamic-oxaloacetic transaminase (SGOT), serum lactic dehydrogenase (LDH), and alkaline phosphatase values (mean ± SEM) for elite (world class) runners, good runners, and non-running controls.

hood found no evidence of increased hemolysis in his 40 male distance runners.[6] We and others have found no abnormalities in red blood cell indices, such as iron, B_{12}, or folate deficiencies, to suggest hemolysis. Although we did not specifically ask for or analyze the dietary supplement intake of the elite runners, Brotherhood has found no differences in the hematological status between runners not on supplements and those taking iron and/or folate.[6] That Brotherhood did not observe any iron or folate deficiencies in his runners plus the normal red blood indices found in our runners argue against the belief that taking iron and/or folate can significantly improve an athlete's hematological status.

While our findings on hemoglobin concentration are somewhat contrary to those of Brotherhood, he did find a 20% higher blood volume and total body hemoglobin content (hemoglobin concentration divided by body weight) in his runners than in nonathletes.[6] We would anticipate similar findings in our runners versus our controls but would not anticipate significant differences between the elite runners and the good runners in total body hemoglobin concentration and would therefore lack an explanation for the superior fitness or physical ability of elite runners simply based on the oxygen carrying capacity of their blood. It is important to note that for both the elite and good runners, and for the runners evaluated by Brotherhood, the hematocrit values can often be at the lower limits of normal or even abnormally depressed when compared to standard laboratory values. It is important to bear this possibility in mind when distance runners participating at the high school or college levels or now during Master's competition (>40 years of age) complain of fatigue and are often considered to be anemic based on their hematocrit values. Not uncommonly this has led to an extensive hematological workup including bone marrow aspirations.

Clinically interesting differences between the runners and their controls appear in some of the eleven different chemical variables analyzed. FIGURE 2 reveals that striking elevations of the enzymes SGOT and LDH were found in the runners, with the elite runners having an SGOT at the upper limits of normal and an LDH abnormally elevated. The differences between the elite and good runners versus controls for SGOT and LDH were significant at the $p < 0.01$ and 0.05 levels, respectively. The world literature is replete with contradictory reports of the effects of acute and short-term exercise on serum enzyme values. However, there appears to be a scarcity of articles reporting enzyme values of chronic high mileage or high level exercisers. Previous studies have shown that LDH remains elevated for 12 to 24 hours after acute exercise, but may have a later secondary rise.[7] For example, Block and colleagues studied the effects of exercise on trained and untrained individuals and looked at not only SGOT and LDH but LDH isoenzymes and CPK levels.[8] They found that trained individuals, because of their ability to perform at higher levels of exercise, had a greater rise in SGOT and LDH and LDH isoenzymes 3, 4, and 5 than untrained individuals. Also of interest was their observation that the LDH fractions derived from red blood cell breakdown were not significantly elevated as were those fractions obtained from muscle and hepatic origin. Whether our observed values reflect the daily high level of activity of these athletes or not is speculative. It is important to note that certain enzymatic values obtained from muscular and liver tissue may be in the upper range of normal and may be frankly elevated. Since LDH and SGOT can also be released in many conditions of cellular damage, especially those of cerebral anoxia, it might facetiously be stated that the finding of a high LDH and SGOT in our distance runners wholly substantiate the claims of nonexercising skeptics who say that distance runners either initially or eventually suffer from cerebral ischemia.

Since SGOT and LDH can be elevated in liver damage, other liver screening parameters were analyzed. It can be seen from FIGURE 3 that total bilirubin was significantly higher in both running groups than for the controls and was just outside the upper limits of this laboratory's normal. No attempt was made to fractionate the bilirubin and thereby distinguish liver from hematolytic abnormalities. However, others have not found an elevated indirect bilirubin suggestive of red blood cell destruction in distance runners.[6] It is important to note that analysis of the alcohol intake of these 28 runners revealed only one ab-

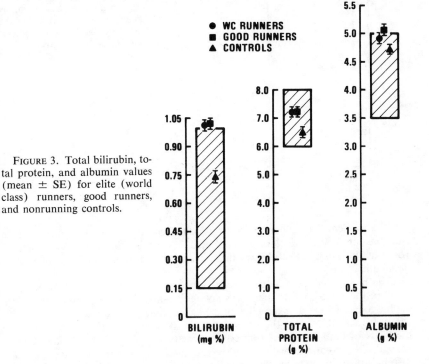

FIGURE 3. Total bilirubin, total protein, and albumin values (mean ± SE) for elite (world class) runners, good runners, and nonrunning controls.

stainer with eight of the runners rarely consuming alcohol, 13 of the runners consuming an average of one to two alcohol beverages per day and six of the runners, all of them in the elite group, consuming greater than three alcoholic beverages per day. Whether these enzyme elevations in runners might be attributed to their alcohol consumption can not be determined from the data available. Other liver function parameters attained, such as the total protein in albumin, were not significantly different between the runners and controls.

FIGURE 4 reveals that the fasting blood sugar for the three groups were entirely within the normal range and there was no significant differences between the lower glucose values obtained for the runners versus the controls. It is interesting to note that the uric acid values obtained were significantly lower in

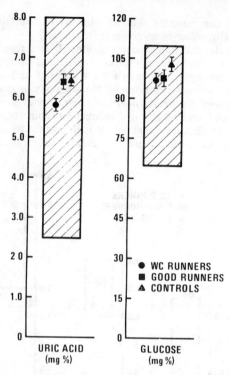

FIGURE 4. Serum uric acid and serum glucose values (mean ± SE) in elite (world class) runners, good runners, and nonrunning controls.

the elite runners than either the controls or the good runners (FIGURE 4). This differs from reports of elevated uric acid in certain highly trained athletes.[7] These findings may reflect dietary differences between runners and other professional athletes.

The blood analyses reflecting renal function, creatinine, and BUN are provided in FIGURE 5. While there was no significant difference between the BUN of the good runners and the elite runners, the good runners did have a significantly higher BUN than the control group. It is important to note that while the BUN of both groups of runners were at the upper end of this laboratory's normal, their creatinine values, with creatinine being a more sensitive indicator of renal function, were at the lower limits of this laboratory's values. The fact that there were no significant differences between the creatinine of the elite and good runners means that whatever differences were seen between the BUN values of these two groups probably cannot be attributed to renal dysfunction.

Considerable evidence has accumulated that supports the concept that in addition to total plasma cholesterol concentration, the manner in which cholesterol is distributed among plasma lipoproteins may be associated with the risk of developing coronary artery disease.[10, 11] Recently much interest has focused on the cholesterol transported as part of the high density lipoprotein (HDL) molecule. In contrast to total LDL or VLDL cholesterol, all of which appear to have a positive relationship to increased risk of coronary atherosclerosis, HDL cholesterol appears to have an inverse relationship.[10, 11] This inverse or negative relationship appears to be independent of total cholesterol level, LDL cholesterol

level, or obesity.[11] A discussion of the evidence currently available relating an
increase in HDL cholesterol to a reduced rate of atherosclerosis and clinical
manifestations of coronary artery disease is included in "Plasma Lipoprotein
Distribution in Male and Female Runners" by Wood and colleagues in this
monograph.

We recently reported that very active male runners, ages 35–59, had significantly lower triglycerides, total plasma cholesterol, LDL cholesterol, and VLDL
cholesterol, and significantly higher HDL cholesterol than age-matched nonrunning controls.[3] With these findings in mind we looked not only at the differences in the lipoprotein profiles between our runners and their controls, but also
at the differences between this group of elite runners, good younger runners, and
those more senior runners and their age-matched controls over the age spectrum
of 20 to 60 years. This comparison was performed with the idea in mind that
if habitual exercise has some beneficial effect in the prevention of coronary
artery disease, then our runners, who have been exercising at a high level for
numerous years, should ideally demonstrate the most beneficial lipoprotein
profile one could expect as a result of altering exercise habits. As can be seen
in FIGURE 6 there was a rather small but readily apparent lower total plasma
cholesterol level in the good and elite runners versus their nonrunning controls.
This difference persists at all ages from 20 to 60 years. These findings are in
agreement with previous works suggesting that a program of increased physical
activity generally results in only minor decreases in total plasma cholesterol
levels. In most studies reporting a reduction in cholesterol with physical activity,

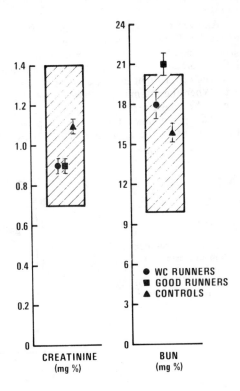

FIGURE 5. Serum creatinine and blood urea nitrogen (BUN) values (mean ± SE) for elite (world class) runners, good runners, and nonrunning controls.

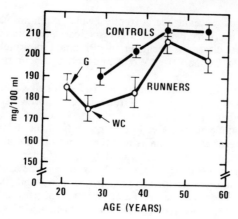

FIGURE 6. Total plasma cholesterol levels (mean ± SE) for runners (G, good; WC, world class or elite) and nonrunning controls.

changes in body weight and possibly in dietary intake have occurred.[13, 14] However, all the runners whose data are included in FIGURE 6 had been exercising at a relatively stable weight for at least several years. Major differences between the runners and their controls do appear when the distribution of their total cholesterol among the various lipoprotein fractions is analyzed (FIGURE 7). The amount of LDL cholesterol was significantly lower in the elite runners and good runners than their controls, again a finding that persists in the older runners.

An even more striking difference is found upon analysis of HDL cholesterol as seen in FIGURE 8. A significantly higher HDL cholesterol was found in all groups of runners versus their controls. It is interesting that the values for HDL cholesterol increased with increasing age in active runners while the controls showed a slight decrease or no change in HDL cholesterol with increasing age. When the plasma HDL cholesterol concentration is expressed as a percentage of the total plasma cholesterol [(HDL cholesterol/total cholesterol) × 100] a greater percentage of the runners' plasma cholesterol is contained in HDL (32%) than in the controls (26%). This relationship, or the relationship of

FIGURE 7. Low density lipoprotein cholesterol (LDL) levels (mean ± SE) for runners (G, good; WC, world class or elite) and nonrunning controls.

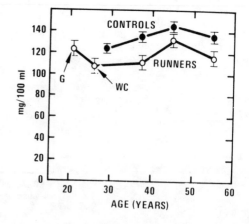

HDL cholesterol to LDL cholesterol concentration, may be important since total or LDL cholesterol may be important determinants in the rate of which lipid is deposited in the arterial wall while HDL cholesterol level may be related to the rate lipid is removed from various tissues including the arterial wall. Miller and Miller have focused on the possible importance of egress of cholesterol from atheroma in arterial walls and or body tissue pools.[10] In other words, they proposed that it may not be only the influx of cholesterol into the arterial walls that is important in the atherosclerotic process, but equally important might be the efflux of cholesterol from body pools back to the liver for catabolism and excretion. To go along with these findings they have reported that total cholesterol pools of the body increased with decreasing plasma HDL concentrations but that total cholesterol pools are unrelated to the plasma concentration of total cholesterol and other lipoproteins. They suggest that these data support the concept that the HDL fraction facilitates the uptake of cholesterol from peripheral tissues and therefore its transport to the liver and catabolism. They suggest that a reduction in plasma HDL cholesterol might accelerate the develop-

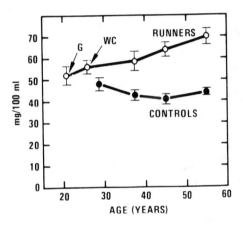

FIGURE 8. High density lipo-protein cholesterol (HDL) levels for runners (mean ± SE) (G, good; WC, world class or elite) and nonrunning controls.

ment of atherosclerosis and hence the manifestations of coronary artery disease. Since only esterified cholesterol can be exchanged between tissue and plasma lipoproteins and since HDL by virtue of its protein structure is a favorable substrate for the enzyme lecithin cholesterol acyltransferase (LCAT), the enzyme responsible for esterification of free cholesterol, an interesting role for HDL in cholesterol migration from the tissue pools to the liver for catabolism and excretion is postulated.

Epidemiological data linking plasma triglyceride concentrations and coronary artery disease prevalence in males is weak at best. Fasting triglyceride concentrations have been found to be lower in physically well-trained men than in their sedentary counterparts;[15] or to be reduced after a program of physical conditioning and to be acutely lowered by vigorous physical activity in hyperlipidemic subjects.[16, 17] Our data on the elite and good runners (FIGURE 9) substantiates these findings of a significantly lower triglyceride in active runners compared to nonrunning controls. It is interesting that in the runners triglyceride levels remain relatively constant with increasing age, while controls showed an age-related increase in plasma triglyceride concentration. These differences in triglycerides do not appear to be due to differences in alcohol intake. Even modest alcohol intake has been shown to increase plasma triglycerides in some individuals.[18] However, runners of all categories and ages reported that the ethanol intake habits were very similar or possibly even exceeded those of similarly aged nonrunners. Even though group comparisons of alcohol intake are very difficult, it is quite evident from the elite runners' data that excellent functional capacity and endurance performance can be achieved despite relatively high chronic alcohol consumption.

One cannot readily attribute the low levels of plasma triglycerides, LDL cholesterol, and VLDL cholesterol and the elevated HDL cholesterol to differences in dietary intake. Dietary questionnaires revealed only one of the 28 runners to be a vegetarian and most of the other elite and good runners consumed a reasonably typical American diet. A recent study of the plasma lipids and lipoproteins in macrobiotic vegetarians versus age-matched controls revealed

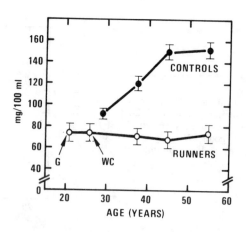

FIGURE 9. Plasma triglyceride levels (mean ± SE) for runners (G, good; WC, world class or elite) and nonrunning controls.

that the vegetarians had remarkably low plasma triglycerides, total cholesterol, LDL cholesterol, and a strikingly lower HDL cholesterol than our runners.[19] Thus, a low-fat diet does not elevate absolute HDL cholesterol levels even though it increases the HDL/total cholesterol ratio.

One characteristic other than the increased level of habitual physical activity that distinguished the runners of all ages from their controls was their lower level of adiposity. It has been postulated that one might reasonably consider this as being responsible, in part, for the decrease plasma triglyceride concentration and increase plasma HDL cholesterol found in runners versus controls. Whereas positive correlations between relative weight and plasma triglycerides have been reported,[20, 21] the correlation between plasma HDL cholesterol concentration and relative weight in the older runners was not significant. That HDL concentration and adiposity are not closely related also has been reported by others.[3] Even if HDL cholesterol is inversely related to degree of adiposity as reported by Rhoades,[11] the relationship of HDL to coronary artery disease manifestation is independent of this relationship.

SUMMARY

In summary, we conclude that the analysis of the blood profiles of elite runners offers no explanation for their superior fitness of physical ability when compared to the good runners. Selected enzymes related to cellular or tissue damage may be elevated in distance runners and could be classified as abnormal on routine clinical evaluation if unaware of their physical lifestyles. It is also important to note that certain blood profile parameters, especially the hematocrit, could be classified as abnormally low. Finally, the high degree of daily physical activity performed by the elite runners and good runners appears to be associated with a lipoprotein profile consistent with a low risk for development of coronary artery disease manifestations. These profiles persist despite increasing age in active running males.

REFERENCES

1. VAN GANSE, W., L. VERSEC, W. EYLENBOSH & K. VUYLSTEEK. 1970. The Electrocardiogram of athletes; comparison with untrained subjects. Brit. Heart J. **32**: 160–166.
2. LOPEZ-S., A., R. VIAL, L. BALART & G. ARROYAVE. 1974. Effect of exercise and physical fitness on serum lipids and lipoproteins. Atherosclerosis **20**: 1–9.
3. WOOD, P. D., W. L. HASKELL, H. KLEIN, S. LEWIS, M. P. STERN & J. W. FARQUHAR. 1976. The distribution of plasma lipoproteins in middle-aged male runners. Metabolism **25**: 1249–1257.
4. POLLOCK, M. L. 1977. Characteristics of elite class distance runners: Overview. Ann. N.Y. Acad. Sci. This volume.
5. LIPID RESEARCH CLINICS MANUAL OF LABORATORY OPERATIONS, VOL. 1. LIPID AND LIPOPROTEIN ANALYSIS. 1974. Department of Health, Education, Welfare Pub. No. (NIH) 75–628. U.S. Government Printing Office. Washington, D.C.
6. BROTHERHOOD, J., B. BROZOVIC & L. G. C. PUGH. 1975. Hematological status of middle and long distance runners. Clin. Sci. Mol. Med. **48**: 138–195.
7. SANDERS, T. M. & C. M. BLOOR. 1975. Effects of repeated endurance exercise on serum enzyme activities of well-conditioned males. Med. Sci. Sport **7**: 44–48.
8. BLOCK, P., M. VAN RIJMENONT, R. BADJOU, A. Y. VON MELSEM & R. VOGELEEK. 1971. The effects of exhaustive effort on serum enzymes in man. Biochemistry of exercise. Med. Sci. Sport **3**: 259–267.
9. HORVATH, G. 1967. Blood-serum level of uric acid in top sportsmen. Acta Rheumatol. Scand. **13**: 308–312.
10. MILLER, A. J. & N. E. MILLER. 1975. Plasma-high density-lipoprotein concentration and development of ischemic heart disease. Lancet **i**: 16–19.
11. RHOADS, G. G., C. L. GULBRANDSEN & A. KAGAN. 1976. Serum lipoproteins and coronary heart disease in a population sudty of Hawaii Japanese men. N. Engl. J. Med. **294**: 294–298.
12. WOOD, P. D., W. L. HASKELL, M. P. STERN, S. LEWIS & C. PERRY. 1977. Lipoprotein distribution in male and female runners. Ann. N.Y. Acad. Sci. This volume.
13. ROCHELLE, R. 1961. Blood plasma cholesterol change during a physical training program. Res. Quar. **32**: 538–550.
14. MILESIS, C. A. 1974. Effects of metered physical training on serum lipids of adult men. J. Sports Med. **14**: 8–13.
15. BJORNTORP, P., M. FAHLEN, G. GRMIBY, *et al.* 1972. Carbohydrate and lipid

metabolism in middle-aged physically well-trained men. Metabolism **21:** 1037–1044.

16. HOLLOSZY, J. O., J. S. SKINNER, G. TORO, *et al.* 1964. The effects of a six month program of endurance exercise on serum lipids of middle-aged men. Amer. J. Cardiol. **14:** 753–760.

17. GOODE, R. C., J. B. FIRSTBROOK & R. J. SHEPHARD. 1966. Effects of exercise and a cholesterol free diet on human serum lipids. Canad. J. Physiol. Pharmacol. **44:** 575–580.

18. GINSBERG, H., J. OLEFSKY, J. W. FARQUHAR & G. M. REAVEN. 1974. Moderate ethanol ingestion and plasma triglyceride levels—A study in normal and hypertriglyceridemic persons. Ann. Int. Med. **80:** 143–149.

19. SACKS, F. M., W. P. CASTELLI, A. DONNER & E. H. KASS. 1975. Plasma lipids and lipoproteins in vegetarians and controls. N. Engl. J. Med. **292:** 1148–1151.

20. STERN, M. P., J. OLEFSKY, J. W. FARQUHAR & G. M. REAVEN. 1973. Relationship between fasting plasma lipid levels and adipose tissue morphology. Metabolism **22:** 1311–1317.

21. ABRAMS, M. E., R. J. FARRETT, H. KEEN, *et al.* 1969. Oral glucose tolerance and related factors in a normal population sample. Brit. Med. J. **i:** 599–602.

BODY COMPOSITION OF ELITE CLASS DISTANCE RUNNERS *

Michael L. Pollock,† Larry R. Gettman, Andrew Jackson,‡
John Ayres, Ann Ward, and A. C. Linnerud§

Institute for Aerobics Research
Dallas, Texas 75230

The percent fat in distance runners has been estimated at 6% to 8%.[1-5] Costill, Bowers, and Kammer,[3] however, have suggested that top quality marathon runners probably have lower values. Limitations in previous investigations that could affect the accuracy of body density (BD) estimation resulted from the researchers' not differentiating distance runners from sprinters or field event athletes, not including elite runners (or mixing elite and average runners in the sample), and not using an accurate laboratory technique for determining percent fat.[1-5] Thus, a precise quantification of BD and percent fat of elite distance runners is needed.

Preliminary results from an investigation on an Olympic gold medal winner (marathon) showed leaner values if BD was measured by the hydrostatic weighing technique rather than by prediction equations using various combinations of anthropometric measures. Forsyth and Sinning [4] concluded that existing prediction equations estimating BD from various combinations of skinfold fat (S), girth (G), and diameter (D) measurements accurately predicted the BD of young sedentary men and athletes, but that the equations might not be valid for a very lean athlete. Likewise, the use of regression equations developed from samples of young men and women systematically resulted in an overestimation of BD for middle-aged men and women;[6,7] this difference was thought to reflect the significantly greater amount of fat found in the middle-aged population. These findings supported the practice of using population-specific equations and questioned the accuracy of predicting BD in a very lean population from equations developed from a normal and/or athletic population with a different body type.

The purpose of this investigation was to measure and predict BD in national and international class distance runners. The questions considered were twofold: what is the BD of elite runners? and can BD of elite runners be estimated accurately with regression equations using anthropometric variables?

Methods

Subjects for this investigation included 20 elite class distance runners described previously by Pollock in the overview section of this symposium. The elite runners were also dichotomized into groups in accordance with their best

* Project supported by the Quinton Instrument Company, Seattle, Washingon.
† Current address: Department of Medicine, Mt. Sinai Medical Center, Milwaukee, Wisc. 53201.
‡ Department of Physical Education, University of Houston, Houston, Texas 77004.
§ Department of Statistics, North Carolina State University, Raleigh, North Carolina 27607.

performance capabilities. The two groups included eight marathon runners and 11 middle–long distance runners (M–LD). One runner (Kardong) was too difficult to classify and was not used in this phase of the data analysis. Three additional samples were included for comparative purposes. These included 95 average young men (average age 19.7 yrs), eight good middle-distance runners from a local university track club (average age 21.3 yrs), and 10 lean but sedentary college males (average age 20.7 yrs).

Upon arrival at the laboratory, the subjects were measured for standing height to the nearest 0.25 inch (0.6 cm) on a standard physician's scale and for body weight to the nearest 10 g on an Acme Scale (Model ACSMIN). Anthropometric determinations included seven S, eleven G, and seven D measures. Then vital capacity (VC), residual volume (RV), and BD by hydrostatic weighing were determined. Experienced technicians administered all tests. Sessions were organized so that the same investigator measured all subjects on the same tests; i.e., one investigator always was assigned to each of the following three stations: anthropometric measurements, spirometry, and hydrostatic weighing.

Skinfold fat was measured at the chest, axilla, triceps, subscapula, abdomen, suprailium, and front thigh locations using a Lange skinfold fat caliper. The caliper had a constant pressure of 10 g/mm², and measures were taken on the right side. Recommendations published by the Committee on Nutritional Anthropometry of the Food and Nutrition Board of the National Research Council were followed in obtaining skinfold fat data.[8] Girth measures were taken with a Lufkin steel tape at the following 11 sites: shoulder, chest (normal), abdomen, waist, gluteus, thigh, calf, ankle, arm, forearm, and wrist. Body diameters were determined with a GPM Swiss-made anthropometer and included the following measures: bideltoid, biacromion, chest width, bi-ilium, bitrochanter, knee, and wrist. Skinfold fat data were measured and recorded to the nearest 0.5 mm; and G and D measures, to the nearest 0.1 cm. The location of the anthropometric sites and the procedures used in measuring were shown and described by Hertzberg et al.[9] and by Behnke and Wilmore.[10]

Vital capacity was determined using a rolling seal spirometer (Model 842, Ohio Medical, Madison, Wisc.) according to the procedures outlined by Kory et al.[11] and W. E. Collins, Inc.[12] Residual volume was determined by the nitrogen washout technique described by Wilmore[13] with a nitrogen analyzer (Model 700, Ohio Medical, Madison, Wisc.). Although RV and hydrostatic weighing determinations were administered separately, the same postural positions (sitting) were used for both.

Hydrostatic weighing was conducted in a $4 \times 6 \times 5$ ft fiberglas tank in which a chair seat was suspended from a Chatillion 15 kg scale. The hydrostatic weighing procedure was repeated six to ten times until three similar readings to the nearest 20 g were obtained.[14] The three values were averaged. Water temperature was recorded after each trial. The technique for determining BD followed the method outlined by Goldman and Buskirk;[15] and the calculation of BD, from the formula of Brožek et al.[16] The percent fat was calculated according to the Siri formula.[17]

The statistical analysis included the calculations of mean values, standard deviations (SD), and a basic correlation matrix of all variables (including BD) for both groups.

Regression analysis was used to test for the homogenity of regression slopes and intercepts. The regression equations reported by several investigators were cross-validated on the sample of elite runners. Multiple stepwise regression analysis was used to isolate the independent variables that accounted for a significant proportion of BD variance and to develop a specific regression equation for predicting BD for the sample of elite runners.[18]

Results and Discussion

The physical characteristics of the elite runners, good runners, untrained lean men and average young men are presented in TABLE 1. The data showed the elite runners to be shorter in stature, lighter in body weight, and higher in BD. These findings are characteristic of trained runners and agreed with previous reports comparing runners to sedentary populations.[3, 10, 19]

The elite runners were 4.7% fat (5.1% using the Brožek and Keys equation [20]), which is a lower value than reported by other investigators.[1-5] The 99% confidence interval of the mean percent fat for elite runners ranged from 0.99 to 5.07. The values reported by other investigators were significantly higher.[1-5] Costill, Bowers, and Kammer[3] found 114 participants at the 1968 U.S. Olympic Marathon Trial to be 7.5% fat; Adams[1] found college distance runners to be 9.8% fat; Behnke and Royce[2] found three long distance runners to be 7.9% fat; and Sprynarova and Parizkova[5] analyzed runners to be 6.3% fat. Comparing these values with the present data, the difference appeared to be related to the previous investigators' mixing of elite runners with good runners, using anthropometric techniques to estimate BD, and/or using runners whose training characteristics were less demanding.

The total body weight of the elite runners was 63.1 kg with a 99% confidence interval that ranged from 59.6 to 66.2 kg. Within this same confidence level, Costill, Bowers, and Kammer[3] reported 64.2 kg; Saltin and Åstrand[21] found 60.0 kg for three elite runners; and deGaray, Levine, and Carter[22] showed 59.8 kg for Olympic middle-distance runners. The 20 Olympic marathon runners also evaluated by deGaray, Levine, and Carter[22] were significantly lower in body weight (56.6 kg). Body weight and fat values of the middle-distance and marathon runners in this investigation showed no significant difference. Although some variance exists, outstanding runners tend to be approximately 60 kg in body weight and 5% fat. The investigation[22] of the 20 Olympic marathon runners included several African and Oriental runners who had lower body weights, but appeared to be similar in body fat. The sum of three S measures (triceps, subscapula, and suprailium) for their runners was 16.8 mm for middle distance runners and 16.7 mm for marathon runners, compared to 16.0 mm for the runners in this investigation.

The descriptive statistics for the anthropometric variables of the elite runners and average young men are presented in TABLE 2. The mean values and standard deviations for the elite runners were smaller than those for the young men, which indicated a homogeneous group.

The product-moment correlations presented in TABLE 2 showed that the relationship between BD and the S, G, and D measurements tended to be negative, while the correlations for the young men were higher. For the runners only three S correlations were significantly different from zero. The significant correlations found for triceps S and thigh S suggested that limb S measurements might be the most appropriate S measurements for this homogeneous population. The lack of variability exhibited by the elite runners was the main reason for these low correlations.

TABLE 1

PHYSICAL CHARACTERISTICS OF ELITE RUNNERS, GOOD RUNNERS, AND UNTRAINED MEN

Subject/Group	Height (cm)	Weight (kg)	Body Density (g/ml)	Body Fat* (%)	Lean Body Weight (kg)	Body Fat Weight (kg)	Residual Volume (liters)	Sum of 7 Skinfolds† (mm)
Elite M-LD Runners (n=11)‡								
Brown	187.3	72.10	1.07428	10.8	64.31	7.79	1.396	53.0
Castaneda	178.6	63.34	1.09102	3.7	61.00	2.34	1.661	32.5
Crawford	171.8	58.01	1.09702	1.2	57.31	0.70	1.625	32.5
Geis	179.1	66.28	1.07551	10.2	59.52	6.76	1.223	49.0
Johnson	174.6	61.79	1.08963	4.3	59.13	2.66	1.963	35.5
Manley	177.8	69.10	1.09642	1.5	68.06	1.04	1.241	32.0
Ndoo	169.3	53.97	1.08379	6.7	50.35	3.62	0.792	33.5
Prefontaine	174.2	68.00	1.08842	4.8	64.74	3.26	1.477	38.0
Rose	175.6	59.15	1.08248	7.3	54.83	4.32	1.538	31.5
Tuttle	176.8	61.44	1.09960	0.2	61.32	0.12	1.640	31.5
11 §	170.5	60.92	1.08916	4.5	58.18	2.74	1.112	34.5
Mean (±SD)¶	176.0 (5.0)	63.10 (5.30)	1.08794 (0.00832)	5.0 (3.5)	59.89 (4.90)	3.21 (2.38)	1.424 (0.320)	36.7 (7.4)
Elite Marathon Runners (n=8)								
Cusack	174.6	64.19	1.08096	7.9	59.12	5.07	1.666	45.5
Galloway	180.9	65.76	1.08419	6.6	61.42	4.34	1.160	43.0
Kennedy	167.0	56.52	1.09348	2.7	54.99	1.53	1.562	37.0
Moore	184.1	64.24	1.09193	3.3	62.12	2.12	1.782	37.0
Pate	179.6	57.28	1.09676	1.3	56.54	0.74	1.599	32.5

Shorter	178.4	61.17	1.09475	2.2	59.82	1.35	1.869	45.0
Wayne	172.1	61.61	1.07859	8.9	56.13	5.48	1.132	42.5
Williams	177.2	66.07	1.09569	1.8	64.88	1.19	2.481	41.5
Mean	176.8	62.11	1.08954	4.3	59.38	2.73	1.656	40.5
(±SD)	(5.6)	(3.66)	(0.00718)	(3.0)	(3.38)	(1.92)	(0.427)	(4.6)
Unclassified (n=1)								
Kardong	191.8	70.20	1.08807	4.9	66.76	3.44	1.893	37.5
Total Elite Runners (n=20)								
Mean	177.0	63.06	1.08859	4.7	60.03	3.03	1.541	38.3
(±SD)	(6.0)	(4.80)	(0.00749)	(3.1)	(4.41)	(2.10)	(0.375)	(6.3)
Good Runners (n=8)								
Mean	181.1	67.48	1.08527	6.1	63.31	4.17	1.590	48.9
(±SD)	(3.9)	(3.77)	(0.00939)	(4.0)	(3.98)	(2.62)	(0.350)	(14.0)
Untrained Lean Men (n=10)								
Mean	180.6	63.23	1.08044	8.2	58.01	5.22	1.460	51.1
(±SD)	(6.4)	(5.54)	(0.00671)	(2.8)	(4.60)	(2.04)	(0.390)	(10.2)
Average Young Men (n=95)								
Mean	179.8	74.60	1.06830	13.4	64.60	10.00	1.50	107.6
(±SD)	(6.4)	(10.90)	(0.01380)	(6.0)	(8.70)	(5.40)	(0.320)	(45.4)

* Percent fat calculated by Siri formula [17]: % Fat = 100 (4.95/density −4.5).
† Sum of 7 skinfolds = chest, axilla, triceps, subscapula, abdomen, suprailiac, and front thigh locations.
‡ Middle-long distance.
§ Subject's name kept anonymous.
‖ SD, standard deviation.

TABLE 2
SKINFOLD, GIRTH, AND DIAMETER MEASURES OF ELITE RUNNERS
AND AVERAGE YOUNG MEN

| | Elite Runners (n=20) | | Average Young Men (n=95) | | Correlation with Density | |
| | | | | | Elite Runners * | Average Young Men † |
Variable	Mean	SD	Mean	SD	r	r
Skinfolds (mm)						
Chest	4.5	1.0	11.4	6.2	−0.30	−0.77
Axilla	4.7	0.8	15.5	7.7	−0.36	−0.75
Triceps	5.0	1.1	13.6	5.7	−0.53	−0.73
Subscapula	6.4	0.9	13.9	5.5	−0.35	−0.73
Abdomen	7.1	2.1	20.6	9.0	−0.40	−0.77
Suprailium	4.6	1.0	15.2	8.5	−0.32	−0.75
Thigh	6.1	1.8	17.4	6.6	−0.82	−0.76
Total of 7	38.0	6.4	107.6	45.4	−0.64	−0.82
Girths (cm)						
Shoulder	106.1	3.9	112.5	7.6	−0.04	−0.16
Chest	91.1	3.4	91.4	6.3	−0.12	−0.29
Abdomen	74.2	3.1	78.8	6.6	−0.32	−0.48
Waist	74.6	3.0	81.0	7.6	−0.34	−0.59
Gluteus	87.8	3.3	94.4	5.4	−0.29	−0.52
Thigh	51.9	2.3	57.1	4.9	−0.38	−0.50
Calf	35.4	1.3	36.5	2.2	−0.36	−0.32
Ankle	21.0	0.9	22.1	1.4	−0.44	−0.33
Arm	28.2	1.0	32.6	3.3	−0.14	−0.16
Forearm	26.4	0.9	28.3	2.1	−0.24	−0.02
Wrist	16.0	0.5	16.7	0.8	−0.13	−0.10
Diameters (cm)						
Bideltoid	44.1	1.9	46.9	2.9	+0.27	−0.14
Biacromion	39.5	1.8	41.1	2.3	+0.39	+0.12
Chest, width	31.3	1.4	31.8	2.4	+0.19	−0.19
Bi-ilium	28.0	1.4	29.6	1.8	−0.19	−0.47
Bitrochanter	32.2	1.2	33.6	1.7	−0.04	−0.44
Knee, width	9.5	0.4	9.8	0.5	−0.29	−0.28
Wrist, width	5.6	0.2	5.9	0.3	−0.29	+0.23

* $r = 0.44$, 18 df, p < 0.05; $r = 0.56$, 18 df, p < 0.01.
† $r = 0.20$, 93 df, p < 0.05; $r = 0.26$, 93 df, p < 0.01.

The homogeneity of regression slopes and intercepts was tested to determine if the anthropometric variables used to develop regression equations for average young men would be appropriate for use with elite runners. The equations selected were from a study conducted previously by the investigators.[7] These six equations had multiple correlations that ranged from 0.81 to 0.88 with standard errors of ±0.0069 to ±0.0082. A random sample of 30 subjects from the 95 average young men was selected for this analysis and the results are presented in TABLE 3. Equations 1 and 2 used only S measurements as independent variables, and the slopes for these equations were not parallel. This result reflected the lack of variability in S measurements. The slopes of the equations that combined S, D, and height were parallel, and the intercepts were within sampling error. Equation 6, which was a combination of S, G, and D measurements, was the only equation with homogeneous slopes, but different intercepts.

To examine more fully the accuracy of regression equations developed on samples of young men, several previously reported equations were applied to the appropriate anthropometric variables of the elite runners.[4, 7, 20, 23-26] The multiple correlations reported for the original equations ranged from 0.80 to 0.87 with the standard errors of measurement ranging from ±0.0050 to ±0.0076. These equations were also used to calculate a predicted BD, means and standard deviations for the predicted BD, the correlations between the predicted BD and determined BD by the hydrostatic technique, and the standard errors. The results are presented in TABLE 4.

With the exception of the Brožek equation, all equations underestimated the true BD mean of the elite runners, and the standard deviations for distributions of predicted BD were smaller than the true standard deviation of 0.0075. The smallest standard deviations were found with the regression equations that used only S measures as independent variables. These small standard deviations supported the current findings that the slopes of regression equations developed from only S variables were not parallel; the use of equations developed from only S measurements tended to reduce the true BD differences that existed among the elite runners.

With the exception of two equations,[4, 24] all correlations between true and predicted BD were significantly different from zero. Also, all the correlations for these investigations were lower than previously reported, but some reduction was expected with cross-validation of regression equations.[27]

A more important statistic for prediction accuracy was the standard error of measurement. Several of the calculated standard errors were larger than the true BD standard deviation of ±0.0075. This finding indicated that these equations, even though significantly correlated, did not provide accurate predictions of BD for elite runners. The calculated standard errors showed that the Sloan [25]

TABLE 3

STATISTICAL COMPARISON OF SLOPES AND INTERCEPTS FOR
ELITE RUNNERS AND AVERAGE YOUNG MEN *

Equation	Variables †	K ‡	Slope F	Slope df	Intercept F	Intercept df
1	S	2	3.14 §	2,44	3.09	1,45
2	S	3	3.21 §	3,39	0.96	1,43
3	S, D, Ht	4	1.62	4,36	1.99	1,41
4	S, D, Ht	5	1.53	5,33	2.06	1,39
5	S, D, Ht	3	0.91	3,39	3.51	1,43
6	S, D, G	8	1.32	8,24	5.33 §	1,33

* Data from Pollock *et al.*[22]
† S, Skinfold fat; D, diameter; Ht, height; G, girth.
‡ Number of variables used in prediction equation.
§ $p < 0.05$.

and Pollock *et al.*[7] equations provided the most accurate prediction models. The original Sloan sample was relatively lean and homogeneous in BD (mean 1.0754 ± 0.200 g/ml) and in percent fat [mean 10.3 (±5.3)%]. The homogeneous characteristics of the sample as well as the use of thigh S as one of the independent variables were important factors in the Sloan equation relating well to the elite runners. The Sloan equation did produce a more homogeneous distribution. The true BD range for the elite runners ranged from 1.0743 to 1,0996 g/ml; BD predicted with the Sloan equation was more restricted and ranged from 1.0806 to 1.0905 g/ml. Using the Sloan equation for estimating body density of elite runners could produce gross errors at the extremes of the distribution.

These findings indicated that elite runners possessed unique body composition characteristics. In order to offer more accurate prediction equations, the

TABLE 4

COMPARISON OF BODY DENSITY PREDICTION EQUATIONS FOR YOUNG MEN

Investigator (Reference)	Variables *	K †	Predicted Density Mean (g/ml)	SD	Correlation of Predicted and Determined Density r	SE ‡
Pollock [22]	S,D,Ht	4	1.0857	0.0042	0.70	0.0060
Brŏzek [4]	S	3	1.0921	0.0018	0.55	0.0074
Pascale [20]	S	3	1.0791	0.0019	0.43	0.0116
Sloan [25]	S	2	1.0878	0.0030	0.80	0.0053
Wilmore [28]	S	2	1.0769	0.0022	0.61	0.0132
Katch [16]	S	3	1.0841	0.0022	0.57	0.0078
Forsyth [12]	S,D	3	1.0819	0.0043	0.36	0.0097

* S, Skinfold fat; D, diameter; Ht, height.
† K, Number of variables used in prediction equation.
‡ Standard error $=[\Sigma(BD'-BD)^2/n]^{1/2}$, where BD' is the predicted body density and BD is the laboratory-determined body density.[11]

data on the elite runners were analyzed by a forward stepwise regression model using several different combinations of independent variables. One equation showed a significant correlation with BD.

$$BD = 1.05637 - 0.00344(\text{thigh S}) + 0.00121(\text{shoulder D}).$$

The multiple correlation was 0.87 with a standard error of ±0.0038. This correlation was significantly different from zero ($F = 27.7$; $df = 2/17$; $p < 0.0001$), and both variables accounted for a significant proportion of BD variance ($t = 7.09$ and 2.59; $df = 17$).

The practice of developing regression equations with a sample size of 20 had obvious statistical limitations. However, the elite runners constituted a unique population, and many of the existing prediction equations were grossly inaccurate for this lean group. The 20 subjects of this investigation constituted the largest sample of elite runners with BD values determined from both anthropometric measurements and the hydrostatic technique reported in the literature.

In order to examine the validity of the regression equation developed from the data on elite runners, the equation was applied to data collected on two additional but different samples tested in the same laboratory. One sample consisted of eight good distance runners, most of whom were middle-distance runners from a local university track team. The second sample was made up of ten lean but sedentary college males. The regression equation developed from the elite runners accurately predicted the means of these two lean groups: 1.0851 (±0.0094) and 1.0810 (±0.0084) g/ml for BD and 6.14% and 7.43% for percent fat for the good runners and young sedentary lean men, respectively. In contrast, if the equation developed on elite runners was applied to the sample of 30 average young men, BD was underpredicted (−0.0131 g/ml) and body fat was overpredicted (5.5%).

These findings showed that the prediction equation developed from anthropometric measures of elite runners estimated BD for both sedentary and active lean samples. The finding of population specific regression equations for predicting BD from anthropometric measures was supported by two previous studies conducted on young and middle-aged men [7] and women.[6]

References

1. ADAMS, W. C. 1968. Effect of a season of varsity track and field on selected anthropometric, circulatory, and pulmonary function parameters. Res. Quart. **39:** 5–15.
2. BEHNKE, A. R. & J. ROYCE. 1966. Body size, shape, and composition of several types of athletes. J. Sports Med. Phys. Fitness **6:** 75–88.
3. COSTILL, D. L., R. BOWERS & W. F. KAMMER. 1970. Skinfold estimates of body fat among marathon runners. Med. Sci. Sports **2:** 93–95.
4. FORSYTH, H. L. & W. E. SINNING. 1973. The anthropometric estimation of body density and lean body weight of male athletes. Med. Sci. Sports **5:** 174–180.
5. SPRYNAROVA, S. & J. PARIZKOVA. 1971. Functional capacity and body composition in top weight-lifters, swimmers, runners, and skiers. Int. Z. Angew. Physiol. **29:** 184–194.
6. POLLOCK, M. L., E. LAUGHRIDGE, B. COLEMAN, A. C. LINNERUD & A. JACKSON. 1975. Prediction of body density in young and middle-aged women. J. Appl. Physiol. **38:** 745–749.
7. POLLOCK, M. L., T. HICKMAN, Z. KENDRICK, A. JACKSON, A. C. LINNURUD & G. DAWSON. 1976. Prediction of body density in young and middle-aged men. J. Appl. Physiol. **40:** 300–304.
8. KEYS, A. (Chairman). 1956. Recommendations concerning body measurements for the characterization of nutritional status. Hum. Biol. **28:** 111–123.
9. HERTZBERG, H. T. E., E. CHURCHILL, C. W. DUPERTUIS, R. M. WHITE & A. DAMON. 1963. Anthropometric Survey of Turkey, Greece, and Italy. Macmillan Company. New York, N.Y.
10. BEHNKE, A. R. & J. H. WILMORE. 1974. Evaluation and Regulation of Body Build and Composition. Prentice-Hall, Inc. Englewood Cliffs, N.J.
11. KORY, R., R. CALLAHAN & H. BOREN. 1961. The veterans administration-army cooperative study of pulmonary function. Amer. J. Med. **30:** 243–258.
12. Clinical Spirometry—Instructions for Use of the Collins Respirometer and for Calculation and Interpretation of Data in Pulmonary Function and Basal Metabolism Testing. W. E. Collins, Inc. Braintree, Mass.

13. WILMORE, J. H. 1964. A simplified method for determination of residual lung volumes. J. Appl. Physiol. **27:** 96–100.
14. KATCH, F. I. 1968. Apparent body density and variability during underwater weighing. Res. Quart. **39:** 993–999.
15. GOLDMAN, R. F. & E. R. BUSKIRK. 1961. Body volume measurement by underwater weighing: Description of a method. *In* Techniques for Measuring Body Composition. : 78–89. J. Brožek & A. Henschel, Eds. National Academy of Science. Washington, D.C.
16. BROŽEK, J., F. GRANDE, J. T. ANDERSON & A. KEYS. 1963. Densitometric analysis of body composition: Revision of some quantitative assumptions. Ann. N.Y. Acad. Sci. **110:** 113–140.
17. SIRI, W. E. 1956. Body composition from fluid spaces and density. Univ. Cal., Donner Lab., Med. Physics Report, 19 March.
18. KERLINGER, F. N. & E. S. PEDHAZUR. 1973. Multiple Regression in Behavioral Research. Holt, Rinehart, and Winston, Inc. New York, N.Y.
19. CURETON, T. K. 1951. Physical Fitness of Champion Athletes. University of Illinois Press. Urbana, Ill.
20. BROŽEK, J. & A. KEYS. 1951. The evaluation of leaness-fatness in man: norms and interrelationships. Brit. J. Nutr. **5:** 194–206.
21. SALTIN, B. & P. O. ÅSTRAND. 1967. Maximal oxygen uptake in athletes. J. Appl. Physiol. **23:** 353–358.
22. DE GARAY, A. L., L. LEVINE & J. E. L. CARTER. 1974. Genetic and Anthropological Studies of Olympic Athletes. Academic Press, Inc. New York, N.Y.
23. KATCH, F. I. & W. D. MCARDLE. 1973. Prediction of body density from simple anthropometric measurements in college-age men and women. Hum. Biol. **45:** 445–454.
24. PASCALE, L. R., M. I. GROSSMAN, H. S. SLOANE & T. FRANKEL. 1956. Correlations between thickness of skinfolds and body density in 88 soldiers. Hum. Biol. **28:** 165–176.
25. SLOAN, A. W. 1967. Estimation of body fat in young men. J. Appl. Physiol. **23:** 311–315.
26. WILMORE, J. H. & A. R. BEHNKE. 1969. An anthropometric estimation of body density and lean body weight in young men. J. Appl. Physiol. **27:** 25–31.
27. DUBOIS, P. 1965. An Introduction to Psychological Statistics. Harper-Row, Publishers. New York, N.Y.

PULMONARY FUNCTION OF ELITE DISTANCE RUNNERS

Peter B. Raven

Institute for Aerobics Research
Dallas, Texas 75230

The inordinately large maximal oxygen uptakes ($\dot{V}_{O_2 max}$) obtained by Olympic class endurance athletes [1] has resulted in extensive investigations into the dimensional differences occurring within the oxygen transport and delivery systems of athletes compared to sedentary normals. One component of these systems receiving attention has been the pulmonary system, yet the results have not proven conclusive. The vital capacity (VC) of athletes has been reported to be larger than in nonathletes by some investigators,[2-4] whereas others have reported no consistent difference.[5-10] However, champion swimmers appear to be a special group of athletes having larger VC than nonathletes.[11-13] Both maximum voluntary ventilation (MVV) and forced expiratory volumes (FEV) of athletes have been reported to be larger than nonathletes,[6, 10, 11] while others found no difference in these measures.[7] In the few investigations that evaluated total lung capacity (TLC) no enlargement was observed.[7, 8]

The athletes examined in the present study represent a unique population of champion endurance runners, whose training regimens alone set them apart from the sedentary or normally active populations. During the course of their clinical screening and underwater weighing procedures, specific lung volumes were determined and it was anticipated that by making selected comparisons, greater insight into the development of the lung with respect to endurance exercise training would be obtained.

Methods

Twenty elite class athletes were scheduled for clinical screening and underwater weighing at which time the specific lung volumes, forced vital capacity (FVC), timed forced expiratory volumes ($FEV_{1.0}$), residual volume (RV), and calculated TLC were obtained. In addition, ten selected Southern Methodist University students were measured at a later date and used as matched controls. These students were matched anthropometrically with the elite runners in terms of height, weight, and lean body mass.

The FVC was determined in the seated position, using a dry rolling-seal spirometer (Model 842, Airco-Ohio Medical, Madison, Wisc.) connected to a digital meter for on-line readout. The largest FVC of three trials, carried out according to the standardized procedures of Kory et al.,[14] was selected for the determination of FVC and $FEV_{1.0}$. Seated residual volumes were determined by the nitrogen washout technique described by Wilmore[15] using a nitrogen analyzer (Model 700, Airco-Ohio Medical) sampling directly at the mouthpiece. Temperatures were measured prior to and following each volume determination and the average temperature was used with the daily barometric pressure to correct the measured volumes to the standard body temperature and pressure, saturated conditions (BTPS).

Data obtained from five of the elite class athletes and one of the matched controls were not used in the comparative analysis. The primary reason for rejecting the data was the inability of the subjects to perform the dynamic volume measurements adequately to trigger the machine computer to obtain reproducible data within the three trials. The pressures of time required that each subject be moved from one station to another as quickly as possible without influencing the technique. In those cases where RV was obtained accurately and in duplicate for underwater weighing, further multiple repeated trials of FVC and $FEV_{1.0}$ were not attempted. Nine of the fifteen elite runners that successfully completed the pulmonary function testing were classified, by reason of running history and performance, as middle–long distance (M–LD) runners, while five were classified as marathon runners. One of the members of the elite group could not be assigned to either grouping based on running history or performance times.

Comparisons of the two types of runners (M-LD and marathon), the sedentary controls, and predicted normative data were made. Absolute volume comparisons and calculated ratios of volume to height were made using Student's t-test.[16] Absolute volumes were standardized with respect to height, as it has been shown that volumes of the lung develop in proportion with the cube of the height,[17] hence it was felt that variations between groups were more comparable when height was accounted for.

Results

TABLE 1 summarizes the comparisons between the elite M-LD and marathon runners. The marathon runners were on the average 4 years older than the M-LD runners ($p < 0.02$), yet had similar absolute values of FVC ($p > 0.05$); however, when height was accounted for, the FVC of the M-LD runners had a 2.6 ml greater volume per centimeter of standing height than the marathon runners ($p < 0.05$). All other comparisons proved nonsignificant. When the elite runners as a group were compared against their matched controls (TABLE 2), it was observed that the controls were 6 years younger than the runners ($p < 0.01$) and had smaller FVCs ($p < 0.05$) and smaller TLCs ($p < 0.01$). These differences were maintained even when individual height differences were accounted for. There were no differences in residual volume (RV), the ratio of residual volume to total lung capacity (RV/TLC) or the ratio of $FEV_{1.0}$ to FVC ($FEV_{1.0}/FVC$). The major differences between the elite runners and the sedentary students (FVC and TLC) were compared further with recently published predicted normative data for a representative population of U.S. males[18] (FIGURES 1 & 2). The mean differences between the actual values obtained for the elite runners and their predicted values were +380 ml and +90 ml for FVC and TLC, respectively. Similarly, the mean difference between the obtained values of the controls and the predicted values was −180 ml and −780 ml for FVC and TLC, respectively. Individual data for the elite runners, in addition to average data of the groups, are summarized in the Appendix for comparative purposes and continuity of format.

Discussion

Initial findings suggest that the pulmonary volumes (TLC and FVC) of elite class athletes were greater than that of the sedentary controls, while dynamic function ($FEV_{1.0}/FVC$) evidenced no consistent difference. However, comparison of the elite class runner's volume data with published normative data [18] indicate that the differences were probably a result of sampling bias. Although matched anthropometrically, the elite runners and the sedentary student population represent the extremes of the distribution of lung volumes of the entire population of young adult males, each group being at diametrically opposite ends of the spectrum. In addition, the student population had average values of FVC and TLC less than predicted for their height and age, whereas

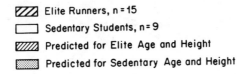

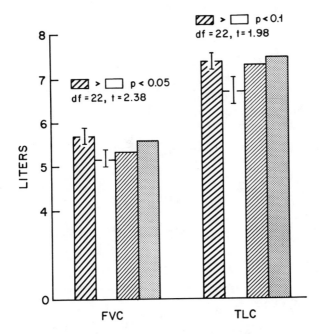

FIGURE 1. Absolute values of forced vital capacity (FVC) and total long capacity (TLC) of elite runners and matched sedentary controls with their predicted values. (After Bates et al.[18])

the elite runners had values greater than predicted (FIGURES 1 & 2). Therefore, it is probable that the observed difference is an example of a Type 2 error (the probability of accepting a hypothesis when it is false) and, hence, is not regarded as being physiologically meaningful.

The significant difference in FVC of 2.6 ml per centimeter of standing height found between the M-LD and marathon runners is similar to those differences observed between various other athletic groups [9, 10, 19-22] (TABLE 3) and is representative of the normal variation found between select groups,

TABLE 1

COMPARISON OF ELITE MIDDLE-LONG DISTANCE
AND ELITE MARATHON RUNNERS *

	Age (yr)	Ht (cm)	FVC (liters)	FEV$_{1.0}$/FVC (%)	RV (liters)	TLC (liters)	FVC/Ht (ml/cm)	TLC/Ht (ml/cm)	RV/TLC (%)
Elite middle-long distance runners (M-LD) (n=9)	24.9 ±0.7	177.3 ±1.6	5.78 ±0.20	78.4 ±1.7	1.53 ±0.08	7.31 ±0.22	32.6 ±0.89	41.2 ±1.09	20.93 ±0.95
Elite marathon runners (n=5)	28.8 ±1.2	180.0 ±1.4	5.40 ±0.18	80.4 ±2.4	1.78 ±0.24	7.18 ±0.18	30.0 ±0.78	39.9 ±1.12	24.6 ±2.84
t (Student's t-test)	2.78	1.36	1.56	0.68	0.99	0.45	2.60	0.79	1.23
df	12	12	12	12	12	12	12	12	12
p value	<0.02	NS	NS	NS	NS	NS	<0.05	NS	NS

* Mean ± standard deviation. FVC, forced vital capacity; FEV$_{1.0}$, forced expiratory volume in 1 sec; RV, residual volume; TLC, total lung capacity.

TABLE 2

SELECTED PULMONARY FUNCTION MEASURES OF ELITE RUNNERS AND A MATCHED SEDENTARY GROUP *

	Age (yr)	Ht (cm)	FVC (liters)	FEV$_{1.0}$/FVC (%)	RV (liters)	TLC (liters)	FVC/Ht (ml/cm)	TLC/Ht (ml/cm)	RV/TLC (%)
Elite runners (n=15)	26.3 ±0.87	179.2 ±1.39	5.72 ±0.15	79.1 ±1.2	1.64 ±0.09	7.35 ±0.17	31.9 ±0.67	41.03 ±0.79	22.22 ±1.07
Sedentary students (n=9)	20.01 ±0.94	180.5 ±2.4	5.16 ±0.18	81.9 ±1.8	1.51 ±0.14	6.67 ±0.30	28.6 ±0.79	36.9 ±1.39	22.34 ±1.13
t (Student's t-test)	4.83	0.47	2.38	1.32	0.75	1.98	3.17	2.58	0.08
df	22	22	22	22	22	22	22	22	22
p value	<0.01	NS	<0.05	NS	NS	<0.10	<0.01	<0.02	NS

* Means ± standard deviation.

where sample size is small. Inspection of this comparative data indicates a remarkable difference in FVC of runners competing in 1924 (Boston marathoners) [9] and those competing in modern day athletics, a change probably reflective of the population as a whole. When height differences were accounted for (FVC/Ht), the differences in volume between the 1924 and the modern day athlete (6 ml/cm) remained tenable, hence the modern day athlete must have had a greater thoracic development than that of 50 years ago. However, these differences indicate that comparisons of data obtained from different generations of athletic populations must be treated carefully.

Åstrand [21] has demonstrated that a significant relationship ($r = 0.95$, $p < 0.01$) exists between FVC and $\dot{V}_{O_2\,max}$ when analyzed over all age groups of the normally active adult (ages ranging from 6 to 71 years). The data of the present investigation form only a small part of Åstrand's continuum, yet a positive relationship ($r = 0.44$, $p < 0.1$) does exist between FVC and $\dot{V}_{O_2\,max}$. As can be seen from the graphical representation (FIGURE 3), the data of elite runners fall within a narrow range at the upper end of the scale and suggest that within this subgroup the relationship between FVC and $\dot{V}_{O_2\,max}$ is different from that observed for the total population ($r = 0.95$ is significantly different from $r = 0.44$, $p < 0.001$). This would suggest that when development is complete and functional capacities are maximized by training, increased size of FVC will have minimal effect on the obtained $\dot{V}_{O_2\,max}$. It is probable, as previously suggested, [22, 23] that at the elite level of athletic ability other factors such

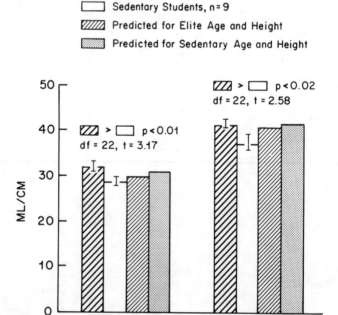

FIGURE 2. Comparisons of FVC and TLC of elite runners and matched sedentary controls with predicted values accounting for height differences.

TABLE 3

COMPARISONS OF ELITE DISTANCE RUNNERS WITH MEAN DATA COLLECTED FROM OTHER ATHLETIC GROUPS

Groups	n	Age (yr)	FVC (liters)	RV (liters)	TLC (liters)	$FEV_{1.0}$/FVC (%)	RV/TLC (%)	FVC/Ht (ml/cm)	TLC/Ht (ml/cm)	Reference
Elite middle–long distance runners	9	24.9	5.78	1.53	7.31	78.4	20.9	32.6	41.2	—
Elite marathon runners	5	28.8	5.40	1.78	7.18	80.04	24.6	30.0	39.9	—
Santa Barbara marathon runners	5	31.4	5.60	2.16	7.76	79.4	27.3	31.9	44.2	25
Fla. Relays marathon runners	11	28.0	5.92	2.15	8.07	81.6	26.3	33.07	45.1	10
Boston marathoners, 1924	66	—	4.25	—	—	—	—	24.9	—	9
Profess. football players	44	—	5.86	1.52	7.42	—	21.0	30.8	39.0	19
Profess. soccer players	18	25.6	5.29	1.39	6.73	—	20.7	30.0	38.2	20
1500 m runners & cross-country skiers	8	—	6.19	—	—	—	—	34.9	—	21
Swedish athletes	8	25.6	6.28	—	—	82.8	—	33.8	—	22

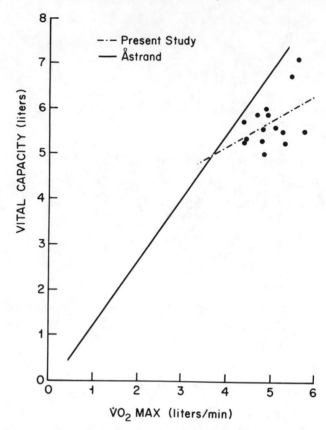

FIGURE 3. Graphical representation of the relationship between FVC and $\dot{V}_{O_2max}$ from Åstrand's study [21] of 97 persons with ages ranging from 6 to 71, where $r=0.95$ and $y=1.423x-0.23$ (———), and from the present study of 15 elite runners (·), where $r=0.44$ and $y=0.571x+2.88$ (- - -).

as pulmonary diffusing capacity (D_L), pulmonary capillary blood volume (V_C), and membrane permeability (D_M) become more important to improved function than pulmonary capacity alone. However, athletic groups at older ages (40–70 years) have shown significantly greater capacities and dynamic capabilities of the lung than that of matched controls; [24] hence, it would prove of value to continue evaluation of the pulmonary function of these elite runners and relate changes to their training regimens on a longitudinal basis. By this means we may be able to determine whether rigorous physical activity throughout life will offset the observed age-related decrement in pulmonary function.

References

1. ÅSTRAND, P-O. & K. RODAHL, Eds. 1970. Textbook of Work Physiology. 1st edit. : 393–395. McGraw-Hill Book Company. New York, N.Y.
2. STUART, D. G. & W. D. COLLINGS. 1959. Comparison of vital capacity and maximum breathing capacity of athletes and nonathletes. J. Appl. Physiol. 14: 507–511.

3. WEST, H. 1920. Clinical studies on respiration: VI. A comparison of various standards for the normal vital capacity of the lungs. Arch. Int. Med. **25:** 306–312.

4. ÅSTRAND, P-O. & K. RODAHL, Eds. 1970. Textbook of Work Physiology. 1st edit. : 202–204. McGraw-Hill Book Company. New York, N.Y.

5. ÅSTRAND, P-O. 1956. Human physical fitness with special reference to sex and age. Physiol. Rev. **36:** 307–330.

6. GRIMBY, G. & B. SALTIN. 1966. Physiological analysis of physically well-trained middle-aged and old athletes. Acta. Med. Scand. **179:** 513–520.

7. NEWMAN, F., B. F. SMALLEY & M. L. THOMSON. 1961. A comparison between athletes and non-athletes in oxygen consumption and pulmonary diffusion at near maximal exercise. J. Physiol. (Lond.) **156:** 7P–8P.

8. NEWMAN, F., B. F. SMALLEY & M. L. THOMSON. 1962. A comparison of exercise, body and lung size on CO diffusion in athletes and non-athletes. J. Appl. Physiol. **17:** 649–655.

9. GORDON, B., S. A. LEVINE & A. WILMAERS. 1924. Observations on a group of marathon runners: with special reference to the circulation. Arch. Intern. Med. **33:** 425–434.

10. KAUFMANN, D. A., E. W. SWENSON, J. FEREL & A. LUCAS. 1974. Pulmonary function of marathon runners. Med. Sci. Sports **6:** 114–117.

11. ÅSTRAND, P-O., L. ENGSTROM, B. O. ERIKSSON, P. KARLBERG, O. NYLANDER, B. SALTIN & C. THOREN. 1963. Girl swimmers. Acta. Pediat. (Uppsula) Suppl. 147.

12. NEWMAN, F., B. F. SMALLEY & M. L. THOMSON. 1961. A comparison between body size and lung function of swimmers and normal school children. J. Physiol. (Lond.) **156:** 9P.

13. SHAPIRO, W., C. E. JOHNSTON, R. A. DAMERON, JR. & J. L. PATTERSON, JR. 1964. Maximum ventilatory performance and its limiting factors. J. Appl. Physiol. **19:** 199–203.

14. KORY, R., R. CALLAHAN & H. CAREN. 1961. The Veterans Administration–Army cooperative study of pulmonary function. Amer. J. Med. **30:** 243–258.

15. WILMORE, J. H. 1964. A simplified method for determination of residual lung volumes. J. Appl. Physiol. **27:** 96–100.

16. GARRETT, H. E., Ed. 1965. Statistics on psychology and education. 5th edit. : 184–209. David McKay Co. Inc. New York, N.Y.

17. BJURE, J. 1971. Ergometry and physical training in pediatrics with special reference to pulmonary function. Acta. Pediat. Scand. Suppl. **217:** 56–59.

18. BATES, D. V., P. T. MACKLEM & R. V. CHRISTIE, Eds. 1971. Respiratory Function in Disease. 2nd edit. : 93. W. B. Saunders Company. Philadelphia, Pa.

19. WILMORE, J. H. & W. L. HASKELL. 1972. Body composition and endurance capacity of professional football players. J. Appl. Physiol. **33:** 564–567.

20. RAVEN, P. B., L. R. GETTMAN, M. L. POLLOCK & K. H. COOPER. 1976. A physiological evaluation of professional soccer players. Brit. J. Sports Med. **10:** 209–216.

21. ÅSTRAND, P-O. 1952. Experimental Studies of Physical Working Capacity in Relation to Sex and Age. : 64. Ejnar Munksgaard. Copenhagen.

22. HOLMGREN, A. & P-O. ÅSTRAND. 1966. DL and the dimensions and functional capacities of the O_2 transport system in humans. J. Appl. Physiol. **21:** 1463–1470.

23. REUSCHLEIN, P. S., W. G. REDDAN, J. BURPEE, J. B. L. GEE & J. RANKIN. 1968. Effect of physical training on the pulmonary diffusing capacity during submaximal work. J. Appl. Physiol. **24:** 152–158.

24. PYORALA, K., A. O. HEINONEN & M. J. KARVONEN. 1968. Pulmonary function in former endurance athletes. Acta Med. Scand. **183:** 263–273.

25. MARON, M. Institute of Environmental Stress, University of California, Santa Barbara, Calif. Personal communication.

APPENDIX

INDIVIDUAL AND GROUP MEAN PULMONARY FUNCTION DATA OF THE ELITE DISTANCE RUNNERS, THE GOOD RUNNERS, AND THEIR CONTROLS

Subject Group	Age (yr)	Ht (cm)	Wt (kg)	BSA (m²)	FVC (liters)	FEV$_{1.0}$/FVC (%)	RV (liters)	TLC (liters)	FVC/Ht (ml/cm)	TLC/Ht (ml/cm)	RV/TLC (%)
Elite M-LD runners, n=9 *											
Brown	22	187.3	74.1	1.99	7.12	82.6	1.40	8.52	38.0	45.6	16.43
Castaneda	23	178.6	62.8	1.79	6.03	84.5	1.66	7.69	33.8	43.1	21.59
Crawford	27	171.8	58.0	1.69	5.31	80.1	1.62	6.93	30.9	40.3	23.38
Geis	21	179.1	66.3	1.83	5.26	80.0	1.22	6.48	29.4	36.2	18.83
Johnson	25	174.6	62.1	1.76	5.87	73.2	1.96	7.83	33.6	44.8	25.03
Manley	32	177.8	69.4	1.86	5.48	71.4	1.24	6.72	30.8	37.8	18.45
Prefontaine	24	174.2	66.3	1.81	5.50	80.0	1.48	6.98	31.6	40.1	21.20
Rose	23	175.6	59.2	1.76	5.87	72.6	1.64	7.41	33.4	42.2	22.65
Tuttle	27	176.8	60.9	1.73	5.60	81.3	1.54	7.24	31.8	41.0	20.79
Mean	24.9	177.3	64.3	1.80	5.78	78.4	1.53	7.31	32.6	41.2	20.93
SD	3.37	4.41	5.18	0.087	0.566	4.76	0.230	0.631	2.51	3.07	2.67
SE	1.19	1.56	1.83	0.031	0.020	1.68	0.081	0.223	0.886	1.086	0.945

Elite marathon runners, n=5											
Galloway	29	181.0	65.0	1.84	5.58	86.4	1.16	6.74	30.8	37.2	17.21
Moore	31	184.2	64.2	1.85	5.30	84.8	1.78	7.08	28.8	38.4	25.14
Pate	28	179.6	57.0	1.72	5.36	76.4	1.60	6.96	29.8	38.8	23.00
Shorter	27	178.4	61.3	1.77	5.74	78.0	1.87	7.61	32.2	42.7	24.57
Williams	29	177.2	66.1	1.82	5.02	76.3	2.48	7.50	28.3	42.3	33.07
Mean	28.8	180.1	62.7	1.80	5.40	80.4	1.78	7.18	30.0	39.9	24.60
SD	1.48	2.70	3.66	0.054	0.276	4.85	0.478	0.367	1.57	2.47	5.683
SE	0.74	1.35	1.83	0.027	0.138	2.42	0.239	0.184	0.78	1.23	2.842
Total elite runners, n=14											
Mean	26.3	178.3	63.76	1.80	5.65	79.11	1.62	7.26	31.66	40.75	22.24
SD	3.38	4.01	4.61	0.075	0.51	4.70	0.34	0.54	2.51	2.85	4.20
SE	0.939	1.113	1.28	0.021	0.14	1.30	0.095	0.15	0.70	0.79	1.17
Good runners, n=7											
Mean	20.57	181.9	67.04	1.87	5.81	80.93	1.68	7.34	31.91	41.14	22.27
SD	1.81	3.28	3.59	0.053	0.18	7.28	0.39	1.16	0.84	2.66	3.62
SE	0.74	1.34	1.46	0.022	0.07	2.97	0.16	0.47	0.34	1.08	1.48
Untrained lean men, n=9											
Mean	20.01	180.50	63.02	1.81	5.16	81.9	1.51	6.67	28.6	36.9	22.34
SD	2.67	6.79	5.78	0.11	0.51	4.98	0.39	0.85	2.23	3.93	3.21
SE	0.94	2.4	2.04	0.039	0.18	1.76	0.14	0.30	0.79	1.39	1.13

* Middle-long distance.

PSYCHOLOGIC CHARACTERIZATION OF THE ELITE DISTANCE RUNNER

William P. Morgan

Department of Physical Education and Dance
University of Wisconsin—Madison
Madison, Wisconsin 53706

Michael L. Pollock

Institute for Aerobics Research
Dallas, Texas 75230

The stress imposed during marathon competition is arduous, to say the least, and marathoners have previously been observed to possess unique anatomical and physiological characteristics. The unique biological nature of the marathoner is further outlined throughout this present volume. However, it has been noted by Costill [1] that ". . . many athletes appear to meet the anatomical and physiological prerequisites for the marathon, while only a select group of men achieve success in this demanding sport." A preliminary study of the personality characteristics of marathoners reported earlier by Morgan and Costill [2] suggested that athletes from this particular subgroup display unique psychological profiles. For example, these marathoners were characterized by introversion, stability, and low anxiety levels. However, none of these variables were found to correlate significantly with marathon performance, and this lack of statistical significance was undoubtedly due in part to the homogeneity of the sample (nine males). As a matter of fact, aerobic power was not found to be correlated with performance either, and this also was related to the "problem" of homogeneity, since Costill *et al.*[3] subsequently demonstrated that aerobic power and endurance performance are significantly correlated in heterogeneous groups.

The study by Morgan and Costill [2] should be replicated for several reasons. First of all, while the marathoners reported on were introverted, as measured by the Eysenck Personality Inventory, one member of the group who had previously won the Boston Marathon, scored very high on the extroversion measure. His extroversion score, as well as his overall psychological profile, was more like that of the world class wrestlers previously described by Morgan.[4] In other words, it would seem imperative that additional data be generated prior to making an attempt at presenting a psychological stereotype intended to characterize marathoners. It should be noted, however, that an extensive body of literature exists in the field of sport psychology suggesting that individual sport athletes (e.g., runners) are more introverted than team sport athletes, and also, noncontact athletes (e.g., runners) have typically been observed to be more introverted than contact athletes.[5] Hence, the earlier findings of Morgan and Costill [2] do fit with theoretical expectations to a certain degree. A second reason why their earlier findings should be viewed with caution, however, is that personality structure in sport may well differ as a function of ability level. Indeed, the recent work of Johnson and Morgan [6] involving successful and unsuccessful college athletes tested during the first week of their college careers reveals that

382

athletic ability is correlated with personality structure. Therefore, the earlier report of Morgan and Costill [2] may not apply to samples comprised solely of elite marathoners. The present paper, unlike the earlier one, is concerned primarily with characterization of elite or world class distance runners.

There are a number of reasons why one might intuitively expect factors of a psychological nature to play an important role in long distance running. First, it appears reasonably clear that endurance performance is governed by both the physical *capacity* and *willingness* of the runner to tolerate the discomfort associated with hard physical work. It appears that substantial differences in both the capacity and willingness to tolerate discomfort exist among marathoners. For example, among finishers of the marathon (26.2 miles or 42.2 km), performance times frequently range from 2 hours 15 minutes to 4 or 5 hours— hence, certainly a considerable difference in capacity, and probably, a fair amount of difference in the willingness to tolerate discomfort. Also, while marathoners perform at approximately 75% of their maximal aerobic power (MAP),[7] the actual range is about 64%–90% of maximum.[8, 9] Of course, the decision to compete at 85% of one's MAP as opposed to 65% obviously represents more than willingness alone. Data presented elsewhere in the present volume clearly attests to the physiological basis of such "decision making." For example, some runners are producing large amounts of lactate at 80% of their MAP whereas others can continue for the full 42.2 km at 85% of their MAP with low lactate levels. Also, the predominant muscle fiber type of the runner is reported elsewhere in this volume to be an important consideration.[10] Therefore, the large individual differences widely observed in marathoners have a substantial physiological basis, and the authors in no way intend to suggest otherwise. An attempt will be made in the present paper, however, to examine the extent to which psychological factors can be useful in characterizing the marathoner.

PROCEDURE

The purposes of this investigation were to (1) compare the psychological characteristics of world class middle-long distance and marathon runners, (2) contrast their psychologic profiles with those of non-world-class runners and athletes from other sports, (3) examine the perceptual processing of "effort sense" information in these runners, and (4) attempt to delineate the factors responsible for *involvement* in competitive running, as well as *adherence* across time.

Subjects

The runners who served as subjects in this investigation consisted of a group of world class athletes ($n = 19$) and a group of college middle distance runners ($n = 8$). The latter runners, while outstanding by college standards, were not of world class caliber. The world class group was further divided into middle-long distance ($n = 11$) and marathon ($n = 8$) subgroups for comparative purposes. Specific details concerning the criteria for subgroup selection are reported earlier in this volume.[11]

Variables

The dependent variables consisted of (1) psychometric test scores obtained from standardized psychological inventories, (2) running histories and race strategies obtained by means of a clinical interview, (3) physiological data obtained during submaximal treadmill running, and (4) ratings of perceived exertion obtained during submaximal running. The details relating to these dependent variables are outlined below.

Psychometric Variables

Each runner completed a battery of psychological inventories during the first evening of the study and prior to the detailed physiological testing described elsewhere in this volume.[11] The inventories consisted of the State-Trait Anxiety Inventory (STAI),[12] Somatic Perception Questionnaire (SPQ),[13] Depression Adjective Checklist (DACL),[14] Profile of Mood States (POMS),[15] Eysenck Personality Inventory (EPI),[16] Physical Estimation and Attraction Scale (PEAS),[17] and the Hidden Shapes Test (HST).[18]

This test battery yielded measures of state and trait anxiety,[12] perception of somatic activity during "stressful" situations,[13] depression,[14] tension, depression, anger, vigor, fatigue, and confusion,[15] extraversion, neuroticism, and conformity,[16] attraction toward physical activity and estimation of physical ability,[17] and field dependence.[18]

Running History and Strategy

A taped clinical interview lasting approximately 45 minutes to 1 hour was carried out with each runner individually. This interview consisted of questions relating to the runner's current training program, occupation, family structure, diet, use of common drugs (e.g., aspirin, alcohol, coffee, and tea), use of tobacco, sleep patterns, and so on. Also, the runner was asked to respond to each of the following questions in 25 words or less: (1) Explain why you first became involved in competitive running. (2) Explain why you continue to run competitively. The runners were encouraged to respond spontaneously, describing the first impressions or thoughts that came to mind. The first question was concerned with the general issue of *involvement* (or gravitation), whereas the second was directed toward the matter of *adherence*—two different but interdependent variables. They were also asked to respond to the following question, but unlike the first two questions there was no limit placed on response length—indeed, the runners were encouraged to elaborate on this question as much as possible: (3) Describe what you think about during a long distance run or marathon. What sort of thought processes take place as a run progresses? There is no limit on the length of your response. Please talk in detail about this matter.

Evaluation of data from the various objective psychological inventories was carried out in accordance with specified scoring procedures described in each of the test manuals. Interpretation of the taped interviews was considerably less objective, but it was possible to identify major thematic processes, as well as answer specific questions posed *a priori*. The following hypotheses were tested in this portion of the study:

(H_1) The motivational forces responsible for *initial* involvement in running would not be characterized by a single thematic dimension.

(H_2) The forces responsible for adherence or continuation in competitive running would be both extrinsic and intrinsic.

(H_3) Dissociation of sensory input would represent the principal "cognitive strategy" employed by these world class distance runners during competition.

Physiological and Perceptual Variables

Maximal and submaximal exercise tests were carried out on each runner as described elsewhere in this volume.[19] Ratings of perceived exertion (RPE) were obtained during submaximal exercise in an attempt to characterize the manner in which these runners processed sensory information relating to physical effort ("effort sense"). The RPE values were obtained using the psychophysical category scale developed by Borg,[20] and the ratings were made during a submaximal test in which the subjects ran at 10 mph (4.5 m/sec) 7 minutes, and 12 mph (5.5 m/sec) for an additional 4 minutes on a motor driven treadmill. The grade was maintained at 0% throughout the run.

The RPE scale ranges from 6 to 20, and the odd numbered categories have verbal anchors (7 = very, very light; 9 = very light; 11 = fairly light; 13 = somewhat hard; 15 = hard, 17 = very hard; and 19 = very, very hard). While the perceptual ratings were being obtained, physiological data were simultaneously acquired. This permitted a comparison of factors such as heart rate, oxygen consumption, ventilatory minute volume, and lactate accumulation in the three groups of runners. More importantly, it was thus possible to study the juxtaposition of perceptual ratings and physiologic responsivity. The physiological data are reported on in detail earlier in this volume.[19]

RESULTS AND DISCUSSION

Psychometric Data

The means, standard deviations, and standard errors for all of the psychological variables appear in TABLE 1 for the total group ($n = 27$). Also, a one-way ANOVA was performed on these data for the three separate groups, and the means and F ratios resulting from these analyses appear in TABLE 2.

This analysis revealed that the world class middle-long distance runners and marathon runners did not differ significantly ($p > 0.05$) on any of the 16 variables, nor did these groups differ from the college runners. Indeed, inspection of the mean data reveals a remarkable similarity for the three groups. Therefore, the three groups were combined for purposes of drawing comparisons with other athlete groups, as well as with published norms for college students.

A comparison of the runners in the present study with previously tested high-level U.S. wrestlers[21] and rowers,[22] appears in FIGURE 1 for data obtained with the POMS.[15] Also, the mean for college students (T score = 50) is represented by the solid line, and the broken lines represent a departure of one standard deviation from the mean. It will be noted that the runners possess

TABLE 1

RAW SCORE MEANS, STANDARD DEVIATIONS, AND STANDARD ERRORS FOR ALL RUNNERS
ON EACH PSYCHOLOGICAL VARIABLE

Variable	Mean ($n=27$)	Standard Deviation	Standard Error
State anxiety	33.50	6.89	1.30
Trait anxiety	31.68	9.27	1.75
Somatic perception	20.93	5.50	1.04
Tension	10.46	5.57	1.05
Depression (POMS)	6.82	7.93	1.50
Anger	7.89	6.03	1.14
Vigor	21.07	5.60	1.06
Fatigue	6.89	5.30	1.00
Confusion	7.43	4.12	0.78
Extraversion	13.43	4.65	0.88
Neuroticism	9.43	5.42	1.02
Exercise attitude	42.64	4.70	0.89
Self esteem	26.89	5.15	0.97
Field dependence	22.75	12.20	2.31
Depression (DACL)	3.96	2.70	0.51
Conformity	3.14	1.82	0.34

TABLE 2

COMPARISON OF RAW SCORE MEANS FOR WORLD CLASS MIDDLE-LONG DISTANCE
AND MARATHON RUNNERS WITH COLLEGE MIDDLE DISTANCE RUNNERS
ON EACH PSYCHOLOGICAL VARIABLE *

Variable	World Class Runners		College Runners ($n=8$)	F
	Middle-Long Distance ($n=11$)	Marathon ($n=8$)		
State anxiety	33.82	32.75	33.75	0.06
Trait anxiety	34.91	26.63	33.00	2.04
Somatic perception	22.18	19.25	20.38	0.66
Tension	10.91	9.75	10.88	0.11
Depression (POMS)	9.18	3.88	6.88	1.01
Anger	8.73	6.75	8.13	0.23
Vigor	19.00	22.75	21.25	1.14
Fatigue	6.81	6.38	7.88	0.16
Confusion	8.82	5.63	7.63	1.40
Extraversion	13.27	12.75	14.88	0.44
Neuroticism	10.27	11.00	6.50	1.66
Exercise attitude	42.27	41.38	43.63	0.46
Self Esteem	26.46	26.38	28.00	0.24
Field dependence	21.27	21.75	25.63	0.30
Depression (DACL)	4.73	4.13	3.13	0.81
Conformity	3.73	2.25	3.38	0.46

* Differences between groups were found not to be significant ($p > 0.05$).

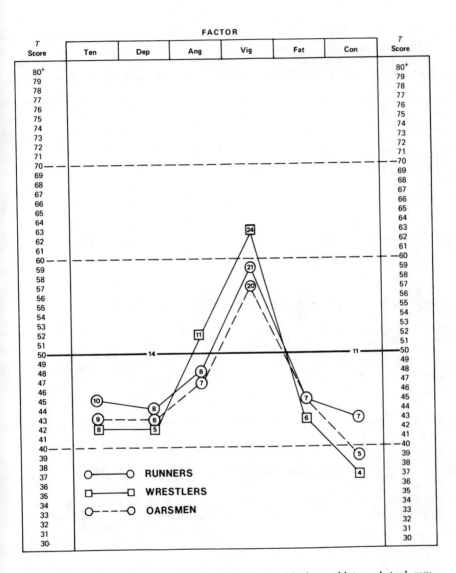

FIGURE 1. The "iceberg" profile identified for world class athletes. Actual raw score units for tension, depression, anger, vigor, fatigue, and confusion as measured by the Profile of Mood States appear in the boxes and circles.

psychological profiles that are quite similar to high-level athletes in wrestling and crew. However, all three groups score appreciably *below* the population mean for tension, depression, fatigue, and confusion, and *above* the mean for vigor. These differences favor the athlete samples in every instance, and the observed group profiles for the athletes can be regarded as positive from a mental health standpoint. The senior author has previously described the observed psychometric configuration as the "iceberg" profile. In other words,

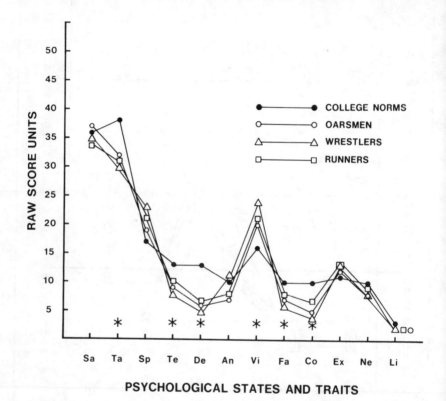

FIGURE 2. Comparison of selected world class athlete groups with college norms for the complete psychological test battery. The variables in abbreviated form are: state anxiety (SA), trait anxiety (TA), somatic perception (SP), tension (Te), depression (De), anger (An), vigor (Vi), fatigue (Fa), confusion (Co), extroversion (Ex), neuroticism (Ne), and conformity (Li).

high-level athletes score below the mean (surface) on the negative psychological constructs contained in the POMS, but above the mean (surface) for the one positively anchored construct (vigor). The actual raw scores for all of the variables appear in FIGURE 2 for the runners tested in the present study and the previously tested wrestlers and oarsmen, as well as means based on published norms. Variables *Te* through *Co* in this figure constitute data obtained from the POMS,[15] and it will be noted that five of the six significant differences (denoted with asterisks) were accounted for with this scale. Also, the only *trait* variable on which differences existed between the athlete samples and the college norms was that of *trait* anxiety in which the athletes were found to score significantly lower ($p < 0.05$). It should also be noted, and emphasized, that these athlete samples *were not* more extroverted (variable *Ex*) or stable (variable *Ne*) than the college norms, which contradicts a substantial portion of earlier research in the field of sport psychology.[5] Also, the earlier finding[2] that marathoners are more introverted than world class wrestlers was not supported in the present comparison. Further, the marathoners were not more introverted than the general population as reported earlier.[2] However, the finding that runners are significantly less anxious and depressed than the general population was in agreement with the earlier report of Morgan and Costill.[2] Whether these consistently observed positive differences in *affect* (or mood) represent the result of years of training, or whether long distance runners differ from the outset on these selected behavioral manifestations remains to be demonstrated with longitudinal research. In the meantime, however, since the runners and other athletes possess extroversion and neuroticism scores (*trait* measures) similar to the college norms, it seems quite likely that low anxiety and depression scores (*state* measures) in runners represent a *consequence* of involvement in distance running rather than reflecting an *antecedent* condition.

The observation that these runners, and athletes from other subgroups as well, scored lower than the college norms on tension (POMS)[15] but not on state anxiety (STAI)[12] warrants comment since these variables are presumably tapping the *same* psychological construct. At first glance this appears to be contradictory. However, the "instructional sets" for these two inventories differ in that the respondent is advised to reply in terms of how he or she *feels at this moment* when completing the STAI[12] whereas the "set" used with the POMS[15] requests the subject to reply in terms of "how you have been feeling during the past week including today." Since the tension scale of the POMS and the state anxiety scale of the STAI are highly correlated, it is fair to assume that a lack of complete concordance in our findings was due to elevated state anxiety in these runners at the time of testing, which was due to the test situation *per se*. This view is supported by the finding that these runners scored significantly lower than the college norms on *trait* anxiety as measured by the STAI.[12] Trait anxiety, however, would not be expected to change in a stressful situation since it represents an enduring as opposed to transient (state) variable. Methodological factors such as those cited above are often useful in explaining the many "controversial" or "contradictory" findings that have been found in the field of sport psychology.

Interview Data

The purpose of the interview data was to (1) test the three hypotheses cited earlier and (2) describe the health behavior of these elite runners. The first hypothesis was *confirmed* in that no single underlying factor or force was responsible for initial involvement in distance running. However, it is noteworthy that none of the runners initially became involved because of the nature of running or its intrinsic appeal. A variety of reasons were given such as (1) peer influence, (2) parental influence, (3) inability to take part in other sports because of body size, (4) a means of getting in shape for another sport such as basketball, and (5) early success in running races held during grade school or junior high school physical education classes.

The second hypothesis was also confirmed in that *adherence* or continuation in competitive running was found to be related to both *extrinsic* and *intrinsic* rewards. The extrinsic rewards related to positive reinforcement resulting from the winning of awards, ability to travel extensively throughout the world, and so on. The intrinsic rewards centered around the sheer joy of running and the sense of well-being resulting from training and competing. Each runner reported that he would continue running for the remainder of his life regardless of whether or not it was possible to continue competing. Hence, the vocational nature of the runner's life style clearly possesses an avocational dimension.

The third hypothesis was rejected, and this represents a major finding in our view. *Dissociation* of sensory input did not represent the principal "cognitive strategy," but rather, these elite marathon runners were found to utilize an *associative* strategy. These runners reported that (1) they paid very close attention to bodily input such as feelings and sensations arising in their feet, calves, and thighs, as well as their respiration; (2) whereas they paid attention to time ("the clock"), pace was largely governed by "reading their bodies"; (3) they identified certain runners they would like to stay with during a given run if possible, but they did not typically employ a "leeching" strategy; (4) during any given marathon they constantly reminded or told themselves to "relax," "stay loose," and so forth; and (5) they typically did not encounter "pain zones" during the marathon, and most of these elite runners dismissed the phenomenon referred to as "the wall" as simply a myth—that is, they did not "come up against the wall" during the marathon run.

Prior work conducted by the senior author [23] revealed that marathon runners characteristically attempt to "dissociate" sensory input during competition. Previous interviews with 20 marathoners, as well as more recent interview data from long distance runners, revealed that these athletes are "cognitively active" during competition, but this cognitive activity seldom, if ever, relates to the actual running. Also, this general finding has since been observed for long distance swimmers and cyclists as well. The cognitive strategy employed by these athletes can best be regarded as "dissociative cognitive rehearsal." Many runners reconstruct images of past events throughout the 42.2 km run. For example, one of the first marathoners interviewed by the senior author routinely rehearsed or reconstructed his entire educational experience during each marathon. During the run he would age regress himself to first grade and attempt to recall as much as possible about the experience (e.g., the teacher's name and face, the names and faces of other boys and girls in the class, various experiences such as learning to read, print, work with crayons, and paste, playing an instrument in the rhythm band, recess, and so on). After a while he would proceed to second grade, recall salient "chunks" of information, and then proceed to third grade. This continued throughout grade school, high school, college, his oral defense, receipt of the Ph.D., as well as his current postdoctoral experiences. This marathoner always reconstructed his educational experience during the marathon; it was always somewhat unique, however, in that he would remember different people, events, and activities each time. In other words, the theme was always the same, but the content varied. Other runners have described remarkably similar approaches, and it would be redundant to proceed with a review of these case studies.[23] Suffice it to say that another runner always builds a house when he marathons; another writes letters to everyone he owes a letter to; another listens to a stack of Beethoven records; another participates in extremely complex mathematical exercises; another steps on the imaginary faces of two co-workers she detests throughout the marathon; another repeatedly sings the Star Spangled Banner in crescendo fashion; another age regresses and becomes a steam locomotive at the base of heartbreak hill; and so on. The various rehearsal themes are rather different, but they all seem to be directed toward the same end—dissociating the painful sensory input. As a matter of fact, most of these runners have reported that use of these techniques helps them negotiate various pain zones and particularly the proverbial (or mythical?) wall.

It is of interest that anthropological reports of Tibetan monks trained in the art of *lung-gom* (swiftness of foot) suggest that a similar form of dissociation may have been used in making possible their alleged, extraordinary runs. For example, it has been reported by Watson[18] that one monk covered more than 300 miles in 30 hours. In other words, he averaged over 10 mph over uneven terrain in a hostile environment (altitude and cold). This performance would equal eleven and a half consecutive marathons at 2:37, or three 100 mile runs of 10 hours each. Such a performance would compare rather favorably with our best marathoners of today running a 12 mph pace at sea level; with moderate temperature ranges; on even road surfaces; and with the best shoes money can buy! The "cognitive strategy" allegedly used by these specially trained monks consisted of the following: While running the monk repeated to himself a secret or sacred phrase (mantra). His respiration was kept in rhythm with the phrase, and his locomotion was put in synchrony with both his respiration and the phrase. The runner fixed his eyes on a distant object, and did not look from side to side, nor did he speak.[18]

In many respects the technique described above is almost identical with the procedure utilized by two marathoners interviewed earlier. Further, portions of the above procedure were used by all of the marathoners in the earlier case studies.

Unfortunately, the validity of such anthropological reports is always open to question. Therefore, the efficacy of such a procedure was recently evaluated under controlled laboratory conditions by Morgan et al.[23] They employed a procedure very similar to that explained earlier for the Mahetang monks with the exception that a "pseudo-mantra," the word *down*, was substituted for the sacred phrase. Using a single-blind, placebo design they found that a simple dissociation strategy of the type described for the Mahetangs resulted in performance gains that averaged 30% over base-line in contrast with both control and placebo treatments. Their subjects were young adult males, and the endurance task consisted of walking to complete exhaustion at 80% of $\dot{V}_{O_2 \text{ max}}$. The enhanced performance, however, was not associated with cardiovascular, metabolic, or endocrine changes. Hence, the gain in performance took place as a result of the subjects willingness to endure or cope with the distress and pain of continued effort.

It has been known for sometime, of course, that endurance performance can be facilitated by means of hypnosis under a variety of conditions.[24] For example, running performance in the 10,000 meters race, bicycle ergometer sprint speed, shoulder and upper arm endurance, and hand endurance have all been facilitated by means of hypnotic suggestion.[24] It has also been demonstrated more recently that perception of effort during standardized bicycle ergometry can be manipulated hypnotically,[25, 26] and exercise heart rate can be increased, as well as decreased during constant work by means of instrumental conditioning using biofeedback techniques.[27] Therefore, it would seem that either through formal (hypnosis or biofeedback) or informal procedures it would be possible for marathoners to facilitate their performances. Hence, it is not surprising that all of the runners interviewed in our earlier case studies employed various self-taught techniques that can best be viewed as dissociative.

The world class marathoners in the present study, however, did not employ such strategies. Indeed, rather than dissociate, these runners characteristically reported a strategy that we feel can best be viewed as *associative* in nature—not *dissociative*. However, it now becomes clear in retrospect that we were dealing with two rather distinct samples from the marathon community. Our first group consisted of average runners who completed the marathon in times ranging from 3 to 4 hours, whereas the present world class group consisted of several runners who had performed below 2:15 and all of them had performed under 2:20.

Additional questions asked during the interview dealt with health-related items such as usage of tobacco, alcohol, coffee, tea, and aspirin; training frequency and duration; reasons for running (not competing); birth order; sleep patterns; and perception of training intensity. A summary of these data are presented below for the elite marathon group.

All of the elite marathoners trained seven days per week, they averaged 100.7 miles per week, and they devoted about 2½ hours daily to training. Also, these runners reported a mean value of 13.6 for training intensity according to the Borg Scale.

The primary reason advanced for running on a regular basis was that it made them "feel good." However, two runners responded that their training was a means to an end, with the end being competition. In other words, these two marathon runners, unlike the other six, did not regard running as an end in itself. On the other hand, both runners reported they would continue running for the remainder of their lives even if they were not able to compete. It is conceivable that these two runners may not have been consciously aware of the primary motivational forces responsible for their involvement in running.

There exists a rather substantial literature dealing with the relationship of ordinal position among siblings and success in various activities. Of the runners in this study, four were firstborn, three mid-born, and one last-born. Unfortunately, the sample size was too small to make meaningful comparisons on this variable, but a ratio of 4:1 for first to last born suggests that ordinal position may be worthy of further study in connection with characterization of distance runners.

Six of the eight marathoners had experimented with the smoking of cigarettes, and the mean age for this initial experimentation was 11 years (range: 10–12). However, only one of the runners *ever* smoked five or more cigarettes on a regular basis and this occurred at the age of 13 years for a brief period in the life of this particular runner. Hence, it is possible to conclude that not only were none of these runners smokers, but for all practical purposes, they had *never* smoked.

Consumption of alcoholic beverages was considered from the standpoint of the number of (1) 12-ounce bottles of beer, (2) 6-ounce glasses of wine, or (3) one 1-ounce shots of liquor consumed per week. Six of the marathon runners did not consume liquor, one consumed an average of one ounce per week, and the last reported a weekly consumption of 18 ounces. Four of the runners did not consume wine, and the remaining four averaged three glasses per week with a range of 1–5. Only one of the runners abstained completely from beer, and the consumption in the remaining seven averaged 9.7 bottles per week. However, the range was 1–30 bottles per week and the mean of 9.7 is skewed as a result of two runners who reported consuming 24 and 30 bottles per week, respectively. It is of some interest that the runner who reported having 24 bottles per week also consumed the largest amount of liquor per week (18 ounces).

Four of the eight marathon runners did not consume coffee, and the remaining four averaged three cups per day (range: 1–5). Also, four of the runners did not consume tea, and the remaining four averaged 4½ cups per day. However, this latter mean is skewed due to one runner who reported a daily consumption of 12 cups.

None of the eight marathoners consumed aspirin, and tension reduction through exercise might be offered as one of the reasons for this observation. Also, these runners averaged 7¾ hours of sleep per night with a range of 6 to 9 hours.

These findings suggest that elite marathon runners are quite homogeneous with respect to (1) the frequency, duration, and intensity of training; (2) the reasons for involvement in running; (3) amount of daily sleep; (4) aspirin utilization; and (5) smoking behavior. However, there is a *tendency* for elite marathoners to be firstborn, and they are extremely heterogeneous with respect to consumption of coffee, tea, and alcohol.

It should also be noted that all of the eight marathoners participated in track and/or cross country during high school. Three of the eight also received varsity letters in basketball during high school, one in cross country skiing, and one in swimming. It is noteworthy that none of these runners had received varsity letters in contact sports such as wrestling or football. Further, all of these athletes went on to earn varsity letters in track and cross country at the college level, but none of them lettered in additional sports as they had in high school. It should be recalled that one of the major reasons why some of the runners went out for cross country during their high school years was to get in shape for another sport such as basketball.

Physiological and Perceptual Data

Physiological data has been reported in detail for the same runners elsewhere in the present volume.[10, 11] The selected data presented here are limited to submaximal exercise responsivity in order to better understand the perception of effort. The means and standard deviations for selected physiological variables appear in TABLE 3. Also, a one-way ANOVA was performed on each variable, and the resulting F ratio and associated probability are given for each comparison. The Newman-Keuls procedure described by Winer[28] was applied when a significant difference for group means occurred.

It will be noted that the three groups did not differ in body weight, percent body fat, or maximal exercise heart rate. A significant difference in groups was observed for maximal aerobic power, and the Newman-Keuls probe revealed that both world class groups scored significantly higher than the college runners. Also, the middle-long distance runners were significantly higher (5 ml/kg·min) than the marathon group. A significant difference was also observed for submaximal exercise lactate, with the elite groups scoring significantly lower than

TABLE 3

COMPARISON OF SELECTED PHYSIOLOGICAL VARIABLES FOR WORLD CLASS
MIDDLE-LONG DISTANCE AND MARATHON RUNNERS AND COLLEGE MIDDLE
DISTANCE RUNNERS

| | World Class Runners | | | | |
| | Middle-Long Distance ($n=11$) | Marathon ($n=8$) | College Runners ($n=8$) | F | p |
Variables					
Body weight (kg)	63.10	61.53	66.85	0.63	NS
Body Fat (%)	5.79	4.63	6.81	0.85	NS
$\dot{V}_{O_2max}$ (ml/kg·min)	78.77	74.10	68.91	20.41	<0.001
Maximum HR (bpm)	198.73	195.75	195.12	0.63	NS
Submaximal exercise lactate level (mg%)	30.73	31.00	69.00	18.66	<0.001

the college runners but not differing from each other. This latter finding is understandable since post-hoc analyses revealed the elite groups were running at 84% of maximum while the college group was performing at 95% of maximum during the same submaximal work bout at 12 mph.

The mean perceived exertion ratings for the three groups across the submaximal runs is illustrated in FIGURE 3. It will de noted that the three groups have very similar RPE values during the first two minutes of exercise at 10 mph, and while the elite groups are lower than the college runners at the fourth and sixth minutes, these latter differences are not significant. However, since the elite runners achieved both a perceptual and physiological steady state at 10 mph, and since the college runners had not achieved such states by the sixth minute, it is quite likely that perceptual differences would have emerged with continued running at 10 mph. Once the treadmill speed was increased to 12 mph all groups experienced a significant increase in perception of effort, and at this higher speed the college runners perceived the exercise intensity to be significantly greater than did the elite runners. Also, it will be noted in FIGURE 3 that the elite distance runners tend to enter a perceptual steady state at this speed, and, of course, many members of this group compete at a 12-mph pace.

Mean data for perceived exertion, heart rate, and ventilatory minute volume appear in TABLES 4 and 5 in connection with the runs at 10 mph and 12 mph, respectively. It is clear that the elite runners encountered a significantly ($p < 0.001$) lower exercise stress at 10 mph when exercise demand is evaluated in terms of heart rate or ventilatory minute volume. However, the fact that the groups did not differ in their perception of effort must be regarded as a major finding in this investigation. In other words, while the runners of lesser ability were exercising at a significantly higher metabolic load, they perceived the cost to be the same. A similar finding was noted in the perceptual responses of candidates for the 1972 U.S. Olympic Freestyle Wrestling Team. While the ten men who eventually made the team were physiologically superior to the thirty who did not, the two groups did not differ in their perception of effort at an absolute work intensity of 750 kpm/min (125 W).[23] The consequences of inaccurately perceiving exercise cost has many readily apparent implications for the competitive situation.

The nature of the physiological differences that existed for the three groups of runners is illustrated in FIGURES 4, 5, and 6. These figures reveal that the elite runners had a significantly lower heart rate and ventilatory minute volume, and they were running at a lower percent of their maximal aerobic power during every minute of exercise at both 10 and 12 mph.

The increase in percent of maximal aerobic power that the runners were forced to work at in going from 10 to 12 mph was essentially the same for all three groups; that is, an increase of about 15% resulted. The mean perceptual ratings, however, differ at 12 mph whereas they did not differ at 10 mph. The RPE values summarized in TABLE 5 reveal that the two elite groups perceived the exercise intensity to be the same, and this agreement is consonant with expectations derived from the measured physiological parameters. The higher RPE values for the less capable runners are also compatible with the physiological observations. A logical question would seem to be why such a difference exists at 12 mph but not 10 mph? One possibility might be that the onset of anaerobisis in the college runners, who were now at 95% of maximum, triggered the perceptual difference. This would appear to be tenable since running at

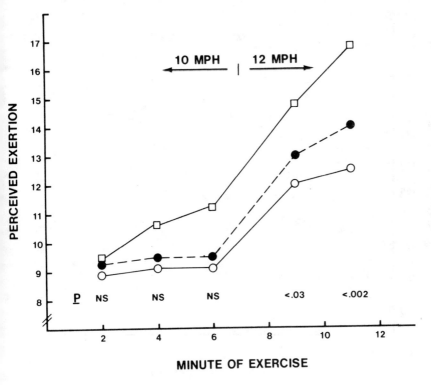

FIGURE 3. Ratings of perceived exertion in the elite marathon (O—O) and middle-long distance runners (●—●) and the college middle distance runners (□—□).

TABLE 4

COMPARISON OF PERCEIVED EXERTION AND SELECTED METABOLIC VARIABLES OF WORLD CLASS MIDDLE-LONG DISTANCE AND MARATHON RUNNERS WITH COLLEGE DISTANCE RUNNERS OBTAINED DURING TREADMILL RUNNING AT 10 mph (4.4 m/sec) AND 0% GRADE

| | World Class Runners | | | | |
Variable	Middle-Long Distance ($n=11$)	Marathon ($n=8$)	College Runners ($n=8$)	F	p
At 2 minutes					
Heart rate (bpm)	157.18	154.50	171.62	8.70	<0.001
Perceived exertion	9.27	8.88	9.50	0.16	NS
At 4 minutes					
Heart rate (bpm)	161.45	154.00	175.00	8.77	<0.001
Perceived exertion	9.45	9.13	10.63	1.57	NS
At 6 minutes					
Heart rate (bpm)	164.27	159.00	178.25	9.44	<0.001
Perceived exertion	10.09	9.50	11.25	1.59	NS
$\dot{V}_E$ (liter/min)	84.18	84.00	107.12	10.66	<0.001

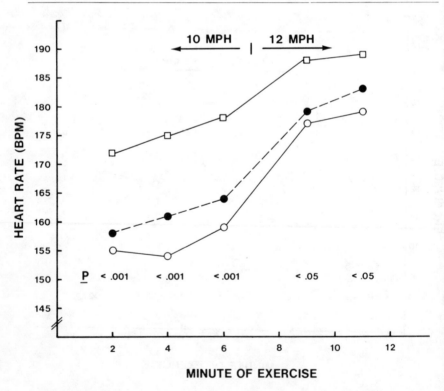

FIGURE 4. Heart rate for the elite marathon (O—O) and middle-long distance runners (●—●) and the college middle distance runners (□—□) during submaximal exercise.

TABLE 5

COMPARISON OF PERCEIVED EXERTION AND SELECTED METABOLIC VARIABLES
OF WORLD CLASS MIDDLE-LONG DISTANCE AND MARATHON RUNNERS WITH
COLLEGE DISTANCE RUNNERS DURING TREADMILL RUNNING AT 12 mph
(5.3 m/sec) AND 0% GRADE *

	World Class Runners		College Runners (n=8)	F	p
Variable	Middle-Long Distance (n=11)	Marathon (n=8)			
At 9 minutes					
Heart rate (bpm)	179.27	177.25	187.62	3.51	<0.05
Perceived exertion	13.00	12.00	14.75	3.92	<0.03
$\dot{V}_E$ (liter/min)	109.80	111.75	144.75	12.71	<0.001
At 11 minutes					
Heart rate (bpm)	182.82	179.12	189.37	3.54	<0.05
Perceived exertion	14.00	12.50	16.75	7.91	<0.002
$\dot{V}_E$ (liter/min)	120.20	120.37	154.12	13.70	<0.001

* First 7 minutes were run at 10 mph, 0% grade.

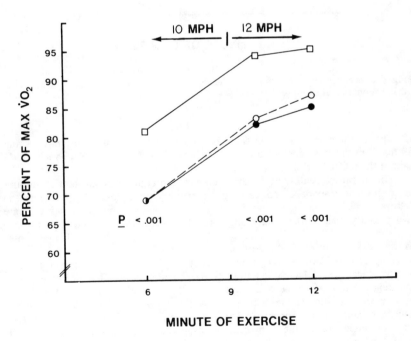

FIGURE 5. Percent of $\dot{V}_{O_2max}$ in the elite marathon (○—○) and middle-long distance runners (●—●) and the college middle distance runners (□—□) during submaximal exercise.

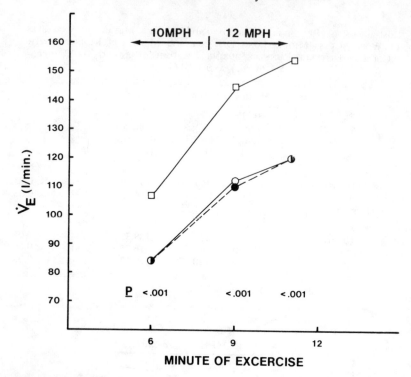

FIGURE 6. Ventilatory minute volume for the elite marathon (○—○) and middle-long distance runners (●—●) and the college middle distance runners (□—□) during submaximal exercise.

12 mph resulted in a mean lactate level of 31 mg% in the elite runners and 69 mg% in the less capable runners. The observed F ratio of 18.66 was significant at the 0.001 level (TABLE 3).

The literature dealing with perceived exertion contains a substantial amount of contradictory evidence concerning the primary physiological input(s) to the "effort sense." Some investigators, for example, have proposed that heart rate is a primary cue,[20] others have suggested that ventilatory minute volume is a key stimulus,[25, 26] and still others have argued that accumulation of metabolites in the working muscles represents a potent input.[23] These arguments have historically centered around the issue of "central" (e.g., heart rate or ventilation) vensus "local" (e.g., lactate accumulation) considerations. In order to evaluate the relationship of perceived exertion with exercise heart rate, ventilatory minute volume and lactate accumulation, these variables were intercorrelated. The correlation matrix appears in TABLE 6. The raw data utilized in this analysis were obtained during the 11th minute of submaximal exercise (12 mph, 0% grade) with the exception that the lactate data were based upon the assay of blood drawn 3 minutes following the exercise bout.

Inspection of TABLE 6 reveals that RPE was significantly correlated with each of the variables, although the magnitude of the correlations differed substantially. Heart rate, for example, accounted for only 18% of the variance, while lactate accounted for 37% or twice as much of the variance. Ventilatory minute volume was intermediary, accounting for 27% of the variance. Hence, while causality in no way can be argued, it is obvious that lactate accumulation is the single best predictor of the runner's subjective estimate of perceptual cost.

SUMMARY

The findings of this investigation can be interpreted in a straightforward fashion for the most part. First, the psychometric data reveal that elite distance runners resemble outstanding athletes in other sports such as wrestling and rowing, and their *affect* (or mood) seems to be consistently superior to that of the general population. Further, since they do not differ from the general population on personality *traits* such as extroversion–introversion and neuroticism stability (enduring qualities), it is theorized that the positive affective profiles (states) reflect the *consequence* of involvement in distance running, not an *antecedent* or selection factor.

Second, the interview data can be interpreted as suggesting that distance runners belong to a rather unique subculture in various ways besides being affectively one standard deviation from the population mean. This uniqueness is reflected in their consummatory behavior as relates to the use of alcohol, tobacco, coffee, tea, and aspirin. Also, their daily investment in running and various forms of training averages 2½ hours, which clearly has vocational connotations. The interview data also suggests that many motivational forces were operative in terms of initial involvement in running, but the most frequently cited explanations were extrinsic in nature. On the other hand, the reasons for adherence were both extrinsic and intrinsic, and there was not a single runner who did not report that he would continue running once the extrinsic rewards were gone.

The major way in which the elite marathoners studied in this investigation differed from those we have interviewed previously (nonelite), was in their cognitive activity during competition. Whereas the nonelite employ a cognitive strategy designed to *dissociate* painful input, the elite runner *associates* and attempts to process this information, or "read his body" and modulate pace

TABLE 6

CORRELATION MATRIX FOR PERCEIVED EXERTION, HEART RATE, VENTILATORY MINUTE VOLUME, AND LACTATE ACCUMULATION DURING SUBMAXIMAL RUNNING AT 12 mph AND 0% GRADE ($n=27$)

Variables	Variables			
	1	2	3	4
1. Perceived exertion	—	0.43 *	0.52 †	0.61 †
2. Heart rate (bpm)		—	0.14	0.44 *
3. $\dot{V}_E$ (liter/min)			—	0.65 †
4. Lactate (mg %)				—

* p $<$0.05.
† p $<$0.01.

accordingly. The elite runner does not place much emphasis on "the wall" or "pain zones," and there are probably at least two reasons why they differ from the nonelite runner in this respect. First, their physiological superiority permits them to run at a greater percentage of their maximum without encountering discomfort. The elite marathoners, for example, had a mean lactate level of 31 mg% in connection with treadmill running at 12 mph, whereas the less capable runners manifested values twice this level. Also, lactate was found to be the best single predictor of "effort sense" in this study. Second, it is quite likely that elite runners avoid pain zones and fail to come up against the wall simply because they *associate,* i.e., monitor sensory input, and adjust their pace accordingly, with the net result that "pain" is avoided. Of course, and this must be kept in mind, the elite runner can afford the luxury of associating, whereas the nonelite cannot. This overall matter is summarized schematically in FIG-URE 7.

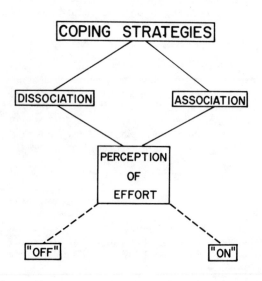

FIGURE 7. Coping strategies used in the perception of effort.

On the basis of our interviews it seems reasonable to propose that mara-thoners might adopt what appears to be two rather divergent "coping strategies." In the one instance it is possible to *dissociate* sensory input because of the dis-comfort it creates, and in the other case it is possible to cope by means of *associating* or "paying attention to 'bodily' signals." In terms of perception of effort these two cognitive strategies are best viewed as rather diverse approaches with the first basically turning the *perceptostat* on, and the latter turning it off. In work with young adult males the efficacy of dissociation has been demon-strated by Morgan *et al.*[23] whereby endurance performance has been consistently facilitated. However, their work was carried out under laboratory conditions with continuous monitoring designed to identify biomedical indices that might contraindicate continued exertion. In this overall context the senior author had occasion to interview a number of casualties following the 1976 "City to Surf" run that is held annually in Sydney, Australia. One young male runner was brought to the medical facility complaining of intense pain in both lower legs.

The runner reported that he experienced pain in one leg at approximately 3 miles into the run and attempted to "run through the pain"; later he experienced similar pain in the opposite limb and attempted to fight through this "pain zone" as well; finally, he had to simply discontinue because the pain became unbearable. It seems reasonable to classify the runner's predominant cognitive strategy as being one of dissociation. Subsequent radiologic examination revealed clean fractures of both the left and right fibula. In all likelihood these injuries could have been prevented had the runner not attempted to dissociate the painful input (signals). Of course, this would have meant dropping out of the run and losing the prior investment of time and training. In other words, while dissociation can facilitate endurance performance [23] under certain conditions, it also carries the attendant risk of tissue, organ, and system(s) trauma.

A simplistic analogy can be drawn between the runner and the household furnace. The furnace is driven by a thermostat, and by analogy we can think of the runner as being driven by his or her *perceptostat* (FIGURE 7). The perceptostat can be viewed as the center of a sensory system that integrates all other sensory systems along with information stores built from past environmental experiences. If one were to turn a thermostat completely on or off when temperature demands operated in opposing directions, there would be a system failure. Also, a thermostat that is not finely tuned will work, but it will be characterized by inefficiency. Most of us have experienced the consequences of a malfunctioning thermostat in that it consistently overshoots and undershoots with the result that it creates an environment that is either hot or cold, and the desired optimum reflected by the actual thermostat is seldom achieved. It is proposed that runners who dissociate resemble such a thermostat in many respects. First, dissociation results in turning the perceptostat off, and it stays off until alerted by a cue to resume functioning. The cut might come in the form of dyspnea or parathesia, or it might be triggered by more serious stimuli such as the onset of heat exhaustion or a bone fracture. At any rate, such an approach would be quite inefficient, and, unlike the elite runner who incurs a deficit at the outset of a run and then achieves a relative steady state through association, the dissociative runner by contrast would incur deficits throughout a run, begin to associate following receipt of "alerting" cues, adjust the pace, repay the deficit, and then return to the dissociative state. The consequence of utilizing such a strategy would be the inefficient utilization of fuel, and the net result would be that such a runner would eventually "come up against the wall," perhaps discontinue the race, or, at best, simply perform at a level below his or her capability.

Since the elite marathon runners consumed significantly less oxygen at the same speed than the middle-long distance runners, and in view of the fact that they did not differ remarkably from a biomechanical standpoint, it would appear that their conscious focus on relaxation, albeit apparently informal, was responsible in part for the lower oxygen consumption. While these differences are small when viewed in terms of ml/kg·min, extension of such a difference across 42 kilometers takes on a significant meaning. At any rate, whether one's chief concern is with performance or avoidance of trauma, an associative strategy would appear to be more efficacious than a dissociative one. A question that remains unanswered relates to the issue of whether the elite runners learn to employ associative techniques or whether they simply possess this quality. This may be an academic point, however, since individuals can readily be taught to either associate or dissociate.[23]

Conclusion

It is concluded that elite marathon runners are very similar from a psychometric standpoint to middle-long distance runners as well as world class athletes in other sports such as wrestling and crew. It is also concluded that elite marathon runners are characterized by positive mental health from an affective standpoint, and this positive affect is regarded as a consequence of training and competition since these world class athletes resemble the general population on most psychological trai... It is further concluded that the major distinguishing psychological dimension of the elite marathoner is in their "effort sense" in that these runners employ an associative cognitive strategy during competition.

References

1. Costill, D. L. 1968. What Research Tells the Coach About Distance Running. AAHPER Publications. Washington, D.C.
2. Morgan, W. P. & D. L. Costill. 1972. Psychological characteristics of the marathon runner. J. Sports Med. Phys. Fitness. **12:** 42–46.
3. Costill, D. L., H. Thomason & E. Roberts. Fractional utilization of the aerobic capacity during distance running. Med. Sci. in Sports. **5:** 248–252.
4. Morgan, W. P. 1968. Personality characteristics of wrestlers participating in the world championships. J. Sports Med. Phys. Fitness. **8:** 212–216.
5. Morgan, W. P. 1971. Sport psychology. *In* Psychomotor Domain: Movement Behavior. 1st edit. R. N. Singer, Ed. : 193–228. Lea & Febiger. Philadelphia, Pa.
6. Johnson, R. W. & W. P. Morgan. (In prep.) MMPI profiles of successful and and unsuccessful university athletes in twelve selected sports.
7. Costill, D. L. & E. L. Fox. 1969. Energetics of marathon running. Med. & Sci. Sports. **1:** 81–86.
8. Pugh, L. G. C., J. L. Corbett & R. H. Johnson. 1967. Rectal temperatures, weight losses, and sweat rates in marathon running. J. Appl. Physiol. **23:** 345–352.
9. Costill, D. L. & E. Winrow. 1970. Maximal oxygen intake among marathon runners. Arch. Phys. Med. Rehabil. **51:** 317–320.
10. Fink, W. J., D. L. Costill & M. L. Pollock. 1977. Submaximal and maximal working capacity of elite distance runners. Part II. Muscle fiber composition and enzyme activities. Ann. N.Y. Acad. Sci. This volume.
11. Pollock, M. L. 1977. Characteristics of elite class distance runners: Overview. Ann. N.Y. Acad. Sci. This volume.
12. Spielberger, C. D., R. L. Gorsuch & R. E. Lushene. 1970. Manual for the State-Trait Anxiety Inventory. Consulting Psychologists Press. Palo Alto, Ca.
13. Landy, F. J. & R. M. Stern. 1971. Factor analysis of a somatic perception questionnaire. J. Psychosom. Res. **15:** 179–181.
14. Lubin, B. 1967. Manual for the Depression Adjective Checklist. Educational and Industrial Testing Service. San Diego, Ca.
15. McNair, D. M., M. Lorr & L. F. Droppleman. 1971. Profile of Mood States Manual. Educational and Industrial Testing Service. San Diego, Ca.
16. Eysenck, H. J. & S. B. G. Eysenck. 1968. Manual for the Eysenck Personality Inventory. Educational and Industrial Testing Service. San Diego, Ca.
17. Sonstroem, R. J. 1974. Attitude testing examining certain psychological correlates of physical activity. Res. Quart. **45:** 93–103.
18. Watson, L. Supernature. 1973. 1st edit. Doubleday. New York, N.Y.
19. Pollock, M. L. 1977. Submaximal and maximal working capacity in elite distance runners. Part I. Cardiorespiratory aspects. Ann. N.Y. Acad. Sci. This volume.

20. Borg, G. A. V. 1973. Perceived exertion: A note on "history" and methods. Med. Sci. Sports. **5:** 90–93.
21. Nagle, F. J., W. P. Morgan, R. O. Hellickson, R. C. Serfass & J. F. Alexander. 1975. Spotting success traits in Olympic contenders. Physician Sportsmed. **3:** 31–34.
22. Morgan, W. P. & R. W. Johnson. 1976. Psychological characterization of national level oarsmen differing in level of ability. Int. J. Sport. Psychol. In press.
23. Morgan, W. P., D. H. Horstman & A. Cymerman. (In prep.) Psychoendocrine responses to vigorous physical activity.
24. Morgan, W. P. 1972. Hypnosis and muscular performance. *In* Ergogenic Aids and Muscular Performance. 1st edit. W. P. Morgan, Ed. : 193–233. Academic Press. New York, N.Y.
25. Morgan, W. P., P. B. Raven, B. L. Drinkwater & S. M. Horvath. 1973. Perceptual and metabolic responsivity to standard bicycle ergometry following various hypnotic suggestions. Int. J. Clin. Exp. Hypnosis. **21:** 86–101.
26. Morgan, W. P., K. Hirota, G. Weitz & B. Balke. 1976. Hypnotic perturbation of perceived exertion: Ventilatory consequences. Amer. J. Clin. Hypnosis. **18:** 182–190.
27. Arnett, A. J. 1974. The influence of contingent reinforcement on heart rate during exercise. M.S. Thesis, University of Wisconsin, Madison.
28. Winer, B. J. 1962. Statistical principles in experimental design. 1st edit. McGraw-Hill Book Co. New York, N.Y.

DISCUSSION

Michael L. Pollock, *Moderator*

Institute for Aerobics Research
Dallas, Texas 75230

K. M. BALDWIN (*University of California, Irvine, Calif.*): What happens to the postexercise diastolic blood pressure in these individuals, since, if blood pressure were lowered it might affect the perfusion of the coronary bed?

M. L. POLLOCK: Postexercise diastolic blood pressures did not fall to abnormal levels. During exercise the diastolic pressures were quite low but were not significantly lower after exercise.

R. SELVESTER (*University of Southern California, Downey, Calif.*): Dr. Gibbons, several of those tracings looked like the QRS was a litttle prolonged. Did you measure the QRS duration and did you tabulate that?

L. W. GIBBONS (*Institute for Aerobics Research, Dallas, Texas*): We did look at the QRS duration, and found it was not significantly prolonged.

R. SELVESTER: What heart rate did these runners get to before they climbed off the treadmill?

L. W. GIBBONS: The average was 196 beats/min.

G. A. SHEEHAN (*Riverview Hospital, Redbank, N.J.*): I think it is all right at the Aerobic Institute to treat this electrocardiogram with the neglect that it should be given, but unfortunately when you are in practice it is a different matter. I happened to have studied the New York Giants for two years and we got similar graphs, though not under stress. At the time when I presented them at a staff conference, someone asked me how one stands legally? I answered, "We are in a bind." People have suggested that athletes get ECGs routinely, and it seems to me that if we do this we are going to end up possibly doing arteriography before we get finished.

L. W. GIBBONS: I think that is a good point to raise. There is a danger in getting routine ECGs in athletes, both in terms of arousing undue concern and in terms of reassuring an athlete with an abnormal ECG that he really is healthy. But hopefully those who are doing ECGs on athletes will become well acquainted enough with the most common abnormalities to reassure the athlete and his personal physician, and rely on clinical judgment to pick out the rare athlete who may really have a problem.

R. A. STEIN (*Downstate Medical Center, Brooklyn, N.Y.*): Were the postexercise tracings administered in the supine or in the upright position?

L. W. GIBBONS: Postexercise tracings were taken in the sitting position.

D. A. ADAMOVICH (*Nassau County Medical Center, East Meadow, N.Y.*): Dr. Underwood, would you comment on your systolic time intervals? I am surprised that the PEP/LVET ratio was not significantly shorter in your world class athletes since they showed a lower heart rate and would have therefore had a longer LVET.

R. H. UNDERWOOD (*Medical City Dallas Hospital, Dallas, Texas*): I am sorry I did not have time to present all of the phonocardiographic data. I would have expected the LVETs to be substantially longer. They were at the upper limit of normal, but they were not pathologically long. Systolic time intervals have fallen into disfavor clinically, perhaps because of the rather wide variations

404

and also the common finding of people who ought clearly to have abnormal measurements, and who when measured often do not. Some of the athletes demonstrated short PEP/LVET ratios, in fact over half, but the difference from group to group was not significant in spite of the difference in heart rates.

H. K. HELLERSTEIN (*Case–Western Reserve University, Cleveland, Ohio*): I think these presentations bring up the unpleasant thought that abnormalities found in otherwise healthy people may or may not be significant. Obviously voltage critria has to be related to the occupation, the sex, and the state of training. In the study of several thousand *Hutterites* (who were farmers) we found that the people who were field workers had voltage criteria that far exceeded the norm, and also ST changes. I would remind you of a study by Erickson on 2,000 or more so-called normal people. He was able to convince 90% of those who had abnormal ST-T changes (which was 115 people) to have a coronary arteriogram; 75% of these people had significant coronary artery disease, meaning one or more vessels had more than 50% stenosis. Others have reported similar data. So I do not believe one can be cavalier and say that we ignore the data because we do not have a complete study.

I would also bring up that I'm a little surprised about the ratio of PEP to LVET, because we have found in measurements of people at rest and after peak effort that the well-trained people with higher aerobic capacity have a shorter PEP/LVET ratio and after exercise it decreases even more. That one fellow whom you thought was hyperkinetic, for example, was his ratio considered lower?

I do believe that one has to harp on the fact that there is occult disease, that disease is silent; the fact that they can perform does not prove by any means that they do not have disease. Maybe with the radionuclides or other methods of investigation one should clarify it. But we do know that football players and other so-called athletes do drop dead; they do have disease. In Korea and World War II, 77% of young people had significant coronary disease of one type or another. So I do not believe that one should say that these are normal variants. We should say statistically they are abnormal, they are out of the range of normal, and they should be further investigated.

R. H. UNDERWOOD: I couldn't agree more. I'm a clinical cardiologist and have a number of patients who have significant coronary disease at a remarkably young age. I have one girl, 27-years-old, who has terrible three-vessel disease. Her blood pressure, heart size, and cholesterol are normal. She does not smoke, and yet she is ravaged by coronary disease. I had the opportunity about 3 months ago to study a marathon runner aged 26 who had echocardiographic evidence of septal hypertrophy, and he had been told that he probably had hypertrophic subaortic stenosis. He was advised that this was the case. His echo was not particularly convincing. A catherterization was done on him and he does in fact has IHSS. I do not know what the finding of septal hypertrophy in some of the athletes means. Certainly it could mean that they do have a problem.

COMMENT: In February of this year a South African marathon runner died during the race. Autopsy showed extensive left ventricular hypertrophy, quite out of keeping with the athlete's state of training. The septum was of a normal size, but the free wall was about 24 mm thick. The slides were reviewed by a British authority and he felt that this was a patient with hypertrophic cardiomyopathy without obstruction, and the suggestion is that this patient may have had an abnormal ECG which responds to training in an abnormal fashion.

P. B. RAVEN (*Institute for Aerobics Research, Dallas, Texas*): Dr. Pollock, did Frank Shorter feel a little disappointed with his low $\dot{V}_{O_2\,max}$ results?

M. L. POLLOCK: I must say when Frank got off the treadmill and found out his results he was disappointed. He was an Olympic champion in the marathon (Munich) and yet had the lowest $\dot{V}_{O_2\,max}$ of all 20 elite runners that were tested. It was explained to him that $\dot{V}_{O_2\,max}$ was only one of many important factors that make up a champion runner. Frank was the most efficient of all the elite runners and thus, it was explained that this was a very important factor in his marathon running success.

COMMENT: Dr. Pollock, with regards to the maximal heart rate data, you ran your athletes at a very high speed on the treadmill compared to what most people do. Dr. Duncan McDougal, while he was at Wisconsin, first noticed that if you put someone on a treadmill at a very high speed you get a heart rate which is higher than what you will record on a maximum treadmill test using a slower speed. In other words, you can get people up to 220 or 230 beats/min by using faster speeds. I wonder if this might be why you observed very high heart rates in these runners.

M. L. POLLOCK: We never had them up quite as high as you suggested, 220 or 230 beats/min. We were a little surprised to see their heart rates this high, but the protocol used in this study is used in many laboratories for testing athletes.

J. H. WILMORE (*University of Arizona, Tucson, Arizona*): I would like to ask you a question with regard to the statement you made concerning the absolute submaximal oxygen consumption value being important in measuring efficiency of running. I would think that maybe it would be best to define efficiency in terms of relative terms, which I think was borne out by the fact that Shorter was less efficient in terms of his having a slightly higher lactate response to that submaximal work level.

M. L. POLLOCK: That's a good point. I think efficiency is looked at in different ways. Actually the 3 mg% difference in the blood lactate of Shorter and Prefontaine would not be considered significant, so we can say lactates were the same. Efficiency, in the case of this study, would best be expressed in terms of one's oxygen uptake (ml/kg·min) at a given running speed. The lactate values found after the submaximal treadmill run test is not as indicative of measuring efficiency.

COMMENT: I think it is a problem when you use enzymes such as succinic dehydrogenase and lactic dehydrogenase to try to get some indication of rates of metabolism through glycolysis, fat oxidation, and so forth. We spent the last 10 years trying to identify principles by which you can use enzyme activity as indicators of maximal flux through pathways, and except for phosphorylase, the other enzymes give you only qualitative information, not quantitative information, unfortunately. If we could have used your data qualitatively there would be no problems. But I would rule against using them for quantitative information. We think now that we have the enzymes that will give us quantitative information without maximum flux through glycolysis, through *glyclogenolysis*, glucose oxidation, the tricarboxylic acid cycle, and indeed fat oxidation. But they are not the usual enzymes that most people measure because, to be quite blunt, they are bloody hard to measure.

M. L. POLLOCK: That is, of course, one of the problems that Costill and Fink had in analyzing the data. They are still in the process of developing techniques at this stage and some of the techniques on hand now were not developed a year and a half ago when the study was conducted.

QUESTION: What is going to be your specific means for disseminating this information to the participating athletes in a means reasonably understandable to them?

M. L. POLLOCK: First of all after the study was completed each of them had personal interviews with the various investigators. Secondly, when the data was initially analyzed each of the particular investigators sent each of the athletes a personal letter with their data explaining what it meant and so forth. When we get through with this meeting each of the athletes will be sent a copy of the complete papers. Finally, a summary article is being prepared that will be published in a track coaches journal. So we're trying to follow through on an educational basis to try and make this information practical for both the coaches and athletes.

J. DANIELS (University of Texas, Austin, Texas): Dr. Cavanagh, I am wondering a couple of things that maybe you can answer for me, which you may have said, but I missed it. One is, were you really comparing people who were training for the same event or were your elite runners training for longer distances than the good runners? I am wondering if any difference you saw in the length or frequency of stride, or ankle flexion was due to a difference of the college people being mostly one-, two-, or three-mile runners?

P. R. CAVANAGH (Pennsylvania State University, University Park, Pa.): The samples were divided as follows: In the elite sample we had five middle-long distance runners and their mean three-mile time was 13:10. We had nine marathon runners with mean marathon times of 2 hours 15 minutes. The good sample was divided into three marathon runners and five middle-long distance runners, so the good sample was slightly biased towards the middle and the elite sample was slightly biased towards the marathon distance runners.

J. DANIELS: My second question then is do you have similar measurements on beginning athletes to see if some of them automatically fall into what seems to be the optimum running style immediately?

P. R. CAVANAGH: Well, I wouldn't claim to know what the optimum running style is.

J. DANIELS: Well, let us say that these runners who have trained for 11 years or so, have found it.

P. R. CAVANAGH: Well, it's a very good question as to whether the human being is a self-optimizing machine. In answer to your question, there is a lot of literature with rather contradictory answers on what people do in relation to their leg length, and I don't think there is, by any means, a concensus of whether there should be or is a good relation between stride length and leg length.

QUESTION: You mentioned asymmetry of running style, what asymmetries are you talking about? Are you talking about the transverse plane deformity, frontal plane deformity, saggital plane deformity in the lower extremity about the subtelar joint range of motion of the midtarsal joint in the knee, the hip? In other words, where do we start with asymmetries as far as efficiency goes in your study?

P. R. CAVANAGH: The single asymmetry that I'm talking about is a difference in the total vertical oscillation of the left foot and right foot of the center of gravity. So if we can consider that when the right foot lands the center of gravity would descend a certain amount, and when the right foot pushes off the center of gravity will rise a certain amount. We take this same value, with the left foot, and if the values are spatially different, we call that an asymmetric pattern of the vertical motion of the center of gravity. I agree with your point that there are many other kinds of asymmetries, both skeletal and dynamic, which I'm not addressing myself to here. We're simply talking about the differences in the vertical motion of the center of gravity.

QUESTION: How confident are you as far as making recomendations to some of these runners to change their style?

P. R. CAVANAGH: That is a crucial question. I've stressed that this is a comparative analysis to date, and I do think though, that the basis is here to really make some progress on what is important in efficient running. There is a tremendous debate about what efficiency really means as the discussion between Pollock and Wilmore today indicated. And I hope that when this is all over the various members of this group can begin in piecing their jigsaw puzzle together from all kinds of data. And I certainly hope to do my part in trying to fit in these biomechanical aspects together with the physiological data.

QUESTION: Dr. Wood, would you characterize the active running males who were not world class who were subjects in this experiment?

P. D. WOOD (*Stanford University, Stanford, Calif.*): Certainly, I planned to do this in somewhat greater length tomorrow in another presentation. However, the older males were running at least 15 miles a week. That was the criterion for having them in the study. In fact, they actually averaged about 39 miles a week. Most I'd say had run a marathon at one time or the other. All of them were in active training at the time they were being tested. The rest of the data concerning their leanness, smoking habits, drinking habits, and so forth, I would like to present tomorrow.

QUESTION: Is it possible that the increases you see in some of your enzymes of the serum and plasma could in fact be due to a decreased rate of breakdown in excretion rather than an increased rate of production?

P. D. WOOD: I think that could be a correct assumption. We do not have any data on that, though.

J. A. DEMPSEY (*University of Wisconsin, Madison, Wisc.*): Dr. Gettman, I'm wondering whether we can really use an assumed simple conversion from body density to percent body fat based on the reference man in the research by Brožek and Keys. In our work with underwater weighing we've seen very lean people with body densities that exceed 1.1, which means 0% body fat, and this is impossible.

L. R. GETTMAN: I agree with you. I think there needs to be more work in this area which, unfortunately, requires cadaver work and that's a problem. But I agree, we're basing it on the the reference man of Brožek and Keys, which may or may not apply to distance runners.

J. A. DEMPSEY: Did you ever see densities exceeding 1.1?

L. R. GETTMAN: Zero percent fat? Yes, we have but when we rechecked our data found some mistakes made in the technique. For example, if residual volume is *predicted* instead of *measured*, it can result in a density over 1.1. Being very accurate in residual volume determination wil increase the validity of using underwater weighing.

R. H. DRESSENDORFER (*Pennsylvania State University, University Park, Pa.*): Your point about residual volume is correct. It should be measured at the time of underwater weighing; otherwise, small differences in residual volume, other than what actually exists underwater at the time of weighing, can result in large errors of calculated percent fat.

L. R. GETTMAN: Right, I agree that residual volume is critical when you're doing this underwater weighing technique. However, within the context of this study, i.e., comparing elite runners with good runners and average young men, all were administered the same technique for measuring residual volume out of water. Therefore, we can at least make the comparison within this study because of the similar technique for all subjects. When you try to compare with other studies then you run the risk of not being exactly comparable because the residual volumes may not be measured in the same way. The measures that you have seen in this study were taken with great care and contain few errors. Our technique is based on administering several repetitions of underwater weighing before accepting the data. This increases the reliability of the procedures and ensures more accurate data.

C. WYNDHAM (*Marshalltown, South Africa*): Dr. Raven, do you know what factors share in the improvement that has been made over the last 50 years? This may really be that we are now selecting from a much wider population and the criteria we are using for success are much more vigorous. That's why you are showing this greater improvement.

P. B. RAVEN: Yes, I think that's possible. However, we may have the same group to study.

R. H. RAHE (*Naval Health Research Center, San Diego, Calif.*): Dr. Morgan, I want to raise a question concerning the dissociative versus associative processes that are going on in runners. Might you not be dealing with a difference between someone who is really concerned about winning a race (elite), and someone who is running a marathon more as a pleasurable distraction? I see that in swimmers for instance, high-level swimmers always dissociate during training. They sing songs to themselves, look at the specks on the bottom of the pool—there are a number of things they do so they can tolerate their training day by day, which is immensely boring unless you think of other things. Then when it comes to the race they concentrate on the race. They concentrate on staying loose because when they are going near 100% capacity and make an error they may tie up and lose the race. But during training you are not going 99% all out, you are down to 80%; it is more leisurely and thus you think of more dissociative things.

W. P. MORGAN (*University of Wisconsin, Madison, Wisc.*): Okay, the position then is one of cognition during competition, not training. So I would agree with the distinction you are making. Secondly, we can extend this now to distance swimmers and the same thing has come through. Our best distance swimmers sing *"The Star Spangled Banner"* during training over and over for the 3 hours or so. So, I would agree 100% with that idea. On the idea of competition, though, we find an interesting thing in terms of the elite runners. One runner for example, who was one of the best middle-distance runners the U.S. has ever had, never did compete for the purpose of winning. In other words, he described himself as an artist. When he ran he created art and it had nothing to do with winning. It was the kind of art that he presented once in a very fleeting kind of way for the baboons who came to the stadium and to the art museum to gawk at art that they do not understand. They must interpret it quickly because he was only going to give it to them in a very fleeting kind of way, but he would have it the rest of his life; the one thing he did not do, though, was to go out with the idea of winning. He went out to create art.

QUESTION: Would you care to speculate what role these studies will have in our elite runners in the future?

W. P. MORGAN: Well, as far as these findings are concerned, I do not think that it should change too much because they are all doing the same thing. If what they are doing is wrong, well, that's another point, I guess.

P. S. JARETT (*Miami, Fla.*): It occurs to me that most runners are able to do faster and more intensive workouts many times when they are working out with someone else who is laboring beside them. I would think that perhaps if you talked to some of the runners long enough you might find some of them were even enjoying the exquisitely sadistic pleasure of knowing that others are suffering. I think Ron Hill mentioned this somewhere one time that he was able to transfer the feeling of suffering, and believe that perhaps I was not suffering as much as others were.

W. P. MORGAN: We had 20 runners. Not one of them reported coming up against the wall; even though our ABC anchorman kept talking about the wall during the Montreal marathon, none of them said they experienced it. There was one runner, he turned out to be the artist I just talked about, who indicated that occasionally he did experience discomfort, but not pain. And any time that ever occurred he turned it on because he knew anyone around him was going to pay for it and he would burn them. So that would fit in with what you are saying. That was his verbalization of that situation. But that was only one out of 20 who felt that way.

H. K. HELLERSTEIN: I think you're rediscovering what many of us who have been observing human behavior have found applies in many other arenas. I studied 47 surgeons who were performing surgery and recorded what was being said, what was being done, and how they were responding in terms of heart rate, blood pressure, and indirect measures of cardiac output. It is of some interest that the coping mechanism is well used by the surgeons as well as other people. For example, some surgeons talk about their boat or many other things, or say, "Yes, dear, pass the hemostat," and so forth. Then, if things start to go badly or a situation arises, they will then go into what you call the associative strategy of let us do this, let us do that, and so forth. So, in observing the different types of people meeting stresses and their ways of avoiding or of focusing upon the problem, I just wonder if you have found that some individuals in the course of long distance running will move from associate to dissociative as a matter of defense. The other idea, of course, is that perception is very poor in other areas; namely, if one tries to find out from a person how hard was the function that they performed—say during surgery, how hard was it on them—they have a very poor idea of how much their blood pressure rose, how high the cardiac output went, how high the heart rate went, whether arrhythmias occurred, and so forth.

W. P. MORGAN: Let me interrupt you for a moment on that point. In a talk like this you cannot go into detail on everything. There is substantial literature, though, indicating that perception of effort is directly related to actual exertional cost in 90% of all subjects tested. It is a perfect linear function.

H. K. HELLERSTEIN: The point is that the rate of perceived exertion holds true in normal people. People who have heart disease do not perceive ischemia; 65% of the people who have ischemic changes do not perceive it as pain.

W. P. MORGAN: Well, heaven forbid if anyone is thinking that I am talking or even suggesting that these findings be generalized to a pathological subgroup such as the coronary patient. We are talking about world class distance runners. That's one point. The second point in that same context is that in our own work, you do not have to go to cardiology to find these individuals. There are 10% in all of our samples who have psychiatric or psychologic elaboration and cannot accurately rate perceived exertion either. In the normal sector that is not the case. It is a very nice function.

ADAPTIVE RESPONSES IN DIFFERENT TYPES OF MUSCLE FIBERS TO ENDURANCE EXERCISE *

K. M. Baldwin

Department of Physiology
University of California
Irvine, California 92717

W. W. Winder

Department of Preventive Medicine
Washington University School of Medicine
St. Louis, Missouri 63110

Regularly performed endurance exercise such as long distance running or swimming can induce major physiological and biochemical adaptations in a variety of organ systems. A number of studies, involving both humans [1, 2] and rodents,[3] have shown that skeletal muscles undergo increases in oxidative potential, which may contribute to the improvement in work capacity that occurs with training. Skeletal muscle fibers in various mammalian and human muscles are distinctly different in terms of (1) their metabolic properties, (2) their recruitment pattern or degree of involvement in performing various activities, and (3) their potential work capacity or resistance to fatigue.[4] A series of studies, summarized herein, were undertaken to investigate the effects of long-term exercise programs on the biochemical properties and patterns of glycogen utilization of three different types of rodent skeletal muscle: (1) fast-twitch, high oxidative, moderate glycogenolytic (FOG); (2) fast-twitch, low oxidative, high glycogenolytic (FG); and (3) slow-twitch, moderate oxidative, low glycogenolytic (SO).[4, 5] Biochemical measurements focused on pathways of respiration, glycolysis, and glycogenolysis and actomyosin ATPase activity, since these systems represent the major pathways of ATP synthesis and hydrolysis during muscle contraction. In addition, glycogen utilization in liver and in different fiber types of skeletal muscle was also examined in trained and nontrained rats subjected to acute bouts of treadmill running.

METHODS

Animal Care and Training Programs

Studies on Enzymatic Adaptations to Training

Male rats, weighing approximately 110 g, were housed in temperature and light controlled quarters and provided with food and water *ad libitum*. They were divided into an exercising group and a sedentary group. The exercising

* This research was supported by Grants from the National Institute of Health (HD01613 and AM05431) and the American Heart Association.

group was trained for a minimum of 12 weeks by means of a program of treadmill running described in detail by Pattengale and Holloszy.[6] At the end of 12 weeks the rats were running continuously 2 hours/day, 5 days/week at a speed of 1.2 mph (0.5 m/sec), 15% grade.

In a separate series of experiments designed to examine time course changes in selected biochemical parameters in skeletal muscle, female rats were trained in a manner similar to the above program (1.0 mph, 25% grade) except that the final attained work duration was 1 hour. Groups of rats were sacrified after 2, 4, 6, and 10 weeks of training.[7] This training program is referred to below as a "steady-state" regimen since workload was held constant during each work bout throughout the program.

Another experiment was designed to determine the effect of intervals of high intensity work bouts on the different types of skeletal muscle fibers. Female rats were subjected to a 9-week program of interval training of progressively increasing intensity and duration. At the end of the 9-week period, rats were running 90 minutes per day up a 6% grade at speeds alternating between 1.2 mph and 2–2.5 mph. The high-intensity running bouts were maintained for 2–3 minute intervals. Groups of rats were killed after 3, 6, and 9 weeks of training.

At the end of the training programs, rats were killed by decapitation and homogenates were prepared from hindlimb muscles. For studies on FOG and FG fiber types, the vastus lateralis muscles were dissected out, freed of fat and connective tissue and separated into two portions: (1) a superficial, white portion (white vastus), which consists entirely of FG fibers;[4, 5, 8, 9] and (2) a deep red portion (red vastus) which consists predominantly of FOG fibers.[4, 5, 8, 9] The soleus muscle was used for studies on SO fibers since this muscle consists of predominantly SO fibers.[8] Homogenates prepared from each of these three muscle samples were used for assays of palmitate-U-^{14}C and pyruvate-2-^{14}C oxidation and for measurements of activity of enzymes of glycolysis, of glycogenolysis, of the citric acid cycle, of the electron transport chain, of fatty acid and ketone oxidation, and of actomyosin ATPase as described previously.[9–12]

Studies on the Effect of Training on Glycogen Depletion during Exercise

For experiments on muscle and liver glycogen depletion patterns in trained and nontrained rats, female rats were subjected to a training regimen consisting of swimming. They initially swam, in groups of 8, in steel barrels filled to a depth of 44 cm with water maintained near 35° C. The duration of swimming was increased by 15 min/day until the rats were swimming continuously 6 hours/day, 5 days/week for a total of 14 weeks.[13] Both swimming-trained and nontrained rats were run 5 days per week on the treadmill for 10 minutes to familiarize them with running. A program of swimming was used to train the rats in order to avoid the factor of running skill affecting the parameters investigated in the exercise test described below. Females were selected for these latter studies since exercising and sedentary female rats gain weight at the same rate, making it possible to control this variable.

At the end of training program, trained (swimming) and nontrained rats were assigned to one of four groups: (1) a resting control group; (2) a group that ran for 15 minutes at 0.8 mph up a 15% grade; (3) a group that ran the same as group 2 plus 15 minutes more at 1.0 mph up a 20% grade; (3) a group that ran the same as group 3 plus an additional 15 minutes at 1.2 mph up a 25% grade. Following the test, the animals were immediately anesthetized with sodium pentabarbital (6 mg/100 g body weight) given i.p., and muscle and liver samples to be used for glycogen analysis were quickly excised and frozen with Wollenberger tongs precooled in liquid nitrogen.[13]

In a separate experiment rats were trained using treadmill running. Intensity and duration of running were gradually increased so that at the end of a 4-week period, rats were running 1.2 mph up a 15% grade for 60 minutes, 5 days/week. The final exercise test consisted of running at 1.2 mph up a 15% grade for 15, 60, or 120 minutes. Rats were anesthetized, and tissues were removed and frozen for glycogen analysis as described above.[14]

TABLE 1

OXIDATION OF PYRUVATE-2-^{14}C AND PALMITATE-U-^{14}C BY HOMOGENATES OF DIFFERENT TYPES OF MUSCLE FIBERS FROM SEDENTARY AND TRAINED ANIMALS *

| | | Fiber Type | | |
	Group	FG	FOG	SO
Pyruvate	Sedentary	96 ± 22	324 ± 56	158 ± 25
(nmoles/g·min)	Trained	207 ± 42 †	832 ± 149 †	376 ± 116 †
Palmitate	Sedentary	5.5 ± 2.5	40.5 ± 5.6	23 ± 3.2
(nmoles/g·min)	Trained	15.6 ± 2.6 †	88.0 ± 16.0 †	48 ± 8.7 †

* Values are means ± standard errors. (Data from Baldwin et al.[9])
† Sedentary versus trained, $p < 0.05$.

RESULTS

Studies on Enzymatic Adaptation to Training

Respiratory Capacity

As shown in TABLE 1, the capacity to oxidize pyruvate-2-^{14}C and palmitate-U-^{14}C increased significantly in FG, FOG, and SO fiber types in response to 12 weeks of endurance running. Further information regarding the effects of exercise on the different fiber types is provided in TABLE 2, which shows that the level of activity of the citric acid cycle enzyme, citrate synthase, the long-chain fatty acid transport enzyme, carnitine palmityltransferase, and the respiratory chain enzyme, cytochrome oxidase, are increased significantly in the three fiber types. However, in absolute quantities, greater net increases in respiratory enzymes occurred in the FOG and SO types as compared to the FG type. This is particularly true for the enzyme 3-hydroxybutyrate dehydrogenase (3-BHDH), which also showed greater relative increases than the other mitochondrial enzymes (TABLE 2). Collectively, the above results provide further evidence to show that both mitochondrial mass and composition are altered with training. There is no evidence of any gross muscle enlargement or of a change in total muscle protein with this training program; thus, the respiratory potential is enhanced as expressed per muscle, per gram of muscle, or per mg of muscle protein.

Hexokinase and Glycogenolytic Enzymes

Hexokinase was increased by 170%, 50%, and 30% above control levels in FOG, SO, and FG fiber types, respectively (TABLE 3). In contrast to the increase in hexokinase activity induced in the FOG fiber type, various enzymes involved in a breakdown of glycogen to pyruvate (glycogenolysis) were decreased by approximately 20% in this fiber type in trained as compared to

TABLE 2

LEVELS OF ACTIVITY OF CITRATE SYNTHASE, CARNITINE PALMITYLTRANSFERASE,
3-HYDROXYBUTYRATE DEHYDROGENASE (3-HBDH), AND CYTOCHROME OXIDASE
IN DIFFERENT FIBER TYPES OF TRAINED AND SEDENTARY ANIMALS *

		Fiber Types		
	Group	FG	FOG	SO
Citrate synthase	Sedentary	10.3 ± 0.9	35.5 ± 3.2	23.2 ± 1.7
(μmole/g·min)	Trained	18.5 ± 0.8 †	69.9 ± 3.7 †	40.9 ± 2.8 †
Carnitine palmityl-transferase	Sedentary	0.11 ± 0.01	0.72 ± 0.06	0.63 ± 0.07
(μmole/g·min)	Trained	0.20 ± 0.02 †	1.20 ± 0.09 †	1.20 ± 0.05 †
3-HBDH	Sedentary	Not detectable	0.14 ± 0.02	0.34 ± 0.03
(μmole/g·min)	Trained	0.03 ± 0.01	0.80 ± 0.05 †	0.88 ± 0.07 †
Cytochrome oxidase	Sedentary	167 ± 8	830 ± 64	621 ± 39
(μl$_{O_2}$/g·min)	Trained	339 ± 21 †	2041 ± 60 †	1347 ± 100 †

* Values are means ± standard errors. (Data from Baldwin et al.[9] and Winder et al.[10])
† $p < 0.05$.

control animals. This is in contrast to the 18%–35% increase in these same enzymes, which occurred in the SO fiber type of the trained group. No distinct changes in the glycogenolytic enzymes occurred in the FG fiber type.

Actomyosin ATPase

As shown in TABLE 4, changes in Mg^{++}-activated ATPase of actomyosin, which is measured with substrate and activating ions (Ca^{++} and Mg^{++}) in the physiological range, paralleled the changes in glycogenolytic enzymes in the different fiber types. This relationship is depicted in FIGURE 1, which shows a high correlation between Mg^{++}-activated ATPase and the level of activity of the rate-limiting enzyme, phosphofructokinase, in different types of muscle in sedentary and trained rats.

TABLE 3

HEXOKINASE, PHOSPHORYLASE, PHOSPHOFRUCTOKINASE (PFK), CYTOPLASMIC
α-GLYCEROPHOSPHATE DEHYDROGENASE (α-GPDH), GLYCERALDEHYDE-3-
PHOSPHATE DEHYDROGENASE (3-PGDH), AND PYRUVATE KINASE ACTIVITIES
IN DIFFERENT TYPES OF SKELETAL MUSCLE OF SEDENTARY AND
TRAINED ANIMALS

Enzyme (μmoles/g·min)	Group	Fiber Types		
		FG	FOG	SO
Hexokinase	Sedentary	0.58±0.04	1.50±0.05	1.57±0.13
	Trained	0.75±0.05 †	4.10±0.29 †	2.39±0.12 †
Phosphorylase	Sedentary	215±15	105±8	27±2
	Trained	220±17	81±7 †	32±2
PFK	Sedentary	96±4	72±3	20±1
	Trained	88±4	58±3 †	24±1 †
α-GPDH	Sedentary	57.3±2.7	26.1±1.3	4.90±0.48
	Trained	55.3±2.1	19.1±1.3 †	7.38±0.31 †
3-PDGH	Sedentary	607±31	432±17	175±8
	Trained	589±32	361±28 †	206±10 †
Pyruvate kinase	Sedentary	473±34	279±26	67±7
	Trained	453±42	232±21	91±9 †

* Values are means±standard errors. (Data from Baldwin et al.[11])

TABLE 4

YIELDS OF ACTOMYOSIN AND MG⁺⁺ AND CA⁺⁺ ACTIVATED ATPASE ACTIVITY OF
ACTOMYOSIN IN DIFFERENT TYPES OF SKELETAL MUSCLE FIBER TYPES OF
SEDENTARY AND TRAINED ANIMALS *

	Group	Fiber Types		
		FG	FOG	SO
Actmyosin	Sedentary	55.1±1.9	51.9±2.8	32.5±4.3
(mg/g)	Trained	51.8±1.8	48.4±1.8	31.4±43.2
Mg⁺⁺ ATPase	Sedentary	0.720±0.03	0.635±0.03	0.209±0.03
(μmole/g·min)	Trained	0.742±0.03	0.529±0.02 †	0.257±0.03 †
Ca⁺⁺ ATPase	Sedentary	0.726±0.09	0.571±0.06	—
(μmole/g·min)	Trained	0.700±0.08	0.421±0.02 †	—

* Values are means±standard errors. (Data from Baldwin et al.[12])
† p<.05.

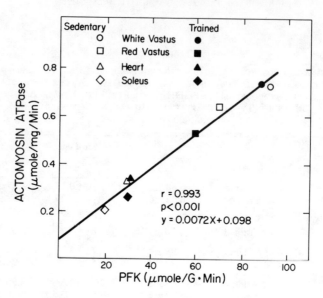

FIGURE 1. Correlation between phosphofructokinase activity and actomyosin ATPase activity in different types of muscle. (After Baldwin *et al.*[12])

Time Course Changes in Marker Enzymes with "Steady-State" and "Interval" Training

As shown in FIGURE 2A, female rats, trained for a period of 10 weeks with a regimen of "steady-state" running (1 mph, 25% grade), responded with increases in citrate synthase activity at each time point in the various fiber types. However, the changes reflect a different pattern for the various fiber types. In FG fibers, there was a 45% increase during the first 2 weeks of training; however, the increases subsequently regressed and plateaued as training continued. A similar pattern was seen for hexokinase activity (FIGURE 2B). In FOG fibers, citrate synthase and hexokinase activities underwent progressive increases during the first 6 weeks of running, finally attaining an approximate 50% increase over control levels after 10 weeks. Similar increases, but of smaller relative magnitude occurred in the soleus muscle.

In contrast to the steady-state running program, a training regimen of high-speed, "interval" running produced a greater relative effect on FG fibers (FIGURE 3A), since citrate synthase activity underwent progressive increases that amounted to nearly a 2-fold change after 9 weeks of running. Surprisingly, increases in citrate synthase activity in FOG and SO fiber types occurred primarily during the latter stages of the training program, at which time the animals exercised for the longest durations (90 minutes).

Interestingly, as shown in FIGURE 3C, PFK activity, in SO and FG fibers, showed responses similar to that seen previously with a steady-state regimen; i.e., no changes occurred in FG fibers, whereas, there was a 25% increase in SO fibers. However, in FOG fibers, the initial reduction in activity, which was similar to previous observations (TABLE 3), was reversed as training continued at the higher speeds of running.

Studies on the Effect of Training on Glycogen Depletion during Exercise

Glycogen Depletion in Skeletal Muscle during Steady-State Exercise

As shown in FIGURE 4, in which 4-week trained rats were run continuously on a treadmill at 1.2 mph, 15% grade, there were sharp decreases (40%–50%) in glycogen content in FOG and SO fiber types during the first 15 minutes of running. Thereafter, the glycogen concentration remained stable. In contrast to FOG and SO muscle, the FG fibers underwent minimal changes in glycogen concentration in response to the exercise. These findings suggest that there was relatively little involvement of FG fibers in the vastus lateralis muscle throughout the exercise bout in these trained animals. Normally, when FG fibers are made

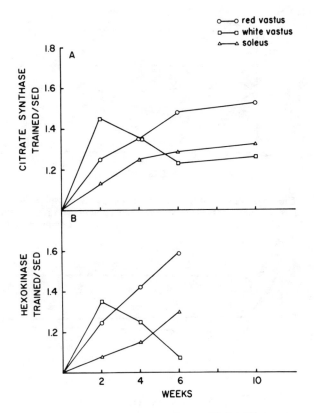

FIGURE 2. Citrate synthase (A) and hexokinase (B) in different types of skeletal muscle, expressed as a ratio of the trained value to the sedentary value at different stages of a 10-week "steady-state" running program. (After Baldwin *et al.*[7])

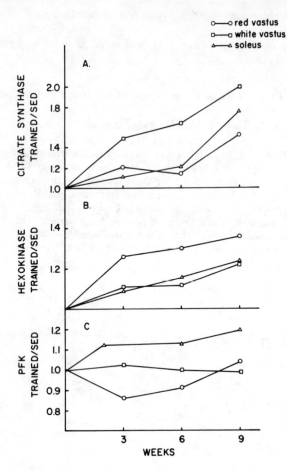

FIGURE 3. Citrate synthase (A), hexokinase (B), and phosphofructokinase (C) activity in different types of skeletal muscle, expressed as a ratio of the trained/ sedentary values at different stages of a 9-week "interval" running program. (After Baldwin *et al.*[7])

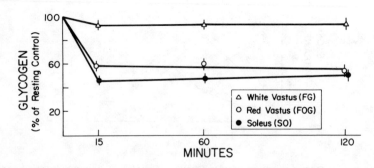

FIGURE 4. Percentage changes in concentration of glycogen in red vastus (FOG), white vastus (FG), and soleus (SO) muscle in response to continuous exercise at 1.0 mph (0.4 m/sec) 15% grade. (After Baldwin *et al.*[14])

to contract electrically or when physiologically activated at high-speed running, marked reductions in glycogen concentration occur in this fiber type.[1]

Glycogen Changes in Skeletal Muscle and in Liver of Trained and Nontrained Rats during Running of Progressive Intensity

FIGURE 5 presents data that compares glycogen depletion patterns in different fiber types of swimming-trained and untrained groups of rats during exercise of progressive intensity. The trained groups had an approximately 35% increase

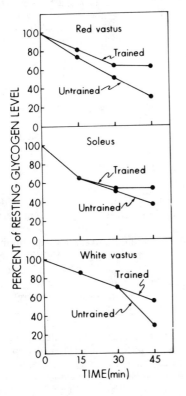

FIGURE 5. Glycogen depletion in red vastus (FOG), soleus (SO), and white vastus (FG) muscles in swimming-trained and untrained rats during an exercise test (see Methods). The figure shows the glycogen concentrations remaining after 15, 30, and 45 minutes of running, expressed as a percent of the resting concentration. For a given fiber type resting glycogen levels were similar in trained and nontrained animals. (After Baldwin *et al.*[13])

in the capacity of gastrocnemius muscle homogenates to oxidize pyruvate plus malate (58 ± 2 versus 43 ± 2 $\mu l_{O_2}/g \cdot min$). In FOG portions, relative glycogen concentration decreased more slowly in trained than in untrained rats throughout the exercise test. As a result, glycogen levels were significantly higher in the trained as compared to the untrained rats after 30 and 45 minutes of running. In soleus, and in FG portions of vastus lateralis muscle, there was a marked difference between trained and untrained rats in rates of glycogen depletion only during the third, most strenuous 15-minute exercise period.

Also, as shown in FIGURE 6, the rate of liver glycogen depletion during each of the three 15-minute periods of running was lower in the trained than in the

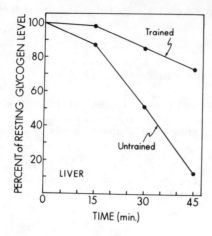

FIGURE 6. Glycogen deple-
tion in liver in swimming-
trained and untrained rats during an exercise test (see Methods). The figure shows the
concentrations of glycogen remaining in the liver after 15,
30, and 45 minutes of running,
expressed as a percent of the
resting concentration, which averaged 72.1 ± 5 and 42.3 ± 7
mg/g in trained and untrained
animals. (After Baldwin *et
al.*[13])

untrained animals. Since resting liver glycogen was 75% greater in the swimmers than in the controls (72 ± 5 versus 42 ± 7 mg/g), at the end of 45
minutes of running, glycogen concentration in the livers of the trained rats was
still higher than the initial, resting level found in the untrained animals.

DISCUSSION

These studies clearly show that all three types of skeletal muscle undergo
adaptations in enzyme concentrations in response to prolonged training. However, of the three primary types, the FG fiber, which normally possesses the
lowest aerobic capacity, adapts the least both quantitatively and qualitatively.
Although increases in respiratory capacity were induced in FG fibers with
training, this fiber type still has less than 50% the capacity for oxidizing various
substrates as normally seen in untrained FOG muscle. Moreover, enzyme
changes in the pathways of glycogenolysis and actomyosin ATPase remained
unaltered. These findings suggest that either the FG fiber type is incapable of
undergoing certain adaptations or this fiber type was used insufficiently during
the training regimen to induce the various adaptations. The latter possibility
seems most likely since glycogen depletion patterns in muscle, which provide
indirect evidence of a given fiber's relative contractile activity, indicate that FG
fibers of trained rats undergo little change in glycogen concentration during
exercise of the same intensity used in the training program. Furthermore, time-
course changes in citrate synthase and hexokinase activity show a regression
following initial increases in FG fibers after as little as 2 weeks of training under
the steady-state regimen (FIGURE 2). These results collectively suggest that as
the training program continues, unless there is a progressive increase in running
speed and/or incline, the animals become capable of performing the daily
exercise task with relatively less participation of FG fibers compared to the
untrained state.

Available evidence suggests that FG fibers are normally recruited when the
excitatory input into the motor neuron pool increases to sufficiently high levels,
i.e., during strenuous work or when FOG fibers possibly fatigue during prolonged continuous exercise.[15, 16] The present results involving trained and un-

trained rats during exercise of progressive intensity (FIGURE 5) suggest that in untrained rats, sufficient glycogen depletion may have occurred in some of the FOG fibers with the consequence that, during the most strenuous 15 minutes of exercise, more FG fibers were additionally recruited in untrained as compared to trained rats. If this is the case, the marked increases in the capacity of FOG fibers to oxidize other substrates, such as free fatty acids and ketones induced by training (TABLES 1 & 2), could play an important role in improving the animal's exercise capacity by promoting a glycogen-sparing effect. In this context, it is also interesting that liver glycogen, which serves as a source of carbohydrate for skeletal muscle, was also depleted to a smaller extent in trained as in untrained rats. Since available evidence suggests that the depletion of glycogen from various depots (liver and muscle) may be an important factor in the development of physical exhaustion during prolonged exercise,[17, 18] the metabolic adaptations induced in FOG muscle and, to a lesser degree, in soleus muscle, may play a dominant role in accounting for the enhancement of submaximal exercise capacity that occurs with training.

In view of the above findings, which collectively suggest that trained rodents rely upon FG fibers to a lesser degree than nontrained rats during submaximal exercise, it is interesting that adaptations in glycogenolytic and actomyosin ATPase enzyme systems also occur in the more frequently recruited FOG and SO types of fibers in response to chronic training. However, it seems puzzling that FOG and SO fiber types respond qualitatively different. One possible explanation for these differential changes is that there may be optimal enzyme levels in the various metabolic pathways of ATP synthesis and degradation to support muscle contraction for prolonged periods of time. In this context, it is interesting that the metabolic capacity of FOG and SO fiber types individually become more in line with the metabolic pattern normally seen in cardiac muscle (high respiratory capacity, high hexokinase activity, and moderately low glycogenolytic and actomyosin ATPase activity). As shown in TABLE 5, endurance training, at intensities normally resulting in marked changes in various enzyme

TABLE 5

CITRATE SYNTHASE, CYTOCHROME C, PHOSPHOFRUCTOKINASE, ACTOMYOSIN ATPASE, AND HEXOKINASE LEVELS IN CARDIAC MUSCLE OF SEDENTARY AND TRAINED ANIMALS

	Sedentary	Trained
Citrate synthase (μmole/g·min)	147±7	142±1
Cytochrome C (nmole/g)	47±1	47±1
PFK (μmole/g·min)	20.9±0.64	22.6±0.89
Actomyosin ATPase (μmole/mg·min)	0.325±0.025	0.335±0.025
Hexokinase (μmole/g·min)	4.40±0.65	4.36±0.68

* Values are means±standard errors. (Data from Winder et al.[10] and Baldwin et al.[12])

systems in skeletal muscle fiber types, produces relatively little change in the metabolic pathways of cardiac muscle. Since the heart contracts continuously and has the highest capacity for aerobic metabolism of any mammalian muscle, it seems reasonable that the enzyme patterns for the generation of ATP and for the hydrolysis of ATP during muscle contraction are the optimal ones for continuous submaximal contractile activity.

Finally, in terms of providing an appropriate stimulus to bring about the various metabolic adaptation in the different fiber types, it would appear, on the basis of these experiments involving the rodent model, that a training program incorporating elements of "steady-state" running at moderately heavy intensity coupled with repeated intervals at high speed would be most suitable. Under these conditions of training, the greatest spectrum of fiber types would be improved metabolically, thus enhancing one's exercise potential during both submaximal and maximal conditions of exercise.

REFERENCES

1. VARNAUSKAS, E., P. BJORNTORP, M. FAHLEN, I. PREROVSKY & J. STENBERG. 1970. Effects of physical training on exercise blood flow and enzymatic activity in skeletal muscle. Card. Res. **4:** 418–422.
2. GOLLNICK, P. D., R. B. ARMSTRONG, B. SALTIN, C. W. SAUBERT IV, W. L. SEMBROWICH & R. E. SHEPHERD. 1973. Effect of training on enzyme activity and fiber composition of human skeletal muscle. J. Appl. Physiol. **34:** 107–111.
3. HOLLOSZY, J. O. & F. W. BOOTH. 1976. Biochemical adaptations to endurance exercise in muscle. Ann. Rev. Physiol. **38:** 273–291.
4. BURKE, R. E. & V. R. EDGERTON. 1975. Motor unit properties and selective involvement in movement. *In* Exercise and Sport Sciences Reviews. Vol. **3:** 31–81. Academic Press. New York, N.Y.
5. PETER, J. B., R. J. BARNARD, V. R. EDGERTON, C. A. GILLESPIE & K. E. STEMPEL. 1972. Metabolic profiles of three fiber-types of skeletal muscle in guinea pigs and rabbits. Biochemistry **11:** 2627–2633.
6. PATTENGALE, P. K. & J. O. HOLLOSZY. 1967. Augmentation of skeletal muscle myoglobin by a program of treadmill running. Amer. J. Physiol. **213:** 783–785.
7. BALDWIN, K. M., D. A. COOKE & W. G. CHEADLE. 1977. Time course adaptations in cardiac and skeletal muscle to different running programs. J. Appl. Physiol. **42:** 267–272.
8. ARIANO, M. A., R. B. ARMSTRONG & V. R. EDGERTON. 1973. Hindlimb muscle fiber populations of five mammals. J. Histochem. Cytochem. **21:** 51–55.
9. BALDWIN, K. M., G. H. KLINKERFUSS, R. L. TERJUNG, P. A. MOLE & J. O. HOLLOSZY. 1972. Respiratory capacity of white, red, and intermediate muscle: Adaptative response to exercise. Amer. J. Physiol. **222:** 373–378.
10. WINDER, W. W., K. M. BALDWIN & J. O. HOLLOSZY. 1974. Enzymes involved in ketone utilization in different types of muscle: Adaptation to exercise. Eur. J. Biochem. **47:** 461–467.
11. BALDWIN, K. M., W. W. WINDER, R. L. TERJUNG & J. O. HOLLOSZY. 1973. Glycolytic enzymes in different types of skeletal muscle: Adaptation to exercise. Amer. J. Physiol. **225:** 962–966.
12. BALDWIN, K. M., W. W. WINDER & J. O. HOLLOSZY. 1975. Adaptation of actomyosin ATPase in different types of muscle to endurance exercise. Amer. J. Physiol. **229:** 422–426.
13. BALDWIN, K. M., R. H. FITTS, F. W. BOOTH, W. W. WINDER & J. O. HOLLOSZY. 1975. Depletion of muscle and liver glycogen during exercise. Protective effect of training. Pflugers Arch. **354:** 203–212.

14. BALDWIN, K. M., J. S. REITMAN, R. L. TERJUNG, W. W. WINDER & J. O. HOLLOSZY. 1975. Substrate depletion in different types of muscle and in liver during prolonged running. Amer. J. Physiol. **225:** 1045–1050.

15. GOLLNICK, P. D., R. B. ARMSTRONG, W. L. SEMBROWICH, R. E. SHEPHERD & B. SALTIN. 1973. Glycogen depletion pattern in human skeletal muscle fibers after heavy exercise. J. Appl. Physiol. **34:** 615–618.

16. GOLLNICK, P. D., K. PIEHL, C. W. SAUBERT IV, R. B. ARMSTRONG & B. SALTIN. 1972. Diet, exercise, and glycogen changes in human muscle fibers. J. Appl. Physiol. **33:** 421–425.

17. AHLBORG, B., J. BERGSTROM, L. G. EKELUND & E. HULTMAN. 1967. Muscle glycogen and muscle electrolytes during prolonged physical exercise. Acta Physiol. Scand. **70:** 129–142.

18. BERGSTROM, J., L. HERMANSEN, E. HULTMAN & B. SALTIN. 1967. Diet, muscle glycogen and physical performance. Acta Physiol. Scand. **71:** 140–150.

THE EFFECTS OF EXERCISE-TRAINING ON THE DEVELOPMENT OF FATIGUE*

Robert H. Fitts †

Department of Biology
Marquette University
Milwaukee, Wisconsin 53233

An increase in endurance is synonymous with a postponement of the development of fatigue. A thorough understanding of the mechanisms by which endurance is increased by exercise-training is therefore dependent on an elucidation of the mechanisms responsible for fatigue. Despite considerable interest in this area, relatively little is known regarding the biochemical events that result in the various symptoms that can force an individual to stop exercising because of fatigue. One point seems clear, however, and that is that fatigue or exhaustion can have various etiologies depending on the intensity and duration of the exercise, the environmental factors, and the individual's condition.

Accumulation of Lactate in Muscle

One factor that has been postulated to cause muscle fatigue during very heavy work of relatively short duration (i.e., in the range of 2–15 min) is the accumulation of lactic acid. Much of the evidence for the hypothesis that high concentrations of lactic acid in muscle cause fatigue came from the studies of Hill and Kupalov,[1] who estimated that frog sartorius muscle stops contracting when the concentration of lactate in the muscle rises to 0.3%, i.e., 33 μmoles/g, and that evidence of fatigue begins to appear at concentrations above 9 μmoles/ g. They calculated that in order to avoid fatigue due to lactate accumulation an interval of 10 seconds should be allowed between twitches when a frog sartorius muscle 0.6 mm thick is stimulated to contract under anaerobic conditions. They estimated, with the use of a diffusion constant for lactate of 1.65×10^5, that sufficient lactate would diffuse out of muscle during the 10-second interval between twitches to keep the lactate concentration below 9 μmoles/g and thus avoid development of fatigue. They found, on testing this calculation, that faster rates of stimulation resulted in rapid development of fatigue, while rates below 6/min could be maintained for long periods until glycogen stores were depleted.[1]

Although these results are persuasive, Hill's hypothesis that lactate accumulation causes muscle fatigue has been seriously questioned on both theoretical and methodological grounds.[2] The major methodological problem was that,

* This work was supported by National Institutes of Health Research Grant AG00425 and by a Muscular Dystrophy Associations of America Neuromuscular Disease Research Center Grant to Washington University Medical School, St. Louis.
† Recipient of a research fellowship from the Muscular Dystrophy Association of America.

because of the lack of simple accurate methods for the determination of lactate, the concentrations of lactate in muscle were not measured. Instead, intramuscular lactate concentrations were estimated from the decreases in muscle tension.[1, 3] Thus, Hill and Kupalov started with the assumption that accumulation of a given quantity of lactic acid results in a fixed reduction in tension.

Somewhat surprisingly, the relationship between intramuscular lactic acid concentration and muscle fatigue had not (as best we could determine in an extensive literature search) been systematically re-evaluated now that simple, accurate assays for lactate are available. Therefore, as a first step in evaluating the role of lactic acid accumulation in muscle fatigue, a study was undertaken to determine whether there is a close correlation between lactic acid concentration and twitch tension in frog sartorius.[4] The frogs in these studies were fed a diet of crickets and mealworms daily for at least 2 weeks to ensure high muscle glycogen concentrations. The isolated sartorius muscles were stimulated at a rate of 30/min with supramaximal pulses while immersed in a glucose-containing Ringer's solution under anaerobic conditions. Muscles were frozen after 2, 6, 10, or 15 minutes of stimulation.

After an initial small increase, isometric twitch tension fell progressively and was only 36% of the initial value after 15 minutes of stimulation. The concentration of lactic acid in the muscles underwent an increase that was inversely proportional to the decrease in contractile force. The increase in lactic acid and the decrease in tension were closely (inversely) correlated ($r = -0.99$, $p < 0.001$). The recovery from fatigue after 15 minutes of stimulation was also investigated; in this study the muscles were allowed to recover in oxygenated solution for either 0.25, 0.50, 1.0, 2.0, 6.0, 10, 20, or 30 minutes, or until isometric twitch tension had returned to the initial, prefatigue level. Complete recovery took 50 minutes. There was also a significant inverse correlation between lactic acid concentration and contractile force during the recovery period ($r = -0.92$, $p < 0.001$).

These findings appear to lend support to Hill's hypothesis that lactic acid accumulation results in muscle fatigue. However, the relationship between lactic acid concentration and twitch tension is by no means as clear-cut as the results of the statistical analysis would suggest, because the return of twitch tension to the control level lagged markedly behind the decrease in muscle lactate. For example, twitch tension was still 23% below the control level after 30 minutes of recovery despite the fact that lactate concentration had fallen to 4.7 μmole/g; at the same lactate concentration after 2 minutes of stimulation at the beginning of the experiment, twitch tension was 103% of control. Thus, muscles having the same concentration of lactate develop different tensions during a twitch early during development of fatigue compared to late during recovery. It is therefore necessary to postulate that if the development of fatigue was largely due to the accumulation of lactate, then some secondary effect induced by increased lactate must persist while lactate concentration is decreasing.

A study of considerably more relevance to the role of lactate in the development of fatigue during normal exercise in man has been reported by Karlsson and Saltin.[5] These investigators measured lactate concentration in quadriceps muscle biopsy samples after exhausting exercise of either 2, 6, or 16 minute duration. Lactate concentration averaged 16.1 mmole/kg of muscle at the point of exhaustion both for the heaviest workload (140% of $\dot{V}_{O_2 \, max}$) and the intermediate workload (100% of $\dot{V}_{O_2 \, max}$), while at the lowest workload (90% of

$\dot{V}_{O_2 max}$) lactate averaged 12.0 mmoles/kg muscle at the point of exhaustion. It was concluded by these investigators that, since the concomitant changes in glycogen and high energy phosphate concentrations could not explain the exhaustion, the high muscle lactate concentrations might have been responsible for the development of fatigue at the two highest workloads.[5]

The concept that accumulation of lactic acid results in fatigue of muscle has considerable theoretical appeal, because evidence exists for at least two mechanisms by which a decrease in intracellular pH could interfere with contractile function. A reduction in pH has been shown to increase the Ca^{++} binding capacity of the sarcoplasmic reticulum[6] and to interfere with Ca^{++} binding to troponin.[7] Both of these mechanisms would function to decrease the number of calcium ions bound to troponin during excitation-contraction coupling and, thus, result in a decrease in contractile force. Furthermore, phosphofructokinase activity is inhibited by a decrease in pH[8]; lactic acid accumulation could by this mechanism result in feedback inhibition of glycolysis during intense muscular work and, thus, result in a decrease in ATP supply. The concept that lactic acid accumulation causes fatigue is particularly attractive, because, as will be discussed in more detail elsewhere in this symposium, it is well documented that training has a protective effect against both lactate accumulation and development of fatigue during exercise.[9] However, while the available evidence is suggestive and the concept has considerable appeal, it still remains to be proved that lactic acid accumulation causes muscle fatigue.

Depletion of Muscle and Liver Glycogen

There is considerable evidence that depletion of body carbohydrate stores results in the development of physical exhaustion during prolonged, strenuous exercise. Studies in which serial biopsies of the quadriceps muscle were obtained from men performing prolonged strenuous exercise have provided evidence that the point of exhaustion coincides with the depletion of muscle glycogen stores.[10-12] The duration for which strenuous exercise, such as long distance running or bicycling can be maintained appears to be determined by the concentration of glycogen in the muscles at the beginning of exercise and the rate at which the glycogen stores are depleted.[10-14] Depletion of liver glycogen stores, resulting in hypoglycemia, can also play an important role in the development of exhaustion.[15, 16]

Trained men deplete their muscle glycogen less rapidly than untrained during a standardized bout of submaximal exercise.[10, 17, 18] Studies on rats have shown that training also protects against liver glycogen depletion during submaximal exercise.[19, 20] Trained muscles compensate for the smaller utilization of carbohydrate by oxidizing a proportionally greater amount of fat; this is reflected in a lower respiratory exchange ratio (R) during the same exercise in the trained as compared to the untrained state.[10, 17, 21] It seems likely that this glycogen-sparing effect is one of the major mechanisms by which exercise-training increases endurance.

One factor that could contribute to the glycogen-sparing effect of exercise-training may involve the cardiovascular adaptations to exercise with, perhaps, a more rapid increase in delivery of blood and O_2 to the working muscles at the onset of exercise. However, it seems unlikely that improved delivery of O_2 to the working muscles plays a significant role in protecting a trained individual against muscle glycogen depletion during prolonged exercise of an intensity that can be maintained for an hour or longer. This interpretation is supported by the evidence that $\dot{V}_{O_2}$ and cardiac output are similar and that muscle blood flow is actually lower during the same exercise in the trained as compared to the untrained state.[22, 23]

On theoretical grounds it seemed reasonable that the increase in muscle mitochondria induced by endurance exercise might play an important role in protecting the trained individual against depletion of body carbohydrate stores during exercise.[9] This possibility was investigated in a recent study in which the relationships between skeletal muscle mitochondrial content, endurance, and depletion of body carbohydrate stores were examined in rats.[19] The animals were exercised on a treadmill for either 10, 30, 60, or 120 minutes per day. As shown in TABLE 1, the mitochondrial content of gastrocnemius, as reflected in a number of mitochondrial markers, increased in proportion to the duration

TABLE 1

EFFECTS OF 10, 30, 60, AND 120 MINUTES OF DAILY RUNNING ON RAT GASTROCNEMIUS MUSCLE MITOCHONDRIAL CONTENT AND ENDURANCE *

Groups	Oxygen Uptake (μl/g·min)	Citrate Synthase μmole/g·min	Cytochrome C (nmole/g)	Run Time to Exhaustion (min)
Sedentary	36.6±0.8	20.0±0.7	10.0±0.5	
Runners (min/day)				
10	39.6±1.3	22.9±1.0	11.6±0.7	22±2
30	44.5±3.2	31.4±2.7	13.1±1.1	41±11
60	57.1±2.0	37.3±2.4	13.8±0.7	50±12
120	75.6±2.3	45.5±2.3	19.2±0.6	111±16

* O_2 consumption of whole muscle homogenates was measured during uncontrolled respiration with pyruvate plus malate as substrate. Citrate synthase and cytochrome C were used as additional markers for evaluating mitochondrial content. For the endurance exercise test, the animals ran at 1.2 mph (0.5 m/sec) up a 15% grade for the first 10 min, and then at 1.5 mph (0.7 m/sec) up a 15% grade until they became exhausted. Values are means ± SE. (Data from Fitts et al.[19])

of the daily running, and varied over a wide range. The exercise tolerance of the animals was investigated both by means of a run to exhaustion and a standard 30-minute long exercise test. The results of the run to exhaustion are shown in TABLE 1. There was a significant correlation between run time to exhaustion and muscle respiratory capacity. Blood lactate levels were not significantly elevated above control in any of the groups after the run to exhaustion. After the 30-minute long exercise test the animals were anesthetized, and their gastrocnemius muscles and livers were frozen and analyzed for glycogen. The glycogen contents of gastrocnemius muscle and liver after the 30 minute exercise test were compared to the glycogen values obtained on some of the trained animals that were not exercised. As shown in FIGURE 1, there is a good correlation between muscle respiratory capacity and the amount of glycogen remaining in liver and muscle at the end of the exercise. Thus, it appears that the rate of carbohydrate utilization is inversely correlated with the concentration of mito-

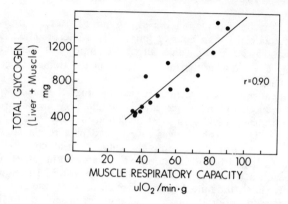

FIGURE 1. Correlation between gastrocnemius muscle respiratory capacity and total glycogen remaining in the liver and muscles of rats after a 30-min exercise test. (Data from Fitts *et al.*[19])

chondria in the animals' leg muscles. Since all the animals performed the same amount of work and, therefore, expended similar amounts of energy, it seems reasonable that the animals that utilized less carbohydrate must have utilized proportionally more fat. This is in keeping with the evidence that oxidation of fatty acids inhibits utilization of carbohydrate in skeletal muscle [24] and that trained individuals have a lower R value than untrained when performing submaximal work of the same absolute intensity.

In contrast to muscle respiratory capacity, which increased in proportion to the duration of the daily exercise sessions, the increase in heart weight in response to training was not significantly greater in the animals that ran one or two hours per day than in those that ran for 30 minutes per day (TABLE 2). This finding does not, of course, prove that maximum cardiac output was not higher in the 120-min/day runners than in the 30-min/day runners. However,

TABLE 2

EFFECTS OF VARIOUS DURATIONS OF DAILY RUNNING ON HEART WEIGHT IN RATS *

Groups	Body Wt (g)	Heart Wt (g)	Heart Wt / Body Wt
Controls	348±3	0.838±0.014	2.41±0.04
Trained (min/day)			
10	340±4	0.902±0.017	2.65±0.03
30	333±5	0.933±0.021	2.80±0.04
60	333±4	0.914±0.011	2.74±0.05
120	335±3	0.944±0.018	2.81±0.05

* Male rats were trained for 5 days/week for 13 weeks on a motor driven treadmill set at a 15% grade and a speed of 1.2 mph (0.5 m/sec). The length of the training sessions were progressively increased, but to different final durations, for the four groups. The final duration of the exercise sessions was either 10, 30, 60, or 120 min/day. Values are means ± SE.

in the absence of cardiovascular pathology, there appears to be a positive correlation between heart size and maximum cardiac output.[25]

Fatigue of Single Muscles in Situ

A simple procedure for evaluating whether or not local adaptations induced in muscle by training result in increased fatigue resistance independent of cardiac adaptations is to study the responses of small muscles stimulated to contract *in situ*. Two studies in which muscles were stimulated to twitch repeatedly *in situ* have shown that twitch tension declines less rapidly in muscles of exercise-trained than in untrained animals.[26, 27] To further evaluate this effect, a study was recently performed to characterize the changes that occur in the mechanical properties of rat soleus muscle as it fatigues and to compare the responses of exercise-trained and untrained animals.[28] Rats were trained by treadmill running 2 hr/day for 18 weeks. The animals were anesthetized, and the soleus was dissected free of surrounding muscles with blood supply intact. The soleus was stimulated to contract via the nerve with tetanic stimuli of 250-msec duration at a rate of 110/min for 30 minutes. After the 30 minutes of stimulation, peak tetanic tension was decreased 31% in the untrained compared to 8% in the trained soleus. These results provide evidence that muscles that have adapted to endurance exercise are more fatigue resistant than controls.

References

1. HILL, A. V. & P. KUPALOV. 1929. Proc. R. Soc. Series B **105:** 313–328.
2. SIMONSON, E. 1971. *In* Physiology of Work Capacity and Fatigue. E. Simonson, Ed. : 9–25. Charles C Thomas, Publisher. Springfield, Ill.
3. HILL, A. V. 1928. Proc. R. Soc. London, Series B **103:** 163–170.
4. FITTS, R. H. & J. O. HOLLOSZY. 1976. Amer. J. Physiol. **231:** 430–433.
5. KARLSSON, J. & B. SALTIN. 1970. J. Appl. Physiol. **29:** 598–602.
6. NAKAMURA, Y. & S. SCHWARTZ. 1972. J. Gen. Physiol. **59:** 22–32.
7. FUCHS, F., V. REDDY & F. N. BRIGGS. 1970. Biochem. Biophys. Acta **221:** 407–409.
8. TRIVEDI, B. & W. H. DANFORTH. 1966. J. Biol. Chem. **241:** 4110–4112.
9. HOLLOSZY, J. O. 1973. *In* Exercise and Sport Sciences Reviews. J. Wilmore, Ed. : 45–71. Academic Press. New York, N.Y.
10. HERMANSEN, L., E. HULTMAN & B. SALTIN. 1967. Acta Physiol. Scand. **71:** 129–139.
11. AHLBORG, B., J. BERGSTROM, L.-G. EKELUND & E. HULTMAN. 1967. Acta Physiol. Scand. **70:** 129–142.
12. BERGSTROM, J., L. HERMANSEN, E. HULTMAN & B. SALTIN. 1967. Acta Physiol. Scand. **71:** 140–150.
13. GOLLNICK, P. D., K. PIEHL, C. W. SAUBERT, R. B. ARMSTRONG & B. SALTIN. 1972. J. Appl. Physiol. **33:** 421–425.
14. COSTILL, D. L., P. D. GOLLNICK, E. D. JANSSON, B. SALTIN & E. M. STEIN. 1973. Acta Physiol. Scand. **89:** 374–383.
15. CHRISTENSEN, E. H. & O. HANSEN. 1939. Skand. Arch. Physiol. **81:** 172–179.
16. PRUETT, E. D. R. 1970. J. Appl. Physiol. **28:** 199–208.
17. SALTIN, B. & J. KARLSSON. 1971. *In* Muscle Metabolism During Exercise. B. Pernow & B. Saltin, Eds. : 289–299. Plenum Press. New York, N.Y.
18. SALTIN, B. & J. KARLSSON. 1971. *In* Muscle Metabolism During Exercise. B. Pernow & B. Saltin, Eds. : 395–399. Plenum Press. New York, N.Y.

19. FITTS, R. H., F. W. BOOTH, W. W. WINDER & J. O. HOLLOSZY. 1975. Amer. J. Physiol. **228:** 1029–1033.
20. BALDWIN, K. M., R. H. FITTS, F. W. BOOTH, W. W. WINDER & J. O. HOLLOSZY. 1975. Pflügers Arch. **354:** 203–212.
21. CHRISTENSEN, E. H. & O. HANSEN. 1939. Skand. Arch. Physiol. **81:** 180–189.
22. GRIMBY, G., E. HAGGENDAL & B. SALTIN. 1967. J. Appl. Physiol. **22:** 305–310.
23. CLAUSEN, J. P. 1976. Prog. Cardiovasc. Dis. **28:** 459–495.
24. RENNIE, M. J., W. W. WINDER & J. O. HOLLOSZY. 1976. Biochem. J. **156:** 647–655.
25. GRANDE, R. & H. L. TAYLOR. 1965. *In* Handbook of Physiology Vol. 3 (Sect. 2) : 2615. Amer. Physiol. Soc. Washington, D.C.
26. BARNARD, R. J. & J. B. PETER. 1971. Amer. J. Physiol. **31:** 904–908.
27. FITTS, R. H., D. R. CAMPION, F. J. NAGLE & R. G. CASSENS. 1973. Pflügers Arch. **343:** 133–141.
28. FITTS, R. H. & J. O. HOLLOSZY. 1976. Fed. Proc. (Abst.) **35:** 378.

EFFECTS OF ENDURANCE EXERCISE ON CYTOCHROME C TURNOVER IN SKELETAL MUSCLE *

Frank Booth

Department of Physiology
School of Medicine
University of Texas Health Science Center at Houston
Houston, Texas 77025

The adaptive responses of skeletal muscle to repeated daily exercise is dependent upon the type of exercise employed. For example, the responses of muscle to distance running and to weight lifting are different. After repeated bouts of distance running, there is an adaptive increase in the concentration of mitochondria within skeletal muscle, but no significant change in muscular mass.[1] In contrast, skeletal muscles adapt to repeated bouts of weight lifting by an increase in mass with little change in the concentration of mitochondria.[1] Thus, adaptations in skeletal muscles are specific to the type of exercise employed during training; and any discussion of the effects of distance running on the turnover of mitochondrial proteins within skeletal muscle must be restricted to those studies that have employed distance running.

Other investigators have reported the final or "near-final" levels of the adaptive increases in enzymes and proteins in response to endurance running.[1] However, few reports exist on the time course of these changes.[2, 3] The major purpose of this paper will be to provide information on the roles that protein turnover and intensity of physical work play on the time course of adaptive changes that occur in the mitochondria of skeletal muscles in response either to detraining or to increasing the daily intensity of running.

It is now well established that all proteins in animal cells endure a continual process of renewal, i.e., a continual process of degradation and replacement by the synthesis of new proteins.[4] Such a process has been termed turnover.[5] Thus, when the level of protein is unchanging or is in steady state, this level is determined by the rates of both synthesis and degradation, as expressed by: $E = k_s/k_d$, in which E is the steady-state level of protein (units mass^{-1}), k_s is the zero-order rate constant for synthesis (units time^{-1} mass^{-1}), and k_d is the first-order rate constant for degradation (time^{-1}).[6] From this equation, it is obvious that the steady-state level of a protein can be altered by changing either k_s or k_d or by changing both. Furthermore, the degradation of a protein is expressed as a first-order rate constant because in all cases studied, except for the red blood cell and hemoglobin, degradation of a protein is proportional to its concentration.[5, 6] For example, if the steady-state level of a protein were 1 unit/mass and k_d were 0.03/day, then 0.03 would be degraded per day. If the steady-state level were to be doubled to 2 units/mass with k_d remaining 0.03, then 0.06 units would be degraded daily. One term frequently employed to express the rate of degradation for a protein is half-life ($t_{1/2}$), which is defined as:

* This work was supported by United States Public Health Service Grant AM-19393 and a grant from the Muscular Dystrophy Associations of America.

431

$t_{1/2} = (\ln 2)/k_d$ in which ln 2 is the natural logarithm of 2 and k_d is the rate constant for degradation.[5] One utilization of this relationship is to obtain $t_{1/2}$ of a protein from the time course of the change in protein levels between two steady states.[7, 8] This is possible because the time course to a new steady state is determined only by the rate constant of degradation, k_d.[7, 8] The following equation demonstrates this point:

$$\frac{E_t}{E_o} = \frac{k_s'}{k_d' E_o} - \left(\frac{k_s'}{k_d' E_o} - 1\right) e^{-k_d' t}$$

in which E_t is the protein concentration at any time t; E_o is the steady-state protein concentration defined by k_s and k_d; and k_s' and k_d' are the new synthesis rate and the new degradation rate constant occurring during the application of the altered physiological stimulus.[5, 6] Thus, only k_d determines the time course between two steady states.[7, 8] Because of this factor, the time course of change between two protein levels can be used to approximate k_d for the protein and thus obtain an estimate of $t_{1/2}$ for this protein.[7, 8] By determining the time course of the change in protein levels (I) from a lower to a higher steady state during the application of a constant physiological stimulus such as distant running repeated daily and (II) from a higher to a lower steady-state level after the removal of stimulus (which would be detraining), an estimate of k_d from these two time courses can be made. When the stimulus of exercise is absent during detraining, the k_d of the protein during detraining is assumed to represent the k_d value for the same protein under basal, sedentary conditions.[8] Consequently, if the k_d values during training and basal conditions are similar, then only an increase in k_s would be responsible for the higher E found at trained steady state.[7] On the other hand, a difference in k_d values in these two conditions would indicate that either a change only in k_d or a change in both k_d and k_s would cause the higher steady-state level of the protein.[7]

By the use of this methodology to obtain k_d and $t_{1/2}$, the time course of the increase in cytochrome c from a lower to a higher steady state was determined during training by distance running. Also, the time course from a higher to a lower steady-state level for cytochrome c was made during detraining. In this report,[9] no significant difference in k_d (and thus $t_{1/2}$) for cytochrome c in skeletal muscle was observed between training and detraining. Thus, it was concluded that a change in k_s must play the major role for the adaptive increases and decreases in cytochrome c levels when the amount of daily distant running is altered.[9] Implicit in these statements are the assumptions that (I) the stimulus to cytochrome c production from distant running ceases relatively abruptly at the start of detraining, (II) the rate of synthesis for cytochrome c immediately, at the onset of detraining, decreases to a synthesis rate that is characteristic of the rate observed in animals that are sedentary and have never undergone training, and (III) the exercise stimulus for cytochrome c to increase during training is applied once in a large amount and this simulus is maintained at the same intensity throughout training. In the experiments performed by us, actual measurements of the time course for the decay in cytochrome c levels did not begin until the second day of detraining.[9] The reasoning for beginning the time course at this time was the assumption that any lag during detraining for the conversion of cytochrome c synthesis rates to basal levels would have ended by the second day of detraining. Thus, it would be possible to assume that the k_d of detraining is reflective of the k_d for cytochrome c in sedentary animals.

The role that the intensity of daily running plays on both the absolute final level of the new steady state and the time course to this new steady state will be discussed next. Duration, speed, and incline contribute to the intensity of the daily run. In our experiments, intensity of distance running has been varied solely by varying the daily duration, while maintaining speed and incline at constant values throughout the training program. Using this experimental protocol, we have observed that the new, apparent steady-state level of cytochrome c after training was a direct function of the intensity of daily running (at the end of training, the daily durations of running varied from 10 to 120 min) [10] (FIGURE 1). From these data, it is possible to suggest a stimulus–response

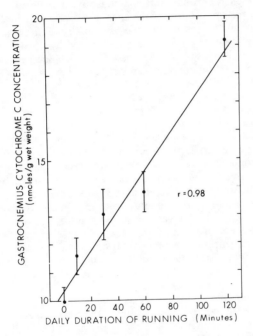

FIGURE 1. Correlation between the final duration of daily running and the level of cytochrome c in the gastrocnemius muscles of rats. All groups ran at 1.2 mph (0.5 m/sec) on a 15% grade. Measurements of cytochrome c were made after 15 weeks of training. (Data from Fitts et al.[10])

relationship between the daily duration of running (stimulus) and the new apparent steady-state level of cytochrome c (response). Similar conclusions have previously been made for other parameters of physical exercise. For example, Nordesjö [11] has concluded that the absolute change in either brief or extended work capacity by humans is directly dependent upon the intensity of training and consequently the total amount of work during training.

The existence of a stimulus–response relationship between the duration of daily running and the resultant steady-state level of cytochrome c in skeletal muscle provides the basis for the next topic, which is whether the rate of change in the intensity of daily exercise plays any role in the time course of the increase in cytochrome c. Previously in this paper it was stated that the k_d or $t_{1/2}$ for cytochrome c between two steady states was the same during training and detraining. However, in this earlier example, the rate by which the intensity of daily exercise was altered was not given. In the earlier training program, the duration of daily running was increased from 15 minutes on the previous day to 100 minutes. Moreover, animals then ran 100 min/day every day for the remainder of the training program (FIGURE 2). Thus, the intensity of exercise was altered by a single, abrupt change. Likewise, there was an abrupt decrease in the intensity of daily exercise for the detraining of the earlier example. Rats did not run any more on the day after running 120 minutes. Since the stimulus to the adaptive change in cytochrome c concentration for both training and detraining was applied abruptly and consequently maintained at this new level of stimulus, then the time course of the change in cytochrome c level in skeletal muscle will be a function of the $t_{1/2}$ (i.e., k_d) of cytochrome c. On the other hand, if the daily duration of running is not altered by a single abrupt change, but is progressively increased (or decreased) on each succeeding day, then the stimulus is progressively increasing (or decreasing) each day (FIGURE 2). In this case, the time for one-half of change of cytochrome c to occur is dependent on the total number of days during which the intensity of daily running (the stimulus) is increased by multiple increments. Thus, the time for one-half of the total increase above pretraining levels is usually much longer than the time of one $t_{1/2}$ of cytochrome c. Obviously, without a single abrupt change in the stimulus, the time course reflects the number of incremental changes rather than the $t_{1/2}$ of cytochrome c. A second approach to consider this concept is to recall that the resultant steady-state level of cytochrome c is caused by the duration (or intensity) of daily running. If the animal runs only a slightly greater duration on a given day, then the stimulus for cytochrome c adaptation is only enough to result in a small increase in steady state if this small stimulus were maintained unchanged for a period of weeks. Increasing the duration only by another small increment on a second day again provides another small increase in stimulus. The final steady-state level that would result from this second small stimulus will be slightly higher than the pretraining steady state. By continually superimposing new stimuli on existing responses, the observed half-time of a response is a function of the number of days the incremental changes in exercise stimulus occur. In FIGURE 3 a comparison of the time courses for the adaptive increases in cytochrome c between (I) the application of an abrupt, large stimulus on a single day, and (II) the application of small stimuli on multiple days is given.

If the $t_{1/2}$ for a protein whose steady-state level adapts to distance running is known, then the time-course of this protein's adaptation can be predicted when the stimulus (i.e., duration) of daily running is abruptly changed on a single day, and this new stimulus is applied on all subsequent days.[7, 8] For example, one-half of the total change in protein content that is to occur with continued application of the new stimulus, will occur after one half-life of this protein. Also, 75% of the total change will occur after two half-lives of this protein (during the second $t_{1/2}$, one-half × the remaining 50% = 25%; so that 50% from first $t_{1/2}$ + 25% from second $t_{1/2}$ = 75%). Then after three half-lives 87.5% of the total change will have occurred, and so forth. This prediction only applies when the $t_{1/2}$ of the protein is relatively long compared to the length of the treatment.[8] Let us apply this information to predict the time course of change in the level of cytochrome c in the skeletal muscle of a runner undergoing detraining, and then undergoing retraining. For this example, let us take a distant runner who has previously undergone endurance training over a period of weeks so that his cytochrome c level in his skeletal muscle has adapted to a

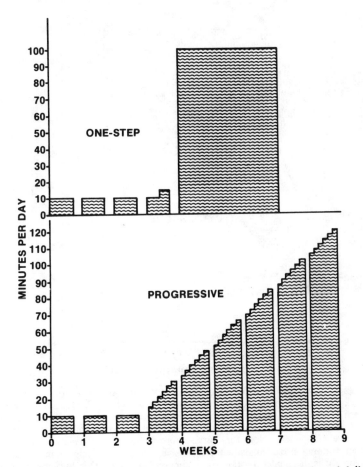

FIGURE 2. Comparison of the application of increases in the duration of daily running for two different training programs for rats. The one-step program involves a single, abrupt change in the duration of daily running from a level of 10–15 min/day for 5 days/week to a level of 100 min each day for 7 days/week. The speed of the treadmill was 1 mph (0.4 m/sec at a 15% grade). The second training program, designated progressive, has been described [18] and involves multiple, 3-min increases in the total duration of running each day. In this program, rats ran at 1 mph up a 10% grade for 6 days/week.

new steady-state level that is twice the level found in the sedentary population. Unfortunately, for the sake of our example, let us consider the consequences of an ankle injury that causes the runner to rest for 7 days, i.e., to undergo detraining for 7 days (FIGURE 4). Furthermore, let us make the assumption

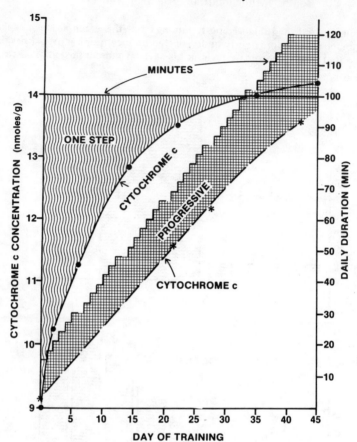

FIGURE 3. Comparison of the time course of increase in the level of cytochrome c in the gastrocnemius muscle of rats undergoing the two types of training programs that were described in FIGURE 2. The increase in the level of cytochrome c for the rats partaking in 100 min of daily running in the one-step program is designated by the upper curve (●——●). Note this curve approximates an exponential increase. For the other training program, called progressive, the rate of change in the level of cytochrome c is designated by the lower curve (*——*). This line approximates a linear change. The cross-hatching is illustrative so as to associate the staircase-like increase in the duration of daily running with the increase of cytochrome c during the progressive program. The wavy lines associate the 100-min daily running and increase in cytochrome c for the one-step training program. (Data from Booth and Holloszy [9] and Terjung et al.[18])

that the $t_{1/2}$ of cytochrome c in the runner's skeletal muscle is similar to the $t_{1/2}$ of cytochrome c in rodent skeletal muscle, which is 7 days.[9] Thus, the runner undergoes detraining for a time period roughly equivalent to 1 half-life of cytochrome c. As previously discussed in this paper, the rate of decay in protein concentration from a higher to a lower steady-state level is solely determined by the $t_{1/2}$ of the protein. Therefore, one-half of the absolute increase in cytochrome c above sedentary levels will be lost in 7 days. To further illustrate this example, the runner has a trained, steady-state level of 20 nmoles of cytochrome c per gram of skeletal muscle while the mean value for cytochrome c in a sedentary population is 10 nmole/g. Thus, after the 7th day of detraining, when the runner has lost one-half the absolute difference between two steady states [½ (20 − 10) =5], the runner would have 15 nmole/g of cytochrome c. Obviously, for simplicity of presentation, a number of assumptions are implicit and will not be discussed in detail. A few such assumptions are that (I) the rate of synthesis for cytochrome c at the onset of detraining immediately returns to values supporting a steady state level of 10 nmoles/g,[8] and (II) the sedentary steady-state level of cytochrome c in the runner of this example would be 10 nmole/g if detraining lasted long enough. Now, if after 7 days of detraining the runner is immediately able to return to an intensity (or duration) daily running, which would be required for a steady-state level of 20 nmole/g cytochrome c, then after 7 days of distance running, his cytochrome c level will have increased one-half of the absolute difference between 20 and 15 [½ (20 − 15) + 15 = 17.5]. Thus, after one

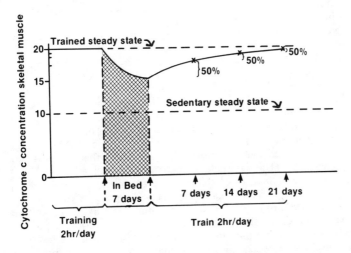

FIGURE 4. The predicted time-course of the change in the level of cytochrome c in the skeletal muscle of a distant runner who undergoes 7 days of detraining and consequently undergoes retraining. Prior to detraining, the runner's steady-state level of cytochrome c in his leg muscle is 20 nmole/g, or twice the steady-state level found in a population of sedentary people. The runner incurs an ankle injury and must not exercise for 7 days (indicated by the cross-hatched area). After these 7 days of detraining, the level of cytochrome c would be predicted to drop one-half of the trained increase (see text for details). Thus, the rate of change of cytochrome c is shown to exponentially decay from 20 to 15 nmole/g during the detraining. On the first day after detraining, it is presumed that the runner can immediately begin to run the same duration as prior to detraining, which is 2 hr/day. Moreover, this 2 hr/day duration is continued daily during retraining. The level of cytochrome c during retraining is predicted every seventh day to exponentially rise one-half of the difference between 20 and the level at the start of each 7-day period. Thus, after 7 days of retraining, it will be 17.5 nmole/g; after 14 days, it will be 18.8; and after 21 days of retraining, 19.4.

week of retraining at this intensity, there would be 17.5 nmole/g cytochrome c in the skeletal muscle of the runner. Likewise, if the runner continued running at the same intensity required for a final steady-state level of 20 nmole/g cytochrome c, then after 14 days of retraining cytochrome c would be 18.8 nmole/g [½ (20 − 17.5) + 17.5 = 18.8]; after 21 days it would be 19.4, and so forth. In summary, although it took only 7 days of detraining for a drop of 5 nmole/g (which is one-half of the difference between 20 and 10), it would take about 28 days of daily running (at a running intensity for a final steady-state level of 20 nmole/g) to regain the lost 5 nmole/g (that is, to increase from 15 to 20).

However, it is often very difficult for a runner to undergo a single, abrupt increase in the intensity of training after many days of detraining. For example, after 7 days of detraining, the runner may not have the fitness level to endure the duration of distance running necessary to stimulate the synthesis rate of cytochrome c necessary to produce the steady-state level of cytochrome c that was present prior to detraining. Therefore, the runner might progressively increase the intensity of daily running until he reached the intensity necessary to stimulate eventually the production cytochrome c at a level equivalent to that existing before detraining. Consequently, the time-course of the increase in cytochrome c when exercise duration is increased in multiple increments will be slower than the time-course for a single, abrupt increase in duration. Therefore, when the duration of daily running is progressively increased, the length of training necessary to regain the 5 nmole/g cytochrome c lost during detraining would be much longer than 28 days.

At this point, it might be good to review the roles that cytochrome c adaptations might play in permitting increased work capacities. Although the exact cause and effect relationships between increased cytochrome c levels in skeletal muscles and increased work capacities have yet to be shown, a number of correlations have been made between (I) parameters that serve as indexes of work capacity and (II) parameters, such as cytochrome c levels in skeletal muscle, that serve as indexes of the capacity of muscle to aerobically produce ATP. For example, a direct relationship between markers for the capacity of skeletal muscle to produce ATP and maximal oxygen uptake of the whole person have been demonstrated in numerous labs.[12-16] Moreover, a direct relationship between running time to exhaustion and cytochrome c levels in rodent skeletal muscle have been shown.[10] Finally, a direct relationship between the amounts of liver and muscle glycogen remaining at the end of a standardized work-bout and the capacity of skeletal muscle to aerobically produce ATP has been reported.[10] Although these correlations do not indicate the direct mode by which cytochrome c levels might play a role in producing increases in work capacity, they do suggest that knowledge of the $t_{\frac{1}{2}}$ of cytochrome c can provide information on the time course of adaptive changes related to work capacity, and can also be used to design training and detraining programs. Furthermore, since most physiological and biochemical processes in the organism are controlled by proteins, then the time-course of the change in maximal oxygen uptake is probably related to the time-course in the adaptations of numerous proteins. For example, a preliminary report indicates that the time-course in cardiac enlargement between sedentary and trained steady states follows first-order kinetics when the duration of daily exercise is altered by a single abrupt change.[17] It would be interesting to determine if the time-course of the increase in maximal cardiac output follows a similar time-course as cardiac enlargement. So, although this paper has dealt with the time-course for the adaptation of a single protein during distance running, the information presented herein might provide models for the time-courses of other adaptations occurring during repeated daily bouts of distance running.

References

1. HOLLOSZY, J. O. & F. W. BOOTH. 1976. Biochemical adaptations to endurance exercise in muscle. Ann. Rev. Physiol. **38:** 273–291.
2. BOSTRÖM, S.-L., G. HÖGBERG & R. G. JOHANSSON. 1974. Enzyme activities in skeletal muscle after contractile activity in vitro. Int. J. Biochem. **5:** 487–494.
3. BENZI, G., P. PANCERI, M. DEBERNARDI, R. VILLA, E. ARCELLI, L. D'ANGELO, E. ARRIGONI & F. BERTÈ. 1975. Mitochondrial enzymatic adaptation of skeletal muscle to training. J. Appl. Physiol. **38:** 565–569.
4. GOLDBERG, A. L. & J. F. DICE. 1974. Intracellular protein degradation in mammalian and bacterial cells. Ann. Rev. Biochem. **43:** 835–869.
5. ARIAS, I. M., D. DOYLE & R. T. SCHIMKE. 1969. Studies on the synthesis and degradation of proteins of the enoplasmic reticulum of rat liver. J. Biol. Chem. **244:** 3303–3315.
6. SCHIMKE, R. T. & D. DOYLE. 1970. Control of enzyme levels in animal tissues. Ann. Rev. Biochem. **39:** 929–976.
7. SCHIMKE, R. T. 1970. Regulation of protein degradation in mammalian tissues. *In* Mammalian Protein Metabolism. H. N. Munro, Ed. Vol. **4:** 177–228. Academic Press. New York, N.Y.
8. SCHIMKE, R. T. 1975. Methods for analysis of enzyme synthesis and degradation in animal tissues. *In* Methods in Enzymology. B. W. O'Mailley & J. G. Hardman, Eds. Vol. **40:** 241–266.
9. BOOTH, F. W. & J. O. HOLLOSZY. 1977. Cytochrome c turnover in rat skeletal muscles. J. Biol. Chem. **252:** 416–419.
10. FITTS, R. H., F. W. BOOTH, W. W. WINDER & J. O. HOLLOSZY. 1975. Skeletal muscle respiratory capacity, endurance, and glycogen utilization. Amer. J. Physiol. **228:** 1029–1033.
11. NORDESJÖ, L-O. 1974. The effect of quantitated training on the capacity for short and prolonged work. Acta Physiol. Scand. (Suppl.) 405.
12. HOPPELER, H., P. LÜTHI, H. CLAASSEN, E. R. WEIBEL & H. HOWALD. 1973. The ultrastructure of the normal human skeletal muscle. Pflügers Arch. **344:** 217–232.
13. COSTILL, D. L., P. D. GOLLNICK, E. D. JANSSON, B. SALTIN & E. M. STEIN. 1973. Glycogen depletion patterns in human muscle fibers during distance running. Acta Physiol. Scand. **89:** 374–383.
14. BOOTH, F. W. & K. A. NARAHARA. 1974. Vastus lateralis cytochrome oxidase activity and its relationship to maximal oxygen consumption in man. Pflügers Arch. **349:** 319–324.
15. KIESSLING, K-H., L. PILSTRÖM, A.-CH. BYLUNG, B. SALTIN & K. PIEHL. 1974. Enzyme activities and morphometry in skeletal muscle of middle-aged men after training. Scand. J. Clin. Lab. Invest. **33:** 63–69.
16. COSTILL, D. L., J. DANIELS, W. EVANS, W. FINK, G. KRAHENBUHL & B. SALTIN. 1976. Skeletal muscle enzymes and fiber composition in male and female track athletes. J. Appl. Physiol. **40:** 149–154.
17. HICKSON, R. C., G. T. HAMMONS, R. K. CONLEE & J. O. HOLLOSZY. 1976. Time course of the development of cardiac hypertrophy with endurance training. Med. Sci. Sports **8:** 55.
18. TERJUNG, R. L., W. W. WINDER, K. M. BALDWIN & J. O. HOLLOSZY. 1973. Effect of exercise on the turnover of cytochrome c in skeletal muscle. J. Biol. Chem. **248:** 7404–7406.

PHYSIOLOGICAL CONSEQUENCES OF THE BIOCHEMICAL ADAPTATIONS TO ENDURANCE EXERCISE *

J. O. Holloszy, M. J. Rennie, R. C. Hickson,
R. K. Conlee, and J. M. Hagberg

Department of Preventive Medicine
Washington University School of Medicine
St. Louis, Missouri 63110

Top level marathon runners maintain a pace of 11 to 12 mph (5–5.5 m/sec) in competition. This is a running speed they could probably not keep up for more than one mile in the untrained state. A question of major importance for this symposium is: What are the adaptations to endurance exercise-training that make it possible for an individual to run at this grueling pace for 26.2 miles?

Biochemical and Structural Adaptations to Exercise

The adaptations to endurance exercise in skeletal muscle and in the heart have been reviewed in detail recently [1, 2] and will therefore be summarized only briefly here to provide a background for a consideration of their consequences. The most important adaptive response of skeletal muscle to endurance exercise such as long distance running or swimming is an augmentation of respiratory capacity with increases in the abilities to oxidize pyruvate,[3, 4] fatty acids,[5, 6] and ketones.[7, 8] As a result of increases in the levels of the enzymes of the malate–aspartate shuttle,[9] there is also an enhancement of the capability for mitochondrial oxidation of the reducing equivalents generated in the cytoplasm during glycolysis. Although a variety of other adaptations occur in muscle in response to endurance exercise, including alterations in glycolytic capacity [10] and actomyosin ATPase activity,[11] these changes appear to be small, and their physiological significance is unclear at present.

The rise in muscle respiratory capacity results from an increase in muscle mitochondria,[4, 12, 13] as well as from an alteration in mitochondrial composition [7, 14–16] that makes skeletal muscle mitochondria more like heart mitochondria in their enzyme pattern. As reviewed elsewhere in this symposium,[82] the increase in mitochondria induced by endurance exercise appears to result from a greater rate of protein synthesis, and can occur in all three types of skeletal muscle fiber.[83] In addition to the increase in muscle mitochondria, the myoglobin concentration in muscle is increased by endurance exercise training.[17]

In contrast to the response to strength exercise such as weight lifting, hypertrophy is not a necessary component of the adaptation to endurance exercise.[2, 3] (Strength exercise does not induce an increase in muscle mitochondria.[18]) The major factor that normally determines the respiratory capacity

* This research was supported by National Institutes of Health Research Grants AG00425 and AM18986 and Training Grant AM05341 and by a Muscular Dystrophy Associations of America Neuromuscular Disease Research Center Grant.

of a muscle fiber appears to be its habitual contractile activity; that is, within wide limits, the more frequently muscle fibers contract, the greater their mitochondrial content, and vice versa.[2] The lower respiratory capacity of white muscle fibers is, at least in large part, a consequence of the fact that they are recruited to contract less frequently than are the red fibers.

While the more detailed studies of the responses of the mitochondrial enzymes in skeletal muscle to endurance exercise have been performed on rats, a number of investigations have firmly established that exercise-training also induces increases in the mitochondrial content and respiratory capacity of skeletal muscle in man.[4, 13, 19, 20] In both species intensive training can result in a 2-fold or greater increase in muscle respiratory capacity.

In contrast to skeletal muscle, there is no increase in the respiratory capacity of heart muscle in response to endurance exercise.[21-23] The concentrations of cytochrome c and of mitochondrial protein as well as the levels of activity of various mitochondrial enzymes, expressed per gram of heart muscle, are not different in trained as compared to untrained rats. There is some evidence that myocardial contractility can be enhanced by training; and it has been reported that the specific activity of actomyosin ATPase is increased in the hearts of rats subjected to programs of swimming.[23] Probably the most important cardiac adaptation to endurance exercise in terms of its physiological consequences is an increase in heart size. In rats subjected to programs of running or swimming the increase in heart weight has been in the range of 15% to 30%.[21, 22] The development of cardiac hypertrophy in rats subjected to a constant exercise stress is a rapid process; the half-times of the increases in heart weight, total protein, and dry weight are in the range of 5 to 6 days.[24] A recent study in which the left ventricular dimensions of endurance athletes were evaluated echocardiographically showed that their cardiac hypertrophy was of the volume overload type, with increased left ventricular end-diastolic volume and mass but with normal wall thickness.[25]

Physiological Manifestations of the Adaptations to Exercise

When previously sedentary individuals are retested at the same absolute submaximal work rate after adapting to endurance exercise, their endurance is found to be markedly increased. (Submaximal work is defined here as exercise requiring less than the individual's $\dot{V}_{O_2max}$.) The cardiovascular response to the same submaximal work (i.e., at the same $\dot{V}_{O_2}$) is considerably modified by training; heart rate is slower, stroke volume is greater, and blood flow to the working muscles is lower.[26, 27] In the trained state a smaller proportion of the cardiac output goes to working muscles, because the decrease in blood flow to the liver and other organs during exercise is less than in the untrained state.[26, 27] The working muscles compensate for the lower blood flow in the trained state by extracting more O_2; this is reflected in an increased arteriovenous O_2 difference.[27] A number of differences in the metabolic response to the same absolute work rate (i.e., at the same $\dot{V}_{O_2}$) are also evident in the trained state. These include a slower depletion of muscle [28-32] and liver [31, 32] glycogen stores, a smaller rise in muscle [29, 30] and blood [28-30] lactate concentration, and a lower respiratory quotient (RQ), indicating a greater reliance on fat oxidation for generation of energy.[28, 30, 33]

Endurance exercise training also results in an increase in the maximum capacity to consume O_2 ($\dot{V}_{O_2max}$); this adaptation makes it possible for an individual to exercise at higher work rates in the trained than in the untrained state. When one takes the trained individual's higher $\dot{V}_{O_2max}$ into account and evaluates the responses to the same relative work rate (i.e., at the same percentage of $\dot{V}_{O_2max}$), heart rate is the same or slightly lower, stroke volume and cardiac output are greater, blood flow per kg of working skeletal muscle is the same, and the arterio-venous O_2 difference is greater in the trained as compared to the untrained state.[26, 27, 34, 35] Despite the fact that a higher work rate is required to attain the same relative $\dot{V}_{O_2}$ in the trained state, the rate of muscle glycogen depletion is the same, muscle and blood lactate concentrations increase less, and the RQ is lower in the trained, as compared to the untrained state at the same relative work rate.[28-30] The latter two findings show that there are qualitative as well quantitative differences in the metabolic response to exercise in the trained as compared to the untrained state. Of particular interest is the finding that no more glycogen is utilized at the same relative work rate in the trained state. It appears, from measurements of the rate of glycogen depletion and of RQ, that the increase in energy requirement caused by the greater work rate needed to attain the same relative $\dot{V}_{O_2}$ following training is met entirely by a proportional augmentation of fat oxidation.[28, 29, 30]

It is well established that endurance is a function of relative work rate; the greater the percentage of one's $\dot{V}_{O_2max}$ required for the performance of an activity, the shorter is the duration for which it can be continued.[36, 37] This relationship applies not only to the whole organism but also to muscle cells. When a muscle, such as the soleus, is stimulated via the nerve with supramaximal shocks so that all the muscle fibers contract, the muscle cells' O_2 consumption varies over a wide range, up to maximum, as a function of stimulation rate (i.e., of the number of contractions per minute) if load is held constant. The greater the stimulation rate and O_2 uptake, the more rapidly the muscle fatigues.

Biochemical Basis for the Increased Endurance for Work of the Same Absolute Intensity after Training

It is not surprising that training that induces an adaptive increase in $\dot{V}_{O_2max}$ also increases endurance, since the same absolute work rate represents a lower relative work intensity (i.e., requires a smaller percentage of $\dot{V}_{O_2max}$) after training. Of the various causes of muscle fatigue, muscle glycogen depletion is the one for which there is probably the best documentation.[28, 38, 39] Glycogen depletion occurs when exercise sufficiently strenuous to cause moderately rapid glycogenolysis is continued for a sufficiently long period. This is just the type of exercise involved in marathon running, in which the competitors generally utilize between 70% and 85% of their $\dot{V}_{O_2max}$.[40, 41] Higher relative work rates can usually not be maintained sufficiently long to result in exhaustion of glycogen stores; at work rates requiring above 75% to 85% of $\dot{V}_{O_2max}$ (there appears to be considerable individual variation) other factors related to the disturbance of cellular homeostasis force the cessation of exercise. Although these factors have not yet been clearly identified, it does seem evident that the extent to which homeostasis is deranged, as measured by such indicators as the rate of lactate production and the rate of development of an O_2 deficit, determines how long work can be continued.[42] Both the rate of glycogen depletion and the extent to which homeostasis is perturbed are a function of the relative, rather than the absolute, submaximal work rate. The biochemical basis for this relationship can best be examined in the context of the mechanisms for gearing ATP production to ATP utilization.

Regulation of ATP Production in Working Muscle. Skeletal muscles can generate the ATP required for work by means of both glycolytic and aerobic phosphorylation of ADP. The relative contributions of these two pathways of energy production depends on work rate relative to the $\dot{V}_{O_2max}$ of the working muscle cells and on substrate availability. The rate at which working muscle cells utilize oxygen is determined by the rate of ATP hydrolysis which, in turn, is determined by the work rate. O_2 can not be utilized unless ADP and P_i are available, because oxidative phosphorylation is tightly coupled to electron transport. This coupling provides the mechanism by which substrate oxidation is geared to ATP utilization. When muscle contracts, ATP is split and the levels of ADP and P_i rise. Of these two compounds, ADP is present in lower concentration and appears to be rate-limiting. There is evidence that the ratio of ATP/ADP, rather than the concentration of ADP alone, determines the rate of O_2 uptake.[43] The increase in ADP with muscle contraction is largely damped by the creatine kinase reaction, which catalyzes the re-synthesis of ATP by transferring the high energy phosphate from creatine phosphate (CP) to ADP. Consequently, CP concentration falls and creatine concentration rises. If work is submaximal, ADP concentration will rise until respiration is turned on sufficiently to balance the rate of ATP splitting.[44] Once a steady submaximal rate of O_2 consumption is attained in a muscle cell, the rate of ATP formation during and between muscle contractions must balance the rate of ATP splitting during the contraction. In the interval between the beginning of work and the attainment of the steady state, before ATP hydrolysis is balanced by oxidative phosphorylation and glycolysis, the high energy phosphate content of the cell drops,[42, 45, 46] resulting in the muscle O_2 deficit. The decrease in high energy phosphate concentration, the increases in P_i and ADP, and the other concomitant changes, which include increases in AMP and ammonium ion concentration, simultaneously result in an acceleration of glycolysis as a result of an increase in phosphofructokinase activity.[47-50] If work is so intense that the rate of ATP utilization exceeds the muscle cell's capacity to regenerate ATP via oxidative phosphorylation, the concentrations of ADP and P_i will continue to rise above the level needed to activate respiration maximally, and CP and ATP levels will drop either until glycolysis is activated sufficiently so that, together with respiration, it generates enough ATP to balance ATP hydrolysis, or until muscle contractile function becomes impaired and work output decreases.

Differences in Response to the Same Absolute Work Rate of Trained and Untrained Muscle. Skeletal muscle that has adapted to endurance exercise has a greater content of mitochondria than untrained; the disturbance in cellular homeostasis that occurs in response to a given submaximal work rate is therefore less. For example, if a "trained" muscle cell contains twice as many mitochondria as an otherwise similar "untrained" muscle cell, the amount of O_2 consumed by each mitochondrion should be only 50% as great in the trained as compared to the untrained muscle at a given submaximal work rate that results in the same O_2 consumption in the two cells. In other words, the greater the number of mitochondrial respiratory chains per unit of muscle mass, the lower must be the O_2 uptake per respiratory chain to maintain a given submaximal level of O_2 consumption. Therefore, it seems reasonable that, in the process of attaining a steady state level of O_2 uptake, the concentration of high energy phosphates must decrease less, and ADP, P_i, and creatine concentrations must increase less in trained than in untrained muscle. Muscles contain large amounts of adenylate kinase, which converts some of the ADP formed to AMP; a portion of this AMP is deaminated by the action of AMP deaminase to form ammonia.[51] With a smaller rise in ADP, it seems likely that AMP and ammonium ion levels are also lower in trained than in untrained muscles.

Glycolysis is to a large extent controlled by the intracellular concentrations of ATP and CP (which inhibit phosphofructokinase) and of P_i, AMP, ADP, and ammonia (which counteract this inhibition).[47-50] Increased oxidation of fatty acids also inhibits glycolysis.[52-56] As will be discussed in more detail later, the adaptive increase in the capacity to oxidize fat results in a shift in the carbon source for the citrate cycle, so that at the same work rate and external fatty acid concentration skeletal muscle that has adapted to endurance exercise obtains more of its energy from fat oxidation and less from carbohydrate.

To summarize, as a result of the adaptive increase in muscle mitochondria, work of the same intensity causes a smaller disturbance of cellular homeostasis and a slower rate of glycogen depletion in the trained than in the untrained state. A smaller decrease in creatine phosphate and ATP concentration helps to explain the smaller O_2 deficit, and, together with increased oxidation of fat, accounts for the slower rates of lactate production and glycogen depletion in the trained state. It is not clear at present whether or not the cardiac adaptations to endurance exercise, which are responsible for the higher maximum cardiac output seen in the trained state, also contribute to the greater endurance at the same absolute work rate. Cardiac output is the same (or less) and blood flow to the working muscles is lower in the trained as compared to the untrained state at the same work rate.[26, 27] It, therefore, seems unlikely that the cardiac adaptations play a role in protecting against the development of skeletal muscle fatigue. On the other hand, there is the possibility that the heart itself might fatigue during prolonged strenuous exercise.[57, 58] If myocardial fatigue does play a role in causing physical exhaustion during prolonged exercise, the physiological cardiac hypertrophy that occurs in response to training could have a protective effect. The role played by the cardiac adaptations is more obvious at a work intensity that requires a $\dot{V}_{O_2}$ higher than the individual's $\dot{V}_{O_2max}$ when he is untrained, but which is submaximal when he is trained; the trained heart can develop a higher output and deliver blood and O_2 to a larger mass of working muscles.

Role of the $\dot{V}_{O_2max}$ in Marathon Running. Good marathon runners maintain a 11 to 12 mph pace in competition. Successful marathon runners are highly efficient in their movements and utilize only about 56 to 60 ml of O_2 per kg per minute at these running speeds.[40, 41, 59] If a marathon runner with a $\dot{V}_{O_2max}$ of 58 ml/kg·min when untrained, and of 75 ml/kg·min when trained, consumes 56 ml O_2/kg·min while running at 11 mph, he would utilize 96% of his $\dot{V}_{O_2max}$ while running at his competitive pace when untrained, and 75% of $\dot{V}_{O_2max}$ when trained. A $\dot{V}_{O_2max}$ of 58 ml/kg per·min is unusually high for an untrained individual; with a more realistic V_{O_2max} of 55 ml/kg·min in the untrained state the marathon runner's competitive marathon pace would require a $\dot{V}_{O_2}$ in excess of his $\dot{V}_{O_2max}$. In either case, it seems clear that he could maintain his competitive pace of 11 mph for only a short distance when he is untrained.

Work of the Same Relative Intensity in the Trained and Untrained States

In order to complete a marathon when he is untrained, a runner would have to maintain a much slower pace than when he is trained. Let us assume that our hypothetical runner could utilize 75% of his $\dot{V}_{O_2max}$ for the same length of time when he is untrained as when he is trained. Let us further assume that running at an 8.5 mph pace requires 75% of his $\dot{V}_{O_2max}$ when he is untrained, and that he has to stop because of exhaustion after 2 hours 23 minutes when he has completed 20.2 miles. In contrast, he can complete the 26.2 mile long marathon in the same length of time in the trained state when his $\dot{V}_{O_2max}$ is 75 ml/kg·min, and he can maintain a 11 mph pace. He would, therefore, actually have to run at a slower pace that requires less than 75% of his $\dot{V}_{O_2max}$ in order to complete the marathon when he is untrained, because he would have to run for a longer period of time. As mentioned earlier, the longer the period of exercise, the lower is the relative work rate that an individual can maintain. Therefore, the lower an individual's level of training (ie., the smaller his $\dot{V}_{O_2max}$), the lower is the percentage of his $\dot{V}_{O_2max}$ that he can utilize while running an entire marathon.

It appears to be the impression of most exercise physiologists who have studied marathon runners that these highly trained individuals can maintain greater relative work rates for longer periods than untrained individuals (or even than trained individuals who do not regularly exercise continually for as long periods in their training programs). However, there is some controversy regarding whether or not training increases an individual's ability to maintain a high relative work intensity.[36, 37] One study that supports the concept that endurance at the same relative work intensity is increased by training has been reported by Gleser and Vogel [60] who tested a group of young men before and after a training program that increased $\dot{V}_{O_2max}$ by 12%. They found that the training resulted in an increase in endurance time on a bicycle ergometer of approximately 21% at a work rate requiring 65% of $\dot{V}_{O_2max}$, of 12% at a work rate requiring 75% of $\dot{V}_{O_2max}$, and of 8% at a work rate requiring 80% of $\dot{V}_{O_2max}$. This question requires further study, particularly in highly trained endurance athletes. If it can be shown that marathon runners are able to maintain work rates requiring 70% to 85% of their $\dot{V}_{O_2max}$ for longer than untrained or moderately trained individuals, the explanation may be in the finding that the increase in muscle mitochondria with intensive prolonged training is proportionally much greater than the increase in whole body $\dot{V}_{O_2max}$.[20, 41] It is conceivable that when a highly trained individual performs the activity in which he is trained, his working muscle cells may utilize a smaller percentage of their maximum capacity to consume O_2 than those of an untrained individual, despite a similar relative whole body $\dot{V}_{O_2}$. If this is so, the disturbance of cellular homeostasis would be milder and fatigue could be delayed.

Although our emphasis has been on the effects of training, it must be kept in mind that successful marathon runners are a highly selected group; it is, therefore, not unlikely that genetic factors contribute to the champion runner's endurance and great work capacity. For example, it seems well documented that the muscles of successful marathon runners contain a higher percentage of slow twitch fibers than average.[18, 41, 61] It seems well documented that the slow twitch muscle fibers are preferentially recruited during work requiring 70% to 85% of $\dot{V}_{O_2max}$.[62-64] When slow twitch fibers are depleted of glycogen during prolonged exercise, fast twitch muscle fibers are recruited to contract.[63] Since glycogen concentration decreases more rapidly in fast twitch white muscle fibers than in slow twitch red fibers in response to contractile activity, the marathon runners' greater pool of slow twitch fibers may provide a significant advantage during prolonged exercise.

Effect of Training on the Proportion of Energy Derived from Oxidation of Fat. Perhaps the most marked difference between trained and untrained individuals in their metabolic responses to the same relative work intensity is in the proportions of fat and carbohydrate utilized. Despite the greater work rate required to attain the same relative $\dot{V}_{O_2}$ after training, the rate of muscle glycogen utilization is similar in the trained and untrained states at the same relative work intensity.[28-30] Measurements of the RQ and of the amount of glycogen utilized have provided evidence that the additional energy required at the same relative work rate in the trained state is provided by oxidation of fat.[28-30] This adaptive increase in fat oxidation has an extremely important glycogen-sparing effect, which plays a major role in accounting for the increase in the capacity for prolonged strenuous exercise that occurs in response to endurance exercise training. If it were not for this adaptation, many marathon runners maintaining a pace requiring 75% of $\dot{V}_{O_2max}$ would probably have depleted the glycogen stores in their slow twitch fibers after completing about three-fouths of the race.

The concentration of fatty acids to which the muscles are exposed and the muscles' capacity to oxidize fatty acids are the two major factors that determine the rate of fatty acid oxidation during submaximal exercise. When the metabolic rate is constant (at rest or during steady-state exercise), the rate of fat oxidation increases linearly with fatty acid concentration.[65, 66] Thus, it appears that the availability of fatty acids to the mitochondria is the rate-limiting factor for fatty acid oxidation at any given $\dot{V}_{O_2}$. However, at any concentration of fatty acids the rate of fatty acid oxidation is highest in the muscles with the greatest capacity to oxidize fat. For example, at the same fatty acid concentration, the heart will oxidize fatty acids more rapidly than skeletal muscle, and red skeletal muscle will oxidize fat more rapidly than white muscle.

It was thought at one time that the trained individual's greater utilization of fat during exercise was the result of a higher plasma concentration of fatty acids.[1] However, there is now considerable evidence showing that plasma fatty acid concentration actually tends to be lower in the trained than in the untrained state during submaximal exercise.[8, 67-69] Thus, the increased oxidation of fat in the trained state appears to be entirely due to the adaptive increase in muscle mitochondria and the increase in mitochondrial enzymes involved in the oxidation of fatty acids.[5, 6]

Since endurance exercise induces comparable increases in the capacities to oxidize fat and carbohydrate in skeletal muscle,[1, 2] it seems reasonable to ask why the trained individual oxidizes proportionately more fat and less carbohydrate than the untrained. It is well documented that glucose uptake, glycolysis, glycogenolysis, and pyruvate oxidation are inhibited in the heart by oxidation of fatty acids,[52-55] and Randle and coworkers in 1963 proposed that inhibition of carbohydrate utilization by oxidation of fatty acids is a general phenomenon.[70] This inhibition is mediated, at least in part, by the accumulation of citrate, which inhibits phosphofructokinase activity.[52, 71, 72] The consequent accumulation of glucose–6–PO_4 in turn inhibits hexokinase.[54, 73] However, studies on skeletal muscle fibers incubated *in vitro*[74] and on perfused rat hindquarter preparations[75-77] failed to show an inhibitory effect of fatty acids on glucose metabolism, leading Reimer *et al.*[77] to conclude that the mechanism proposed by Randle *et al.*[73] is confined to heart muscle and does not occur in skeletal muscle.

However, this conclusion is not consistent with the observation that the progressive increase in plasma free fatty acid concentration during prolonged exercise[78-80] is associated with a decrease in RQ,[33, 79, 81] which indicates a change in the carbon source for oxidation from carbohydrate to fat. It is also not in keeping with the finding that trained individuals derive more of their energy from fat oxidation than do untrained during submaximal exercise. We have, therefore, re-examined the effects of fatty acids on carbohydrate utilization in skeletal muscle. In our first study we compared the responses of rats in which plasma free fatty acids were increased (by feeding a fat meal followed by administration of heparin) with those of control rats during a standardized bout of treadmill running.[56] It was found that elevation of plasma fatty acids slowed the rate of glycogen depletion in the red types of muscle, and partially inhibited uptake of plasma glucose.[56] Subsequent studies on soleus muscle stimulated to contract *in situ* in anesthetized rats have provided evidence that these effects of fatty acids are mediated, at least in part, by accumulation of citrate, with inhibition of phosphofructokinase.[84] Thus, it appears clear that, as in the heart, fatty acids have a glycogen-sparing effect in the red types of skeletal muscle fibers, which are selectively recruited to contract during prolonged exercise. If, as postulated above, the glycogen-sparing effect of an enhanced oxidation of fatty acids contributes importantly to the increased endurance of trained individuals, then an artificial elevation of plasma fatty acid concentration should mimic this effect of training. This hypothesis was confirmed in a recent study in which the effects of elevation of plasma fatty acids on endurance was examined in rats subjected to an exhausting treadmill run. It was found that animals in which plasma fatty acids were raised, by feeding a fat meal followed by injection of heparin, were able to run approximately 50% longer than control rats before becoming exhausted.[85]

In summary, endurance exercise training induces an increase in the rate of myocardial protein synthesis, which results in a physiological cardiac hypertrophy. Endurance exercise also induces an adaptive increase in the mitochondrial content and respiratory capacity of skeletal muscle. These two adaptations result in an increase in $\dot{V}_{O_2,max}$ and make it possible for an individual to exercise at higher absolute work rates for prolonged periods when he is trained than when he is untrained. As a result of the increase in the respiratory capacity of skeletal muscle, submaximal exercise of the same absolute intensity causes a smaller disturbance in homeostasis and a slower utilization of glycogen in the working muscle cells of trained as compared to untrained individuals. The adaptive increase in the capacity to oxidize fatty acids also results in a greater reliance on fat oxidation for energy during work of the same relative intensity in the trained state; this adaptation helps to protect against the rapid depletion of glycogen stores.

References

1. HOLLOSZY, J. O. 1973. Exercise and Sport Sciences Reviews. J. Wilmore, Ed. : 45–71. Academic Press. New York, N.Y.
2. HOLLOSZY, J. O. & F. W. BOOTH. 1976. Ann. Rev. Physiol. **38:** 273–291.
3. HOLLOSZY, J. O. 1967. J. Biol. Chem. **242:** 2278–2282.
4. MORGAN, T. E., L. A. COBB, F. A. SHORT, R. ROSS & D. R. GUNN. 1971. In Muscle Metabolism During Exercise. B. Pernow & B. Saltin Eds. : 87–95. Plenum Press. New York, N.Y.
5. MOLÉ, P. A., L. B. OSCAI & J. O. HOLLOSZY. 1971. J. Clin. Invest. **50:** 2323–2330.
6. HOLLOSZY, J. O., P. A. MOLÉ, K. M. BALDWIN & R. L. TERJUNG. 1973. In Limiting Factors of Physical Performance. J. Keul, Ed. : 66–80. Georg Thieme Verlag. Stuttgart, West Germany.
7. WINDER, W. W., K. M. BALDWIN & J. O. HOLLOSZY. 1974. Eur. J. Biochem. **47:** 461–467.
8. WINDER, W. W., K. M. BALDWIN & J. O. HOLLOSZY. 1975. Can. J. Physiol. Pharmacol. **53:** 86–91.
9. HOLLOSZY, J. O., F. W. BOOTH, W. W. WINDER & R. H. FITTS. 1975. In Metabolic Adaptation to Prolonged Physical Exercise. H. Howald & J. R. Poortmans, Eds. : 438–446. Birkhauser Verlag. Basel, Switzerland.
10. BALDWIN, K. M., W. W. WINDER, R. L. TERJUNG & J. O. HOLLOSZY. 1973. Amer. J. Physiol. **225:** 962–966.
11. BALDWIN, K. M., W. W. WINDER & J. O. HOLLOSZY. 1975. Amer. J. Physiol. **229:** 422–426.
12. GOLLNICK, P. D. & D. W. KING. 1969. Amer. J. Physiol. **216:** 1502–1509.
13. HOPPELER, H., P. LUTHI, H. CLAASSEN, E. R. WEIBEL & H. HOWALD. 1973. Pflügers Arch. **344:** 217–232.
14. HOLLOSZY, J. O. & L. B. OSCAI. 1969. Arch. Biochem. Biophys. **130:** 653–656.
15. HOLLOSZY, J. O., L. B. OSCAI, I. J. DON & P. A. MOLÉ. 1970. Biochem. Biophys. Res. Commun. **40:** 1368–1373.
16. OSCAI, L. B. & J. O. HOLLOSZY. 1971. J. Biol. Chem. **246:** 6968–6972.
17. PATTENGALE, P. K. & J. O. HOLLOSZY. 1967. Amer. J. Physiol. **213:** 783–785.
18. GOLLNICK, P. D., R. B. ARMSTRONG, C. W. SAUBERT, K. PIEHL & B. SALTIN. 1972. J. Appl. Physiol. **33:** 312–319.
19. VARNAUSKAS, E., P. BJORNTORP, M. FAHLEN, I. PREROVSKY & J. STENBERG. 1970. Cardiovasc. Res. **4:** 418–422.
20. GOLLNICK, P. D., R. B. ARMSTRONG, B. SALTIN, C. W. SAUBERT, IV, W. L. SEMBROWICH & R. E. SHEPHERD. 1973. J. Appl. Physiol. **34:** 107–111.
21. OSCAI, L. B., P. A. MOLÉ, B. BREI & J. O. HOLLOSZY. 1971. Amer. J. Physiol. **220:** 1238–1241.
22. OSCAI, L. B., P. A. MOLÉ & J. O. HOLLOSZY. 1971. Amer. J. Physiol. **220:** 1944–1948.
23. SCHEUER, J., S. PENPARGKUL & A. K. BHAN. 1974. Amer. J. Cardiol. **33:** 744–751.
24. HICKSON, R. C., G. T. HAMMONS, R. K. CONLEE & J. O. HOLLOSZY. 1976. Med. Sci. Sports **8:** 55 (Abst.).
25. MORGANROTH, J., B. J. BARON, W. L. HENRY & S. E. EPSTEIN. 1975. Ann. Intern. Med. **82:** 521–524.

26. ROWELL, L. B. 1974. Physiol. Rev. **54:** 75–159.
27. CLAUSEN, J. P. 1976. Prog. Cardiovasc. Dis. **82:** 459–495.
28. HERMANSEN, L., E. HULTMAN & B. SALTIN. 1967. Acta Physiol. Scand. **71:** 129–139.
29. SALTIN, B. & J. KARLSSON. 1971. *In* Muscle Metabolism During Exercise. B. Pernow & B. Saltin, Eds. : 395–399. Plenum Press. New York, N.Y.
30. SALTIN, B. & J. KARLSSON. 1971. *In* Muscle Metabolism During Exercise. B. Pernow & B. Saltin, Eds. : 289–299. Plenum Press. New York, N.Y.
31. BALDWIN, K. M., R. H. FITTS, F. W. BOOTH, W. W. WINDER & J. O. HOLLOSZY. 1975. Pflügers Arch. **354:** 203–212.
32. FITTS, R. H., F. W. BOOTH, W. W. WINDER & J. O. HOLLOSZY. 1975. Amer. J. Physiol. **228:** 1029–1033.
33. CHRISTENSEN, E. H. & O. HANSEN. 1939. Skand. Arch. Physiol. **81:** 180–189.
34. GRIMBY, G., E. HAGGENDAL & B. SALTIN. 1967. J. Appl. Physiol. **22:** 305–310.
35. EKBLOM, B., P.-P. ASTRAND, B. SALTIN, J. STENBERG & B. WALLSTROM. 1968. J. Appl. Physiol. **24:** 518–528.
36. ÅSTRAND, P.-O. & K. RODAHL. 1970. *In* Text Book of Work Physiology. : 291–293. McGraw-Hill Book Company. New York, N.Y.
37. SALTIN, B. 1971. Scand. J. Rehab. Med. **3:** 39–46.
38. BERGSTROM, J., L. HERMANSEN, E. HULTMAN & B. SALTIN. 1967. Acta Physiol. Scand. **71:** 140–150.
39. AHLBORG, B., J. BERGSTROM, L.-G. EKELUND & E. HULTMAN. 1967. Acta Physiol. Scand. **70:** 129–142.
40. COSTILL, D. L. & E. L. FOX. 1969. Med. Sci. Sport **1:** 81–86.
41. COSTILL, D. L., W. J. FINK & M. L. POLLOCK. 1976. Med. Sci. Sport **8:** 96–100.
42. KARLSSON, J. & B. SALTIN. 1970. J. Appl. Physiol. **29:** 598–602.
43. DAVIS, E. J. & L. LUMENG. 1975. J. Biol. Chem. **250:** 2275–2282.
44. JOBSIS, F. F. & J. C. DUFFIELD. 1967. J. Gen. Physiol. **50:** 1009–1047.
45. PIIPER, J., P. E. DI PRAMPERO & P. CERRETELLI. 1968. Amer. J. Physiol. **215:** 523–531.
46. HULTMAN, E., J. BERGSTROM & N. MCLENNAN ANDERSON. 1967. Scand. J. Clin. Lab. Invest. **19:** 56–66.
47. PASSONNEAU, J. V. & O. H. LOWRY. 1963. Biochem. Biophys. Res. Commun. **13:** 372–379.
48. UYEDA, K. & E. RACKER. 1965. J. Biol. Chem. **240:** 4689–4693.
49. WILLIAMSON, J. R. 1966. J. Biol. Chem. **241:** 5026–5036.
50. KRAZANOWSKI, J. & F. M. MATSCHINSKY. 1969. Biochem. Biophys. Res. Commun. **34:** 816–823.
51. LOWENSTEIN, J. M. 1972. Physiol. Rev. **52:** 382–414.
52. GARLAND, P. B., P. J. RANDLE & E. A. NEWSHOLME. 1963. Nature (London) **200:** 169–1970.
53. GARLAND, P. B. & P. J. RANDLE. 1964. Biochem. J. **93:** 678–687.
54. NEWSHOLME, E. A. & P. J. RANDLE. 1964. Biochem. J. **93:** 641–651.
55. NEELY, J. R. & H. E. MORGAN. 1974. Ann. Rev. Physiol. **36:** 413–459.
56. RENNIE, M. J., W. W. WINDER & J. O. HOLLOSZY. 1976. Biochem. J. **156:** 647–655.
57. HARTLEY, L. H., B. PERNOW, J. HAGGENDAL, J. LACOUR, J. DELATTRE & B. SALTIN. 1970. J. Appl. Physiol. **29:** 818–823.
58. MAHER, J. T., A. L. GOODMAN, R. FRANCESCONI, W. D. BOWERS, L. H. HARTLEY & E. T. ANGELAKOS. 1972. Amer. J. Physiol. **222:** 207–212.
59. COSTILL, D. L. 1970. J. Appl. Physiol. **28:** 251–255.
60. GLESER, M. A. & J. A. VOGEL. 1973. J. Appl. Physiol. **34:** 438–442.
61. COSTILL, D. L., J. DANIELS, W. EVANS, W. J. FINK, G. KRAHENBUHL & B. SALTIN. 1976. J. Appl. Physiol. **40:** 149–154.
62. GOLLNICK, P. D., K. PIEHL, C. W. SAUBERT, R. B. ARMSTRONG & B. SALTIN. 1972. J. Appl. Physiol. **33:** 421–425.

63. GOLLNICK, P. D., R. B. ARMSTRONG, C. W. SAUBERT, W. L. SEMBROWICH, R. E. SHEPHERD & B. SALTIN. 1973. Pflügers Arch. **344:** 1–12.
64. COSTILL, D. L., P. D. GOLLNICK, E. D. JANSSON, B. SALTIN & E. M. STEIN. 1973. Acta Physiol. Scand. **89:** 374–383.
65. PAUL, P. & B. ISSEKUTZ. 1967. J. Appl. Physiol. **22:** 615–622.
66. PAUL, P. 1970. J. Appl. Physiol. **28:** 127–132.
67. JOHNSON, R. H., J. L. WALTON, H. A. KREBS & D. H. WILLIAMSON. 1969. Lancet **ii:** 452–455.
68. JOHNSON, R. H. & J. L. WALTON. 1972. Quart. J. Exp. Physiol. **57:** 73–79.
69. RENNIE, M. J., S. JENNETT & R. H. JOHNSON. 1974. Quart. J. Exp. Physiol. **59:** 201–212.
70. RANDLE, P. J., P. B. GARLAND, C. N. HALES & E. A. NEWSHOLME. 1963. Lancet **i:** 785–789.
71. PASSONNEAU, J. V. & O. H. LOWRY. 1963. Biochem. Biophys. Res. Commun. **13:** 372–379.
72. PARMEGGIANI, A. & R. H. BOWMAN. 1963. Biochem. Biophys. Res. Commun. **12:** 268–273.
73. RANDLE, P. J., E. A. NEWSHOLME & P. B. GARLAND. 1964. Biochem. J. **93:** 625–665.
74. BEATTY, C. H. & R. M. BOCEK. 1971. Amer. J. Physiol. **220:** 1928–1934.
75. JEFFERSON, L. S., J. O. KOEHLER & H. E. MORGAN. 1972. Proc. Nat. Acad. Sci. U.S.A. **69:** 816–820.
76. GOODMAN, M. N., M. BERGER & N. B. RUDERMAN. 1974. Diabetes **23:** 881–888.
77. REIMER, F., G. LÖFFLER, G. HENNIG & D. H. WIELAND. 1975. Hoppe-Seyler's Z. Physiol. Chem. **356:** 1955–1966.
78. COSTILL, D. L., R. BOWERS, B. BRANAM & K. SPARKS. J. Appl. Physiol. **31:** 834–838.
79. PAUL, P. 1971. Muscle Metabolism During Exercise. B. Pernow & B. Saltin, Eds. : 225–247. Plenum Press. New York, N.Y.
80. RENNIE, M. J. & R. H. JOHNSON. 1974. Eur. J. Appl. Physiol. **33:** 215–226.
81. COSTILL, D. L., K. SPARKS, R. GREGOR & C. TURNER. 1971. J. Appl. Physiol. **31:** 353–356.
82. BOOTH, F. W. 1977. Ann. N.Y. Acad. Sci. This volume.
83. BALDWIN, K. M. & W. W. WINDER. 1977. Ann. N.Y. Acad. Sci. This volume.
84. FITTS, R. H., J. O. HOLLOSZY & M. J. RENNIE. 1976. J. Physiol. **263:** 160.
85. HICKSON, R. C., M. J. RENNIE, R. K. CONLEE, W. W. WINDER & J. O. HOLLOSZY. Unpublished results.

DISCUSSION

John O. Holloszy, *Moderator*

Department of Preventive Medicine
Washington University School of Medicine
St. Louis, Missouri 63110

M. Skinner: Dr. Booth, how long was the training period till they reached their steady state?

F. W. Booth (*University of Texas, Houston, Texas*): Between 3 and 4 weeks.

M. Skinner: And then you stopped them at that point?

F. W. Booth: No, they kept running for an additional period to insure that they were in steady state. Cytochrome c concentration did not increase further between 28 and 35 days.

M. Skinner: The reason I ask the question is that in the work reported a number of years ago by Mueller from West Germany on isometric strength of muscle, he found out that if the person adapted very rapidly, i.e., got a large increase in strength very rapidly and then stopped, the drop-off would be much faster than if he had developed over a long period of time and maintained it; the rate of drop-off would be less. My question is whether or not you considered doing that kind of work to find out whether in fact the half-time or the rate of decay after training depends on how long the person has been training because if he's been training like a marathon runner for 5 or 10 years and then has an accident and can't run for one week, I would think that the drop-off would be much less than a person who just started last month.

F. W. Booth: That may be possible; we have not compared the time course of the decrease in respiratory enzyme levels after different periods of training.

D. S. Kronfeld (*University of Pennsylvania, Philadelphia, Pa.*): The first and last speakers on this panel showed us some evidence that training enhances the oxidation of fatty acids and ketone bodies and this will tend to conserve muscle glycogen and hence delay fatigue. The last speaker showed us some brief strategies to try and make available more fatty acids. I wonder whether the group has studied any longer-ranged strategies intended to favor the oxidation of fatty acids and ketone bodies and hence spare the utilization of muscle glycogen.

J. O. Holloszy (*Washington University, St. Louis, Mo.*): We have been unable to alter muscle enzyme levels by dietary means. We've kept rats on high fat diets for long periods of time, and this has had no effect on the capacity of the muscles to utilize fat.

D. S. Kronfeld: Have you studied any dietary regimes that would influence the availability of fatty acids and ketone bodies to the muscle?

J. O. Holloszy: Well, the animals in the study I just mentioned were on a diet containing about 70% fat and were ketotic.

D. S. Kronfeld: So you haven't been studying any carbohydrate-loading diets that might show you a difference?

J. O. Holloszy: There's a species difference here. Carbohydrate loading does not result in supercompensation to any great extent in the rat. I don't

451

know why. But you can't increase glycogen concentration in rat muscle beyond about 12 mg/gram muscle, whereas in the human you can increase the glycogen levels to 40 or 45 mg/gram muscle.

R. HUGHSON (*McMaster University, Hamilton, Ont.*): Just another possible continuation in this species variation. I suppose you chose your rats very carefully because I found in training rats that if I just randomly assigned them to groups, which is obviously the best way to do it, you have a terrible time getting some rats to train. I suppose you are not using Sprague Dawley rats for one thing, but how do you allow for this in your experimental design?

K. M. BALDWIN (*University of California, Irvine, Calif.*): First of all, we used rats of a Wistar strain as you pointed out. In most of these experiments we would start with more than twice the number of animals that we would be dealing with for the training program. So we would collect animals that were willing to run and then randomly assign the runners to a sedentary or an exercising group. So I don't think we've done anything to remove the randomization.

QUESTION: Dr. Holloszy, in regard to the increase in maximum $\dot{V}_{O_2}$, you mentioned you found in the trained rats that the two responsible factors were the increased cardiac output or cardiac adaptations and the mitochondrial density increase. Would you care to put a percentage on one or the other, which was most important? Can you divide the total increase into those two categories. Which would be the most important or limiting factor?

J. O. HOLLOSZY: This hasn't been studied in rats. What information is available was obtained on humans. On the average, in people who have trained 3 or 4 days a week for 8 to 12 weeks, about half of the increase in $\dot{V}_{O_2 \, max}$ is due to an increase in maximum cardiac output, and the other half is due to an increase in the arterio-venous oxygen difference. In other words the trained muscles are extracting more oxygen. I think most people working in this field would say that in the marathon runner who has been training for years a greater proportion is due to an increase in maximum cardiac output, but I don't think that this has been established.

QUESTION: Which of the two would be the limiting factor. I mean which is going to peak out?

J. O. HOLLOSZY: It is dangerous to talk about limiting factors unless you define your conditions very carefully. I think that the cardiac output, blood flow, and respiratory capacity, are rather closely geared to each other. However, I suspect that during very heavy exercise involving a large muscle mass the limiting factor probably is delivery of oxygen to the muscles.

K. E. ELLINGWOOD (*University of Florida, Gainesville, Fla.*): Dr. Booth, I realize that you apparently measured enzyme decay and once you have a certain level present the decline follows an exponential decay. Does enzyme induction follow the same pattern? In other words once you start training do you increase logarithmically? Have you measured that directly?

F. W. BOOTH: Yes, the increase in cytochrome c concentration and respiratory enzyme levels does follow an exponential course. However, this only occurs when the exercise stimulus is kept constant throughout the training period. It depends on the way you manipulate your training program. The increase is exponential only if the speed and duration of the daily running, and the incline of the treadmill, are constant throughout the training program.

K. E. ELLINGWOOD: Then the enzyme induction also follows an exponential increase?

F. W. BOOTH: That's correct, under conditions where you apply the stimulus abruptly and then maintain it as constant. It should be pointed out that's not the way people normally train. Most training programs are of the progressive type.

K. E. ELLINGWOOD: My second question is in relation to the capacity to oxidize fats. Which type of fats were fed to the rat and has any type of fat been studied in human beings as a diet supplement that would preferentially be used in metabolism when you're trying to switch someone from glycogen to fatty acid metabolism?

J. O. HOLLOSZY: Fatty acids turn over with a half-time of about 2 or 3 minutes or even faster, probably much faster during exercise, and it is not possible, therefore, to elevate fatty acids by feeding fatty acids. The only practical way that's known for raising fatty acids is to give a meal containing triglycerides, in the form of oil or fat, wait until the plasma is grossly lipemic, which takes 2 or 3 hours, and then activate lipoprotein lipase. Fatty acids are maintained at a high level for a considerably period because triglycerides are continually absorbed from the gut and then hydrolyzed.

K. E. ELLINGWOOD: Then from a practical view what diet would you suggest to elevate fatty acids.

J. O. HOLLOSZY: I don't think this study has any practical application. This is just an experimental tool. It would be dangerous and inappropriate to administer heparin to athletes to activate lipoprotein lipase.

S. J. MANN (*Montefiore Hospital, The Bronx, N.Y.*): Given exogenously supplied carbohydrate and free fatty acids supplied to the muscle, which would result in greater endurance?

J. O. HOLLOSZY: I think that muscle glycogen is the essential factor. I suspect that, under normal condition, neither glucose nor fatty acids from the blood can get into muscle cells sufficiently rapidly to provide the mitochondria with enough substrate to support a rate of O_2 consumption in excess of about 50% of maximum. Blood glucose is of course important during exercise because if it falls below a certain level you become hypoglycemic and develop a variety of central nervous system symptoms. It is, therefore, essential to maintain blood glucose in the normal range.

S. J. MANN: And what is the limiting factor in the use of the free fatty acids that are mobilized for example during the long duration of a marathon?

J. O. HOLLOSZY: They have a glucose and glycogen sparing effect so that you don't use up your muscle glycogen rapidly.

S. J. MANN: Right. Over that long time, what is the limiting factor in the use of the free fatty acids that are mobilized?

J. O. HOLLOSZY: The muscles' capacity to utilize fatty acids.

S. J. MANN: Mitochondrial?

J. O. HOLLOSZY: Yes.

J. CLARE (*Oakland, Calif.*): Mr. Chairman, you mentioned as others have the existence of cardiac hypertrophy with training and yet I think Dr. Baldwin showed no change in the cardiac muscle enzyme systems. It seems to me surprising that there's a stimulus for one change and apparently no stimulus for the other. So I wonder what thought you have as to the mechanism that accounts for hypertrophy of cardiac muscle?

J. O. HOLLOSZY: There are two different types of cardiac hypertorphy.

One is pressure overload and the other is volume overload hypertrophy. What you see with endurance exercise training is a volume overload type of hypertrophy. In other words, you get an increase in left ventricular volume. The stimulus responsible for development of hypertrophy appears to be increased tension or stretching of the muscle fibers. I think that the mitochondrial enzyme level, that is—the mitochondrial content of the heart, is already at the upper limit. The heart contracts continually and its respiratory capacity is probably maximal. During development of hypertrophy, there is growth of all the components of the cardiac cell. As a result, the cell gets bigger. The total mitochondrial content of the heart is increased, but per gram of heart there is no increase in mitochondria.

J. CLARE: When you refer to volume overload you are still retaining the idea of hypertrophy as an increase of cell mass and not merely meaning volume distention?

J. O. HOLLOSZY: Right. There is increase in the mass of the heart. In a recent study published in the Annals of Internal Medicine,* in which cardiac size was evaluated in marathon runners and other endurace athletes using echocardiography, the cardiac mass appeared to be increased by about 50%.

* MORGANROTH, J., B. J. BARON, W. L. HENRY & S. E. EPSTEIN. 1975. Ann. Int. Med. **82:** 521–524.

CHARACTERISTICS OF POSTCORONARY MARATHON RUNNERS

Terence Kavanagh, Roy J. Shephard, and Johanna Kennedy

Toronto Rehabilitation Centre
Toronto, M4G 1R7, Ontario
Canada

Department of Preventive Medicine and Biostatistics
University of Toronto
Toronto, Ontario
Canada

Previous papers from this laboratory discussed the participation of small groups of our "postcoronary" patients in marathon running events.[1-6] The main focus of these reports was upon the immediate problems of nutrition, fluid and mineral balance, and temperature homeostasis. Further analysis of the data seems warranted to determine to what extent we are dealing with an atypical subsample of the general population of patients with ischemic heart disease. Accordingly, we have now traced the course of training in 13 postcoronary patients who have each completed from one to eight marathon events, comparing results with those for 610 unselected cases of ischemic heart disease attending an exercise-based rehabilitation program.

METHODS

Subjects. The marathoners were all patients who had sustained a myocardial infarction; the larger unselected sample of 610 patients were also mainly uncomplicated infarcts, although 47 cases of angina and 24 by-pass operations were also included in the sample. Laboratory data were collected on enrollment at the Toronto Rehabilitation Centre, and at intervals of 3–6 months thereafter. In the larger sample, the training results were obtained after an average of 22 months conditioning.

Personality Measurements. The Minnesota Multiphasic Personality Inventory was completed under the supervision of a psychologist 16–18 months postinfarction, with repetition of the test 2 years later.

Body Composition. Height, weight, and skinfold thickness (triceps, subscapular and suprailiac folds) were measured by standard anthropometric techniques.[7] Body fat and thus lean body mass were predicted using the equations of Durnin & Rahaman.[8]

Exercise Tests. Maximal treadmill stress tests were carried out on all members of the marathon group from 1972. However, for comparative purposes they were also assessed at the same times as the general group by the following submaximal test. Exercise was performed on a Fleisch ergostat at a constant pedal speed of 60 rpm. A three-stage progressive test format was used, with three minutes of exercise at each stage, loadings being adjusted to bring subjects to a final 75% of aerobic power. The heart rate and electrocardiogram were monitored throughout, using standard chest leads (CM_5). Expired gas was collected by a standard open-circuit technique during the final minute at each work load, with analysis of oxygen (paramagnetic method) and carbon dioxide (infrared analysis) for determination of oxygen consumption. The maximum oxygen intake was predicted from the oxygen scale of the Astrand nomogram;[9] previous work has shown a good concordance between such estimates and direct measurements of aerobic power in our postcoronary patients.[10]

Systemic blood pressures were measured by a standard clinical cuff, with the subjects sitting at rest on the bicycle ergometer; readings were obtained prior to exercise and during the final 15 seconds at each work load; the exercise figure to be discussed is that obtained at the 75% loading.

ST segmental sagging was determined using an analog computer to average 16 successive ECG complexes; the results to be discussed are again those obtained at the 75% loading.

RESULTS

Clinical Status

In most respects, the marathoners were typical of patients attending the Toronto Rehabilitation Centre. The average period of hospital stay following infarction was 28 days. Complications were few, but one patient was found to have extensive 3 vessel disease that was unsuitable for an aortocoronary by-pass and so a Vineberg procedure was carried out. Three of the 13 men had suffered two distinct infarctions, five had been troubled by dysrythmia at various times, and five had some degree of hypertension (diastolic pressure greater than 90 mmHg in two cases, and greater than 100 mmHg in three cases.) Almost all types of infarct were represented, five being posterior, five inferior, and six anterior in site; ten of the 16 episodes were transmural infarctions. We were unable to obtain quantitative estimates on infarct size; nevertheless, all episodes were accompanied by substantial elevations of SGOT levels, the average recorded peak being 172 units (TABLE 1).

All of the marathoners had been heavy smokers prior to their attack. None of the group had any experience of distance running prior to their infarction.

Personality

The personality, as assessed by the MMPI, showed somewhat lower depression (D) scores for the marathoners than in some of the postcoronary patients,[11] average normalized scores amounting to 58 and 63 units, respectively. Nevertheless, the marathoners were significantly depressed relative to the general population. Compared with the 44 depressed postcoronary patients discussed elsewhere in this issue,[15] the marathoners had low scores for hysteria (Hy), hypochondriasis (Hs), psychasthenia (Pt), and social introversion (Si). On the other hand, neither hypomania (Ma) nor masculinity (Mf) was very different from scores attained by the 44 depressed patients.

Training did not produce large changes in personality scores for the marathoners (TABLE 2). Average readings for hysteria, hypochondriasis, and social introversion all showed an insignificant decline, while psychopathic deviation (Pd), schizophrenia (Sc), and hypomania showed small and in-

TABLE 1

CLINICAL CHARACTERISTICS OF MARATHON PATIENTS

	Electrocardiographic Findings	Enzymes Elevated	Characteristic Chest Pain at Infarction	History of Angina	Complications		
					Pump Failure	Dysrhythmia	Hypertension
A	1st Non-TM posterior	Yes	Yes	No	No	No	No
B	2nd TM posterior	Yes	Yes	Yes	No	Yes	150/110
	Non-TM anterior	Yes	Yes	Yes	No	No	160/90
C	TM anterior-septal	Yes	Yes	Yes	VP*	No	160/90
D	Non-TM posterior-lateral	Yes	Yes	No	No	No	No
E	TM inferior	Yes	Yes	No	No	No	No
F	1st TM posterior	Yes	Yes	Yes	No	Yes	No
	2nd Non-TM inferior	Yes	Yes	No	No	No	No
G	TM inferior	Yes	Yes	No	No	No	No
H	1st Non-TM anterior	Yes	Yes	Yes	No	No	No
	2nd TM anterior	Yes	Yes	No	No	Yes	160/105
I	non-TM anterior	Yes	Yes	Yes	No	Yes	150/110
J	TM anterior-lateral	Yes	Yes	No	No	Yes	No
K	TM inferior	Yes	Yes	No	No	No	No
L	TM posterior-lateral	Yes	Yes	No	No	No	No
M	TM inferior	Yes	Yes	No	No	No	No

* VP, Vineberg procedure.

TABLE 2

MINNESOTA MULTIPHASIC PERSONALITY INVENTORY *

	Hs	D	Hy	Pd	Mf	Pa	Pt	Sc	Ma	Si
Normal score	11.3	16.7	16.5	19.0	20.7	8.0	23.0	22.0	17.0	25.0
Marathoners' scores 1974	12.4 (±5.8)†	20.7 (±5.1)	18.6 (±4.2)	19.1 (±4.3)	25.9 (±5.8)	8.6 (±3.3)	24.7 (±5.9)	19.9 (±5.9)	18.6 (±2.4)	31.9 (±12.9)
Marathoners' scores 1976	10.3 (±2.9)	20.7 (±1.7)	16.7 (±3.1)	21.7 (±4.0)	25.6 (±5.9)	7.7 (±4.2)	25.4 (±1.5)	22.0 (±3.7)	20.7 (±3.5)	26.3 (±14.9)
Change, 1974 to 1976	-2.1 (±5.8)	0.0 (±5.8)	-1.9 (±3.0)	+2.6 (±3.8)	-0.3 (±5.6)	-0.9 (±2.4)	+0.7 (±6.4)	+2.1 (±5.6)	+2.1 (±3.8)	-5.6 (±10.6)
Subject H.B., change, 1974 to 1976	-2	+2	0	0	+2	-1	-3	0	0	+2

* Raw scores obtained in marathon participants in 1974 and 1976, compared with normal (50th percentile) scores. Subject H.B. was able to run a full marathon in 1973, but only a half marathon in 1976.
† Standard deviation (SD).

significant increments. One subject who completed a full marathon in 1973 but was reduced to a half marathon in 1976 (H.B.) showed changes in the opposite direction to the remainder of the group for most of these variables.

Body Composition

The body build of the marathoners was unremarkable and indeed in some instances unfavorable to distance running (TABLE 3). Stature was above the average for our postcoronary group, and the weight was also at least average, one of the marathoners weighing an initial 91.2 kg. However, initial skinfold readings (average 13.5 ± 4.1 mm) were lower than in the general sample of postcoronary patients (15.6 ± 5.0 mm). The percentage of body fat averaged 19.6% in the marathoners; this was similar to data for other postcoronary patients, and more typical of a sedentary young man than a distance runner.

TABLE 3

A COMPARISON OF BODY COMPOSITION BETWEEN 13 MARATHON PARTICIPANTS AND 610 UNSELECTED MEN ATTENDING A POSTCORONARY REHABILITATION PROGRAM *

	Marathon			Total Sample	
	Mean	SD	Range	Mean	SD
Age (yr)	45.5	±5.8	35–57	48.6	±7.8
Height (cm)	176.0	±6.8	167.6–189.2	173.3	±6.9
Weight (kg)	75.1	±10.3	61.1–91.2	75.9	±8.4
Excess weight (kg)	4.8	±6.9	−4.5–+20.0	7.6	±7.2
Skinfold (mm) (average for 3 folds)	13.4	±4.1	7.3–16.9	15.6	±5.0
Percent fat	19.2	±3.4	12.5–24.0	19.7	±3.4
Lean body mass (kg)	60.5	±7.2	50.3–71.1	59.9	±6.1
Lean body mass per cm	0.343	±0.030	0.299–0.397	0.345	±0.028

* Data obtained on entry to the rehabilitation program.

Lean mass per cm of standing height was also close to the anticipated figure for a sedentary young man.

Training did not lead to significant changes of body composition in either the marathoners or the general postcoronary group (TABLE 4).

Exercise Tests

The initial aerobic power of the marathoners (28.0 ± 4.7 ml/kg·min) was slightly greater than in the unselected cases of ischemic heart disease (25.1 ml/kg·min). Training of the marathon group led to a progressive increase of $\dot{V}_{O_2max}$ to a peak of 43.5 ± 10.4 ml/kg·min (155% of initial value, 125% of age-matched Toronto normal [12]) over an average of 2 years of conditioning. Some of the subjects who were frequent marathon participants showed even larger changes (FIGURE 1), four of the group progressing from

TABLE 4

CHANGES IN BODY COMPOSITION WITH TRAINING. A COMPARISON BETWEEN
13 MARATHON RUNNERS AND 610 MEN ATTENDING POST-CORONARY PROGRAM.
CHANGE FROM INITIAL TO MOST RECENT DATA

	Marathon		Total Sample	
	Mean	S.D.	Mean	S.D.
Body weight (kg)	+0.52	±4.8	+0.19	±3.73
Excess weight (kg)	+0.58	±5.0	+0.15	±4.18
Skinfold thickness (mm)	+0.2	±2.4	−0.20	±4.62
Percentage fat	+0.16	±3.4	−0.29	±3.06
Lean body mass (kg)	+0.3	±5.9	+0.3	±2.9
Lean body mass per cm	−0.002	±0.20	+0.002	±0.059

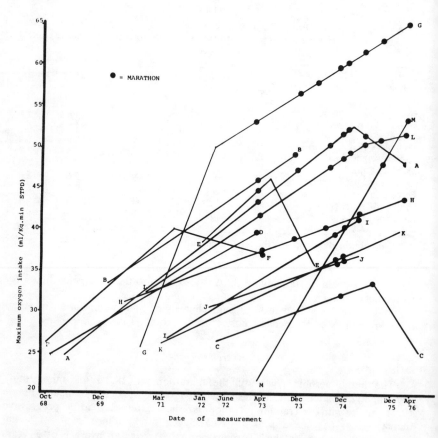

FIGURE 1. Development of maximum oxygen intake in 13 postcoronary patients.
Marathon participation indicated by ●.

an initial average of 26.6 ml/kg·min to 56.0 ml/kg·min over 2 to 4 years; two of the four realized almost a half of their gains in the first 6 months of training, but one took a year to attain 50% of his final gain, and the fourth runner (with a final score of 54.4 ml/kg·min) showed almost no improvement until the fourth year of training. Two of the 13 who ceased vigorous conditioning showed substantial losses of aerobic power (8–10 ml/kg·min) over the following year of observation.

Hemodynamic Variables

When first seen, the marathoners had a larger resting systolic pressure and a larger pulse pressure than the general sample (TABLE 5). With training, the large pulse pressure remained, but there were significant diminutions of

TABLE 5

HEMODYNAMIC RESPONSES TO EFFORT. A COMPARISON BETWEEN 13 MARATHON PARTICIPANTS AND 610 MEN ATTENDING THE POSTCORONARY PROGRAM *

	Marathon			Total Sample	
	Mean	SD	Range	Mean	SD
Rest blood pressure (*mmHg*)					
Systolic	138.5	±13.3	120–160	128.6	±16.8
Diastolic	87.5	±10.5	70–100	87.7	±9.0
Exercise blood pressure (*mmHg*)					
Systolic	174.6	±22.2	140–210	167.9	±25.2
Diastolic	90.1	±12.5	70–125	96.4	±14.4
ST segmental depression					
Voltage, at 75% load					
(heart rate 133.9±8.8)†	−0.116	±0.15	−0.47–+0.03	−0.10	±0.13

* Data obtained on entry to the program.
† The actual heart rate attained was closer to 70% load.

resting systolic and diastolic pressures (TABLE 6). In contrast, conditioning of the general postcoronary group led to a widening of the resting pulse pressure, with a small but significant increase of systolic pressure, and a small but significant decrement of diastolic pressure. During initial exercise at the 75% loading, the marathon runners again developed a higher systolic pressure and a wider pulse pressure than the general postcoronary population (TABLE 4). With training, both groups improved the systolic pressure that they could sustain at the 75% loading (TABLE 5).

The extent of the initial ST segmental sagging was rather comparable in the two groups (Table 4). In six of the 13 marathoners, the initial response to the 75% loading was an ST sagging of more than 0.1 mV. With training, both groups tended towards less negative ST segmental voltages, although there was a suggestion of a somewhat greater improvement in the marathon participants. At the final testing, only two of this group had an ST depression of more than 0.1 mV, and in one of these two (J.R.) there had nevertheless been a very large improvement, from −0.47 to −0.12 mV. Part of the explanation in this patient was that he had been a heavy smoker. With marathon participation, he was persuaded to stop smoking; however, he later resumed the habit, to die during his sleep and two years after his last marathon; postmortem did not reveal any evidence of recent coronary occlusion or myocardial infarction and the cause of death was termed "electrical failure."

TABLE 6

CHANGES IN HEMODYNAMIC RESPONSE WITH TRAINING. COMPARISON BETWEEN 13 MARATHON PARTICIPANTS AND 610 MEN ATTENDING THE POSTCORONARY PROGRAM. CHANGE FROM INITIAL TO MOST RECENT DATA

	Marathon		Total Sample	
	Mean	SD	Mean	SD
Resting blood pressure (mmHg)				
Systolic	−8.9	±14.9	+3.9	±20.8
Diastolic	−9.1	±12.6	−1.0	±9.2
Exercise blood pressure (mmHg)				
Systolic	+13.4	±21.3	+14.8	±24.9
Diastolic	−2.5	±14.0	+1.5	±14.2
ST segmental depression (mmHg)				
Voltage, at 75% load				
(heart rate 132.8±9.8)*	+0.08	±0.17	+0.03	±0.16

* The actual heart rate attained was closer to 70% load.

DISCUSSION

Specificity of Sample

In terms of their clinical history and previous experience of running, there is little evidence that the marathon team of the Toronto Rehabilitation Centre differs from our general postcoronary population.

However, the marathon runners show less evidence of depression and development of the neurotic triad (hysteria, hypochondriasis, and psychasthenia) than is the case for our general sample. Since changes of personality scores in response to marathon preparation and participation were quite limited, we must conclude that relative to the average infarct victim the marathoners had either a less drastic psychological reaction to the acute episode or a more favorable response to early rehabilitation. None of the distance competitors had a D score higher than 23 (a STEN value of 65 units). If this is indeed the maximum depression compatible with successful preparation for a marathon contest, we would conclude that about a half of the patients with myocardial infarction could not undertake such activity.

The physiological data supports the idea that the marathoners were in some respects a selected segment of our postcoronary population. The initial estimated percentage of body fat and lean mass were much as in the general sample, but the marathoners had some advantage with respect to pulse pressure, maximum tolerated systolic pressure, and aerobic power. The poorest scores found in the marathon team were an initial body fat of 24%, a lean body mass of 0.299 kg/cm, and an aerobic power of 21.7 ml/kg·min. On each of these criteria, a proportion of our general sample would have been eliminated.

Gains from Marathon Running

Granted that the marathon sample had some initial advantages of mood and physiological status relative to the general postcoronary population, it is still plain that the long distance runners made enormous physiological gains over their period of training. The most striking change was in aerobic power, the improvement in this variable averaging 55%, compared with a gain of only 20% in the general postcoronary population. The infarct victim does not die of a low maximum oxygen intake as such. However, if he can improve his physical condition, then the heart rate and thus the cardiac workload for a given task is reduced. This in turn lessens the occurrence of myocardial ischemia and thus the risk of sudden death from cardiac arrest or ventricular fibrillation.

The data also suggests that in marathoners conditioning lessens ST segmental sagging during exercise at 75% loadings, despite an associated increase of systolic blood pressure and an unchanged heart rate. However, this is not categoric proof that exercise has improved the myocardial blood supply through the development of collateral blood channels—other possibilities include an improvement of coronary flow secondary to the cessation of smoking, and a reduction in cardiac workload through myocardial hypertrophy or an alteration of ventricular dimensions.

The favorable influence of distance running upon other "risk factors" is well established.[13] The decision to engage in distance running can be a significant factor in a successful smoking withdrawal program. It is debatable whether there is much advantage in correcting abnormal blood lipids after a heart attack has occurred; however, if a patient is helped to give up smoking, this can have a major impact on the likelihood that his infarct will recur.

There is no doubt that participation in the long distance contests gave these men a tremendous psychological boost. However, this is not reflected in large differences of personality scores between the marathoners and other participants in our program. This is partly because it is easier to reduce the D score in a grossly depressed patient than to change the same variable in a person whose score is only a little above the population average. Another important consideration is that the runners have seen their marathon participation as a triumph for the Centre's program as well as for themselves; because of their unselfish attitudes, the happy experience has been shared with other more disabled patients, to the point where all have enjoyed a vicarious elevation of mood.

Dangers of Marathon Participation

Since it is well established that unusual, unaccustomed, and prolonged activity can increase the immediate risks of a heart attack,[14] it is most important that intending marathon participants prepare themselves thoroughly, undertaking systematic, gradual, medically supervised, and progressive long slow distance training for a number of years before considering formal competition. Each time that a substantial training distance is to be covered, a brief check must be made for warning signs such as increasing angina or unusual dysrhythmia. In our program, a complete physical examination, including a 12-lead electrocardiogram and maximal treadmill stress test is mandatory before and after a formal marathon. During the run itself, the runners must keep to a predetermined pace that has been ascertained to be within safe limits. Individual participants must be advised to compete only against themselves, stopping if there are any unusual symptoms or sensations. To date, 22 of our patients have participated in marathon events in Boston, Hawaii, and Toronto, some with times as good as 190 minutes for the 26¼ mile course. Happily, over 50 races have been completed without complications, either immediate or late. However, this record will be maintained only by scrupulous attention to the precautions outlined above.

The one occasional disadvantage encountered by our distance runners is domestic. A wife put it in these terms: "I married a man who would spend each night in front of the television with a six-pack of beer. Now I find myself living with a running enthusiast, and I'm not sure I like it." This woman is perhaps the exception. The majority of the wives are proud of the new achievements of their husbands. Nevertheless, the case cited does stress the importance of involving other members of the family in any program of treatment that has major social implications. Compliance with long periods of prescribed exercise is much more likely if this can be pursued as a family.

SUMMARY

The characteristics of 13 postcoronary patients who have each completed one to eight marathon events were compared with data obtained on a larger sample of 610 infarct victims attending the Toronto Rehabilitation Centre.

In clinical terms, the marathon group was composed of typical postcoronary patients, but personality assessments by the Minnesota Multiphasic Personality Inventory showed less depression than in many of our general sample (average normalized D scores 58 and 63, respectively). None of the marathoners had previous experience of running before their infarction, and body build was not particularly advantageous for distance events [stature (176.0 ± 6.8 cm) was above average and body weight (75.1 ± 10.3 kg) was average although skinfolds (13.5 ± 4.1 mm) were lower than the 15.6 ± 5.0 mm found in the larger sample].

The initial aerobic power (28.0 ± 4.7 ml/kg·min) of the marathoners was marginally higher than that of the larger sample (25.1 ml/kg·min). Training led to a progressive increase of $\dot{V}_{O_2 max}$, so that after 2 years the marathoners attained an average of 43.5 ml/kg·min, a 55% increase over their initial value and a 25% increase over the age-matched sedentary Toronto normal. In contrast, the main sample of postcoronary patients increased their $\dot{V}_{O_2 \, max}$ by only 20% with training.

Both at rest and during exercise at 75% of aerobic power, the initial systolic blood pressure and pulse pressure were some 10 mmHg larger in the marathoners than in the general sample. Training induced a 9 mmHg fall of resting pressure in the marathoners, but both the marathoners and the larger sample showed an increase of the exercise systolic pressure. ST segmental sagging was reduced in both groups over the training period, although the change in the marathoners (0.08 ± 0.17 mV) was somewhat larger than in the main sample (0.03 ± 0.16 mV).

Marathon participation did not induce any large changes in personality scores.

REFERENCES

1. KAVANAGH, T., R. J. SHEPHARD & V. PANDIT. 1974. Marathon running after myocardial infarction. J. Amer. Med. Assoc. **229**(12): 1602–1605.
2. SHEPHARD, R. J. & T. KAVANAGH. 1975. Biochemical changes with marathon running—Observations on post-coronary patients. *In* Metabolic Adaptations to Prolonged Physical Activity. H. Howald & J. Poortmans, Eds. Birkhauser Verlag. Basel, Switzerland.
3. KAVANAGH, T. & R. J. SHEPHARD. 1975. Maintenance of hydration in post-coronary marathon runners. Brit. J. Sports Med. **9**: 130–135.
4. KAVANAGH, T. & R. J. SHEPHARD. Hydration of middle-aged marathon runners. Brit. J. Sports Med. In press.
5. SHEPHARD, R. J. & T. KAVANAGH. 1976. Fluid and mineral balance on post-coronary distance runners. Studies on the 1975 Boston Marathon. Proceedings, International Conference on Nutrition, Dietetics and Sport, Bordighera.
6. SHEPHARD, R. J., T. KAVANAGH, S. CONWAY, M. THOMSON & G. H. ANDERSON. 1975. Nutritional demands of sub-maximum work: marathon and Trans-Canadian events. *In* Proceedings of International Symposium on Athletic Nutrition, Warsaw.
7. WEINER, J. S. & J. A. LOURIE. 1975. Human Biology: A Guide to Field Methods. Blackwell Scientific Publishers. Oxford, England.
8. DURNIN, J. V. G. A. & M. M. RAHAMAN. 1967. The assessment of the amount of fat in the human body from measurements of skinfold thickness. Brit. J. Nutrit. **21**: 681–689.
9. ASTRAND, I. 1960. Aerobic work capacity in men and women with special reference to age. Acta Physiol. Scand. **49** (Suppl. 169): 1–92.
10. KAVANAGH, T. & R. J. SHEPHARD. 1976. Maximum exercise tests on post-coronary patients. J. Appl. Physiol. **40**: 611–618.
11. KAVANAGH, T., R. J. SHEPHARD & J. A. TUCK. 1975. Depression after myocardial infarction. Canad. Med. Assoc. J. **113**: 23–27.
12. SHEPHARD, R. J. 1977. Endurance Fitness. 2nd edit. University of Toronto Press. Toronto, Canada.
13. MORGAN, P., M. GILDINER & G. W. WRIGHT. 1976. Smoking reduction in adults who take up exercise: A survey of a running club for adults. Canad. Assoc. Health. Phys. Ed. Recreat. J. **42**: 39–43.
14. SHEPHARD, R. J. 1974. Sudden death—A significant hazard of exercise? Brit. J. Sports Med. **8**: 101–110.
15. KAVANAGH, T., R. J. SHEPHARD & J. A. TUCK. 1977. The effects of long distance running program on depression and psychological profile. Ann. N.Y. Acad. Sci. This volume.

METABOLIC ADJUSTMENTS TO MARATHON RUNNING IN CORONARY PATIENTS *

Rudolph H. Dressendorfer,† Jack H. Scaff, Jr.,
John O. Wagner, and James D. Gallup

Department of Physiology
University of Hawaii
School of Medicine
Honolulu, Hawaii 96822

Honolulu Medical Group
Honolulu, Hawaii 96813

How well do trained heart patients respond to the physiological demands of marathon running? As part of a long-range project investigating the efficacy of long-distance running (≥ 10 km) in the treatment and prevention of coronary artery disease, the present study was undertaken to quantify physiological adjustments of five trained coronary patients to running the 1974 Honolulu Marathon (42.2 km). The study provides supportive and additional data on the above question regarding the physiology and safety of marathon running by myocardial infarct patients.[1] Reported findings include cardiorespiratory, thermal, biochemical, and metabolic measurements made before, during, and after the marathon run.

PATIENTS AND METHODS

Subjects

Five moderately to well trained middle-aged men were selected from volunteers in a group of coronary patients who had undergone 6 months of marathon training. On the average, these subjects were quite typical of patients in our cardiac rehabilitation program who show improvement with physical conditioning. The selection was made to provide a range in type and severity of coronary artery disease on the basis of diagnostic tests made one year earlier.

A description of subjects is presented in TABLE 1. Subject 1 showed electrocardiographic signs of ischemia with chest pains during maximal treadmill stress testing and was presumed to have coronary artery disease. Subjects 2–5 had healed myocardial infarcts (MI), which occurred 1.5 to 4 years before the race. The MIs were diagnosed and quantified with electrocardiographic changes,

* This work was supported in part by a grant from the Honolulu Medical Group Research Foundation.

† Present address: Human Performance Laboratory, Department of Physical Education, University of California at Davis, Davis, Calif. 95616.

serum enzyme levels, angiograms, and vectorcardiography. Subject 5 underwent surgical bypass revascularization of three coronary arteries 1 year before the race. TABLE 1 also shows measurements of average skinfold thickness, resting pulse rate, and blood pressure. Percent body fat, predicted from triceps, subscapular, and umbilical skinfolds,[2] averaged 18.7%. Subject 4, estimated as 32% fat, was classified obese despite a substantial weight loss during training. Subject 3 was a finisher in the 1973 Honolulu and 1974 Boston marathons. Smoking and alcohol consumption had been discontinued for about 1 year.

TABLE 2 shows fasting serum levels for cholesterol, triglycerides, uric acid, glucose, sodium, and potassium as determined 2 weeks before the race. Mean values were within the clinical range of normal. Before exercise reconditioning, subject 5 had serum cholesterol and triglyceride levels of 344 and greater than 1200 mg/dl, respectively.

In the month preceding the marathon race, training distance for the group averaged 60 to 75 km·wk^{-1} at a mean velocity of about 150 m·min^{-1}. Subject 1, however, consistently averaged 140 km·wk^{-1}, whereas subjects 4 and 5 were bothered by minor leg injuries that prevented their training mileage from increasing beyond a level of 60 km·wk^{-1}. Longest training runs before the race were 25 to 30 km. During these long runs no subject experienced angina pectoris.

Design of Experiment

Measurements of oxygen uptake ($\dot{V}_{O_2}$) and heart rate (HR) were made 1 to 3 weeks before the race during road running tests at various velocities to a maximum. The observed relationships between $\dot{V}_{O_2}$ and running velocity and $\dot{V}_{O_2}$ and HR for each subject were subsequently used in estimating $\dot{V}_{O_2}$ during the race.

Fifteen days before the race, each subject performed a 15-minute treadmill run at 80%–85% of his highest observed HR (HR$_{max}$) while respiratory metabolism and the electrocardiogram (ECG) were obtained. Determinations of systolic time intervals (STI), measured in the supine position, were made before and approximately 5 minutes postexercise. In addition, rectal temperature (T_{re}) was measured and blood and urine were collected before and 5 to 10 minutes after the treadmill run.

Urine samples and body weights were taken within 10 minutes before the race. During the race each subject was accompanied by a cardiac nurse who bicycled alongside. Whenever the subject stopped to consume fluids, the nurse palpated his pulse and recorded time, place, and quantity of fluid consumed. Immediately after completing the race, the subject was escorted to an air-conditioned room located 100 m from the finish line where body weight, T_{re}, and blood and urine samples were obtained within 10 minutes. The subject then performed a second treadmill test at the target HR level obtained in the first treadmill test. Respiratory metabolism, ECG, and recovery STI were determined as before.

TABLE 1

DESCRIPTION OF SUBJECTS *

Subject No.	Age (yr)	Height (cm)	Weight (kg)	Subcutaneous Fat † (mm)	Sitting Pulse Rate (b·min⁻¹)	Sitting Blood Pressure (mmHg)	History of Coronary Disease (years before marathon race)
1	48	169	56.9	14.2	50	108/72	S-T segment depression (>2 mm) during treadmill stress test; presumed coronary artery disease (1 yr)
2	45	168	62.1	11.7	60	128/84	3–4 cm anterior transmural MI with dyskinetic segment and presumed ventricular aneurism (4 yr)
3‡	43	175	60.4	8.4	64	140/84	4–5 cm inferior transmural MI (2 yr)
4	47	175	77.9	26.2	54	130/84	4–5 cm inferior transmural MI (2 yr)
5	47	170	62.1	18.7	68	100/70	MI (1.5 yr); triple bipass aorto-coronary transplant (1 yr)
Mean	46	171	65.1	15.8	59	121/79	4 patients post-MI, 1 patient asymptomatic

* Measurements made two weeks before marathon race.
‡ Completed two previous marathon races (42.2 km) within preceding year.
† Unweighted average skinfold thickness measured at seven sites: triceps, subscapular, suprailiac, umbilical, chest, axillary, and front thigh.

Measurement Techniques

Field testing to determine the energetics of road running was conducted along a flat, approximately 800 m circuit after the subjects had completed training runs of 10 to 15 km. The subject ran 1 m beside a car at self-paced running velocities up to a voluntary maximum. At each velocity, expired gas was collected in a 200-liter meteorological balloon over the second 400 m using portable respiratory equipment designed for this purpose.[3] Duplicate gas samples were drawn in glass syringes and measured for O_2 and CO_2 concentrations with a micro-gas analyzer (Scholander, Rutledge, Pa.). Gas volume and temperature were measured after each run in a gasmeter (Type CD4, Parkinson-Cowan, Blue Bell, Pa.). Maximal O_2 uptake ($\dot{V}_{O_2\,max}$) was defined as the highest V_{O_2} observed, which typically leveled off at maximum velocities. Exercise HR was estimated by timing 15 carotid pulses in the immediate recovery.

TABLE 2

FASTING SERUM LEVELS *

Subject No.	Cholesterol (mg/dl)	Triglycerides (mg/dl)	Uric Acid (mg/dl)	Glucose (mg/dl)	Na (meq/l)	K (meq/l)
1	215	90	8.2	109	142	4.1
2	185	196	6.7	120	146	4.6
3	250	83	5.1	103	147	4.8
4	305	100	5.9	122	145	5.0
5	205	273	8.8	105	143	5.3
Mean	232	150	6.9	112	145	4.8

* Blood samples taken 2 weeks before marathon race, 12 to 16 hours after eating, with the subjects being well rested.

Zero grade was used in both treadmill tests. Expired gas was collected and analyzed as discussed above. Heart rate was determined from the ECG obtained using bipolar chest leads placed in the V_5 and manubrium positions. STI values before and after exercise were measured according to the method and procedures described in detail by Maher *et al.*[4]

Body weight was measured on a platform scale accurate to ±50 g. Sweat loss during the race was estimated from changes in body weight after correcting for fluid intake and respiratory weight losses.[5] Fluid intake, which included water and sundry solutions of sugar and electrolytes, was measured by using containers of known volume. Rectal temperature was measured with a mercury-in-glass thermometer inserted 8 cm.

Blood samples were drawn by syringe from an antecubital forearm vein at rest before and then 8 to 10 minutes following the first treadmill test, and also 8 to 10 minutes after the race. Technical difficulties precluded blood sampling before the race. All determinations were made on serum except for hematocrit (Hct), hemoglobin (Hb), and lactate, which were made on whole blood. Analysis for total protein, albumin, cholesterol, calcium, inorganic phosphorous, glucose, creatinine, uric acid, total bilirubin, alkaline phosphatase (Enzyme Code 3.1.3.1), lactate dehydrogenase (LDH, E.C. 1.1.1.27), and aspartate aminotransferase (GOT, E.C. 2.6.1.1) were performed on a sequential multiple automatic analyzer (Type 12/60, Technicon Instruments Corp., Tarrytown, N.Y.). Hct, calculated as mean corpuscular volume times red blood cell count, and Hb were determined with a cell counter (Model S, Coulter, Hialeah, Fla.). Lactate was analyzed by the enzymatic method using a commercially available test kit (Sigma Chemical Co., St. Louis, Mo.). Osmolality was determined by freezing point depression. Triglycerides were measured by a fluorometric procedure.[6] Sodium, potassium, and magnesium were determined by atomic absorption. Alphahydroxybutyrate dehydrogenase (α-HBDH, E.C. 1.1.1.27) was determined with a commercial test kit (Boehringer, Indianapolis, Ind.). Creatine phosphokinase (CPK, E.C. 2.7.3.2) was analyzed according to Rosalki.[7] All serum enzyme determinations were done spectrophotometrically at 25° C by measuring either the appearance or disappearance of NADH or NADPH.

A full report on the methods and results of urine analysis will be published elsewhere.

Marathon Race

The subjects were among 19 cardiovascular patients who completed the 1974 Honolulu Marathon, a certified road course measuring 42,195 m. Most of the course was flat, but a hill 38 m in vertical elevation had to be climbed at 8.4 km (average grade of 2.4% for 1400 m) and again at 36.9 km (average grade of 1.0% for 3000 m). Thus, hill-running on two gradual slopes comprised 20% of the race. The course record as of 1975 was 2:17.24 (J. Foster, New Zealand).

Ambient conditions at the start (6:30 AM) to when the last subject finished (12:40 PM) ranged as follows: T_a, 22° to 28° C; RH, 79% to 58%; wind velocity, 3.6 to 6.7 m·sec⁻¹; cloud cover, about 50%. Runners were resisted by an average 4.0 m·sec⁻¹ headwind for 7.5 km and aided by an equally strong tailwind for 3 km.

Physicians and nurses were available at 11 first aid and refreshment stations along the course beginning at 5 km.

RESULTS

Subjects were numbered according to their sequence of finishing the race.

O_2 Uptake during Road Running

FIGURE 1 shows curves relating $\dot{V}_{O_2}$ (ml·kg⁻¹·min⁻¹) to running velocity (m·min⁻¹) for each subject. Oxygen uptake was a linear function of velocity before plateauing at an apparent $\dot{V}_{O_2 max}$, which averaged 2.66 liter·min⁻¹ (41.3

ml·kg^{-1}·min^{-1}). Regression analysis of grouped data excluding points after $\dot{V}_{O_2}$ began leveling off resulted in the least squares best fit equation: $\dot{V}_{O_2} =$ 0.158(velocity) + 6.0. This relationship had a highly significant correlation coefficient of 0.97. Although resting $\dot{V}_{O_2}$ was not used in the linear regression analysis, the value of 6.0 ml·kg^{-1}·min^{-1} at the y intercept approximated standing $\dot{V}_{O_2}$ prior to running. Individual curves relating HR to $\dot{V}_{O_2}$ are shown in FIGURE 2. Peak values for HR averaged 176 b·min^{-1}. For subjects 1, 3, and 4 only, $\dot{V}_{O_2\,max}$ was also measured during uphill treadmill running and results were within ±3 ml·kg^{-1}·min^{-1} of their road running values.

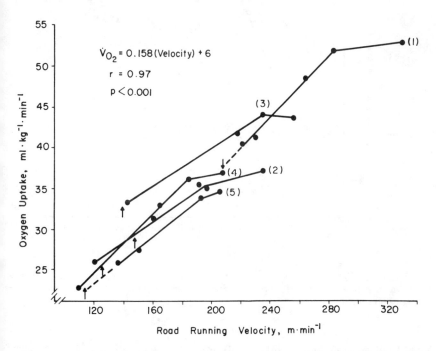

FIGURE 1. Relationship between road running velocity and O_2 uptake in five coronary patients. Subject numbers are shown in parentheses. Arrows indicate average velocity during the marathon race.

Observations during the Marathon Race

Observed and derived data for each subject are presented in TABLE 3. Finishing times averaged 299 minutes and ranged from 205 to 370 minutes.

Estimation of $\dot{V}_{O_2}$

Running velocity was determined at 7 to 10 locations on the course and averaged 147 m·min^{-1}. For descriptive purposes, the race was arbitrarily subdivided into the following three stages: start to 16 km, 16 to 32 km, and 32

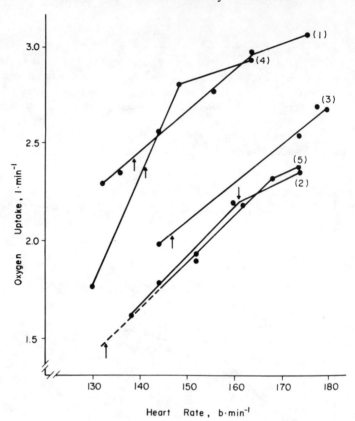

FIGURE 2. Relationship between heart rate and the O_2 uptake during road running shown in FIGURE 1. Arrows indicate average heart rate for each subject during the marathon race.

km to finish. FIGURE 3 shows velocity, $\dot{V}_{O_2}$, HR, and $\% \dot{V}_{O_2\,max}$ for each stage. Average velocity for each stage was 156, 149, and 129 m·min⁻¹, respectively.

From the start to 16 km, $\dot{V}_{O_2}$ was 30.7 ml·kg⁻¹·min⁻¹ and HR averaged 150 b·min⁻¹. The hill climb at 8.4 km increased HR to 163 b·min⁻¹, which predicted a $\dot{V}_{O_2}$ of 2.53 liter·min⁻¹ (39.2 ml·kg⁻¹·min⁻¹) or 95% of $\dot{V}_{O_2\,max}$. If we assume the runners maintained their velocity, the predicted $\dot{V}_{O_2}$ is very similar to that observed in treadmill studies.[8] Uphill running, therefore, increased the average $\dot{V}_{O_2}$ for this stage to 31.4 ml·kg⁻¹·min⁻¹.

From 16 to 32 km, $\dot{V}_{O_2}$ was 29.5 ml·kg⁻¹·min⁻¹ while HR was 141 b·min⁻¹. During this part of the race, however, the subjects were confronted by a steady 4.0 m·sec⁻¹ headwind for 7.5 km, which according to Pugh[9] should have increased $\dot{V}_{O_2}$ by 0.14 liter·min⁻¹ to about 31.6 ml·kg·min⁻¹. Thus, the adjusted average $\dot{V}_{O_2}$ for this stage was 30.4 ml·kg⁻¹·min⁻¹.

Except for subject 2 who maintained his pace, average velocity decreased

15% in the last 10.2 km. Subject 3 developed severe leg cramps and was forced to walk several km. Subjects 4 and 5 fatigued considerably and could only manage a fast walk alternating with brief periods of jogging. $\dot{V}_{O_2}$ estimated from velocity dropped to 26.4 ml·kg^{-1}·min^{-1} while HR remained at 140 b·min^{-1}. No attempt was made to correct $\dot{V}_{O_2}$ for the 3 km uphill portion of this stage since the grade was slight (1.0%) and subjects 3, 4, and 5 walked much of the way.

The overall adjusted $\dot{V}_{O_2}$ was 29.8 ml·kg^{-1}·min^{-1} (about 1.92 liter·min^{-1}) or 72% of $\dot{V}_{O_2\,max}$ (TABLE 3). It should be noted that this method of estimating $\dot{V}_{O_2}$ did not consider downhill running for 4.4 km, nor running with an aiding wind ($\sim$4.0 m·sec^{-1}) for about 3 km. Had HR been used to estimate $\dot{V}_{O_2}$ throughout the race, predicted $\dot{V}_{O_2}$ would have averaged 2.10 liter·min^{-1} (79% of $\dot{V}_{O_2\,max}$). However, the value of 1.92 liter·min^{-1} is believed more accurate because HR tends to rise during prolonged exercise.

Energy Expenditure

The calculated mean energy cost was 2770 kcal (TABLE 3). This value can also be expressed as 1.0 kcal·kg^{-1}·km^{-1}, which is identical to that found by Margaria *et al.*[10] for brief bouts of treadmill running.

TABLE 3

OBSERVATIONS ON FIVE CORONARY PATIENTS DURING ROAD RUNNING
AND A MARATHON RACE (42.2 km)

	Subject No.					
	1	2	3	4	5	Mean
Road Running						
$\dot{V}_{O_2max}$						
liter·min^{-1}	3.03	2.33	2.67	2.91	2.35	2.66
ml·kg^{-1}·min^{-1}	53.2	37.4	44.2	37.3	34.5	41.3
HR$_{max}$ b·min^{-1}	176	175	180	165	174	174
Marathon Race						
Finishing Time, min	205	285	302	335	370	299
Velocity, m·min^{-1}	205	148	140	126	114	147
O$_2$ uptake, ml·kg^{-1}·min^{-1} *	37.6	29.6	33.1	25.7	23.0	29.8
O$_2$ uptake, liter·min^{-1} *	2.19	1.85	1.98	1.97	1.60	1.92
% of $\dot{V}_{O_2max}$	72	79	74	68	68	72
Energy expenditure, kcal	2200	2584	2930	3234	2901	2770
Mean heart rate, b·min^{-1}	139	161	147	141	133	144
% of HR$_{max}$	79	92	82	85	78	83
Peak heart rate, b·min^{-1}	160	164	164	160	168	163
Fluid intake, ml	840	1400	1540	850	2140	1350
Rectal temp., ° C	39.0	38.5	38.6	38.6	38.4	38.6
Weight loss, kg	1.8	2.4	2.2	2.6	1.4	2.1

* Estimated from running velocity (FIGURE 1).

Fluid Exchange

Fluid intake during the race averaged 1350 ml and the observed weight loss was 2.1 kg, or 3.1% of prerace body weight (TABLE 3). Thus, the total weight loss was 3.45 kg, of which 0.45 kg (13%) represented respiratory losses, and the remaining 3.0 kg was sweat. The calculated rate of sweating was $0.6 \text{ kg} \cdot \text{hr}^{-1}$ ($340 \text{ ml} \cdot \text{m}^{-2} \cdot \text{hr}^{-1}$).

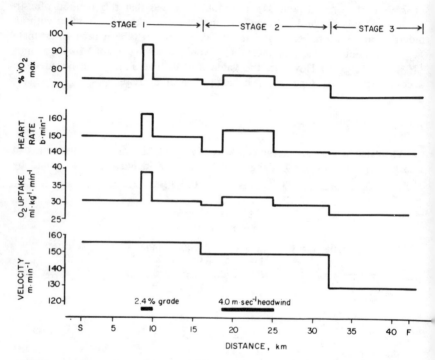

FIGURE 3. Observations of running velocity, estimated O_2 uptake, and heart rate during the marathon race.

Rectal Temperature

Postrace T_{re} averaged 38.6° C (TABLE 3) under ambient conditions that can be considered thermally stressful for long distance running.

Subjective Responses

The major source of discomfort during the race was leg fatigue in the last 10 km. Following the race, subjects 1 and 2 were seemingly well recovered after only 10 minutes. On the other hand, subjects 3, 4, and 5 complained of leg cramps and stiffness. Aside from the leg cramps, there were no symptoms related to heat exhaustion. There were also no symptoms of dypsnea or angina.

Treadmill Testing

The results of treadmill tests held two weeks before and immediately after the race are compared in TABLE 4.

Cardiorespiratory Responses

Heart rates were not significantly different since the HR obtained in the prerace test was used as a target level for the test after the race. At a mean HR of 139 b·min⁻¹ there was a 17% reduction in treadmill speed and a significantly lower $\dot{V}_{O_2}$ by 0.11 liter·min⁻¹ during the postrace test. Predictions of $\dot{V}_{O_2}$ using treadmill speed in the equation derived from measurements of $\dot{V}_{O_2}$ during road running were close to observed values in the prerace test but underestimated $\dot{V}_{O_2}$ after the race by 10%. The predicted $\dot{V}_{O_2}$ for the postrace treadmill test was, however, in agreement with findings by Jankowski *et al.*[11] Thus, it appears that muscular fatigue from the race resulted in decreased mechanical efficiency for treadmill exercise and an elevated HR for a given $\dot{V}_{O_2}$. Mean HR values for both tests were similar to mean HR during the race (TABLE 3).

Electrocardiogram

Subjects 1 and 3 had normal records for both tests. Subject 2 had >2 mm S-T segment depression with occasional premature ventricular beats during and after the prerace treadmill test. His S-T depression was 1 to 2 mm after the race and also during the postrace test he had fewer premature beats. Subjects 4 and 5 had minimal (0 to 1 mm) S-T depression during the first test but no depression after the race.

Systolic Time Intervals

Recovery HR was significantly higher after the race. Comparisons against normalized STI values corrected for HR were therefore required (TABLE 4). Subjects 1, 2, and 5 had normal left ventricular ejection time (LVET) and pre-ejection period (PEP) for both tests. Subjects 3 and 4 had prolonged LVET that were borderline normal for both tests.

Biochemical Results

FIGURES 4 through 8 show the results of blood analysis. Hct, Hb, and total protein, which may be used to indicate changes in hemoconcentration,[12] were not significantly different from resting values either after the prerace treadmill run or after the marathon race (FIGURE 4). Compared to treadmill running for 15 minutes at a similar percent of $\dot{V}_{O_2 \, max}$, the 205 to 370 minute marathon run had no statistically significant effects on Hct, Hb, total protein, and albumin (FIGURE 4), triglycerides, cholesterol, and glucose (FIGURE 5), sodium, potassium, magnesium, and phosphorus (FIGURE 6); alkaline phosphatase and GOT (FIGURE 7), and total bilirubin (not shown).

TABLE 4

CARDIORESPIRATORY RESPONSES TO TREADMILL RUNNNING IN FIVE TRAINED
CORONARY PATIENTS BEFORE AND AFTER A MARATHON RACE (42.2 km)*

	15 Days before Race	15 Minutes after Race	p †
Weight, kg	65.1±8.2	64.4±7.6	NS
Treadmill speed, m·min⁻¹	142±26	118±17	NS
Heart Rate, b·min⁻¹	142±9	139±7	NS
% of HRmax	81±4	80±3	NS
O₂ uptake			
liter·min⁻¹	1.84±0.10	1.73±0.16	<0.025
ml·kg⁻¹·min⁻¹	28.3±3.6	27.2±4.4	NS
% of $\dot{V}_{O_2max}$	70±7	66±6	<0.025
Expired min vol, liter·min⁻¹			
(BTPS)	64.3±9	57.3±9	<0.05
CO₂ output, liter·min⁻¹	1.68±0.13	1.33±0.20	<0.01
Resp. exchange ratio	0.91±0.03	0.77±0.06	<0.025
Rectal temp, ° C	38.1±0.1	38.5±0.2	<0.05
Blood pressure, mmHg	165/84±19/9	— ‡	—
Systolic time intervals §			
HR, b·min⁻¹	69±14	88±18	<0.05
LVET, msec	284±22 (296±25)	255±23 (263±30)	NS
PEP, msec	117±15 (103±6)	88±9 (96±7)	NS

* Values are means ± standard deviations. Ambient temperature during both tests was 25° C.
† Paired t-test. NS=not significant (p >0.05).
‡ Inadvertently omitted on two subjects.
§ Measured in supine position during recovery (LVET, left ventricular ejection time; PEP, pre-ejection period). Since supine HR was significantly higher after the race, before and after values for LVET and PEP were compared by absolute difference from normal values (shown in parenthesis), which are corrected for HR.

The only significant biochemical change from resting levels after the 15-minute treadmill run was a 2-fold increase in lactate (FIGURE 8). Following the marathon run, however, lactate was close to resting levels and significantly lower than after the treadmill test (FIGURE 8). After the race, significantly higher values were found for osmolality and calcium (FIGURE 6), CPK, LDH, and α-HBDH (FIGURE 7), creatinine and uric acid (FIGURE 8), as compared to after the 15-minute run.

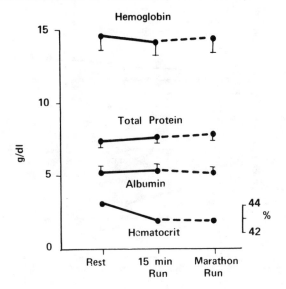

FIGURE 4. Effects of running for 15 min versus running for 205 to 370 min at equal average intensities on serum total protein, serum albumin, hemoglobin, and hematocrit ratio of five trained coronary patients. Values are means ± standard deviations. Asterisks indicate significant differences (p <0.05) between the 15-min. run and the marathon run, which were separated by 2 weeks (broken line).

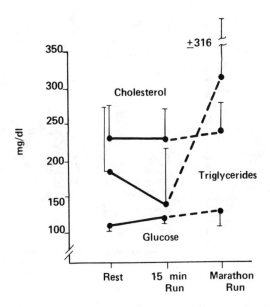

FIGURE 5. Effects of running for 15 min versus running for 205 to 370 min at equal average intensities on serum lipids and glucose of five trained coronary patients.

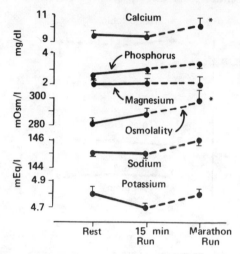

FIGURE 6. Effects of running for 15 min versus running for 205 to 370 min at equal average intensities on serum electrolyte levels and osmolality of five trained coronary patients.

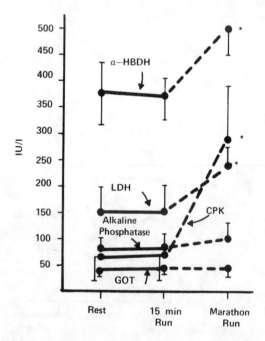

FIGURE 7. Effects of running for 15 min versus running for 205 to 370 min at equal average intensities on serum enzyme levels of five trained coronary patients.

DISCUSSION

The mean, weight-adjusted $\dot{V}_{O_2\,max}$ during road running of the four subjects with healed MIs was 38.4 ml·kg⁻¹·min⁻¹. This value is about the same as that for active, healthy men of similar age,[13] but considerably higher than typical values for coronary patients following physical conditioning.[14] It is tempting to attribute the relatively high $\dot{V}_{O_2\,max}$ of the present subjects to their regular participation in the marathon training clinic. Unfortunately, measurements of $\dot{V}_{O_2\,max}$ were not made early in rehabilitation. However, long distance running as a method of post-MI rehabilitation has been shown effective in increasing $\dot{V}_{O_2\,max}$ to levels above that of our subjects, i.e., above average for North American men of comparable age.[1][15]

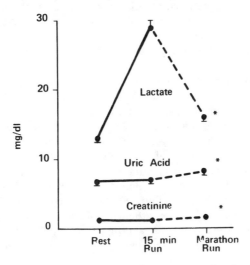

FIGURE 8. Effects of running for 15 min versus running for 205 to 370 min at equal average intensities on blood lactate, uric acid, and creatinine of five trained coronary patients.

It is well established that $\dot{V}_{O_2}$ is linearly related to running velocity.[10,16] This relationship has been used previously to estimate the O_2 cost of marathoning in runners who averaged 217 m·min⁻¹,[17] 254 m·min⁻¹,[16,18] and 145 m·min⁻¹.[1] Costill and Fox [16] estimated that national class long distance runners utilized 75% of $\dot{V}_{O_2\,max}$ (range: 68% to 82%) in their best races and Adams *et al.*[18] found a similar value. The present findings are also within this range (67% to 79%). Seven post-MI patients studied by Kavanagh *et al.*[1] completed the Boston Marathon at an average velocity equal to the present subjects. Using Shephard's nomogram [8] these authors estimated the fraction of $\dot{V}_{O_2\,max}$ utilized averaged 81%. Thus, relative to $\dot{V}_{O_2\,max}$, O_2 transport and utilization during marathon running in trained coronary patients appears similar to healthy, competitive runners.

While the percentage of $\dot{V}_{O_2 \, max}$ derived from average velocity may indicate the overall metabolic strain of marathon running, it does not reveal acute cardiorespiratory demands imposed enroute. For example, our subjects averaged 72% of $\dot{V}_{O_2 \, max}$, but early in the race they were able to utilize approximately 95% during uphill running (FIGURE 3). This distinction may be essential with certain coronary patients since work rates eliciting 72% of $\dot{V}_{O_2 \, max}$ are usually below the threshold of undesirable ECG changes, whereas exercise at 95% might exceed it and be contraindicated. Our subjects had no ill effects.

For a given $\dot{V}_{O_2}$, heart rate was elevated 6 b·min⁻¹ during the postrace treadmill test and was possibly up to 15 b·min⁻¹ higher in the last stage of the race as compared to the two earlier stages (FIGURE 3). Increased HR is a common finding during prolonged steady-state work and generally accompanies increasing body temperature.[18, 19] The use of running velocity to estimate $\dot{V}_{O_2}$ during the race was, therefore, preferred to using HR. However, the increase in the ratio of $\dot{V}_{O_2}$ to speed observed during the post-race treadmill test, indicating reduced work efficiency, suggests that this indirect method may have underestimated $\dot{V}_{O_2}$ slightly during the last stage of the race when fatigue was pronounced.

Fluid intake averaged 1350 ml and replaced approximately 45% of the 3.0-liter sweat loss. Consequently, weight loss was only 3.1% of prerace body weight, whereas without fluid replacement it would have been 5.1%. The actual free water deficit was probably closer to 2% since metabolic water production and release of water bound to glycogen must have contributed to total body water. Fluid deficits on the order of 2% are well tolerated during exercise and result in only small increases of equilibrium T_{re}.[18, 20, 21] In fact, postrace T_{re} was similar to predicted values of equilibrium T_{re} for exercise at 72% of $\dot{V}_{O_2 \, max}$ in unstressful ambient conditions.[22] The observed sweat loss had little effect on serum electrolyte balance although osmolality was 3% higher (p < 0.05) than prerace resting values. Again, the importance of fluid replacement in avoiding dehydration hyperthermia during long distance running should be emphasized.[23]

The lower respiratory exchange ratio after the race agrees with previous findings [18, 24] and provides evidence of a metabolic shift to fatty acids as glycogen storage is reduced, despite unchanged serum glucose levels. This conclusion is supported by the lower lactate accumulation after the race as compared to a brief bout of running (FIGURE 2).

Mean values for all biochemical determinations at rest were essentially normal except for α-HBDH, which was 2.5 times higher than the upper limit of normal. Elevated α-HBDH activity is commonly used in clinical practice along with other serum enzymes such as GOT, LDH, and CPK to confirm suspected cases of acute MI.[25] However, increased serum enzyme levels have also been found in healthy subjects after long distance running [26-28] and can remain elevated at rest during training.[29] The high resting α-HBDH levels in the present subjects undoubtedly had a functional, nonpathologic cause such as training.

Compared to running for 15 minutes, the 299-minute marathon run resulted in increased serum activities for α-HBDH, LDH, and CPK of 39%, 59%, and

296%, respectively (FIGURE 7). Since the runs were performed at equal average intensities (% of $\dot{V}_{O_2 \, max}$), the 20 times longer duration of marathoning appears to have promoted the increases, and perhaps those observed for creatinine (36%) and uric acid (17%) as well. Elevated uric acid levels after endurance exercise have been previously reported.[26]

The data are too limited to specify which tissues were responsible for the increased serum enzymes because they can originate from many cell types. Origin from red blood cell hemolysis is unlikely since GOT did not also increase, and lack of change in alkaline phosphatase suggests sources other than bone, digestive organs, or the liver.‡ Several investigators have hypothesized that distance running may cause hyperpermeability of the cell membrane of skeletal muscle enabling a greater efflux of large cytoplasmic substances.[26-28, 30] However, the mechanism by which prolonged muscular activity might increase permeability is not clear. One concept proposes that tissue hypoxia in the active muscles during high intensity work reduces the amount of ATP available for maintaining the integrity of the cell membrane.[29] Findings that training reduces serum enzyme levels at a given work load support this concept.[26, 29, 31] On the other hand, it is unlikely that there was muscular hypoxia in the present subjects during the marathon since the energy requirement must have been satisfied aerobically. Also, previous research has shown that untrained subjects had adequate oxygen delivery to working muscles while exercising to exhaustion at a percentage of $\dot{V}_{O_2 \, max}$ similar to our subjects.[32]

Another possible explanation for reduced ATP availability and cell membrane integrity during prolonged exercise is depletion of muscle glycogen. Costill[33] has suggested that selective depletion of muscle glycogen in slow-twitch fibers is the primary cause of muscular exhaustion experienced by runners in the final stage of marathon races. The diminished carbohydrate energy reserves of slow-twitch fibers could explain reduced availability of ATP for maintaining membrane integrity.

All of the subjects except one (subject 2) showed decreased running velocity in the final stage of the race and decreased work efficiency after the race. Muscular exhaustion was clearly evident in subjects 3, 4, and 5. Costill[33] listed six popular theories to explain the observed muscular exhaustion: (1) lactic acid accumulation, (2) hypoglycemia, (3) dehydration, (4) excessive electrolyte losses, (5) hyperthermia, and (6) depletion of muscle glycogen. Our results indicate that after the race blood lactate levels were low, serum glucose was normal, dehydration was minimal, serum electrolytes were mostly unchanged, and body temperature was well regulated. The data indirectly support Costill's point that muscle glycogen depletion is the most likely cause of muscular exhaustion during marathon running in moderate ambient conditions. Furthermore, since the ECG and STI measurements were not significantly altered by the marathon race, it can be concluded that left ventricular performance was adequate. Thus, factors not related to cardiac function, such as depletion of

‡ Serum glutamate pyruvate transaminase (GPT) concentration was determined on postmarathon blood samples and was within normal limits for all subjects. This finding also suggests that liver cells did not release the observed enzymes.

muscle glycogen reserves, were responsible for the decreased performance of the active limb muscles.

In summary, the findings of this study show that five patients with recent histories of asymptomatic to severe coronary artery disease were capable, after a program of long distance running, of completing the 1974 Honolulu Marathon (42.2 km). The patients utilized 72% of $\dot{V}_{O_2 \, max}$ much like competitive marathon runners and expended 2770 kcal in 5 hours. The data indicate that the patients made suitable physiological adjustments to the stresses of marathon running and myocardial function was unimpaired. After further training, subjects 1, 4, and 5 improved their times by 17, 24, and 42 minutes while running the same race a year later. It is concluded that the coronary patients of this study acquired a high level of endurance fitness and responded favorably to the heavy physiological demands of marathon running. It should be emphasized that these patients had undergone an extensive aerobic conditioning program prior to the marathon race, and they responded well to this training. Moreover, these patients were under the close supervision and coaching of medical personnel who were marathon runners themselves. We can recommend marathon running only for similarly trained and supervised coronary patients.

ACKNOWLEDGMENTS

The authors are indebted to the many physicians and nurses who donated their time and skills in making this study possible. We acknowledge with gratitude the expert technical assistance of the following persons: Tom Ferguson (Race Director), Andrea Yap, M.A., Kathy Nekomoto, M.A., Kathy Brown, R.M.T., Jeanie Hoepfel, R.N., and Jo Schroeder, R.N.

REFERENCES

1. KAVANAGH, T., R. J. SHEPHARD & V. PANDIT. 1973. Marathon running after myocardial infarction. J. Amer. Med. Assoc. 229: 1602–1605.
2. EDWARDS, K. & H. WHYTE. 1962. The simple measurement of obesity. Clin. Sci. 22: 347–352.
3. DANIELS, J. 1971. Portable respiratory gas collection equipment. J. Appl. Physiol. 31: 164–167.
4. MAHER, J. T., G. A. BELLER, B. J. RANSIL & L. H. HARTLEY. 1974. Systolic time intervals during submaximal and maximal exercise in man. Amer. Heart J. 87: 334–342.
5. MITCHELL, J. W., E. R. NADEL & J. A. J. STOLWIJK. 1972. Respiratory weight losses during exericse. J. Appl. Physiol. 32: 474–476.
6. BLOCK, W. D. & K. J. JARRETT. 1969. An automated technique for the quantitative determnination of serum total triglycerides. Amer. J. Med. Tech. 35: 1–10.
7. ROSALKI, S. B. 1967. An improved procedure for serum creatine phosphokinase determination. J. Lab. Clin. Med. 69: 696–705.
8. SHEPHARD, R. J. 1969. A nomogram to calculate the oxygen cost of running at slow speeds. J. Sports Med. 9: 10–16.
9. PUGH, L. G. C. E. 1970. Oxygen intake in track and treadmill running with observations on the effect of air resistance. J. Physiol. 207: 823–835.
10. MARGARIA, R., P. CERRETELLI, P. AGHEMO, et al. 1963. Energy cost of running. J. Appl. Physiol. 18: 367–370.

11. JANKOWSKI, L. W., R. J. FERGUSON, M. LANGELIER, L. N. CHANIOTIS & G. CHOQUETTE. 1972. Accuracy of estimating O_2 cost of walking in coronary patients. J. Appl. Physiol. **33**: 672–673.

12. VAN BEAUMONT, W., J. E. GREENLEAF & L. JUHOS. 1972. Disproportional changes in hematocrit, plasma volume, and proteins during exercise and bed rest. J. Appl. Physiol. **33**: 55–61.

13. DEHN, M. M. & R. A. BRUCE. 1972. Longitudinal variations in maximal oxygen intake with age and activity. J. Appl. Physiol. **33**: 805–807.

14. FERGUSON, R. J., R. PETITCLERC, G. CHOQUETTE & L. W. JANKOWSKI. 1974. Effect of physical training on treadmill exercise capacity, collateral circulation, and progression of coronary disease. Amer. J. Cardiology. **34**: 764–768.

15. KAVANAGH, T., R. J. SHEPHARD, H. DONEY & V. PANDIT. 1973. Intensive exercise in coronary rehabilitation. Med. Sci. Sports **5**: 34–39.

16. COSTILL, D. L. & E. L. FOX. 1969. Energetics of marathon running. Med. Sci. Sports **1**: 81–86.

17. PUGH, L. G. C. E., J. L. CORBETT & R. H. JOHNSON. 1967. Rectal temperatures, weight losses, and sweat rates in marathon running. J. Appl. Physiol. **23**: 347–352.

18. ADAMS, W. C., R. H. FOX, A. J. FRY & I. C. MACDONALD. 1975. Thermoregulation during marathon running in cool, moderate, and hot environments. J. Appl. Physiol. **38**: 1030–1037.

19. ROWELL, L. B. 1974. Human cardiovascular adjustments to exercise and thermal stress. Physiol. Rev. **54**: 75–159.

20. GISOLFI, C. V. & J. R. COPPING. 1974. Thermal effects of prolonged treadmill exercise in the heat. Med. Sci. Sports **6**: 108–113.

21. GREENLEAF, J. E. & B. L. CASTLE. 1971. Exercise temperature regulation in man during hypohydration and hyperhydration. J. Appl. Physiol. **30**: 847–853.

22. KAMON, E. 1975. Ergonomics of heat and cold. Texas Rep. Biol. Med. **33**: 145–182.

23. AMERICAN COLLEGE OF SPORTS MEDICINE POSITION STATEMENT ON PREVENTION OF HEAT INJURIES DURING DISTANCE RUNNING. 1975. Med. Sci. Sports **7**: vii–ix.

24. COSTILL, D. L. 1970. Metabolic responses during distance running. J. Appl. Physiol. **28**: 251–255.

25. WITTEVEEN, S. A. G. J., H. C. HEMKER, L. HOLLAAR & W. TH. HERMENS. 1975. Quantification of infarct size in man by means of plasma enzyme levels. Brit. Heart J. **37**: 795–803.

26. MAGAZANIK, A., Y. SHAPIRO, D. MEYTES & I. MEYTES. 1974. Enzyme blood levels and water balance during a marathon race. J. Appl. Physiol. **36**: 214–217.

27. ROSE, L. I., S. L. LOWE, D. R. CARROLL, *et al.* 1970. Serum lactate dehydrogenase isoenzyme changes after muscular exertion. J. Appl. Physiol. **28**: 279–281.

28. ROSE, L. I., J. E. BOUSSER & K. H. COOPER. 1970. Serum enzymes after marathon running. J. Appl. Physiol. **29**: 355–357.

29. HUNTER, J. B. & J. B. CRITZ. 1971. Effect of training on plasma enzyme levels in man. J. Appl. Physiol. **31**: 20–23.

30. FOWLER, W. M., S. R. CHOWDHURY, C. M. PEARSON, *et al.* 1962. Changes in serum enzyme levels after exercise in trained and untrained subjects. J. Appl. Physiol. **17**: 943–946.

31. SANDERS, T. M. & C. M. BLOOR. 1975. Effects of repeated endurance exercise on serum enzyme activities in well–conditioned males. Med. Sci. Sports **7**: 44–47.

32. THOMPSON, J. M., J. A. DEMPSEY, L. W. CHOSY, *et al.* 1974. Oxygen transport and oxyhemoglobin dissociation during prolonged muscular work. J. Appl. Physiol. **37**: 658–664.

33. COSTILL, D. L. 1974. Muscular exhaustion during distance running. Phys. Sportsmed. **36** (Oct.): 41.

LIMITATIONS OF MARATHON RUNNING IN THE REHABILITATION OF CORONARY PATIENTS: ANATOMIC AND PHYSIOLOGIC DETERMINANTS *

Herman K. Hellerstein

School of Medicine
Case Western Reserve University
Cleveland, Ohio 44106

University Hospitals of Cleveland
Cleveland, Ohio 44106

INTRODUCTION

Rehabilitation has been defined as the process by which a patient is returned realistically to his optimal physiologic, mental, psychologic, emotional, social, vocational, and economic usefulness and if employable is provided an opportunity for gainful employment in a competitive industrial world.[1] Rehabilitation also includes efforts to reverse or to prevent the progression of the underlying disease process. Successful rehabilitation in this modern sense is not restricted to economic or vocational rehabilitation alone, rather it is the complete development of a pattern of living that will enable the individual to enjoy the fullest physical and mental capacities with due allowances for his disabilities. Exercise training and conditioning has been shown to play an important role in the rehabilitation of selected coronary patients. In our initial studies, begun 17 years ago and subsequently confirmed by others, emphasis was placed upon the enhancement of physical fitness of coronary patients.[2-5] However, physical conditioning was part of a comprehensive program that also involved weight control, diet therapy, cessation of smoking, regular performance of supervised prescribed exercise, continuation of gainful employment and of a normal social mode of life, adequate recreation, and rest. In addition, essentially normal male subjects with many coronary risk factors were included, predicated upon the findings of prospective epidemiologic surveys that certain host factors are consistently associated with a high risk of developing coronary artery disease prematurely. The predisposing factors include elevated serum lipids, hypertension, obesity, cigarette smoking, physical inactivity and unfitness, and abnormal carbohydrate metabolism. The wisdom of including asymptomatic coronary-prone subjects was confirmed by the findings in these asymptomatic subjects of ischemic ST-T responses to exercise in more than 5%; of this 5%, 75% have a significant coronary arteriosclerosis.[6, 7]

Exercise Prescription. Prior to entry into an exercise program a detailed evaluation of each individual was made, including psychologic, nutritional, anthropologic, and physiologic tests. The chronotropic, power, mechanism,

* This work was supported in part by grants from the Rehabilitation Services Administration, Department of Health, Education and Welfare, Award No. ORD-RD-P 55917/5, contributions by Mr. & Mrs. Harry Mann, Cleveland, Ohio, and by Messrs. David and Arthur Genshaft, Massillon, Ohio.

and aerobic capacities were determined from peak performance of multistage exercise tests. Each exercise prescription was compounded to stress each subject to approximately 60% to 70% of his aerobic capacity, during three 1-hour training periods each week. At this relative load many physiological and biochemical changes transpire: the respiratory exchange ratio approaches unity and there are increases in blood lactate, fibrinolytic activity, urinary catecholamine excretion, capacity to oxidize fatty acids, release of fatty acids from adipose tissue, capacity to regenerate ATP by oxidative phosphorylation, and so forth, desirable changes that are associated with favorable adaptation and improvement.[8] Each exercise session consisted of 30 minutes of calisthenics for development of strength, 15 minutes of run-walk sequences for endurance, and recreational exercise (games, etc.) for fun. The capacity to complete 2 or 2½ miles in 15 minutes was considered to be a satisfactory attainment. Participants were not encouraged to run longer distances.

Effects of Non-Long Distance Training Program. A majority (75%–85%) of patients with myocardial infarction have responded to the carefully supervised comprehensive reconditioning program in a multitude of fashions: improvement of subjective well-being, lowering of the scores of depression, hypochondriasis, hysteria, and psychasthenia scales of the Minnesota Multiphasic Personality Inventory Test, marked improvement of work capacity, lessening of the ST-T segment displacement, reduction of hypertensive blood pressure responses and of peripheral vascular resistance during exercise diminution of the heart rate at rest, during sleep, and during exercise in submaximal effort, lowering of serum lipid levels, reduction of adipose tissue and body weight, enhanced extraction of oxygen by the peripheral tissues, and a suggestive reduction in mortality rate.[2–5]

Determinants of Improvement to Physical Conditioning Programs. The occurrence and the magnitude of improvement of functional aerobic capacity depended primarily on the severity of the anatomic lesions in the coronary arteries and the extent of myocardial involvement[9] and on adherence to a properly supervised, quantitated exercise program. Adherence was favorably influenced by the program design, attitude of the spouse, the variety of acceptable and pleasurable activities, and accessibility of training personnel and facilities in a nearby community center.[2–4]

Are More Vigorous Training and Marathon Running Desirable and Valuable in the Rehabilitation of Coronary Patients? In the past decade considerable publicity and emphasis have been placed upon long distance running, and more recently on marathon running, as the primary conditioning method, not only for normal but also for cardiac subjects. In the past several years marathon running by a handful of coronary men in several communities[10] has been given much publicity and in my considered opinion has aroused unrealistic expectations for the vast majority of coronary patients.

In the present report, I will discuss (1) the limited cardiovascular value of lower extremity training by long distance running (marathon) for the performance of the majority of occupations, (2) the influence of age and severity of underlying heart disease on the aerobic capacity and its enhancement, which limits the applicability of marathon running to the general coronary population, and (3) the hazards of high-level-activity-induced cardiac arrest, which is reversible and thus mandates available of cardiopulmonary resuscitative equipment and personnel in the *immediate* vicinity of *all* subjects undertaking long distance (marathon) running.

Limited Cardiovascular Value of Lower Extremity Training for the Majority of Occupations and Vocations. Generally speaking the aim of physical conditioning is to increase muscle strength or endurance or both. Clausen, Hollosczy, and others have demonstrated convincingly that the adaptation induced by exercise training occurs predominantly in the working skeletal muscle.[11-13] These changes include decreased blood flow, increased arteriovenous oxygen extraction, increases in myoglobin concentration, mitochondral changes with increases in respiratory enzymes and oxidation of NADH succinate, increased citric acid cycle enzymes, and increased substrate oxidation of pyruvate, palmitate, oleate, and fatty acids. In contrast, effects of training on myocardium of humans or experimental animals have been unimpressive, with little change in respiratory capacity, cytochrome c or mitrochondral protein.[12] However, Scheuer has reported an increase of actinomycin ATPase of the myocardium of trained normal rats.[14] Our recent preliminary studies have demonstrated that myocardial contractility as well as peripheral arteriovenous oxygen extraction by skeletal musculature may improve with training.[15] Measurement of systolic intervals before and after xeercise tests and training have shown that the ratio of the pre-ejection period to the left ventricular ejection time (PEP/LVET) became lower at rest and decreased even more after exercise as functional aerobic capacity improved.[15] These changes are consistent with an improvement of the ventricular ejection fraction.[16]

However, the predominant view is that the chief effects of training are on the skeletal muscles used for training and that the heart and central circulation are effected only indirectly if at all. The importance of training effects on the heart has not been resolved.

Lack of Cross-Adaptation of Upper and Lower Extremity Training Effects. The importance of peripheral adaptions to training has been well documented.[11] For example, Clausen, Trap-Jensen, and Lassen trained two groups of men, one group exercised using the arms and the other using the legs. In tests after training, both groups alternated between arm and leg exercise using the same protocol. This investigation demonstrated that the training of the arm muscles effected the heart rate response only during arm exercise and vice versa. The lack of cross-over benefits was recently confirmed by a study of kayak ergometer performance after kayak and after leg bicycle ergometer training.[17] The kayak-ergometer-trained subjects increased by 50% the number of kilopond meters per minute able to be performed during kayak testing in contrast to approximately 6% improvement in leg exercise after kayak ergometer training.

The limitations of restrictions of training to the lower extremities can be readily demonstrated by two examples shown in TABLE 1. The cross-country runner had an upper extremity exercise maximal oxygen uptake 54.8% of that of the lower extremities, viz., 28.9 and 52.7 ml/kg·min, respectively. In contrast, the swimmer who was also a cycler had a maximal arm exercise oxygen uptake 84.2% of that of the legs (48.0 and 57.0, respectively). The greater volume of the upper extremities of the second subject could account for 6.4 of the 19.1 ml/kg·min difference in the oxygen uptake with maximal arm exercise of the two subjects.

Application to Rehabilitation and Counselling of Cardiac Patients. The lack of cardiovascular cross-over benefits of training of the lower extremities or upper extremity efforts and vice versa has a significant implication for counselling of cardiac patients for return to occupations and vocations. In our previous studies my associates and I found few occupations that require significant walking even at a slow rate; practically none required jogging or running, except for protective service personnel, police officers, their fugitives, and marathon buffs.[1, 18-20]

The principle of muscle specificity is important in planning exercise training programs in cardiac rehabilitation. An individual who relies principally upon the arm musculature in daily activity needs to be concerned primarily with training these muscle groups, with the expectation that heart rate and blood pressure response will decrease with training. These favorable changes are particularly important for the coronary patients who develop angina pectoris as a result of a high heart rate and systolic blood pressure product at a lower work level than with legs. Since one of the principal objectives of cardiac rehabilitation is to prepare an individual for a return to occupation

TABLE 1

EFFECTS OF UPPER AND LOWER EXTREMITY TRAINING ON MAXIMAL ARMS AND LEGS PERFORMANCE

	Cross Country Runner			Swimmer & Cycler		
	Arms	Legs	Legs at Max Arms	Arms	Legs	Legs at Max Arms
$\dot{V}_{O_2 max}$ (ml/kg·min)	28.9	52.7	22.5	48.0	57.0	42.6
Blood Pressure (mmHg)						
Systolic	154	216	174	160	170	186
Diastolic	84	90	88	70	70	78
Heart Rate	186	203	114	192	198	170
Volume (liters)	2.7	8.4		3.3	9.0	
Arms/Legs Volume (%)		32.1			36.3	
Body Fat (%)		14.3			10.5	

* Legs working at a rate equal to the maximal work rate of the arms.

and leisure-time physical activities, a physical training program needs to include exercise for arms as well as for the legs and torso.

Prescription of Intensity of Exercise Training of Upper Extremities. It is necessary to test the maximal or peak performance of the upper extremities in order to develop insight into the magnitude of the training intensity. Recently my associates and I have studied the cardiorespiratory responses of arm and leg exercise during submaximal and maximal physical exertion.[21, 23] Maximal oxygen uptake ($\dot{V}_{O_2 max}$), minute ventilation ($\dot{V}_E$), heart rate (HR), systolic blood pressure (SBP), the product of HR and SBP (a measure of myocardial oxygen need), and the respiratory exchange ratio (R) were significantly greater during arm exercise compared to leg exercise at the same submaximal work load and when compared at the level of maximal arm exercise. The response to maximal exercise, the oxygen uptake, $\dot{V}$, and the

HR × SBP product were significantly higher during leg exercise. The maximal oxygen uptake with arm exercise was approximately 60% of that of leg exercise. However, since the volume of the upper extremities was approximately 30% of that of the lower extremities and since the maximal oxygen uptake with the upper extremity exercise was 60% of that of the lower extremity exercise when considered per unit volume, the $\dot{V}_{O_2\,max}$ for arm exercise was twice that of the legs.

Since heart rate and oxygen uptake are related in a linear fashion at moderate to maximal work loads the heart rate can serve as an indication of the individual's oxygen utilization. Arbitrary heart rates or approximated energy costs should not be used as criteria for training intensity. Since maximal heart rates decrease with age, a fixed training heart rate will not elicit the same physiological responses. The regression equations between the $\%\,HR_{max}$ and $\%\,\dot{V}_{O_2\,max}$ revealed no difference between arm and leg exercise compared at the same [8, 22] relative work load $y = 1.2x - 29.3$, $r = 0.96$ and $y = 1.3x - 36.3$, $r = 0.97$. The clinical significance of this relationship is that relative to maximum, exercise prescriptions can be based upon the same regression equations regardless of the muscle groups involved and the condition of the subjects.

The concept of arm exercise testing and training is relatively new and deserves to be explored further. Submaximal arm work is performed at a greater physiologic cost than leg work at the same work level. Maximal physiologic responses are significantly greater in leg than arm work.

Other Limitations of Lower Extremity Training. Low extremity exercise may be limited in patients who have skeletal musculature difficulties, particularly arthritis and arthralgias with skeletal muscle involvement, and even more important in patients with coronary artery disease and associated peripheral vascular disease. In our recent experiences at least 8% of the subjects entered into the National Exercise and Heart Disease Project have significant restrictions due to peripheral arteriosclerosis. Fortunately by design the training program includes upper and lower extremity training. In subjects with intermittent claudication due to atherosclerosis the maximal heart rate that can be attained with lower extremity exercise is considerably less than that of upper extremity exercise, contrary to the situation of subjects with normal peripheral circulation.

APPLICABILITY OF LONG DISTANCE MARATHON RUNNING TO THE POPULATION WITH CLINICAL CORONARY ARTERIOSCLEROTIC HEART DISEASE

Influence of Age and Disease on the Aerobic Capacity and Its Modification. Cross-sectional and longitudinal studies have demonstrated that the aerobic capacity decreases with age [23] and even more with the development of clinical heart disease.[24] To gain insight into the potential attainment of the functional aerobic capacity of coronary patients to complete a marathon even at a noncompetitive time of 5 hours, I have made an analysis of the age, sex, and severity of coronary disease patients discharged from our cardiac monitoring unit (CMU) in the past year and the response of selected subjects to intensive training.

The average age of men discharged from our CMU was 60.4 years (± 10.94 years, standard deviation) for the men and 64.5 ± 12.97 years for the women;

5.3% were less than 45 years of age, and potentially could be eligible to develop a functional aerobic capacity of 38 to 42 ml/kg·min, values of normal sedentary and active subjects.[24]

A brief review of the oxygen required to complete the marathon at various speeds is graphically presented in FIGURE 1 (a modification of the elegant report by Margaria).[25] The time to complete the marathon can be accurately estimated, taking into account whether from 70% to 100% of the maximal aerobic capacity was used. For an individual with a $\dot{V}_{O_2 max}$ of 50 ml/kg·min. at 70% capacity, the time is 241 minutes; at 80%, 213 minutes; and at 90%, 179 minutes. The impossibility of 100% capacity for 1 hour has been amply demonstrated but theoretically at such a rate a marathon could be accomplished in

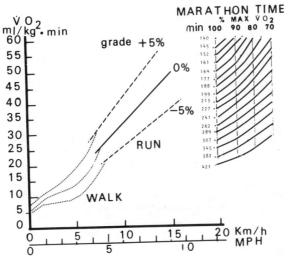

FIGURE 1. Energy expenditure in milliliters of oxygen per kilogram body weight per minute (ml/kg·min), as a function of speed in kilometers or miles per hour, in walking and running on the level or uphill and downhill at a 5% grade. (After Margaria et al.[25]) In the upper right hand corner, estimated times in minutes to complete a marathon race, at 70% to 100% of maximal oxygen uptake. (Discussed in text.)

169 minutes. Astrand and others have indicated about 85% of maximal aerobic capacity can be used for 1 hour but not much longer.[26] For cardiac patients a maximal oxygen uptake of 40 to 42 ml/kg·min would be required to complete the run in 300 minutes at 70% capacity, or 260 minutes at 80% capacity. The maximal oxygen uptake of active normal subjects of 45 years of age is approximately 40 ml/kg·min body weight. In my review I found 5.3% of subjects discharged from the CMU were less than 45 years of age. Furthermore, analysis of our experiences in 1959–1968 with training indicates that the average $\dot{V}_{O_2 max}$ uptake in the coronary subjects of this age group before and after was 24.7 and 29.2 ml/kg·min, respectively. Similar data have been reported by others.[4, 27] In our recent experience of 74 subjects who had trained at a more intense level, maximal oxygen uptake increased from 24.9 to 34.8 ml/kg·min. However,

only 10.8% of the latter group of subjects were able to attain a maximal oxygen uptake of more than 39 ml/kg·min. Stated otherwise, of 53 of 1000 subjects discharged from a CMU 10.8%, i.e., 5 or 6 can potentially be trained to attain an aerobic capacity sufficient to complete, if motivated, a marathon run in 300 minutes. In the present conference Kavanagh confirmed that relatively few coronary subjects, i.e., 22 of 600 men with coronary disease enrolled in a training program can complete a marathon run.[10]

The validity of estimating the potential marathon time from a determination of maximum $\dot{V}_{O_2}$, and an assumption that approximately 70% of the maximum $\dot{V}_{O_2}$ will be employed is substantiated by my own experience with private patients and by the preceding presentation by Dr. Dressendorfer.[28]

Case Illustration. On April 9, 1970, one of my patients, then 51 years old,

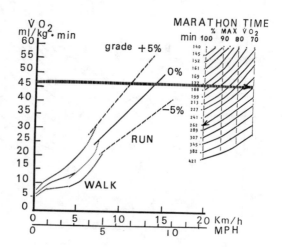

FIGURE 2. Estimation of the time to complete the Boston Marathon by a man with maximal oxygen uptake of 46 ml/kg·min, at 70% $\dot{V}_{O_2 max}$. The estimated time was 262 minutes, actual time was 262 minutes, actual time was 255 minutes. (Discussed in text.)

completed the Boston Marathon in 4 hours 15 minutes. In March 1965 he had sustained an acute inferior myocardial infarct. His convalescence was uneventful, and approximately 6 weeks later he entered a program of physical training at the local Y.M.C.A. In December 1965 he ran his first mile, in 1966 he ran three miles at one time, in early 1967 six miles, and in November seven miles at one session. By December 1967 he reached the 1000 mile mark. In the subsequent 3 years his overall endurance improved sufficiently to undertake a marathon run. His performance was remarkable in view of his completing the run within the first 35% of the participants who finished the 1970 Boston Marathon. His maximal oxygen uptake determined in my laboratory was 46.3 ml/kg·min. According to the diagram of FIGURE 2 his estimated time would have been 262 minutes if he had averaged an expenditure of 70% of his maximal aerobic capacity. The subsequent clinical history of this remarkable patient is noteworthy. He continued to maintain his training program. However, during a 6-week period in February and March of 1971 he experienced five episodes of Stokes-Adams syndrome with complete loss of consciousness and required emergency treatment. Electrocardiograms on various occasions documented ventricular tachycardia and atrial fibrillation with a very rapid ventricular rate. Coronary arteriograms revealed left ventricular pressure 128/14 mmHg, complete occlusion of the proximal third of the right coronary artery, 90% stenosis of the proximal third of the left anterior descending coronary artery, 30% stenosis of the left circumflex artery, abundant collateral flow to the distal right coronary artery; enlargement and impaired contractility of the left ventricle, moderately severe. Stated otherwise, his entire circulation was based upon flow through the left circumflex artery, itself narrowed by 30%. This patient has continued to run long distances, and has logged 18,000 miles from 1970 to October 1976.

This experience demonstrated the potential hazard of severe arrhythmias occurring *during* a marathon run, at which time immediate resuscitative efforts might not be available. For this reason, and because of the lack of substantial proof of the medical value of such athletic virtuosity, I have subsequently discouraged other similarly trained coronary men from marathon running. The time to complete the marathon race by the five coronary subjects studied by Dr. Dressendorfer similarly could be predicted with remarkable precision.[28] According to the diagram modified after Margaria (FIGURE 1), with a $\dot{V}_{O_2 max}$ of 41.3 ml/kg·min., and assuming 70% of max capacity was used, the race time would be approximately 300 minutes, more than 289 and less than 307 minutes.

Recapitulation. Of 1000 subjects discharged from a CMU, five to seven potentially have the capacity to attain a $\dot{V}_{O_2 max}$ sufficient to complete, if motivated, a marathon run in 5 hours or less. Obviously marathon running can not be applied in the rehabilitation of a significant number of coronary patients.

Influence of Severity of the Disease. The aerobic capacity decreases with the severity of the underlying lesions in the coronary arteries and the extent of myocardial involvement.[9, 24] Even more important than adherence to a training program was the severity of the anatomic involvement of the coronary arteries and myocardium. In the previously cited study of 55 men with occlusive coronary disease, the $\dot{V}_{O_2 max}$ after training varied directly with the coronary score (5, complete occlusion; 4, 75% to 99% stenosis; 3, 50% to 75% stenosis).[8] The subjects with coronary score of 8.3, 9.7, and 11.9 attained a $\dot{V}_{O_2 max}$ of 33.5, 30.3, and 25.5 ml/kg·min, respectively.[9]

HAZARDS OF HIGH-LEVEL-ACTIVITY-INDUCED CARDIAC ARREST THAT IS REVERSIBLE

The risk and reversibility of "mechanism death," mainly ventricular fibrillation and cardiac arrest, at rest and associated with high levels of physical activity have been amply documented.[29, 30] The reversibility of mechanism death mandates the availability of cardiopulmonary resuscitation equipment and personnel in the *immediate* vicinity of known coronary patients and normal subjects with occult or undiagnosed coronary or other heart disease (cardiomyopathy, myocarditis, etc.). The need for immediate resuscitative equipment is highlighted by the fact that over 60% of coronary patients who die do so before they can get to the hospital. Many of these deaths have been shown to be reversible if effective CPR measures are instituted immediately. The tragic death of a 1976 marathoner in whom CPR was unsuccessful,[31] and of a veteran marathoner with previously undiagnosed stenosis of the left anterior descending coronary artery, for whom CPR was *not* applied, highlights the need for such emergency care for normals and cardiacs. The ready availability of CPR in the Seattle Heart Watch Program accounts for their success.[30] The danger of cardiac arrest is particularly great in coronary patients. In our experience approximately 9% of coronary subjects entered into our training program had experienced ventricular fibrillation, cardiac arrest or complete AV block in the onset of their myocardial infarct. Follow-up data from the Framingham study indicates that approximately 30% of patients who have been successfully resuscitated in the early phase of their infarct have the expectation of recurrence of such complex and fatal arrhythmias within the subsequent year. Thus, the coronary patient who enters into a long distance training exercise program is at high risk of developing ventricular arrhythmias.

Because of the hazards of sudden death, coronary patients and individuals with suspected occult coronary disease and/or with several risk factors should be advised, in my opinion, to run only in an environment where resuscitative equipment and personnel are immediately available. On no occasion should they run alone or with groups of people in an unsupervised, unmonitored environment.

Other potential hazards that may be lethal for the coronary patient include the competition that is engendered by running in a group and the adverse effects of environment, particularly humidity and high temperatures, which can change blood viscosity and be particularly lethal by producing heat stroke. Other important complications of running by older subjects may involve the skeletal musculature and central nervous systems.

In addition, coronary patients with an average age of 60 years cannot be expected, except under unusual circumstances, to complete a marathon in less than 5 hours. The heroic legendary DeMar completed the marathon at the age of 66 years.[32] This is a remarkable feat and implies that his maximal aerobic capacity was at least 42 ml/kg·min. Older champion athletes in the age range of coronary patients have attained remarkable $\dot{V}_{O_2 max}$, but their potential marathon time can be estimated to be 3 or more hours. In a recent report older champion track athletes at an age of 45 years had an average $\dot{V}_{O_2 max}$ of 57.5; age 55 years, 54.4; and age 65 years, 51.4 ml/kg·min, indicating the potential marathon time (using 70% of maximal aerobic capacity), of 199, 218, and 230 minutes, respectively.[33]

OTHER COMMENTS

As yet, no substantial data have been accumulated prospectively to indicate that the high levels of $\dot{V}_{O_2 max}$ required for marathon running can be attained by a significant number of coronary patients. In addition, there is no evidence that marathon running provides immunity to development of or to the progression of coronary artery disease already present, as documented by coronary arteriography.

Although the quality of life, (vigor, enthusiasm, and cardiovascular improvement with leg exercise) can be enhanced by marathon running of a few cardiac subjects, as yet there is no evidence in prospective studies that the "quantity" (longevity) is similarly enhanced.

The question as to whether physical conditioning of lesser intensity prolongs life as well as increasing the quality of living may be answered by the ongoing multicentered National Exercise and Heart Disease Project in which subjects are randomized into control and long-term exercise groups with prescribed and supervised exercise.[34]

SUMMARY

Prescribed, supervised exercise training has proved valuable in the rehabilitation of selected coronary patients. However, long distance (marathon) running has limited cardiovascular value in the rehabilitation of patients for a majority of occupations, which involve predominantly upper extremity effort. The age of patients with coronary heart disease and the severity of the lesions preclude the wide application of marathon running to the general coronary heart disease population. Less than 6/1000 subjects with coronary heart disease have been estimated as potentially being able to achieve by high-level training a maximum $\dot{V}_{O_2}$ sufficient to complete a marathon race in 5 hours. The hazards of high-level-activity-induced cardiac arrest that is reversible mandates the availability of CPR equipment and personnel in the *immediate* vicinity of all coronary patients and most coronary-prone patients who are undertaking such heroic activity.

Over-publicized marathon running by a few subjects has aroused unrealistic expectations for the majority of coronary heart disease subjects and probably similarly for a considerable number of coronary-prone subjects, many of whom have "silent" coronary disease.

REFERENCES

1. HELLERSTEIN, H. K. & A. B. FORD. 1957. J. Amer. Med. Assoc. **164:** 225–231.
2. HELLERSTEIN, H. K., E. Z. HIRSCH, W. CUMLER, L. ALLEN, S. POLSTER & N. ZUCKER. 1963. *In* Coronary Heart Disease. Likoff, W. & J. H. Moyer, Eds. : 448–454. Grune & Stratton. New York, N.Y.
3. HELLERSTEIN, H. K. 1968. Bull. N.Y. Acad. Med. **44:** 1028–1047.
4. HIRSCH, E. Z., H. K. HELLERSTEIN & C. A. MACLEOD. 1972. *In* Exercise & the Heart. R. L. MORSE, Ed. : 106–187. Charles C Thomas, Publisher. Springfield, Ill.
5. NAUGHTON, J. P. & H. K. HELLERSTEIN, Eds. 1973. Exercise Testing & Exercise Training in Coronary Heart Disease. Chapters **10:** 129–168; **16:** 253–262; **29:** 421–426. Academic Press. New York, N.Y.
6. ERIKSSEN, J. 1976. Circulation **54:** 371–376.
7. FROELICHER, V. F., JR., A. J. THOMPSON, M. R. LONGO, J. H. TRIEBWASSER & M. C. LANCASTER. 1976. Prog. Cardiovasc. Dis. **18:** 265–276.
8. HELLERSTEIN, H. K., E. Z. HIRSCH, R. ADLER, N. GREENBLOTT & M. SIEGEL. 1973. *In* Exercise Testing & Exercise Training in Coronary Heart Disease. J. P. Naughton & H. K. Hellerstein, Eds. Chap. **10:** 129–167. Academic Press. New York, N.Y.
9. HELLERSTEIN, H. K. 1972. Das Chronisch Kranke Herz. H. Roskamm & H. Reindell, Eds. Section **4:** 513–520. F. K. Schattauer. Verlag-Stuttgard. New York, N.Y.

10. KAVANAGH, T. 1976. This volume.
11. CLAUSEN, J. P., J. TRAP-JENSEN & N. A. LASSEN. 1970. Scand. J. Clin. Lab. Invest. **26:** 295–301.
12. HOLLOSZY, J. O. 1975. Med. Sci. Sports **7:** 155–164.
13. DETRY, J., M. ROUSSEAU, G. VANDENBROUCKE, F. KUSUMI, L. A. BRASSEUR & R. A. BRUCE. 1971. Circulation **44:** 109–118.
14. SCHEUER, J. 1973. Circulation **47:** 677–680.
15. HELLERSTEIN, H. K. Unpublished observations.
16. LEWIS, R. P., H. BOUDOULAS, T. G. WELCH & W. F. FORESTER. 1976. Amer. J. Cardiol. **37:** 787–796.
17. RIDGE, B. R. 1976. Med. Sci. Sports **8:** 18–22.
18. FORD, A. B. & H. K. HELLERSTEIN. 1958. Circulation **18:** 823–832.
19. FORD, A. B., H. K. HELLERSTEIN & D. J. TURELL 1959. Circulation **20:** 537–548.
20. HELLERSTEIN, H. K. & A. B. FORD. 1959. *In* Work and the Heart. F. F. Rosenbaum & E. L. Belknap, Eds. Chap. **14:** 122–131. Hoeber. New York, N.Y.
21. HELLERSTEIN, H. K. 1976. Physician Sports Med. **4:** 58–62.
22. FARDY, P. S., D. WEBB & H. K. HELLERSTEIN. 1976. In press.
23. ROBINSON, S. 1938. Arbeitsphysiologie **10:** 251–323.
24. BRUCE, R. A. 1973. *In* Exercise Testing & Exercise Training in Coronary Heart Disease. J. P. Naughton & H. K. Hellerstein, Eds. Chapt. **4:** 45–59. Academic Press. New York, N.Y.
25. MARGARIA, R., P. CERRETELLI, P. AGHEMO & G. SASSI. 1963. J. Applied Physiol. **18:** 367–370.
26. ÅSTRAND, P. O. 1963. J. Applied Physiol. **18:** 619–622.
27. FRICK, M. H. 1968. Amer. J. Cardiol. **22:** 417–425.
28. DRESSENDORFER, R. H. 1976. Ann. N.Y. Acad. Sci. This volume.
29. BECK, C. S., W. H. PRITCHARD & H. S. FEIL. 1947. J. Amer. Med. Assoc. **135:** 985–986.
30. BRUCE, R. & W. KLUGE. 1971. J. Amer. Med. Assoc. **216:** 653–658.
31. GREEN, L. H., I. C. STAFFORD & G. KURLAND. 1976. Ann. Intern. Med. **84:** 704–706.
32. CURRENS, J. H. & P. D. WHITE. 1961. N. Eng. J. Med. **265:** 988–993.
33. POLLOCK, M. L., H. S. MILLER, JR. & J. WILMORE. 1974. J. Gerontol. **29:** 645–649.
34. The National Exercise & Heart Disease Project Common Protocol. 1975. The Coordinating Center. The George Washington University Med. Center. Washington, D.C.

EFFECTS OF EXERCISE TRAINING ON PROGRESSION OF DOCUMENTED CORONARY ARTERIOSCLEROSIS IN MEN *

R. Selvester, J. Camp and M. Sanmarco

Rancho Los Amigos Hospital
Downey, California 90242

INTRODUCTION

In the hierarchy of coronary risk factors in the various prospective studies [1-7] a sedentary overweight subject had an increased risk ratio ranging from 1.0 to 1.5. These studies had been done by occupational stratification into sedentary, active, strenuous, and very strenuous levels. A number of studies have been attempted in primary prevention of coronary artery disease (CAD) by multiple risk factor intervention trials, and definitive results are yet to be published. A number of secondary prevention trials are under way and have shown a consistent reduction in mortality from recurrent infarction in the active, exercising, fit subjects when compared to less active controls and a less certain change in the incidence of new coronary events.[8, 9]

We have been doing serial angiograms in a group of patients with angina and/or a prior myocardial infarct. This has the distinct advantage over epidemiological studies of looking at the target organ (the coronary arteries) directly instead of the more indirect endpoints of new events, documented infarction or mortality, which are the secondary effects on the end organ. It has the disadvantage that the target population being studied is not the apparently well population but the patient who has already suffered some direct consequence of serious disease. Thus, the study can be related directly only to this diseased subset of the whole population.

All subjects were given a baseline battery of noninvasive and biochemical studies including fasting and 2-hour-postprandial blood sugar and serum lipids tests, PA and lateral chest X rays, high-fidelity, high-gain ECG/VCG, exercise stress tests, and routine history and physical examinations. These were repeated at 3 to 6-month intervals to objectify change. Selective coronary angiograms and biplane ventriculograms were done on entry to the protocol and were repeated usually within 18 months.

After initial work-up, as many as would accept it were entered into an outpatient program of progressive exercise and risk factor reduction. In the initial phase a level of exercise was chosen that would not necessarily produce a physical conditioning effect, i.e., general physical activity such as walking, calisthenics, group games, and so forth. This activity was progressively increased to high levels (70% of predicted maximal or more) over several weeks.

Weekly education classes were conducted in the physiology of exercise and the anatomy and physiology of coronary disease with class and individual counseling on weight reduction, low-cholesterol, low-saturated-fat diet, smoking, and blood pressure control. Individual and group sessions were maintained for

* This work was supported in part by Grants HL–14138–05/S1 and NIH 5 501 HL 13524–05 from the National Institutes of Health.

support of and exploration of emotional, family, sexual, and social adjustment problems.

From these data the question can thus be asked, does adherence to a strict protocol of exercise, no smoking, low cholesterol diet, and good blood pressure control influence the rate of progression of atherosclerotic lesions in serial coronary angiograms? Since biplane ventriculograms were recorded on all, the question can also be explored, does good adherence to the protocol decrease the incidence or extent of new infarctions as measured by regional wall motion studies, and by serial high-fidelity ECG and VCG? In regard to the possible protective effect of exercise in this group of patients, the following hypotheses are subject to direct test by these data:

   (1) Active exercise increases collateral in the heart, especially in areas made ischemic by high-grade occlusive coronary artery disease, and if atherosclerosis continues to progress:

      (a) Progression to total occlusion should be associated with a decreased incidence of clinical coronary events in the active subjects as compared to the inactive.

      (b) Ventriculograms in such patients should show less deterioration of ventricular function in follow-up angiograms.

      (c) ECG/VCGs should show a decreased incidence of "new events."

   (2) Active exercise retards atheroma production, and the incidence of clear-cut progression in coronary angiograms is decreased.

The same outcome variables can be tested independently for how they have been affected by the various risk factor interventions such as weight loss, decreased serum cholesterol, cessation of smoking, and blood pressure.

METHODS

A total of 104 test subjects who had repeat angiograms at a mean interval of 20 months are the basis of this report. Of these, 56 came as part of a larger group that responded to media and newspaper stories about the Rancho Cardiac Rehabilitation program and an invitation to participate in ongoing studies of secondary prevention of coronary atherosclerosis. All had had a previous myocardial infarct and were, in general, asymptomatic; 48 were subjects with angina pectoris with and without prior infarction. All had agreed with informed consent on initial interview to repeat angiograms and to join ongoing studies of risk factor reduction and/or revascularization surgery.

Initial work-up consisted of high-gain, high-fidelity 12-lead ECG and Cube and McFee VCG, PA and lateral chest X-rays, a history and physical examination with special attention to family history and risk factors, an exercise stress test (treadmill) with a modified Bruce protocol and a submaximal 85% endpoint, and a fasting and 2-hour-postprandial blood sugar and lipid profile including serum cholesterol, total lipids and triglycerides. Also, right and left heart pressures and cardiac output, before and after contrast material were recorded routinely. Ventriculograms were recorded in right and left anterior oblique projections. Left ventricular volumes and ejection fractions were calculated by the method of Sandler and Dodge, as modified by Sanmarco. Selective cine coronary angiograms were recorded on 35-mm film using the Judkins technique and were recorded in at least five projections in the left coronary artery and three in the right. Patients with left main disease, i.e., 70% or more obstruction, were advised urgent surgery as were those with left main equivalent (FIGURE 1), which is defined as 70% narrowing of the left anterior descending *and* the circumflex at their take off before any branches. Operated patients are not included in this report.

All films were reviewed by two experienced angiographers independently. Drawings were made of the right and left coronary artery and its branches in RAO and LAO projections. Location and extent of narrowing was marked on each drawing. Each local obstructive coronary lesion was graded as to the percent of narrowing of cross sectional area deemed to be present. Differences of less than 10% were considered insignificant differences and the average of the two numbers was used in the analysis (85% of all identified lesions fell into this category). Differences in readings of more than 10% narrowing were

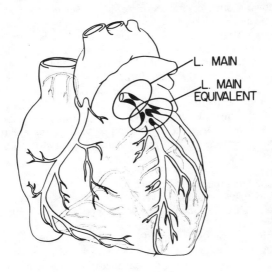

FIGURE 1. Diagram of the heart showing left main disease and left main equivalent disease in the left main coronary artery.

resolved by a conference between the two primary reviewers. Five sets of films where one set or the other was deemed unsatisfactory in technical quality for adequate comparison were rejected. For the purpose of the analysis of this report, an increase of 30% or more, or progression to total occlusion as a consensus reading was considered as true progression.

RISK FACTOR REDUCTION PROGRAM

All subjects were offered the program of progressive exercise and risk factor reduction described above. Safety precautions included telemetry and blood pressure monitoring as needed. This need was usually identified in the original stress test and work-up. A cardiologist was in the area but not necessarily in attendance at each exercise session.

When the target heart rate had been established and the supplementary information gathered, the patient was given an initial exercise prescription by the physician and physical therapist with team inputs, and begun on an exercise program. The initial exercise periods were used to establish the proper intensity of exercise. This process is best described as a series of trial periods beginning at low levels of stress. The patient and physical therapist constantly monitor for signs of poor adaptability to the exercise stress. Telemetry of ECG is used along with the noting of heart rate, blood pressure, angina, and dyspnea. Walking was used most often as the initial type of exercise, but other activities such as riding a stationary bicycle and treadmill were also used. As a general rule, the period of walking is set at five intervals. Prior to exercise intervals, a brief period of calisthenics was undertaken to assist in warm up and prevention of musculoskeletal complications. Each interval is separated by 30-second to 1-minute periods to check pulses and the intervals are organized into a warm-up, peak, cool-down sequence. For example, a typical sequence of intervals would be 2, 5, 15, 5, and 2 minutes. This provides a progressive warm-up and cool-down period allowing adequate opportunity for patients with impaired cardiovascular function to adapt to increasing and decreasing work demands. The middle interval (stress interval) is used for increasing the exercise stress. The heart rate should reach target rate during the stress (middle) interval. At the end of the last interval (cool-down) the heart rate should approximate the heart rate at the end of the initial pre-warm-up interval. If the patient has no trouble accomplishing this, the intervals are adjusted to provide more stress until the intermediate target heart rate and/or symptoms are reached.

There are three basic ways to manipulate the intervals to reach the protocol target levels of exercise:

(1) By changing the target heart rate.
(2) By changing the length of time or distance for any one interval, and/or
(3) By changing the pace (speed) at which the patient walks.

The number of intervals and the length or distance of each interval is determined by the physical therapist. The target heart rate in this initial phase is determined by physician and physical therapist. The patient is instructed to alter his pace within each interval in order to effect a pulse change and reach his target rate.

Progressing the Patient

Initially when the patient's exercise tolerance is low, many intervals of short duration and comfortable pace are used. With improvement, the number of intervals is decreased and the duration of intervals and pace increased. This flexibility allows the program to be held to a reasonable length of time. For example, an initial sequence would be 2, 5, 15, 5, and 2 minutes at a slow pace. A more advanced one would be 2, 5, 30, 5, and 2 minutes at a fast pace.

When the patient's heart rate at the stress interval is lower than target rate, he has physiologically accommodated to the exercise stress and his program requires upward adjustment. Using this method of progression, the exercise program is continually adjusted to provide increasing stress in accordance with the patient's exercise tolerance, and/or his study protocol category.

Patient Grouping by Average Level of Exercise

Patients in this study group who had a second angiogram were classified into each of four groups based on an assessment of their exercise diary, a personal interview by a physical therapist, and an evaluation of exercise tolerance testing. The goal here is to classify patients by their average level of training in the interval between angiograms.

Group 1 (Inactive): No regular recreational or planned exercise.

Group 2 (Low level): Habitually exercised some each week, in general below 50% of predicted maximum (at a pulse rate of >110, only occasionally to levels approaching 70% of predicted maximum).

Group 3 (Moderate): Exercised an average of one to two times per week for 20 to 30 minutes to 60% to 70% or more of predicted maximum at a pulse rate of 120 to 130, or sporadically to 75% or more. Consistently exercised more actively than the low level group described above, they were usually targeted for Group 4 training levels (below) but only achieved these levels intermittently.

Group 4 (Trained): Exercised at least three times a week for at least 30 minutes to 70% or more of predicted maximum. Pulse 135 to 150.

RESULTS

Self-selection at the onset was clearly apparent. Although a randomized protocol was attempted, some subjects refused to join the classes for instruction and programmed activity, but did come back in for repeat catheterization and provided a reference or control group, having experienced no significant change in life-style or in any of the intervention variables. Others made half-hearted attempts at adherence to the protocol, but in spite of intense team efforts to maintain adherence, made only minor changes in the intervention variables. Others would become exercise enthusiasts but refused to change their dietary habits and made only minor changes in their smoking. Still others stopped smoking completely while being only modestly interested in diet change or exercise, and so forth, and so forth. Upon review of the data, it was seen that the scatter of adherence to each of the intervention variables was such that it seems reasonable for the purposes of this report to assume, that, in fact, self-selection was the primary operant control in spite of rigorous team attempts to gain adherence to the randomization protocol.

There were more heavy smokers with less severe coronary disease in subjects who remained noncompliers to exercise than there were in those who became reasonably good compliers to fitness levels of endurance exercise training. Other risk factors were scattered across groups without significant differences in these variables between groups.

Age and Progression of Coronary Disease

The age profile is shown in FIGURE 2 for the 104 test subjects with a record of progression. As reported previously [10] there was, in the asymptomatic younger group (under 50 years), a much more rapid progression in patients who had overt CAD documented before 45 years of age. These data are con-

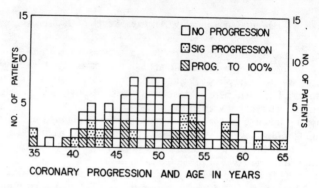

FIGURE 2. Age profile of 104 test subjects with progressive coronary disease.

sistent with the hypothesis that the younger one is when he develops angina and/or documented myocardial infarction, the more likely he is to show progression of the disease in his coronary arteries. In the group with early onset of infarction, this probability is highly significant ($p < 0.001$).[10]

Number of Progressible Coronary Artery Lesions and Progression

Since vessels with minor lesions were only rarely noted to progress and since vessels with 100% occlusions were also not seen to progress, it seems useful to look at two additional notions:

(1) "Progressible" vessels, i.e., major coronary arteries with 50% or more, but less than 100% narrowing visible on initial angiogram, and

(2) Critical lesions, i.e., vessels with 75% or more narrowing.

Of the 104 subjects, 18 patients had no progressible vessels on their initial angiograms by this definition (FIGURE 3) and only two of which showed a change in any vessel of their follow-up angiogram and both of these occurred after 4 years; 33 had one progressible vessel, 13 (39%) of which showed significant progression, 6 (18%) to complete occlusion; 42 patients had two progressible vessels of whom 27 (64%) showed progression in one or more of these diseased vessels on the second angiogram, 17 (40%) of the 27 having gone on to total occlusion in at least one vessel. The remaining 11 patients had three progressible vessels each and 8 (66%) went on to progress, 5 of which to total occlusion in at least one vessel. Of the original 104 patients surviving to and agreeing to a repeat angiogram, 86 had one or more progressible vessels for a total of 149 vessels at risk; 51 (34%) of these vessels showed progression at follow-up angiogram, and of these, 29 vessels (19%) had gone on to total occlusion. Of these 29 vessels, 24 (16%) had associated visible new myocardial damage on follow-up angiograms and 15 had been related to a known "clinical infarct"; 9 therefore were related to a "silent infarct."

The average follow-up period was 20 months, and, based on these data, the average risk of significant progression is 20% per year per vessel at risk and the risk of total occlusion is 12% per year per vessel at risk. There is a 10% chance per year per vessel at risk of having significant new myocardial damage associated with this occlusion, and a 6% chance per year per vessel at risk of a new "clinical infarct." One would project therefore a mortality of approximately 6% per year per vessel at risk as well in this group of patients at high risk of progression. This possibility is the subject of a natural history study underway at this institution at the present time.

"Critical" Coronary Narrowing and Progression

Lesions greater than 75% of the lumenal area but less than 100% were defined as "critical." It would seem reasonable to assume that these high-grade lesions would progress to total occlusion at a more rapid rate than lesser degrees of "progressible" vessels. This hypothesis was tested by comparing the number with various degrees of narrowing that went on to total occlusion. There was indeed further concentration of the risk of total occlusion in this group. The risk of total occlusion and new infarct was four times as high in the 92 vessels with greater than 75% narrowing as it was in the 57 vessels with progressible lesions but with lumenal narrowing to 50% to 70%.

The risk of death in these two groups is also considered from other data to approximate that of clinical infarct but these data do not speak directly to this point, since these studied patients are survivors.

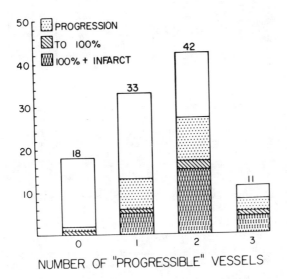

FIGURE 3. Of 104 subjects, 18 patients had one or more totally occluded vessels and insignificant disease in the other vessels and thus no "progressible" vessels, 11 patients had three progressible vessels, with significant but subtotal occlusion. Clearly the rate of progression in serial angiograms is a function of how many progressible vessels are present.

Exercise Training and Coronary Artery Disease Progression

The goal of the progressive exercise program was to attain a true training effect as measured by improved exercise test performance and improved muscle efficiency. The number of hours per week of exercise and the level of that exercise was assessed by an exercise diary and an interview by the physical therapists. Patients were divided into four categories based on level of exercise as described above. The level of exercise habitually observed during the interval between angiograms ranged from none to high levels of fitness and endurance training. Nine (8%) of the subjects attained the latter levels; 20 subjects (19%) were actively attempting fitness training but complied less than 100%, achieving a moderate level of fitness training; 39 more subjects were considered

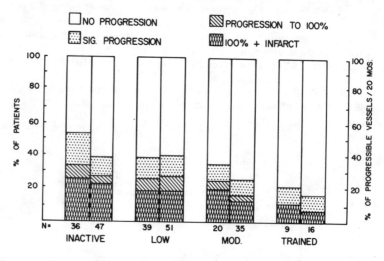

FIGURE 4. Exercise activity and progression. The left hand set of bar graphs shows coronary progression rate related to average activity level between angiograms in 104 patients. The right hand bars normalize the data in each subset to the percentage of progressible vessels and the mean follow-up period for the whole group of 20.0 months.

to be working at a low level of exercise that would not produce a training or fitness effect; and 36 (35%) were totally sedentary in the study interval. The average activity level was related to the presence or absence of coronary progression in serial coronary angiograms and to the degree of progression and/or infarction seen in biplane ventriculograms. These results are shown in FIGURES 4, 5, and 6. These data show that increased exercise, especially to fitness levels, is associated with a decreased incidence of progression of atherosclerosis in coronary arteries, 21 of 47 (45%) in inactive as compared to three of 16 (19%) for high-level training subjects, ($p < 0.06$). When one combines the moderate and trained subjects into one group and the inactive low level into another, and compares the incidence of progression, the more active patients have less progression (11 of 51 vessels; 22%) as compared to 40 of 98 (41%)

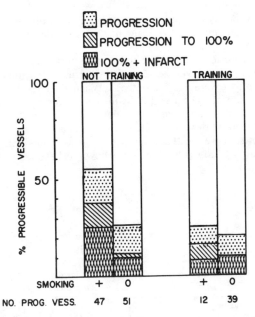

FIGURE 5. The effects of smoking and/or training on the progression of coronary artery disease. Smokers are represented by left bars; nonsmokers by right bars.

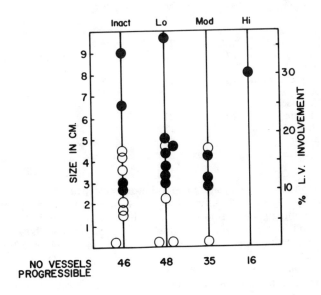

FIGURE 6. Activity level and infarct size. Open circles are total occlusions without clinical infarct. There were nine patients with visible new infarcts on their ventriculogram, i.e., "silent infarct." Closed circles total occlusions with clinical infarct.

for the low-level inactive group. This difference is significant (p < 0.02). No differences were identified in the incidence of total occlusion or new infarct between these two groups.

However, as described above, the follow-up interval was longer in the inactive and low-level group (average 21 months) than in the moderate and high-level activity group (average 17 months). When one normalizes each to the expected progression at the mean follow-up period for the whole group of 20 months, the level of significance falls below the 0.05 level (p < 0.06). The incidence of smokers as described below was twice as high in the sedentary and low level groups as it was in the patients exercising at moderate or high levels of endurance training. Since smoking was shown to have a significant effect on

TABLE 1

PROGRESSION OF CORONARY ARTERY DISEASE: EFFECT OF EXERCISE
TRAINING PROGRAM

	Activity Level				
	Inactive (n=36)	Low (n=20)	Moderate (n=20)	High (n=9)	Total Average (n=104)
Average interval between angiogram in months	23.7	18.5	17.2	16.8	20.0
Progressible Vessels	47	51	35	16	149
Prog. vessels per patient	1.31	1.31	1.75	1.78	1.43
Vessels with progression	21	19	8	3	51
	45%	37%	23%	19%	34%
Vessels with progression, normalized to 20 months	18	20	9	3	50
	38%	39%	26%	19%	34%
Progressible vessels in smokers	27	20	11	1	60
Vessels with progression in smokers	15	11	3	0	29
	56%	55%	25%		48%
Progressible vessels in nonsmokers	20	31	24	15	89
Vessels with progression in nonsmokers	6	8	5	3	22
	30%	26%	22%	20%	25%

progression in the sedentary and low-level groups independent of exercise levels, the possibility exists that the effect shown here between these groups of training versus nontraining patients is in fact due to the difference seen in their smoking. FIGURE 5 and TABLE 1, which tabulate progressible vessels, show that in the nonsmokers, the rate of progression was higher (14 of 51 or 27%) in the sedentary, low-level group than it was in training patients (8 of 39 or 21%). While this would give an increased risk ratio of 1.3 for sedentary nonsmoking subjects, these differences are not significant. In the smokers the rate of progression was even greater in nontraining (sedentary or low-level activity) patients, occurring in 26 of 47 (55%) of vessels than it was in the training subjects where three of 12 (25%) progressed (p < 0.05). This gives an increased risk in sedentary smokers of 2.2, suggesting that endurance training levels of exercise may exert an independent protective effect against coronary progression.

Regarding the possibility that habitually active persons, particularly those who exercised to fitness levels of endurance training, would increase coronary collateral and decrease the incidence or the size of recurrent infarction, we examined the data to see if this had occurred. The incidence of the new ECG/VCG changes and the extent of these changes were compared in the four groups: sedentary nonactive, low-level active, moderately active, and athletically trained subjects. Biplane ventriculograms were also examined in each group. The incidence of visible new infarct in each group and the size of the new infarct was examined (FIGURE 6). The incidence of new clinical coronary episodes in each group was recorded. A high-gain, high-fidelity ECG showed significant infarct changes in 25 of 104 subjects, and the biplane ventriculograms showed a significant new infarct in 24, with one of these showing two new infarcts. Overt clinical infarct was documented in 15 patients; one of these had had two clinical infarcts. These numbers are too small to establish a statistical significance but show that when stratified into four groups according to activity, there is the same percentage decrease of new clinical episodes or documented new infarcts in the active subjects (FIGURES 4, 5 & 6). One large infarct, however, has been observed in the trained subjects and subtotal coronary progression has been seen in two of the nine subjects. There was no significant difference between groups in the size of these infarcts.

Smoking and Coronary Artery Disease Progression

Some 60 of the 104 subjects (58%) were nonsmokers before the onset of overt coronary artery disease or became nonsmokers after they had sustained a documented infarct and/or clinically typical anginal syndrome and joined the study. There were, therefore, 44 of 104 (42%) who continued to smoke. The progression rate was two times as high in those who continued to smoke even if they had decreased their cigarette consumption. Specifically, those patients who continue to smoke show a 60% incidence overall of significant progression in their coronary arteries as compared to a 32% for those who were nonsmokers ($p < 0.004$ by the Fisher exact test). No difference was seen between decreased cigarette (light smoking) and continued heavy smoking.

It was noted that the incidence of smoking was higher (36 of 75 or 48%) in the sedentary and low-level activity groups than it was in the patients who maintained moderate or high levels of endurance training (seven of 29 or 24%) in the interval between angiograms. The possibility therefore exists that all or part of the increase in progression in the smokers was attributable to the fact that more smokers were also sedentary. These comparisons are shown in FIGURE 5 and tabulated as progressible vessels in TABLE 1. In the 47 progressible vessels occurring in the low-level and inactive smokers, 26 (55%) showed significant progression while only 14 of 51 (27%) of such vessels in low-level inactive nonsmokers showed this degree of progression. This difference was significant ($p < 0.05$ by Fisher exact test). However, in the 51 progressible vessels in patients who were participating in moderate to high levels of endurance training, the rate of progression was similar in smokers (three of 12 or 25%) as it was in nonsmokers (eight of 39 or 21%). These differences are not significant. Thus, the probability exists that endurance training decreased the risk in smokers.

Diet, Serum Cholesterol, and Coronary Artery Disease Progression

Average cholesterol levels over the interval between angiograms was measured; dietary compliance as evaluated by a diet diary and interview, and changes in cholesterol levels were examined as related to progression of coronary disease. The average cholesterol between angiograms was related to the angiogram and coronary progression in an inverse way but the correlation was low and will be the subject of a separate report.

Blood Pressure and Coronary Artery Disease Progression

Systolic and diastolic pressures at rest and at peak of exercise were examined by treadmill stress testing at serial intervals, usually every 3 months between angiograms. The best discriminator appears to be the resting diastolic pressure with the patient standing quietly before the start of the exercise test. The lower resting diastolic blood pressures seem to be associated with a lowered incidence of progression, even in patients that are normotensive at rest. That is, the higher the resting diastolic pressure on the initial or subsequent examinations, the higher the probability of progression. These data were not analyzed in detail for this report, but are being reported elsewhere.

DISCUSSION

The major question of relevance to this symposium relates to the effects of endurance training and the risk of progression of coronary artery disease. Any postinfarction training program is a combined program and fitness training, diet, weight reduction, and cessation of smoking as a minimum. If the patient trains to fitness levels of conditioning, the risk of progression is independently reduced by a factor of 1.7; if he is a nonsmoker or stops smoking, the risk of progression is decreased by a factor of 2; and the lower his resting diastolic blood pressure is, the less likely is progression. It is clear from these data that the younger he is when overt coronary artery disease appears, the more likely he is to progress on serial angiograms. The more extensive the disease is, as identified on initial angiograms, the more likely it is to progress. It is not clear whether the malignant form of the disease seen in younger subjects is a product of their personality type and habitual stress levels (94% of these interviewed by the Friedman-Rosenman Interview and by the Jenken questionnaire were type A) or is constitutional. Both of these possibilities are being explored by a retrospective interview and by detailed family profiles. The data to date do not discriminate these possibilities and will be reported subsequently.

It may be inappropriate to generalize from this study group to patients with recent onset coronary artery disease because of the self-selection problems mentioned earlier. It is even less appropriate to generalize to the population at large. Nonetheless, a few tentative observations seem warranted. In the secondary prevention of recurrent infarction, these studies suggest that the control of smoking is perhaps the most important risk factor and that diet, cholesterol levels, blood pressure and fitness training programs assume a somewhat more secondary role in the prevention of the disastrous progression of coronary artery disease. *These data also suggest that exercise training programs, to be effective, should aim at true fitness levels of endurance training.*

The major impact of postcoronary rehabilitation programs may indeed be that due to the multipronged attack at the reducible risk factors. No small effect in this group has been the change in self-esteem, self-image and self-confidence induced by the successful accomplishment of the goals of fitness, weight reduction, cessation of smoking, control of resting or exercise hypertension. It is also clear from the data presented here that the more accurately one knows the coronary and ventricular anatomy, the more accurately one can prognosticate the risk of progression and subsequent morbidity and mortality. This information is also of paramount importance in assessing the cardiac functional reserve and expected physical exercise capacity.

Epidemiology studies of risk factors and coronary disease, as well as primary intervention trials, require large numbers of subjects followed for long periods of time to establish significance of results, and hence, are time-consuming and expensive. This is because the incidence rate is low and the end points used for evidence of change in the atherosclerotic process is that of end-organ damage, i.e., strokes, new coronary events, documented myocardial infarcts, major ECG change and death. Secondary prevention trials that do not include coronary angiography and coronary change as a measured variable have a similar problem. In this instance the incidence of the disease is high because of starting with population that has evidence of atherosclerotic disease. The attack rate of "clinical infarct," however, is 8% per year as compared to an attack rate of 15% per year for total occlusion and an attack of 24% per year for significant progression of arterial occlusive disease. It is noteworthy that in this and other series the Proband group defined as having a documented recent myocardial infarct have 10% of subjects with no documentable coronary occlusive disease on coronary angiography. If not excluded, these subjects would further dilute the sample.

Since the smaller atherosclerotic lesions in experimental atherosclerosis are more likely to regress, it would seem sensible to give more attention to quantitation of the minor lesions in coronary angiograms, with particular attention to quantitating change. With major changes occurring in 21 months in nearly half of these patients, it is likely that minor changes occurred in smaller lesions and other large lesions in most, if not all, of these patients. Image-processing methods, such as computer reconstruction from multiple angiographic projections of three dimensional vessels with details of lumenal narrowing and irregularities offer real promise of providing this quantitation. Development of such image-processing and image-enhancement techniques would clearly provide the tools required to answer the questions in living man about the efficacy of multiple risk factor reduction, and the relative merit and cost-effectiveness of such interventions. Once such quantitative assessment of the coronary vessels is in hand, it is likely to provide definitive information early regarding atheroma regression/progression and the secondary prevention of new clinical episodes. It should also provide the basis for establishing the relative importance in this patient group of each so-called primary and secondary risk factor.

It is our view that in institutions where the angiographic skills are well developed and the risk to the patient is low, that serial angiograms are the most cost-effective way to follow these patients in secondary prevention trials.

SUMMARY AND CONCLUSIONS

The following are associated with a high risk of rapid progression and/or new myocardial damage in patients with angiographically proven coronary disease, as seen in serial coronary angiograms and biplane ventriculograms: (1) Young age at onset. (2) Severe two- and three-vessel disease with two or more critically narrowed progressible vessels. (3) Cigarette smokers.

The following may have beneficial effects on progression:

(1) Exercise training to endurance fitness levels.
(2) Lowering of serum lipids—less certain.
(3) Lowering of blood pressure—less certain.

REFERENCES

1. KANNEL, W. B., T. R. DAWBER, M. KAGAN, et. al. 1961. Factors of risk in the development of heart disease—Six year follow-up experience. The Framingham study. Ann. Int. Med. **55:** 33–50.
2. KANNEL, W. B., P. SORLIE, P. M. McNAMARA. 1971. The relation of physical activity to the risk of coronary disease: the Framingham study: *In* Coronary Heart Disease and Physical Fitnesss. O. A. Clarksen & A. O. Malmborg, Eds. : 256–272. University Park Press. Baltimore, Md.
3. CHAPMAN, J. M. & F. J. MASSEY. 1964. The inter-relationship of serum cholesterol, hypertension, body weight, and the risk of coronary heart disease: Results of the first ten year follow-up in Los Angeles Heart Study. J. Chronic Dis. **17:** 922–999.
4. EPSTEIN, F. H., L. D. OSTRANDER, B. C. JOHNSON, et al. 1965. Epidemiological studies of cardiovascular disease in a total community—Tecumseh, Michigan. Ann. Int. Med. **62:** 1170–1187.
5. MORRIS, J. N., C. ADAMS, S. P. W. CHAVE, C. SHIREY, L. EPSTEIN & D. J. SHEEHAN. 1973. Vigorous exercise in leisure time and the incidence of coronary heart disease. Lancet **i:** 333–339.
6. PAFFENBARGER, R. S., JR. 1975. Work activity and coronary heart mortality. N. Eng. J. Med. **292:** 545–550.
7. RABKIN, D. E., A. L. MATHEWSON, P. HSU. 1977. Relation of body weight to development of ischemic heart disease in a cohort of young North American men after a 26 year observation period. The Manitobe Study. Amer. J. Cardiol. **39:** 452–458.
8. HELLERSTEIN, H. J., T. R. HORSTEN, A. GOLDBERG, A. G. BURLANDO, E. H. FRIEDMAN, E. Z. HIRSCH & S. MARIK. 1967. The influence of active conditioning upon subjects with coronary artery disease. Can. Med. Assoc. J. **96:** 901–903.
9. BRUNNER, D. & N. MESHULMAN. 1969. Prevention of recurrent myocardial infarction by physical exercise. Israel J. Med. Sci. **5:** 783–785.
10. SANMARCO, M. D., R. H. SELVESTER, S. H. BROOK & D. J. BLAKNSHORFN. 1976. Risk factors reduction and changes in coronary arteriography (Abstract). Circulation **54** (Suppl. II): 140.

DISCUSSION

Herman K. Hellerstein, *Moderator*

School of Medicine
Case Western Reserve University
Cleveland, Ohio 44106

H. K. HELLERSTEIN: The question that we have discussed tonight is the place of marathon running in rehabilitation of cardiacs. Is marathon running practical? Is it feasible? Is it beneficial? What are the evidences to support this view?

Let us start with definitions. Rehabilitation is the process by which a person is returned realistically to his or her optimal physiologic, mental, psychologic, emotional, social, vocational, and economic usefulness, and if employable is provided an opportunity for gainful employment in our competitive industrial world. Rehabilitation also includes efforts to reverse or prevent the progression of the underlying disease process. In this modern sense rehabilitation is not restricted to physiologic rehabilitation alone or to economic rehabilitation, but rather its a complete development of a way of living that will enable the individual to enjoy the fullest physical and mental capacity with due allowances for impairments.

Exercise training and conditioning unequivocally have been shown to have an important role in the rehabilitation of coronary patients. The question then is what is the role of long distance marathon running, which requires higher levels of physical fitness, and can it be applied to patients with clinical coronary disease?

D. JORDAN (*York College, City University, New York, N.Y.*): Dr. Kavanagh, relative to the ST segment changes did you also happen to calculate estimated myocardial oxygen consumption as that's been shown sometimes to reflect some of the ST changes?

T. KAVANAGH (*Toronto Rehabilitation Centre, Toronto, Ont.*): The answer is no.

R. STEINMULLER (*Albert Einstein College of Medicine, The Bronx, N.Y.*): I was surprised that there wasn't a change in the D scale considering how these people looked in the slides. Are there any psychosocial parameters of improved mental functioning in terms of better return to work, improvement in sex life, or other variables that might reflect improvement more than MMPI score?

T. KAVANAGH: Yes. We have done other tests, Cattell, Taylor, and, body image type of tests. These have all shown great improvement. The reason we stay with the MMPI is because our clinical psychologists assure us that this has more validity than the others. He describes some of the others as pen and paper polygames. And I think he has some support from his fellow psychologists in this regard. However, your point is a good one and it may well be that the D score doesn't alter too much because, as some psychologists believe, these scores are inherent and part of the person's personality, and extraneous events don't vary them very much. But I agree with you. We were surprised to find that the D score didn't go up, didn't improve that much. However, it wasn't too bad to start with. They weren't too severely depressed to start with. That may be the reason.

H. K. HELLERSTEIN: Dr. Kavanagh, I would like to interject that in our Cleveland studies on exercise training of cardiacs there was a more significant decrease in the D scale than in the Hs (hypochondriasis) and Hy (hysteria) scales, the so-called neurotic triad.* Such a change implies an improvement in coping capacity since D scale higher than Hs and Hy scales generally means inadequate defenses against depression. In addition, the Pt scale (psychasthenia) scale also shows similar improvement. The cultural and other characteristics may account for the differences in the result of the U.S.A. and Canadian studies.

In reference to the question about psychosocial parameters, very definitely work performance, attitudes toward work and spouse, and also conjugal sexual activity showed favorable changes. R. A. Stein likewise has reported similar improvement, viz., after training there is an increase in the frequency and the quality of conjugal sexual activity.

T. E. KENNEDY (*University of Massachusetts, Amherst, Mass.*): I just have three short questions for you: How long after the original myocardial infarct did they start this training program? What was the progression you used to get them up to be able to run 3 miles? Was there any other negative after effects besides the Achilles tendon strain?

T. KAVANAGH: In regard to the first question, we take patients 8 weeks post-MI. The earliest marathon run in that group was 15 months post-MI. In answer to your second question, we developed a series of training tables. They are available in a book that we have published entitled *Heart Attack, Counter Attack*. It may take up to a year or more to get them to that level. As to the third question about the side effects other than the Achilles tendon, they occur but are surprisingly few. We feel that is so because the level of training is quite low. We believe as many others do in the audience, certainly with these types of patients, in duration rather than intensity. I would rather a man run 5 miles at 12-minute mile pace than try and run 2 miles at an 8-minute mile pace if that's too much for him. We base our starting level on his $\dot{V}_{O_2 \, max}$ predicted from the stress test.

QUESTION: What is the rationale for a maximal stress test both before and after the marathon?

T. KAVANAGH: I think it was really to reassure me. I wanted to be sure that the patient could actually go to physiological maximum as measured by analysis of expired gases flat out before I would let them subject themselves to a situation where not only were they going to be under some degree of physical stress, but for the first time anyway a fair degree of psychological stress. You know what it's like the day of the race, the shouting, the squealing, the gong goes off, the catecholamine surges through the blood. I wanted to be sure that they could take a maximum effort on the treadmill because they would be running of course at less than maximum effort. But the additional factors would have to be allowed for.

QUESTION: Dr. Dressendorfer, I was rather interested in the lack of change

---

* HELLERSTEIN, H. K. & T. R. HORNSTEN, *et al.* 1967. *In* Atherosclerotic Disease, A. M. Brest & J. H. Moyer, Eds. : 115–128. Appleton-Century-Crofts Meredith Publishing Co. New York, N.Y.

in the serum magnesium. We've made some measurements of magnesium loss in the sweat and have found quite substantial amounts of magnesium are being lost that way in a marathan race. I wonder do you think it's coming out of the bone or some other depot in the body?

R. H. DRESSENDORFER (*Pennsylvania State University, University Park Pa.*): Well, I'm not completely happy with the electrolyte results because these blood samples were taken between 5 and 10 minutes after the race and I think a lot happens between zero and 5 minutes.

QUESTION: Dr. Hellerstein, there are a couple of things that I wonder if you could clarify. I don't quite see how the individual that Dr. Kavanagh described who is running 35 to 50 miles a week is somehow getting less exercise or is somehow going to be incapable of doing the arm exercise that a typist or physician requires. It seems to me that this guy is exercising plenty. Another point I had a question about is that is there any reason to think that a post-myocardial-infarct patient who is not in an exercise program should feel any assurance in going to a football game and getting excited or having sexual relations with his wife without a defibrillator at the bedside?

H. K. HELLERSTEIN: First of all sexual activity is the safest thing in the world to do with your own wife. Dr. Ueno in Japan and the study in Cleveland showed that less than three out of 500 nontraumatic sudden cardiac deaths occur in sexual activity. When they do occur, at least in the studies in Japan, they occurred in geisha houses or with other extramarital liaisons.† So be faithful.

In reference to running as the means of rehabilitation, patients with coronary disease and the "shoulder-hand syndrome" or equivalent often experience angina while performing arm work in a factory even though they can run well. When placed in an arm training program, the blood pressure and heart rate responses (an indirect measure of myocardial oxygen demands) will decrease and angina will subside. In other words, metabolic adaptations occur in the specific muscles that are trained.‡ In regard to the concern about sudden death at a football game or during sexual activity your concern is justified. Probably the coronary patient should carry a syringe loaded with antiarrhythmic medications, as recommended by Dr. Stanley Sarnoff, or should have an indwelling cardiac catheter electrode, an electronic sensor, which would turn on a DC shock if ventricular fibrillation appears. Hopefully more facilities will be available in many areas, i.e., shopping centers, recreational areas, and so forth, where cardiac emergencies may occur.

T. J. BASSLER (*Centinela Valley Community Hospital, Inglewood, Calif.*): Have you ever known of ischemic heart disease killing a single marathon runner?

H. K. HELLERSTEIN: Yes. In *Runner's World* a physician reported that Mr. Shettler, a well-known runner, died while running. Autopsy revealed severe stenosis of the left anterior descending artery.

T. J. BASSLER: Yes, he started and dropped out in three marathons. But you don't know anyone who has finished one marathon who's died of a heart attack.

† HELLERSTEIN, H. K. & E. H. FRIEDMAN. 1970. Arch. Int. Med. **125:** 987–999.

‡ CLAUSEN, J. P., J. TRAP-JENSEN & N. A. LASSEN. 1970. Scand. J. Clin. Lab. Invest. **26:** 295–301.

H. K. HELLERSTEIN: In my presentation I mentioned the patient who completed the Boston Marathon, but required resuscitative therapy. At a later time, effectively, he would have died had emergency care not been effective.

T. J. BASSLER: He's still running today?

H. K. HELLERSTEIN: He only ran again because there was somebody there to resuscitate him.

T. J. BASSLER: I know, but he's still running today.

H. K. HELLERSTEIN: But he's not running marathons. He runs within a protected environment.

T. J. BASSLER: And for what reason we should all have an indwelling catheter?

H. K. HELLERSTEIN: No, as yet that is not feasible. However, we must emphasize that silent coronary disease and sudden death are realities. Of patients with coronary artery disease who die from their disease, 60% never get to the hospital in their terminal episode. Many of these deaths are potentially reversible. I have received a recent report from New Zealand with similar data. Mechanism death is what kills the majority of these patients who die before they get to the hospital.

QUESTION: Dr. Kavanagh, it's well established that the normal myocardium can metabolize almost any substrate; however, there is a large body of evidence that in experimental myocardial ischemia free fatty acids, ketone bodies, and catecholamines are deleterious and may increase the size of a myocardial infarction. Later I'm presenting data on myocardial infarction occurring in marathon runners during marathon races. Now we can only speculate at the moment whether these factors, a rise in free fatty acids, possibly a rise in catecholamines, and cardiovascular drift are instrumental in promoting conditions favorable to myocardial infarction. I'd like to know why you feel that a maximal exercise test before a marathon race can in fact predict what is going to happen during the race at the myocardial level. Is it not possible that there are two stresses here? That a maximal exercise stress tests one thing? In fact, in a marathon race your myocardium is being stressed by other factors that are not tested in your maximal exercise test.

T. KAVANAGH: I agree. I couldn't agree more. But then you use the tools that are readily available and that is the most obvious tool for us to use, the maximal stress tests. There are bound to be factors that that particular test is not going to uncover, but then unless you can suggest an equally efficacious test that will cover the particular factors you're interested in, then we don't have any alternative.

D. ADAMOVICH (*Nassau County Medical Center, East Meadow, N.Y.*): Dr. Selvester, I think your study points out a very important thing, that even though patients are showing significant lesions in their coronary artery, that's an anatomic finding and it does not necessarily reflect impairment in their ability to perform and that their physiology is still intact.

Dr. Hellerstein, I would like to comment on something in your presentation. In one of your slides by Clausen and Trap-Jensen on specificity of arm versus leg training, I believe they have subsequently reviewed that data and agreed that they were wrong in what they originally presented, and that in fact leg training does carry over somewhat to arm work. I do see a great benefit of jogging for the cardiac patient.

R. SELVESTER (*University of Southern California, Downey, Calif.*): I personally don't disagree with what you just said. I think the important thing to see from this data is that one must try to remain somewhat objective in all of this. There is a lot of this kind of arm waving going on at the moment. But it's really pretty important I think to really ask the hard question and to stick with these patients, watch them for a while and see what happens. If one of these patients starts to deteriorate functionally then at that point we reassess their angiograms, if they have serious progression then they are offered bypass surgery. One patient progressed, was offered a bypass, and refused it. I'm still waiting to see what happens with this fellow. I would be very interested to know if he could really protect himself with 90%, 90%, and 100% blockage, and he's gone two years. According to the statistics in general he's surpassed the statistics by ten to one as far as what we would have expected from him, but he has not progressed.

R. H. RAHE (*Naval Health Research Center, San Diego, Calif.*): I just wanted to mention, I'm surprised I haven't heard it yet, that there is a masters program in running as well as in swimming. We've been hearing that the cardiac patient shouldn't go out and become a marathon runner; that's like trying to deny your disease entirely and identify with a useful group of which this room is mostly composed. Then we hear you have to stay on a track and just run around with a defibrillator and a little cart behind you, and that reaffirms psychologically that the runner is an invalid and that rather destroys the whole psychological rehabilitation we heard about in the first paper. There is an intermediate road. The masters program is age-restrictive so when you run with masters runners, you run with people in your own age group. This way you don't have to compete with Frank Shorter. It's controlled in that sense. It is more medically supervised. I think it is a good happy intermediate. The other thing I like about it is that psychologically it has all of the trappings of the real thing. Everybody does wear a number and in fact the swimmers all wear numbered swimsuits, and they all wear the little patches that we've seen. They walk into the hotel lobby and they're accorded as athletes just as we've been. They go out and run at lunch. They can have all the good psychological inputs about being healthy and vigorous normal people again, but they are in a situation that is more regulated, yet certainly not as restricted as running around with a defibrillator.

R. SELVESTER: My concern about the masters program and that level of exercise is very explicit in those slides I think, and I would have agreed with you a year ago before I got this data together. From this data it looks like we offered very little in the way of protection, maybe some protection from progression but not certainly from new infarction or the size of the infarct from those patients who are operating at those levels. I would also like to comment on your comment about the defibrillator. I totally agree with that attitude. I think the most important single thing we do for these patients is to define the risk. There are those who are at high risk, and they need to know that. Many of them are not at high risk, and they need to know that as well. One of the worst thinks we do as doctors, and particularly internists and worst of all cardiologists, is treat these people all as if they're the same. That's the most mindless thing we can do because there is a whole batch of these people who carry no risk at all—60% or 70% of those patients gave a very small risk. If you looked at that first slide, and I didn't have time to deal with it at length, those three-vessel diseases other than left main equivalent, two-vessel diseases that do not have a poor ejection fraction, and single-vessel diseases have a 1% or 2% 3-year mortality. That's really a modestly low mortality. The real mortality is carried by a subset. The important thing in my view is to identify that subset and to put this intense attention on that group, not on the other groups. And I think the most important thing we do for the rest of them is to get them unhooked from the anxiety. We do not carry a defibrillator around in our hip pocket and we send these people on bike-athons and long trips without a defibrillator. We're going to lose one someday, I have no doubt about that, but the risk in my mind is well worth taking.

QUESTION: I'll address my question to Dr. Selvester and to Dr. Hellerstein if it's appropriate. We've seen evidence of some improvement with three-vessel disease and Dr. Hellerstein has alluded to no improvement. In your experience what is the potential of post-coronary-bypass people?

R. SELVESTER: We have probably 50 or 60 people who are post-bypass at the present time in our program, and I think the trainability of the patient as far as I can tell hasn't got much to do with how bad the disease was in this sense. There is something about these angiograms that is very incomplete when a guy with an 80% and a 90% or 100% block can really be running 5 or 6 miles a day every day with an ejection fraction of 68% or 70% and doing very well. These numbers do not tell the whole story. There must be some collateral we're not seeing; some perfusion of that myocardium that we're not seeing. In our experience it doesn't make much difference. The most important single parameter was the one that Dr. Hellerstein alluded to, the amount of damage to the myocardium. People who have an ejection fraction below 40% who have an infarct that's greater than 8 or 9 cm along its curvilinear dimension on the wall of an LAO ventriculogram or that represents roughly 30% of their left ventricular involvement of the left ventricular wall, have an upper limit of what their pump can do and they're the ones that we have trouble training. The rest of these people, even those with angina, or ST segments do much better. One of our patients has 5–6 mm of ST segment depression every time we test him. Still we have to push him clear up to the top and we take these people to maximal routinely as part of our routine test now. He has to get to pretty high levels before he gets that 5 mm. The bypass patients are equally trainable. I think they get to it a little quicker because they have had a fairly dramatic increase in perfusion in some of their vessels.

H. K. HELLERSTEIN: After bypass surgery many patients are highly de-conditioned just by their very experience. They are rapidly retrainable. Many times they have midsternal incisional pains that they have to overcome.

R. BECKER (*Allegheny Valley Hospital, Natsona Heights, Pa.*): Dr. Heller-stein has indicated that the presence of collaterals are more or less an indi-cation of severity of the disease. I wondered if Dr. Selvester has looked at the people who have occluded to 100% without infarct and if he's looked for the presence of collaterals.

R. SELVESTER: I'm sure no good angiographer wouldn't look for the presence of collaterals. But as far as we can tell those visible collaterals haven't got a thing to do with what's going on. That's what everybody else has found. But the fascinating thing is there is a group of people who de-veloped total occlusion, who do not develop visible collaterals from any other vessel, and yet have good ventricular function. Now this is only 20% of all those who totally occlude. I think I made that point. If you totally occlude, you've got an 80% chance of developing an infarct. Half of these infarcts are under 3 cm., so there is not very much damage associated with them. The rest of them are small enough you can't see them on a ventriculo-gram and they don't show on an electrocardiogram, and I assume therefore there was no damage, no significant damage at all to the myocardium.

They're not necessarily associated with increased collateral. I do not know exactly how that squares with what Dr. Hellerstein was saying earlier.

H. K. HELLERSTEIN: Now is the time for recapitulation and resumé. This evening the essayists have asserted that a small number of coronary patients are able to attain a high level of physical performance. In Dr. Kavanagh's experience, 22 of 600 people (about 4%) achieved that level. My calculation is that in our coronary population potentially 10% could develop an aerobic capacity sufficient to complete a marathon "slog" (instead of run) in 5 hours. Dr. Selvester has reported that a similar percentage of his coronary subjects advanced to a high level of training. We certainly agree that the question as to whether arteriosclerosis is regressible has not been resolved because of the factor of self-selection. For this reason, the ongoing National Exercise and Heart Disease Project and the Canadian Collaborative Project have randomized patients to obviate the problem of self-selection.

The unequivocal fact is that coronary artery disease tends to progress at variable rates, unpredictable in individual patients. The mechanism of benefit remains unresolved. It's obvious that the lack of gross changes in the coronary arteriograms is not sufficient to explain why coronary patients can improve so much after physical training. The studies on myocardial uptake of catecholamines § and on serum levels of catecholamines suggest that training changes catecholamines metabolism. The limitations of present day coronary arteriograms must be emphasized, i.e., failure to visualize vessels below 100 μm. Postmortem injection studies of the hearts of patients with obstructive large coronary artery disease have shown a plethora of capillary anastomoses and/or collaterals that are not seen with angios.

Unresolved is the matter of risk of jogging and long distance running, which can kill in certain circumstances. There is a medical/legal problem. Mechanism death is a reality. Dr. Robert Bruce of Seattle, Washington has accumulated a total of 15 cases of exercise-induced mechanism death. All have been successfully reversed. None of them died because they were exercising and developed ventricular fibrillation *in a controlled environment*.

The question of how to deal with the coronary patients who are at high risk of fatal arrhythmias is unresolved. Should the risk be ignored and denied? Should they only exercise in supervised and closely monitored areas? Does this produce unnecessary iatrogenic disability? Emotionally I agree that the height of successful rehabilitation is to remove the label of the cardiac. However, the undeniable truth is they remain cardiacs and ultimately about 90% of them will die from heart disease; 50% to 60% will die before they ever get to the hospital. While the bravado expressed by several of the discussants is attractive and admirable ("get them unhooked from anxiety," "forget about it, let them run," "Go on long trips without a defibrillator," etc.), nevertheless cardiacs do "die" suddenly. They develop exercise induced arrhythmias, which are irreversible and lethal unless emergency facilities and trained personnel are *immediately* available.

When the controlled and randomized studies of the National Exercise and Heart Disease Project and the Canadian Collaborative study are completed in another 4 or 5 years perhaps the New York Academy of Sciences may sponsor another such meeting, at which time we will have hard data untainted by the confounding factor of self-selection.

§ SALZMAN, S. H., E. Z. HIRSCH, H. K. HELLERSTEIN & J. H. BRUELL. 1970. J. Appl. Physiol. **29:** 92–95.

INTRODUCTORY REMARKS

Paul Milvy

Environmental Sciences Laboratory
Mount Sinai School of Medicine
New York, New York 10029

Permit me to open this session devoted to epidemiological studies of prolonged aerobic exercise by quoting at length from the letter I sent to each participant of this session several months ago:

". . . Epidemiological methods can discover and discern hidden relationships and associations, but to determine if they are causal relationships is a much more difficult task. Thus a study in 1964 [1] showed greater cardiovascular problems among those who have higher sucrose intake (not saturated fats, but sugar). A reinvestigation showed probably no causal relationship but did show that those with high sugar intakes also had higher cigarette consumption.[2, 3] Why this relationship exists was not explored but the cause and effect relationship shown by many other studies (animal, histopathological, epidemiological, etc.) is most probably between nicotine and carbon monoxide (and possibly the tars) and coronary heart disease.

"A second example: Morris's classic 1953 study of London bus drivers and conductors concluded that physical exercise increased life expectancy.[4] Yet, a follow-up paper by him in 1956 (subtitled 'Epidemiology of Uniforms')[5] demonstrated that the bus drivers had greater girth, and indeed, were heavier when initially hired, as reflected in the size of their first uniform. So self-selection is a constant threat to the validity of all epidemiological studies (if it were to be shown that runners, for example, live longer, on an average than the general population, this would be interesting, perhaps even important, but also predictable, since runners are thinner, generally don't smoke, etc.).

"And it is not at all clear that runners refrain from overeating and smoking by virtue of their running. Other subgroups of our population don't overeat or smoke: perhaps such a group must be or should be used as a control in studies of runners. (Incidentally, industrial workers have a lower mortality than the general population; all that this indicates is that the general population includes a group of infirm people who cannot work; self-selection again. Nor could these infirm people run, again biasing the data when comparing runners to the general population.)

"In any event, I suppose I'm belaboring the point. The only point I'm trying to make is that statistical and epidemiological studies are tricky, contain many uncertainties and often only sophisticated techniques can assure valid conclusions. There is probably no such thing as a completely definitive epidemiological study of anything. Nor can I reasonably expect the participants of our session to be the first to achieve one since studies in this decade still suffer from confounding variables, self-selection, and so forth. But what I do hope—and this is the motivation for this letter—is that each speaker prepare a careful paper and that each author be aware of the inherent and inevitable areas of weakness of the study he is reporting upon. Thus, perhaps in the submitted manuscript, it would be most desirable that the author concern himself, however briefly, with the possible inadequacies in his choice of the control group he may use, biases of the investigators if subjective data is employed, preselection, confounding variables, mathematical handling of the data and the adequacy of these algorithmic techniques, and so forth.

"I am sure you will agree that really sophisticated epidemiological studies of the implications of physical exercise and activity on health, morbidity, and mortality are inherently extremely difficult to achieve. I am also certain that you would agree that each author should try to achieve a high level of epidemiological sophistication. More than this, I cannot require! . . ."

I think this session promises to be an interesting one. It includes a presentation by a doctor who has asserted in his widely read book entitled *Type A Behaviour and Your Heart* that jogging is "a miserable post-collegiate athletic travesty (that) has already killed at least scores, possibly hundreds."[6] It includes a pathologist who has asserted that "a search of the literature failed to document a single death due to coronary arteriosclerosis among marathon finishers,"[7] and, "when the level of vigorous exercise is raised high enough, the protection [from coronary heart disease] appears to be absolute."[8] A paper will be presented that is coauthored by the greatly admired physiologist, D. B. Dill, who for 20 years was Director of Research at Harvard's Fatigue Laboratory, and for the last 11 years has been active at the University of Nevada's Laboratory of Environmental Pathophysiology. Still an active researcher, during the first 85 years of his life, Dr. Dill conducted research in the areas of the physiology of exercise, environmental physiology, and the physiology of aging.

Dr. Leon has published extensively in the areas of fundamental studies of exercise training in rodents as well as man. Working in the well-known Laboratory of Physiological Hygiene at the University of Minnesota, he has also written several reviews of this general field. Ken Cooper, whose book *Aerobics* appeared at a time when jogging was just beginning to become a national phenomenon, if not a national pasttime, heads an active "running lab" in Dallas. His book was probably motivated in part by this national phenomenon, but certainly in its own right has played a role in motivating additional thousands to begin to run and jog.

Maarti Karvonen is internationally known and highly regarded for his many epidemiological studies, spanning several decades, of lumbermen, elite cross-country skiers, and of athletes in general. These studies were conducted among a population in which the incidence of coronary heart disease, like our own, is terribly high, and thus these studies are relevant to us today. Dr. Rose, a sociologist by training who specializes in gerontology, is the author of a fascinating book[9] that involved the outpatients at Boston's Veterans Administration. Tim Noakes, a cardiologist from the University of Capetown, South Africa, is a colleague of L. H. Opie, who has been carrying on in the letter columns of several medical and scientific journals, a running (pun intended!) argument over CHD and marathoning with Tom Bassler. Dr. Noakes, like at least six of the other participants in this session, is a marathoner and has twice run the famed 52-mile Comrades race. Finally, Terry Kavanagh, Medical Director of the Toronto Rehabilitation Centre in Canada, has done careful work that involves an exercise program for postcoronary patients. He has become an annual fixture at the Boston Marathon, running the full marathon with a handful of his "A+ students."

In conclusion, I would remind you that, because we will hear many points of view today concerning the relationship between physical activity and CHD, to assume some golden mean midway between the extreme points of view here presented cannot be justified. It would be a little like the man who, listening to two friends argue, one holding that grass is green, the other that it is shocking pink, concludes that the truth must lie somewhere in between!

References

1. YUDKIN, J. 1964. Dietary fat and dietary sugar in relation to ischaemic heart disease and diabetes. Lancet. ii: 4.
2. ELWOOD, P. C., S. MOORE, W. E. WATERS & P. SWEETMAN. 1970. Sucrose consumption and ischaemic heart disease in the community. Lancet i: 1014–1016.
3. BENNETT, A. E., R. DOLL & R. W. HOWELL. 1970. Sugar consumption and cigarette smoking. Lancet i: 1011–1014.
4. MORRIS, J. N., J. A. HEADY, P. A. RAFFLE, C. G. ROBERTS & J. W. PARKS. 1953. Coronary heart disease and physical activity of work. Lancet ii: 1053–1057, 1111–1120.
5. MORRIS, J. N., J. HEADY & P. A. RAFFLE. 1956. Physique of London busmen. Lancet ii: 566–570.
6. FRIEDMAN, M. & R. H. ROSENMAN. 1974. Type A Behavior and Your Heart. Alfred A. Knopf, Inc. New York, N.Y.
7. BASSLER, T. J. 1972. Letter. Lancet ii: 711.
8. BASSLER, T. J. 1973. Letter. Science 128: 1083.
9. ROSE, C. L. & B. BELL. 1971. Predicting Longevity. D. C. Heath & Co. Lexington, Mass.

A CRITICAL REVIEW OF EPIDEMIOLOGICAL STUDIES OF PHYSICAL ACTIVITY

Paul Milvy

Department of Community Medicine
Mount Sinai School of Medicine
New York, New York 10029

W. F. Forbes and K. S. Brown

Faculty of Mathematics
University of Waterloo
Waterloo, Ontario
Canada N2L 3G1

INTRODUCTION

Early this century, medical opinion held that excessive physical activity was detrimental to health, but it is now widely believed that physical activity has a protective effect against cardiovascular diseases and hence may increase lifespan. However, the presumed health consequences of intensive and prolonged physical activity are often based on anecdotal evidence, and hard data from well-designed studies are difficult to obtain. This paper outlines some of these difficulties, together with a critical review of the more important studies in this rapidly growing field.

THEORETICAL CONSIDERATIONS OF CAUSE AND EFFECT RELATIONS

Suppose X represents an independent variable (e.g., physical inactivity) and Y a response or dependent variable (e.g., premature development of coronary heart disease, CHD), and it is required to establish that X causes Y. Then, if X and Y are associated, the alternatives (Y has caused X; an extraneous variable Z has caused both X and Y; or the association between X and Y is due to chance) must be dismissed.

The basic requirement for a cause-and-effect relationship is that X precedes Y in time, and that the relationship is asymmetrical. The degree to which extraneous variables can be assumed to be similar between comparison groups depends on the research design, and these design considerations are therefore essential for establishing the strength of any inference. That is, Z and X may be statistically associated so that when Z and Y are associated, X and Y will be associated. Any observed changes in Y could, therefore, have been caused by a change in Z or by a change in X. The control of confounding or extraneous variables by means of an appropriate research design allows the investigator to protect himself from misleading inferences.

The possibility that the association between X and Y may result from chance is removed by requiring that any observed association be reproducible.[36] In the physical sciences reproducibility is generally not difficult to achieve, but the epidemiologist frequently must rely on evaluating the consistency of data that have been obtained with different research designs and methods.

Although information on the nature of associations between variables may be obtained in the analysis phase, it is during the design phase that control of confounding variables is exercised most effectively. For example, a relationship between variables that cannot be untangled during analysis is provided by the following two hypothetical models, entirely different in their inference but for which the results, on analysis, would be similar:

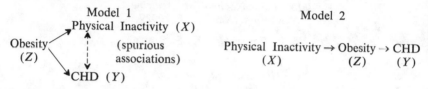

In both models, when obesity is controlled during analysis, the association between physical inactivity and coronary heart disease will disappear. Thus the analysis is unable to settle the question of the relevance of the variable Z in the association between X and Y. If the question of the role of Z cannot be resolved by a suitable design, information may have to be obtained from other sources, such as the logical order of the variables with respect to time.

In investigating the relationship between X and Y the epidemiologist must therefore assess the research design that gave rise to the collected data, and, in this connection, it is useful to define three basic types of observational methods and to examine the strength of inference possible from each.

Types of Observational Methods

The three classes of observational methods are anecdotal reports, the passive or observational method, and the experimental method.

Anecdotal reports represent unplanned observations that might be suggested either by data in isolation or by data obtained through either of the other two methods, but which are fragmentary, isolated, or incomplete. Data of this type are useful for suggesting hypotheses, which might then be verified by experiment or at least checked for consistency by considering alternative sources of information. They are incapable, on their own, of establishing any type of cause-and-effect relationship.

The passive or observational method involves data collected via surveys or historical records. Conditions are not varied by the experimenter but are studied essentially in the form in which they are available. Such a method may produce evidence for hypotheses consistent with an association between two or more variables, such as illustrated in Models 1 and 2, but this method again is not capable of demonstrating cause and effect. For example, in investigations of physical activity and mortality, the self-selection of individuals into occupations and/or leisure time activities involving physical exercise represents one condition over which the investigator may have little control. That is, individuals who are obese, who smoke and/or drink heavily, or in general who are less "health conscious," might be expected to select occupations or life styles that do not involve physical activity. Similarly, individuals with histories of cardiovascular disease, emphysema or bronchitis or with any physical impairment would be expected to be underrepresented in self-selected physically active groups. Thus, any of a number of health-related differences might exist between groups that select physical activity and groups that do not, between groups that continue to exercise late in life, and those that do not, or between groups that adhere to prescribed exercise programs and groups that do not. Hellerstein [60] emphasizes that point strongly: "There are no data . . . to show that exercising middle-aged, sloppy, overweight, cigarette smoking, paunchy men, 20% of whom are hypertensive, and 7% of whom are diabetic will make a bit of difference in survivorship. There are no data because there is self-selection."

With the experimental method, in contrast to the above, control over the independent variable (X) is exercised and the behavior of the dependent variable (Y) is then observed. Such control is essential to the demonstration of cause and effect.

Research Designs

In this section five basic epidemiological research designs as identified by Clark and Hopkins [22] will be discussed with respect to their ability to demonstrate cause and effect.

The field study represents the classical cross-sectional or "snapshot" study in which a population is examined and measurements are taken at one time. No evidence of cause and effect can be determined from such studies since causes and effects are observed simultaneously. That is, the lack of a time dimension makes it generally impossible to determine if the supposed cause preceded the supposed effect.

The prospective study involves measurement of a set of postulated "causes" (X) in a cohort that is then followed in time until the "effects" (Y) are noted or the study terminates. It is thus possible to make inferences about an association between X and Y and about their ordering in time. However, proof of causation is difficult because of the possible influence of confounding variables or self-selection, and because the change with time in many variables might be quite different in those subgroups for which the effect is noted.

The retrospective, or case-control study involves matching an individual in which the dependent variable is present with one in which it has not been observed and examining past information to determine if the independent variable occurs with a greater or lesser frequency or to a greater or lesser degree in cases relative to controls. The results can again provide evidence of an association but while the matching procedure may remove some sources of extraneous variation, in a multifactor disease process it is unlikely that all sources can be controlled. Further, as Susser [154] indicates, the information on which a pair is matched may be imprecise, particularly when the matching variable varies with time. For example, the matching of a CHD case with a suitable control would be difficult if variables such as blood pressure and serum cholesterol were chosen as matching variables, since even if the relevant data were available, the change of these variables with time may differ between cases and controls.

The historical prospective study is prospective in historical time though retrospective in real time and is equivalent to the prospective study but displaced in time so that the end point is the present. The comments regarding cause and effect, which were made for the prospective, and retrospective studies, also apply to the historical prospective studies.

The clinical trial represents the only design in which the experimenter exercises control and hence is capable of demonstrating cause and effect. Because he exercises control the experimenter is able, by matching treatment and control groups with respect to characteristics thought to affect the dependent variable, to systematize the effects of these known sources of variation. These effects may then be estimated and removed from experimental error during analysis. The random assignment of subjects to treatment and control groups ensures, as much as possible, that observed variation in the dependent variable is attributable to the treatment and not to confounding variables that the experimenter has been unable to control directly. It is this random assignment of subjects to treatment and control groups that is the necessary criterion for demonstrating cause and effect. Since if X (the independent variable) is assigned by a randomization device, this technique precludes Y (the dependent variable) or Z (some extraneous factor) causing X, although they may appear to do so.

TABLE 1

APPROXIMATE TOTAL SAMPLE SIZES REQUIRED TO DETECT A DIFFERENCE OF THE GIVEN MAGNITUDE BETWEEN TREATMENT AND CONTROL GROUPS *

Ratio Sample Size Control/ Treatment	Reduction in Proportion of Cases in Treatment Group *	Approximate Total Sample Size Required			
		Proportion of Cases in Control Group			
		0.05	0.10	0.15	0.20
9	5%	722,000	360,000	240,000	182,000
	10%	172,000	85,600	57,200	43,200
	25%	23,500	11,700	7,790	5,880
3	5%	344,000	168,000	110,000	80,600
	10%	82,500	40,400	26,300	19,400
	25%	11,500	5,650	3,700	2,730
1	5%	254,000	121,000	76,100	53,800
	10%	62,000	29,400	18,600	13,200
	25%	9,060	4,330	2,750	2,000

* 5% level of significance, one tailed; power of test, 90%. Sample sizes were computed from the formula of Patnaik [106] and assume with the assumption of no drop-outs or nonadherents in either group.

† $[(P_C - P_T)/P_C] \times 100$, where P_C and P_T are the proportions of cases in the control and treated groups.

In the study of the possible link between physical inactivity and increased mortality, or CHD, it would be difficult to perform clinical trials that meet the proper criteria. Even with the random assignment of subjects to treatment and control groups, the trial generally could not be conducted "blind" or "double-blind," and the assumption implicit in a clinical trial, that the only difference between groups is the treatment, would not be justified. During the trial relatively high drop-out rates in treatment groups, possibly as a consequence of health-related factors such as obesity or smoking habits (or merely as a result of loss of interest) and the presence of individuals in the control group who nevertheless participate in exercise programs, could reduce such a trial to the status of a prospective study, implying that the inference, because of this self-selection, would become one of association rather than causation.

With regard to the number of subjects required for a clinical trial, TABLE 1 gives approximate total sample sizes necessary to be 90% certain of detecting, at the 5% level of significance, a difference in proportions of cases (e.g., of CHD) between treatment and control groups when the treatment has the indicated effect, i.e., a 5%, 10%, or 25% reduction. These sample sizes assume no nonadherents, or loss to follow-up, which would further increase the required sample sizes.[138] Thus, for example, if development of CHD in initially healthy males were chosen as the endpoint of such a trial, the proportion of CHD cases in 8 years for average males of ages 35, 45, and 55 would be 0.016, 0.060, and 0.116 respectively.[164] (These "average" males would include individuals who exercise and, for a sedentary population, the proportions could be somewhat higher.) The appropriate approximate sample sizes can be inferred from TABLE 1, which, together with the duration of the study, probably make such a trial a practical impossibility. For a thorough discussion of sample size, see Taylor *et al.*[162]

On the other hand, from smaller clinical trials of shorter duration, information on the relevance of exercise programs can be obtained if a different endpoint is chosen. For example, a beneficial risk factor change, such as an increase in work capacity and cardiovascular efficiency,[6] in exercise groups could suggest a decrease in eventual CHD incidence. However, such extrapolations may be tenuous since there is little evidence that risk factor modification will lead to increased life expectancy (see Morris [99]).

SPECIFIC EPIDEMIOLOGICAL STUDIES

The earliest study that will be discussed is that by Morris *et al.*,[97] published in 1953. This well-known paper examined three groups of workers, namely, London transport workers, postal workers, and civil servants. The authors observed that the bus conductors had less CHD and that the disease seemed to appear later and was less severe than that experienced by the more sedentary bus drivers. They briefly discussed several of the possible confounding factors, and with the above conclusion serving as a hypothesis, also examined postal workers and civil servants in different job classifications. Somewhat similar results were obtained, although it was found that angina was more pronounced and frequent in the active postmen than in the more sedentary grades such as drivers and telephonists. The CHD mortality among skilled, semiskilled, and unskilled workers from England and Wales who died between 1930 and 1932 was also investigated. These workers were divided into heavy, intermediate, light, and doubtful activity groups. The coronary mortality of the groups of heavy-activity workers was found to be less than half that of the light-work group, consistent with the hypothesis that physical activity offers protection from CHD. This study has been referred to frequently, although its weaknesses in terms of confounding variables and self-selection diminish the strength of its conclusions. However, its authors indicate the complexities of such studies and discuss the theoretical approaches required for competent epidemiological studies. In particular, they examine the possible occupational or social class factors that might introduce bias. Three years later, Morris *et al.*[95] specifically identified and examined one of the confounding factors and showed that the drivers had greater girth (measured by waistline and jacket size) than the conductors. This might be anticipated, since the drivers were involved in more sedentary work. However, the drivers' first uniforms, issued when their employment as drivers started, were also larger than that of the conductors, implying that their girth was larger when they were first hired. Interestingly, although the conductors were thinner, a subset of conductors who transferred to the job classification of driver had a "girth profile" that was more like the drivers group than the conductors group; that is, they were from the outset, as conductors, more like drivers in build. Other confounding factors were not analyzed.

In 1962, after a number of papers had appeared [11, 12, 21, 35, 82, 96, 98, 101, 147] that discussed Morris's study and their conclusions, Taylor et al.[160] reported an extensive study of active and sedentary white men aged 40 to 64 years, that were employed in the railroad industry. This historical prospective study found that the age-adjusted rates for all deaths and for deaths from arteriosclerotic heart disease were significantly lower in the most active versus most sedentary categories in three and four of the 5-year age groups, respectively. Taylor mentioned several confounding variables including personal characteristics that may lead to self-selection, but no method to obviate these problems was provided. Four years later Taylor et al.[158] reported on a cohort of 8,053 clerks, switchmen, and executives drawn from 20 northwestern U.S. railroad companies. Data were presented that "illustrate the problems of estimating the true prevalence of CHD in the physically active as compared to the sedentary occupations. The observed prevalence of CHD was influenced by greater withdrawal of younger switchmen with CHD as compared to clerks and selection against the experiment by switchmen with CHD." Taylor concluded that "a majority of the (known) factors affecting observed prevalence rates operate to exaggerate any true excess that may exist in an active population over that in a sedentary population." However, the question as to how many factors, yet unknown, operate similarly, remains obscure. In 1967 Taylor [157] discussed his own data in relationship to physical activity and CHD, with attention to the general problems of sample size, occupational withdrawals, physical activity classification, self-selection of occupation, and other epidemiological problems. He noted that "the incidence ratio between physically active [and] sedentary occupations is closer to one than that observed in the bus drivers and conductors (studied by Morris)." (See also Taylor et al.[161] for a 5-year follow-up of this study and Menotti and Puddu [87] for a comparable Italian study.

In 1966 Morris et al.[100] reported that 7% of 667 healthy middle-aged London busmen who had been followed for 5 years developed ischemic heart disease and that the rate was higher in the drivers than in the conductors. The smokers, the obese, the short men, the men with family histories of CHD, with high systolic blood pressure, and with high plasma cholesterol were at considerably greater risk, and the latter two risk factors were the best predictors of disease. In 1967 Oliver [104] studied the physiques and serum lipid concentrations of the young recruits for the jobs of bus conductors and bus drivers before any occupational factors resulting from these two job categories could manifest themselves. He found that "it is apparent that British men with certain physical characteristics choose or are chosen to become drivers as opposed to conductors" and that the "study supports the view that inherited characteristics, one of which may be susceptibility to heart disease, may predispose to a particular occupation."

The following year Malhotra [83] reported that mortality from ischemic heart disease in a southern Indian railway workers population was seven times higher than that in a northern railway population. Sedentary clerks had a much lower mortality than physically active fitters and sweepers, although mortality in the socioeconomic group of executives was nearly 7 times greater than in the lower socioeconomic group, designated class IV following the British convention. The fact that consumption of sugar and fat and cigarette smoking was about an order of magnitude higher in the North, where mortality was lower, than in the South is a striking feature. The observation that sweepers had a mortality rate 15 times greater in the South than in the North, with age, physical activity, and bilirubin levels (a reflection of rate and route of fat digestion and fat profile) remaining matched, led the author to infer that cooking and masticatory habits, which were considered to be quite different in the North and the South, may account for these large variations in mortality.

Beginning in 1970, Paffenbarger [108-111] reported on a 3,262-man cohort of San Francisco longshoremen that have been followed since 1951. These papers showed that with high versus low levels of physical activity (nearly 1000 more kilocalories are expended per workday by cargo handlers than by men in less active work categories) stroke fatalities were independent of levels of work activity, but death rates from CHD were about 26% lower in the active workers. In the 1975 paper [110] Paffenbarger finds attractive the arguments advanced by Fox and Haskell,[41] Morris *et al.*,[94] the W.H.O.,[168] and Cooper *et al.*[25] in terms of the efficiency of high intensity exercise producing a "training effect," and he suggests that it is the repeated "bursts" of great effort rather than the total integrated work effort that leads to the protective effect of the expenditure of the extra 1000 calories per work shift. However, all the epidemiological studies including these studies by Paffenbarger that address themselves to the proposed inverse correlation of CHD mortality and physical activity have only looked at the overall physical activity levels. Insofar as "intense bursts of physical" activity have not been studied directly, this form of energy expenditure must be regarded in a sense as a confounding variable. However, since other variables (smoking, systolic blood pressure, and weight) also seem to be related to activity, the relationship between physical activity and the mortality from CHD ought to be examined for different subgroups. In this connection it may be noted that the data of Paffenbarger *et al.*[111] indicate that in the group in which weight for height was less than the mean, the CHD death rate was only 7% less in the more active longshoremen. One can of course assume that increased physical activity represents the independent variable and the resulting dependent variables of lower mortality from CHD and lower weight preclude the isolation or separation of these two factors, but Morris' study on "the epidemiology of uniforms" [95] may be cited to argue that self-selection accounts for the correlation of thinner and more active, or fatter and more sedentary. Perhaps the greater prevalence of additional risk factors that a sedentary, emotionally and intellectually numbing job might entail that were not considered by Paffenbarger (such as work satisfaction, the lack of any intellectual or mental exertion, etc.) also represent confounding variables.[66, 133, 166] Finally, since longshoremen do not die only from stroke and CHD, not dying from these two diseases may imply dying from other diseases. The question then arises how mortality from all causes is influenced by the extra 1000 kcal of physical activity per day expended by the physically active longshoremen.

In a multinational study of the incidence of CHD in middle-aged men, Keys *et al.*[74] studied 2404 U.S. railway men and 8728 European men grouped in 13 cohorts from five European countries. He investigated the relationship of CHD and age, blood pressure, serum cholesterol, smoking, physical activity, and weight. It was found that CHD risk within a population "is well predicted from the results of the multivariate analysis of the experience of men in other far-distant populations differing in circumstance, language, and ethnic background"; that is, European data could be used to predict American CHD incidence and vice versa. Although the first four variables mentioned identify men much above average risk in terms of mortality from CHD, because of the large unexplained intranational variation, it was concluded that one or more unknown variables unrelated to the risk factors considered were also influential as predictors of CHD mortality.

Hickey et al.[65] examined 15,171 Irish men for coronary risk factor, and evaluated their leisure and work activities. The mean levels of five coronary risk factors tended to decrease with increasing leisure activity but no similar trend was observed for work activity. The authors state, however, that "possibly those men who are physically active during their leisure time may smoke less and eat more prudently for personality, psychological, or cultural reasons. And possibly, because of their better health, they may be enabled to take more exercise. Intuitively, we may postulate that the psychological factors that motivate men to perform heavy leisure activity may also cause them to adopt other means of maintaining good health."

Two rural male populations from East and West Finland were followed for 15 years by Karvonen,[119] and significant differences between the incidence of CHD in these regions were observed. These men were also classified in four activity levels, with lumberjacks, representing the most physically active group with an energy expenditure of 4,500–8,000 kcal per day. Although the sedentary category, through self-selection was "unduly loaded with men having CHD . . . it is of special interest that initially healthy lumberjacks, i.e., men who were free of CHD and engaged in extremely heavy work activity, fared no better but rather worse as regards to the development of CHD than men with a less heavy occupation," and only slightly better than men in the most sedentary category. The possibility was therefore raised that habitual physical activity that *exceeds* a certain threshold is deleterious, or at least does not further reduce the risk of CHD."

The general point should also be made that sociological studies indicate that those who are physically active on the job are often inactive off the job—longshoremen don't jog—and vice versa. This factor may be relevant in every study that evaluates mortality versus leisure activity, or mortality versus job-related activity, but does not try to assess both; the effect of this might be to reduce differences between physical activity groups.

The point that psychosocial factors may be confounded with physical activity is also illustrated, for example, by reference to a study by Palmore.[112] In addition to evaluating the levels of physical functioning and health (in which the risk factors cholesterol, smoking and obesity were grouped) of 268 elderly men (median age 70), many parameters indicative of intelligence, daily on-job and off-job activities and attitudes, and socioeconomic status were also considered. In general, work satisfaction and physical functioning were the most important predictors of longevity, but the two measures of socioeconomic status (education and occupation) were poorly correlated with longevity. It can also be anticipated that work satisfaction and physical functioning are related since poor physical functioning presumably decreases the satisfaction derived from activities.

Other social and psychological factors that correlate with longevity must also be borne in mind when studying physical activity and mortality, especially off-job physical activity (sports, hobbies, etc.), since it is entirely possible that self-selection and confounding variables based upon these factors are particularly relevant. The number of "psychological and sociological param- eters" that possibly might exert a real influence on mortality analysis is large, and thus, any attempt to examine other risk factors without an attempt to control for these factors is probably simplistic. This has been well il- lustrated by animal studies since, for example, Henry *et al.* have shown that overcrowding mice from the same litter produces quantitatively less pathological disease (hypertension and aggresive behavior) than overcrowding nonlitter- mates.[63] With human populations, the situation is much more complicated and remains obscure.[18] In this connection, it has been observed [53] that Japanese- Americans who remain in the Japanese community within the territorial U.S. suffer less CHD and other diseases known to occur more frequently in the U.S. than in Japan, although for those Japanese-Americans who are more dis- persed among the U.S. Caucasian population the incidence of these diseases rises sharply even when other variables remain constant. This also suggests that the belief that overcrowding gives rise to some (noncontagious) diseases is an oversimplification. Moreover, Hong Kong and Holland, which represent areas of high population density, both enjoy high levels of mental and physical health.[31] Further, studies by Syme *et al.*[155, 156] demonstrated that the prevalence of CHD is higher among occupationally and residentially mobile people than among stable populations, and Tyroler and Cassel [164] have shown that not only groups in flux (social, geographical), but groups that are stable, but are surrounded by a matrix of populations in social flux (e.g., undergoing ur- banization) exhibit relatively greater death rates from CHD. For general discussions, both theoretical and phenomenological, of those social influences on health and disease, see Cassel,[18, 20] Jenkins,[66] Rose,[130] Van Dijl,[166] and Rose and Bell.[131] In addition, the papers by Rosenman [134] and Brand *et al.*[10, 11] on type A–type B personality (discussed later in this review) are pertinent in this regard.

EPIDEMIOLOGICAL STUDIES INVOLVING COMMUNITIES

The studies described in the previous section can be classified as epi- demiological studies in a population generally representing a single trade or occupational group. The following studies concern themselves with popula- tions drawn from entire communities, or from specific geographic areas.

Chapman *et al.*[21] studied a 1949 working population of Los Angeles City civil service employees that varied in age from 18 to 70 and were employed in 399 different job classifications. Preliminary findings on the incidence of CHD versus physical exertion were at variance with almost all other epidemiological studies (25% more new CHD and deaths from CHD in the two highest levels of physical activity as compared with the two lowest levels). The authors also observed CHD incidence versus ponderal index (a 6-fold increase in new CHD and deaths from CHD in the lowest ponderal index category than in the highest index for men aged 40–54 years, and 1.5 times for men aged 55–70 years), and CHD incidence versus blood pressure (nearly 4 times higher for men 40–54 with diastolic pressure of 95 or systolic of 145 and over versus lower pressures, although this difference in health risk disappeared for men 55–70). However, the numbers of men observed with new CHD and new

CHD deaths were extremely small and consequently of doubtful statistical significance.

An epidemiological study of CHD in a population of 106,000 males 33 years or older in six counties of North Dakota was made by Zukel [172] who found that farmers had less CHD than men in other occupations, although diets were essentially identical. Physical inactivity was an apparent risk factor but interview information on physical activity was unreliable and a tendency existed for men to report less heavy physical work in their usual occupation if they described this work after they had experienced an MI than if they had not experienced one.

Reports of a study by the Health Insurance Plan of Greater New York (HIP) [46–48, 139, 140] discuss the results of research initiated in 1961. In this multi-risk-factor study, physical activity (combined on-job and off-job activities) was graded at three levels. It was found that men with "light" activity had an elevated risk of myocardial infarction, men with "heavy" physical activity had a higher risk of angina, and that the risk of fatality from a first myocardial infarction (MI) was much greater in the lower activity group. However, the study suffers from the usual problems of self-selection, as the authors acknowledge. In addition, in Shapiro et al. [139] it is shown that for those in the classification "physical activity unknown" the incidence of CHD was more than 5 times lower than in the physically most active. An additional HIP study by Weinblatt et al. [167] evaluated the prognosis of men who have survived a first MI, and it concluded that the severity of the MI appears to have little influence on long-term prognosis. In addition, even if high levels of physical activity offer some protection against a first MI, the level of physical activity appears to bear only a weak relationship to the probability of experiencing a second MI. Similarly, the Framingham Study [67] evaluated the role of physical activity, measured "crudely" by taking a 24-hour history from 5,127 people and measured "objectively" from physiological tests of weight gain, vital capacity, and resting pulse, and concluded that the more sedentary fraction of the population had a "distinctly worse outlook" vis-á-vis CHD.

The incidence of CHD in a northern Indian town was investigated by Sarvotham et al. [136] by examining 2030 persons above the age of 30. The incidence of CHD (roughly half of that found in Framingham) increased with age, with socioeconomic status, with sedentary life-style, with hypertension, with obesity, and with subscapular skin-fold thickness.

Hammond and Garfinkel [57] reported in 1969 on the results of a prospective study of more than 800,000 men and women 40–79 years of age who were followed for 6 years and who, at the start of the study, had no history of heart disease, stroke, or cancer. The usual risk factors for CHD, stroke, and nonsyphilitic aortic aneurysm (and in addition several other variables, e.g., hours of sleep, subjective evaluation of nervous tension, and weight loss during previous decade) were related to mortality experience based on nearly 20,000 deaths. Dividing their data into two extreme groups, a low-risk and high-risk group, the latter group was categorized by heavy smoking, overweight, little exercise, and fewer hours of sleep per night. The death rates from these three diseases, even in the low-risk group, were not low in an absolute sense, suggesting that some other etiological factors in the U.S. may be of equal or greater importance. In this connection, it should also be remembered that the CHD mortality is higher in the U.S. than in many other countries. A similar study by Belloc [2] employing 6,928 adults of Alameda County, California also related mortality after 5½ years to a number of risk factors and, with the exception of weight, mortality was found to vary in accord with what might be termed "good health practices."

A study in 1965 by McDonough *et al.*[86] and a follow-up study of 91% of the original cohort by Cassel *et al.* published in 1971,[19] concluded that in Evans County, Georgia, white farmers had a significantly lower incidence of CHD than nonfarmers. Further, Blacks had a lower incidence of CHD in every occupational category, except share-cropping, than whites. The authors consider that the physical activity differential between farmers and nonfarmers is the most likely distinguishing characteristic, and this characteristic was suggested as the causal factor.

Rosenman,[134] reporting on the incidence of CHD in men participating in the Western Collaboration Group Study (WCG, a prospective study of 3154 healthy men aged 39–59 in 1960–61) found that men with type A behavior patterns who exercised regularly had a CHD incidence that was 60% of those who did not. However, for type B men no such differences was discerned, and type B men as a group, irrespective of exercise levels, had a CHD incidence that was 60% of the regularly exercising type A's, or 37% of the inactive type A's. Brand *et al.*[10] continued this study and in 1976 reported that the multivariate prediction of CHD using the WCGS data correlates strongly with data from the Framingham Study at 12 years follow-up using the Framingham logistic equation. This type of analysis gave an approximate relative risk of 2.0 for type A compared to type B men aged 30–59 years, representing a 31% additional risk from CHD from the factors inherent in type A–type B behavior.

In 1973 Morris *et al.*[94] published a study of the effects of vigorous exercise during leisure time in a cohort of nearly 17,000 male executive-grade British civil service office workers over 40 years of age, who in 1968–70 had been screened by a questionnaire. In the vigorous activity group, only one-third the rate of CHD was manifest compared with the sedentary leisure time controls. Smoking habits were similar in both groups. The authors admit their reluctance to enter into the "triangular debate on how much such findings are attributable to what the men are (their inheritance and experience), how much to what they currently do, how much the latter accounts for the former and how much both are molded by the environment," although they add the caveat that, through exercise, "the fit will thus preserve and enhance fitness."

The Statistical Bulletins of January, June, and September 1975 [149, 151, 152] are of ancillary interest. The June bulletin [151] reported that between 1962 and 1973 heart disease mortality among white insured men decreased about 21.5% (7.6% for white men in the general population), and for insured white women, 2.4% (15.6% for white women in the general population). This differential rate between the general and insured populations is evaluated and discussed by Blackburn [7] who found selective factors operating in the insured population and in the initial risk underwriting process that make this population not representative of the general population. The January Bulletin [149] shows that there exists a mortality ratio of 230% between the lowest and highest social classes (using a total of 5 classes) and also, that the mortality ratio differential between one or more years of college versus less than 8 years of school for white U.S. males aged 25–64 is 50%. Thus, if physical exercise confers some protection against a high mortality, one must be able to demonstrate this possibly small perturbation within the larger effect of social class, since as mentioned previously, "longshoremen don't jog." Finally, a 50% reduction of diseases of the heart has been estimated to result in a 2.9 year potential gain in longevity for the average 45-year-old U.S. male,[152] illustrating the type of estimate that can be made by theoretically altering the risk profile of the general population.

AUTOPSY STUDIES

A number of epidemiological and clinical evaluations of the role of physical exercise in CHD have relied on postmortem studies. In 1958 Reindell, Musshoff, and Klepzig [125] studied the hearts of 34 athletes and 78 controls, and reported the average heart volumes to be 965 and 733 ml, respectively. Karvonen [71] found that the average heart volume of well-trained skiers was 50% greater than that of controls, while Reindell et al.[126] had demonstrated previously that among athletes endurance runners have especially large heart volumes, whereas sprinters have average heart sizes. Spain [144] examined all the deaths caused by artery diseases in a 7-year period in Westchester County, New York and concluded that the men who had engaged in sedentary occupations tended to die from coronary occlusions at a younger age than those whose occupations involved considerable physical activity. Nearly twice the incidence of death from this cause was observed among sedentary men aged 55 as compared with strenuously active men of the same age. Morris et al.[98] reviewed about 5000 reports of deaths from CHD, deaths from diseases associated with CHD, and deaths not normally associated with CHD. The conclusion was reached that those in inactive jobs have less CHD during middle age, and that the disease is less severe and develops later in life. However, Spain and Bradess [143] in a 1960 autopsy study of 207 "normal" white men between the ages of 30 and 60 years, who died suddenly from accident, homicide, or suicide found no significant differences in degree of coronary atherosclerosis in those engaged in sedentary occupations versus physically active occupations.

Currens et al.[27] performed the autopsy on the marathoner Clarence De Mar who died of cancer at the age of 69 and observed his coronary arteries to be about 2 or 3 times the normal cross-sectional area. Whether he became a long distance runner by virtue of this advantage, or whether the large coronary arteries derived from and developed from De Mar's running is not known. A study by Rose et al.[132] comparing autopsy samples from men from light, active, and heavy occupational groups who died from infarcts, with suitable controls, indicated that in the active and heavy occupational groups, arteries were 75% greater in cross-sectional areas than in the controls.

Rissanen [128] studied 172 adult Finnish men who died from violence, accident, suicide, or homicide and evaluated fatty streaks, raised lesions, calcification, and coronary obstructions in different portions of the coronary arteries and the aorta. Although the results were ambiguous, there was a tendency for more severe atherosclerotic involvement of the coronary arteries in the moderately active and sedentary men, in contrast to the active men. The degree of aortic atherosclerosis, however, did not correlate with levels of physical activity, in contrast to recent papers by Mitrani et al.,[91] Morris *et al.*,[98] Möttönen,[102] and Spain *et al.*[143] Raissenen also reported fewer myocardial scars in the hearts of sedentary men than in the more active men, which is in opposition to Morris'[98] findings. The authors did not control for possible differences in smoking habits, social class, and other life habits, but this is not unusual in this type of study, several of which are summarized by the authors.

ATHLETIC STUDIES

It might seem that the proper starting point of studies of physical activity would be the athlete himself, but it is in the area of sports medicine and sports epidemiology that many methodological problems arise. For example, a control group for marathon runners probably should be a cohort that is thin, that does not smoke, that is educationally above average, that consults doctors with above average frequency, and that is probably more careful about their eating habits and general health than the general population. In addition probably few marathoners are employed at jobs entailing high levels of physical activity nor do they work in areas of high levels of occupational exposure to dust and noxious gases. Finally, marathoners almost certainly do not have congenital or rheumatic heart disease, emphysema, neuropathic conditions, diseases of the musculature, nor a host of other debilitating diseases, which the general population does suffer from to some degree. The absence of several other risk factors, be they lower socioeconomic status or congenital heart disease, generally would also be associated with marathon runners. All these considerations invalidate the use of the general population * as the control group for an epidemiological study of marathoners. Hence, self-selection in a study of marathoners represents an intractable problem. The point in mentioning that marathoners in general are probably not exposed to several risk factors is also to emphasize again that the absence of these factors may or may not be a *consequence* of their marathoning. Nevertheless, an estimate of the number of marathoners expected to die from coronary heart disease has been made. Milvy[89] has estimated that the number of deaths per annum expected among the 10,000 U.S. male 1975 marathoners is not statistically different if 0%, 50%, or 100% "protection" from CHD diseases resulted from their participation in this sport.

In specific studies, Dublin[30] in 1932 studied 38,269 men who graduated 27 to 57 years previously, and showed that major athletes, who presumably did not include "students of relatively feeble constitution" had the same life expectancy as their nonathletic colleagues (at age 22), although their life expectancy was about a half a year less at age 42. Academic honor graduates had an increased life expectancy vis-á-vis student controls of 2.0 and 1.6 years at age 22 and 42, respectively. However, the relative "salubrious and sheltered occupations chosen by them (honor graduates) after leaving college" also may be of importance and this and other differences between the athletes

---

* Incidentally, the general population, which of course includes paupers and bankers, has a lower life expectancy than industrial workers, who although exposed to all types of dangerous materials[153] do not include those who are too sick to work. Those that are too sick to be employed represent a subgroup in the general population obviously at increased mortality risk.

and "controls" may be partly responsible for the fact that these college graduates as a group had a 2.4 year greater life expectancy at age 22 as compared with white males from 27 representative U.S. states. On the other hand, a study of 834 Cambridge sportsmen by Rook [129] showed no difference in life expectancy compared with controls, intellectuals or honor list members lived 1.5 years longer, and "heavily built" (this term includes heavily "girthed") men might have shorter lifespan than "light" or "thin" athletes, although the results did not differ significantly. In 1956 Montoye et al.[93] reported that the life expectancy of 629 respondents to a questionnaire sent to 1130 former Michigan State University athletes was not different than that of the controls, although the former athletes smoked and drank considerably more frequently than the control group. A recent article by Montoye [92] reviews various studies of the health and longevity of former athletes. Karvonen [71] reported that champion skiers lived 7 years longer than the corresponding Finnish male population of 15 years of age in 1931–34. Karvonen points to the intensity of this type of exercise, as well as to the many years of participation in the sport that typically characterizes its athletes as possible explanations. A similar study by Karvonen in 1974,[72] which studied the mortality of 396 Finnish championship skiers born between 1845 and 1910, concluded that their life expectancy was nearly 3 years longer than the general population's, that 77% of those still surviving in 1957 continued to ski, and that they had low blood pressure and seldom smoked although they did have the same serum cholesterol and EKG ischemic abnormalities as their matched controls. Karvonen [70] also investigated the effects of vigorous exercise on the heart (volume, EKG conduction times, and voltages) using Finnish male champion skiers as his subjects. Former Finnish champion cross-country skiers, as well as endurance runners aged 40 or over, constitute the group examined by Pyörälä et al.[121, 122] for a host of physiological and epidemiological parameters. The control group was (roughly) matched Helsinki male residents (see also Karvonen[62]). Among a large number of findings it was noted that "Ischemic changes occur with the same frequency in former athletics and the general population."

In the study of Polednak and Damon [114] of 2090 Harvard students, it was found that letter winners in "major" varsity sports had the lowest life expectancies, athletes who did not win letters in these same sports had the longest life expectancies, and the nonathletic controls had intermediate life expectancies. The incidence of major diseases was similar for all three categories. It was also found that men with three or more letters died slightly earlier and significantly more frequently from cardiovascular disease and CHD than men with one or two letters. Although this study also showed lettermen to be fatter, more muscular, and stockier than the other group, this variable was more carefully examined in three papers by Polednak [115-117] using the same cohort. The data suggest that life-style and psychosocial factors may be important.[115] However, these data [116] suggest that "differences in all studies are small, but the consistency in trend is impressive [and] may be explained in part if not entirely by physique." Polednak [117] also discusses a paper by Schnohr [137] on Danish male athletic champions, which reported that mortality after age 50 is unaffected by past athletic performance, but prior to this age it is reduced significantly. Self-selection might be particularly manifest here: "the group of athletic champions contained only individuals in excellent health." Prout's 1972 article [118] on Life Expectancy of College Oarsmen also observed increased life expectancy (6.3 years) in the athletes (compared with randomly selected classmates) and notes that "obviously the oarsmen were in good condition to begin with, otherwise they would not have been picked." A study by the Statistical Bureau of the Metropolitan Life Insurance Company [150] shows that major league baseball players had a favorable mortality significantly below that for men born in the same years in the general population. Somewhat curiously, those players who played less than 5 years had a mortality ratio 18% lower than those who had played 5 years or longer, raising the suspicion that other variables may well be important.

STUDIES OF MI AND CHD PATIENTS—MI DURING EXERCISE

The studies of medical treatment of physically active men who suffer an MI during exercise, of controlled physical exercise in the rehabilitation of MI patients, and of the treatment of CHD patients are distinct from studies that set as their goals the assessment of the role of physical exercise in postponing and retarding the development of CHD. Nevertheless, these investigations are related to the more general area under review, and are derived from the epidemiological studies that were first to focus on the problem of the possible significance to mortality of relative physical inactivity.

Weinblatt *et al.*[167] in the 1960s evaluated the prognosis of men enrolled in New York HIP after they had experienced a first MI. A total of 881 predominantly white men with a first MI during a 4-year period were observed in terms of their overall mortality and their first MI recurrence. This cohort was followed for 4.5 years and it was observed that 31% died within 24 hours of the first MI, an additional 5% within the next month and 48% of the cohort had died by 4.5 years postinfarct. Men who were physically active had about twice the likelihood of surviving 1 month post-MI as did the physically inactive men. After the initial 1 month post-MI interval, no long-term disadvantages were observed among physically inactive men.

A program for the rehabilitation of cardiac patients (preponderantly patients with ischemic heart disease) through graded exercise had been conducted in Israel since 1955 by Gottheimer.[54] A total of 1,103 trainees, half of whom had experienced an MI and half with coronary insufficiency, formed the basis of the data gathered after 5 years of observation. The mortality rate was 3.6% for the 5-year interval compared with 12% in a "comparable" series of physically inactive "postinfarction" patients. Whether a group of postinfarction patients are comparable to a group of patients only half of whom had experienced an MI seems dubious, but this study does suggest the efficacy of physical exercise in the management of post-MI patients. Wilhelmsen *et al.*[169] also analyzed the influence of supervised physical training on death and nonfatal reinfarction in a nonselected series of 315 patients 55 years or younger hospitalized for a myocardial infarction. After one year, the exercise group had improved physical working capacity, their blood pressure was lower, but their blood lipids were not different. During 4 years of follow-up, although patients who attended the training program showed lower mortality than matched controls, the differences were not statistically significant.

Space does not permit the discussion of several papers written prior to Gottheimer's paper, but a paper by Hirsch *et al.*[61] reporting experiences with a group of 656 white, middle-aged, middle-class males, including 254 with atherosclerotic heart disease (angina and/or documented MI) should be mentioned, since the design of a rehabilitation program is discussed. Hellerstein [61] also reports on an 8-year prospective study to enhance the physical fitness of a cohort of 656 middle-aged men, one third of whom had CHD. Relevant general questions and approaches to exercise in health and disease are considered in another paper by Hellerstein.[62] More recently, Taylor et al.,[159] Pyörälä et al.,[121, 122] and Taraslinna et al.[163] also studied the propriety of exercise in the prevention of CHD. A case report of cardiac arrest suffered during exercise rehabilitation after a history of 2 MIs is discussed by Pyfer et al.,[120] and two other similar incidents are discussed by Cantwell et al.,[16] prompting an editorial addressed to the theme of joggers and CHD.[127] A chapter by Lown and Kosowsky in Exercise and the Heart [82] discusses several of the lethal complications of exercise, while Cooper [23, 24] outlines guidelines for the management of the exercising patient. Bruce and Kluge [14] present seven cases of exertional cardiac arrest and discuss the defibrillatory procedures to which all the patients responded successfully. Rechnitzer et al.[124] discuss the design of a prospective study of an exercise program designed to improve the survival rate of a group of 285 men (140 in a lower intensity exercise control group) who had survived a first MI.

A recent article by Green et al.[55] discusses the case history of a 44-year-old trained marathoner who collapsed during the 1973 Boston marathon and died after 50 days of coma. EKG evidence of extensive MI was documented. The suspicion exists that the relatively high temperature (23° C) and "high" humidity produced hyperthermia and that this condition precipitated the collapse and concurrent massive MI. A number of letters in 1975 and 1976 bearing on the subject of exercise, particularly running, and sudden death among athletes have also appeared.[17, 28, 105-107]

Scientific and Medical Studies

The papers in this section, although several are epidemiological in design, concentrate on the physiological and biological mechanisms that operate in the development of the disease processes themselves and the modification of these mechanisms in the presence (or absence) of risk factors.

Research studies on animals are extensive and a few may be mentioned: the experiments of Leon and Bloor [79, 80] on the effect of daily and intermittent exercise (swimming) and its cessation on body weight, heart size, cross-sectional luminal area of extracoronary collateral and coronary arteries, and capillary-ventricular muscle fiber ratios in young male rats demonstrated that exercise resulted in reduced body weight and in cardiac hypertrophy, increased myocardial capillary density and in increased cross-sectional luminal areas during the initial 10 weeks of training. Subsequent and partial deconditioning was then compared with complete deconditioning and continued conditioning. The continued conditioning did not suppress weight gain, but did prevent excessive weight gain associated with deconditioning. The full exercise program was required for maintenance of cardiac hypertrophy, although more modest exercise sessions permitted the maintenance of extracoronary collateral arteries. The effects of age on these parameters was also investigated by observing the effect of several exercise regimens on young, adult, and old male rats.[9] In all exercise groups body weight was less than in the controls; cardiac hypertrophy, present in intermittently and daily exercised young animals, appeared only in the intensively exercised adults; and cardiac muscle mass was lost in the old exercised animals. Extracoronary collateral artery areas developed in all age groups with exercise, but in all age groups this development was maximal in the intermediate exercise groups. On the other hand, Leon *et al.*[81] have reported that norepinephrine levels did not change in exercised rats, although exercise results in hypertrophied hearts. Apparently conflicting results had been reported previously. Saltzman *et al.*[135] reported that mice exercised for 9 weeks on activity wheels had, in addition to a greater heart/body weight ratio than the unexercised controls, decreased epinephrine uptake per milligram of ventricular tissue, although total ventricular uptake was not different. The inference was advanced that dilution of cardiac binding sites for epinephrine occurs, concomitantly with ventricular hypertrophy.

The physiological, morphological, metabolic, and hemodynamic changes that occur in the heart and its vasculature during prolonged physical exercise or in its absence, or as a consequence of other risk factors, are discussed in several surveys. Cumming's review[26] concentrates on the response of the cardiovascular system to exercise. Fox,[40] in addition to reviewing cardiovascular mechanisms, also briefly reviews blood chemistry, clotting and fibrinolytic activity, autonomic regulation, psychic stress, and other parameters; and Mitchell,[90] in a review of exercise training in the treatment of CHD, discusses many of these same physiological categories in the normal heart and in the heart already suffering from CHD. Two papers on stress EKGs[15, 29] address themselves to the analysis of ST segment responses and their hemodynamic determinants during physical exercise in patients with CHD before and after physical training and in healthy middle-aged American and Chinese (Taiwan) men. The first paper involves the quantitization of EKG data while the second paper reports that physical training, unlike nitroglycerin, does not alter the relationship of the magnitude of ST segment depression during exercise to the blood-pressure heart rate product. The study concluded that ST segment changes result not from changes in myocardial blood supply, but from changes in the hemodynamic responses of the heart to exercise. A recent book titled *Stress Testing* by Ellestand[32] discusses stress testing in the coronary patient. An interesting report of ST depression at moderate work load in a young athlete with normal coronary arteries led Frick *et al.*[50] to employ myocardial scintigraphy to discern a perfusion defect.

A review article by Katz in 1967[73] examined the benefits of a physical training program, enumerating benefits to several body systems. Katz accepts that there is no proof that exercises reduces human morbidity and mortality, and he raises a number of interesting questions related to the efficacy of physical training.

Frick[49] reviews changes in several indices of cardiac function involving the hemodynamic effects of physical training and concludes that training affects cardiac oxygen requirements so that in any given stressful situation the oxygen requirements of the trained heart are less than those of the untrained heart. Frick believes "that there is no effect on mortality statistics, except for the possibility that in the trained subject with chronic CHD more time elapses before the oxygen supply/demand ratio of the heart becomes critical," and "the results from prevalence studies are influenced, since with the same coronary artery status the trained heart is less liable to show signs of ischemia . . . [especially if] the diagnosis of CHD is made on the basis of a history of angina. . . . If the lower exercise heart rate of the physically fit subjects in the [epidemiological] sample is neglected, a false picture is likely to be obtained of the relation between physical activity and CHD." This latter point would seem to be important and appears to have been inadequately investigated. The mean total vital capacity was shown by Friedman *et al.*[51] to be a predictor of a subsequent first MI. Raskoff *et al.*[123] have evaluated the prevalence and importance of physiological left ventricular hypertrophy (LVH) in 30 long distance runners and used echocardiographic, EKG, and treadmill evidence to distinguish this type of LVH from pathological LVH when ischemic ST segment depression was observed during treadmill stress. Cooper *et al.*,[25] in a cross-sectional study, documented an inverse relationship between levels of physical fitness as measured by treadmill performance and a variety of physiological measurements. However, the effect of physical activity on some of these risk factors has also been summarized recently,[1] and it was stated "there appears to be little or no effect of physical activity on serum cholesterol or blood pressure but other results suggest that leisure time physical activity lowers serum triglycerides; this may be important in view of the recent emphasis being placed on elevated triglycerides as a coronary risk factor. On the other hand the protective effect of physical activity may be mediated via an improvement in cardiopulmonary conditioning." Mann[84] discussed the amount of exercise necessary to achieve and then maintain fitness in adults, where fitness is defined as the ability to do work, at maximal treadmill levels. An extensive review of the literature relevant to an assessment of the comparative cardiovascular adaptation to exercise in animals and men and its relevance to CHD is provided by Leon.[78] The use of the supine 12-lead EKG in conjunction with the exercise stress test to predict the future incidence of CHD among men 40–59 years of age was reported by Blackburn *et al.*[8] in 1970. These workers related the future risk of CHD to major and minor Q and QS complexes, T-wave abnormalities, block patterns, atrial fibrillation, sinus tachycardias, and other irregularities. In the absence of exercise, certain large Q and QS patterns (1.1 by the Minnesota code criteria) correlate well with future CHD and are accepted as indicative of new CHD events. ST segment depression during stress testing, with none at rest, was shown to be predictive of future CHD in U.S. men, but not in non-U.S. men.

REVIEW OF REVIEWS

Although research in the area of prevention of, and therapy for CHD through physical activity is only about a decade old, and although the accumulation of the evidence that points—tenuously—to physical inactivity as a risk factor in the development of CHD has occurred mainly during the last two decades, this area of scientific and medical investigation ·and practice is well established, viable, and active. Several dozen reviews have now appeared. The following listing and review will present the early review articles primarily published in the later 1960s, and will also attempt to categorize in terms of purpose and sophistication the review articles of this present decade.

A review entitled "The Epidemiology of Coronary Heart Disease" by Epstein[34] gives a presentation of the risk factors that have been associated with the incidence of CHD and mortality, and also discusses mortality studies, pathology, prevalence, and preventive approaches. A historical approach to the etiology of CHD by Michaels[88] appeared in 1966, suggesting that it was not the inadequate sophistication of the medical profession that led to its failure to record the existence of CHD until the publication of Heberden's paper[59] in 1772,† but rather the lack of a population at significant risk until the present century. Michaels also attempts to isolate the risk factor most probably responsible for the development of the disease. He argues against the relevance of physical activity in the etiology of CHD.

In 1966, Karvonen[69] reviewed the limited literature that directly concerned itself with the relationship of habitual physical activity to diseases of the cardiovascular system, citing epidemiological studies of mortality and morbidity. Reviewing similar studies is a paper by Fox and Haskell,[41] and Fox and Paul[45] present the arguments on the relationship between physical activity and CHD. Fox *et al.*[44] in 1971 and Fox *et al.*[42] in 1972 published similar reviews, which contain summaries of existing epidemiological data and discuss the possible mechanisms for the protection effect and, finally, provide two useful appendices (Appendix 1 contains the criteria to be used for allowing middle-aged individuals to begin strenuous activity after an extended sedentary existence and Appendix 2 provides approximate metabolic intensities for different physical activities). A similar review by Fox *et al.*[43] appeared in 1972, while in 1974 Haskell and Fox[58] again reviewed the pertinent literature with a view towards evaluating active intervention designed to introduce sedentary adults to a more physically active life. Morris[99] gives a skeptical review of 25 years of modern research into the etiology of CHD and the guidelines that have developed for its prevention. Citing the "appallingly difficult [CHD] prevention experiments" in which several risk factors in addition to physical inactivity are removed, Morris states that "there is no proof that by altering behavior in accord with the results of the observational studies which have been carried out . . . individual risk and population incidence will be lowered." Morris concludes that although it would not be "pusillenimous" to suggest that in view of this we do nothing, nevertheless perseverance may eventually provide knowledge that can be of practical applicability and benefit.

The analysis of 35 epidemiological studies on the possible association between CHD and physical inactivity is presented by Froelicher and Oberman.[52] All studies are discussed in terms of experimental design, methodology for assessing levels of physical activity, evaluation of risk factors, and diagnostic criteria. The authors conclude that "analysis of the data regarding physical inactivity as a risk factor, although suggestive, remains tenuous and should not supersede efforts directed towards the major risk factors" (of hypercholesterolemia, smoking, and hypertension). A general review, not detailed, but presented with an adequate discussion of pertinent ancillary and peripheral areas, is presented in Chapter 17 of Shepherd's *Alive Man*.[141] However, only general references are cited.

An extensive review by Bruce[13] of the literature that focuses on the possible benefits of a physical training regimen to the CHD patient has appeared re-

---

† The first mention of CHD disease, the medical description of a new disease entity designated "angina pectoris," was made by William Heberden[59] in the Medical Transactions of the Royal College of Physician of London in 1772. It was based on about 20 cases of this disease seen by Heberden over several decades. Heberden accurately describes the symptoms of the disease, identifies those that are at risk (men over 50 years of age, "inclined" to be fat), and inaccurately suggests that it "may partly proceed" from an "ulcer," and that "the heart is not affected by it"; he did not "see anyone who had died of it." (See also Michaels.[88])

cently. The review summarizes animal studies that observed cardiovascular changes with activity, epidemiological studies, physiological studies, and studies of changes in personality and psychological profile that result from activity, and it presents the clinical experience of exercise programs in cardiac rehabilitation programs, and finally presents clinical guidelines and criteria for the physical training of cardiac patients. The review concludes that although physical training of coronary patients is a plausible approach to the treatment of ischemic heart disease, "lacking appropriately controlled studies, long-term effects on life expectancy are not well established." Stamler et al.[146] present the findings of eight studies undertaken during the years beginning in 1951, in which they review the possible role of physical activity and fitness in the prevention of CHD. These studies lead the authors to conclude that these types of "first generation primary prevention studies seem to suggest an apparently positive prophylactic effect on mortality" but warn that these conclusions are "preliminary, tentative and guarded." In another recent paper, Stamler[145] reviews the design, data, and conclusions of four "first generation" studies of primary prevention of CHD. The four studies, the New York Anti-Coronary Club, the Finnish Mental Hospital Study, the Los Angeles Veterans Administration Domicillary Center Study, and the Chicago Coronary Prevention Evaluation Programme, indicate that changes in living habits, particularly changes in diet and smoking, are associated with a decreased incidence and/or mortality from myocardial infarction and CHD. These studies do not emphasize the role of physical inactivity as a risk factor.

Blackburn[4] in a review of the literature relevant to the use of exercise therapy after MI cites many studies and presents evidence and arguments that can be used to conclude that such therapy is disadvantageous, at worst, or impotent and benign at best. Thus, although short-term therapy seems promising, long-term studies are less clear-cut. For example, although increased coronary collaterals are cited in one study of chronically exercised dogs, a more recent experiment could not duplicate these findings; and, although some studies show less ST segment depression at a particular work load in coronary patients, in general this is not observed. Blackburn raises a number of questions concerning the propriety of exercise therapy for post-MI patients, but these questions can only be answered by hard data, requiring by Blackburn's estimate the cooperation of 2,665 post-MI, 5-year-exercised surviving patients.

A general review of ischemic heart disease by Fejfar[35] outlines many of the problems of past studies and indicates how current studies and plans for future studies are attempting to confront these problems, often by using multinational and multivariate approaches. This review is general, but the pertinence of physical activity is not ignored (see also Blackburn[5] ‡).

Several reviews of the literature of physical activity and its relationship to mortality in general and to CHD in particular can be regarded as in a class by themselves. Thus, in a 1966 review of the problems inherently associated with epidemiological studies, Taylor et al.[162] noted that a morbidity and mortality ratio in physically active compared with sedentary groups is perhaps of the order of 0.5, small enough that the many confounding variables, which too often unavoidably (although sometimes unnecessarily) intrude themselves on

---

‡ A book devoted to the role of exercise in the prevention diagnosis and treatment of CHD has also appeared recently.[38]

the data, may strongly influence the conclusions of the studies. Also, since the U.S. CHD incidence (one of the highest in the world) is still low compared with the number of middle-aged men at risk (approximately 4 MIs and 4 new anginas per year, per 1000 males at age 50), small errors in techniques can too easily obscure, or reverse, the findings and conclusions of a study. Considerations of sample size, duration of observations, and withdrawal and retirement rates (which may differ in the active and sedentary subsamples of the study) are all discussed, with data drawn from Taylor's 1962 U.S. railway employees study,[160] as well as from other studies. Two critical reviews by Keys [75, 76] discuss many of the best known studies of physical activity and CHD and demonstrate that "at best it [is] extremely difficult to evaluate the influence of physical activity on susceptibility to CHD. The task [is] impossible, unless such evidence as may be available is analyzed more critically than has characterized too many investigations." Thus, problems of job transfers (almost invariably from active to less active positions), failure to consider racial and ethnic compositions of populations at risk, assumptions that observed blood pressure and cholesterol differences are caused by differential physical activities, cohorts that are statistically too small, unduly loading populations with prime candidates for heart attacks, and inaccurate indices of physical activity are some of the weaknesses Keys identifies in the studies he evaluates in his 1970 paper.[75] His 1975 review [76] is more general in focus and attempts to summarize the current epidemiological knowledge of CHD. The different frequencies of CHD in different populations are presented and possible explanations for these different frequencies are examined. The various risk factors including physical inactivity are also considered. Critical evaluations of a substantial number of well-known studies in this field are made, all too often demonstrating the serious weaknesses that are evident in many of these studies. Some of these shortcomings are inherent in the subject matter, others only in the conception, design, and realization of the experimental approach. The most recent review of "physical activity and CHD" appeared as Chapter 16 in *Controversy in Cardiology* by Fox.[39] It provides evidence for and against the hypothesis that physical activity is a significant risk factor, cites studies that are particularly relevant to angina, reviews autopsy studies, studies of athletic training and CHD, levels of physical activity and CHD, and postinfarct physical training and regimens, and devotes an extensive section to the physiological effects of physical training. Fox concludes that "although the hypothesis that such (physical) activities are capable of postponing or decreasing coronary morbidity and mortality remains unproven, the practitioner can recommend participation on the basis of data indicating almost predictable improvement in performance and feeling states with an acceptably low hazard to those properly screened."

DISCUSSION

The relationship between physical activity and health represents an interesting and important problem, and the earlier discussion along with the literature cited illustrate the difficulties of designing the appropriate experiments to establish a cause-and-effect relationship. In fact, such experiments are almost impossible to carry out. Therefore a critical evaluation of the available evidence must be relied upon to arrive at a reasonable judgment.

In this regard, it is worthwhile to note that this is a problem that is also faced with respect to other epidemiological studies when controlled experiments are not feasible. For example, although the relationships of smoking and health have been fully investigated over many years [56, 165, 170] and the adverse effects of smoking on health are now generally accepted, the relationships between smoking and some specific disease entities, such as specific clinical manifestations of arteriosclerosis, are not clear. Also, there remains the possibility that subgroups of populations exist for whom smoking may not be especially harmful. For example, the risk of CHD for an older population, whose levels of other risk factors are relatively low, may not be raised appreciably by smoking. Also in younger populations the possibility exists that the lack of certain detoxifying enzymes might, because of genetic variability, be at very low levels in lung tissue, thus placing these smokers at a decreased risk of lung cancer.

Similarly, the physiological and pathological consequences of exercise in subgroups of a population may be very different, and also the type of exercise undertaken may have different effects for different subpopulations. This point has been hinted at in a number of studies such as those of Paffenbarger [110] and Morris.[94]

Because of the inherent difficulty of defining and measuring physical activity and health, various hypotheses can be formulated, which again are difficult to test quantitatively. One can illustrate this by an example: Longshoremen, athletes, and in general individuals involved in any strenuous occupations or activity will expend more calories per day on average than will those involved in sedentary activities. The form in which this extra food energy is obtained represents an effect that is confounded with the effect of physical activity, and moreover, could account for the lower CHD incidence in certain physically active groups. In this connection, it may be noted that Keys [76] suggests that physically active kibbutzim workers may obtain extra energy by increasing their intake of food high in carbohydrates. Hence, the possibility that the physically active increase the ratio of dietary carbohydrates to saturated fats (by increased carbohydrate consumption) and by virtue of this *relative* decrease in fats are protected from CHD, may be put forward as an hypothesis that may account for the assumed inverse relationship between physical activity and CHD. Such a hypothesis is consistent with studies of certain native groups (e.g., New Guineans [142] who consume diets consisting almost entirely of carbohydrates and for whom atherosclerosis and related disorders (e.g., hypertension, hypercholesterolemia) are rare. However, it should be noted that the hypothesis, in this form, and without further defining the type of carbohydrate (simple or complex) is vague since there is evidence that excessive dietary carbohydrates will produce hypertriglyceridemia, although different carbohydrates may have different effects.[77, 103] Also, there is some evidence that a relatively low consumption of food generally may protect against CHD, irrespective of the type of food.[85] Finally there are studies that conclude that sugar consumption itself may represent a CHD risk factor [171] although sugar consumption and cigarette consumption are positively correlated.[1, 3, 33] In addition, there are many confounding factors, which have been stressed in the previous discussion, such as that more active persons may smoke less, may be less obese, and may have a better life-style than other subgroups of a population, and such factors may be more important than the relative amounts of carbohydrates in the diet. Indeed, their concern for a better life-style may be the independent variable that motivates these individuals to eat better, not to smoke, and to be more active. Hence the indefiniteness of the hypothesis, like the hypotheses postulating a causal connection between a stressful style of living and CHD, which have been mentioned previously, makes it extremely difficult to test quantitatively. These considerations illustrate the difficulty of testing a reasonable hypothesis. That is, the multifactorial causes of heart disease and their interactions make it easy to postulate a hypothesis but difficult to affirm or refute it since data from properly designed trials are not available. Consequently, one must frequently rely on the criteria that a hypothesis is judged reasonable if the assumptions required to be consistent with it are minimal.

In summary, there are a number of factors that may explain the association between physical inactivity and CHD mortality, many of which have been mentioned in this paper. A number of these factors are highly correlated but arguing from cause to effect in the absence of appropriate clinical trials is tenuous. One important point that has been stressed by many authors is that those who engage in regular physical activity represent a self-selected group who may be, in some sense, genetically different and/or may follow a more favorable life-style. However, the question whether a particular subgroup of a population would be better off in terms of life expectancy or reduced morbidity if they were to engage in running or any other specific type of physical activity is much less clear. Also, it might be argued that, from the point of view of reducing CHD incidence, it may be more desirable to reduce the well-established risk factors, particularly those that lend themselves to active intervention such as cigarette smoking; of course one approach does not preclude others.

Although the evidence can probably never be entirely clear-cut as to whether a specific type of exercise for a particular person will exert a protective effect against CHD, at some stage it is necessary to make a decision on the basis of the available data so that appropriate advice can be given to real people living in the real world. Such advice should also be in relative terms, in the sense that priorities can be attached to the various benefits that might be expected from altering a person's life-style. For example, on the basis of available evidence, it is generally agreed that cessation of smoking is beneficial for human health, although it is not clear whether cessation of smoking is beneficial to every member of a population, and the statement is known to be more valid for cigarette smoking than, for example, for pipe smoking. The case for physical activity would seem to be much weaker. This follows partly because the relationship between smoking and health, compared with the relationship of physical inactivity and health is more precise: There are not too many forms of smoking, and these are relatively easy to define and measure. In addition, many of the effects of smoking are fairly specific, such as the occurrence of lung cancer. And lung cancer is statistically rare in a nonsmoking population: it is basically not caused by exposure to other environmental entities.

With respect to the relationship between physical activity and mortality (specifically mortality from CHD), perhaps the balance of the evidence indicates that exercise may well be beneficial to most members of the population. It must be emphasized, however, that this inference is based upon evidence that has accumulated—much of it reviewed in this paper—that demonstrates the existence of correlations and not causal relationships between mortality and physical inactivity.

REFERENCES

1. AUSTRALIAN ACADEMY OF SCIENCE. 1975. Diet and Coronary Heart Disease. Netley, South Australia.
2. BELLOC, N. B. 1973. Relationship of health practices and mortality. Preventive Med. **2:** 67–81.
3. BENNET, A. E., R. DOLL & R. W. HOWELL. 1970. Sugar consumption and cigarette smoking. Lancet **i:** 1011–1014.
4. BLACKBURN, H. 1974. Disadvantages of intensive exercises therapy after myocardial infarction. *In* Controversy in Internal Medicine. F. J. Ingelfinger, R. V. Ebert, M. Finland & A. S. Relman, Eds. Vol. **2:** 162–172. W. B. Saunders Co. Philadelphia.
5. BLACKBURN, H. 1976. Concepts and controversies about the prevention of coronary heart disease. *In Cardiovascular Problems.* H. I. Russek, Ed. : 123–137. University Park Press. Baltimore, Md.
6. BLACKBURN, H. 1972. Multifactor preventive trails (MPT) in coronary heart disease. *In* Trends in Epidemiology. G. T. Stwart, Ed. Charles C Thomas, Publisher. Springfield, Ill.
7. BLACKBURN, H. & R. W. PARLIN. 1966. Antecedents of disease: Insurance mortality experience. Ann. N.Y. Acad. Sci. **134:** 965–1017.
8. BLACKBURN, H., H. L. TAYLOR & A. KEYS. 1970. The electrocardiogram in prediction of five year coronary heart disease. Circulation **41** (Suppl. 1): 154–161.
9. BLOOR, C. M. & A. S. LEON. 1970. Interaction of age and exercise on the heart and its blood supply. Lab. Invest. **22**(2): 160–165.
10. BRAND, R. J., R. H. ROSENMAN, R. I. SCHOLTZ & M. FRIEDMAN. 1976. Multivarite prediction on coronary heart disease in the Western Collaborative Group Study compared to the findings of the Framingham Study. Circulation **53:** 348–355.
11. BRESLOW, L. & P. BUELL. 1960. Mortality from coronary heart disease and physical activity of work in California. J. Chronic Dis. **11:** 421–444.
12. BROWN, R. G., L. A. G. DAVIDSON, T. McKEOWN & A. G. W. WHITFIELD. 1957. Coronary artery disease. Influences affecting its incidence in males in the seventh decade. Lancet (Nov. 30) : 1073–1077.
13. BRUCE, R. A. 1974. The benefits of physical training for patients with coronary heart disease. *In* Controversy in Internal Medicine. F. J. Ingelfinger, R. V. Ebert, M. Finland & A. S. Relman, Eds. Vol. **2:** 145–161.
14. BRUCE, R. A. & W. KLUGE. 1971. Defibrillatory treatment of exertional cardiac arrest in coronary disease. **216:** 653–658.
15. BRUCE, R. A. & J. A. MAZZARELLA. 1966. Computer quantiation of ST responses to maximal exercise in middle-aged American and Chinese men. *In* International Symposium on Physical Activity in Health and Disease. K. Evang & K. L. Anderson, Eds. : 90–102. The Williams and Wilkins Company. Baltimore, Md.
16. CANTWELL, J. D. & G. F. FLETCHER. 1969. Cardiac complications while jogging. J. Amer. Med. Assoc. **210:** 130–131.
17. CARRUTHERS, M., P. DIXON & A. MURRAY. 1975. Safe Sport. Lancet **i:** 447 (letter).
18. CASSEL, J. 1974. Psychosocial processes and "stress": Theoretical formulation. Int. J. Health Serv. **4:** 471–482.
19. CASSEL, J., S. HEYDEN & A. G. BARTEL, B. H. KAPLAN, H. A. TYROLER, J. C. CORONI & C. G. HAMES. 1971. Occupational and physical activity and coronary heart disease. Arch. Intern. Med. **128:** 920–928.
20. CASSEL, J. 1974. An epidemiological perspective of psychosomal factors in disease etiology. Amer. J. Public Health **64:** 1040–1043.

21. CHAPMAN, J. M., L. S. GOERKE & W. DXON. 1957. Measuring the risk of coronary heart disease in adult population group IV. Clinical status of a population in Los Angeles under observation for two or three years. Amer. J. Pub. Health **47** (Special Suppl): 33.

22. CLARK, V. A. & C. E. HOPKINS. 1967. Time is of the essence (editorial). J. Chronic Dis. **20:** 565–569.

23. COOPER, K. H. 1970. Guidelines in the management of the exercising patient. J. Amer. Med. Assoc. **211:** 1663–1667.

24. COOPER, K. H. 1968. A means of assessing maximum oxygen intake. Correlation between field and treadmill testing. J. Amer. Med. Assoc. **203:** 201–204.

25. COOPER, K. H., M. L. POLLOCK, R. P. MARTIN, S. R. WHITE, A. C. LINNERUD & A. JACKSON. 1976. Physical fitness levels vs. selected coronary risk factors. J. Amer. Med. Assoc. **236**(2): 166–169.

26. CUMMING, G. R. 1963. The heart and physical exercise. Can. Med. Assoc. J. **88:** 80–85.

27. CURRENS, J. H. & P. D. WHITE. 1961. Half of a century of running. Clinical physiologic and autopsy findings in the case of Clarence De Mar ("Mr. Marathon") N. Eng. J. Med. **265:** 988–993.

28. DAYTON, S. 1975. Long distance running and sudden death (Letter). (Other letters by Lionel H. Opie). N. Eng. J. Med. **293**(18): 941.

29. DENTRY, J. M. & R. A. BRUCE. 1971. Effects of physical training on exertional S–T segment depression in coronary heart disease. Circulation **44:** 390–396.

30. DUBLIN, L. I. 1932. College honor men long-lived. Statist. Bull. **13:** 5–7.

31. DUBOS, R. 1968. The human environment in technological societies. Rockefeller Rev. July–Aug.

32. ELLESTAND, M. H. 1975. Complications of exercise. *In* Stress Testing. : 212–215. F. A. Davis Co. Philadelphia, Pa.

33. ELWOOD, P. C., S. MOORE, W. E. WATERS & P. SWEETMAN. 1970. Sucrose consumption and ischaemic heart-disease in the community. Lancet **i:** 1014–1016.

34. EPSTEIN, F. H. 1964. The epidemiology of coronary heart disease. Prepared for the Second National Conference on Cardiovascular Diseases. Washington, D.C. November, 1964.

35. FEJFAR, Z. 1975. Prevention against ischaemic heart disease: A critical review. *In* Modern trends in Cardiology, M. F. Oliver, Ed. Vol. **3:** 465–499. Butterworths. Boston, Mass.

36. FISHER, R. A. 1966. The Design of Experiments. 8th edit. Hafner. New York, N.Y.

37. FJORSSMAN, O. & B. LINDEGÅRD. 1958. The post-coronary patient. J. Psychosom. Res. **3:** 89–169.

38. FLETCHER, G. F. & J. D. CANTWELL. 1974. Exercise and Coronary Heart Disease in Prevention, Diagnosis, Treatment. Charles C Thomas, Publisher. Springfield, Ill.

39. FOX, S. M. III. 1976. Physical activity and coronary heart disease. *In* Controversy in Cardiology. E. K. Chang, Ed. : 201–219. Springer Verlag. New York, N.Y.

40. FOX, S. M. III & W. L. HASKELL. 1966. Physical activity and health maintenance. J. Rehab. **32:** 89–92.

41. FOX, S. M. III & W. L. HASKELL. 1968. Physical activity and prevention of coronary heart disease. Bull. N.Y. Acad. Med. **44:** 950–967.

42. FOX, S. M. & J. P. NAUGHTON. 1972. Physical activity and the prevention of coronary heart disease. Prevent. Med. **1:** 92–120.

43. FOX, S. M. III, J. P. NAUGHTON & P. A. GORMAN. 1972. Physical activity and cardiovascular health. Modern Concepts of Cardiovascular disease. Amer. Heart Assoc. **41**(4): 17–20.

44. FOX, S. M. III, J. P. NAUGHTON & W. L. HASKELL. 1971. Physical activity and prevention of coronary heart disease. Ann. Clin. Res. **3:** 404–432.

45. Fox, S. M. III & O. Paul. 1969. Physical activity and coronary heart disease. Amer. J. Cardiol. **23:** 298–306.
46. Frank, C. W. 1968. The course of coronary heart disease factor relating to prognosis. Bull. N.Y. Acad. Med. **44:** 900–914.
47. Frank, C. W., E. Weinblatt, S. Shapiro & R. V. Sager. 1966. Physical inactivity as a lethal factor in myocardial infarction among men. Circulation **34:** 1022–1033.
48. Frank, C. W., E. Weinblatt, S. Shapiro & R. V. Sager. 1966. Myocardial infarction in men. J. Amer. Med. Assoc. **198**(12): 103–107 and 1241–45.
49. Frick, M. H. 1968. Coronary implications of hemodynamic changes caused by physical training. Amer. J. Cardiol. **22:** 417–425.
50. Frick, M. H., O. Korhola, M. Neiminen & J. Valle. 1975. Ischaemic electocardigraphic changes in an athlete with normal coronary arteries. Ann. Clin. Res. **4:** 264–268.
51. Friedman, G. D., A. L. Klatsky & A. M. Siegelbaum. 1976. Lung function and sudden cardiac death. N. Eng. J. Med. **294:** 1071–1075.
52. Froelicher, V. P. & A. Oberman. 1972. Analysis of epidemiologic studies in physical inactivity as risk factor for coronary artery disease. Prog. Cardiovasc. Dis. **15**(1, July/August): 41–65.
53. Giger, H. J. 1976. The tasks of community medicine. The Sciences **16**(3): 23–26.
54. Gottheiner, U. 1968. Long-range strenuous sport training for cardiac reconditioning and rehabilitation. Amer. J. Cardiol. **22:** 426–435.
55. Green, L. H., L. C. Stafford & G. Kurland. 1976. Fatal myocardial infarction in marathon racing. Ann. Intern. Med. **84:** 704–706.
56. Hammond, E. C. 1966. Smoking in relation to death rates in one million men and women. NCI Monograph 19. January, 1966.
57. Hammond, E. C. & L. Garfinkel. 1969. Coronary heart disease, stroke and aortic aneurysm. Arch. Env. Health **19:** 167–182.
58. Haskell, W. & S. M. Fox, III. 1974. Physical activity in the prevention and therapy of cardiovascular disease. *In* Science and Medicine of Exercise and Sport. 2nd edit. W. R. Johnson & E. R. Buskirk, Eds. : 455–468. Harper and Row. New York, N.Y.
59. Heberden, W. 1772. Some accounts of a disorder of the breast. Med. Trans. R. Coll. Phys. London **2:** 59–67.
60. Hellerstein, H. K. 1976. Phys. Sports Med. (August) : 68.
61. Hellerstein, H. K. 1969. Exercise and treatment of heart disease. J. South Carolina Med. Assoc. (December Suppl.) : 45–56.
62. Hellerstein, H. K. 1969. Relation of exercise to acute myocardial infarction. Circulation **39–40** (Suppl. IV): 124–129.
63. Henry, J. P., J. P. Meeham & P. M. Stephens. 1967. The use of psychosocial stimuli to induce prolonged hypertension in mice. Psychosom. Med. **29:** 408–432.
64. Hirsch, E. Z., H. K. Hellerstein & C. A. McLeod. 1969. Physical training and coronary heart disease. *In* Exercise and the Heart. R. L. Morse, Ed. : 106. Charles C Thomas, Publisher. Springfield, Ill.
65. Hickey, N., R. Mulcany, G. J. Bourke, I. Grahan & K. Wilson–Davis. 1975. Study of risk factors related to physical activity in 15,171 men. Brit. Med. J. : 507–509.
66. Jenkins, C. D. 1976. Recent evidence supporting psychologic and social risk factors for coronary disease. N. Eng. J. Med. **294**(18): 987–774.
67. Kannel, W. B. 1967. Habitual level of physical activity and risk of coronary heart disease. Canad. Med. Assoc. J. **96:** 811.
68. Karvonen, M. J. 1975. Sports and longevity. 3rd Pavlo Nurmi Symposium. : 18–20.
69. Karvonen, M. J. 1966. The relationship of habitual physical activity to diseases in the cardiovascular system. *In* International Symposium on Physi-

cal Activity in Health and Disease. K. Evang & K. L. Anderson, Eds. : 81–89. Williams and Wilkins. Baltimore, Md.

70. KARVONEN, M. J. 1959. Effects of vigorous exercise on the heart. *In* Proc. of Conference on Work and the Heart. F. F. Rosenbaum & E. L. Belknap Eds. : 199–210. Hoeber. New York, N.Y.

71. KARVONEN, M. J. 1976. Sports and longevity. Adv. Cardiol. **18:** 243–248.

72. KARVONEN, M. J., H. KLEMOLA, J. VIRKAJARVI & A. KEKKONEN. 1974. Longevity of endurance skiers. Med. Sci. Sports **6:** 49–51.

73. KATZ, L. N. 1967. Physical fitness and coronary heart disease. Circulation **35:** 405–415.

74. KEYS, A., C. ARAVANIS, H. BLACKBURN, F. S. P. VAN BUCHEM, R. BUZINA, B. S. DJORDJEVIC, F. FIDANZA, M. J. KARVONEN, A. MENOTTI, V. PUDDY & H. L. TAYLOR. 1972. Probability of middle-aged men developing coronary heart disease in five years. Circulation **45:** 815–828.

75. KEYS, A. 1970. Physical activity and the epidemiology of coronary heart disease. *In* Medicine and Sport. Vol. 4. Physical Activity and Aging. D. Brunner & E. Jokl, Eds. : 250–266. University Park Press. Baltimore, Md.

76. KEYS, A. 1975. Coronary heart disease—The global picture. Atherosclerosis **22:** 149–192.

77. LANG, C. M. & C. H. BARTHEL. 1972. Effects of simple and complex carbohydrates on serum lipids and atherosclerosis in non-human primates. Amer. J. Clin. Nutr **25:** 470–475.

78. LEON, A. S. 1972. Comparative cardiovascular adaptation to exercise in animals and man and its relevance to coronary heart disease. Comparative Patholphysiology of Circulation Disturbances. Colin M. Bloor, Ed. : 143–174. Plenum Press. New York, N.Y.

79. LEON, A. S. & C. M. BLOOR. 1976. The effect of complete and partial deconditioning on exercise-induced cardiovascular changes in the rat. Exercise and Coronary Heart Disease Symposium, Finland, Sept. 1971. Adv. in Cardiol. Ser. **9**.

80. LEON, A. S. & C. M. BLOOR. 1968. Effects of exercise and its cessation on the heart and its blood supply. J. Appl. Phys. **24**(4): 485–490.

81. LEON, A. S., W. D. HORST, N. SPIRT, E. B. WIGGAN & A. H. WOMELSDORF. 1975. Heart norepinephrine levels after exercise training in the rat. Chest **67:** 341–343.

82. LOWN, B. & B. KOSOWSKY. 1969. Lethal complications of exercise. *In* Exercise and the Heart. R. L. Morse, Ed. : 200–212. Charles C Thomas, Publisher. Springfield, Ill.

83. MALHOTRA, S. L. 1967. Epidemiology of ischaemic heart disease in India with special reference to causation. Brit. Heart J. **29:** 895–905.

84. MANN, G. V., L. GARRET & A. LONG. 1971. The amount of exercise necessary to achieve and maintain fitness in adult persons. South. Med. J. **64:** 549–553.

85. MASIRORI, R. 1970. Dietary factors and coronary heart disease. Bull. World Health Org. **42:** 103–114.

86. MCDONOUGH, J. R., C. G. HAMES, S. C. STULB & G. E. GARRISON. 1965. Coronary heart disease and Negroes and Whites in Evans County, Georgia. J. Chron. Dis. **18:** 443–468.

87. MENOTTI, A. & V. PUDDU. 1976. Death rates among Italian railroad employees, with special reference to coronary heart disease and physical activity at work. Environ. Res. **11:** 331.

88. MICHAELS, L. 1966. Aetiolog. of coronary artery disease: A historical approach. Brit. Heart J. **28:** 258.

89. MILVY, P. 1977. Statistical analysis of deaths from coronary heart disease anticipated in a cohort of marathon runners. Ann. N.Y. Acad. Sci. This volume.

90. MITCHELL, J. H. 1975. Exercise training in the treatment of coronary heart disease. Adv. Intern. Med. **20:** 249–272.

91. MITRANI, Y., H. KARPLUS & D. BRUNNER. 1970. Coronary atherosclerosis in cases of traumatic death. *In* Medicine and Sport. Vol. 4. Physical Activity and Aging. D. Brunner & E. Jokl, Eds. : 241–248. University Park Press. Baltimore, Md.

92. MONTOYE, H. L. 1974. Health and longevity of former athletes. *In* Science and Medicine of Exercise and Sport. 2nd edit. W. R. Johnson & E. R. Buskirk, Eds. : 366–376. Harper and Row. New York, N.Y.

93. MONTOYE, H. J., W. D. VAN HUSS, H. W. OLSON & A. J. HUDEC. 1956. The longevity and morbidity of college athletes. J. Amer. Med. Assoc. **162**: 1132–1134.

94. MORRIS, J. N., S. P. W. CHAVE, C. ADAM *et al.* 1973. Vigorous exercise in leisure time and the incidence of coronary heart disease. Lancet **i**: 333–339.

95. MORRIS, J. N., J. N. HEADY & P. A. RAFFLE. 1956. Physique of London busmen. Lancet **ii**: 566–570.

96. MORRIS, J .N. 1959. Health and social class. Lancet **i**: 303–305.

97. MORRIS, J. N., J. A. HEADY, P. A. RAFFLE, C. G. ROBERTS & J. W. PARKS. 1953. Coronary heart disease and physical activity of work. Lancet **ii**: 1053–1957 and 1111–1120.

98. MORRIS, J. N. & M. D. CRAWFORD. 1958. Coronary heart disease and physical activity of work-evidence of a national necropsy survey. Brit. Med. J. (Dec.) : 1486–1496.

99. MORRIS, J. N. 1975. Primary prevention of heart attack. Bull. N.Y. Acad. Med. **51**(1): 62–74.

100. MORRIS, J. N., A. KAGAN, D. C. PATTISON & M. S. GARDNER. 1966. Incidence and prediction of ischaemic heart disease in London busmen. Lancet **ii**: 553–559.

101. MORRISON, S. L. 1957. Occupational mortality in Scotland. Brit. J. Indust. Med. **14**: 130–132.

102. MÖTTÖNEN, M. 1970. Myocardial infarction and coronary atherosclerosis among and comparison between intellectual and manual workers in Finland. Beitr. Pathol. **141**: 148–154.

103. NIKKILÄ, E. A. 1972. Influence of dietary fructose and sucrose on serum triglycerides in hypertriglyceridemia and diabetes. *In* Sugars in Nutrition. H. L. Sipple & K. W. McNutt, Eds. **26**: 439–448. Academic Press. New York, N.Y.

104. OLIVER, R. M. 1967. Physique and serum lipids of young London busmen in relation to ischaemic heart disease Brit. J. Indust. Med. **24**: 181–186.

105. OPIE, L. H. 1976. Heart disease in marathon runners. New Engl. J. Med. **294** (19): 1067.

106. OPIE, L. H. 1975. Long distance running and sudden death (letter). New Engl. J. Med. **293**(18): 941–942.

107. OPIE, L. H. 1975. Sudden death and sport. Lancet **i**: 678.

108. PAFFENBARGER, R. S. 1972. Factors predisposing to fatal stroke in longshoremen. Prevent Med. **1**(4): 522–527.

109. PAFFENBARGER, R. S., A. GIMA, M. E. LAUGHLIN & R. A. BLACK 1971. Characteristics of longshoremen related to fatal coronary heart disease and stroke. Amer. J. Pub. Health **61**(7): 1362–1370.

110. PAFFENBARGER, R. S. & W. E. HALE. 1975. Work activity and coronary heart mortality. N. Engl. J. Med. **292**(11): 545–550.

111. PAFFENBARGER, R. S., M. E. LAUGHLIN, A. S. GIMA & R. A. BLACK. 1970. Work activity of longshoremen as related to death from coronary heart disease and stroke. New Engl. J. Med. **282**: 1109–1114.

112. PALMORE, E. G. 1969. Physical, mental and social factors in predicting longevity. Gerontologist **9**: 103–108 and 247–250.

113. PATNAIK, P. B. 1948. The lower function of the test for the difference between two proportions in a 2×2 table. Biometrika **35**: 157–175.

114. POLEDNAK, A. P. & A. DAMON. 1970. College athletics, longevity and cause of death. Human Biol. **42:** 28–46.
115. POLEDNAK, A. P. 1972. Longevity and cardiovascular mortality among former college athletes. Circulation **46:** 649–654.
116. POLEDNAK, A. P. 1972. Longevity and cause of death among Harvard College athletes and their classmates. Geriatrics **27**(10): 53–64.
117. POLEDNAK, A. P. 1972. Previous health and longevity of male athletes (letter). Lancet **ii:** 711.
118. PROUT, C. 1972. Life expectancy of college oarsmen. J. Amer. Med. Assoc. 1709–1710.
119. PUNSAR, S. & M. J. KARVONEN. 1976. Physical activity and coronary heart disease in populations from East and West Finland. Adv. Cardiol. **18:** 196–207.
120. PYFER, H. R. & B. L. DOANE 1969. Cardiac arrest during exercise testing. J. Amer. Med. Assoc. **210:** 101–102.
121. PYÖRÄLÄ, K., M. J. KARVONEN, P. TASKINEN, J. TAKKUNEN, M. TAKKUNEN, H. KYRÖNSEPPA & P. PELTOKALLIO 1967. Cardiovascular studies of former endurance athletes. Amer. J. Cardiol. **20:** 191–205.
122. PYÖRÄLÄ, K., M. J. KARVONEN, P. TASKINEN, J. TAKKUNEN & H. KRYÖNSEPPÄ. 1966. Cardiovascular studies on former endurance athletes. *In* Physical Activity and the Heart. M. J. Karvonen & A. J. Barry, Eds. : 301. Charles C Thomas, Publisher. Springfield, Ill.
123. RASKOFF, W. J., S. GOLDMAN & K. COHN 1976. The "athletic heart" J. Amer. Med. Assoc. **236**(2): 158–162.
124. RECHNITZER, P. A., D. A. SAUGAL, G. R. CUNNINGHAM, *et al.* 1975. A controlled prospective study of the effect of endurance training on the recurrence rate of myocardial infarction. Amer. J. Epidemiol. **102:** 358–365.
125. REINDELL, H., K. MUSSHOFF & H. KLEPZIG 1958. Die physiologische und Krankhafle Hervergrösserung. *In* Die Functions diagnostik des Herzens. H. Klepzig Ed. : 128–144. Springer Verlag. Berlin.
126. REINDELL, H., R. WEYLAND, H. KLEPZIG, K. MUSSHOFF & E. SCHILDGE. 1954. Das Sportherz (athletic heart). Erg. Inn. Med. Kinderh. **5:** 306–359.
127. RESNEKOR, L. 1969. Jogging and coronary artery disease (editorial). J. Amer. Med. Assoc. **210:** 126.
128. RISSANEN, V. 1975. Coronary and aortic atherosclerosis in relation to occupational physical activity in male violent deaths. Ann. Clin. Res. **7:** 394–401.
129. ROOK, A. 1954. An investigation into the longevity of Cambridge sportsmen. Brit. Med. J. **i:** 773–777.
130. ROSE, C. L. 1964. Social factors in longevity. Gerontologist **4:** 27–37.
131. ROSE, C. L. & B. BELL 1975. The interdisciplinary study of life span. *In* Understanding Aging. G. Spencer & C. Dorr, Eds. 54–66. Appleton-Century-Crofts. New York, N.Y.
132. ROSE, G., R. PRNEAS & J. MITCHELL 1967. Myocardial infarction and the intrinsic calibre of coronary arteries. Brit. Heart J. **29:** 548–552.
133. ROSE, C. L. & B. BELL. 1971. Predicting Longevity. D. C. Heath and Co., Lexington, Mass.
134. ROSENMAN, R. H. 1970. The influence of different exercise patterns on the incidence of coronary heart disease in the Western Collaborative Group Activity and Aging. *In* Medicine and Sport. Vol. 4. Physical Activity and Aging. D. Brunner & E. Jokl, Eds. : 267–273. University Park Press. Baltimore, Md.
135. SALZMAN, S. H., E. Z. HIRSCH & H. K. HELLERSTEIN 1970. Adaptation to muscular exercise, myocardial epinephrine-^{3}H uptake. J. Appl. Phys. **29:** 92–95.
136. SARVOTHAM, S. G. & J. N. BERRY 1968. Prevalence of coronary heart disease in urban population in Northern India. Circulation **37:** 939–953.

137. SCHNOKR, P. 1971. Longevity and causes of death in male athletic champions. Lancet ii: 1364–1365.

138. SHURK, M. R. & R. O. REMINGTON 1967. The determination of sample size in treatment-control comparisons for chronic disease studies in which drop-out or non-whereabouts is a problem. J. Chronic Dis. **20:** 223.

139. SHAPIRO, S., E. WINBLATT, C. W. FRANK & R. V. SAGER 1965. The H.I.P. Study of incidence and prognosis of coronary heart disease. J. Chronic Dis. **18:** 527–558.

140. SHAPIRO, S., E. WEINBLATT, C. W. FRANK, et al. 1969. Incidence of coronary heart disease in a population insured for medical care (H.I.P.). Myocardial infarction, angina pectoris and possible myocardial infarction. Amer. J. Pub. Health **57** (Supp. II): 1–101.

141. SHEPHARD, R. J. 1972. Alive Man. : 501–528. Charles C Thomas, Publisher. Springfield, Ill.

142. SINNETT, R. F. & H. M. WHYTE 1973. Epidemiological studies in a total highland population, Tukisenta, New Guinea. Cardiovascular disease and relevant clinical, electrocardiographic, radiological and biochemical findings. J. Chronic Dis. **26:** 265–290.

143. SPAIN, D. M. & V. A. BRADESS 1960. Occupational physical activity and the degree of coronary arteriosclerosis in "normal" men. A postmortem study. Circulation **22:** 239–242.

144. SPAIN, D. M. & V. A. BRADESS. 1957. Sudden death from coronary arteriosclerosis. Age, race, sex, physical activity and alcohol. Arch. Intern. Med. **100:** 228–231.

145. STAMLER, J. 1971. Acute myocardial infarction—Progress in primary prevention. Brit. Heart J. **33**(Suppl.): 145–161.

146. STAMLER, J., D. M. BERKSON et al. 1970. Long-term epidemiologic studies on the possible role of physical activity and physical fitness in the prevention of premature clinical coronary disease. In Medicine and Sport. Vol. 4. Physical Activity and Aging. D. Brunner & E. Jokl, Eds. White Plains, N.Y.

147. STAMLER, J., M. KJELSBURG & Y. HALL 1960. Epidemiologic studies in cardiovascular-renal diseases: I. Analysis of mortality trends by age-race-sex-occupation. J. Chronic Dis. **12:** 440–455.

148. Statistical Bulletin. 1959–1960. Overweight, its prevention and significance. Metropolitan Life Insurance Company. A series of articles reprinted from Statistical Bulletin. : 3–19.

149. Statistical Bulletin. 1975. Socioeconomic mortality differentials. Metropolitan Life Insurance Company. January : 3–5.

150. Statistical Bulletin. 1975. Longevity of major league baseball players. Metropolitan Life Insurance Company. April, : 3–4.

151. Statistical Bulletin. 1975. Recent trends in mortality from heart disease. Metropolitan Life Insurance Company. June : 3–6.

152. Statistical Bulletin. 1975. Potential gains in longevity after midlife. Metropolitan Life Insurance Company. Sept. : 8–10.

153. STELLMAN, J. M. & S. D. DAUM. 1973. Work is Dangerous to Your Health. Pantheon Books, New York, N.Y.

154. SUSSER, M. 1972. Procedures for establishing casual associations. In Trends in Epidemiology. Charles C Thomas, Publisher. Springfield, Ill.

155. SYME, S. L., M. M. HYMAN & P. E. ENTERLINE 1964. Some social and cultural factors asssociated with the occurrence of coronary heart disease. J. Chronic Dis. **17:** 277–289.

156. SYME, S. L., N. O. BORHANI & R. W. BUECHLEY 1966. Cultural mobility and coronary heart disease in an urban area. Amer. J. Epidemiol. **82:** 334–346.

157. TAYLOR, H. L. 1967. Occupational factors in the study of coronary heart disease and physical activity. Canada. Med. Assoc. J. **96:** 825–831.

158. TAYLOR, H. L., H. BLACKBURN, J. BROZEK, R. W. PARLIN & T. PUCHNER. 1966. Railroad employees in the U.S.A. Acta Med. Scand. (Suppl.) **460:** 55–115.

159. TAYLOR, H. L., E. R. BUSKIRK & R. D. REMINGTON. 1973. Exercise in controlled trials of the prevention of coronary heart disease. Federation Proceedings. **32**(5): 1623–1627.

160. TAYLOR, H. L., E. KLEPETAR, A. KEYS, W. PARLIN, H. BLACKBURN & T. PUCHNER 1962. Death rates among physically active and sedentary employees of the realroad industry. Amer. J. Pub. Health **52**: 1697–1707.

161. TAYLOR, H. L., H. BLACKBURN, A. KEYS, R. W. PARLIN, C. VASQUEZ & T. PUCHNER 1970. Five Year followup of employees of selected U.S. railroad companies. Suppl. I to Circulation **41–42**(Suppl. I): 120–139.

162. TAYLOR, H. L., R. W. PARLIN, H. BLACKBURN & A. KEYS. 1966. Problems in the analysis of the relationship of coronary heart disease to physical activity or its lack, with special reference to sample size and occupational withdrawal. *In* Physical Activity in Health and Disease. K. Evang & K. L. Anderson, Eds. : 242–261.

163. TERASLINNA, P., T. PARTANEN, K. PYÖRÖLÄ, S. PUNSAR, R. KARAVA, P. OJA & A. KOSELA. 1969. Work-Environ.-Health **6**: 25.

164. TYROLER, H. A. & J. CASSEL. 1964. Health consequences of culture change II. The effect of urbanization on coronary heart mortality in rural residence. J. Chronic Dis. **17**: 167–177.

165. U.S. Department of Health, Education and Welfare. 1973. The Framingham Study. Epidemiological Investigation of Cardiovascular Disease. W. B. Kannel & T. Gordon, Eds. Section 28 (NIH 1466).

166. VAN DIJL, H. 1975. Myocardial infarction patients and work attitudes—An empirical study. J. Psychosom. Res. **19**: 197–202.

167. WEINBLATT, E., S. SHAPIRO, C. W. FRANK & B. SAGER 1968. Prognosis of men after first myocardial infarction: Mortality and first recurrence in relation to selected parameters. Amer. J. Pub. Health **58**(8): 1329–1347.

168. World Health Organization. 1973. Second working group methodology of multifactor preventive trials. Copenhagen.

169. WILHELMSEN, L., H. SANNE, D. ELMFELDT, G. GRIMBY, G. TIBBLIN & H. WEDEL. 1975. A controlled trial of physical training after myocardial infarction. Prevent Med. **4**: 491–508.

170. WILHELMSSON, C., J. S. VEDIN, D. ELMFELDT, *et al.* 1975. Smoking and myocardial infarction. Lancet **i**: 415–420.

171. YUDKN, J. 1964. Dietary fat and dietary sugar in relation to ischaemic heart disease and diabetes. Lancet **ii**: 4.

172. ZUKEL, W. J., R. H. LEWIS, P. E. ENTERLINE, *et al.* 1959. A short-term study of the epidemiology of coronary heart disease. Amer. J. Pub. Health **49**: 1630–19639.

A PHYSIOLOGICAL PROFILE OF A JOGGING CLASS: YOUNG AND OLD, MALE AND FEMALE *

A. Goldman †

Mathematics Department
University of California
Davis, California 95616

D. B. Dill

Laboratory of Applied Physiology
Desert Research Institute
Boulder City, Nevada 89005

Get your facts first and then you can distort them as much as you please.

Mark Twain

INTRODUCTION

Six jogging classes sponsored by the continuing education department at the University of Nevada, Las Vegas (UNLV) had been conducted from the period September 1973 to May 1976. A total of over 200 students took part; however, because of a lack of facilities on campus, a complete physiological test was accomplished only on 40 men and 35 women. This includes the results of a special study involving seven women from ages 63 to 88. The jogging class was conceived as a temporary effort until a human performance laboratory could be incorporated in the University system. At that time students would become involved in physiological studies on an informal basis. Despite limited data, a statistical analysis of the class data showed some interesting results worthy of investigation. The "experiment" may be looked upon as a pilot study and shows a need for follow-up research. It is hoped that the given statistical procedures can also be used as a guide for future endeavors.

A statistical method known as stepwise regression was used in determining the "best" subset of ten variables that could predict $\dot{V}_{O_2 \max}$ for men, women, and women excluding the seven elderly. In addition a psychological test displaying 18 personality traits were given to some of the subjects. A summary of these results and a statistical analysis will be presented. An explanation of the terms used in this report is given as an appendix.

TESTING

Each student was subjected to various tests during the 8-week course. The class met four times per week for 30 minutes per session. Each person was

* This work was supported in part by National Institutes of Health Grant AG 00437–04A1 and by a University of Las Vegas research grant.

† Permanent address: Mathematics Department, University of Nevada Las Vegas, Las Vegas, NV 89154.

categorized by ability and given a compatible jogging program to follow. The following is a breakdown of the tests and measurements given during the session:

Blood. Analysis was conducted by the pathology division of the Sunrise Hospital in Las Vegas. Measurements included hemoglobin (Hb), hematocrit (hct), triglycerides (Trigl), and cholesterol (chol).

Body Fat. Analysis was conducted by the health division of the Environmental Protection Agency located on the UNLV campus. Observations were made with the use of a whole-body counter that measured potassium. Body fat was computed from these observations using standard procedures.

Physiological Measurements. Analysis and results were compiled by the Laboratory of Environmental Patho-Physiology, Desert Research Institute, at Boulder City, Nevada. Measurements included height (ht), weight (wt),

TABLE 1

PHYSIOLOGICAL STATISTICS FOR MEN

Variable	Mean	Standard Deviation	No. of Cases
Age (yr)	43.50	12.80	40
	41.74	11.04	116
Wt (kg)	80.22	10.85	40
	78.15	10.35	116
RQ	1.15	0.09	40
	1.17	0.12	116
$\dot{V}_{O_2 max}$ (ml/min·kg)	39.49	9.26	40
	37.61	8.11	116
Ht (cm)	177.38	6.30	40
	177.19	7.27	116
Hb (g/100 ml)	15.27	0.97	40
Trigl (mg/100 ml)	104.60	57.45	40
Chol (mg/100 ml)	240.85	52.60	40
Hct (%)	45.19	2.72	40
VC (liters)	5.15	1.09	40
Body fat (%)	23.35	5.82	40

respiratory quotient (RQ), aerobic capacity ($\dot{V}_{O_2 max}$), and vital capacity (VC).

Personality Traits. Results were compiled by the Psychology Department at UNLV. A detailed description will be presented later.

ANALYSIS OF PHYSIOLOGICAL TESTING

In order to gain a descriptive insight as to the class composition, lists of the sample means and standard deviations of the 11 observed variables for men and women are presented in TABLES 1 and 2. Notice that information available on 116 men does not appear to be significantly different from that on 40 men. Unfortunately measurements such as body fat were made on just 40 of the 116 participants. The effect of missing data on $\dot{V}_{O_2 max}$ shows only a small decrease in mean and standard deviation. On the other hand, rather large differences in statistics occur when the older women's data are removed. When the seven elderly are discarded, sharp drops in mean and standard deviation occur for both triglycerides and of course, age. Notice also that there was a drop in the average body fat.

Simple correlations (*r* values) were examined among the variables. Not surprisingly, hematocrit and hemoglobin scored the largest, $r = 0.933$. Absolute

TABLE 2

PHYSIOLOGICAL STATISTICS FOR WOMEN

Variable	Mean	Standard Deviation	No. of Cases
Age (yr)	36.89	10.40	28
	43.71	17.00	35
	41.78	13.84	64
Wt (kg)	62.55	11.29	28
	62.59	10.44	35
	63.93	10.70	64
RQ	1.06	0.15	28
	1.05	0.14	35
$\dot{V}_{O_2\,max}$ (ml/min·kg)	26.31	3.58	28
	24.77	4.82	35
	25.91	4.88	64
Ht (cm)	163.98	6.35	28
	163.55	6.13	35
Hb (g/100 ml)	13.39	0.74	28
	13.35	0.95	35
Trigl (mg/100 ml)	83.18	46.15	28
	105.51	85.25	35
Chol (mg/100 ml)	225.11	42.35	28
	238.17	53.10	35
Hct (%)	40.56	2.48	28
	40.32	2.84	35
VC (liters)	3.83	0.89	28
	3.60	0.94	35
	3.67	0.88	54
Body fat (%)	25.01	7.32	28
	26.83	7.85	35

values of correlations greater than 0.49 are presented for comparative purposes in TABLE 3.

Simple correlations with $\dot{V}_{O_2\,max}$ are given in TABLE 4. Notice that body fat, triglycerides, and age have the three largest *r* values for men, but we shall see that this does not imply that these variables when taken together comprise the best set of multiple predictors. Age, body fat, and cholesterol have the highest correlations for total women ($n = 35$) and hematocrit, body fat, and weight

TABLE 3

CORRELATIONS BETWEEN VARIABLES *

Men Variables	r	Total Women ($n=35$) Variables	r	Young and Middle-Aged Women ($n=28$)	r
Hct and Hb	0.933	Hct and Hb	0.824	Hct and Hb	0.708
Body fat and $\dot{V}_{O_2 \, max}$	−0.561	Age and $\dot{V}_{O_2 \, max}$	−0.674	Body fat and wt	0.703
Body fat and wt	0.557	Trigl and chol	0.647	Age and Hb	−0.544
Age and chol	−0.545	Wt and body fat	0.635	Trigl and chol	0.516
$\dot{V}_{O_2 \, max}$ and Trigl	−0.543	Age and VC	−0.620	Ht and VC	0.504
Age and $\dot{V}_{O_2 \, max}$	−0.524	Age and body fat	0.593	Hct and body fat	−0.491
Ht and VC	0.514	Age and chol	0.516		
Age and Trigl	0.506	Body fat and $\dot{V}_{O_2 \, max}$	0.514		
Age and VC	−0.505				
$\dot{V}_{O_2 \, max}$ and hct	0.492				

* Only correlations greater than 0.49 are presented.

TABLE 4

SIMPLE CORRELATIONS WITH $\dot{V}_{O_2\ max}$

Variable	Men ($n=40$)	Young and Middle-Aged Women ($n=28$)	Total Women ($n=35$)
Age	−0.524	−0.315	−0.674
Wt	−0.245	−0.330	−0.190
RQ	0.182	0.234	0.371
Ht	0.323	−0.136	0.055
Hb	0.019	0.270	−0.004
Trigl	−0.543	0.208	−0.359
Chol	−0.408	−0.022	−0.452
Hct	−0.042	0.448	0.163
VC	0.492	−0.152	0.248
Body fat	−0.561	−0.435	−0.514

have the largest values for young and middle-aged women ($n=28$). It is interesting that body fat is the only variable that appears in the top three for all sets.

Stepwise regression is an appealing method for determining the best set of predictors in a linear model. For instance, in order to investigate all possible linear prediction models for $\dot{V}_{O_2\ max}$, a total of 1024 different regression curves would have to be examined. By using the F-ratio test, the stepwise analysis includes or excludes a variable based upon its "amount" of contribution. The results of applying this technique are given in TABLE 5. For men, the significant

TABLE 5

MULTIPLE COMPARISONS

	Observed Data			Ranks		
	Variables	R	R^2	Variables	R	R^2
Men ($n=40$)	BF	0.5606	0.31	Trigl	0.5974	0.36
	BF,Trigl	0.7327	0.54	BF,Trigl	0.7278	0.53
	BF,Trigl,ht	0.8027	0.64	BF,Trigl,ht	0.7803	0.61
	BF,Trigl,ht,RQ	0.8321	0.69			
	BF,Trigl,ht,RQ, chol	0.8568	0.73			
Total women ($n=35$)	Age	0.6737	0.45	Age	0.6386	0.41
	Age,RQ	0.7315	0.54	Age,RQ	0.7467	0.56
	Age,RQ,ht	0.7551	0.57	Age,RQ,BF	0.7955	0.63
Young and middle-aged women ($n=28$)	hct	0.4485	0.20	wt	0.5603	0.31
	Hb,BF	0.5119	0.27	wt,RQ	0.6260	0.39
	Hb,BF,Trigl	0.5905	0.35	wt,RQ,BF	0.6855	0.47
	BF,Trigl (Hb removed)	0.5472	0.30	RQ,BF (wt removed)	0.6735	0.45
				RQ,BF,Age	0.7084	0.50

variables contributing to $\dot{V}_{O_2 max}$ include body fat, triglycerides, height, respiratory quotient, and cholesterol. The rather small sample size might be reason for deleting the latter two variables. In general, three variables might be sufficient for explaining $\dot{V}_{O_2 max}$ when the sample size numbers around 50. Stepwise regression was also performed on ranks of the observations in lieu of the measurements. This was done in order to standardize the data. The three influential variables were the same and R^2 values were in agreement. A similar comparison was conducted for women and with $n = 35$, age and RQ were significant in both the conventional and rank cases; however body fat replaced height with a somewhat larger R^2. When the eight elderly women were removed, only body fat and triglycerides were important, but RQ, body fat, and age were found important for ranked data. The value of R^2 was 0.50 for ranks contrasted with 0.30 for measurements, indicating the ranked data may be more pertinent. It is of academic interest to note that the stepwise procedure discarded hematocrit and weight as being important contributors for measurements and ranks, respectively. Sharp contrasts in $\dot{V}_{O_2 max}$ between men and women precluded the combining of data for overall prediction purposes.

The results may be examined in another way. Assume that the linear equation is adequate for prediction purposes and assume further that the derived $\dot{V}_{O_2 max}$ can be used as a standard for a person having "average" $\dot{V}_{O_2 max}$. The following equations were found:

Men: $\dot{V}_{O_2 max} = -19.46370 + 0.48355(ht) - 0.07341(Trigl) - 0.82016$
$$\text{(body fat)} \qquad (1)$$

Women ($n = 35$): $\dot{V}_{O_2 max} = 50.60303 - 0.20375(age) +$
$$8.97567(RQ) - 0.16093(ht) \qquad (2)$$

Women ($n = 28$): $\dot{V}_{O_2 max} = 30.51592 + 0.02669(Trigl) -$
$$0.25676(\text{body fat}) \qquad (3)$$

Suppose a 42-year-old male has measured his height at 187 cm (approx. 6′1″), body fat 16.1%, triglycerides 82 mg/100 ml, and $\dot{V}_{O_2 max} = 54$ ml/min·kg. Equation 1 would predict that his $\dot{V}_{O_2 max}$ should be 51.7, a favorable comparison.

Consider a second example. A 35-year-old female has an RQ of 1.18, is 175 cm tall, and has a $\dot{V}_{O_2 max} = 27.3$. Equation 2 would predict her $\dot{V}_{O_2 max}$ to be 25.90. Her triglycerides were 47 mg/100 ml and body fat $= 25\%$; then Equation 3 would yield 25.351.

These examples are presented for pedagogical purposes. The necessary assumptions are subject to criticism. In the first place, 40 subjects do not constitute a sample size adequate for making accurate predictions. In addition, it may be necessary to examine other variables. A third cause for caution is that the prediction model may be something other than linear. Further, one might feel more comfortable about making predictions when R^2 is greater than 0.70.

Special Study

A class consisting of ten women ranging in age from 63 to 88 were involved in a project sponsored by a UNLV research grant. Each woman was paid for attending a 10-week walk-jog session. Any possible randomness was destroyed by virtue of the fact that only those in a reasonable state of fitness could enroll. The women worked out for approximately 30 minutes 4 days a week. Seven of the ten managed to complete the program. The improvements in some cases were remarkable. For example, E. L., a 72-year-old, started by walking and jogging one mile in 20 minutes and at the end of the class, she could jog 3 miles in under 40 minutes. The enthusiasm and spirit displayed by this group indicates that more effort should be placed on providing group jogging and walking programs for those over 60. Some results of the testing to exemplify improvement in $\dot{V}_{O_2 \text{ max}}$ are given in TABLE 6.

TABLE 6

IMPROVEMENT IN $\dot{V}_{O_2\text{max}}$ IN WOMEN AGED 63–88 AFTER TRAINING *

Subject		Age	wt	RQ	ht	Hb	Trigl	chol	hct	VC	Body Fat	$\dot{V}_{O_2\text{max}}$
L.L.	Pre	68	66.7	0.94	159	13.4	74	265	39.4	2.9	35.3	16.1
	Post		67.0	1.02						3.2		18.8
L.E.	Pre	63	76.7	1.05	170	12.7	145	272	37.1	3.3	41.3	24.4
	Post		75.7	1.05						3.5		28.8
E.S.	Pre	67	66.2	1.02	159	12.6	489	347	37.7	3.4	34.5	18.7
	Post		63.6	0.87						2.7		19.3
M.H.	Pre	71	54.2	0.88	168	14.8	207	380	44.2	3.1	26.8	16.8
	Post		58.9	0.83						2.9		17.3
A.C.	Pre	68	67.7	0.88	162	13.9	223	270	41.6	2.3	37.4	13.4
	Post		68.3	0.98						2.2		17.6
E.L.	Pre	72	53.4	1.05	159	10.1	83	188	32.5	2.5	26.3	22.5
	Post		53.2	1.03						1.3		22.7
C.W.	Pre	88	58.8	1.03	156	14.8	143	311	43.5	2.1	37.2	15.4
	Post		—	—						—		—

* Approximately 30 minutes, 4 times a week.

To illustrate the inadequacy of Equation 3 when used for predicting those over 60, consider M. H. ($\dot{V}_{O_2 \text{ max}} = 17.3$). The following result is found:

Estimated $\dot{V}_{O_2 \text{ max}} = 30.51592 + 0.02669(207) - 0.25676(26.8) = 29.2$.

On the other hand, Equation 2 when $n = 35$ yields

$50.60303 - 0.20375(71) + 8.97567(0.88) - 0.16093(168) = 17.0$.

These results point out the need for more data involving older ages.

PERSONALITY TESTS

The California Personality Inventory Tests were given to some of the subjects. The tests involve 18 personality traits, which are scored on a percentile basis. Equations 1 and 2 were used to separate subjects into either "good" or "poor" fitness, while the personality trait was judged "high" or "low" depending upon whether the score was greater or less than the median. A total of 33 men and 16 women took part, which means that the results can be looked at as being more indicative than conclusive. The breakdown is given in TABLE 7. There is not enough information about women who were physically fit to utilize statistical tests. On the other hand, the hypothesis may be stated that of 12 women who were not physically fit, six should respond above and six below the median. The binomial test statistic was used to determine that the hypothesis was rejected at the 0.05 level in four cases indicating that physically-unfit women are (1) not self-confident, (2) have a low personal worth, (3) do not attempt to create a good impression, and (4) have high feminine interests. A similar test indicated that unfit men are irresponsible and do not attempt to create a good impression. Borderline acceptances (probability level = 0.0768) indicate that unfit men were intolerant and socially immature, and had a low personal worth. In addition, the tests indicated that fit men were self-confident, independent, and interested in others. The assumption was made that the test results are statistically independent. There was one response removed from the data when a subject scored below the 20th percentile in communality, a check on whether the questions were answered consistently.

SUMMARY AND CONCLUSIONS

The measurements from tests given to a jogging class were analyzed by statistical methods involving stepwise regression and the binomial distribution. The conclusions in the text were stated in a guarded manner allowing for small sample sizes, and small values of R^2. The need for including elderly people in a study of the prediction of $\dot{V}_{O_2 \, max}$ was dramatically illustrated by stepwise regression. The variables selected for women were age, respiratory quotient, and height when seven women over the age of 63 were included and body fat and triglycerides when the remaining 28 were analyzed. The differences in $\dot{V}_{O_2 \, max}$ for men and women quite obviously represented two distinct populations and the data treatment was handled accordingly. The prediction variables for men included height, triglyceride, and body fat. There seems to be good agreement that for both men and women between the ages of 20 and 60 that body fat and triglycerides play a role in ascertaining $\dot{V}_{O_2 \, max}$. Triglycerides could be subjected to discredit because of the tremendous variation in the measurements (standard deviation is over one-half of the mean). The psychological tests given to the class indicated some personality traits that might be related to a person's physical condition. For example, both unfit men and women tend not to create a good impression and have a low personal worth. The binomial distribution was used to test the hypothesis that an equal number of persons in a categorized physical condition fell above or below the median (50th percentile) for a given personality trait. The statistical tests involving 16 unfit men is analogous to testing the hypothesis that the probability of obtaining a head equals ½ when tossing a coin 16 times. Further studies involving a much larger group of subjects is necessary to substantiate the results presented here.

TABLE 7

PSYCHOLOGICAL TEST RESULTS

	Men		Women	
Trait *	Poor	Good	Poor	Good
1. Dominance				
H (dominant)	9	7	3	2
L (retiring or unassuming)	7	10	9	2
2. Capacity for Status				
H (striving for increased social status)	7	7	3	2
L (not striving)	9	10	9	2
3. Sociability				
H (outgoing, competitive)	5	7	3	2
L (detached, quiet)	11	10	9	2
4. Social Presence				
H (self-confident)	7	13 ‡	2 ‡	3
L (not self-confident)	9	4 ‡	10 ‡	1
5. Self-Acceptance				
H (high personal worth)	4 §	10	2 ‡	1
L (feelings of guilt and self-blame)	12 §	7	10 ‡	3
6. Sense of Well Being				
H (few complaints or worries)	7	11	3	1
L (many complaints or worries)	9	6	9	3
7. Responsibility				
H (responsible)	2 ‡	9	3	2
L (not responsible)	14 ‡	8	9	2
8. Socialization				
H (socially mature)	4 §	11	3	1
L (socially immature)	12 §	6	9	3
9. Self-Control				
H (deliberate, thoughtful)	8	8	3	1
L (impulsive, uninhibited)	8	9	9	3
10. Tolerance (Permissive, accepting social beliefs)				
H (tolerant)	4 §	11	4	2
L (intolerant)	12 §	6	8	2
11. Good Impression				
H (attempts to create good impression)	2 ‡	7	1 ‡	0
L (distant from others, aloof)	14 ‡	10	11 ‡	4
12. Communality				
H (test questions answered consistently)	9	9	9	1
L (test questions answered inconsistently)	7	8	3	3
13. Achievement via Conformance				
H (striving to achieve in a group)	7	11	5	1
L (not striving to achieve in a group)	9	6	7	3
14. Achievement via Independence				
H (striving to achieve alone)	7	15 ‡	8	2
L (not striving to achieve alone)	9	2 ‡	4	2
15. Intellectual Efficiency (*NOT* an IQ score)				
H (a high interest in intellectual efficiency)	8	12	4	2
L (no interest in intellectual efficiency)	8	5	8	2

TABLE 7—*Continued*

PSYCHOLOGICAL TEST RESULTS

	Fitness †			
	Men		Women	
Trait *	Poor	Good	Poor	Good
16. Psychological-Mindedness				
H (interested in others)	8	15 ‡	7	2
L (not interested in others)	8	2 ‡	5	2
17. Flexibility (thinking and social behavior)				
H (flexible)	8	11	7	2
L (rigid)	8	6	5	2
18. Feminity				
H (more feminine interests)	9	6	10 ‡	2
L (more masculine interests)	7	11	2 ‡	3

* H, scored higher than median (50th percentile) on psychological trait; L, scored less than median (50 percentile).

† Good, measured $\dot{V}_{O_2max}$ greater than computed value. Poor, measured V_{O_2max} less than computed.

‡ Indicates significant departure from expected at 0.05 level.

§ Indicates significant departure from expected at 0.08 level.

ACKNOWLEDGMENTS

Institutional support was provided by the Pathology Section of the Sunrise Hospital, by the Environmental Protection Agency, and by Continuing Education, UNLV, all of Las Vegas. In addition the following were very helpful collaborators: Drs. John B. Connolly, M. K. Yousef, and Lars F. Soholt; also Thomas P. Davis, Mary Greeley, Jan Miller, Mary Loughran, Tom Drost, Deanna McLean, Bret Foreman, Daniel S. Morris, Jr., and Terry Goudy.

APPENDIX

Aerobic capacity, $\dot{V}_{O_2\ max}$, is the amount of oxygen that can be supplied to the body in all-out exercise. It was measured with the subject walking or running on the treadmill at a constant rate with the grade increased each minute until the subject finds he has reached his limit. It is expressed in milliliters of oxygen per minute and per kg of body weight (ml/kg·min).

Respiratory quotient (RQ) is the ratio of carbon dioxide output to oxygen used when the aerobic capacity has been reached.

Vital capacity (VC) is the volume of air that can be expelled from the lungs after a maximum inspiration. It is measured in liters.

Hemoglobin (Hb) the oxygen-carrying blood pigment is expressed in grams per 100 ml of blood (g/100 ml).

Hematocrit (hct) measures the percent by volume of red blood cells. It is expressed in percent.

Cholesterol (chol) is a normal constituent of blood that tends to increase with age. Unusually high values may be found in cardiovascular disease. It is expressed in milligrams per 100 ml of blood (mg/100 ml).

Triglycerides (Trigl) are normally present in the blood and may increase in cardiovascular disease. Concentration is measured in milligrams per 100 ml of blood (mg/100 ml).

Body fat is an essential component. The minimum value is above 5%. The usual value in young men is 12% to 15% and in young women 20% to 25%. Increases beyond these ranges generally and unfortunately occur in middle age. Body fat generally declines above age 80. Body fat is measured in percent.

Preliminary observations included in most cases resting systolic and diastolic blood pressure and an electrocardiogram both in rest and immediately following a stressful brief ride on a bicycle ergometer. These records were examined by our consulting physician John R. Connolly. Aerobic capacity was measured only on those rated in good cardiovascular health by Dr. Connolly.

THE RELATIONSHIP OF PHYSICAL ACTIVITY TO CORONARY HEART DISEASE AND LIFE EXPECTANCY

Arthur S. Leon and Henry Blackburn

Laboratory of Physiological Hygiene
School of Public Health
and
Department of Medicine
Medical School
University of Minnesota
Minneapolis, Minnesota 55455

Exercise and General Health

Historically, physical exercise has been praised as an adjunct to good health, at least since the time of the ancient Greeks. Studies during the past quarter century have confirmed its value. This is especially true in light of the World Health Organization's modern definition of health as "physical, mental, and social well-being, not merely the absence of disease or infirmity." The physical component of this definition includes the positive quality of physical fitness, "the ability to carry out daily tasks with vigor and alertness without undue fatigue and with ample reserve energy to enjoy leisure pursuits and meet unforseen emergencies."

Beneficial physiological adaptations resulting from endurance exercise conditioning observed in athletes, sedentary people, coronary heart disease (CHD) patients and animals have recently been reviewed,[1,2] and include the following: (1) A reduction in heart rate and blood pressure and morphological changes in skeletal and cardiac muscle, resulting in improved physical work capacity, enhancement of cardiovascular efficiency in delivering oxygen and nutrients to the tissues, and a reduction in myocardial oxygen requirements for any given amount of work; (2) Increased muscular endurance; (3) Possible increased myocardial vascularity, including capillary density, coronary collaterals, and size of the coronary artery tree as demonstrated by animal studies; (4) Reduced blood coagulability and a transient increase in fibrinolysis; (5) Reduction in weight and adiposity and increased lean body mass; (6) Increased cellular sensitivity to insulin, reducing requirements at any given glucose load;[3] (7) Blood lipid changes including a reduction in serum triglycerides and an increase in the amount of cholesterol carried by high-density (alpha) lipoprotein,[4,5,115] low levels of which are reported in population studies to be related to development of CHD.[6,7]

Psychological benefits of regular exercise are difficult to measure; however, there is no doubt that exercise helps relieve muscular tension, makes one feel better and sleep better, and may aid motivation for improving health habits including cessation of cigarette smoking.[1,8,9] In contrast, limitation of physical activity results in a progressive deterioration of cardiovascular performance and efficiency, metabolic disturbances, difficulty in maintaining normal body weight, increased sympathetic nervous system activity, and possibly emotional disturbances.[10-12]

There is no question that the physiological and psychological benefits of regular exercise can improve the quality of life. Let us consider next whether it also protects against CHD and increases the quantity of life.

Exercise and CHD

CHD is by far the major adult health problem and the primary cause of premature death in the United States and other industrialized nations in the world. At least three aspects of the modern mode of living have been demonstrated to play a role: (1) a diet high in animal fat, calories, and salt, frequently associated with elevated blood lipids, obesity, hypertension, and glucose intolerance; (2) cigarette smoking; and (3) a low level of physical activity resulting from extensive automation and mechanization on the job and in the home and emphasis on television and spectator sports for leisure time activity. The adaptations accompanying physical fitness can be expected to modify the course of CHD. Additional evidence in favor of this are demonstrations of the association of exercise and high levels of physical fitness with lower levels of coronary risk factors.[12-14] However, Mann et al.[15] feel that, based on their studies the direct effects of physical fitness are more important in protecting against CHD.

Rigorous experimental evidence of the protective effects of exercise in man is not available. Under this circumstance, careful analysis and interpretation of epidemiological studies of "natural experiments" are useful for a better understanding of the possible relationship of physical inactivity to CHD. A forerunner of such studies was a report in 1864 of a higher mortality rate in people with sedentary occupations compared to those who are physically active.[16] In the first systematic study of this relationship undertaken in 1939, Hedley[19] reported a lower annual death rate from coronary occlusion in middle-aged laborers in Philadelphia as compared to professional men and other nonmanual workers. However, little attention was paid to this report and the relationship between occupational physical activity and CHD was not studied further until the 1950s. Since then there have been more than 50 published reports. Most of these have been recently reviewed in detail elsewhere,[2, 17, 18] and will only be briefly surveyed here without a specific critique of each. Physical activity has in most of these studies been assessed by occupation, with subjects classified into 3 or 4 categories such as light, medium, and heavy work. Only recently have recreational activities been taken into consideration.

The method of classifying these studies was adapted from Froelicher and Oberman.[17] The results are expressed in terms of whether or not a positive or negative relationship was found between physical inactivity and CHD mortality and/or morbidity as shown in TABLES 1–4.

Discussion

The positive studies revealed an inverse relationship between physical activity levels and CHD, with the active subjects having about ½ the incidence of CHD and ⅓ the associated mortality.

Let's consider now some of the problems that must be considered in interpreting these studies. Study limitations include the following:

(1) Individuals may have selected or been selected for different types of work or recreational activities because of physical constitution (e.g., body build), and/or psychological factors. These variables in turn may have their

own independent influence on the course of the atherosclerotic process and CHD. For example, in the London transport workers study there were different height standards for conductors and drivers with hiring records indicating that the drivers were considerably fatter than the conductors prior to beginning on the job.[93]

(2) Subjects with different activity levels may also differ in other coronary risk factors, ethnic and social backgrounds, diet habits, home and work environments and other factors. For example, the London bus drivers in follow-up study were found to have higher serum cholesterol and blood pressure levels than conductors and the difference in CHD incidence may actually have been due to this rather than physical activity levels.[58] In the Masai [38] an apparent inherited propensity for hypocholestremia coupled with low blood pressure and their nonsmoking and extremely lean body build, rather than their high physical activity and fitness levels may account for the reported low incidence of CHD.[94] However, differences in major risk factors could not explain the apparent lower incidence of CHD in Finnish lumberjacks.[36] The lumberjacks had similar serum cholesterol levels and cigarette smoking habits and only slightly lower systolic and diastolic blood pressures than men in other less active occupations from the same area. In the Evans County, Georgia studies [69] the greatest difference in CHD incidence was associated with differences in race, i.e., Black versus White, and between farmers and nonfarmers.

In general in large population studies it is difficult if not impossible to separate physical activity levels from socioeconomic factors. Many of the confounding variables were excluded in the studies involving the Israeli kibbutzim in which the population had a similar ethnic origin, socioeconomic status, stress of daily living, medical care, body weight, and ate in a common dining facility receiving similar meat rations. Recent reports from that group suggests that the job activity risk gradient persists after adjustment for major coronary risk factors.[95] However, as Keys [94] has observed, it can be safely predicted that the men doing heavier work had a larger caloric intake in the form of bread and other carbohydrate foods thereby reducing the percent of calories from animal fat. Also the kibbutzim members were not randomly assigned to jobs, but to those which they were best suited.

It also appears from prospective population studies that other risk factors, especially serum cholesterol, cigarette smoking, and blood pressure have a much more potent influence on the progress of CHD than does physical activity level.

(3) Individuals change from more active to less active occupations and reduce vigorous recreational activities because of health reasons. Thus CHD may be concentrated among the least active men. In the long-term (22-year) study involving longshoremen, Paffenbarger [64] took into account change of occupational activity in analyzing his data, assuming that the protective effects of physical activity would be short-lived (<6 months). This study showed that the high-activity men had a reduced mortality rate from CHD, sudden coronary death, and strokes. This relationship persisted after adjustments for age, smoking habits, and blood pressure levels.

(4) There are difficulties in assessing physical activity levels. Job title may be inadequate for assessing physical activity. For example, Taylor et al.[60] observed that some supposedly sedentary railroad clerks were apparently as physically active as sectionmen.

Interview information on physical activity also may be unreliable. In one study, information could only be replicated 50% of the time. Moreover there

TABLE 1

RETROSPECTIVE AND CROSS-SECTIONAL (PREVALENCE) STUDIES

Primary Investigator	Population	Relationship of Physical Inactivity to CHD
Large general population groups with activity levels from job title on death certificate and CHD diagnosed from death certificate		
Hedley [19]	Philadelphia	Positive
Morris [20]	Britain and Wales	Positive
Lilienfeld [21]	Baltimore	Negative
Stamler [22]	Chicago	Negative
Breslow [23]	California	Positive
Population groups with activity levels from job title and questionnaire and CHD diagnosed from death certificates or medical records		
Zukel [24] and Fox [25]	North Dakota	Positive
Occupational groups with activity level from job classification or salary level and CHD diagnosed from death certificate or industrial records/or medical records.		
Morris [20]	London busmen and postmen	Positive
Brunner [26, 27]	Israeli kibbutzim	Positive
Taylor [28]	U.S. railmen	Positive
Kahn [29]	U.S. Postmen	Positive
Adelstein [30]	South African railmen	Negative
Mortensen [31] and Hinkle [32]	Bell Telephone	Negative
McDonough [33]	Evans County, Ga. (farmers vs non-farmers)	Positive
Pell [34]	Dupont Chemical	Negative
Stamler [35]	Peoples' Gas	Positive
Occupational group with activity level from job title and CHD diagnosed by ECG (rest and/or exercise)		
Karvonen [36]	Finnish lumberjacks vs. nonlumberjacks	Positive
Occupational group with activity level (duration of walk to work) from questionnaire and diagnosis of ischemia by ECG records		
Rose [37]	British Civil Service Workers	Positive
Population group with physical fitness level by physiological evaluation (exercise test) and CHD diagnosed by clinical evaluation		
Mann [38]	Masai	Positive
Population group with activity level of job and leisure time from questionnaire and CHD diagnosed from medical records		
Frank [39, 40]	Health Insurance Plan of Greater New York	Positive
Hospital groups with activity level of job from job title or a questionnaire and diagnosis of CHD from medical records		
Shanoff [41]	Toronto V.A.	Negative
Forsmann [42]	Malmo (Sweden)	Negative

TABLE 1—*Continued*

RETROSPECTIVE AND CROSS-SECTIONAL (PREVALENCE) STUDIES

Primary Investigator	Type of Athlete	Reduced Cardiovascular Disease	Increased Longevity
Comparisons of cause of death and differences in life expectancy among former athletes and nonathletes using questionnaires, letters to relatives, college records and death certificates			
Morgan [43]	College oarmen	—	Positive
Dublin [44]	College	Negative	Negative
Rook [45]	College	Positive	Negative
Montoye [46]	College	Negative	Negative
Karvonen [47]	Finnish skiers	—	Positive
Pomeroy [48]	College football	Positive	—
Paffenbarger [49]	College	Positive	—
Polednak [50,51]	"Major" college sports "Minor" college sports	Negative	Negative
Schnohr [52]	Danish champions	Negative	Positive
Prout [53]	College oarmen	Negative	Positive
Bassler [54,55]	Marathon runner	—	Positive
Metropolitan Life [56]	Ex-Major League Baseball Players	Positive —	— Positive

appears to be a tendency for men after they have had a heart attack to report less heavy physical work in their usual occupation. Thus an important attribute for good epidemiology, a valid and reliable measuring instrument, was not met.

(5) The physical activity gradient among jobs in some industries may be too small to be significant, for example, the Peoples' Gas Co.,[57] the Bell Telephone Co.,[31, 32] and Civil Service workers [62] studies. Because of wide-spread mechanization and automation that has reduced physical activity in industry, future studies will have to concentrate on leisure-time activity in relating activity to CHD as have Morris *et al.*[72, 73] The latter studies suggest that relatively high exercise intensity levels of 7.5 kcal/min or more may be required for protection from CHD. There is need for further assessment and validation of questionnaires on habitual leisure time activity suitable for large population studies. Little data exists on the relationship between questionnaire classification and direct physiological measurements of physical activity. This is currently being evaluated in the Laboratory of Physiological Hygiene.[96]

(6) Physiological measures used to assess habitual physical activity and fitness levels, such as vital capacity and resting heart rate, have not been vali-

TABLE 2

PROSPECTIVE (LONGITUDINAL) STUDIES INVOLVING INITIALLY CHD-FREE MEN

Primary Investigator	Population	Relationship of Physical Inactivity to CHD
Occupational groups with activity levels from job title and/or job evaluation and CHD diagnosed from medical records		
Stamler [57]	Peoples' Gas	Negative
Morris [58]	London busmen	Positive
Paul [59]	Western Electric	Negative
Taylor [60]	U.S. railmen	Negative
Taylor [61]	Italian railmen	Negative
Chapman [62]	L.A. civil servants	Negative
Paffenbarger [63,64]	Longshoremen	Positive
Population study in which physical activity status (job and leisure) evaluated by questionnaire and diagnosis of CHD obtained from death certificates		
Hammond [65]	American Cancer Society volunteers	Positive
Population studies involving initially CHD-free people with activity (job and leisure) by questionnaire and CHD diagnosed by medical evaluation		
Keys [66]	7 Countries	Negative
Kannel [67]	Framingham	Negative
Rosenmann [68]	Western Collaborative	Positive
Cassel [69]	Evans County (Ga.)	Positive
Werko [70] and Wilhelmsen [71]	Götesborg (Sweden)	Positive
Occupational Group of Initially CHD-Free Men with Leisure Time Activity Level from Questionnaire and CHD Diagnosed by Medical Evaluation		
Morris [72] and Epstein [73]	British Civil Service Workers	Positive
Population and occupational groups with physical fitness assessed by physiological data and CHD diagnosed by medical evaluation		
Kannel [74]	Framingham	Resting HR, vital capacity, weight change	Positive
Stamler [57,75]	Peoples' Gas	Resting and exercise HR, oxygen consumption, vital capacity, weight change	Positive
Karvonen [76]	Finland	Exercise HR and blood pressure	Positive
Taylor [77]	U.S. Railmen	Resting and exercise HR	Positive
Bruce [78]	Seattle	Exercise HR and blood pressure	Positive

TABLE 2—*Continued*

PROSPECTIVE (LONGITUDINAL) STUDIES INVOLVING

INITIALLY CHD-FREE MEN

Primary Investigator	Population	No. Subjects	Duration (Years)
Effect of physical conditioning programs on CHD in middle-aged men at high risk for CHD			
Stamler [57]	Chicago	519	8
Pyörala [79]	Helsinki	424	1.5
Taylor [80]	Minneapolis, U. of Wisconsin Penn State U.	385	1.5

TABLE 3

PATHOLOGICAL STUDIES

Primary Investigator	Population	Relationship of Physical Inactivity to CHD
Postmortem studies in men dying of CHD correlating activity level from job titles with severity coronary artery lesions and coronary size		
Spain [81]	Westchester County (N.Y.)	Positive (Sedentary men died younger from CHD)
Rose [82]	Oxford (England)	Negative (No difference in size of coronaries)
Postmortem studies in men dying of noncardiac causes correlating activity level from job titles with severity of coronary atherosclerosis and/or myocardial ischemic changes		
Spain [83]	Westchester County (N.Y.)	Negative
Morris [84]	British Hospitals	Similar coronary atherosclerosis but less coronary occlusions and ischemic myocardial damage in physically active
Rose [82]	Oxford	Similar in coronary atherosclerosis but larger coronaries in physically active
Currens [85]	Clarence DeMar	Positive
Mitrani [86]	Israel	Negative

dated. The heart rate and systolic blood pressure during exercise (and their products), the duration of exercise on a standard test protocol, and maximal oxygen uptake are better measures of fitness. However these measurements are influenced by "natural endowment."

(7) The diagnoses of CHD in many of these studies were not standardized and often depended upon unreliable death certificate data, the diagnoses of many different physicians, and information collected for other reasons. The data are especially tenuous prior to the mid-1940s before objective criteria from electrocardiograms became available.

(8) Studies on the cause of death of former athletes have many inherent problems. These include selection for particular sports because of particular physical and psychological makeup, inadequate control groups for comparison, possible unreliable diagnosis of CHD, and lack of information on other coronary risk factors and habitual physical activity levels. Pomeroy and White [48] noted that a small subsample of former Harvard football players who habitually

TABLE 4

REHABILITATION (SECONDARY PREVENTION) STUDIES

Primary Investigator	Population (Coronary Patients)	Relationship of Physical Inactivity to CHD
Effects on myocardial infarct survivors of physical conditioning programs on recurrence of myocardial infarction and CHD mortality		
Hellerstein [87]	Cleveland	Positive
Göttheiner [88]	Israel	Positive
Brunner [89]	Israel	Positive
Rechnitzer [90]	Canada	Positive
Bruce [91]	Seattle	Positive (reduced mortality only)
Wilhelmsen [92]	Götesborg	Negative

maintained heavy physical activity throughout their lifetime remained free of CHD.

A search of the literature and review of reports of deaths of marathon runners by Bassler [54, 55] "failed to document a single death due to coronary atherosclerosis" among active marathoners or within 6 years of having completed a marathon by runners of any age. However, because of the relatively small number of marathoners, most of whom are young, lean, and nonsmoking, CHD would be expected to be rare. Green et al. [97] recently reported a death associated with myocardial infarction in a trained runner during the Boston Marathon; however, the autopsy revealed normal coronary arteries. Heat stroke may have been a contributing factor. Cantwell [98] recently showed that well-conditioned long distance runners are not immune to ventricular arrhythmias, presenting case reports on three who developed ventricular tachycardia during exercise. He postulated that sudden bursts of ventricular tachycardia-fibrillation may be the mechanism for the sudden death that occasionally occurs in joggers. However, a study in the Laboratory of Physiological Hygiene showed a decreased incidence of ventricular premature beats during exercise stress testing in men following an exercise conditioning program.[99]

(9) Pathological studies are limited by difficulties in assessing physical activity status after death (obtained from job title or questioning survivors) as well as limitations in methodology of measuring coronary atherosclerosis and myocardial damage.

(10) Because of an insufficient sample size, the exercise intervention studies reported in the literature lack the power to answer the question of whether increased physical activity can protect middle-aged men at high risk for CHD. Although CHD is a common condition in the United States, the number of new clinical cases appearing annually in a middle-aged population is only a small proportion of the number of people at risk. In planning an investigation to compare the incidence of CHD between an exercise group and a control group, randomization has to be used to equally distribute other coronary risk factors (known and unknown). Decisions have to be made regarding the sample size of the two groups taking into consideration the expected incidence of new CHD cases annually, the number of expected nonadherers ("dropouts" and shifting between groups), and the length of time the groups will be studied. The investigative manpower requirements, facilities available, and the cost are among other factors to be considered. These problems have been analyzed in detail elsewhere, and the estimated sample size necessary for a 5-year exercise study under various "dropout" patterns has been calculated.[100, 101] It is clear from this data that thousands of subjects would be required for such a study, necessitating a multicenter approach.

A pilot study was carried out in the Laboratory of Physiological Hygiene in the late 1960s in which middle-aged men at high risk for coronary heart diseases were randomly assigned to a supervised physical activity program or a control group for 18 months.[80] Because of the high dropout rate (50% in the first 6 months) and the large expense for facilities, equipment, and supervising personnel, it was concluded that a national primary CHD prevention trial using exercise was not feasible.

(11) Rehabilitation of survivors of myocardial infarction using exercise conditioning has been established as an effective means of improving quality of life, through physiological and psychological benefits.[102, 103] However, reported cardiac rehabilitation studies are inadequate to determine whether exercise can reduce the recurrence rate of myocardial infarction and premature mortality. The number of patients studied are too few to answer the above questions, and except for the study by Wilhelmsen et al.,[92] lacked an adequately matched control group. This Swedish study was the first large scale trial to involve randomization of subjects into an exercise conditioning and control group. However, 25% of the 188 selected were excluded because of contraindication to exercise, and only 25% remained on the exercise program for the full 4 years of the study.

It has been estimated that 3,000 or more eligible myocardial infarct survivors would have to be randomized and studied for 5 years in order to demonstrate a significant reduction in mortality rate among the group receiving exercise therapy as compared to the control group.[102] A pilot study involving 6 centers is currently underway in the United States (The National Exercise and Heart Disease Project of the Social Rehabilitation Service, Department of Health, Education and Welfare). A multicenter prospective study is also being carried out in Canada.[104] Such studies may be the best chance for more definitively demonstrating the possible value of physical activity in reducing severity of CHD.

Exercise and Longevity

Male and female rats subjected to a lifelong program of 10 minutes per day of walking exercise on a motor-driven drum were demonstrated by Retzlaff *et al.*[105] to live about 25% longer than nonexercised litter mates. The effect of exercise on human longevity is more difficult to determine. Attempts to evaluate this relationship has focused primarily on determining the longevity of men who were athletes in college or champions in their sports. The studies cited above yielded equivocal results. There is also a question of their applicability since in most of these studies apparently relatively few subjects habitually exercised, and it is well known both from human and animal studies that the physiological benefits of exercise conditioning rapidly regress upon cessation of training.[1, 106] An exception to the latter criticism is the study of Karvonen [47] who found that Finnish skiers, most of whom had participated in their sport throughout life, had a life expectancy that exceeded the general male population by several years. In a prospective study involving a California population, Belloc [107] found that physical activity (determined by questionnaire) was among those health habits related to reduced mortality and improved life expectancy.

An additional clue to the effects of heavy physical activity on longevity comes from studies on the life-styles of certain long-lived isolated populations. Such populations include the Abkhazia Republic in the foothills of the Caucasus Mountains in Southern Russia, Vilcabamba in the Andes Mountains in Equador, and Hunza, a municipality in the Himalaya Mountains of Southern Pakistan on the Chinese border.[108-110] These three regions are characterized by having a relatively large percentage of vigorous elderly people in the population including a much higher percentage of people over 100 years of age than in the United States. In all three cultures the people are physically active throughout life, being primarily farmers who labor by hand and walk a great deal in mountainous terrain instead of riding. However, other environmental factors, including diet, being cut off from the mainstream of modern life, and living in the mountains, as well as good genetic endowment certainly must contribute towards their longevity.

It is now clear that physical inactivity contributes to the reduced work and cardiorespiratory capacity previously attributed to aging. This is evidenced by the fact that the reduction in aerobic capacity (maximal oxygen consumption) associated with aging can be slowed or reversed by endurance exercise conditioning.[111] Physically active elderly people have been shown to have levels of aerobic capacity ordinarily attributed to much younger people, the end result of which is more energy and vitality, making it possible to pursue a more vigorous life style. Thus, while it is not presently possible to determine from existing data whether habitual life long exercise adds years to life, it appears certain that it adds "life to years."

Amount of Exercise Necessary

Many of the epidemiological studies cited above suggest that relatively small increases in habitual physical activity levels are adequate to reduce the incidence and severity of coronary heart disease. In several studies in which energy expenditure has been assessed between various occupational activity groups, the difference in daily caloric expenditure in sedentary and physically active workers ranged from 400 to 1000 kilocalories.[1] Moreover, it appeared that a sedentary individual might have to increase his activity by no more than 100 kilocalories per day to be placed in a more favorable intermediate activity group. In several studies, the greatest difference in coronary heart disease frequency or mortality was noted among those classified as inactive and slightly more active. Zukel [24, 25] found that as little as 1 hour daily of heavy physical activity was associated with a lower incidence of coronary heart disease. Morris and coworkers [72] found that a minimum of 30 minutes of vigorous physical activity per week requiring peak energy output of 7.5 kilocalories per minute or more was associated with "protection" against coronary heart disease. In terms of physiological benefits, studies performed on healthy individuals and subjects with physical disabilities or coronary heart disease have revealed that endurance exercise training such as provided by walking, cycling or jogging (2 to 4 times for 30 to 60 minutes a session) significantly improves working capacity and cardiovascular endurance,[112] and may reduce coronary risk factors. Associated lifestyle changes may contribute to risk factor reduction. It also appears likely that the cardiovascular benefits achieved by such exercise programs can be maintained with less frequent and/or intense exercise sessions. The key to obtaining a beneficial cardiovascular adaptation to exercise is that it should produce a sustained increase in cardiorespiratory and metabolic function. Attention has been focused on the work heart rate as a means of determining whether sufficient training stimulus of the cardiovascular respiratory system has taken place.

Physiologic adaptive changes can be expected to occur when the training heart rate is about 70% of the maximal heart rate of the individual. Apparently, older people need not be stressed to the same extent as younger to bring about training effects. A progressive multistage exercise electrocardiographic test on a treadmill or bicycle ergometer may be used to establish the appropriate exercise intensity level for individuals 35 or over. By the use of such tests, exercise can be prescribed on an individualized basis at an intensity and heart rate range appropriate to the individual's functional capacity, although subjective sensations are useful personal guidelines. Recreational interests and skills appropriate to observed physiological capacity have to be considered in selecting exercise activities to which a person will adhere as part of life-style. More work is needed on how to motivate different types of people to adhere to physical activity programs. In prescribing exercise, one should be aware of contraindications and precautions and the possibility of harmful effects. Training programs should be initiated at an exercise intensity and duration lower than test limits and gradually increased over a period of a few weeks, in order to minimize the possibility of musculoskeletal injuries. Exercise sessions should include warm-up and cool-down periods.

Recommendations

The current Joint British Cardiac Society report [113] provides clear-cut recommendations for individual behavior and professional prescriptions in the area of physical activity. Broad social recommendations are needed, however. We agree with one of its principal authors, Professor J. Morris [114] of London, who insists that a health policy of increasing physical activity requires no further justification because of the following:

(1) It is commendable in its own right because of the physiological and psychological benefit (in terms of improvements in emotional and general physical well-being, functional efficiency, self-image, body mobility, and weight control).

(2) The balance of benefits of physical activity appears favorable over the risks associated with inactivity and sensible exercise programs.

(3) Physical activity is a universal cultural attribute and thus is appropriate in applying to the universal problem of CHD.

(4) Intervention on physical activity of patients is economical and has little affect, if any, on the cost of health services.

(5) The idea of habitual physical activity is timely, topical, socially acceptable and largely uncontroversial.

Summary and Conclusions

Physiological, metabolic, and psychological adaptations accompanying regular endurance exercise increase cardivoscular capacity and efficiency, promote general health, improve the quality of life, retard the deterioration in physical work capacity that occurs with aging, and may attenuate several coronary risk factors. Such changes may be expected to favorably modify the course of CHD and increase functional and actual longevity. Numerous retrospective, cross-sectional, and prospective epidemiological studies involving population and occupation groups have considered the relationship of activity levels on the job and/or at leisure on CHD incidence, prevalence, and/or mortality. The consensus from this evidence is that physically active persons have a lower incidence of myocardial infarction and associated mortality and that an inverse relationship exist between physical activity and CHD. However, these studies have serious flaws including job and leisure activity changes by subjects due to disease, confounding independent variables, too small a gradient in physical activity within some populations, and difficulties in assessing habitual activity levels as well as in confirming the diagnosis of CHD. The few reported postmortem studies failed to demonstrate any significant reduction in the severity of coronary atherosclerosis in the physically active, although larger coronary artery lumen size, fewer occlusions and less ischemic myocardial damage were observed. These pathologic studies have many of the same problems mentioned above.

Exercise is currently being widely used to help rehabilitate patients after uneventful recovery from myocardial infarction. Although the pioneer uncontrolled studies suggest that exercise programs can reduce the recurrence of myocardial infarction and associated mortality, this has not yet been confirmed by a controlled study. A multicenter collaborative controlled secondary prevention trial may be the best approach to answer the question of whether habitual physical activity can alter CHD morbidity and/or mortality. Animal studies and evaluation of the life-styles of certain populations with unusual longevity suggest that exercise helps promote this increased longevity, independent of its effect on CHD; however, epidemiologic studies relying primarily on follow-up information on former college athletes are inadequate to answer the question. Based on current knowledge it is prudent for the practitioner to prescribe regular exercise as part of a hygienic CHD prevention program, to include elimination of cigarette smoking, a diet lower in saturated fats and calories, and control of elevated blood pressure. The exercise program should be based on an individualized prescription, following an exercise stress test, and should be carried out at least 2 to 4 times per week for 30 to 60 minutes a session.

References

1. LEON, A. S. 1973. Comparative cardiovascular adaptations to exercise in animals and man and its relevance to coronary heart disease. *In* Comparative Pathophysiology of Circulatory Disturbance. C. M. Bloor, Ed. : 143–174. Plenum Publishing Corporation. New York, N.Y.
2. FLETCHER, G. F. & J. D. CANTWELL. 1974. Exercise and Coronary Heart Disease. Charles C Thomas, Publisher. Springfield, Ill.
3. BJÖRNTORP, B. P., M. FAHLEN, G. GRIMBY, A. GUSTAFSON, J. HOLM, P. RENSTRÖM & T. SCHERSTEN. 1972. Carbohydrate and lipid metabolism in middle-aged physically well trained men. Metabolism **21:** 1037–1044.
4. LOPEZ-S, A., R. VIAL, L. BELFORT & G. ARROYAVE. 1974. Effect of exercise and physical fitness on serum lipids and lipoproteins. Atherosclerosis **20:** 1–9.
5. WOOD, P. D., P. D. KLEIN, S. LEWIS & W. L. HASKELL. 1974. Plasma lipoprotein concentrations in middle-aged male runners (Abstract). Circulation **49** (Suppl. 3): 115.
6. LEWIS, B., A. CHAIT, C. M. O. OAKLY, I. D. P. WOOTON, D. M. KRIKLER, A. ONITIRI, G. SIGURDSSON & A. FEBRUARY. 1974. Serum lipoprotein abnormalities in patients with ischaemic heart disease; comparisons with a control population. Brit. Med. J. **iii:** 489–493.
7. MILLER, G. J. & N. E. MILLER. 1975. Plasma high-density lipoprotein concentration and development of ischaemic heart disease. Lancet **i:** 16–19.
8. HEINZELMANN, F. 1973. Social and psychological factors that influence the effectiveness of exercise programs. *In* Exercise Testing and Exercise Training in Coronary Heart Disease. J. P. Naughton & H. K. Hellerstein, Eds. : 275–287. Academic Press. New York, N.Y.
9. BAHR, R. 1975. This doctor prescribes movement. Runners World **10**(Nov.): 40–42.
10. TAYLOR, H. L., A. HENSCHEL, J. BROZEK & A. KEYS. 1949. Effects of bed rest on cardiovascular function and work performance. J. Appl. Physiol. **2:** 223–239.
11. KOTTKE, F. J. 1966. The effects of limitation of activity upon the human body. J. Amer. Med. Assoc. **196:** 825–830.
12. SALTIN, B., G. BLOMQUIST, J. H. MITCHELL, R. L. JOHNSON, JR., K. WILDENTHAL & C. B. CHAPMAN. Response to exercise after bed rest and after training. Circulation **38**(Suppl. 12): 1–55.
13. HICKEY, N., R. MULCAHY, G. J. BOURKE, I. GRAHAM & K. WILSON-DAVIS. 1975. Study of coronary risk factors related to physical activity in 15,171 men. Brit. Med. J. **ii:** 507–509.
14. COOPER, K. H., M. L. POLLACK, R. P. MARTIN, S. R. WHITE, A. C. LINNERUD & A. JACKSON. 1976. Physical fitness levels vs. selected coronary risk factors. A cross-sectional study. J. Amer. Med. Assoc. **236:** 116–169.
15. MANN, G. V., H. L. GARRETT, A. FARHI, H. MURRAY & F. T. BILLINGS. 1969. Exercise to prevent coronary heart disease. An experimental study of the effects of training on risk factors for coronary disease in man. Amer. J. Med. **46:** 12–27.
16. SMITH, E. 1864. Report on the sanitary circumstances of tailors in London. *In* Rep Med Officer Primary Council with Appendix. 6th edit. : 416–430. H. M. Stationary Office. London, England. (Cited in Reference 2.)
17. FROELICHER, V. F. & A. OBERMAN. 1972. Analysis of epidemiologic studies of

physical inactivity as risk factor for coronary artery disease. Prog. Cardiov. Dis. **15:** 41–65.

18. Fox, S. M. III & J. P. Naughton. 1972. Physical activity and the prevention of coronary heart disease. Prev. Med. **1:** 92–120.

19. Hedley, O. F. 1939. Analysis of 5,116 deaths reported as due to acute coronary occlusion in Philadelphia, 1933–1937. U.S. Weekly Pub. Health Rep. **54:** 972. (Cited by Clarke, H. H. 1972. Physical activity and coronary heart disease. Physical Fitness Res. Digest **2:** 1–13.)

20. Morris, J. N., J. A. Heady, P. A. B. Raffle, C. G. Roberts & J. W. Parks. 1953. Coronary heart disease and physical activity of work. Lancet **265:** 1053–1057, 1111–1120.

21. Lillienfeld, A. M. 1956. Variations of mortality from heart disease. Public Health Rep. **71:** 545–552.

22. Stamler, J., M. Kjelsberg & Y. Hall. 1960. Epidemiological studies on cardiovascular-renal diseases: I. Analysis of mortality by age-race-sex-occupation. J. Chron. Dis. **12:** 440–455.

23. Breslow, L. & P. Buell. 1960. Mortality from coronary heart disease and physical activity of work in California. J. Chron. Dis. **11:** 428–444.

24. Zukel, W. J., R. H. Lewis, P. E. Enterline, R. C. Painter, L. S. Ralston, R. M. Fawcett, A. P. Meredith & B. Peterson. 1959. A short-term community study of the epidemiology of coronary heart disease. Amer. J. Pub. Health **49:** 1630–1639.

25. Fox, S. M., III & W. L. Haskell. 1966. Physical activity and health maintenance. J. Rehab. **32:** 89–92.

26. Brunner, D. & G. Manelis. 1960. Myocardial infarction among members of communal settlements in Israel. Lancet **ii:** 1049–1050.

27. Brunner, D. & G. Manelis. 1970. Physical activity at work and ischemic heart disease. *In* Coronary Heart Disease and Physical Fitness. O. A. Larsen & R. O. Malmborg, Eds. : 244–250. University Park Press. Baltimore, Md.

28. Taylor, H. L., E. Klepetar, A. Keys, W. Parln, H. Blackburn & T. Puchner. 1962. Death rates among physically active and sedentary employees of the railroad industry. Amer. J. Publ. Health **52:** 1697–1707.

29. Kahn, H. A. 1963. The relationship of reported coronary heart disease mortality to physical activity of work. Amer. J. Publ. Health **53:** 1058–1067.

30. Adelstein, A. M. 1963. Some aspects of cardiovascular mortality in South Africa. Brit. J. Prev. Soc. Med. **17:** 29–40.

31. Mortensen, J. M., T. T. Stevensen & L. H. Whitney. 1959. Mortality due to coronary disease analyzed by broad occupational groups. Arch. Indust. Health **19:** 1–4.

32. Hinkle, L. E., L. A. Whitney, E. W. Lehman, J. Dunn & B. Benjamin. 1968. Occupation, education, and coronary heart disease. Science **161:** 238–246.

33. McDonough, J. R., C. G. Hames, S. C. Stulb & G. E. Garrison. 1965. Coronary heart disease among Negroes and whites in Evans County, Georgia. J. Chron. Dis. **18:** 443–468.

34. Pell, S. & C. D'Alonzo. 1970. Chronic disease morbidity and income level in an employed population. Amer. J. Publ. Health **60:** 116–129.

35. Stamler, J., H. A. Lindberg, D. M. Berkson, A. Shaffer, W. Miller & A. Poindevter. 1960. Prevalence and incidence of coronary heart disease in strata of the labor force of a Chicago industrial corporation. J. Chron. Dis. **11:** 405–420.

36. Karvonen, M. J., P. M. Rautaharju, E. Orma, S. Punsar & J. Takkunen. 1961. Heart disease and employment. Cardiovascular studies on lumberjacks. J. Occup. Med. **3:** 49–53.

37. Rose, G. 1969. Physical activity and coronary heart disease. Proc. R. Soc. Med. **62:** 1183–1188.

38. Mann, G. V., R. D. Shaffer & A. Rich. 1965. Physical fitness and immunity to heart disease in Masai. Lancet **ii:** 1308–1310.

39. FRANK, C. W., E. WEINBLATT, S. SHAPIRO & R. V. SAGER. 1966. Physical inactivity as a lethal factor in myocardial infarction among men. Circulation 34: 1022–1033.
40. FRANK, C. W. 1968. The course of coronary heart disease: Factors relating to prognosis. Bull. N.Y. Acad. Med. 44: 900–915.
41. SHANOFF, H. M. & J. A. LITTLE. 1961. Studies of male survivors of myocardial infarction due to "essential" atherosclerosis. I. Characteristics of the patients. Canad. Med. Assoc. J. 84: 519–530.
42. FORSSMAN, O. & B. LINDEGARD. 1958. The post-coronary patient. J. Psychosom. Res. 3: 89–169.
43. MORGAN, J. E. 1873. University Oars. (Cited in KARPOVICH, P. V. 1941. Longevity and athletics. Res. Quart. 12: 451–455.)
44. DUBLIN, L. I. 1932. College honormen long-lived. Statis. Bull. Metropolitan Life Insur. Co. 13: 5–7.
45. ROOK, A. 1954. Investigation into longevity of Cambridge sportsmen. Brit. Med. J. i: 773–777.
46. MONTOYE, H., W. D. VAN HUSS, H. OLSON, A. HUDEE & E. MAHONEY. 1956. Study of the longevity and morbodity of college athletes. J. Amer. Med. Assoc. 162: 1132–1134.
47. KARVONEN, M. J., J. KIHLBERG, J. MAATA & J. VIRKAJARVI. 1956. Longevity of champion skiers. Duodecim 72: 893–903. (In Finnish, abstact in English.)
48. POMEROY, W. C. & P. D. WHITE. Coronary heart disease in former football players. J. Amer. Med. Assoc. 167: 711–714.
49. PAFFENBARGER, R. S., J. NOTKIN, D. E. KRUEGER, P. A. WOLF, M. C. THORNE, E. J. LA BAUER & J. WILLIAMS. 1966. Chronic disease in former college students. II. Methods and observations on mortality from coronary heart disease. Amer. J. Publ. Health 56: 1026–1030.
50. POLEDNAK, A. P. & A. DAMON. 1970. College athletics, longevity and cause of death. Human Biol. 42: 28–46.
51. POLEDNAK, A. P. 1972. Longevity and cardiovascular mortality among former college athletes. Circulation 46: 649–654.
52. SCHNOHR, P. 1971. Longevity and causes of death in male athletic champions. Lancet ii: 1364–1366.
53. PROUT, C. 1972. Life expectancy of college oarmen. J. Amer. Med. Assoc. 220: 1709–1711.
54. BASSLER, T. J. 1972. Previous health and longevity of male athletes (Letter). Lancet ii: 711.
55. BASSLER, T. J. 1976. Marathon running and myocardial infarction (Letter). Ann. Intern. Med. 85: 389.
56. METROPOLTAN LIFE INSURANCE CO. 1975. Longevity of major league baseball players. Statis. Bull. (September.).
57. STAMLER, J., D. M. BERKSON, H. A. LINDEBERG, T. T. WHIPPLE, W. MILLER & Y. HALL. Long-term epidemiologic studies on the possible role of physical activity and physical fitness in the prevention of premature clinical coronary heart disease. 1970. In Medicine and Sports. Vol. 4. Physical Activity and Aging. D. Brunner & E. Jokl, Eds. : 274–300. University Park Press. Baltimore, Md.
58. MORRIS, J. N., A. HAGAN, D. C. PATTESON & M. J. GARDNER. 1966. Invidence and prediction of ischaemic heart disease in London busmen. Lancet ii: 553–559.
59. PAUL, O., M. H. LEPPER, W. H. PHELAN, G. W. DUPERTUIS, A. MACMILLAN, H. MCKEAN & H. A. PARK. 1963. A longitudinal study of coronary heart disease. Circulation 28: 20–31.
60. TAYLOR, H. B., H. BLACKBURN, A. KEYS, R. W. PARLIN, C. VASQUEZ & T. PUCHNER. 1970. IV. Five-year follow-up of employees of selected U.S. railroad companies. Circulation 41(Suppl. I): 120–139.
61. TAYLOR, H. L., A. MENOTTI, V. PUDDU, M. MONTI & A. KEYS. 1970. XI. Five

years of follow-up of railroad men in Italy. Circulation **41**(Suppl. I): 113–122.

62. CHAPMAN, J. M. & F. J. MASSEY. 1964. The interrelationship of serum cholesterol, hypertension, body weight, and risk of coronary disease. Results of the first ten years' follow-up in the Los Angeles heart study. J. Chron. Dis. **17**: 933–949.

63. PAFFENBARGER, R S., JR., A. S. GIMA, M. E. LAUGHLIN, E. MARY & R. A. BLACK. 1971. Characteristics of longshoremen related to CHD and stroke. Amer. J. Pub. Health **61**: 1362–1370.

64. PAFFENBARGER, R. S., JR. & W. E. HALE. 1975. Work activity and coronary heart mortality. New Engl. J. Med. **292**: 545–550.

65. HAMMOND, E. C. 1964. Smoking in relation to mortality and morbidity. Findings in first thirty-four months of follow-up in a prospective study started in 1959. J. Nat. Cancer Inst. **32**: 1161–1188.

66. KEYS, A., Ed. 1970. Coronary heart disease in seven countries. Circulation **41**(Suppl. I): 1–211.

67. KANNEL, W. B. 1966. The Framingham Heart Study, Habits, and Coronary Heart Disease. Public Health Service Publication No. 1515. Washington, D.C., U.S. Department of Health, Education, and Welfare.

68. ROSENMAN, R. H. 1970. The influence of different exercise patterns on the incidence of coronary heart disease in the Western Collaborative Group Study. *In* Medicine and Sports. Vol. 4. Physical Activity and Aging. D. Brunner & E. Jokl, Eds. : 267–273. University Park Press. Baltimore, Md.

69. CASSEL, J., S. HEYDEN, A. G. BARTEL, B. H. KAPLAN, H. A. TYROLER, J. C. CORONI & C. G. HAMES. 1972. Occupation and physical activity and coronary heart disease. Arch. Intern. Med. **128**: 920–928.

70. WERKO, L. 1971. Can we prevent heart disease? Ann. Intern. Med. **74**: 278–288.

71. WILHELMSEN, L., G. TIBBLIN & L. WERKO. 1972. A primary prevention in Götesborg, Sweden. Prev. Med. **1**: 153–160.

72. MORRIS, J. N., S. P. W. CHAVE, C. ADAM, C. SIREY, L. EPSTEIN & D. J. SHEEHAN. 1973. Vigorous exercise in leisure-time and the incidence of coronary heart disease. Lancet **i**: 333–339.

73. EPSTEIN, L., G. J. MILLER, F. W. STITT & J. N. MORRIS. 1976. Vigorous exercise in leisure time, coronary risk factors, and resting electrocardiogram in middle-aged male Civil Servants. Brit. J. **38**: 403–409.

74. KANNEL, W. B. 1967. Habitual levels of physical activity and risk of coronary heart disease. The Framingham Study. Canad. Med. Assoc. J. **96**: 811–812.

75. BIRKSON, D. M., T. J. STAMLER, H. A. LINDBERG, W. A. MILLER, E. L. STEVENS, R. SOYUGENC, T. J. TOKICH & R. STAMLER. 1970. Heart rate: An important risk factor for coronary mortality—10-year experience of the Peoples' Gas Company epidemiologic study (1958–68). *In* Atherosclerosis, 2nd International Symposium. R. J. Jones, Ed. : 382–389. Springer/Verlag. New York, N.Y.

76. KARVONEN, M. 1976. Physical activity of occupation and coronary heart disease. *In* Advances in Cardiology Vol. 18. 3rd Paavo Nurmi Symposium. Exercise and Coronary Heart Disease, Porvooo (Finland), September 1975. P. Halonen & E. Louhija, Eds. : 243–248. S. Karger, New York, N.Y.

77. TAYLOR, H. L. & H. BLACKBURN. Unpublished findings in U.S. Railroad Employees Study. Laboratory of Physiological Hygiene. Minneapolis, Minn.

78. BRUCE, R. A. June 1976. Presentation at the International Congress of Electrocardiology. Brussels, Belgium.

79. PYÖRALA, K., R. KARAVA, S. PUNSAR, P. OJA, P. TERASLINNA, T. PARTANEN, M. JAASKELAINEN, M. PEKKARINEN & A. KOSKELA. 1971. A controlled study of the effects of 18 months physical training in sedentary middle-aged men with high indicies of risk relative to coronary heart disease. *In* Coronary Heart

Disease and Physical Fitness. O. A. Larsen & R. O. Malmborg, Eds. : 261–265. University Park Press. Baltimore, Md.

80. TAYLOR, H. L., E. R. BUSKIRK & R. D. REMINGTON. 1973. Exercise in controlled trials of the prevention of coronary heart disease. Fed. Proc. **32:** 1623–1627.

81. SPAIN, D. & V. A. BRADESS. 1957. Sudden death from coronary atherosclerosis. Age, race, sex, physical activity and alcohol. Arch. Intern. Med. **100:** 228–231.

82. ROSE, G., R. J. PRINEAS & J. R. A. MITCHELL. 1967. Myocardial infarction and the intrinsic calibre of coronary arteries. Brit. Heart. J. **29:** 548–552.

83. SPAIN, D. M. & V. A. BRADESS. 1960. Occupational physical activity and the degree of coronary atherosclerosis in "normal" men. A postmortem study. Circulation **22:** 239–242.

84. MORRIS, J. N., J. A. HEADY, P. A. B. RAFFLE, C. G. ROBERTS & J. W. PARKS. 1953. Coronary heart disease and physical activity of work. Lancet **ii:** 1053–1057.

85. CURRENS, J H. & P. D. WHTE. 1961. Half century of running. Clinical, physiologic, and autopsy findings in the case of Clarence DeMar ("Mr. Marathon"). N. Eng. J. Med. **265:** 988–993.

86. MITRANI, Y., H. KARPLUS & D. BRUNNER. 1970. Coronary atherosclerosis in cases of traumatic death. *In* Medicine and Sport. Vol. 4. Physical Activity and Aging. D. Brunner & E. Jokl, Eds. : 241–248. University Park Press. Baltimore, Md.

87. HELLERSTEIN, H. K. 1968. Exercise therapy in coronary disease. Bull. N.Y. Acad. Med. **44:** 1028–1043.

88. GÖTTHEINER, V. 1968. Long-range strenuous sports training for cardiac reconditioning and rehabilitaiton. Amer. J. Cardiol. **22:** 426–435.

89. BRUNNER, D. & N. MESHULAM. 1969. Prevention of recurrent myocardial infarction by physical exercise. Israel J. Med. Sci. **5:** 783–785.

90. RECHNITZER, P. A., H. A. PICKARD, A. V. PAIVO, M. S. YUHASZ & D. CUNNINGHAM. 1972. Long-term follow-up study of survival and recurrence rates following myocardial infarction in exercising and control subjects. Circulation **45:** 853–857.

91. BRUCE, E. H., K. FREDRICK, R. A. BRUCE & L. D. FISCHER. 1976. Comparison of active participants and dropouts in Capri cardiovascular rehabilitation programs. Amer. J. Cardiol. **37:** 53–60.

92. WILHELMSEN, L., H. SANNE, D. ELMFELDT, G. GRIMBY, G. TIBBLIN & H. WEDEL. 1975. A controlled trial of physical training after myocardial infarction. Effects on risk factors, nonfatal reinfarction and death. Prev. Med. **4:** 491–508.

93. MORRIS, J. N., J. A. HEADY & P. A. RAFFLE. 1956. Physique of London busmen. Epidemiology of uniforms. Lancet **ii:** 569–570.

94. KEYS, A. 1975. Coronary heart disease. The global picture. Atherosclerosis **22:** 149–192.

95. BRUNNER, D., G. MANELS, M. MODAN & S. LEVIN. 1974. Physical activity at work and the incidence of myocardial infarction, angina pectoris and death due to ischemic heart disease. An epidemiological study in Israeli collective settlements (kibbutzim). J. Chron. Dis. **27:** 217–233.

96. LEON, A. S., G. DE BACKER, D. R. JACOBS, JR. & H. L. TAYLOR. 1976. Relationship of life habits and physical characteristics to work capacity on treadmill. Circulation **53** (Suppl. II)**:** 52.

97. GREEN, L. H., S. I. COHEN & G. KURLAND. 1976. Fatal myocardial infarction in marathon racing. Ann. Intern. Med. **84:** 704–706.

98. CANTWELL, J. D. 1976. Marathon racing and myocardial infarction (letter). Ann. Intern. Med. **85:** 391–392.

99. BLACKBURN, H., H. L. TAYLOR, B. HAMRELL, E. BUSKIRK, W. C. NICHOLAS & R. D. THORSEN. 1973. Premature ventricular complexes induced by stress testing. Amer. J. Cardiol. **31:** 441–448.

100. TAYLOR, H. L., R. W. PARLIN, H. BLACKBURN & A. KEYS. 1966. Problems in the analysis of the relationship of coronary heart disease to physical activity or the lack with special reference to sample size and occupational withdrawal. Proc. of the Beitostolen Symposium in 1966. K. Evang & K. L. Anderson, Eds. : 242–261. Williams & Wilkins Company. Baltimore, Md.

101. REMINGTON, R. & M. A. SCHORK. 1967. Determination of number of subjects needed for experimental epidemiologic studies on the effect of increased physical activity on incidence of coronary heart disease—preliminary consideration. In Phyical Activity and the Heart. Proc. of a Symposium, Helsinki, Finland. M. J. Karvonen & A. J. Barry, Eds. : 311–319. Charles C Thomas, Publisher. Springfield, Ill.

102. LEON, A. S. & H. BLACKBURN. 1974. Exercise and coronary heart disease. Minn. Med. 57: 106–107.

103. LEON, A. S. 1976. How much exercise? Med. World News 17: 51–53.

104. RECHNITZER, P. A., S. SANGAL, D. A. CUNNINGHAM, G. ANDREW, C. BUCK, N. L. JONES, T. KAVANAGH, J. O. PARKER, R. J. SHEPARD & M. S. YUHACZ. 1975. A controlled prospective study on the effects of endurance training on the recurrence rate of myocardial infarction. A description of the experimental design. Amer. J. Epid. 102: 358–364.

105. RETZLAFF, E., J. FONTAINE & W. FURUTA. 1966. Effect of daily exercise of life-span of albino rats. Geriatrics 21: 171–177.

106. LEON, A. S. & C. M. BLOOR. 1976. The effects of complete and partial deconditioning on exercise-induced cardiovascular changes in the rat. In Advances in Cardiology, Vol. 18. 3rd Paavo Nurmi Symposium on Exercise and Coronary Heart Disease. Porvoo (Finland) September 1975. P. Halonen & A. Louhija, Eds. : 81–92. S. Karger. New York, N.Y.

107. BELLOC, N. B. 1973. Relationship of health practices and mortality. Prev. Med. 2: 67–81.

108. LEAF, A. 1973. Getting old. Sci. Amer. 229: 45–52.

109. LEAF, A. 1973. Scientists visit some of the world's oldest people. Every day is a gift when you are over 100. National Geographic 143: 92–119.

110. WRENCH, G. T. 1972. The Wheel of Health. The Sources of Long Life and Health Among the Hunza. 2nd edit. Schocken Books, New York, N.Y.

111. TAYLOR, H. L. & H. L. MONTOYE. 1972. Physical fitness, cardiovascular function and age. In Epidemiology of Aging. A. M. Ostfeld, D.C. Gibson & C. P. Donnelly, Eds. : 223–241. U.S. Government Printing Office. Washington, D.C.

112. POLLOCK, M. L. 1973. The quantification of endurance training programs. In Exercise and Sports Science Reviews. J. W. Wilmore, Ed. Vol. 1: 155–188. Academic Press. New York, N.Y.

113. Report of the Joint Committee of the Royal College of Physicians and the British Cardiac Society. 1976. Brit. Heart J. In press.

114. MORRIS, J. 1977. Exercise: health and prevention. In The Strategy of Postponement of Ischemic Heart Disease. P. Schnohr, Ed. Danish Heart Foundation. Copenhagen, Denmark. In press.

115. LEON, A. S., J. CONRAD, D. HUNNINGHAKE, D. JACOBS & R. SERFASS. 1977. Exercise effects on body composition, work capacity, and carbohydrate and lipid metabolism of young obese men. Med. Sci. Sports 9: 60.

MARATHON RUNNING AND IMMUNITY TO ATHEROSCLEROSIS

Thomas J. Bassler

Department of Pathology
Centinela Hospital
Inglewood, California 90307

Atherosclerosis (ASCVD) is a specific term limited to the lipid-related arterial lesion that accounts for half of the adult deaths in the urban centers of advanced countries. Many factors, the so-called "benefits" of civilization, have been associated with this increased incidence of ASCVD. These include: refined tobacco use,[1] lack of exercise,[2] and a rich diet. The urban diet is suspect because it lacks food "fiber," [3] unsaturated fats,[4] ascorbic acid,[5] and tocopherols.[6]

Immunity to atherosclerosis has been reported in the Masai warriors who herd cattle on foot [7] and the Tarahumara Indians who take part in ceremonial runs.[8] These populations are primitive. They lack the refined foods found in our urban diet. Their tobacco is coarse and in short supply. It has a harsh smoke that is difficult to inhale. They cover a great deal of ground on foot routinely, averaging 20 kilometers and burning 1,200 kcals each day.

Marathon runners (42-km men) have much in common with these primitive populations.[9] They avoid inhaling tobacco smoke. They cover a great deal of ground on foot, often in the range of 50 to 100 kilometers a week; and their diet contains conspicuous amounts of unsaturated fats, food fiber, and the vitamins C and E. At autopsy, their coronary arteries have been described as "enlarged" and "widely patent." [10] Mann observed this same enlargement in the coronary arteries of Masai warriors and attributed it to their high degree of fitness.[11] Marathon running is "addictive." [12] Few of the 42-km men have discontinued their sport. Thus, in marathoning, we have a "low-risk" life-style with high adherence. Also, the marathon races, themselves, give us a clear record of who the 42-km men are, and their level of fitness at the time of the race. Therefore, the American Medical Joggers Association (AMJA) considers these runners to be the ideal population to study the effects of their multifactoral life-style in the prevention of a high-incidence multifactoral disease, atherosclerosis.

METHODS

Reports of deaths in marathon runners are reviewed, world-wide. An excess of 200 reports have been received during the past 10 years. Many are duplicates. Most were below the 42-km threshold.

RESULTS

To date, there have been no reports of fatal ASCVD, histologically proven, among 42-km men.

DISCUSSION

Heart Attack

The popular euphemism for any sudden death is "heart attack." There is no justification for this diagnosis in 42-km men unless it is confirmed by autopsy, since the first case has yet to be reported. Myocardial infarction due to causes other than ASCVD has been seen. There are many such causes.[13] Such lesions as anomalies, trauma, thrombocytosis, and arteritis are not related to life-style.

These other causes of cardiac death may mimic ASCVD at gross autopsy examination. Microscopic studies are necessary for identification of coronary mural thickening due to arteritis, metabolic diseases, and dissection.

Nonfatal cardiac emergencies have also been reported in 42-km men. However, when the patient is a "regular distance runner with no recognizable risk factors" the coronary angiogram is usually normal. Such a case has been reported by Cantwell.[14]

Race Documentation

"Low-mileage" runners have often been mistaken for 42-km men. This is understandable when they have produced championship performances at middle-distances (5 km–10 km). However, the same mistake is often made for slow joggers if they have been unusually visible at running events.

Case No. 1. A man in his 30s collapsed in a race, falling near the 12-km mark. Death was instantaneous. Autopsy showed fatal ASCVD (FIGURE 1) with a marked inflammatory reaction around the lipids in the wall of the coronary arteries (FIGURE 2). Prior to death, he had been discussing his two previous marathon runs with a racing partner. However, his heart showed none of the usual signs of marathon training. His coronary arteries were small, and his plaques were inflamed.

Comment: The race directors of the two marathons mentioned by the deceased were contacted and had "no record" of him. Training partners in his home town confirmed that his training was "low mileage." His next of kin were aware of his ASCVD.

Jogging Deaths

10,000 autopsies have been studied by Orselli, Carroll, Roberts, and myself.[15] Deaths while wearing athletic gear are not rare. Most of these weekend sportsmen smoke and engage in activities that require great strength or speed, not endurance. The runners usually confined their distances to 5 km or less, well under the "threshold" described as "protective" by Morris.[2]

Autopsy Documentation

Deaths in 42-km men have a statistical pattern similar to the teenage population: 50% traffic accidents, 25% "other accidents," homicide or suicide; and 25% "natural deaths other than ASCVD."

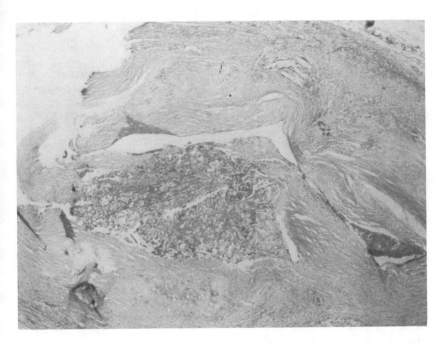

FIGURE 1. Nonmarathoner: Anterior descending branch of left coronary artery with hemorrhage into ASCVD plaque, rupture of plaque and thrombosis of lumen. (H & E stain; × 10.)

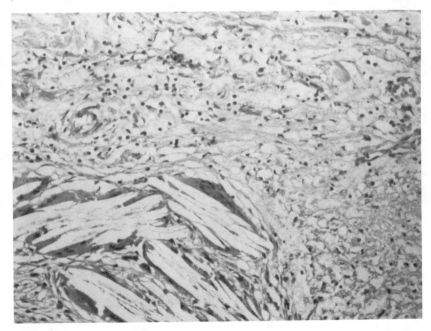

FIGURE 2. Same lesion as shown in FIGURE 1, at higher magnification: Marked inflammatory reaction to lipids in plaque. (H & E stain; × 245.)

581

The death certificates of some 42-km men state that fatal ASCVD was present, but these have been unsupported by autopsy evidence so far.

Case No. 2. A 35-year-old man ran 84 km in under 7 hours. He died with chest pain while still a well-conditioned runner. The first report stated that autopsy showed "ischemic heart disease with a number of small infarcts." [16] However, no autopsy was performed. [17]

Case No. 3. A 19-year-old man died while running in his second marathon. The single word "atheroma" has survived as the verbal autopsy report. There was no written record of the autopsy, and histological studies were not done. [17]

Case No. 4. Gross autopsy showed fatal ASCVD in a nonmarathoner who had been taking long training runs. [16]

Comment: The original reports [16] of these three cases strongly suggests that 42-km men have died of fatal ASCVD. They have been widely circulated in the medical and running literature. However, they are clearly unsubstantiated histologically.

Case No. 5. A popular myth states that a messenger named Pheidippides died after a run from Marathon to Athens in 490 B.C. [18]

Comment: Messengers were professional runners. A single individual could probably cover distances over 200 km if we can apply our observations of the modern Tarahumara Indians. [8] Fatal ASCVD has not been reported among these Indian runners, so to speculate that this disease might have killed Pheidippides is unwarranted. Re-enactment of his legendary run suggests that environmental heat stress would have been the greatest threat. [19]

Nonatheromatous Disease

Deaths by accidents, homicide, or suicide are rarely confused with ASCVD. The exceptions occur, however. Asphyxia due to food aspiration, occult electric shock, heat stroke, and unwitnessed drug overdose can simulate a fatal heart attack. Correct diagnosis requires meticulous, thorough autopsy in these cases.

Cases Nos. 6 through 12. Seven 42-km men have died "in their sleep" during the past 10 years. Five of the hearts were examined at autopsy. None showed fatal ASCVD.

Details: There was one case of viral myocarditis, one case of coronary anomaly, and in two of the cases toxicologic studies were positive.

The fifth case was "undetermined." The autopsy was not complete, and toxicologic studies were not done.

Comment: 42-km men, like teenagers, should have toxicologic studies when gross autopsy findings do not explain the cause of death. This is especially true of unwitnessed deaths where overdose is a possibility.

Neoplasms

Schmid reports an increased incidence of malignant tumors in former athletes. [20] This may be a statistical artifact since he excluded all deaths that were not due to natural causes. (This would exclude some 75% of the deaths in 42-km men.) He does review animal studies which showed that exercise *reduced* the incidence of malignancy.

Besides exercise, several other factors in the 42-km man's life-style may reduce the incidence of tumors: antioxidants,[21] specifically vitamins E [22] and C; [23] and a full-fiber diet.[3] Also, the very low incidence of tobacco use should reduce the number of tumors by eliminating cancer of the respiratory tract.

Marathoner Clarence de Mar did die of cancer.[10]

Case No. 13. A 62-year-old nonmarathoner died while jogging. "Heart attack" was given as the cause of death. There was no autopsy. He did not smoke.

Comment: He had jogged about 10 km per day for 40 years and had a normal stress test. Five years prior to death a malignant melanoma was removed from his arm. There was no evidence of recurrence, clinically. He drank about 20 cups of coffee per day.

Speculation about the cause of death in such a case should include the possibility of occult metastases from the melanoma. ASCVD is a remote possibility in view of the normal stress test, no smoking, and the impressive number of 10-km runs.

Case No. 14. A man in his 60s was under medical care for myeloproliferative syndrome when he took up marathon training. He completed several 42-km runs and a 50-km run. He stopped running for two weeks for a minor surgical procedure and died suddenly. Autopsy showed brain hemorrhage due to thrombocytosis. ASCVD was not a factor in his death.

Comment: Coronary arteries were widely patent with areas of resorption of calcium plaques (FIGURES 3, 4, 5 & 6). This is consistent with his 3 years of marathoning.

Congenital Anomalies

Anomalies are a rare cause of death in adults. However, when present, they can mimic ASCVD. They are not related to life-style.

Case No. 15. A track coach in his 60s died while jogging. Autopsy showed brain hemorrhage due to a ruptured berry aneurysm. ASCVD was not a factor.

Comment: The newspaper accounts carried this case as "another heart attack in a jogger."

Case No. 16. A heavy smoker in his 50s died in sleep. Ten years prior to death he recovered from a myocardial infarct. Two years prior to death he ran 42 km in 5½ hours. Only the heart was examined at autopsy.

The remote heart attack consisted of highly vascular scar tissue in the myocardium and a recanalized occlusion in the right coronary artery (FIGURE 7). Resorption of fibrous plaque was present (FIGURE 8). "Small vessel disease" (FIGURES 9 & 10) and "ischemic microlesions" (FIGURES 11 & 12) were also noted. There was an anomaly of the coronary arteries with the left circumflex arising from the right sinus of Valsalva.[24]

Comment: Sudden, unexpected death has been associated with double coronary arteries arising from the same sinus of Valsalva.[13] The "ischemic microlesions" are consistent with the reported cause of death: arrhythmia. ASCVD was not considered a factor. There was no evidence of thrombosis or infarction. The small-vessel disease may have been due to smoking, and may have played a role in the ischemic changes. The vascular scar and recanalized artery may have been part of the increased collateral circulation, perhaps induced by the marathon training.

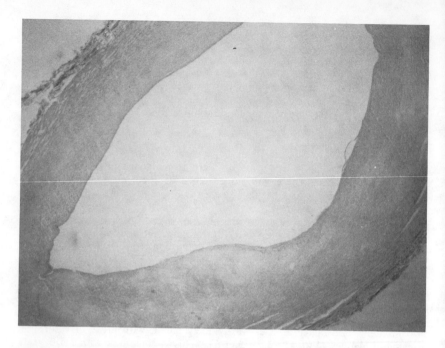

FIGURE 3. Marathoner: Coronary artery with characteristic widely patent lumen and minimal ASCVD. (H & E stain; × 10.)

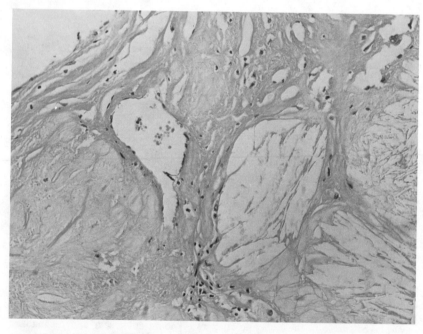

FIGURE 4. Same vessel as shown in FIGURE 3, at higher magnification: Mild inflammatory reaction to lipids in plaque. (H & E stain; × 245.)

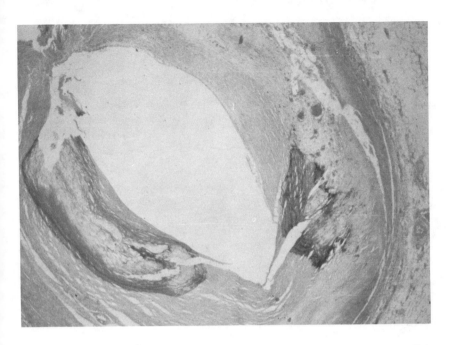

FIGURE 5. Marathoner: Calcified plaques in coronary artery. (H & E stain; × 10.)

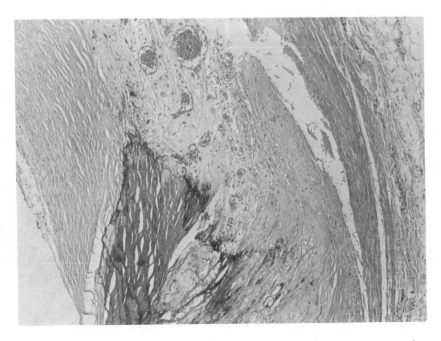

FIGURE 6. Same lesion as shown in FIGURE 5, at higher magnification: Resorption of calcium plaque by cellular granulation tissue. (H & E stain; × 70.)

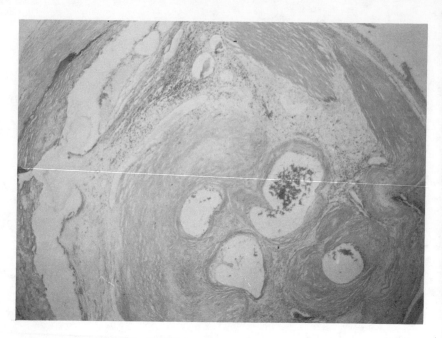

FIGURE 7. Marathoner: Right coronary artery with four new channels 10 years after myocardial infarction. "Recanalization." (H & E stain; × 10.)

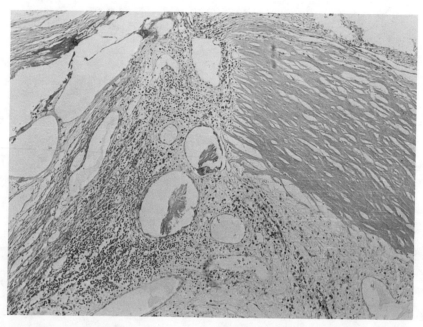

FIGURE 8. Same lesion as FIGURE 7, at higher magnification: Resorption of fibrous plaque by granulation tissue. (H & E stain; × 105.)

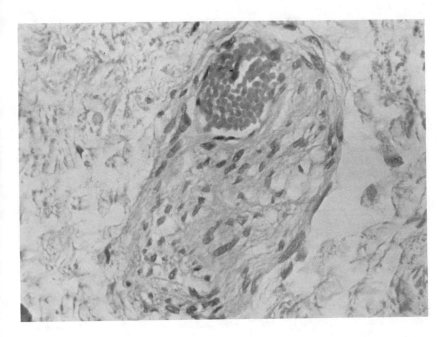

FIGURE 9. Cigarette smoker: "Small vessel disease." Intramural coronary artery narrowed by hyperplasia of endothelial and muscle cells. (H & E stain; × 245.)

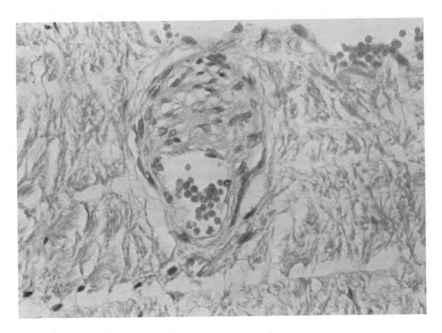

FIGURE 10. Cigarette smoker: Small vessel disease." (H & E stain; × 245.)

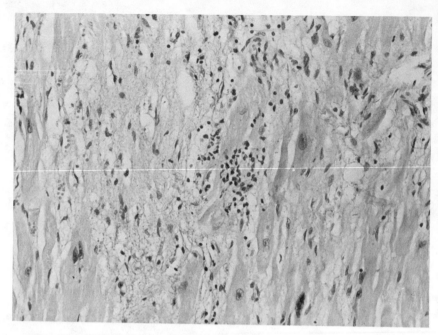

FIGURE 11. Marathoner: "Ischemic microlesions." Single muscle cell injury with small inflammatory infiltrate. (H & E stain; × 210.)

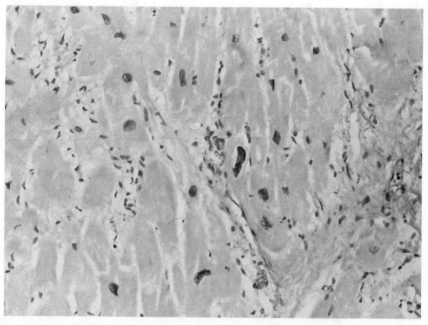

FIGURE 12. Marathoner: "Ischemic microlesions." (H & E stain; × 210.)

Hazards of Racing

Marathon training is possible in the presence of coronary atherosclerosis. Rehabilitation programs now turn out "cardiac athletes" specifically trained for the 42-km distance. Several former patients have finished 80-km events. The best example of this is the Cardiac Division in the December Honolulu Marathon, which includes runners with severe triple-vessel disease, with and without infarction, and with and without by-pass surgery. The periods of training are less than a year in some cases. One post-myocardial-infarction patient completed 42 km 9 months after infarction. A triple-by-pass patient completed 42 km 10 months after surgery.

Nonfatal cardiac emergencies do occur in 42-km men.[25] These events have been associated with smoking, fluid and electrolyte problems, heat stress, viral infections, spasm, and dietary "fat loading" prior to a race.

Case No. 17. A cardiac patient in his 50s developed chest pain in bed the night before his first marathon. He had spent the day consuming vast amounts of fatty foods in an effort to "load fuel for the race." Six hours after the onset of pain he ran 42 km in 5½ hours. He attributed the pain to "heartburn." Two weeks later he ran 42 km in 5 hours. EKG studies confirmed the presence of an infarct.

Comment: The infarct occurred at rest in a man with documented triple vessel disease. He had stopped running his usual 20 km per day at the same time that he markedly increased his fat intake.

Other 42-km men have been admitted to hospital for "possible heart attack," but most are back running 10 km in a few days and 42 km in a few weeks. Usually angiograms in such cases show enlarged coronary arteries.

Case No. 18. A 42-km man in his early 30s survived infarction due to coronary spasm. The first angiogram showed spasm with complete occlusion of the left anterior descending coronary artery and 80% narrowing of the right coronary artery by thrombus. Several weeks later the thrombus was absent on angiogram and all three vessels were open. There was no evidence of ASCVD. Lipids were normal. He did not smoke. He is still alive.

Case No. 19. A well-conditioned marathoner suffered brain death while racing under hot and humid conditions. The coronary arteries were enlarged and widely patent at autopsy.[26]

Comment: Traffic accidents and environmental heat stress are hazards of road racing. Deaths from hypothermia have been reported by Sutten.[27] Such deaths should not be confused with deaths due to natural causes such as ASCVD.

Low-Mileage Runners

Olympic 10-km men have died of ASCVD.

Case No. 20. Paavo Nurmi. *Case No. 21.* Vladimir Kuts. Both of these athletes won Olympic gold medals and set world records. However, they did die of ASCVD after they stopped running and developed risk factors.

Comment: Middle-distance events require carbohydrates for energy substrate, while the longer 42-km event uses fats.[28] The winning times for 5 km and 10 km are under the 30-minute threshold found to be protective by Morris.[2] Part of this protection may be due to the different energy substrates required by the longer events. Preferential utilization of unsaturated fatty acids (UFAs) occurs during the 42-km race.[30] This is reflected in the diet of the runners. Our observations have shown that items rich in linoleic (18:2) acid are consumed more avidly by the 42-km men than by the 10-km men in the Seniors Track Club.[29] These supplements included vegetable oils such as wheat germ oil and peanut oil. Tocopherols were also taken.

Adding UFAs to the diet does lower the degree of saturation of body tissues, and this lowers the death rate due to ASCVD.[4] This agrees with the autopsy studies of Tuna and Mangold[31] who reported that the ASCVD lesions lower in linoleic acid were more likely to cause death. The triglyceride fractions of atheromatous plaques were analyzed for linoleic acid. Those who did not die of ASCVD had levels three times higher than those who did die of ASCVD. By eating UFAs 42-km men can provide fuel for their races and protect their ASCVD lesions. The inflammatory reaction is less in the plaque of the 42-km man (FIGURE 4) than the 10-km man (FIGURE 2), in spite of the fact that the 42-km man is twice the age of the 10-km man. This difference is probably related to the content of UFAs.[31]

Case No. 22. A 43-year-old hobby jogger ran 20 minutes a day for 8 years, completing 2 miles in 13 minutes on one occasion. He died while jogging. Autopsy showed ASCVD.

Comment: Hobby joggers who die of ASCVD usually train at distances that require carbohydrate for energy substrate. The UFAs are not conspicuous in their diets. Most smoke up to the time of death.[15] The plaques are similar to FIGURE 2.

SUMMARY

This is an interim report of an on-going study of deaths in 42-km men. The absence of fatal ASCVD in these athletes can not be construed as evidence for the protective role of exercise alone. The ability to run 42 km depends on many factors. Exercise is only one. Avoiding tobacco is another. Dietary factors also play a role. It has not been feasible to remove one of these factors while maintaining the ability to cover the 42 km distance. Some 42-km men claim that megadoses of ascorbic acid protect them from collagen injury. This is supported by animal studies that show increased collagen synthesis proportional to ascorbic acid intake up to dosage levels that would equal 10 grams per day for humans.[32] Their self-selected macrobiotic diet contains a high ratio of peanuts:steak resulting in a high P/S ratio (polyunsaturates/saturates). Dietary manipulation quickly effects their ability to train. Smoking is so rare among these runners that it must be related to specific effects, such as a catalytic agent in tobacco smoke converting linoleic acid into a toxic lipid oxide.

Noakes and Opie recently confirmed again (May, 1976) that *no* cases of "death due to coronary atherosclerosis" have been recorded in marathon finishers.[35] If this holds true for the second 10-year period of this study, then marathon runners will have joined the longshoremen[33] by earning life-long protection against ASCVD. These longshoremen burned 1,876 kcals on the job, equivalent to a 30-km run. Roberts and Straus[34] suggest that many factors can cause atherosclerosis. Only time will tell whether the marathoner is protected from all of them.

ACKNOWLEDGMENTS

The author acknowledges assistance in case-finding by: B. Balke, W. Bortz, J. Boyer, J. D. Cantwell, A. Catts, K. Cooper, B. Cruickshank, M. Ellestad, S. M. Fox, V. F. Froelicher, E. Jokl, T. Kavanagh, T. Kostrubala, T. D. Noakes, L. H. Opie, J. Scaff, G. Sheehan & J. Ullyot; assistance in case-analysis by: O. Atkins, F. Bisignano, J. Burgasser, F. Cardello, R. Closson, D. Cronin, A. Corwin, G. Davall, G. DeWitt, J. Donan, B. Filler, J. Harper, M. Hattem, R. Herman, D. Jones, T. Jones, R. Leach, W. Marano, A. Monk, C. Paulson, M. Reeder, B. Rosin, J. Rudberg, R. Sanford, L. Sanza, R. Steiner & R. Ullrich; for his observations on the Tarahumara Indians, R. W. Davies; and for his observations on the Masai, J. C. Roberts.

REFRENCES

1. ARONOW, W. S. 1974. Tobacco and the heart. J. Amer. Med. Assoc. **229:** 1799–1800.
2. MORRIS, J. N., S. P. W. CHAVE, C. ADAM, C. SIREY & L. EPSTEIN. 1973. Vigorous exercise in leisure-time and the incidence of coronary heart-disease. Lancet **i:** 333–339.
3. BURKITT, D. P., A. R. P. WALKER & N. S. PAINTER. 1974. Dietary fiber and disease. J. Amer. Med. Assoc. **229:** 1068–1074.
4. MIETTINEN, M., O. TURPEINEN, M. KARVONEN, R.. ELOSUO & E. PAAVILAINEN. 1972. Effect of cholesterol-lowering diet on mortality from coronary heart-disease and other causes. Lancet **ii:** 835–838.
5. TURLEY, S. D., C. E. WEST & B. J. HORTON. 1976. The role of ascorbic acid in the regulation of cholesterol metabolism and in the pathogenesis of athero-sclerosis. Atherosclerosis **24:** 1–18.
6. SINCLAIR, H. M. 1973. Deficiency of vitamin E and myocardial infarction. Lancet **ii:** 500–501.
7. BISS, K., K. J. HO, B. MIKKELSON, L. LEWIS & C. B. TAYLOR. 1971. Some unique biological characteristics of the Masai of East Africa. N. Engl. J. Med. **284:** 694–699.
8. GROOM, D. 1971. Cardiovascular observations on Tarahumara Indian runners— the modern Spartans. Amer. Heart J. **81:** 304–314.
9. BASSLER, T. J. 1975. Marathon running and immunity to heart disease. Phys. Sports. Med. **3:** 77–80.
10. CURRENS, J. & P. D. WHITE. 1961. Half a century of running. N. Engl. J. Med. **265:** 251–255.
11. MANN, G. V., A. SPOERRY, M. GRAY & D. JARASHOW. 1972. Atherosclerosis in the Masai. Amer. J. Epidemiol. **95:** 26–37.
12. KOSTRUBALA, T. 1976. The Joy of Running. J. B. Lippincott Company. New York, N.Y.
13. CHEITLIN, M. D., H. A. McALLISTER & C. M. DE CASTRO. 1975. Myocardial infarction without atherosclerosis. J. Amer. Med. Assoc. **231:** 951–959.
14. CANTWELL, J. D. 1976. Ann. Intern. Med. **85:** 391-392.
15. Most of the autopsy material was handled through the Los Angeles County Medical Examiner's Office, Los Angeles, California in the years 1961–1969. An estimated 3,000 cases were sudden, unexpected deaths due to atherosclero-sis. This office serves a population in excess of 6 million people, mostly urban.
16. OPIE, L. H. 1975. N. Engl. J. Med. **293:** 941–942.
17. OPIE, L. H. 1976. N. Engl. J. Med. **294:** 1067.

18. STOKES, J. 1976. Ann. Intern. Med. **85:** 393.
19. I am grateful to Mr. Wm. Zappas for his observations during his run from Marathon to Athens in 1975.
20. SCHMID, L. 1975. Malignant tumours as causes of death of former athletes. J. Sports Med. **15:** 117–124.
21. SHAMBERGER, R. J., F. F. BAUGHMAN, S. K. KALCHERT, C. E. WILLIS & G. C. HOFFMAN. 1973. Carcinogen-induced chromosomal breakage decreased by antioxidants. Proc. Nat. Acad. Sci. U.S.A. **70:** 1461–1463.
22. HABER, S. L. & R. W. WISSLER. 1962. Effect of vitamin E on carcinogenicity of methylcholanthrene. Proc. Soc. Exp. Biol. Med. **111:** 774–775.
23. SCHLEGEL, J. U., G. E. PIPKIN, R. NISHIMURA & G. N. SHULTZ. 1969. The role of ascorbic acid in the prevention of bladder tumor formation. Trans. Amer. Assoc. Genito-Urinary Surg. **61:** 85–89.
24. HAEREM, J. W. 1975. Myocardial lesions in sudden, unexpected coronary death. Amer. Heart J. **90:** 562–568.
25. BASSLER, T. J. 1976. Runner's World **11** (3): 6.
26. GREEN, L. H., S. I. COHEN, G. KURLAND. 1976. Ann. Intern. Med. **84:** 704–706.
27. SUTTON, J. 1972. N. Engl. J. Med. **286:** 951.
28. BLEICH, H. L. & E. S. BORO. 1975. Fuel homeostasis in exercise. N. Engl. J. Med. **293:** 1078–1084.
29. Ten year observation of the 200 marathoners in the Seniors Track Club, Los Angeles, Calif.
30. HUNTER, R., J. SWALE, M. A. PEYMAN & C. W. H. BARNETT. 1972. Some immediate and long-term effects of exercise on the plasma lipids. Lancet **ii:** 671–675.
31. TUNA, N. & H. K. MANGOLD. 1963. Fatty acids of the atheromatous plaque. *In* Evolution of the Atherosclerotic Plaque. R. J. Jones, Editor. University of Chicago Press. Chicago, Ill.
32. YEW, M. S. 1973. "Recommended daily allowances" for vitamin C. Proc. Nat. Acad. Sci. U.S.A. **70**(4): 969–972.
33. PAFFENBARGER, R. S. & W. E. HALE. 1975. Work activity and coronary heart mortality. N. Engl. J. Med. **292:** 545–550.
34. ROBERTS, J. C. & R. STRAUS, Eds. 1965. Comparative Atherosclerosis. Harper & Row. New York, N.Y.
35. NOAKES, T. D. & L. H. OPIE. 1976. Lancet **i:** 1020.

CORONARY HEART DISEASE
IN MARATHON RUNNERS *

Tim Noakes, Lionel Opie, and Walter Beck

*MRC Ischaemic Heart Disease Research Unit
and the Cardiac Clinic
Department of Medicine
University of Cape Town Medical School
Observatory 7925, South Africa*

John McKechnie

*Department of Medicine
University of Natal
Durban, South Africa*

Alberto Benchimol and Kenneth Desser

*Institute for Cardiovascular Diseases
Good Samaritan Hospital
Phoenix, Arizona 85062*

Unforeseeing one! Yes, he fought on the Marathon day: So, when Persia was
dust, all cried "To Akropolis! Run Pheidippides, one race more! The meed is
thy due! "Athens is saved, thank Pan," go shout! He flung down his shield,
And Athens was stubble again, a field which a fire runs through,
Till in he broke "Rejoice, we conquer!" Like wine through clay,
Joy in his blood bursting his heart, he died—the bliss!

"Pheidippides"
Robert Browning
1879

INTRODUCTION

The marathon race commemorates the immortal run of an unknown soldier,
fully armored and "hot from battle," to Athens to inform the Greek capital
that the invading Persians had been defeated on the plains of Marathon. Had
the Athenians in their unguarded capital remained ignorant of the Persian
defeat, they might have surrendered without resistance to a direct seaborne
invasion; thus the reason for the run.

Legend has it that, having delivered his news "Rejoice, rejoice, Victory is
ours!", the messenger died suddenly from what Browning considered to be a
cardiac death. Thus, in legend at least, the marathon race links extreme physical
exertion with sudden cardiac death.

A recent hypothesis suggests this relationship to be unproven because "there
are no documented deaths from coronary heart disease among marathon
finishers of any age."[1] Thus far this hypothesis has been characterized by
repetitive statement[1-27] but without any published documentation. In addition,

* This work was supported by the South African Medical Research Council and the
Chris Barnard Fund.

it has not always been entirely clear what this "Bassler hypothesis" entails [28] because marathon running has variously been described as providing immunity to coronary heart disease,[1-10] to ischemic heart disease,[11, 12] to fatal myocardial infarction,[13-15] to "loafers heart," [16] and to coronary atherosclerosis.[17-26]

In this paper we report six cases of myocardial infarction in highly-trained marathon runners. Four of these athletes had coronary artery disease demonstrated angiographically and considered indistinguishable from coronary atherosclerosis.

CASE REPORTS

Case 1

A 35-year-old man had been running for at least 10 years before his death in February 1974. His athletic achievements included a best standard marathon time of 2 hours 33 minutes in April 1973, a time of 3 hours 24 minutes in April 1972 for 33 miles, and in May 1971 he finished the 56 mile Comrades Marathon in 45th position out of 925 competitors in a time of 6 hours 51 minutes. During 1972 and 1973 he ran a total of 4783 miles.

There was no family history of heart disease. His running logbook records that he went running on 11 occasions during the first three weeks of January 1974. On six of these runs reference is made to the presence of chest pain and/or pain between the shoulder blades. This was severe enough to force him to stop running on a number of occasions. During one 4½-mile time trial, at which his wife was present, she recalls that he was forced to stop running five or six times. A friend advised him to see a doctor but he declined attributing his problems to "unfitness." In this period he ran 27- and 40-mile training runs. During this longer run he had severe chest pain that frequently forced him to stop.

On the day of his death, he went to work as usual but telephoned home at 4 P.M. to say he was going surfing. However, he arrived home 50 minutes later saying that he was "too breathless" to surf properly. He went inside the house and 20 minutes later asked his wife to take him to the doctor immediately as he had severe chest pain. His wife recalled that he looked pale but was not sweating and did not complain of nausea. During the car ride to the doctor he requested his wife to drive faster as the chest pain was getting worse and that it was now present in his left hand, which felt paralyzed.

He was seen by a general practitioner who gave him an injection and informed his wife that he had had a heart attack. The patient was driven to hospital immediately where he was admitted to the Intensive Care Unit. A diagnosis of acute myocardial infarction was made on the clinical features and the absence of signs of rupture of aortic aneurysm or massive pulmonary embolus or other causes of acute severe chest pain.

The patient died at 6:40 P.M. and the diagnosis on the death certificate was coronary thrombosis. No postmortem was performed and an incorrect report in a letter [29] was discounted on further investigation.

An electrocardiogram was taken on admission to hospital (FIGURE 1) and later reported as showing changes of acute inferior subendocardial ischemia.

In view of the clinical picture and the supportive evidence of the ECG, it is believed that this constitutes a fatal myocardial infarction occurring in an active marathon runner. Scaff's claim [30] that the ECG was that of heat stroke could readily be discounted because the patient had not been running on the day of his death. Our case thus disproves at least one of Bassler's statements.[13-15]

As no autopsy was performed, Bassler rejected this case as disproving his hypothesis. He modified his previously ambiguous statements by clarifying that marathon running provided immunity only to coronary atherosclerosis.[23, 27] However, coronary atherosclerosis need not present only as sudden death. Thus, for his hypothesis to be epidemiologically valid, marathon runners who develop other clinical manifestations of coronary atherosclerosis such as exertional chest pain or myocardial infarction must be shown to be free of this disease. In four

CASE 1

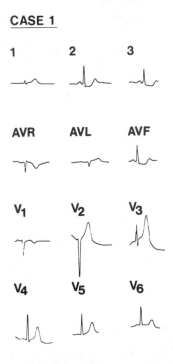

FIGURE 1. Case 1. ECG taken shortly before death showing ST changes compatible with acute inferior subendocardial ischaemia.

marathon runners with myocardial infarction we have shown the presence of significant coronary artery disease considered angiographically indistinguishable from coronary atherosclerosis. A fifth runner who has sustained a documented myocardial infarction, has an ischemic response to submaximal exercise but declined coronary angiography.

Case 2

A 39-year-old White male participated in rugby football and amateur boxing in which he was nationally ranked until the age of 18, after which he became physically inactive. Apart from occasional acute attacks of gout from 1963 onwards (for which he took allopurinol), he had no cause to seek medical attention. In January 1974 he took up long distance running and in the course of the following 27 months completed two Comrades Marathons, a number of standard marathons and had run 4050 miles in training. By the end of March 1975, he was in full training for the Comrades Marathon and was running more miles at a faster pace than at any previous time in his life. However, having completed his usual Sunday morning run of 26 miles uneventfully, he became aware of a sharp stabbing pain in his right elbow after he had run about 1 mile of a planned 8-mile training run on Monday, March 28. The pain persisted and after a further 2 miles was followed by the onset of moderately severe, cramping, anterior chest pain. These pains became progressively worse until he was forced to walk. Within a minute of walking these pains disappeared only to reappear immediately on jogging. The patient returned home and although he felt sluggish, he had no further chest pain. On the following 2 days the patient walked and ran a total of 18 miles and was again troubled by the same pains. On Thursday morning, the patient was awakened by severe, crushing precordial chest pain radiating to the right elbow. There was associated sweating and nausea.

He was seen in Casualty at Bloemfontein National Hospital where the electrocardiogram showed a hyperacute inferolateral myocardial infarction with marked ST-segment elevation in leads II, III, AVF, V5, and V6, with pathological Q waves in III, AVF, and V6. On admission to the Intensive Coronary Care Unit, the only abnormal findings were a jugular venous pressure raised 2 cms above the manubrium sterni and a third heart sound. He was treated with digoxin, furosemide, and supplemental potassium for mild right ventricular failure.

Cardiac enzymes were elevated the day after admission, creatine phosphokinase 510 units/ml (normal up to 50); lactate dehydrogenase 283 units/ml (normal up to 90). Enzymes returned to normal values within 4 days. He was discharged from hospital on propranolol (40 mgs three times daily) and on sulphinpyrazone.

On the day of his hospital discharge (against his physician's advice) he walked half a mile without chest pain and returned to work the following morning, 12 days after myocardial infarction.

Over the next 3 weeks he increased his daily walking distance to 2 miles at which stage he resumed jogging. For a period he developed elbow and chest pain when jogging, but always walked immediately when any chest pain started. By the end of June he was jogging without symptoms up to a distance of 6 kilometers. In mid-July 1976 he was admitted to Groote Schuur Hospital for assessment of coronary risk factors and evaluation of the desirability of his continued marathon running.

There was no family history of heart disease or hypertension, but one maternal aunt had died from diabetes in her forties. He abstained from alcohol but had smoked three pipefuls of tobacco and two to three cigarettes from the age of 18 until one month after his myocardial infarction.

The patient was a small (5'6"), muscular White male (somatotype 2:6½:1 Heath-Carter, percentage body fat 13.6%). There were no stigmata of hyperlipidemia. The patient was normotensive (blood pressure 110/70 mmHg) and the resting heart rate was 50 beats per minute. The apex beat was not displaced and there were no abnormal auscultatory findings. All peripheral pulses were present. Other features, including urine and blood count were normal, and the ESR was 5 mm/hr (Westergren).

The glucose tolerance test was normal, serum uric acid was greater than 12 mgs per 100 ml, and a fasting lipogram was classified as a type IIb hyperlipidemia; cholesterol 265 mg/100 ml, triglyceride 235 mg/100 ml (normal up to 150 mg/100 ml), chylomicrons 16 mg/100 ml (normal up to 12 mg/100 ml), pre-beta-lipoproteins 177 mg/100 ml (normal up to 150 mg/100 ml),

CASE 2

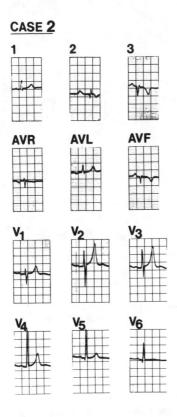

FIGURE 2. Case 2. Resting ECG 3 months after acute myocardial infarction showing Q waves in leads 2, 3, and AVF. The tall T wave in V_2 and V_3 is normal for athletes.[56] Heart rate: 52/min.

and beta-lipoproteins 513 mg/100 ml (normal up to 480/100 ml). Chest X ray was normal and a resting electrocardiogram showed an old inferior myocardial infarction (FIGURE 2). The effort electrocardiogram did not reveal any symptoms, arrhythmias or ST changes up to a heart rate of 130 per minute while on propranolol 40 mg *b.d.*

The echocardiogram showed normal sizes and movement of heart chambers and no thickening of the posterior ventricular wall. The patient was Holter-monitored during a 30-minute jog, and no arrhythmias were found.

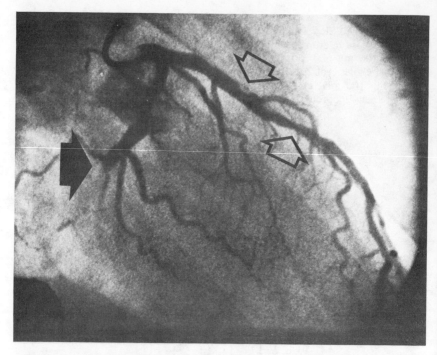

FIGURE 3. Left coronary angiogram in right anterior oblique (R.A.O.) showing complete occlusion of the circumflex artery (black arrow) and luminal irregularities in the anterior descending coronary artery (open arrows).

Left heart catheterization showed an increased left ventricular end-diastolic pressure (20 mmHg).

Angiography revealed complete occlusion in the distal circumflex artery just after the origin of the obtuse marginal branch (FIGURE 3), with a small segment of the more distal vessel filling later by means of bridge collateral. The left anterior descending artery had minor luminal irregularities (FIGURE 3). There was a 50% narrowing of the right coronary artery, which involved the origin of the right ventricular branch; the rest of the vessel was of good caliber with some luminal irregularities (FIGURE 4). Cineangiography of the left ventricle showed good contraction except for an area of inferior and infero-basal hypokinesia.

Treatment for the patient's gout and hyperlipidemia was instituted and the patient was advised against running extreme distances such as the 56-mile Comrades Marathon.

Case 3

A 48-year-old White male had been physically active throughout his life and was a nonsmoker. There was a family history of heart disease, his father had died suddenly at the age of 60 and a paternal uncle had died of "heart failure."

There was no past history of significance. He had been a long distance runner for 10 years and during this period had completed seven Comrades Marathons and more than 20,000 miles in training. After completing the 1975 Comrades Marathon in 9¾ hours, he maintained a heavy training schedule until the end of October 1976 when he traveled to Greece to run the Sacred Marathon on the course over which the legendary Marathon was run. For 6 weeks prior to this event he had been training 80–90 miles a week, including 25 mile runs at the weekend. He had never trained as hard as this in his life.

This Sacred Marathon was run in adverse environmental conditions, it being dry and hot, with the race starting at 1 PM. Facilities to supply the runners with fluid replacement were inadequate and in contrast to his usual practice, the patient was forced to drink very little fluid during the first 20 miles of the race. At about this point the patient began to feel nausea and was aware of a dull pain, feeling like a wind, in the epigastrium. The pain forced him to walk and he soon began vomiting. There was no chest pain.

Despite this discomfort and the regular occurrence of vomiting, the patient insisted on completing the last 6 miles of the course, which he did in two hours.

After the race the patient returned to his hotel where he continued to vomit and was unable to eat or drink. Four hours after finishing the

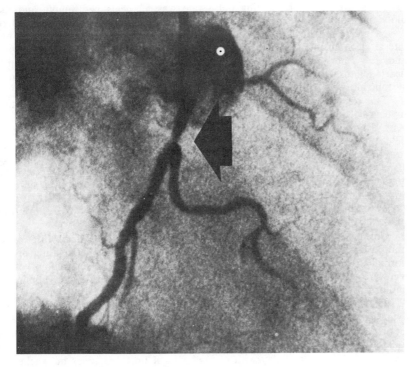

FIGURE 4. Case 2. Right coronary angiogram showing stenosis of the proximal right coronary artery (black arrow).

marathon, the patient was pain free and was seen by a marathon-running physician (J.M.) who prescribed an antiemetic to control the vomiting and advised the patient to drink fluids as he was dehydrated. During the night he passed urine but remained ill. For the next 24 hours his condition remained unchanged, but on the evening of the following day the epigastric pain radiated up both sides of the chest and into the back. A cardiologist was called and a diagnosis of acute myocardial infarction was made; the patient was admitted to the Intensive Care Unit of a local Athens hospital where an ECG showed an anteroseptal myocardial infarction. The patient was given two liters of intravenous fluid rapidly as he was dehydrated and anuric; this treatment relieved both the epigastric and chest pains. His further course was uncomplicated and he flew back to South Africa 4 days later in the company of J.M. From the plane he went to a hospital where he remained for 8 days.

Four days after discharge (against medical advice) he began walking 4 to 5 miles a day, and within a further 3 weeks he commenced jogging again. In January 1976 he was running 25 miles a week and by the beginning of March he had doubled this and thereafter continued at this level of activity.

In August 1976 he was admitted to Groote Schuur Hospital for investigation. Systemic interrogation did not reveal any additional features. On physical examination there were no stigmata of hyperlipidemia. The patient's somatotype was endo-mesomorphic (4:5½:2 Heath Carter) and he had an estimated 22.5% body fat indicating more adiposity than is usually associated with marathon runners. The resting pulse rate was 52 beats per minute and the blood pressure 130/90 mmHg. While the apex beat was not displaced there was a palpable fourth heart sound and on auscultation at the apex, in the lateral decubitus position, a systolic click and a late systolic murmur were audible. Phonocardiography at the mitral area showed third and fourth heart sounds, and there was an intermittent nonejection click. No definite systolic murmur was recorded.

The electrocardiogram showed the pattern of an old transmural anterior myocardial infarction with lateral T wave abnormality (FIGURE 5). The chest X ray showed mild cardiomegaly with a cardiothoracic ratio 52%. The lung fields were clear. A glucose tolerance test was within normal limits. The fasting lipogram showed cholesterol of 268 mg/100 ml and triglycerides of 107 mg/100 ml. Echocardiography showed that the left ventricular internal diameter was increased; the percentage of fractional shortening was normal; and no increased thickening of the posterior left ventricular wall was detected.

At cardiac catheterization, the left ventricular end-diastolic pressure was markedly elevated (30 mmHg at rest).

Coronary angiography showed a 2-cm area of 50%–75% narrowing in the mid-portion of the left anterior descending artery, but with good filling of the normal distal vessel (FIGURES 6a & b). The mainstem and circumflex vessels were free of disease. The right coronary artery was unobstructed, dominant, and of large caliber.

The left ventricular angiogram showed an enlarged left ventricle with an extensive akinetic area involving the apical, anterolateral, and inferior surfaces.

The patient easily ran 18 miles with one of us (T. N.) without the development of symptoms or undue fatigue. In view of this, he was advised to maintain running up to 8 miles a day with a single run of up to 15 miles on weekends. He was advised how to avoid dehydration while running [31] and was dissuaded from running in competitive marathons.

Case 4

A 50-year-old White male had been running for 10 years and had participated in competitive long distance running since 1969. He had completed 18 standard marathons and on average, had run more than 40 miles a week during this period.

His best marathon time was 3 hours and 36 minutes and in October 1974 he ran the Albuquerque, New Mexico Marathon in an attempt to qualify for

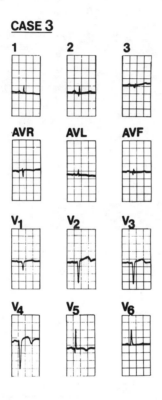

CASE 3

FIGURE 5. Case 3. Resting ECG 9 months after acute myocardial infarction showing Q waves and loss of R amplitude in V leads.

the 1975 Boston Marathon (Qualifying Standard: 3 hrs 30 mins). After 15 miles of this marathon he became aware of vague chest discomfort which he attributed to altitude and dehydration. Although he did not feel particularly ill, he was reduced to walking the last 7 miles of the race and finished in 5 hours and 10 minutes.

After the race he continued to feel ill and in the plane flying home, he again felt chest discomfort, which was not severe enough to cause him alarm. At work the next day he was troubled by a vague malaise and at noon on the following day, 48 hours after the marathon, he developed severe precordial

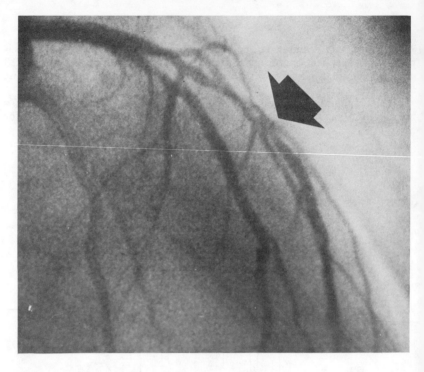

FIGURE 6a. Case 3. Left coronary angiogram in R.A.O. showing a 2-cm segment (arrowed) of the anterior descending coronary artery with 50%–75% narrowing and good distal filling.

chest pain radiating down the left arm into the fingers, associated with marked dyspnoea.

He went immediately to the local hospital where he was admitted to the Coronary Care Unit. On admission, the patient was normotensive (110/80), and except for a prominent fourth heart sound, a gallop rhythm, and a pericardial friction rub, the cardiovascular examination was normal. The chest X ray was normal and the electrocardiogram was compatible with acute inferior myocardial infarction. Serial enzyme and electrocardiographic changes confirmed this diagnosis. Serum lipids were normal (cholesterol 216 mg/ml, triglycerides 114 mg/ml). The patient's hospital course was uncomplicated and he was discharged from hospital on the ninth day post-infarction. The following day, against medical advice, he recommenced jogging.

In November 1974, one month after myocardial infarction, the athlete was admitted to the Good Samaritan Hospital for assessment of his cardiovascular status. Five years previously, the patient had been admitted to hospital with severe chest pain, but as the electrocardiogram and serum enzymes were normal, a firm diagnosis could not be established.

Additional interrogation revealed that the patient was a nonsmoker, that his father had suffered from hyperlipidemia and had died from a heart attack; his mother had suffered from hypertension and had died from a cerebrovascular accident.

A maternal uncle suffers from diabetes.

The patient was normotensive. On palpation at the apex a systolic bulge was noted, and on auscultation a third and fourth heart sound was heard. Phonocardiography confirmed these findings. The remainder of the cardiovascular examination was normal.

The electrocardiogram showed the pattern of an old transmural inferolateral myocardial infarction (FIGURE 7). The chest X ray was reported as normal. Echocardiography showed both the left ventricular internal diameter and the posterior wall thickness to be normal.

At cardiac catheterization, the right atrial, right ventricular, the pulmonary arterial and pulmonary "wedge" pressure were all normal as was the left ventricular end-diastolic pressure. Parameters of left ventricular function, specifically cardiac output and the tension-time index were all normal.

Selective coronary angiography showed the left coronary artery to be normal (FIGURE 8). The right coronary artery was dominant with only minor segmental lesions in its proximal extent (FIGURE 9a), but there was an area of significant stenosis more distally (FIGURE 9b).

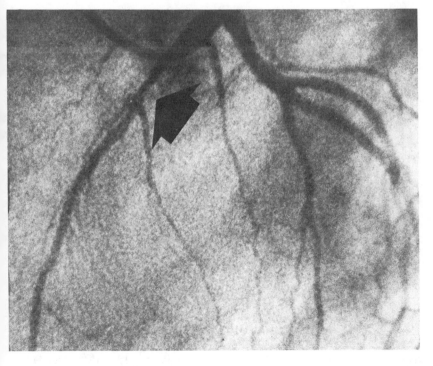

FIGURE 6b. Case 3. Left coronary angiogram in left anterior oblique (L.A.O.) showing narrowed segment (arrowed).

CASE 4

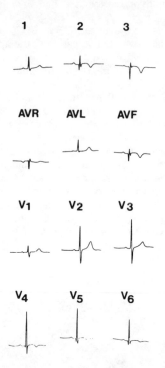

FIGURE 7. Case 4. Resting ECG one month after acute myocardial infarction showing Q waves in leads 2, 3, and AVF and anterolateal T wave inversion.

After nitroglycerin administration, there was no change in the luminal diameter of the coronary arteries.

The left ventricular angiogram showed a normal-sized left ventricle, but a dyskinetic area was shown at the apex of the left ventricle (FIGURES 10a & 10b).

In January 1975, two months after myocardial infarction, the patient completed the Fiesta Bowl Marathon in 4 hours 13 minutes. He has subsequently completed a further five marathon races and has returned to his preinfarction training status.

Case 5

A 37-year-old White male, who was a nonsmoker and who had no family history of heart disease, began jogging regularly in 1967 in order to improve his health and to lose weight. At the urging of a friend, in late 1971, he increased his training mileage with a view to running the 1973 Comrades Marathon. In 1972 he ran approximately 1500 miles in training.

During 1972 a routine medical examination for insurance purposes revealed

T-wave inversion in the inferior leads (leads 2, 3, & AVF). He received insurance only at a loaded premium and was told that he had the Billowing Mitral Leaflet Syndrome (Barlow's Syndrome).

In 1973 and 1974 he completed the Comrades Marathon in 7 hr 17 min and 7 hr 20 min, respectively. During this period he ran about 2000 miles in training annually. His best time for the standard marathon was 2 hr 51 min. In the 5 months before the 1976 Comrades Marathon he had run a further 1200 miles.

During the race itself, he passed the halfway mark of the course in 3 hr 19 minutes and was lying amongst the top 100 runners. He was feeling "strong" and considered it very likely that he would complete the distance in under 7 hours. However, after a further 6 miles of running, he suddenly felt very tired, nauseous and noted that he was sweating profusely. He chose to walk for a period of 20 minutes after which he was again able to run. This sequence recurred three times but there was no chest pain nor did he vomit.

He completed the race in 7 hr 33 min but as he continued to feel ill after the race, he was referred for admission to a local hospital. Overnight he was treated with intravenous fluids and the following morning was found to be grossly edematous, with a jugular venous pressure raised 8 cm above the manubrium sterni, a third heart sound, dullness to percussion at both lung bases, and a 3-cm hepatomegaly with gross abdominal ascites. An ECG at the time showed an acute inferior myocardial infarction and serial enzyme changes were compatible with this diagnosis. The patient responded well to conservative therapy and was discharged from hospital 11 days later.

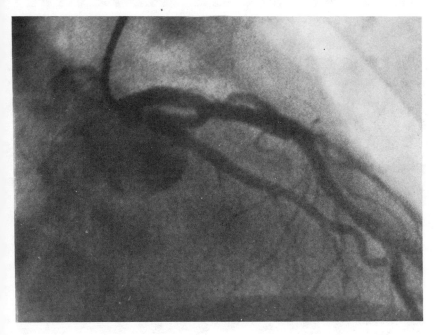

FIGURE 8. Case 4. Left coronary angiogram showing a normal left coronary artery in R.A.O. view.

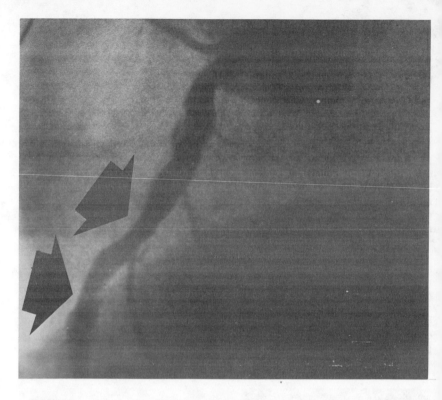

FIGURE 9a. Case 4. Right coronary angiogram in R.A.O. showing dominant right coronary artery with minor segmental irregularities in its proximal and middle thirds.

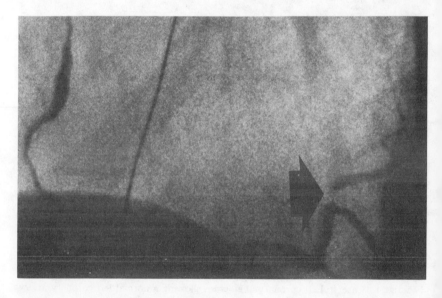

FIGURE 9b. Case 4. Right coronary angiogram in L.A.O. showing a distal stenotic lesion in the late filling phase (arrow).

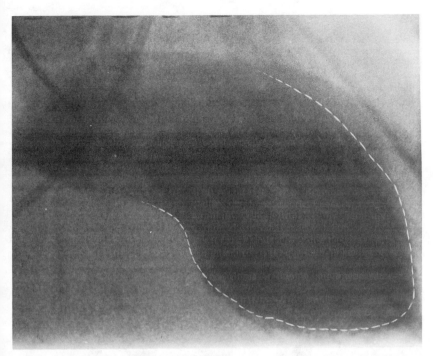

FIGURE 10a. Case 4. Ventriculogram during diastole. Part of the apex and inferior surface of the ventricle has been outlined in white.

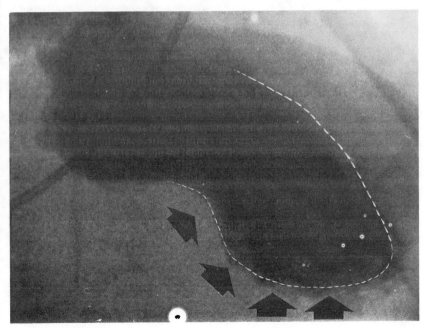

FIGURE 10b. Case 4. Ventriculogram during systole showing an area of inferior and apical dyskinesia (black arrows).

He commenced regular walking on discharge from hospital and two months later began jogging 3 to 5 miles, four times a week.

He was seen at Groote Schuur Hospital 19 months after his initial hospitalization. An ECG confirmed an old transmural inferior myocardial infarction (FIGURE 11). Clinical examination was entirely normal, there being no stigmata of hyperlipidemia; the patient's blood pressure was 130/90, the heart sounds were normal, and all pulses were present. The chest X ray was normal.

Echocardiography revealed all the heart chambers to be of normal size. The movement of the mitral valve was also normal, and was not considered compatible with Barlow's Syndrome.

During the exercise stress test, segmental ST depression first appeared at a heart rate of 160 beats/min and became progressively more severe in the anterior lead up to a heart rate of 190.

Immediately after exercise, ST depression was present in leads V4, V5, and V6 (FIGURE 12). Together with the inferior myocardial infarction, this could suggest diffuse coronary artery disease.

The patient declined to have coronary angiography performed.

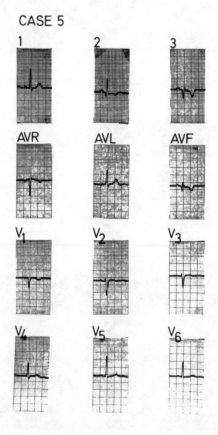

CASE 5

FIGURE 11. Case 5. Resting ECG, 19 months after inferior myocardial infarction.

CASE 5

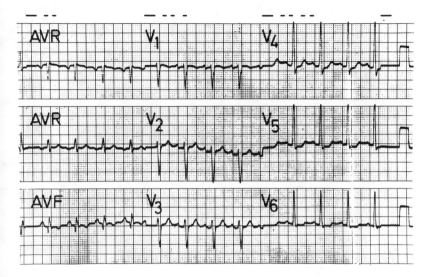

FIGURE 12. Case 5. ECG 5 minutes after exercise showing ST depression in leads V4, V5, and V6.

Case 6

A 46-year-old White male athlete was first seen in 1972 with a complaint of pain in the left groin while running. He was fully examined, including an ECG (FIGURE 13) and no cardiovascular abnormality was reported.

The patient was next seen in December 1974 with the complaint that while running 5 days previously, he had developed a severe pain across the front of his chest. On this occasion he had refused to stop and, despite chest pain, had run on 3 of the following 4 days, including a 10-mile time trial. An ECG at the time showed changes of anteroseptal myocardial infarction (FIGURE 13). The patient refused hospitalization. He was allowed to rest at home but persisted in physical activity, including mowing his lawn, for 5 hours, with severe chest pain.

In February 1975, an effort electrocardiogram, a glucose tolerance test, a fasting lipogram, and serum uric acid estimation were all normal. The patient was allowed to start careful jogging but was advised against any future competitive running. However, in September 1975, he completed a 17-mile road race without difficulty and in April 1976 he ran 93 miles in a 3-day race.

Two years after the original diagnosis of myocardial infarction, the patient was admitted to Groote Schuur Hospital for cardiac evaluation as he wished to run his 15th Comrades Marathon in 1977.

Special interrogation revealed that the patient was known to have retinitis pigmentosa, leaving him with moderately impaired vision. There was a family history of heart disease, his father dying suddenly at the age of 51 from myocardial infarction. His mother had died at 53 from diabetes and was a carrier of an X-linked gene for retinitis pigmentosa.

The patient was a teetotaler and had never smoked. He had always been extremely physically active, representing his Province at swimming while still a schoolboy. Failing vision forced him to turn to rowing, and in 1958 he was selected to represent South Africa as an oarsman at the Empire Games. In 1960 he took up long distance running and between 1961 and 1974 had completed 14 consecutive Comrades Marathons and had run more than 30,000 miles in training.

Systemic interrogation revealed only that the patient frequently developed exertional chest pain, particularly when running uphill or before he had "warmed up." When on the flat he was able to "run through" his chest pain, but was often reduced to a walk on the uphill. On physical examination, there were no stigmata of hyperlipidemia. The pulse rate was 65 beats per minute with the occasional irregular beat. The blood pressure was 130/90. The apex was impalpable and there were no abnormal auscultatory findings. All peripheral pulses except the dorsalis pedis on both sides were present and there were no bruits.

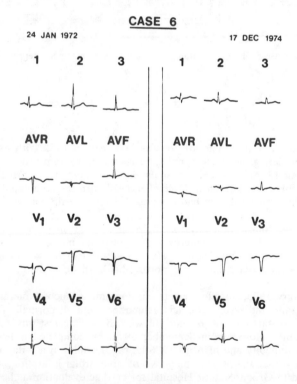

CASE 6

FIGURE 13. Case 6. Resting ECGs taken 2 years apart. The 1972 tracing shows diminishing R waves in V1–V2 and narrow Q waves in V3 suggestive of old anterior infarction. The more recent tracing, taken 4 days after the onset of chest pain, shows Q waves with loss of R waves in V2–V4.

CASE 6

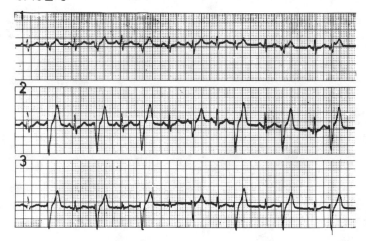

FIGURE 14. Case 6. ECG taken 4 minutes after exercise showing ventricular bigeminy.

The chest X ray was normal and the resting ECG was unchanged from that shown in FIGURE 13.

An effort electrocardiogram was unchanged up to a heart rate of 174 beats per minute but at 4 minutes postexercise, a run of ventricular bigeminy appeared lasting for 1 minute (FIGURE 14).

Left heart catheterization showed all the pressures to be normal.

Coronary angiography revealed a dominant right coronary artery with mild proximal disease and a 70% area of narrowing in the posterior descending artery (FIGURE 15). The distal left anterior descending coronary artery was seen to fill retrogradely.

The mainstem left coronary artery was free of disease but the circumflex artery had mild, diffuse disease (FIGURE 16a). The left anterior descending artery was narrowed by approximately 80% in at least three areas of its proximal and midportions with the distal vessel filling late (FIGURE 16b). A large diagonal branch, supplying a significant area of myocardium, was present (FIGURES 16a and 16b).

The left ventricular angiogram showed a large akinetic area involving the anterolateral, apical, and diaphragmatic segments with good contraction of the inferobasal and anterobasal segments (FIGURES 17a and 17b).

DISCUSSION

Marathon Running and Immunity to
Coronary Atherosclerosis

Strong epidemiological evidence exists to suggest that regular physical activity may be beneficial in terms of favorably altering coronary risk profile,[32] in reducing the incidence of ECG abnormalities compatible for myocardial

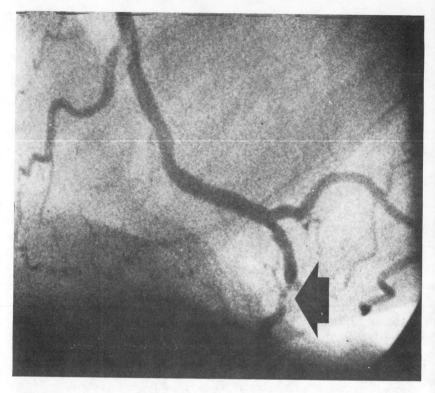

FIGURE 15. Case 6. Right coronary angiogram showing the right coronary artery in L.A.O. with mild proximal disease and a 70% area of narrowing in the posterior descending artery (arrow).

ischemia,[33] and in reducing coronary mortality [34, 35] and, in particular, the incidence of sudden death.[36]

This report of coronary heart disease amongst highly-trained marathon runners in no way refutes these important studies nor does it alter the belief stated previously by two of the present authors, in the benefits of regular physical activity.[37, 38] However, neither the mechanism whereby exercise may protect nor the amount of exercise required for protection has been established. The Bassler hypothesis has had the unfortunate effect of promoting marathon running as the method by which anyone, regardless of precursor pathology or risk factors for coronary heart disease, can achieve total immunity to coronary atherosclerosis. In addition, it has left many with the impression that other less vigorous sports may have no place in coronary heart disease prevention.

We report six cases of myocardial infarction in highly-trained marathon runners. Four of these athletes had coronary artery disease demonstrated

FIGURE 16b. Case 6. Left coronary artery in R.A.O. showing an area of stenosis in the circumflex branch (open arrow). The anterior descending coronary artery is narrowed by approximately 80% in at least three areas (black arrows).

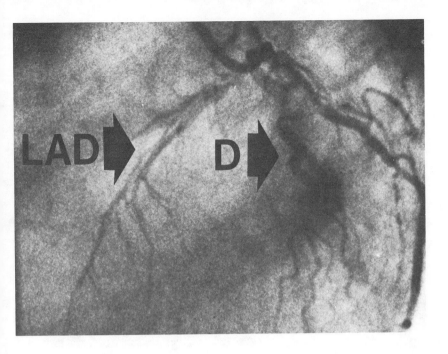

FIGURE 16a. Case 6. Left coronary artery in L.A.O. showing a severely diseased left anterior descending artery (L.A.D. in diagram), a large diagonal branch (D in diagram) and diseased circumflex artery.

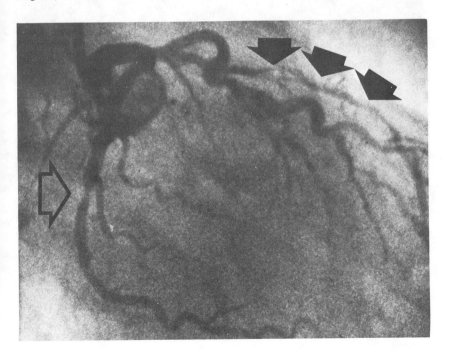

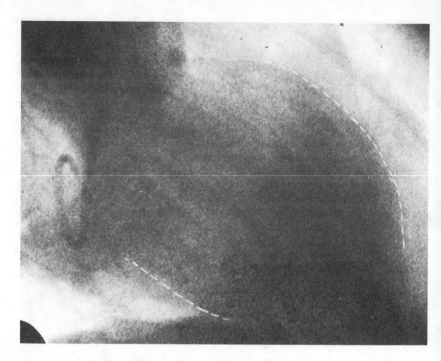

FIGURE 17a. Case 6. Ventriculogram during diastole.

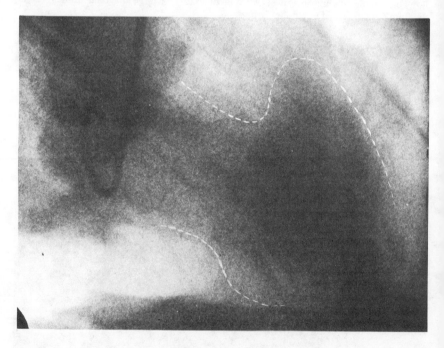

FIGURE 17b. Case 6. Ventriculogram during systole showing a large apical akinetic area.

angiographically and considered indistinguishable from coronary atherosclerosis. All athletes developed myocardial infarction despite continued high levels of physical activity. This contrasts with Bassler's statement that "immunity to heart disease is synonymous with physical fitness" [1] and is in accord with the findings of Vouri and his colleagues [39] and Jokl [40] that high levels of physical fitness do not guarantee the absence of significant cardiovascular disease.

Recently the sudden death of a veteran long distance runner has been reported. Although technically not a marathon runner, he had completed a 23-mile training run the day before his death, he had been running regularly since his teens, he was a nonsmoker, and within the year before his death he had won the National A.A.U. Masters 25-kilometer race. The finding of significant coronary atherosclerosis of the anterior descending coronary artery at autopsy supplies additional evidence against the Bassler hypothesis. [41]

Exertional Symptoms

All six athletes had warning symptoms. Four athletes developed exertional chest pain but in two the onset of predominantly gastrointestinal symptoms caused a delay in diagnosis.

Despite symptoms, three athletes completed marathon races, one athlete ran more than 20 miles after the onset of exertional discomfort to complete the 56 mile Comrades Marathon. The athlete who died continued training for 3 weeks, including a 40-mile run, with chest pain which he ascribed to "unfitness." Two other athletes continued to train with chest pain.

It is possible that the exaggerated claims for the protective effect of marathon running, widely publicized in lay athletic journals, may have contributed to athletes continuing running despite symptoms.

Competitiveness appeared to be a factor, in that four athletes were undergoing particularly rigorous training in attempts to improve on their previous best marathon times. In a previous study of sudden death amongst sportsmen, both competitiveness and a denial of symptoms were apparent. [42] Thus marathon runners, like other sportsmen, [42] need to be warned of the serious significance of the development of exertional symptoms. It is possible that competitiveness and over-training may have contributed to the subsequent development of myocardial infarction in some of these runners.

Marathon Running and "Normal Coronary Arteries"

An over-emphasis of the role of marathon running might play in the prevention of coronary heart disease may have obscured important facts about the dangers of marathon running in persons with apparently normal or mildly diseased coronary arteries. Thus Green et al. [43] have reported a fatal myocardial infarction occurring during a marathon race in an athlete with normal coronary arteries at autopsy, while Frick and his colleagues [44] report a runner with angiographically normal coronary arteries, ischemic electrocardiographic changes during exercise testing, and a demonstrable area of myocardial underperfusion. Cantwell [45] has recently described a veteran marathon runner who collapsed during exercise and required cardiopulmonary resuscitation. A subsequent exercise stress test provoked couplets of ventricular premature beats at a heart rate of 100 beats per minute. At angiography, the coronary arteries of this athlete were reported to be normal.

Myocardial Infarction during Marathon Racing

The absence of coronary artery occlusion in two athletes (Cases 3 & 4) who developed infarction during marathon racing, raises questions regarding the mechanisms by which transmural myocardial infarction can occur without coronary artery occlusion. It has been argued [46] that recanalization of an occluding thrombus may occur in the period between infarction and coronary angiography; thus at angiography the vessels may appear patent. Case 4, who had mild coronary artery disease, underwent coronary angiography only 1 month after infarction suggesting that if this was the mechanism, recanalization occurred rapidly. Case 3 first underwent coronary angiography three months after infarction and at that stage, his angiogram was unchanged from that reported here and done 6 months later. (We thank Professor E. Chesler of Durban for details.)

Coronary artery spasm has been evoked to explain why some persons with angiographically normal coronary arteries can develop angina pectoris or even myocardial infarction [47, 48] and this mechanism has been offered to explain this association in the Billowing Mitral Leaf Syndrome. [49]

The third explanation postulates biochemical factors in the myocardium leading to an imbalance of adenosine triphosphate (ATP) supply and demand. [50] ATP production is dependent on an adequate oxygen supply to maintain oxidative phosphorylation (which is presumably normal in persons without coronary artery disease), but the rate of ATP breakdown (hydrolysis) may be influenced by factors other than the rate of mechanical work. Thus during marathon running a continual rise in heart rate, in body temperature, in circulating free fatty acids, and in catecholamines might all be expected to exert a deleterious effect on the myocardium or to increase myocardial oxygen consumption or to "waste ATP." [42, 51]

In addition, dehydration, which occurs to an alarming extent in marathon runners, [52] might increase viscosity and decrease coronary blood flow, thus reducing myocardial oxygen delivery or predispose to coronary thrombosis. [53]

Regardless of the mechanism, the finding of transmural myocardial infarction occurring during marathon running in athletes without occlusive artery disease re-emphasizes the complexity of the relationship of exercise, coronary atherosclerosis, and sudden death ór myocardial infarction.

Conclusions

Firm evidence for the benefits of marathon running in the prevention of coronary heart disease will only result, as has been suggested by Werkö, [54] from carefully controlled epidemiological studies that take into account all the factors discussed in this section of the Marathon Symposium. Only then will it become apparent whether it is marathon running by itself or the favorable alteration in the other coronary risk factors, simultaneously advocated by Bassler, that influences coronary mortality. Until such time as this data is available, we strongly support Dayton [55] in calling for a moratorium on public assertions that marathon running prevents coronary heart disease.

Summary

Six highly trained marathon runners developed myocardial infarction. One of the two cases of clinically diagnosed myocardial infarction was fatal, and there were four cases of angiographically-proven infarction. Two athletes had significant arterial disease of two major coronary arteries, a third had stenosis of the anterior descending and the fourth of the right coronary artery.

All these athletes had warning symptoms. Three of them completed marathon races despite symptoms, one athlete running more than 20 miles after the onset of exertional discomfort to complete the 56 mile Comrades Marathon. In spite of developing chest pain, another athlete who died had continued training for three weeks, including a 40 mile run. Two other athletes also continued to train with chest pain.

We conclude that the marathon runners studied were not immune to coronary heart disease, nor to coronary atherosclerosis and that high levels of physical fitness did not guarantee the absence of significant cardiovascular disease. In addition, the relationship of exercise and myocardial infarction was complex because two athletes developed myocardial infarction during marathon running in the absence of complete coronary artery occlusion. We stress that marathon runners, like other sportsmen, should be warned of the serious significance of the development of exertional symptoms.

Our conclusions do not reflect on the possible value of exercise in the prevention of coronary heart disease. Rather we refute exaggerated claims that marathon running provides complete immunity from coronary heart disease.

ACKNOWLEDGMENTS

We are indebted to all our patients for their enthusiastic cooperation and to Professor P. H. T. Kleynhans of Bloemfontein, to Drs. R. Morris and R. D. K. Tucker of Johannesburg, and to Professor E. Chesler, Drs. R. Hart, and D. Gentin, all of Durban, for their generous assistance with the case histories. We gratefully acknowledge the assistance of Dr. J. E. Stevens who performed the echocardiographic and phonocardiographic examinations, Dr. B. Margolis who helped with the coronary arteriograms, and Professor P. Beighton for genetic consultation regarding Case 6. We thank the Medical Superintendent, Groote Schuur Hospital for permission to publish.

[NOTE ADDED IN PROOF. Against our advice, Cases 2, 3, and 6 have all subsequently completed marathon races. Thus of the 6 runners, only Case 1 (deceased) and Case 5 (jogging 20–30 miles per week) have not returned to marathon running.]

REFERENCES

1. BASSLER, T. J. 1975. Marathon running and immunity to heart disease. Phys. Sports Med. 3(April): 77–80.
2. BASSLER, T. J. 1973. Physician deaths (letter). J. Amer. Med. Assoc. **223**: 1391.
3. BASSLER, T. J. 1973. Long-distance runners (letter). Science **182**: 113.
4. BASSLER, T. J. 1974. Prevention of coronary heart disease (letter). J. Amer. Med. Assoc. **228**: 565.
5. BASSLER, T. J. 1974. Prevention of heart disease (letter). Lancet **i**: 626.
6. BASSLER, T. J. & J. H. SCAFF. 1974. Can I avoid heart-attack? (letter). Lancet **i**: 863–864.
7. BASSLER, T. J. 1974. Prevention of coronary heart disease (letter). Lancet **i**: 1106–1107.
8. BASSLER, T. J. 1974. Marathoning (letter). Science **183**: 256–257.

9. BASSLER, T. J. & F. P. CARDELLO. 1975. Jogging and health (letter). J. Amer. Med. Assoc. **231:** 23.

10. BASSLER, T. J. 1975. Life expectancy and marathon running (letter). Amer. J. Cardiol. **36:** 410–411.

11. BASSLER, T. J. & J. H. SCAFF. 1975. Exercise running and the heart (letter). N. Engl. J. Med. **292:** 302.

12. BASSLER, T. J. & J. H. SCAFF. 1975. Marathon running after myocardial infarction (letter). J. Amer. Med. Assoc. **233:** 511.

13. BASSLER, T. J. 1973. Cardiac rehabilitation (letter). J. Amer. Med. Assoc. **226:** 790.

14. BASSLER, T. J. 1974. Coronary heart disease prevention (letter). Circulation **49:** 594–595.

15. SCAFF, J. H. & T. J. BASSLER. 1974. Inputs into coronary care (letter). Ann. Intern. Med. **81:** 862.

16. BASSLER, T. J. 1976. Quality of life (letter). West. J. Med. **124:** 343.

17. BASSLER, T. J. 1972. Athletic activity and longevity (letter). Lancet **i:** 712–713.

18. BASSLER, T. J. 1972. Jogging deaths (letter). New. Engl. J. Med. **287:** 1100.

19. BASSLER, T. J. & J. H. SCAFF. 1974. Mileage preferable to medication (letter). N. Engl. J. Med. **291:** 1192.

20. BASSLER, T. J. & J. H. SCAFF. 1975. Immunity to atherosclerosis in the marathon runner. Exercise and dietary factors (letter). Artery **1:** 188.

21. BASSLER, T. J. & J. H. SCAFF. 1976. Impending heart attacks (letter). Lancet **i:** 544–545.

22. BASSLER, T. J. & F. P. CARDELLO. 1976. Fiber-feeding and atherosclerosis (letter). J. Amer. Med. Assoc. **235:** 1841–1842.

23. BASSLER, T. J. 1976. Marathon racing and myocardial infarction (letter). Ann. Intern. Med. **85:** 389.

24. BASSLER, T. J. 1976. Is atheroma a reversible lesion? (letter). Atherosclerosis **25:** 141.

25. BASSLER, T. J. 1976. Risk factors and coronary heart disease (letter). Amer. Heart J. **92:** 266.

26. BASSLER, T. J. 1976. Heart disease and athletics (letter). Phys. Sports Med. **4**(Oct.)**:** 11.

27. BASSLER, T. J. 1976. Marathon vs distance running (letter). N. Engl. J. Med. **294:** 114.

28. OPIE, L. H. 1976. Heart disease in marathon runners (letter). N. Engl. J. Med. **294:** 1067.

29. OPIE, L. H. 1975. Long distance running and sudden death (letter). N. Engl. J. Med. **293:** 941–942.

30. SCAFF, J. H. 1976. Heart disease in marathon runners (letter). N. Engl. J. Med. **295:** 105.

31. KAVANAGH, T. & R. J. SHEPHARD. 1975. Maintenance of hydration in "postcoronary" marathon runners. Brit. J. Sports Med. **9:** 130–135.

32. COOPER, K. H., M. L. POLLOCK, R. P. MARTIN, S. R. WHITE, A. C. LINNERUD & A. JACKSON. 1976. Physical fitness levels vs selected coronary risk factors. J. Amer. Med. Assoc. **236:** 166–169.

33. EPSTEIN, L., G. V. MILLER, F. W. STITT & J. N. MORRIS. 1976. Vigorous exercise in leisure time, coronary risk-factors and resting electrocardiogram in middle-aged male civil servants. Brit. Heart J. **38:** 403–409.

34. FOX, S. M. 1973. Relationship of activity habits to coronary heart disease. In Exercise Testing and Exercise Training in Coronary Heart Disease. 1st edit. J. P. Naughton, H. K. Hellerstein & I. C. Mohler, Eds. : 3–22. Academic Press, New York, N.Y.

35. MORRIS, J. N., C. ADAM, S. P. W. CHAVE, C. SIREY & L. EPSTEIN. 1973. Vigorous exercise in leisure-time and the incidence of coronary heart disease. Lancet **i:** 333–339.

36. PAFFENBARGER, R. S. & W. E. HALE. 1975. Work activity and coronary heart mortality. N. Engl. J. Med. **292:** 545–550.
37. NOAKES, T. D. & L. H. OPIE. 1976. The cardiovascular risks and benefits of exercise. Practitioner **216:** 288–296.
38. OPIE, L. H. 1974. Exercise training, the myocardium, and ischemic heart disease. Amer. Heart. J. **88:** 539–541.
39. VUORI, I., M. SARASTE, M. VIHAVA & A. PEKKARINEN. 1975. Feasibility of long distance ski hikes (20–90 km) as a mass sport. *In* Proceedings of the 20th World Congress in Sports Medicine. : 530–544. Congress Secretariat. Carlton, Australia.
40. JOKL, E. 1971. Exercise and cardiac death (letter). J. Amer. Med. Assoc. **218:** 1707.
41. ULLYOT, J. 1976. The Medical Report. Runners World **11**(Sept.): 16.
42. OPIE, L. H. 1975. Sudden death and sport. Lancet **i:** 263–266.
43. GREEN, L. H., S. I. COHEN & G. KURLAND. 1976. Fatal myocardial infarction in marathon racing. Ann. Intern. Med. **84:** 704–706.
44. FRICK, M. H., O. KORHOLA, M. NIEMINEN & M. VALLE. 1975. Ischaemic electrocardiographic changes in an athlete with normal coronary arteries. Ann. Clin. Res. **7:** 264–268.
45. CANTWELL, J. D. 1976. Marathon racing and myocardial infarction (letter). Ann. Intern. Med. **85:** 391–392.
46. ARNETT, E. N. & W. C. ROBERTS. 1976. Acute myocardial infarction and angiographically normal coronary arteries. An unproven combination. Circulation **54:** 395–400.
47. ENDO, M., K. HIROSAWA, H. KANEDO, K. HASE, Y. INOUE & S. KONNO. 1976. Prinzmetal's variant angina. Coronary arteriogram and left ventriculogram during angina attack induced by methacholine. N. Engl. J. Med. **294:** 252–255.
48. CHENG, T. O., T. BASHOUR, B. K. SINGH & G. A. KELSER. 1972. Myocardial infarction in the absence of coronary arteriosclerosis. Result of coronary spasm (?). Amer. J. Cardiol. **30:** 680–682.
49. CHESLER, E., R. E. MATISONN, J. B. LAKIER, W. A. POCOCK, I. W. PROMUND OBEL & J. B. BARLOW. 1976. Acute myocardial infarction with normal coronary arteries. A possible manifestation of the Billowing Mitral Leaflet Syndrome. Circulation **54:** 203–209.
50. HARRIS, P. 1975. A theory concerning the course of events in angina and myocardial infarction. Europ. J. Cardiol. **3:** 157–163.
51. OPIE, L. H. 1975. Metabolism of free fatty acids, glucose and catecholamines in acute myocardial infarction. Relation to myocardial ischemia and infarct size. Amer. J. Cardiol. **36:** 938–953.
52. WYNDHAM, C. H. & N. B. STRYDOM. 1969. The danger of an inadequate water intake during marathon running. S. Afr. Med. J. **43:** 893–896.
53. BURCH, G. E. & N. P. DE PASQUALE. 1962. Haematocrit, blood viscosity, and myocardial infarction. Amer. J. Med. **32:** 161–163.
54. WERKÖ, L. 1976. Risk factors and coronary heart disease (letter). Amer. Heart J. **92:** 266–267.
55. DAYTON, S. 1975. Long distance running and sudden death (letter). N. Engl. J. Med. **293:** 941.
56. RASKOFF, W. J., S. GOLDMAN & K. COHN. 1976. The "athletic heart." Prevalence and physiological significance of left ventricular enlargement in distance runners. J. Amer. Med. Assoc. **236:** 158–162.

STATISTICAL ANALYSIS OF DEATHS FROM CORONARY HEART DISEASE ANTICIPATED IN A COHORT OF MARATHON RUNNERS

Paul Milvy

Environmental Sciences Laboratory
Department of Community Medicine
Mount Sinai School of Medicine
New York, New York 10029

Introduction

Many reports have appeared in the last decade that describe epidemiological studies of the relationship between physical activity and mortality, especially mortality from coronary heart disease (CHD). (For recent general reviews, see References 1–6). The methodological and epidemiological problems encountered by these studies are extreme, and valid conclusions are notoriously difficult to achieve.[7-10] In particular, controversy has developed over the point of view, expressed by Bassler in the most extreme form in 1972, that "a search of the literature failed to document a single death due to coronary arteriosclerosis among marathon finishers"[11] and in 1973, "when the level of vigorous exercise is raised high enough, the protection appears to be absolute. The American Medical Joggers Association (AMJA) has been unable to document a single death resulting from coronary heart disease among marathon finishers of any age."[12] The implication seems to be that after completing a 26.2 mile marathon at some point in one's life, the individual is then protected from death from CHD for the remainder of his life. The controversy engendered by this assertion has continued in the last several years, as may be seen by consulting several recent letters to the editors of several medical and scientific journals.[13-17] We do not know what significance we are to place upon Bassler's communications: we do not know how many deaths of marathoners—from all causes—was revealed by the search of the literature conducted by Bassler, nor do we know the number of autopsies performed or reviewed by the AMJA; both crucial facts for establishing statistical significance to their findings.

In general, epidemiology utilized two general approaches to establish an association between variables that may be involved in human disease: the prospective study and the retrospective (or retrospective-prospective) study (causation, as opposed to association, can only be rigorously proven by the clinical trial, where randomization of variables can be achieved). The following analysis demonstrates the futility of informally applying these epidemiological approaches to a cohort of U.S. marathoners with the expectation of arriving at an evaluation of the influence of marathoning on the incidence of mortality from ischemic and related heart disease.

Materials and Methods

In 1975, 10,482 men and women completed a marathon road race.* [18] Approximately 5% of these runners were women, and have not been included

---

* This includes AAU certified and uncertified marathon courses. In 1976, 20% more completed one.

in the data base, leaving 9,958 male marathoners. In the remainder of this article an estimate is made of the number of men expected to die from ischemic and related heart disease for a cohort of 9,958 white American males whose age distribution is the same as these marathoners, but whose relative weight and smoking habits are the same as the general American male population. The two factors of weight and cigarette consumption place the general male population at substantial risk from CHD. However, marathoners, as a group, are almost invariably thin and not addicted to smoking. It is well known that marathoners have certain characteristics in common. Almost to a man (or to a woman) they do not smoke, they drink little alcohol and they are very thin. The average sub-3-hour marathoner who is under 35 years old weighs in pounds about twice the numerical measure of his height in inches. This is on the order of 15% to 20% less than the weight of the average American man of similar age. Older marathoners although slightly heavier are proportionally even lighter than men of similar age in the general population. Thus, two important risk factors in CHD are absent in virtually all marathoners. But it must be stressed that it has never been established that running *causes* men to be thin and not to smoke. Many men who have never run are still thin and do not smoke, and it is acknowledged that this is likely to be the result of multiple causation, which may but does not necessarily include running. The motivation to run is complex. Several motives that suggest themselves are certainly sheer pleasure; probably competitiveness and agression; and possibly hostility, masochism, vanity, conceit, or public recognition. In addition, concern for one's health and well-being is probably a motivation for many. This would require the ancillary belief by the runner in the widely accepted but basically unproven proposition that running helps achieve good health to a greater degree than is achieved from participation in any other hobby that one enjoys and which may be said to add to the quality of one's life. The same concern for health and well-being is a motivation not to smoke and not to become overweight. The non-smoking thin runner may achieve this status by virtue of a complex of causal factors. The scheme that suggests that running is the independent variable, and nonsmoking and thin body the dependent variable cannot be easily demonstrated. There may also be other risk factors affecting most Americans that are substantially absent among marathoners. For example, the poorer social classes (classes 4 and 5) are very under-represented among marathoners, and marathoners to a greater degree carry life insurance than the typical American, both of which are factors that place the runner in a lower mortality risk category.[19, 20]

Appropriate corrections will be applied to the estimated mortality for a cohort of men that is reasonably equivalent to the 9,958 male marathoners, save that they do not run or engage in physical exercise more than does the general insured American male population. Thus, an estimate will be made of the number of marathoners that would be expected to die per year in this cohort, independent of any postulated "protection" that marathoning per se might afford.

Procedure

TABLE 1 presents the distribution of the mean relative body weight of male smokers and nonsmokers in a population of over 900,000 men and women studied by Hammond and Garfinkel.[21] The distribution of weights for the two primary smoking categories is seen not to differ substantially. TABLE 2 presents

TABLE 1

DISTRIBUTION OF MEAN RELATIVE WEIGHTS AND CIGARETTE CONSUMPTION FOR MALES

Smoking Habits (Cigarettes per Day)	Relative Weight Distribution				Mean Relative Weight
	<90%	90%–109%	110%–119%	≥120%	
Never smoked regularly	13.2	62.8	16.7	7.3	102.0%
1–9	20.2	61.7	12.8	5.3	99.3%
10–19	26.4	60.3	9.8	3.5	97.0%
20–39	24.5	60.7	11.1	3.7	97.6%
40+	17.8	60.3	15.1	6.8	100.6%
Average all smokers	23.6	60.7	11.5	4.2	98.0%

* Relative weight $= (w/<w>) \times 100\%$, where w is a subject's weight and $<w>$ is the average weight of all subjects normalized for height.

a profile of the smoking habit of the American male population. This table was extracted from the data contained in the NCI Monograph No. 19.[22]

TABLE 3 presents data from Hammond and Garfinkel[21] that has been recalculated to show mortality normalized to 1.00 for the "non or slight cigarette smoker" of weight at least 10% under the average weight for this large cohort. The first three columns of TABLE 4 show the distribution by age of the 9,958 male marathoners and the percent in each age category. The annual mortality is given in column 4 and is taken from the Statistical Bulletin data on mortality for ischemic and related heart disease in 1973 for metropolitan standard ordinary policy holders.[19] Column 5 shows the number of deaths expected per annum for each age category in this cohort, without adjustment for smoking or weight factors. Columns 6 and 7 show the smoking–weight combined risk factors, which were presented in TABLE 3 columns A and B, respectively, with the conservative assumption that all men are in the 90%–109% relative weight category. For these columns the assumption that cigarette consumption is 20

TABLE 2

PERCENT OF MEN WHO SMOKE ONLY CIGARETTES, BY AGE *

Cigarette Consumption (Cigarettes per Day)	Age			
	35–44	45–54	55–64	65–74
Never smoked regularly	25.1	25.3	31.4	48.4
1–9	5.2	5.3	7.1	9.6
10–19	11.7	12.0	14.5	15.3
20–39	48.5	48.1	40.2	24.4
40+ †	10.4	11.2	7.3	3.1
Average	21.3	21.4	18.2	11.6

* Data from Appendix Table 2a and Appendix Table 3a from Hammond[22] were used to construct this table.

† For calculation of the average number of cigarettes, the category "40+" was arbitrarily (but reasonably) set equal to 50.

per day to age 59 and "intermediate" at older ages is also made. The two extreme right columns "Adjusted Mortality" (np/f where f represents the smoking–weight risk factors) present the annual mortality expected from 9,958 men who do not smoke and are less than 90% of average adjusted weights. That is, this is the mortality per annum that might reasonably be expected in 1976 from the real 9,958 man cohort that completed a marathon in 1975, without consideration of physical inactivity as a risk factor.

TABLE 3

NORMALIZD MORTALITY RATIOS

| Cigarette Consumption per Day | Age | Relative Weight * | | | |
| | | <90% | | 90%–109% | |
		A †	B †	A †	B †
None or slight	40–49	1.00 ‡	—	1.70	—
	50–59	1.00	1.00	1.54	1.54
	60–69	1.00	1.00	1.06	1.06
	70–79	1.00	1.00	1.06	1.06
Intermediate	40–49	4.00	2.51	3.84	—
	50–59	4.00	2.51	4.12	2.59
	60–69	4.00	2.51	4.36	1.74
	70–79	4.00	2.51	3.16	1.99
20.0 (Average of "Intermediate" and "20+")	40–49	4.28	—	6.27	—
	50–59	4.28	2.76	4.96	3.21
	60–69	4.28	2.76	4.55	2.94
	70–79	4.28	2.76	3.72	2.40
20+	40–49	4.56	—	8.71	—
	50–59	4.56	3.01	5.79	3.82
	60–69	4.56	3.01	4.74	3.13
	70–79	4.56	3.01	4.28	2.83

* See Table 1.
† Column A is normalized to the death rate for the 40–49-year-old nonhypertensive male who smokes slightly or not at all and weighs <90% of the mean relative weight. Because the death rate for 40–49, none or slight smoker, is not known accurately, column B' is presented, normalized to the 50–59-year-old male with other variables remaining the same. This data is taken from Table 7 of Reference 21.
‡ Too little data to determine accurately.

Discussion

The last two columns of TABLE 4 present the deaths per year expected from a cohort equivalent in age distribution, smoking habit, and in weight to the 9,958 males who ran a marathon in 1975 in the United States. But these columns reflect the mortality for a cohort that *did not* run a marathon and were no more physically active than the metropolitan ordinary insured policy holders. From this group we may anticipate one or two deaths per annum from ischemic and related heart disease. (From a 9,958 cohort whose weight and smoking profiles were similar to the weight and smoking distributions of the *insured* population, but who were similar in age distribution to the marathoners, we would anticipate 5.37 deaths from ischemic and related heart disease, as shown in TABLE 4 column 5.) To detect the relatively rare event of one or two such deaths per year against a background of over 330,000 U.S. men who die annually from ischemic and related heart disease is a formidable task for the epidemiologist, even were he to have access to the best national registry.

In summary, if marathoning conferred absolute protection from death from ischemic and related heart disease, we would expect no CHD deaths per year from the 10,000 cohort of male marathoners. If it provided 50% protection, we would expect about one runner per year would die from this disease, while

TABLE 4

EXPECTED MORTALITY FOR COHORT

Age	n	%	Mortality p *	np	Risk Factors † f_1	Risk Factors † f_2	Adjusted Mortality np/f_1	Adjusted Mortality np/f_2
≤ 29	5540	56.0	1.8 ‡	0.10	8.4 §	5.00 §	0.012	0.020
30–39	2393	24.0	20.5	0.49	7.3 §	4.50 §	0.067	0.109
40–49	1439	14.0	122.0	1.71	6.27	4.00 §	0.273	0.428
50–59	463	4.6	403.0	1.85	4.96	3.21	0.373	0.576
60–64	79	0.8	841.0	0.66	4.36 ¶	1.74 ¶	0.151	0.379
64–69	32	0.3	1234.0	0.39	3.76 ¶	1.87 ¶	0.104	0.208
≥ 70	12	0.1	1704.0	0.17	3.16 ¶	1.99 ¶	0.054	0.158
Total	9958	99.8		5.37			1.02	1.89
All ages **	9958		237.0	23.6				

* Mortality is per 10^5 persons.

† f_1, based up TABLE 3 column A; f_2, based upon TABLE 3 column B. For explanation, see text.

‡ Estimated mortality; too few deaths to compute accurately.

§ Risk factors estimated based upon observed trend with age. Note that total adjusted mortality in columns 8 and 9 is insensitive to variations in these risk factors: they contribute less than 8% to the total mortality.

¶ Based upon "intermediate" category of cigarette consumption from Table 3.

** Distribution of ages reflecting general insured public.

if it provided no protection, we would expect an average of one or two runners per year to die. In addition to the formidable problems of discovering these deaths, were death to occur at all, it is clear that the statistics, which under alternative initial conditions achieve only a difference of at most 2 deaths per year, are not able to assess meaningful differences (in risk factors) in the two cohorts, let alone provide evidence that marathoning prevents CHD. It is no wonder that Tom Bassler has not observed a single infarct among American marathoners. If he had, the proposition that marathoning might be deleterious to general health must be entertained, and I might seriously consider ending my marathon career forthwith, in spite of the tremendous pleasure and gratification that it has given me.

Conclusion

What we seek to assess, the validity of the proposition that marathoning may confer absolute, limited, or no protection from CHD to the American male, cannot be easily proven without a formal marathon cohort and recourse to formal epidemiological methods. By formal, we intend to convey the concept of a study in which several thousand marathoners are maintained under observation for a number of years as in conventional prospective epidemiological studies. Clearly under such conditions in which the study is maintained for many years with a carefully selected matched control group in which no known confounding factors complicate the analysis, it would be anticipated that valid data can be collected and valid conclusions achieved. But this is a formidable task.

References

1. BLACKBURN, H. 1974. Disadvantages of intensive exercises therapy after myocardial infarction. *In* Controversy in Internal Medicine. F. Ingelfinger, Ed. Vol. 2: 162–172. W. B. Saunders Co. Philadelphia, Pa.
2. BRUCE, R. A. 1974. The benefits of physical training for patients with coronary heart disease. *In* Controversy in Internal Medicine. F. Ingelfinger, Ed. Vol. 2: 145–161. W. B. Saunders Co. Philadelphia Pa.
3. FEJFAR, Z. 1975. Prevention Against Ischaemic Heart Disease. A Critical Review, Modern Trends in Cardiology, 3, pp. 465–499. Ed. by M. F. Oliver, Butterworths, Boston.
4. FOX, S. M., III, J. P. NAUGHTON & W. L. HASKELL. 1971. Physical activity and prevention of coronary heart disease. Ann. Clin. Res. 3: 404–432.
5. FROELICHER, V. F. & A. OBERMAN. 1972. Analysis of epidemiologic studies in physical inactivity as risk factor for coronary artery disease. Prog. Cardiovasc. Dis. 15 (1, July/August): 41–65.
6. MILVY, J., W. F. FORBES & K. S. BROWN. 1977. A review of epidemiological studies of physical exercise and its relationship to health and mortality. Ann. N.Y. Acad. Sci. This volume.
7. TAYLOR, H. L., R. W. PARLIN, H. BLACKBURN & A. KEYS. 1966. Problems in the analysis of the relationship of coronary heart disease to physical activity or its lack, with special reference to sample size and occupational withdrawal. *In* Physical Activity in Health and Disease. E. Evang & K. L. Anderson, Eds. : 242–261.
8. KEYS, A. 1970. Physical activity and the epidemiology of coronary disease. *In* Physical Activity and Aging. Medicine and Sport. D. Brunner, Ed. Vol. 4: 250. University Park Press. Baltimore, Md.
9. KEYS, A. 1975. Coronary heart disease—The global picture. Atherosclerosis 22: 149–192.
10. FOX, S. M., III. 1972. Physical activity and coronary heart disease. *In* Controversy in Cardiology. E. K. Chang, Ed. : 201–219. Springer Verlag. New York, N.Y.
11. BASSLER, T. J. 1972. Letter to the editor. Lancet ii: 711.
12. BASSLER, T. J. 1973. Long distance runners. Science 128: 1083.
13. BASSLER, T. J. 1970. Marathon vs. distance running (letter). New Eng. J. Med. 294(2): 114.
14. CORDELLO, F. 1976. Letter to the editor. New Eng. J. Med. 294(2): 115.
15. STEINER, R. 1976. Letter to the editor. New Eng. J. Med. 294(2): 115.
16. BASSLER, T. J. 1975. Marathon running and immunity to heart disease. Phys. Sports Med. 3: 77–80.

17. OPIE, L. H. 1976. Heart disease in marathon runners. New Eng. J. Med. **294** (19): 1067.
18. YOUNG, K. 1975. U.S. Distance Rankings for 1975. National Running Data Center, University of Arizona, Tucson, Ariz.
19. STATISTICAL BULLETIN. 1975. Socioeconomic Mortality Differentials. Metropolitan Life Insurance Co., January.
20. BLACKBURN, H. & R. W. PARLIN. 1966. Antecedents of disease: Insurance mortality experience. Ann. N.Y. Acad. Sci. **134**: 965–1017.
21. HAMMOND, E. C. & L. GARFINKEL. 1969. Coronary heart disease, stroke and aortic aneurysm. Arch. Env. Health **19**: 167–182.
22. HAMMOND, E. C. 1966. Smoking in relation to the death rates of one-million men and women. National Cancer Institute Monograph #19. : 127–204. January.

A 4-YEAR PROSPECTIVE STUDY OF THE RELATIONSHIP OF DIFFERENT HABITUAL VOCATIONAL PHYSICAL ACTIVITY TO RISK AND INCIDENCE OF ISCHEMIC HEART DISEASE IN VOLUNTEER MALE FEDERAL EMPLOYEES *

Ray H. Rosenman, Richard D. Bawol, and Mark Oscherwitz

Harold Brunn Institute
Mount Zion Hospital and Medical Center
San Francisco, California 94120

A sedentary life-style has been strongly implicated if not established as a risk factor for coronary heart disease (CHD). Although not conclusive to date, the evidence has led to widespread interest in programs for improvement of physical fitness that, among other things, may prove beneficial for both primary and secondary prevention of CHD.

The hypotheses that enhanced physical activity may diminish several other risk factors for CHD and/or have a direct preventive effect for the incidence of CHD, are being investigated in a prospective study of volunteer federal employees in the San Francisco Bay area. Some of the preliminary results of this study are presented in this paper.

Methods and Materials

This is a prospective study of 2,635 volunteer male federal employees of postal, health, aerospace and other agencies. The men were aged 35–59 years at intake in 1970. The study excluded 95 subjects who were found to exhibit manifest CHD at intake. The 2,540 initially well men included 270 Blacks, 181 Asian-Americans, 2,065 Whites, and 24 others. There were 903 postal employees (191 supervisors, 277 clerical workers, 58 mail handlers, 242 mail carriers, and 135 others) and 1,637 employees of NASA, Letterman General Hospital, and the Federal Building in San Francisco (453 supervisors, 1,010 technicians, 39 craftsmen, and 135 service workers).

The present paper is concerned only with the 2,065 Whites, of whom 356 were aged 35–39 years, 1,035 aged 40–49 years, and 674 aged 50–59 at intake. The subjects were followed annually for 4 years during which clinical CHD was observed in 65 subjects (as well as in 14 of the 475 ·on-White population at risk), in whom the initial CHD event was symptomatic myocardial infarction (MI) or CHD death in 35 subjects, silent or clinically unrecognized MI in four subjects, and angina pectoris without infarction in 26 subjects. Three of the CHD cases occurred in the intake 35–39-year-old age group, 36 in the 40–49-year group and 26 in the 50–59-year group.

Intake studies included a questionnaire dealing with health status, age, education, annual income, details of occupation, physical activity at work, the number of hours per week in such activities, and smoking habits. Intake exami-

* This study was supportd by grants from the National Dairy Council and the National Heart and Lung Institutes, National Institutes of Health, Bethesda, Maryland (Research Grant HL–03429).

nation included measured height, weight and blood pressure, 12-lead ECG, and determination of serum cholesterol by the Ness method (which gives values 27–29 mg/100 ml higher than by the Liebermann-Burchard method in the range of 150–300 mg/100 ml). Relative body weight is calculated as the percent of median weight for each height to the nearest inch in this population.

An intake physical activity questionnaire provided an interviewer-assisted, self-assessed division of vocational activity into *sedentary* workers (mainly seated at work: including most administrators, clerical, and technical workers); *moderate* activity (mainly standing at work: including most supervisory and various clerical and technical workers); and *heavy* activity (mainly mail handlers, mail carriers, and craft and service workers). A detailed physical activity questionnaire concerned with all vocational and avocational physical activity also was completed by the subjects and from this was calculated the annual caloric expenditure spent in each respective activity [1] (see Appendix). However, this was not administered until the first annual resurvey examination in 1971, thus reducing the number of subjects at risk to 1,741 and the number of CHD cases to 41 for the analyses involving this measure of physical activity. The subjects also were divided by occupation type into "white collar" (supervisors, administrators, clerical, and technical workers) and "blue collar" (all others) workers.

Individual variables were studied by comparing the relative frequencies for categorical variables and the means for continuous variables. The chi-squared test was used to assess the associations, and analysis of variance (ANOVA) was used to test the differences between means. The Framingham equations for risk of CHD [2] were applied to the data in order to compare the CHD risk as predicted by multiple variables. The composite CHD risk score combines the predictive effects of serum cholesterol, systolic blood pressure, relative body weight, ECG abnormality, and cigarette smoking, using previously cited maximum likelihood coefficients [3] that are different for each age group. However, the age and hemoglobin terms of each equation have been omitted. In the present analyses age is a nuisance variable and its direct predictive effect on CHD risk is not relevant to the comparisons that are made. This omission appears acceptable because the Framingham study coefficients were estimated separately for each age group and the comparisons in this report are only made within age groups. The omission of hemoglobin, which was not measured in this study, appears to be unimportant since this emerged as a weak predictor of CHD in Framingham. [2]

Composite risk scores are studied by one- and two-way analysis of variance (ANOVA). One-way ANOVA is used to test for differences in observed mean composite risk between groups subdivided on the basis of either vocational physical activity or socioeconomic status (SES). Since composite risk scores are based on the multiple logistics model, differences between means can be interpreted as differences in mean log odds of risk. These differences can be converted into estimates of odds ratios, which approximate relative risk between groups. Two-way ANOVA is used to study two factor (vocational physical activity and SES) effects on composite risk using an additive model. Main effects can be interpreted as additions to log odds. These additions can be converted into estimates of odds ratios and dence relative risk between levels of each factor.

Analysis of the strengths of the associations of the risk factors for the incidence of CHD used the multiple logistic model [2] for the combined subjects.

Since age is included in the logistic model, adjustment for the effect of age trends is provided by the analysis. The strengths of the associations of the factors to the incidence of CHD are shown by estimates of relative risk. These "standardized" relative risks or odds ratios are the approximate relative risks corresponding to changes in the risk factor scores by amounts equal to their respective standard deviations and give an impression of the relative importance of the various risk factors for the observed incidence of CHD. Details of the multiple logistic risk analysis methodology have been previously provided.[4, 5]

Vocational physical activity, socioeconomic status (SES), and type of occupation are thus studied in relation to risk of CHD by two methods of assessment. In the first method, traditional risk factors for CHD are combined via Framingham risk equations [2, 3] to provide a composite risk score. This method is therefore based entirely on data obtained from the intake findings in this population. It gives some indication of the extent to which the physical activity and SES measures may be related to predictive pathways for CHD. The second method uses incidence data obtained during 4 years of follow-up of the subjects in this population. These data, although limited by the relatively small number of subjects who exhibited CHD during follow-up, provide an indication of the predictive strengths of these measures after adjustment for the effects of the traditional CHD risk factors.

Results

The findings for the intake variables for the three age groups are shown in TABLE 1 in which the subjects have been divided by the three levels of self-assessed vocational physical activity. There are marked differences in the distributions of the hours of vocational activity for the three groups, supporting the belief that these represent very different amounts of vocational activity. The differences in the occupations included in each group additionally suggest that not only the amount but also the intensity of the physical work activity varies significantly between groups. As can be seen, there is a distinct tendency for subjects with heavy work activity to exhibit higher levels of the CHD risk factors. Thus, mean serum cholesterol, blood pressures and relative weight and percent of subjects with abnormal ECGs and the percent of current cigarette smokers tend to increase from sedentary to moderate or from moderate to heavy activity groups, although the differences are not always statistically significant. Little or no differences are found among the three groups for mean age, amount of avocational exercise or amount smoked by current smokers. The most striking associations with vocational activity are found with education and income. Thus, the sedentary group is dominated by men with greater education and higher annual income and the heavy activity group is dominated by men with lower education and lower annual income.

Education and income are two measures of SES and these are highly associated in the subjects of all three age groups. For purposes of simplification the relationship between education and income is shown for all ages combined in TABLE 2 and is combined into a single categorization of SES which is arbitrarily defined in TABLE 3.

The findings for the intake variables for the three age groups are shown in TABLE 4, in which the subjects have been divided by the three levels of SES, and are similar to those observed in TABLE 1. Thus, mean serum cholesterol,

TABLE 1

INTAKE VARIABLES BY AGE AND VOCATIONAL ACTIVITY

Variables at Intake	Age 35-39				Age 40-49				Age 50-59			
	Vocational Activity *			Signifi-cance *	Vocational Activity			Signifi-cance	Vocational Activity			Signifi-cance
	Light	Moderate	Heavy		Light	Moderate	Heavy		Light	Moderate	Heavy	
No. subjects	204	106	46	(p)	505	350	179	(p)	309	236	128	(p)
Age (yrs)	37.0±0.1†	37.1±0.1	37.3±0.2	0.246	45.1±0.1	45.2±0.2	45.2±0.2	NS	52.3±0.1	52.3±0.1	52.6±0.2	0.206
Education (%)												
16+ yrs	80.9	49.1	17.4	<0.001	65.0	35.1	5.1	<0.001	47.9	20.8	4.7	<0.001
13-15 yrs	14.7	22.6	28.3		17.2	23.7	19.8		23.6	26.3	17.2	
1-12 yrs	4.4	28.3	54.3		17.8	41.1	75.1		28.5	53.0	77.3	
Income (%)												
$20,000 and over	19.1	10.4	0.1	<0.001	31.1	14.6	0.0	<0.001	29.4	8.9	4.0	<0.001
$10-19,999	75.0	61.3	15.2		60.8	58.3	19.0		61.2	57.6	28.1	
$10,000 and under	5.9	28.3	84.8		8.1	27.1	81.0		9.4	33.5	71.9	
No. years in job	6.5±0.3	6.7±0.5	7.3±0.8	NS	7.6±0.4	7.5±0.4	9.6±0.6	0.001	8.0±0.4	8.8±0.5	11.1±0.9	0.001
Exercise (hrs/week)												
Vocational	4.4±0.3	12.7±0.9	25.5±1.1	<0.001	5.0±0.2	13.5±0.5	24.3±0.7	<0.001	6.0±0.4	15.0±0.7	23.9±0.9	<0.001
Avocational	8.2±0.4	10.7±0.9	9.7±1.7	0.030	8.9±0.3	9.7±0.4	7.7±0.5	0.005	9.4±0.4	9.1±0.5	7.9±0.6	0.118
Smoking (%)												
Current	27.9	39.6	37.0	0.042	36.0	37.7	42.4	NS	35.9	37.3	41.4	NS
Former	44.6	28.3	43.5		39.2	38.9	32.4		40.8	38.1	32.8	
Never	27.5	32.1	19.6		24.6	23.4	24.6		23.0	24.6	25.8	
Current: Cigs/Day	26.8±2.0	25.1±2.1	19.3±3.3	0.186	25.6±1.3	25.4±1.2	25.5±1.6	NS	26.5±1.8	25.6±1.8	25.1±1.6	NS
Relative Weight (%)	99.8±0.8	97.5±1.1	106.1±2.2	0.001	100.4±0.5	101.1±0.6	102.6±1.0	0.002	100.6±0.7	101.5±0.8	101.6±1.1	NS
Abnormal ECG (%)	4.9	5.7	8.7	NS	6.9	9.1	7.3	0.476	12.9	12.3	14.8	NS
Blood Pressure (mmHg)												
Systolic	133.0±0.1	132.6±1.7	137.3±2.9	0.210	134.1±0.7	135.3±0.9	137.4±1.4	0.086	140.4±1.1	140.9±1.3	141.1±1.7	0.404
Diastolic	84.1±0.7	84.3±1.2	87.2±1.7	0.231	85.8±0.5	86.2±0.7	87.4±0.9	0.333	88.7±0.7	88.3±0.8	89.2±1.2	NS
Serum Cholesterol (mg/100 ml)	237.3±3.4	239.7±4.4	252.7±7.5	0.145	247.2±2.2	245.1±2.5	259.5±5.4	0.009	247.3±2.6	242.0±3.1	259.1±4.9	0.006

* NS = Not significant at p > 0.50
† Mean values ± standard deviation (SD).

TABLE 2

DISTRIBUTION OF INCOME BY EDUCATION

Annual Income	No. Years Education		
	16+	13–15	1–12
No. of subjects	888	429	745
Annual income (%)			
$20,000 and over	34.3	4.4	2.6
$10,000–19,999	58.1	51.9	39.6
Under $10,000	7.6	43.7	57.8

blood pressures, relative weight, and the percent of current smokers tend to increase from high to middle to low SES, although the differences again, are not always statistically significant. The strongest association is found between SES and the amount of vocational physical activity.

TABLE 5 shows the findings for intake variables for the three age groups in which the subjects have been divided by their type of occupation. In comparison with the "white collar" workers, the "blue collar" workers exhibit higher mean serum cholesterols, blood pressures, and relative weight, greater frequency of cigarette smoking, less education, higher annual income and are more often in jobs associated with moderate or heavy physical activity.

Estimates of the composite risk scores for CHD are shown in TABLES 6–8. TABLE 6 shows the findings for the three age groups in which the subjects have been divided by the three levels of vocational physical activity, with CHD risk as unity for subjects with sedentary work activity. A consistent increase in relative risk is observed from sedentary to moderate to heavy activity groups in all age categories, although the magnitude of the increase diminishes with age. The lack of statistical significance for the youngest age group is probably a reflection of the smaller sample size for this group.

TABLE 7 shows the findings for the three age groups in which the subjects have been divided by levels of education, annual income, and the SES categorization (TABLE 3). As with vocational activity, a consistent pattern is observed for all three measures. The relative CHD risk is observed to increase from higher to lower levels of education, annual income, and SES, and again, the magnitude of these increases diminishes with age.

The above analyses found that higher CHD risk is associated with greater vocational physical activity and with lower SES. It was therefore important to do a two-way analysis of CHD risk in which both vocational physical activity and SES levels are simultaneously considered. The results of such an analysis

TABLE 3

SOCIOECONOMIC STATUS (SES) IN TERMS OF EDUCATION AND INCOME

Annual Income	No. Years Education		
	16+	13–15	1–12
$20,000 and over	High	High	Middle
$10,000–19,999	High	Middle	Low
Under $10,000	Middle	Low	Low

TABLE 4

INTAKE VARIABLES BY AGE AND SOCIOECONOMIC STATUS (SES)*

Variables At Intake	Age 35–39				Age 40–49				Age 50–59			
	High	SES Middle	Low	Significance†	High	SES Middle	Low	Significance	High	SES Middle	Low	Significance
No. subjects	211	52	93	(p)	454	147	432	(p)	202	130	341	(p)
Age (yrs)	36.9±0.1‡	37.3±0.2	37.2±0.1	0.104	44.9±0.1	45.4±0.2	45.3±0.1	0.064	52.2±0.1	52.4±0.2	52.4±0.1	NS
No. years in job	6.9±0.3	5.2±0.6	7.0±0.6	0.037	8.2±0.3	7.6±0.6	7.7±0.3	NS	9.0±0.6	7.6±0.6	9.2±0.5	0.157
Exercise (hrs/week)												
Vocational	4.6±0.3	12.6±1.3	19.3±1.1	<0.001	5.3±0.3	10.9±0.8	17.5±0.5	<0.001	5.2±0.3	11.9±0.9	17.1±0.6	<0.001
Avocational	8.9±0.5	9.4±1.0	9.6±1.1	NS	9.3±0.3	9.5±0.5	8.4±0.3	0.042	9.7±0.4	8.7±0.6	8.7±0.4	0.247
Smoking (%)												
Current	24.2	42.3	46.2		31.6	37.4	44.3		31.8	37.7	40.5	
Former	43.6	40.4	30.1	0.001	38.0	47.6	35.0	<0.001	36.8	43.8	37.5	0.034
Never	32.2	17.3	23.7		30.5	15.0	20.6		31.3	18.5	22.0	
Current: cigs/day	24.9±2.0	26.9±2.9	24.6±2.3	0.003	25.4±1.5	28.5±2.3	25.3±1.0	<0.001	27.5±2.4	25.6±2.9	25.4±1.2	0.031
Relative weight (%)	98.5±0.8	99.2±1.8	103.6±1.5	0.003	99.1±0.5	103.0±1.0	102.3±0.6	<0.001	99.5±0.8	103.1±1.0	101.4±0.7	0.031
Abnormal ECG (%)	5.2	9.6	4.3	0.380	7.3	3.4	9.7	0.041	16.3	7.7	13.2	0.074
Blood Pressure (mmHg)												
Systolic	132.1±1.0	133.7±2.2	136.4±1.9	0.093	133.1±0.7	133.4±1.2	137.7±0.9	<0.001	138.5±1.3	141.1±1.8	141.9±1.1	0.165
Diastolic	83.3±0.8	85.9±1.6	86.7±1.1	0.034	84.8±0.5	85.6±0.9	87.9±0.6	<0.001	87.3±0.8	88.9±1.0	89.4±0.7	0.160
Serum Cholesterol (mg/100 ml)	236.5±3.3	246.2±7.1	244.4±4.8	0.254	242.6±2.2	249.3±3.6	254.7±2.9	0.003	248.1±3.3	237.6±4.0	251.1±2.7	0.023

* Defined in Table 3.
† NE = Not significant at p > 0.50.
‡ Mean values ± SD.

VARIABLES BY AGE AND TYPE OF OCCUPATION

Variables At Intake	Age 35-39			Age 40-49			Age 50-59		
	Type of Occupation		Signifi-cance	Type of Occupation		Signifi-cance	Type of Occupation		Signifi-cance
	White Collar	Blue Collar		White Collar	Blue Collar		White Collar	Blue Collar	
No. subjects	302	54	(p)	825	210	(p)	539	135	(p)
Age (yrs)	37.0±0.1	37.4±0.2	0.058	45.1±0.1	45.3±0.2	0.248	52.3±0.1	52.6±0.2	0.040
Education (%)									
16+ yrs	71.9	14.8	<0.001	53.3	9.6	<0.001	35.5	8.9	<0.001
13–15 yrs	14.2	44.4		19.8	20.2		25.7	14.1	
1–12 yrs	13.9	40.7		26.9	70.2		38.8	77.0	
Income (%)									
$20,000 and over	16.6	0.0	<0.001	24.8	1.4	<0.001	20.6	0.7	<0.001
$10,000–19,999	71.5	16.7		60.1	23.8		61.0	23.7	
$10,000 and under	11.9	83.3		15.0	74.8		18.4	75.6	
No. years in job	6.6±0.2	7.2±0.8	0.375	7.6±0.2	9.1±0.6	0.007	8.2±0.3	11.5±0.9	<0.001
Exercise (hrs/week)									
Vocational	7.5±0.5	21.2±1.3	<0.001	8.9±0.3	20.3±0.8	<0.001	10.7±0.4	19.6±1.1	<0.001
Avocational	9.1±0.4	9.6±1.4	NS	9.0±0.2	8.5±0.5	0.311	9.2±0.3	8.2±0.7	0.114
Smoking (%)									
Current	29.5	30.0	0.011	36.3	43.5	0.155	37.0	39.3	NS
Former	41.1	31.5		39.0	34.4		38.3	39.3	
Never	39.5	18.5		24.8	22.0		24.7	21.5	
Current: Cigs/Day	26.3±1.6	21.5±2.5	0.124	26.4±0.9	24.3±1.4	0.240	26.4±1.3	24.0±1.6	0.345
Relative Weight (%)	99.4±0.1	102.9±2.2	<0.001	100.3±0.4	103.8±0.9	<0.001	100.8±0.5	102.3±1.1	0.195
Abnormal ECG (%)	6.0	3.7	NS	7.5	8.6	NS	13.9	9.6	0.186
Blood Pressure (mmHg)									
Systolic	132.8±0.9	137.1±2.4	0.061	133.9±0.6	139.7±1.3	<0.001	140.5±0.9	141.2±1.6	NS
Diastolic	84.2±0.6	86.4±1.5	0.186	85.3±0.4	89.6±0.8	<0.001	88.3±0.5	39.9±1.1	0.170
Serum Cholesterol (mg/100 ml)	238.5±2.7	248.4±6.9	0.164	246.1±1.7	258.1±4.8	0.003	243.4±2.0	264.8±4.4	<0.001
Vocational Activity (%)									
Sedentary	65.6	11.1	<0.001	57.3	15.7	<0.001	53.6	14.9	<0.001
Moderate	28.1	38.9		35.7	26.7		35.6	32.8	
Heavy	6.3	50.0		7.0	57.6		10.8	52.2	

TABLE 6

ESTIMATED RELATIVE RISKS OF VOCATIONAL ACTIVITY GROUPS *

Age	Vocational Activity †			F Statistic	Significance (p)
	I	II	III		
35–39	1.00	1.13	1.56	$F_{2,353} = 2.24$	0.108
40–49	1.00	1.09	1.27	$F_{2,1031} = 6.66$	0.001
50–59	1.00	1.00	1.20	$F_{2,670} = 3.21$	0.041

* Relative to sedentary mass: derived by one-way ANOVA of composite risk score.
† I=sedentary, II=moderate, III=heavy.

are shown in TABLE 8. When the composite risk of CHD is thus studied simultaneously in relation to vocational physical activity and the three measures of SES, the level of vocational physical activity is not found to be associated with the CHD risk. However, the relationship between composite CHD risk and the three measures of SES persists in these two-way analyses. In each instance there is an increase of relative CHD risk in going from high to middle to low education, income, or SES. These associations again tend to diminish with age. However, with the exception of the association with education in the older age group, the findings are statistically significant for each indicator in each age group.

Although the data are not shown here, the above associations are supported by an examination of the relative CHD risk for blue collar and white collar workers, in which the composite risk of the white collar worker is held as unity.

TABLE 7

ESTIMATED RELATIVE RISKS OF SOCIOECONOMIC GROUPS *

Age	Years of Education			F Statistic	Significance (p)
	16+	13–15	1–12		
35–39	1.00	1.52	1.61	$F_{2,353} = 6.32$	0.002
40–49	1.00	1.26	1.45	$F_{2,1029} = 24.27$	<0.001
50–59	1.00	1.05	1.19	$F_{2,669} = 4.38$	0.013
	Annual Income				
	>20,000	12–20,000	<10,000		
35–39	1.00	1.05	1.82	$F_{2,358} = 5.87$	0.003
40–49	1.00	1.25	1.59	$F_{2,1029} = 22.58$	<0.001
50–59	1.00	1.08	1.33	$F_{2,669} = 8.10$	<0.001
	Education-Income Class (SES)				
	High	Middle	Low		
35–39	1.00	1.71	1.82	$F_{2,353} = 8.79$	<0.001
40–49	1.00	1.27	1.43	$F_{2,1029} = 25.61$	<0.001
50–59	1.00	0.96	1.18	$F_{2,669} = 5.09$	0.006

* Relative to highest education, income, or education-income classification: derived by one-way ANOVA of composite risk score.

TABLE 8

ESTIMATED RELATIVE RISKS OF VOCATIONAL ACTIVITY AND SOCIOECONOMIC GROUPS IN COMBINATION *

	Ages 35–39					Ages 40–49					Ages 50–59				
	Factor Level			F to remove	Significance (p)	Factor Level			F to remove	Significance (p)	Factor Level			F to remove	Significance (p)
	I	II	III			I	II	III			I	II	III		
Model 1															
Vocational activity †	1.00	0.97	1.18	$F_{2,835}=0.36$	NS	1.00	0.99	1.03	$F_{2,1027}=0.36$	NS	1.00	0.96	1.23	$F_{2,097}=1.76$	0.173
Education ‡	1.00	1.65	1.67	$F_{2,835}=4.37$	0.013	1.00	1.24	1.43	$F_{2,1027}=17.72$	<0.001	1.00	1.05	1.18	$F_{2,097}=2.77$	0.063
Model 2															
Vocational activity	1.00	0.99	1.01	$F_{2,851}=0.01$	NS	1.00	1.01	1.00	$F_{2,1027}=0.01$	NS	1.00	0.93	1.03	$F_{2,097}=1.03$	0.358
Income ‡	1.00	1.05	1.82	$F_{2,851}=3.57$	0.029	1.00	1.25	1.58	$F_{2,1027}=15.96$	<0.001	1.00	1.11	1.37	$F_{2,097}=5.71$	0.003
Model 3															
Vocational activity	1.00	0.90	0.94	$F_{2,851}=0.21$	NS	1.00	0.98	1.00	$F_{2,1027}=0.09$	NS	1.00	0.95	1.09	$F_{2,097}=1.50$	0.224
Education–income cross-classification ‡	1.00	1.75	1.92	$F_{2,851}=6.65$	0.001	1.00	1.27	1.43	$F_{2,1027}=19.01$	<0.001	1.00	0.97	1.15	$F_{2,097}=3.21$	0.041

* Relative to Class I within each age group: Derived by 2-way ANOVA additive model of composite risk score.
† I = sedentary; II = moderate; III = heavy.
‡ I = high; II = middle; III = low (see TABLE 5).

The estimated composite relative risk for blue collar workers for the three age groups, respectively, is 1.54 (p = 0.026), 1.32 (p < 0.001), and 1.23 (p = 0.002), again showing an association that diminishes with age.

The physical activity of the subjects was assessed by the three levels of vocational physical activity used for the above analyses and, additionally, by a questionnaire that explored all types of both vocational and nonvocational activity, and from which was calculated the annual caloric expenditure in each type of activity.[1] The correlations between the different measures of physical activity are shown in TABLE 9. For all three age groups the level of vocational

TABLE 9

CORRELATIONS BETWEEN PHYSICAL ACTIVITY VARIABLES

	Occupation Type	Vocational Caloric Expenditures	Avocational Caloric Expenditures	Total Caloric Expenditures
Ages 35–39 ($n=302$)				
Vocational activity *	0.510 †	0.578 †	−0.008	0.474 †
Occupation type §	—	0.456 †	−0.029	0.363 †
Vocational caloric expenditures	—	—	0.036	—
Ages 40–49 ($n=861$)				
Vocational activity	0.495 †	0.628 †	−0.040	0.472 †
Occupation type	—	0.413 †	−0.074 ‡	0.281 †
Vocational caloric expenditures	—	—	−0.007	—
Ages 50–59 ($n=578$)				
Vocational activity	0.406 †	0.534 †	−0.155 ‡	0.326 †
Occupation type	—	0.353 †	−0.068	0.237
Vocational caloric expenditures	—	—	−0.037	—

* Vocational activity coded: 1=sedentary, 2=moderate, 3=heavy.
† Significant at p=0.01 (critical values: $R=0.147$ for $n=302$, $R=0.088$ for $n=861$, $R=0.107$ for $n=578$).
‡ Significant at p=0.05 (critical values: $R=0.112$ for $n=302$, $R=0.067$ for $n=861$, $R=0.081$ for $n=578$).
§ Occupation type coded: 0=white collar; 1=blue collar.

physical activity (i.e., sedentary, moderate, and heavy) is significantly correlated with both the type of occupation (i.e., white or blue collar worker) and with the calculated annual vocational caloric expenditure. However, only small correlations are observed between nonvocational caloric expenditure and either the level of vocational physical activity or caloric expenditure or the type of occupation, and these are generally not statistically significant.

The correlations between the calculated annual caloric expenditures for vocational and nonvocational activity and the intake variables and composite CHD risk scores are shown in TABLE 10. The vocational caloric expenditure is significantly but inversely correlated with level of education and annual in-

TABLE 10

CORRELATIONS BETWEEN CALORIC EXPENDITURES (1971) AND CHD RISK VARIABLES (1970) BY AGE GROUP

	Age (Within age group)	Height	Weight	Body Mass Index	Relative Weight	Smoking (0, 1)	No. of Cigs * (Smokers Only)	ECG (0, 1)	Systolic Pressure	Diastolic Pressure	Serum Cholesterol	Education (1–16)	Income	Composite Risk Framingham
Ages 35–39 (n = 302)														
Vocational caloric expenditures	0.080	−0.182†	−0.013	0.091	0.095	0.065	−0.187	−0.005	0.039	0.037	0.053	−0.332†	−0.478†	0.059
Avocational caloric expenditures	0.025	−0.019	−0.110	−0.113‡	−0.113‡	0.029	−0.111	−0.119‡	0.083	0.040	−0.044	0.124‡	0.094	−0.007
Total caloric expenditures	0.080	−0.161†	−0.069	0.016	0.019	0.070	−0.219	−0.067	0.076	0.052	0.021	−0.209†	−0.346†	0.046
Ages 40–49 (n = 861)														
Vocational caloric expenditures	0.015	−0.147†	−0.024	0.073‡	0.077‡	0.030	0.044	0.011	0.016	0.035	0.049	−0.400†	−0.461†	0.087‡
Avocational caloric expenditures	0.024	0.021	0.022	0.007	0.015	−0.062	−0.082	0.026	0.010	0.029	−0.082‡	0.115‡	0.143‡	−0.113†
Total caloric Expendiures	0.026	−0.104†	−0.006	0.062	0.070‡	−0.014	−0.010	0.024	0.019	0.046	−0.012	−0.246†	−0.277†	−0.001
Ages 50–59 (n = 578)														
Vocational caloric expenditures	0.006	−0.094‡	0.014	0.075	0.076	0.000	−0.095	0.010	−0.003	−0.010	0.086‡	−0.249†	−0.398†	0.055
Avocational caloric expenditures	0.001	−0.001	−0.041	−0.045	−0.046	−0.074	0.079	0.009	−0.039	−0.015	−0.043	0.104‡	0.171‡	−0.079
Total caloric expenditures	0.006	−0.075	−0.015	0.031	0.032	−0.047	−0.041	0.013	−0.027	−0.018	0.041	−0.132†	−0.208†	−0.006

* Correlations with No. of Cigarettes based on subgroup of $n = 70,218$, and 136 smokers for ages 35–39, 40–49, and 50–59, respectively
† Significant at $p = 0.01$ (critical values: $R = 0.147$ for $n = 302$; $R = 0.088$ for $n = 861$; $R = 0.107$ for $n = 578$).
‡ Significant at $p = 0.05$ (critical values: $R = 0.112$ for $n = 302$; $R = 0.067$ for $n = 861$; $R = 0.107$ for $n = 578$).

come, as previously found for vocational physical activity by the three-level self-assessment. An interesting inverse association is found between height and vocational caloric expenditure in all three age groups. The remaining correlations are generally of small magnitude and not significant.

TABLE 11

MULTIPLE LOGISTIC COEFFICIENTS FOR RISK FACTORS FOR CORONARY HEART DISEASE IN 4 YEARS

	Inter-cept	Age	Choles-terol	Systolic Pres-sure	Ciga-rette Smok-ing	Additional Variable
Model 1						
Log coefficient	−10.523	0.084	0.005	0.013	0.219	None
Factor Std Dev	—	5.72	50.76	17.88	1.10	—
Odds ratio *	—	1.62	1.26	1.26	1.27	—
p Value	—	0.001	0.024	0.041	0.029	—
Model 2						Vocational activity †
Log coefficient	−10.555	0.084	0.005	0.013	0.219	−0.107
Factor Std Dev	—	5.72	50.76	17.88	1.10	0.38
Odds ratio	—	1.62	1.27	1.26	1.27	0.96 (1.04)
p Value	—	0.001	0.023	0.040	0.029	0.748
Model 3						Type of occu-pation ‡
Log coefficient	−10.519	0.084	0.005	0.013	0.219	0.012
Factor Std Dev	—	5.72	50.76	17.88	1.10	0.39
Odds ratio	—	1.62	1.26	1.26	1.27	1.00
p Value	—	0.001	0.026	0.042	0.029	0.969
Model 4						Total daily caloric expendi-tures
Log coefficient	−10.365	0.090	0.003	0.006	0.214	0.0004
Factor Std Dev	—	5.72	51.05	17.28	1.06	428.72
Odds ratio	—	1.68	1.17	1.11	1.26	1.19
p value	—	0.005	0.265	0.470	0.098	0.226

* Standardized relative risk or approximate relative risk for a change in the risk factor by an amount equal to its standard deviation.
† 0=sedentary or moderate, 1=heavy.
‡ 0=white collar, 1=blue collar.

The relationship between the risk factors and the incidence of CHD is shown in TABLE 11. Multivariate risk analysis is motivated by the need for methods that assess the direct predictive strength associated with each member of a cluster of possibly interrelated risk factors. The essence of multiple risk analysis is to examine the changes of risk with varying levels of one factor at various fixed levels of the remaining factors. The present analysis utilized the multiple logistic risk model as described elsewhere,[2-5] with age, serum cholesterol, systolic blood pressure, and cigarette smoking as the CHD risk factors. As can be seen in TABLE 11, each of these factors is significantly associated with the incidence of CHD in this population (Model 1). When the additive logistic model also separately included the level of vocational physical activity (Model 2), the type of occupation (Model 3), and the level of caloric expenditure (Model 4), none of the latter measures are found to be associated with the CHD incidence. Moreover, the strengths of the associations between the four CHD risk factors and the CHD incidence are not altered by addition of the measures of vocational activity or type of occupation. They were decreased in the additive logistic model that included total caloric expenditure, but this is probably a reflection of the smaller number of CHD cases available for this particular analysis.

Discussion

These appears to be little question about the beneficial effects of physical fitness on general well-being, psychologic outlook, and cardiovascular function. The latter appears to be related primarily to a more optimal heart rate and blood pressure response to exertion. Thus, the trained cardiovascular response to the same work load is characterized by a lesser increase of heart rate and blood pressure and a decreased calculated tension-time index. It does not appear to be related to any proven effects of physical conditioning on the size of either the coronary or intercoronary collateral circulation.

The fundamental questions are whether physical conditioning significantly alters other risk factors for CHD, prolongs life, or reduces the incidence of primary or recurrent clinical CHD.

The extensive data concerning these questions have been critically reviewed elsewhere [6-8] and no attempt will be made herein to review the relevant literature. Retrospective and prospective population studies have not established the level of physical activity as a risk factor of comparable magnitude to serum cholesterol, blood pressure, type A behavior pattern, or cigarette smoking, nor have they shown that enhanced physical fitness substantially alters these other risk factors or protects against development and progression of coronary atherosclerosis.[6, 7] There are suggestive findings that enhanced physical activity exerts a beneficial effect on the primary and recurrent incidence of CHD and on the severity of their clinical manifestations, but the findings to date are not conclusive.[8]

The present study is a prospective investigation of middle-aged males with very different habitual vocational physical activity. The level of vocational physical activity in this population is not found to be related either to other risk factors for CHD or to the incidence of clinical CHD occurring during four years of annual follow-up. The findings do not speak to the issue of whether purposeful physical conditioning programs that aim at achieving cardiovascular training have a beneficial effect on the incidence of CHD.

Summary

A prospective study of coronary heart disease (CHD) was done in 2,635 volunteer male federal employees of postal, health, aerospace, and other agencies, aged 35–59 years at intake. The present annalysis is concerned with 2,065 initially well whites, of whom 65 suffered clinical CHD during 4 years of annual follow-up. The subjects differed markedly in their levels of habitual vocational physical activity, which is classified (1) by division into sedentary, moderate, and heavy activity groups, (2) by blue collar or white collar type of occupation, and (3) by calculated annual caloric expenditure for both vocational and non-vocational physical activities.

Intake variables that were studied in relation to physical activity and the CHD incidence include age, serum cholesterol, systolic blood pressure, relative body weight, ECG abnormality, and cigarette smoking. Socioeconomic status (SES) is assessed by levels of education and income and by a combined SES categorization based upon both. Estimated composite CHD risk scores are based upon Framingham equations.

The CHD risk factors, singly, as well as in a derived composite risk score, are higher for men with heavy compared to sedentary or moderate habitual physical activity. However, this is a spurious association found to be induced by differences of SES. Thus, when physical activity and SES are studied in a concurrent analysis, a higher CHD risk is significantly associated with lower SES status but not with differences of vocational physical activity.

The CHD incidence in this population is studied in relationship both to the risk factors and physical activity by multivariate analysis, using the multiple logistic risk model. The incidence of CHD is significantly associated with age, serum cholesterol, systolic blood pressure, and cigarette smoking. It is not found to be associated with the type of occupation (i.e., blue or white collar), the level of reported habitual vocational physical activity, or the calculated total vocational plus nonvocational caloric expenditure in physical activity.

Appendix

The determination of caloric expenditure in physical activity is derived from a self-administered questionnaire based on a 1-year recall and developed by Pascarella.[1] In this the subjects recorded the number of hours per week of vocational time spent in sitting, light activities (e.g., walking, filing, drafting) and heavy activities (e.g., pushing, lifting, carrying) in both primary and other jobs. Average daily vocational caloric expenditure was calculated from annual amounts using expenditure rates of 2 kcal/min for sitting, 4 kcal/min for light activities, and 6 kcal/min for heavy activities.

The subjects also recorded the estimated number of times in the past year and average number of hours (to nearest ¼ hour) of time spent in each of 26 types of nonvocational physical activities. These included 20 types of sports and athletics and six types of home physical activities. The average daily nonvocational caloric expenditures were calculated from kcal/min expenditure rates provided by Passmore and Durnin.[9]

References

1. PASCARELLA, E. A. 1969. An analysis of the relationship between 2 measures of obesity derived from selected anthropometric dimensions and the occurrence of coronary heart disease. Doctoral Thesis, Dept. of Epidemiology, School of Public Health, University of North Carolina, Chapel Hill, N.C.

2. TRUETT, J., J. CORNFIELD & W. KANNEL. 1967. A multivariate analysis of the risk of coronary heart disease in Framingham. J. Chronic Diseases **20:** 511–524.
3. HALPERIN, M., W. C. BLACKWELDER & J. I. VERTER. 1971. Estimation of the multivariate logistics risk function: A comparison of the discriminant function and maximum likelihood approaches. J. Chronic Diseases **24:** 125–158.
4. BRAND, R. J., R. H. ROSENMAN, R. I. SHOLTZ, *et al.* 1976. Multivariate prediction of coronary heart disease in the Western Collaborative Group Study compared to the findings of the Framingham Study. Circulation **53:** 348–355.
5. ROSENMAN, R. H., R. J. BRAND, R. I. SHOLTZ & M. FRIEDMAN. 1976. Multivariate prediction of coronary heart disease during 8.5 year follow-up in the Western Collaborative Group Study. Amer. J. Cardiol. **37:** 903–910.
6. FROELICHER, V. F. & A. OBERMAN. 1972. Analysis of epidemiologic studies of physical inactivity as risk factors for coronary artery disease. Prog. Cardiovasc. Dis. **15:** 41–65.
7. BLACKBURN, H. 1974. Disadvantages of intensive exercise therapy after myocardial infarction. *In* Controversy in Internal Medicine. F. J. Ingelfinger, *et al.,* Eds. Vol. **2:** 162–172. W. B. Saunders Co., Philadelphia, Pa.
8. FROELICHER, V. F. 1976. The effects of exercise on the heart and on coronary atherosclerotic disease: Literature survey. *In* Cardiovascular Clinics, A. Brest, Ed. F. A. Davis Co., Philadelphia, Pa.
9. PASSMORE, M. & M. DURNIN. 1955. Physiol. Rev. **35:** 801–840.

THE IMPORTANT ROLE OF FITNESS DETERMINATION AND STRESS TESTING IN PREDICTING CORONARY INCIDENCE

Kenneth H. Cooper, Betty Ullman Meyer, Richard Blide,
Michael Pollock, and Larry Gibbons

Institute for Aerobics Research
Dallas, Texas 75230

Recent reports from the National Center for Health Statistics show that there has been a decline in death from ischemic heart disease since at least 1970.[1] Dr. Robert I. Levy, director of the National Heart, Lung and Blood Institute, in attempting to explain this turnaround, mentioned voluntary efforts to switch to more prudent patterns of diet, reduce smoking, and increase exercise.[2]

Many studies have been concerned with the relationship of various indicators, such as lipid levels and health habits, to the development of coronary heart disease (CHD).[3-5] These variables, which frequently are associated with incidence of the disease, have become known as risk factors and include the following items: elevated blood pressure, hyperlipemia (mainly serum cholesterol and triglycerides), cigarette smoking, obesity, physical inactivity, glucose intolerance, excessive emotional stress, previous family history of CHD, and certain electrocardiogram (ECG) abnormalities at rest. Furthermore, findings from population studies such as Framingham have shown not only that the manifestation of CHD is influenced by certain risk factors, but that the incidence rate increases dramatically with additive numbers of risk factors.[6]

A recent study by Kannel, McGee, and Gordon showed that six risk factors could significantly predict incidence of CHD.[7] Their risk factor profile included the following variables: age, serum cholesterol, systolic blood pressure, cigarette smoking, glucose intolerance, and left ventricular hypertrophy (LVH). It appears that a profile such as this would provide important information to both the physician and patient in helping to identify persons at high risk.

Recently, two additional factors have been isolated that show diagnostic and/or prognostic value in predicting morbidity and mortality from CHD: first, the results of exercise stress testing with ECG monitoring and, second, the level of cardiorespiratory fitness (endurance performance capacity), precisely quantified. Each was found to relate to the incidence of myocardial infarction and to survival.[8-9] In another investigation, endurance performance was significantly associated with lowered values of risk function variables.[10]

In a review of the sensitivity and specificity of the stress test ECG to predict the presence of CHD, Ellestad observed a significant relationship. He reported that the predictive value of such a test was improved by using multi-lead monitoring systems and having patients perform to maximum or near maximum levels.[8] Cooper et al.[10] in a cross-sectional study of 3,000 men found a significant relationship between measured levels of physical fitness and selected CHD risk factors. In addition, Margolis et al.[9] found that the treadmill performance capacity of patients with coronary artery disease was significant in its prognostic value for prediction of mortality. Thus, it appears that the inclusion of the two additional variables, presence or absence of stress-test ECG abnormalities, and level of physical fitness, may further increase the sensitivity of the Framingham risk factor profile.

The purpose of this investigation was to explore that possibility in a preliminary study involving patients at the Cooper Clinic.

Methods

Over 9,000 men and women have been medically examined and stress-tested one or more times at the Cooper Clinic since 1971.

The subjects reported for morning testing in a 12-hour postabsorptive state; they were asked not to smoke prior to reporting to the laboratory. Tests were conducted in air-conditioned rooms with an ambient temperature of $22° \pm 1.7° C$. Prior to testing, the subjects completed an extensive medical history questionnaire that included the following: general information, occupation, purpose for coming to the clinic, present and past medical history, family history, and smoking and exercise habits.

A 15-ml sample of blood was drawn from the antecubital vein after 15 to 20 minutes of sitting and was analyzed for serum cholesterol and triglycerides, glucose, and uric acid. Cholesterol, glucose, and uric acid values were determined on an automated system of chemical analysis, and the methods described by Huang *et al.*,[11] Bittner and McCleary,[12] and Musser and Ortigoza [13] were followed. Serum triglyceride values were determined on a single-channel automated system, according to the method described by Kessler and Lederer.[14] The blood analyzers were checked daily with standard samples, and monthly with a quality control check.

Body height and weight were measured on a standard physician's scale with subjects in the nude. Body density was determined by the underwater displacement technique as described by Allen;[15] in order to facilitate the accuracy of this measure, each subject underwent multiple trials. By use of the equation of Brožek *et al.*[16] percent body fat was calculated from the body density measurement. Residual volume was estimated from both height and age as outlined by Goldman and Becklace [17] and was used in the equation for estimating body density.

A 12-lead resting ECG was recorded after a rest period of approximately 10 minutes. Abnormal resting ECGs were evaluated carefully, and patients with severe problems were excluded from the study, i.e., those for whom stress testing would be dangerous.[18] Resting heart rates were obtained from a 6-second recording of standard lead II while the patient was at rest in the supine position. Systolic and diastolic blood pressure readings were taken using an aneroid sphygmomanometer which was calibrated at 3-month intervals.

Cardiorespiratory endurance was determined from a maximal treadmill stress test (MTST), according to a modified Balke and Ware protocol.[19] The speed of the treadmill was held constant at 90 m/min (3.3 mph). The grade of the treadmill was set at 0% for the first minute, was raised 2% at the end of the first minute, and then was increased 1% every minute until the 25th minute.

A single-channel electrocardiograph and scope were used to monitor each subject during MTST. By switching from lead to lead, a continuous multilead ECG was recorded in all tests by either a five- or seven-lead patient-cable. When the five-lead system was used, leads I, II, III, aV_R, aV_L, aV_F, and V_5 were recorded. The seven-lead system was used for all subjects over 50 years of age and for any subject suspected of having heart disease; for this system, the seven electrical leads were recorded, as well as V_1 and V_3 by using a multiplexer switch.

The subjects were instructed to continue the MTST as long as possible. The endpoints for the MTST were either volitional exhaustion, ECG abnormality,[18, 20] or a minimum of 85% of the age-adjusted predicted maximal heart rate.[21]

Criteria for exercise ECG abnormality are essentially those of Ellestad,[8] with abnormal defined as ST segment depression of at least 1.0 mm, and equivocal defined as ST segment depression at least 0.05 mm, but less than 1.0 mm. In each case, the duration must be no less than 0.08 second. Determination of LVH by ECG was according to the criteria of Romhilt and Estes.[22]

For this investigation a matched study design was used. The "cases" consisted of 27 males, healthy when examined at the Cooper Clinic, but later experiencing fatal (7 cases) and non-fatal (11) myocardial infarctions (MI), or undergoing coronary by-pass procedures (9). These men ranged from 39–68 years of age when examined, with mean age 54. The time period between examination and coronary events averaged 17 months, and varied between one and 53 months; median time was 14 months.

For comparison, three controls were selected for each "case." They were matched from the entire group of patients seen at the Cooper Clinic for whom complete data were available, who were without CHD at any examination and were not known to have died or to have developed heart disease since their last visit. Matching was based on age, year of examination, and on probability of developing CHD in a 2-year period. This information was calculated using formulae derived from the Framingham study.[23, 24]

The "risk function," from which the Framingham formulae were derived, is a particularly useful description. It relates cholesterol, blood pressure, smoking, glucose intolerance, LVH, and age to the probability (risk) of developing CHD or particular manifestations of CHD. In addition to its use as a concise summarization of past observations, the risk function can be used predictively. Based on values of the characteristics mentioned above, probability of disease in an individual, or more meaningfully, in a group of individuals, can be calculated.

Two different risk functions were used: for the 21 patients who experienced MI or CHD death, or had coronary by-pass surgery without previous symptoms of angina pectoris (AP), the risk of CHD *other than AP* was calculated. For the remainder who reported AP before by-pass surgery, risk of CHD *including AP* was used. Controls were required to have a probability within ±10% for the same clinical disease endpoint as the "case," i.e., the same formula was applied to calculate risk for the control as for the case to be matched.

Formulae used were:

$$P = [1 + \exp (9.69136 - 0.04592 \times age - 0.00571 \times cholesterol - 0.01035 \times SBP - 0.02102 \times cigarettes/day - 0.57015\ LVH1 - 0.62724 \times glucose\ intolerance)]^{-1} \times 1000$$

for the first group, and

$$P = (1 + 24.386803 - 0.506622 \times age + 0.003357 \times age \times age - 0.023038 \times cholesterol - 0.010494 \times SBP - 0.550991 \times cigarette\ habit - 0.883188 \times LVH2 - 0.510296 \times glucose\ intolerance + 0.000315 \times age \times cholesterol)^{-1} \times 1000$$

for the second group, where P = probability of developing CHD in two years, per thousand persons; age is measured in years; cholesterol in mg%; SBP in mmHg; cigarettes/day is number currently smoked; LVH1 = 0 for LVH absent, 1 for probable LVH, 2 for definite LVH; LVH2 = 0 for LVH absent or probable, 1 for definite LVH; glucose intolerance = 1 if glucose value $\geq$ 120 or diabetes reported, 0 otherwise; cigarette habit = 1 if cigarettes smoked currently, 0 otherwise.[24, 25]

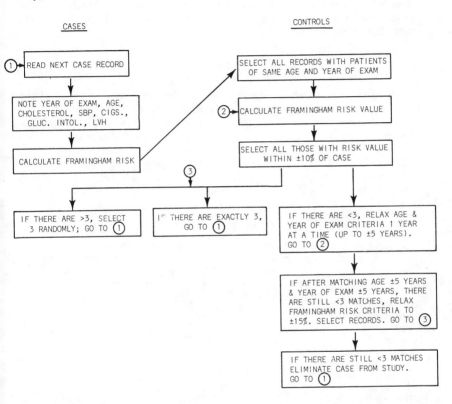

FIGURE 1. Flow chart for case-control match.

Exclusion criteria for cases and controls were the same as described for the Framingham incidence study,[25] i.e., those who had pre-existing CHD identified as definite AP, definite history of MI, definite MI by ECG, doubtful MI by ECG, or definite coronary insufficiency by ECG and history.

When comparison of risk yielded more than three persons in the healthy population for a particular "case," three were chosen randomly. If fewer than three were available, matching criteria were relaxed slightly, first by allowing age and year of examination to vary within one year and then, if necessary, to allow the risk for the control to be within $\pm 15\%$ of the risk calculated for the "case." A schematic flowchart of the matching process is displayed in FIGURE 1. Matching of cases with controls was accomplished for all but two potential study subjects. They had to be eliminated from the investigation because the only matching noncases that could be found had died of causes other than CHD, and/or had had pre-existing heart disease.

Statistical analysis consisted of calculations of means and standard deviations of the quantitative variables measured on the cases and controls by age group, disease classification, and total group. For qualitative variables, percentage in each category was computed. Hypothesis tests for differences in means and proportions were carried out. Use of univariate methods was consistent with the preliminary nature of this report of work in progress. Future analyses will consider age trends, interrelationships, adjustments, and other multivariate approaches.

Results

All cases were matched with at least one control within one year of their age; six cases had one or more controls whose age differed from theirs by 2 years, and one case had a control 3 years younger. All but two cases had controls examined within 2 years of their examination year. Eight controls were examined either three or four years apart from their matched case.

Comparison of cases and controls on Framingham risk, variables included in the calculation of Framingham risk, and some related variables are shown in TABLE 1. Age and risk agree to within 0.1 year (0.2%) and 0.3 (1.5%),

TABLE 1

COMPARISON OF CASES AND CONTROLS

	Cases ($n=27$)	Controls ($n=81$)
Mean Values		
Age * (yrs)	54.2	54.3
Height (in.)	68.7	69.8
Weight (lbs)	173.2	176.5
Body fat (%)	23.8	22.9
Cholesterol * mg%	254.4	234.1
Glucose mg%	105.1	113.7 †
Triglycerides mg%	146.3	152.7
Uric acid mg%	6.8	6.7
SBP * mmHg	133.9	133.7
DBP mmHg	87.7	85.1
Framingham risk (incidence/ 1000 in 2-year period)	19.7	19.4
Percent Having		
Cigarette habit *	15	25
Glucose intolerance * (glucose ≥ 120 or diagnosed diabetes)	22	37
Left ventricular hypertrophy *	0	0
Relatives with heart disease:		
Total	71	49
Aged < 50	15	11
Aged > 50	56	38

* Variables used in the calculation of Framingham risk.
† Case control difference significant, p > .05.

TABLE 2

CASE VERSUS CONTROL COMPARISON OF FITNESS VARIABLES, BY AGE

	Mean Treadmill Performance			
	Cases		Controls	
Age	*n*	Time (min)	*n*	Time (min)
39–49	8	15.6	24	14.7
50–59	10	11.3 *	30	14.6 *
60+	9	11.5	27	12.1
Total	27	12.6	81	13.8

	Exercise ECG			
	Cases		Controls	
Age	*n*	% Abnormal or Equivocal	*n*	% Abnormal or Equivocal
39–49	8	25.0	24	4.2
50–59	9	77.8 †	30	6.7 †
60+	9	33.3	27	40.7
Total	26	46.1	81	17.3

* Case and control differences significant with p <0.05.
† Case and control differences significant with p $\ll 0.001$.

respectively. Among the variables used to calculate risk, a significant difference was found in cholesterol, with mean for cases being 20.3 mg% greater than for controls. Compensating for this was a difference favoring the controls of 10% in cigarette habit and 15% in glucose intolerance. Systolic blood pressure and presence of LVH showed no significant difference between the groups. Other variables thought to affect coronary incidence showed nonsignificant small differences, with uric acid and diastolic blood pressure being higher for cases and serum triglycerides higher for controls. The small difference shown in body height and weight and percent fat were found to be nonsignificant.

Having matched the cases and controls for the risk factors generally associated with CHD, a comparison of cardiorespiratory fitness and ECG status resulting from MTST can explore the question of whether there is an additional contribution to be made by them in the prediction of CHD incidence. TABLE 2 shows the differences of treadmill performance time and exercise ECG abnormalities in the cases and controls. Overall, the comparison implies that exercise ECG and physical fitness are additional predictors of coronary incidence, beyond that shown by use of the Framingham risk formula. The percentage with an abnormal or equivocal exercise ECG is 2½ times as great in the cases as in the controls. The differences between groups was 7-fold and 10-fold for those in the fourth and fifth decades of life, but was not significant for those over 60 years of age.

Similarly, while the difference in treadmill performance time for the entire group was not statistically significant, the difference for those between 50 and 59 years of age was significant at the 0.05 level. The differences in body weight and percent body fat of the two groups was insufficient to account for the observed difference in treadmill time.

Another outcome of this study was the observation that the two groups differed in the proportion reporting heart attacks in first-degree relatives; 70% of cases and 49% of controls report one or more such events. In both groups, approximately one-fifth of the heart disease occurred in relatives less than 50 years old.

The important differences observed between cases and controls in exercise ECG abnormalities occurred in the 50–59-year-old age group, and a much smaller difference was observed in those over 60. The difficulty of predicting CHD in the older age groups is common in other studies.

Again in treadmill performance time, the difference between groups is mainly attributable to those 50–59 years of age. A more detailed analysis of this measure of endurance capacity was carried out. Although controls had been chosen without regard to whether they had been seen at the Cooper Clinic any particular number of times (each patient visit was equally likely to be

TABLE 3

TREADMILL PERFORMANCE TIME: COMPARISON OF CASES WITH CONTROLS
WHO HAD MADE FOLLOW-UP VISITS

Age	Cases		Controls	
	n	Time (min)	n	Time (min)
39–49	5	16.6	11	15.0
50–59	8	10.1 *	13	15.9 *
60+	7	11.6	13	13.7
Total	20	12.2 †	37	14.9 †

* Case and control differences significant with p <0.01.
† Case and control differences significant with p <0.05.

selected for the control, except that no patient could be used more than once), the possible variation in follow-up resulting from this method was seen as a shortcoming. Of all the 81 controls selected, 36 had been seen only once in the Clinic, with the remaining 45 having had between two and sixteen visits. The mean follow-up time for them was 22 months. It was hoped that a group more comparable to the cases would result using only those controls who had been seen at least once again after the examination used for the study. A new analysis was carried out, comparing 20 cases to 37 controls, with a weighting scheme employed for balancing the groups. This analysis is reported in TABLE 3. Differences between cases and controls have increased for the entire group and for each age group, except for those under 50.

The possibility that those patients who return to the Clinic are those who are making a greater effort at improvement of endurance capacity was considered. Actually, of the 37 utilized in the study, 11 had decreased treadmill performance time at a subsequent visit, 23 showed an increase, with the remainder either staying the same or omitting the test for endurance at their visit.

Discussion

The design for the present study was intended to investigate whether physical fitness and exercise ECG abnormalities influence prediction of CHD independently of the risk factors of blood pressure, cholesterol, glucose, smoking, LVH, and age, already evaluated in many other studies. The preliminary findings in this report, based on a small number of cases and using a matched design, demonstrate that an independent effect of treadmill performance time and stress ECG abnormalities does exist.

Separately, each of the risk factor variables has proved predictive of coronary incidence. Correlations between them have confounded the determination of relative contribution.

A number of studies have reported the diagnostic importance of abnormal exercise ECG.[26-30] Recent advances have continued to increase the sensitivity and specificity of this tool.[31-33] Treadmill testing used to evaluate ST segment responses, now has itself been shown to provide another independent prognostic measure.[9] Endurance performance capacity, estimated by number of minutes before patients were forced to stop exercise, related closely to presence and extent of anatomic coronary artery disease and with severity of ventricular dysfunction. Furthermore, even after controlling for these factors, and for ST segment response, endurance performance was strongly associated with survival for patients with coronary artery disease.

Various investigations have correlated one or more of the other risk factors with measures of fitness and physical activity.[34-39] The more active generally have lower values of cholesterol and blood pressure and tend to smoke less. In the Cooper study,[10] levels of fitness were related to most of the risk factors identified by the American Heart Association. Differences of risk factor values between high and low fitness groups were significant with $p \leq 0.05$.

In the Framingham study,[10] physical activity was evaluated by self-reported, 24-hour history of usual activity. In spite of the possible inaccuracies in this assessment, analysis confirmed the impression that physical activity contributed to risk of CHD independently of other factors, but the relationship was considered to be uncertain. However, the correlations of physical activity index with blood pressure and cholesterol were near zero, and this perhaps reflects on the inadequacy of the index used.

Many other studies have examined the relationship between physical activity and CHD. Some have failed to show any association; others have demonstrated beneficial effects but have been criticized for various shortcomings.[41-44] Most comments relate to problems related to measurement of physical activity, to diagnosis of disease and/or cause of death, to bias in population selection, to inattention to other possibly correlated risk factors and to confounding factors such as socioeconomic and environmental differences.

This study attempts to consider most of the deficiencies in the other studies. Physical fitness was quantified precisely, and definite endpoints of CHD were used. Comparisons were made within a homogeneous population and all known risk factors were considered concurrently.

Summary

The question of whether there is some effect of status of cardiorespiratory fitness and exercise ECG abnormalities on occurrence of CHD other than their effect on the risk factors of serum cholesterol, blood pressure, glucose, and smoking seems to have been answered in the affirmative by this study. The relative prognostic importance of the measures considered here, the role of exercise, and the interrelationships between fitness, exercise, other risk factors, and CHD provide many interesting hypotheses for continued study.

A future investigation will involve a large prospective study in which the risk function to be derived would include stress ECG and treadmill performance as predictor variables. The retrospective approach reported in this paper had certain limitations. It did, however, permit demonstration of new results because, essentially for the first time, all of the important risk factors are measured in the study population and can be evaluated simultaneously.

References

1. Monthly Vital Statistics Report. 1976. **24**(13): 26.
2. Heart disease deaths drop below one million. New York Times. 1976. (September 2).
3. Heart Facts. 1972. American Heart Association. New York, N.Y.
4. HEYDEN, S. 1969. Epidemiology. *In* Atherosclerosis. F. G. Schettle & G. S. Boyd, Eds. : 169–329. Elsevier Publishing Co. Amsterdam, The Netherlands.
5. DAWBER, T. R. 1973. Risk factors in young adults: The lessons from epidemiologic studies of cardiovascular disease: Framingham, Tecumseh, and Evans County. J. Amer. Coll. Health Assoc. **22**: 84–95.
6. KANNELL, W. 1966. The Framingham Heart Study: Habits and Coronary Heart Disease, Public Health Service Publication No. 1515. U.S. Government Printing Office.
7. KANNEL, W. B., D. McGEE & T. GORDON. 1976. A general cardiovascular risk profile: The Framingham Study. Am. J. Cardiol. **38**: 46–51.
8. ELLESTAD, M. H. 1975. Stress Testing: Principles and practice. F. A. Davis. Philedelphia, Pa.
9. MARGOLIS, J. R., J. A. KISSLO, R. H. PETER, Y. KONG, V. S. BEHAR, R. ROSATI & A. G. WALLACE. 1976. Treadmill exercise capacity: its diagnostic, prognostic, and therapeutic implications in the context of coronary artery disease. Presentation at North Carolina Heart Association, May 27.
10. COOPER, K. H., M. L. POLLOCK, R. P. MARTIN, S. R. WHITE, A. C. LINNERUD & A. Jackson. 1976. Physical fitness levels vs. selected coronary risk factors: a cross-sectional study. J. Amer. Med. Assoc. **236**(2): 166–169.
11. HUANG, T. C., C. P. CHEN, V. WEFLER, *et al.* 1961. A stable reagent for the Liebermann-Burchard reaction: Application to rapid serum cholesterol determination. Anal. Chem. **33**: 1405–1407.
12. BITTNER, D. L. & M. L. McCLEARY. 1963. Cupric phenantaroline chelate in the determination of monosaccharides in whole blood. Amer. J. Clin. Pathol. **40**: 423–424.
13. MUSSER, A. W. & C. ORTIGOZA. 1966. Automated determination of uric acid by the hydroxylamine method. Tech. Bull. Regist. Med. Technol. **36**: 21–25.
14. KESSLER, G. & H. LEDERER. 1966. Fluorometric measurement of triglycerides. *In* Automation in Analytical Chemistry, Technicon Symposia, 1965. L. T. Skeggs, Ed. : 341. Mediad, Inc. New York, N.Y.
15. ALLEN, T. H. 1963. Measurement of human body fat: A quantitative method suited for use by aviation medical officers. Aerosp. Med. **34**: 907–909.
16. BROŽEK, J., F. GRANDE, J. ANDERSON, *et al.* 1963. Densitometric analysis of body composition: Revision of some quantitative assumptions. Ann. N.Y. Acad. Sci. **110**: 113–140.
17. GOLDMAN, H. I., & M. R. BECKLAKE. 1959. Respiratory function tests: Normal

values at median altitudes and the prediction of normal results. Am. Rev. Tuber. Resp. Dis. **79:** 457–467.

18. COOPER, K. H. 1970. Guidelines in the management of the exercising patient. J. Amer. Med. Assoc. **211:** 1663–1667.

19. BALKE, B. & R. WARE. 1959. An experimental study of physical fitness of Air Force personnel. U.S. Armed Forces Med. J. **10:** 675–688.

20. Exercise Testing and Training of Apparently Healthy Individuals: A Handbook for Physicians. 1972. American Heart Association. New York, N.Y.

21. ROBINSON, S. 1938. Experimental studies of physical fitness in relation to age. Arbeitsphysiol. **10:** 251–323.

22. ROMHILT, D. W. & E. H. ESTES, JR. 1968. A point score system for the ECG diagnosis of left ventricular hypertrophy. Amer. Heart J. **75:** 752–758.

23. GORON, T. 1976. Personal communication.

24. KANNEL, W. B. & T. GORDON, Eds. 1974. The Framingham Study: An Epidemiological Investigation of Cardiovascular Disease. Section 27. U.S. Government Printing Office. Washington, D.C.

25. KANNEL, W. B. & T. GORDON, Eds. 1974. The Framingham Study: An Epidemiological Investigation of Cardiovascular Disease. Section 30. U.S. Government Printing Office. Washington, D.C.

26. DOYLE, J. T. & S. KINCH. 1970. The prognosis of an abnormal electrocardiographic stress test. Circulation **41:** 545–553.

27. SHEFFIELD, L. T., D. ROITMAN & T. REEVES. 1969. Submaximal exercise testing. J. S. C. Med. Assoc. **65:** 18–25.

28. HARRISON, T. R. & T. J. REEVES. 1968. Principles and Problems of Ischemic Heart Disease. Year Book Medical Publishers. Chicago, Ill.

29. BLACKBURN, H., H. L. TAYLOR, C. L. VASQUEZ & T. C. PUCHNER. 1966. The electrocardiogram during exercise: Findings in bipolar chest leads of 1,449 midle-aged men, at moderate work levels. Circulation. **34:** 1034–1043.

30. SHEFFIELD, L. T., J. H. HOLT & T. J. REEVES. 1965. Exercise graded by heart rate in electrocardiographic testing for angina pectoris. Circulation **32:** 662.

31. ELLESTAD, M. H. 1976. Can stress testing predict the severity of coronary disease? Chest **69:** 708–710.

32. GOLDMAN, S., S. TSELOS & K. COHN. 1976. Marked depth of ST-segment depression during treadmill exercise testing. Chest **69:** 729–733.

33. MCCONAHAY, D. R., B. MCCALLISTER & R. SMITH. 1971. Postexercise electrocardiography: Correlations with coronary arteriography and left ventricular hemodynamics. Amer. J. Cardiol. **28:** 1–9.

34. MORRIS, J. N., J. HEADY & P. RAFFLE. 1956. Physique of London busmen. Lancet **ii:** 569–570.

35. KAGAN, A., D. PATTISON & M. GARDNER. 1966. Incidence and prediction of ischaemic heart disease in London busmen. Lancet **ii:** 553.

36. MANN, G .V., H. GARRETT, A. FARHI, H. MURRAY & F. BILLINGS. 1969. Exercise to prevent coronary heart disease. An experimental study of the effects of training on risk factors for coronary disease in man. Amer. J. Med. **46:** 12–27.

37. MCDONOUGH, J. R., C. HAMES, S. STULB & G. GARRISON. 1965. Coronary heart disease among negroes and white in Evans County, Georgia. J. Chronic Dis. **18:** 443.

38. ROSENMAN, R. H. 1970. The influence of different exercise patterns on the incidence of coronary heart disease in the western collaborative group study. *In* Medicine and Sport. D. Brunner & E. Jokl, Eds. Vol. **4:** 267–273. S. Karger. White Plains, N.Y.

39. HICKEY, N., R. MULCAHY, G. BOURKE, I. GRAHAM & K. WILSON-DAVIS. 1975. Study of coronary risk factors related to physical activity in 15,171 men. Br. Med. J. **iii:** 507-509.

40. KANNEL, W. B., T. GORDON, P. SORLIE & P. MCNAMARA. 1971. Physical activity and coronary vulnerability: The Framingham Study. Cardio. Dig. (Jun) : 28–40.

41. FROELICHER, V. F. & A. OBERMAN. 1972. Analysis of epidemiologic studies of physical inactivity as risk factor for coronary artery disease. Prog. Cardiovasc. Dis. 15(1): 41–65.
42. KEYS, A. 1970. Physical activity and the epidemiology of coronary heart disease. In Medicine and Sport. D. Brunner & E. Jokl, Eds. Vol. 4: 250–266. S. Karger. White Plains, N.Y.
43. FOX, S. M. & J. SKINNER. 1964. Physical activity and cardiovascular health. Amer. J. Cardiol. 14: 731–746.
44. FOX, S. M., J. NAUGHTON & W. HASKELL. 1971. Physical activity and the prevention of coronary heart disease. Ann. Clin. Res. 3: 404–432.

ENDURANCE SPORTS, LONGEVITY, AND HEALTH

Martti J. Karvonen

Headquarters of the Defence Forces
Helsinki, Finland

The modern sports movement has its origin among the Anglo-Saxon nations. The sports practiced traditionally among the British upper class were direct descendants of the medieval education of the gentry in the arts of battle and chivalry. These obviously had been considered favorable for survival, at least when they emerged. As the industrial revolution moulded the society, the sports of the aristocracy met the traditional sports and games of the farm village. Classic scholars added something of the Greek heritage of Olympia. The spirit of the nineteenth century was utilitarian: Even sport had to serve some useful purpose. The enthusiasts claimed that sport was useful for health and longevity. Generations of children and youth have now been educated in this belief.

Sports became an integral part of student life early in the British and American universities. Their student populations also afforded an opportunity for follow-up studies during a period when general population registers were rather incomplete. The first follow-up study of longevity was published in 1873;[1] its subjects were oarsmen. College oarsmen have then for hundred years remained a favorite subject of studies of longevity.[2-4] The outcome of these studies has been favorable for rowing: The oarsmen have lived longer than their nonrowing controls.

Rooks[5] studied the longevity of British student athletes with special attention to the type of sport practiced. Runners tended to reach a higher age than throwers, independently of the distance run: 57% of the sprinters, 56% of the long distance runners and only 34% of the hammer throwers and shot-putters attained the age of 70 years.

Several extensive studies have shown that on an average the student athlete does not gain or lose much in longevity.[3, 6-8] As the student leaves the university, he often also stops practicing athletics. Life-long addicts to athletics, if such people exist, should indeed be expected to manifest any effects of sports on longevity more clearly than college athletes do.

Marathon running comes close to being a life-long sport. At the Olympic Games of 1952 in Helsinki, the youngest participant of the marathon race was 21 years, the oldest 44 years old; the median age was 37 years.[9] Among the track and field events, the marathon regularly shows the widest age range of the participants. With advancing age, a runner may proceed from shorter to longer distances. The famous Finnish runner Paavo Nurmi ran his best time for 800 meters at the age of 26, but his best marathon when he was 35 years old.

Another sport to stay with the man for years is cross-country skiing. In order to attain international success, a cross-country skier has to train some 7 years, he may stay in the international class for another 7 years, and thereafter he still is able to compete with success in national events for perhaps 7 years.

Long-distance running and skiing are popular sports in Finland. Skiing competitions have been organized longer, and thus data for a longevity study cover a longer period. From the year 1889, the Oulu race was the most important annual skiing event. It was run on a level course, on the sea ice. In the 1920s and 30s, cross-country skiing became popular, and the Oulu races vanished in 1930. The present-day Finns are a skiing nation: up to 100,000 Finns yearly take part in organized day-long ski tours.

For a study of longevity, a group of skiers was compiled from the best participants of the Oulu races of 1889–1930, and other champion skiers of the same era were added. The mortality of the series was followed until 1967.[10] The group of skiers comprised 396 men born from 1845 to 1910. Of them 57 were still living, 325 had died, and 14 had disappeared in wars or emigrated. The median year of birth was 1882 and that of death 1947.

The skiers were compared to the general male population, 15 years or older, by using a life-table analysis. Their median length of life was 73.0 years. The longevity of the reference population was 4.3 years shorter, 68.7 years. Over the period of the study, from 1889 to 1967, the longevity of the reference population varied. In 1956–60, which period corresponds to the third quartile of the years of death among the skiers, the median age at death of the reference population had risen to 70.2 years, which still was 2.8 years less than the longevity of the skiers.

It is by no means unique to find subgroups who live longer than the general population. The U.S. major league baseball players of the years 1876 to 1973 had a total mortality of only 72% of that of U.S. white males of similar age.[11] As a sport, baseball certainly is very different from cross-country skiing. On the other hand, it is of interest that an occupation requiring unusually heavy work, such as lumbering, is not similarly associated with long life expectancy.[12] Heavy physical activity for leisure and for living, respectively, seem to have quite different relations to health.

Former endurance athletes, both long-distance runners and cross-country skiers, may still in old age differ in many health-related parameters from a nonathletic reference population. In a study of 61 former champions of whom nine had won a Gold Medal in the Olympic Games, the athletes, whose mean age was 56 years, had significantly lower blood pressure (137/87 mmHg) than their controls (147/92 mmHg). The ex-athletes also smoked less and exercised more than their nonathletic controls, but there was no difference in the serum cholesterol. Electrocardiographic changes due to coronary heart disease (CHD) had roughly the same prevalence in both groups, but the nonathletic controls tended to report more often symptoms of CHD.[13] The athletes also had larger lung volumes and a greater pulmonary diffusing capacity than the controls.[14]

Within a nation, differences in longevity may be revealed by stratification according to sex, ethnic origin, social class, religion, occupation, and other criteria. The choice of a reference population for any subgroup is more or less arbitrary. To ascribe an observed difference in longevity to this or that particular causative factor is always problematic.

As an example, let us examine the longevity of the medical profession. Up to 1945, the age-standardized mortality of the Finnish physicians had been the same as that of the general male population. From the latter half of the 1940s onwards, the doctors have progressively gained in longevity, as compared with their patients, and during the latter half of the 1960s their mortality reached only 72% of the reference value.[15] Doctors in Britain and in the United States also have smaller mortality than the general population does, but the published figures show a smaller difference than in Finland.

Why do the Finnish physicians today live so much longer than their patients? An obvious reason is that many doctors have stopped smoking. However, some Finnish doctors have also acquired the habit of jogging. Every year, approximately 300 doctors take part in a special 10,000 meters competition in the Helsinki Olympic Stadium. They are approximately 5% of the total medical profession. These 5% obviously are "the top of the iceberg;" many more doctors jog outside the Stadium walls.

In trying to understand the complexities of human behavior and their effects on health, conclusions are seldom self-evident. Endurance sports appear to be associated with long life, while physically heavy occupations may show the opposite. Endurance training changes several physiological parameters, some of them in a direction opposite to that due to aging. Training also makes one feel better and less sensitive to pains and aches. However, it still is no panacea against atherosclerotic disease. In judging the merits of endurance sports for leisure, their psychological effects may be even more important than their physical implications.

REFERENCES

1. MORGAN, J. E. 1873. University Oars 20: 300, cited by Hartley and Llewellyn, Reference 3.
2. KNOLL, W. 1938. Welches Lebensalter erreichen die Ruderer von "Oxford-Cambridge". Med. Klin. 34: 464–466.
3. HARTLEY, P. H.-S. & G. F. LLEWELLYN. 1939. The longevity of oarsmen. A study of those who rowed in the Oxford and Cambridge boat race from 1829 to 1928. Brit. Med. J. i: 657–662.
4. PROUT, C. 1972. Life expectancy of college oarsmen. J. Amer. Med. Assoc. 220: 1709–1711.
5. ROOK, A. 1954. An investigation into the longevity of Cambridge sportsmen. Brit. Med. J. i: 773–777.
6. MONTOYE, H. J., W. D. VAN HUSS, H. OLSON, A. HUDEC & E. MAHONEY. 1956. Study of longevity and morbidity of college athletes. J. Amer. Assoc. 162: 1132–1134.
7. MONTOYE, H. J., W. D. VAN HUSS, H .W. OLSON, W. R. PIERSON & A. J. HUDEC. 1957. The Longevity and Morbidity of College Athletes. Michigan State University Press. Ann Arbor, Mich.
8. POLEDNAK, A. P. & A. DAMON. 1970. College athletics, longevity and cause of death. Hum. Biol. 42: 28–46.
9. JOKL, E., M. J. KARVONEN, J. KIHLBERG, A. KOSKELA & L. NORO. 1956. Sports in the Cultural Pattern of the World. A Study of the 1952 Olympic Games at Helsinki. Institute of Occupational Health, Helsinki.
10. KARVONEN, M. J., H. KLEMOLA, J. VIRKAJÄRVI & A. KEKKONEN. 1974. Longevity of endurance skiers. Med. Sci. Sports 6: 49–51.
11. Longevity of major league baseball players. 1975. Statistical Bulletin, Metropolitan Life Insurance Co. April 2–4.
12. PUNSAR, S. & M. J. KARVONEN. 1976. Physical activity and coronary heart disease in populations from East and West Finland. Adv. Cardiol. 18: 196–207.
13. PYÖRÄLÄ, K., M. J. KARVONEN, P. TASKINEN, J. TAKKUNEN, H. KYRÖNSEPPÄ & P. PELTOKALLIO. 1967. Cardiovascular studies on former endurance athletes. Amer. J. Cardiol. 20: 191–205.
14. PYÖRÄLÄ, K., A. O. HEINONEN & M. J. KARVONEN. 1968. Pulmonary function in former endurance athletes. Acta Med. Scand. 183: 263–273.
15. HEINONEN, P. K., K. FRIMAN, K.-O. SÖDERSTRÖM & J. PIETILÄ. 1976. Mieslääkärien kuolleisuus Suomessa vuosina 1956–70. Suom. Lääk. L. 31: 850–854.

THE EFFECTS OF CONTINUED TRAINING ON THE
AGING PROCESS

Terence Kavanagh

Toronto Rehabilitation Centre
Toronto, Ontario
M4G 1R7 Canada

Roy J. Shephard

Department of Preventive Medicine and Biostatistics
University of Toronto
Toronto, Ontario, Canada

Several previous reports [1-6] have described the physiological characteristics of small samples of middle-aged and elderly athletes. At least one report [1] has claimed that aerobic power ages more slowly in the continuing athlete than in the general population, although this view seems based mainly on an unusually rapid deterioration of the control sample, the annual loss of maximum oxygen intake among the athletes being much as seen in other large cross-sectional surveys of average citizens. [7, 8]

Until recently, only a small proportion of athletes have continued to participate in international competitions after the age of 40 years. Those tested in middle and later life have thus been a highly selected subsample of the original athletic population, including varying proportions of star competitors and subjects no longer engaged in rigorous training. The development of age-specific contests has greatly increased the popularity of track and field events for elderly competitors, to the point where cross-sectional data on such subjects can be used to explore the probable response of the average person to a lengthy period of hard physical training.

The hosting of the World Masters' Championships in Toronto in August, 1975 provided us with the opportunity to question and examine a substantial number of middle-aged and elderly track competitors. The results obtained form the basis of the present report.

METHODS

Subject Selection and Experimental Plan

A total of 1,308 men and 77 women competed in the 1975 World Masters' Championships in Toronto. All participants were invited to complete a questionnaire relating to training habits, injuries, and the use of dietary supplements, and to attend a clinic for assessment of body composition, performance of a submaximal bicycle ergometer test with electrocardiogram, and measurement of heart volume by thoracic radiography.

The complete test battery was carried out by 128 men (9.8% of male participants) and 7 women (9.1% of female participants). There was some bias in sampling. Although contestants came from many parts of the world, the majority of those tested were from English-speaking nations (the United Kingdom, Australia, and New Zealand, with smaller numbers from Canada and the U.S.). This reflects our more ready communication with the Anglo-phone contestants. The preponderance of recruits from the United Kingdom, Australia, and New Zealand rather than Canada and the U.S. may imply that facilities for exercise testing are less readily available to athletes from countries outside of North America; certainly, the overseas competitors seemed more intrigued by the tests than were their sophisticated North American counter-parts.

The age distribution of the sample is illustrated in TABLE 1. Irrespective of event, the typical competitor was aged about 50 years, and had begun serious competitive training about 20 years earlier. Twenty-seven men were partici-pants in events of less than 400 meters distance (hereafter described as sprint-ers); their average age was 51.3 ± 11.4 years, with 26.5 ± 15.3 years of experi-

TABLE 1

AGE, HEIGHT, AND WEIGHT OF MASTERS' ATHLETES RELATIVE TO A RANDOMLY SELECTED SAMPLE OF CANADIAN ADULTS [7] (MEAN±SD)

Class	n	Age (yr)	World Masters Sample		Saskatoon Sample [7]	
			Height (cm)	Weight (kg)	Height (cm)	Weight (kg)
Male competitors						
Sub-Masters	8	34.8±3.7	175.2±6.9	69.9±9.6	176.7±5.5	80.0±10.9
1 (40–50 yr)	64	44.4±1.3	174.7±6.4	69.4±8.3	176.2±5.9	81.7±10.4
2 (50–60 yr)	34	54.7±1.4	172.6±6.9	66.0±7.1	173.1±6.1	77.1±9.4
3 (60–70 yr)	18	63.6±1.3	172.3±6.3	68.7±11.6	171.5±7.3	77.4±11.5
4 (70+ yr)	4	81.5±8.4	165.3±8.9	61.0±11.7	—	—
Female com-petitors	7	43.1±12.4	164.9±8.1	57.1±6.1	161.8±6.1	62.0±8.6

ence. Nineteen were entered in middle-distance events (800–3000 meters); their average age was 49.6 ± 8.2 years, with 19.5 ± 13.5 years of experience. Seventy-seven men were competing in long distance events (5000 meters and more); their average age was 50.7 ± 10.4 years, with 18.9 ± 13.3 years of experience. The sample was completed by five engaged in other field events and seven women.

The standing of the competitors was assessed by expressing their perfor-mance as a percentage of the current age- and distance-specific world record. The majority of those tested were average rather than outstanding competitors (TABLE 2), achieving between 80% and 90% of record performances; older competitors over short and medium distances had even poorer results (60%–80% of world records for their age).

Laboratory Techniques

Standing height, body weight, and the thickness of three skinfolds (triceps, subscapular, and suprailiac) were determined by standard anthropometric techniques.[9] Body fat percentages were determined using the tables of Durnin & Rahaman.[10]

A standard three-stage progressive bicycle ergometer test was performed on a Monark bicycle ergometer. The subjects exercised for 3 minutes at each of three increasing work loads, the final intensity of effort being adjusted to develop a heart rate equivalent to 75% of the individual's anticipated aerobic power.[11] The electrocardiogram was recorded from standard chest leads (CM-5),[8] and the maximum oxygen intake (aerobic power) was predicted from the work scale of the Åstrand nomogram.[12] A standard clinical sphygmomanometer cuff was used to measure the systemic blood pressures. Readings were taken in

TABLE 2

PERFORMANCE OF MALE CONTESTANTS RELATIVE TO CURRENT WORLD RECORD SPEED
FOR THEIR AGE AND DISTANCE
MEAN PERCENT ± SD

Age (yr)	Sprint	Middle Distance	Long Distance
<40	88.8±5.1	—	86.1±10.3
40–50	86.4±5.7	88.3±7.2	82.8±8.1
50–60	88.2±4.6	87.3±6.6	82.9±10.0
60–70	76.6±3.9	73.1±7.1	81.1±6.7
70–90	63.8±3.1	—	—

the sitting position, immediately prior to exercise and during the final 30 seconds at each work load.

The heart volume was determined from standard PA and lateral chest films, using the technique of Reindell et al.[13]

RESULTS

Training Patterns

The total mileage covered per week was substantial (TABLE 3); it was apparently well sustained through the sixth decade, decreasing in older competitors. The older age groups also relied more upon long slow distance work and less upon fast and interval training. The female competitors used more fast training, and covered a lower weekly mileage than men of the same age. Fast and interval type training were naturally more popular with the sprinters, while the distance men concentrated on long slow distance work (TABLE 4).

TABLE 3

TRAINING DISTANCE (MILEAGE/WK) AND FORMAT OF TRAINING
MEAN ± SD

| Age (yrs) | Training Pattern | | | |
	Mileage (per week)	Percent Fast	Percent Slow	Percent Interval
Male competitors				
< 40	27.6±9.1	25.0±22.6	30.0±24.5	45.0±46.4
40–50	42.0±25.5	23.5±21.1	57.7±28.6	18.2±15.8
50–60	38.4±17.3	19.0±23.3	62.8±30.5	18.1±20.6
60–70	26.6±14.8	15.6±22.9	63.3±32.3	21.0±26.3
Female competitors	23.3±16.3	43.4±34.8	42.0±40.8	14.6±16.0

Dietary Supplements

Many of the athletes were taking dietary supplements (TABLE 5), this practice being particularly common among those enrolled for middle and long distance events. The items taken included vitamin C, vitamin B mixtures, wheat germ oil, yoghurt, vitamin E, and yeast extract. A number, particularly among the English contestants, were also keeping to a vegetarian diet.

Injuries

A very large proportion of the contestants had suffered an injury sufficient to interrupt training during the previous year; 39.6% of those injured had experienced at least one week of disability, a further 26.7% had been incapacitated for 1–4 weeks, and 33.7% had been affected for more than 4 weeks. Injuries were sustained by contestants in all three categories (sprinters, 26.1%, middle distance runners, 21.0%, and long distance runners, 52.9%) with the greater number being in the long distance runners.

Those taking dietary supplements, with 63.1% injuries, fared somewhat worse than those who did not supplement their diet (48.8% injuries). Of the first group, 51 were taking megadoses of vitamin C (more than 500 mg/day);

TABLE 4

TRAINING PATTERN OF MALE CONTESTANTS CLASSIFIED BY EVENT
MEAN ± SD

| Event | Training Pattern | | | |
	Mileage (per week)	Percent Fast	Percent Slow	Percent Interval
Sprint	16.8±9.5	25.2±27.6	47.6±32.5	27.2±25.1
Middle distance	32.7±15.9	19.1±13.5	52.3±27.2	28.5±22.8
Long distance	47.1±21.3	19.8±21.8	64.9±28.1	15.2±19.7

TABLE 5

THE USE OF DIETARY SUPPLEMENTS BY MALE COMPETITORS IN TRACK EVENTS

Event	Yes	No	No Response
Sprint	6	15	6
Medium distance	10	5	4
Long distance	41	15	21

their injury experience (64%) was slightly higher than those subjects who were taking no supplements (48.8%).

Body Build

The average standing height of the sample was unremarkable (TABLE 1). Relative to a random sample of the general population,[7] the athletes perhaps lost height a little more slowly up to the age of 65 years, but there was a marked decrease of stature in the oldest category of participant. The female competitors were slightly taller than their age-matched contemporaries from the general population.

The men were 10–12 kg lighter than average Canadians of the same age (TABLE 1). However, in the women, the weight disparity was smaller (about 5 kg). Relative to modified actuarial standards,[14] the athletes did not develop the excess weight seen in normal middle-aged sedentary individuals.[8] The estimated percentage of body fat (TABLE 6) was greater than in young track athletes,[15] but remained relatively constant over the period of observation; figures for both men and women were substantially lower than for the general population of the same age.[15]

In contrast to the situation in the general population,[16] lean mass was well preserved to the age of 65 years, although there was some decrease in the oldest age category.

TABLE 6

BODY COMPOSITION AND AGE DATA FOR MASTERS' ATHLETES

Age (yr)	Excess Weight (kg)	Percent Fat	Lean Mass (kg)	Lean Mass (kg/cm height)
Male competitors				
<40	−0.3±6.6	13.9±2.6	59.7±7.6	0.339±0.033
40–50	0.7±5.3	14.5±3.6	59.1±5.8	0.339±0.028
50–60	−1.3±6.2	14.4±4.3	56.5±5.0	0.327±0.023
60–70	+1.3±8.8	14.4±4.0	58.5±7.6	0.339±0.036
70–90	−5.7±3.1	11.1±5.1	53.9±8.2	0.325±0.032
Female competitors	−1.3±3.3	22.8±4.8	44.3±7.2	0.268±0.033

When the subjects were classified by event (TABLE 7), the sprinters were found to be relatively heavier than the distance competitors. Although the sprint performers carried a slightly greater percentage of body fat than the distance men, the major part of this additional mass was attributable to lean tissue. As in samples of younger athletes,[15] the middle distance men tended to be taller than either the sprinters or the long distance performers.

Cardiorespiratory Variables

Resting systemic blood pressures (TABLE 8) were slightly lower than the normal values cited by Master et al.,[17] the advantage amounting to 3–15 mmHg (average 9 mmHg) for systolic pressure, and −1 to +7 mmHg (average 4 mmHg) for diastolic pressure.

The heart rates attained during exercise (TABLE 8) were well up to the required 75% loadings, and the work loads sustained at these heart rates were

TABLE 7

BODY BUILD AND COMPOSITION OF MALE COMPETITORS CLASSIFIED BY EVENT
(MEAN ± SD)

Event	Height (cm)	Weight (kg)	Excess Weight (kg)	Percent Fat	Lean Mass (kg)	Lean Mass (kg/cm height)
Sprint	173.4±6.9	73.0±11.2	+4.8±9.3	15.3±4.3	61.5±7.9	0.354±0.027
Middle distance	175.3±6.4	68.2±6.6	−1.2±5.5	13.4±2.3	59.0±4.9	0.336±0.024
Long distance	173.0±6.9	66.3±7.7	−2.3±7.7	13.9±3.9	56.8±5.6	0.329±0.025

far larger than would have been tolerated by the general population of the same age. Nevertheless, the exercise blood pressures were approximately the same as in sedentary individuals exercising at the same relative work loads. Predicted maximum oxygen intakes were substantially larger than in average Torontonians,[8] the discrepancy increasing from 22.5% in the women and 25.5% in the youngest men tested to 55.2% in the 60–70-year-old athletes. Maximum oxygen intakes were no greater in those competitors who were taking dietary supplements than in those who were not.

Heart volumes were in general larger than would have been anticipated in sedentary adults, 12 of the 135 contestants having values of over 14 ml/kg. Furthermore, group averages were not only maintained but even increased as the contestants became older.

Classifying the cardiorespiratory data by event (TABLE 9), the middle distance and long distance men developed a higher work load for a given heart rate than did the sprinters. As might have been anticipated, many of the sprinters had no more than an average aerobic power, high values being concentrated among the middle and long distance competitors. However, exercise blood pressures at the target heart rates were comparable for all three classes of

TABLE 8

CARDIORESPIRATORY VARIABLES CLASSIFIED BY AGE (MEAN±SD)

| Age (yr) | Resting Blood Pressure | | Maximum Attained Effort | | | | | | | |
| | Syst. (mmHg) | Diast. (mmHg) | Heart Rate (min^{-1}) | Work Load (watts) | Blood Pressure | | Predicted $\dot{V}_{O_2}$ | | Heart Volume | |
					Syst. (mmHg)	Diast. (mmHg)	liter/min STPD	ml/kg·min STPD	ml	ml/kg
Male competitors										
<40	124±18	79±10	154±13	197±21	185±12	81±4	3.39±0.57	49.6±9.8	720±248	12.0±2.3
40–50	120±16	77±8	142±11	194±19	194±17	82±10	3.43±0.70	49.9±10.0	856±121	12.5±1.7
50–60	127±16	77±8	139±12	183±18	191±17	82±11	3.02±0.57	46.0±8.3	804±163	12.4±1.7
60–70	128±19	77±11	135±13	169±14	199±18	88±12	2.80±0.66	41.6±11.1	916±127	13.9±2.8
70–90	140±36 *	83±10	124±22	106±59	185±37	78±13	1.75±0.50	29.0±9.0	790±141	13.2±3.0
Female competitors										
	111±9	77±10	150±17	132±19	176±10	86±10	2.49±0.84	43.0±10.8	—	—

*Two of the four subjects in this category were mildly hypertensive, with blood pressures of 180/90 and 160/90 mmHg, respectively.

TABLE 9

CARDIORESPIRATORY VARIABLES FOR MALE CONTESTANTS CLASSIFIED BY EVENT (MEAN±SD)

| Event | Maximum Attained Effort | | Blood Pressure | | Predicted Aerobic Power (ml/kg·min STPD) | Heart Volume | |
	Heart Rate (min⁻¹)	Work Load (watts)	Syst. (mmHg)	Diast. (mmHg)		(ml)	(ml/kg)
Sprint	144±17	171±34	195±17	88±11	38.8±8.8	881±130	12.5±1.9
Middle distance	139±15	196±21	198±18	82±10	51.8±12.0	841±183	12.2±2.0
Long distance	139±11	187±22	192±18	81±10	48.9±9.7	839±135	12.7±2.0

competitor, and there were no significant interclass differences of cardiac volume.

Electrocardiograms

Seventeen of the athletes showed occasional ventricular premature systoles at rest, but in all except two of the group these disappeared during the exercise test. Four athletes showed other minor abnormalities of the resting electrocardiogram; none were considered contraindications to endurance exercise.

The principal abnormality encountered during exercise was a substantial (>0.1 mV) depression of the ST segment. Fifteen of 135 exercise tracings showed this abnormality (TABLE 10), a somewhat smaller proportion of the

TABLE 10

ELECTROCARDIOGRAPHIC FINDINGS AT REST (SITTING) AND EXERCISING
AT A TARGET HEART RATE EQUAL TO 75% OF AEROBIC POWER

Age (yrs)	Abnormal Resting ECG	Abnormal Exercise Test	Average Depression in Abnormal Records (mV)	Average Depression of Total Group (mV)
Male competitors				
<40	0	2 (25%)	−0.11	−0.044±0.064
40–50	2	4 (6.3%)	−0.16	−0.034±0.052
50–60	1	6 (17.1%)	−0.17 *	−0.056±0.074
60–70	1	3 (16.7%)	−0.25	−0.079±0.091
70–90	0	0	0	−0.090±0.074
Female competitors	0	0	0	−0.084±0.052

* Excluding one case with known myocardial infarction, −0.40 mV.

sample than would have been anticipated in the general population of the same age (TABLE 11), despite the fact that the athletes were working at a much higher absolute work load.

DISCUSSION

Details of the present results can be compared with findings on three previous samples of elderly athletes. Saltin & Grimby [3] reported data for participants in the sports of orienteering and cross-country skiing, events that tax endurance even more than distance running.[15] Pollock [2] examined a population of American track athletes that apparently included some sprinters; all were said to be national champions for their age. Asano et al.[6] described a more average group of men who had been running at least one hour per day for 2 years or more, covering a weekly training distance of at least 50 km; some of this group were entrants in a Japanese veterans marathon race.

TABLE 11

REPORTED FREQUENCY OF ISCHEMIC ST CHANGES
IN THE EXERCISE ELECTROCARDIOGRAM OF NORMAL OLDER SUBJECTS *

Age Category (yrs)	Åstrand (men) %	Åstrand (women) %	Bruce (men) %	Lester (men) %	Goldberg et al. (men) %	Cumming (men) %	Cumming (women) %	Sidney & Shephard (men) %	Sidney & Shephard (women) %
<40	<10	—	2	—	0	2	—	—	—
40–50	15	20	9	4	7	7	—	—	—
51–60	20	30	25	2	27	17	—	—	—
61–65	35	55	46	18	—	30	37	29	36

* For sources of data, see Cumming;[18] the results of Sidney & Shephard are as yet unpublished.

TABLE 12

A COMPARISON OF BODY BUILD BETWEEN THE PRESENT SAMPLE
OF MALE MASTERS' COMPETITORS (M), AND OTHER SAMPLES
STUDIED BY POLLOCK [2] AND ASANO et al.[6]

Age (yr)	Height (cm)			Body Fat (%)		Lean Mass (kg/cm)		Weekly Mileage	
	M	Pollock	Asano	M	Pol-lock	M	Pol-lock	M	Pol-lock
<40	175.2	—	—	13.9	—	0.339	—	27.6	—
40–49	174.7	180.7	162.6	14.5	11.2	0.339	0.352	42.0	40.4
50–59	172.6	174.7	163.9	14.4	10.9	0.327	0.343	38.4	42.0
60–69	172.3	175.7	162.9	14.4	11.3	0.339	0.339	26.6	29.7
>70	165.3	175.6	156.6	11.1	13.6	0.325	0.329	—	20.0

Our subjects were covering a similar weekly mileage to the U.S. track athletes, but they were shorter, with a higher percentage of body fat, a smaller lean mass per unit height, and a lower aerobic power (TABLES 12 & 13). The discrepancy in aerobic power may arise in part from the comparison of predicted and directly measured maximum oxygen intake values. Furthermore, our sample included 27 sprint performers who had a relatively low average maximum oxygen intake (TABLE 9). Nevertheless, the greater percentage of body fat and the smaller lean mass of the Toronto sample of athletes support the view that they were more poorly endowed and/or had trained less intensively than the group tested by Pollock.[2] The track times of our sample were not outstanding, and in terms of aerobic power, they were more comparable with the shorter Japanese runners studied by Asano et al.[6] Asano et al. were apparently examining average individuals who had decided to undertake vigorous training in middle age, and discussion with the Masters' contestants often revealed an analogous situation.

By virtue of their average endowment and many years of regular endurance training, our sample may give some indication of the pattern of aging to be

TABLE 13

A COMPARISON OF AEROBIC POWER (ml/kg·min STPD) BETWEEN THE PRESENT
SAMPLE OF MALE MASTERS' COMPETITORS (M) AND OTHER SAMPLES STUDIED
BY POLLOCK,[2] ASANO et al.,[6] AND SALTIN & GRIMBY [3]

Age (yr)	Present Study *	Pollock †	Asano †	Saltin & Grimby †
<40	49.6	—	—	—
40–50	49.9	57.5 (46–64)	49.7	57
50–60	46.0	54.4 (49–57)	45.1	53
60–70	41.6	51.4 (40–61)	42.2	43
>70	29.0	40.0 (38–41)	38.9	—

* Predicted value.
† Directly measured value.

anticipated when middle-aged patients adhere faithfully to prescribed programs of progressive physical activity. Unfortunately, the wide age-spread of our sample (six decades), coupled with the inclusion of some middle and short distance competitors militates against the precise definition of aging curves. Favorable trends were seen in a number of variables, including standing height, percentage of body fat, lean tissue mass, maximum oxygen intake, heart volumes, resting blood pressures, and exercise electrocardiograms. However, in most instances differences from the general population were small and of doubtful statistical significance. Furthermore, we have no categoric proof that such differences as were demonstrated did not arise from either an initial process of self-selection or a subsequent selective attenuation of the athletic sample, men with problems such as hypertension ceasing to participate in competition.

Standing height normally decreases with age, due to a combination of the secular trend (up to 1 cm/decade) and changes in the configuration of the vertebral column (kyphosis and compression of intervertebral discs, most apparent from the sixth decade onwards). Exercise as an adult cannot modify the secular trend, but by strengthening the back muscles and improving posture, it could conceivably delay the onset of kyphosis. It may thus be significant that the Masters' athletes show a slightly smaller decrease of stature than the Saskatoon population from age 35 to 65, with a substantial 7 cm diminution from age 63.6 to 81.5 years.

Sedentary subjects show a progressive increase of body fat with aging. Some 10 kg of excess adipose tissue accumulate by 45 years of age,[8] and fat accounts for 28%–30% of body weight in the elderly man. It is well recognized that endurance running is an effective method of reversing this trend,[16] and it is thus not surprising that the average Masters' competitor has less body fat than a sedentary man aged 25 years. Nevertheless, there is still scope to improve body composition. Both in the present sample and in the data of Pollock,[2] the sprinters were fatter than the distance competitors, and our average Masters' contestants were fatter than Pollock's national champions of the same age.

The lean body mass of the sedentary person decreases progressively after the age of 45 years. Again, there is good evidence that this trend can be reversed by a progressive increase of endurance-type activity.[16] In the present sample, lean tissue was well-preserved except in the oldest age category, where there was probably a decrease in both the volume and the intensity of the training undertaken. Interestingly, not all athletes fare as well as our sample. The continuing orienteers of Saltin & Grimby[3] showed a 6 kg loss of weight from age 45 to 55 years, and a 7 kg loss from 45 to 65 years.

The aerobic power of the average individual shows a rather steady decline of 4–5 ml/kg·min per decade between the ages of 25 and 65 years.[7, 8, 15] The loss in the Masters' competitors, only 8 ml/kg·min from age 35 to 65, seems appreciably less. However, this may reflect the habitual activity patterns of the two populations rather than any more direct effect of endurance training upon the aging of aerobic power. In the general population, there is a substantial decline in voluntary activity between 25 and 65 years of age;[15] in contrast, many of the Masters' competitors first became interested in competition around 35 years of age. In the younger groups, we are thus comparing a Masters' candidate who may have initiated training recently with a general population that is itself taking some recreational activity, whereas in subsequent decades the comparison is between a well-trained veteran runner and an average citizen who is taking no voluntary activity. Irrespective of mechanisms, the Masters' competitors develop a substantial advantage over the general population in terms of their capacity for endurance work. The 65-year-old competitor has a maximum oxygen intake that is close to the average anticipated in a sedentary university student aged 25 years.[8]

Reindell and his colleagues [19] suggest that the heart volume is normally rather constant at 11 ml/kg between the ages of 35 and 65 years. By this standard, most of the Masters' runners had some cardiac enlargement, and in the twelve with volumes >14 ml/kg, the increase of volume was substantial. The high values in the sub-Masters' category could be construed as an effect of selection, but the apparent further increase of volume from 12 ml/kg at age 35 to 13.9 ml/kg at 65 years suggests that much of the difference from the general population is a response to training. Unfortunately, the radiographic estimate gives no indication as to whether the increased volume represents cardiac muscle or an increased blood content.

TABLE 14

A COMPARISON OF RESTING SYSTEMIC BLOOD PRESSURES (mmHg) BETWEEN THE PRESENT STUDY, THE DATA OF POLLOCK [2] AND ASANO et al.[6] FOR ELDERLY RUNNERS, AND THE VALUES OF MASTER et al.[17] FOR THE GENERAL POPULATION

Age (yr)	Present Study		Pollock		Asano et al.		Master et al.	
	Syst.	Diast.	Syst.	Diast.	Syst.	Diast.	Syst.	Diast.
<40	124	79	—	—	—	—	127	80
40–50	120	77	117	76	117	70	130	82
50–60	127	77	129	81	132	79	137	84
60–70	128	77	122	78	135	82	143	84
>70	140	83	141	83	157	78	146	82

Opinions have varied as to whether the resting blood pressures are modified by endurance training. The current concensus seems that while there may be decreases in patients who are initially hypertensive, any changes induced in the general population are small and of no practical significance. Our data for the Masters' candidates (TABLE 14) agrees with that of Pollock [2] and of Asano et al.[6] in showing values marginally lower than the published norms [17] at all ages.

The frequency of abnormal electrocardiograms in endurance athletes with large hearts is also controversial. Some authors have reported a high incidence of ST segmental abnormalities in former competitors,[20] but others have found a normal or even a low incidence.[3, 21] Discrepancies in such reports may relate to differences in training intensities sustained as the athletes have become older. One previous study of elderly subjects [22] indicated that the initiation of regular endurance training of sufficient vigor could reduce the extent of ST depression at a given heart rate. The relatively low incidence of abnormalities in the present sample of Masters' athletes is thus not surprising. Possible explanations include not only the development of the coronary collateral circulation, but also a lessening of the hyperkalemia of effort, and a reduction in the work load per unit mass of myocardium secondary to hypertrophy or a change in the average dimensions of the heart.

Perhaps the most disappointing aspect of the present study was the high incidence of muscular injuries. Several previous reports have stressed that in the first few months of training, geriatric exercise programs can encounter musculo-skeletal problems in as many as 50% of participants. However, it is disturbing to note that the frequency of such injuries is not much lower when elderly runners have 20 years experience of techniques, presumably with associated conditioning of the muscles and tendons. Plainly, there is still great scope for preventive medicine in this area. It may be unavoidable that the older person will push himself to the point of frequent injury if he wishes to excel in inter-national competition. Nevertheless, in many instances, faulty techniques are to blame. Certainly, if the objective is to improve cardiorespiratory condition, an individually prescribed program can produce dramatic gains in 65-year-old men and women with no more than the occasional mild muscle pull,[23] and until the contrary is proven, it would be wrong to accept the current injury rates for Masters' competitors as inevitable.

SUMMARY

Many of the participants in the World Masters' Championships were average individuals who have continued to train over substantial distances (up to 40 miles per week) until reaching an advanced age. The present report describes physiological data on 128 men and 7 women participating in the 1975 competi-tions in Toronto. The average weekly training mileage did not diminish in the older age categories, but fast and interval-type training tended to be replaced by long slow distance work. Age-related changes in a number of variables apparently proceed a little more slowly than in the general population. The sub-Masters' (<40 yr, SM) and Masters' category 1 (40–50 yr, M-1) were of average height (175.2, 174.7 cm) and weight (excess relative to actuarial standards, −0.3 and −0.7 kg). Over the next two decades, the loss of height was less than in the general population (M-2, 50–60 yr, 172.6 cm; M-3, 60–70 yr, 172.3 cm), but there was a rapid decline in the oldest category (M-4, 70–90 yr, 165.3 cm at a mean age of 81.5 years). Women contestants (W, average age 43.1 ± 12.4 years) were fairly tall (164.9 cm). Body fat was less than in the general population, accounting for about 14% of body weight in the men and 23% in the women. Lean tissue was well preserved except in advanced age (SM 59.7 kg; M-1, 59.1 kg; M-2, 56.5 kg; M-3, 58.5 kg; M-4, 53.9 kg; W, 44.3 kg). Aerobic power showed a smaller decrease than in the general popula-tion between the ages of 35 and 65 years, with a more rapid decline in the oldest category (SM, 49.6 ml/kg·min; M-1, 49.9; M-2, 46.0; M-3, 41.6; M-4, 29.0; W, 43.0). Heart volumes were larger than 14 ml/kg in 12 of the 135 contestants, and did not decline with age (SM, 12.0 ml/kg; M-1, 12.5; M-2, 12.4; M-3, 13.9; M-4, 13.2). Resting blood pressures were marginally lower than in the general population, but exercise blood pressures were normal at a given relative work load. Electrocardiographic abnormalities were less frequent than in the general population of comparable age, only 15 of the 135 subjects showing significant ST segmental depression (≥ 0.1 mV). Muscular injuries were disturbingly frequent, with no protection being gained from megadoses of vitamin C (>500 mg/day) or other types of dietary supplement.

REFERENCES

1. GRIMBY, G. & B. SALTIN. 1966. Physiological analysis of physically well-trained middle-aged and old athletes. Acta Med. Scand. **179:** 513–529.

2. POLLOCK, M. L. 1974. Physiological characteristics of older champion track athletes. Res. Quart. **45:** 363–373.
3. SALTIN, B. & G. GRIMBY. 1968. Physiological analysis of middle-aged and old former athletes. Comparison with still active athletes of the same ages. Circulation **38:** 1104–1115.
4. HOLLMANN, W. 1965. Korperliches Training als Pravention von Herz-Kreislauf Krankherten. Hippokrates Verlag. Stuttgart, W. Germany.
5. DEHN, M. & R. A. BRUCE. 1972. Longitudinal variations in maximal oxygen intake with age and activity. J. Appl. Physiol. **33:** 805–807.
6. ASANO, K., S. OGAWA & Y. FURUTA. 1976. Aerobic work capacity in middle and old-aged runners. International Congress of Physical Activity Sciences, Quebec City, Canada.
7. BAILEY, D. A., R. J. SHEPHARD, R. L. MIRWALD & J. A. MCBRIDE. 1974. Current levels of Canadian cardio-respiratory fitness. Canad. Med. Assoc. J. **111:** 25–30.
8. SHEPHARD, R. J. 1977. Endurance Fitness, 2nd edit. University of Toronto Press. Toronto.
9. WEINER, J. S. & J. A. LOURIE. 1969. Human Biology. A guide to field methods. Blackwell Scientific Publications. Oxford, England.
10. DURNIN, J. V. G. A. & M. M. RAHAMAN. 1967. The assessment of the amount of fat in the human body from measurements of skinfold thickness. Brit. J. Nutr. **21:** 681–689.
11. SHEPHARD, R. J. 1971. Standard tests of aerobic power. *In* Frontiers of Fitness. R. J. Shephard, Ed. Charles C Thomas, Publisher. Springfield, Ill.
12. ÅSTRAND, I. 1960. Aerobic work capacity in men and women with special reference to age. Acta Physiol. Scand. **49**(Suppl. 169)**:** 1–92.
13. REINDELL, H., K. KÖNIG & H. ROSKAMM. 1966. Funktionsdiagnostik des gesunden und Kranken Herzens. Thieme Verlag. Stuttgart, W. Germany.
14. SHEPHARD, R. J. 1974. Men at Work. Applications of Ergonomics to Performance and Design. Charles C Thomas, Publisher. Springfield, Ill.
15. SHEPHARD, R. J. 1977. Human Physiological Work Capacity. I.B.P. Synthesis Vol. 4. Cambridge University Press. London. In press.
16. SIDNEY, K. H., R. J. SHEPHARD & J. E. HARRISON. 1977. Endurance training and body composition of the elderly. Amer. J. Clin. Nutr. **30:** 326–333.
17. MASTER, A. M., E. J. VAN LIERE, H. A. LINDSAY & W. S. HARTROFT. 1964. Arterial blood pressure. *In* Biology Data Book. P. L. Altman & D. S. Dittmer, Ed. Federation of American Societies for Experimental Biology. Washington, D.C.
18. CUMMING, G. R. 1972. The frequency and possible significance of ischaemic S-T changes in the exercise electrocardiogram. *In* Training, Scientific Basis and Application. A. W. Taylor, Ed. Charles C Thomas, Publisher. Springfield, Ill.
19. ROSKAMM, H., H. REINDELL & K. KÖNIG. 1966. Korperliche Aktivität and Herz-und Kreislauferkrankungen. J. A. Barth. Munich, W. Germany.
20. HOLMGREN, A. & J. STRANDELL. 1959. Relationship between heart volume, total hemoglobin and physical working capacity in former athletes. Acta Med. Scand. **163:** 149.
21. PYÖRÄLÄ, K., M. J. KARVONEN, P. TASKINEN, J. TAKKUNEN & H. KYRÖNSEPPÄ. 1967. Cardiovascular studies on former endurance athletes. *In* Physical Activity and the Heart. M. J. Karvonen & A. J. Barry, Eds. Charles C Thomas, Publisher. Springfield, Ill.
22. SIDNEY, K. H. & R. J. SHEPHARD. Training and ECG abnormalities in the elderly. Brit. Heart J. In press.
23. SIDNEY, K. H. & R. J. SHEPHARD. 1977. Frequency and intensity of exercise training for elderly subjects. Manuscript submitted to Med. Sci. Sports.

RELATIVE IMPORTANCE OF PHYSICAL ACTIVITY FOR LONGEVITY *

Charles L. Rose and Michel L. Cohen

Normative Aging Study
Veterans Administration Outpatient Clinic
Boston, Massachusetts 02108

INTRODUCTION

There has been general agreement in the folklore for many centuries [1] and in the scientific literature of more recent vintage [2] that ordinary exercise is good for you. The interest of the Conference on the Marathon is on a rather extreme and esoteric form of exercise, namely, long distance running. The present paper, however, addresses itself to the garden variety physical activity indulged in by ordinary citizens, and investigates its relationship to length of life.

I published a book in 1971 entitled *Predicting Longevity: Methodology and Critique,*[3] a refined and expanded version of a belated doctoral dissertation. In this work I investigated over 200 variables that might possibly be related to longevity, and of course I included a number of physical activity variables. The findings relative to physical activity were impressive enough to get me an invitation to present at this scholarly conference. This caused me to revisit the original data.

At first I was also impressed with the physical activity findings. Later, I concluded that I had to add some new analyses not included in the original book. Still later I realized that I couldn't use any of the original findings; I had to reanalyze from scratch. There were two reasons for this. First, the question asked in the original analyses was a general one: What predicts longevity? The question in the present paper is more circumscribed: What is the role of physical exercise in all this? To answer the more limited question required a different analytic strategy. Secondly, and more important, I was chagrined that I hadn't thought of certain statistical approaches to some methodological problems that I had originally left unsolved. So this paper became my second chance to build a better mouse trap.

Here is the background of the original study: I was associated beginning in 1963 with the design of a large-scale longitudinal study of aging.[4, 5] The plan called for enrolling 2,000 initially healthy males across all adult ages, and following them until death. Under this plan it would take 40 years for the younger participants to die off. Therefore, we had on our hands a rather long-range study, and it would be most important to make sagacious decisions early in the game with respect to what data we wished to collect, in order to relate them to the longevity of the subjects as well as to illuminate aging processes in general. This gave rise to the notion of a one-shot study of a community population that had just died, with comprehensive data comprising better than 200 variables, which were collected from the surviving next-of-kin. The results

* This work was supported by the Veterans Administration Medical Research Service, Washington, D.C., and by The Council for Tobacco Research, New York, N.Y.

of this "quickie" study could then be folded into the data collection of the longitudinal study.

The optimal method for arriving at predictors of longevity is the longitudinal method, and the role of the preliminary study was to ensure better pay off from the tremendous investment in research over the 40-year period. But perhaps more important for immediate purposes, a longevity study was a substantive and contributory piece of research in its own right. Actually, because of the immense complexities in predicting longevity, I gave priority to the development of methodology, particularly data analytic methodology. But as necessary as it was to emphasize methodology, some substantive findings did manage to peep through.

The Secular Effect

Unfortunately, a nagging problem haunted the original data analysis, the secular contamination of the data. This was due to the following chain of circumstances: (1) The need for age at death made it necessary for all subjects to be dead, and for information to be collected from a survivor-informant. (2) In order to have an available informant, who turned out in most cases to be the wife, it was necessary to interview her within a few months of the death, otherwise the chances were good that she would be changing her address from that indicated on the death certificate, and it would be difficult to locate and interview her. (3) In order to complete the data collection within a year's time, it would also be necessary for all subjects to die within a year's time. (4) Since all subjects had to die during a given year, the longer lived ones had to be born earlier. (5) This introduced the secular effect into many of the variables.

An example is education. Those who lived longer and were therefore born earlier, had less education since there was less education available at the earlier period. It therefore turned out that those who lived longer had less education. This was patently spurious, since it is well known that those of higher education live longer.[6] Actually any variable which is sensitive to changing times may be secular. Examples are social-class-related variables such as number of children, income, parental education, weight, number of siblings, and occupational level. The secular trend has been for number of children to go down from one generation to the next, and income and occupational levels to go up. As a result, in the present design, longer life would have been associated with larger number of children, lower income, and lower occupational level. Such findings would have been spurious.

I therefore expunged such secular variables from the original variable set. However, some variables were less obviously secular or were partly secular. An example was cigarette smoking. This was found to have a strong inverse relationship with age at death. However, since there has been an increase in cigarette smoking,[7] those born later and therefore dead at an earlier age smoked more cigarettes. Thus, the inverse relationship between cigarette smoking and age at death was at least in part due to the secular shift in cigarette smoking.

For the original analysis I had selected 69 variables as being the least secular. These included the physical activity variables on which we are focusing today. In drawing up a list of variables for the present analysis, I realized that even the exercise variables could be secular. There certainly has been a shift from blue collar to white collar occupations that involve less physical activity.[8] This would tend to relate the later born and less long lived to less on-job physical activity, and thereby weaken the usual relationship between shorter life and manual occupation. Also, with the shift to nonmanual occupation there could well be a shift to more off-job physical activity. This would tend to relate more off-job activity to shorter life, which again could be misleading.

Adjusting for the Secular Effect

The challenges for the present paper, then, were to reanalyze the data focusing on the special question of physical activity and if possible to do something about the secular problem within the constraints of the original study design. I accomplished the former by inserting into the analysis the best correlating variables with physical activity and/or length of life. I accomplished the latter by a partial correlation approach as follows: I started with the two most obviously secular variables, education and occupational level. With respect to education, the secular effect not only wiped out the positive correlation with age at death, it drove it into a spurious negative correlation (-0.21). Occupational level was expected to show a substantial positive correlation with longevity, but it in fact showed a reduced correlation of 0.10. This was apparently due to a neutralizing secular relationship between higher occupational level and later birth–shorter life, a result of the shift over time toward higher occupational levels in the occupational structure.

Since the secular effect actually reversed the sign of the correlation between education and longevity, I reasoned that controlling for education might at least partly correct for the secular contaminant. These partial correlations are therefore offered as a truer picture of the relationships between independent variables and age at death. As will be seen, the shift in correlation with education controlled is in the hypothesized direction. This would appear to validate the procedure.

Please don't misunderstand. I do not claim that the partial correlation technique gives secular-free results. It gives results closer to the truth. There is another method available that allows a one-shot approach with individuals all born at the same time. Under this method, an age cohort is examined at a later point in time as to who is alive and who is dead, and the differences between the two groups are taken as predictors of shorter versus longer life.[9, 10] Such investigation could be carried out for live-dead groups of successive age cohorts. This design requires an entirely new data collection and is an important next step in longevity prediction research. But lacking such new data, we must content ourselves at the moment with the analysis of the data that we have.

Additional Analyses

In addition to looking at a whole series of longevity predictors including physical exercise and thus determining its relative importance, I also looked at the predictors of exercise themselves. I felt this would deepen our knowledge since we would learn which predictors were related to exercise and not longevity and which were related to longevity but not exercise. I now raised a similar question as the one raised in connection with predicting age at death: perhaps there was a secular effect in connection with predicting exercise, in which case

I could perhaps use a partial correlation technique to control for it. Now I could partially correlate out age at death, which is the perfect index of birth year and therefore of the secular effect. I couldn't partially correlate controlling for age at death when age at death was also the dependent variable, but I could certainly use it to determine the correlates of physical activity. So I did.

With this strategy I could bring back into the independent variable set the all-important social class predictors of longevity. These had previously been excluded because they were highly secular.

Also, I had previously excluded a number of categorical variables which were not suitable for complicated multivariate analyses. For the present analyses I related categorical variables to longevity and exercise by one-way analyses of variance (ANOVA), and adjusted for the secular effect by co-varying, respectively, for education and longevity.

Procedures

The data on which I base this paper was drawn from the original monograph published in 1971.[3] I therefore need not repeat here the rationale and details of population selection, selection of measures, and data collection and data analytic procedures. The monograph also contains an extensive literature review, so that selected references will suffice here.

Very briefly, the population consisted of 500 white males whose deaths were recorded in the Boston City Hall during 1965 and met the following conditions: (1) death not earlier than age 50; (2) exclusion of deaths by accident, suicide, and homicide; (3) availability of an informant residing in the Boston area; and (4) a rectangular age-at-death distribution with equal numbers (125) in the age at death ranges, 50–59, 60–69, 70–79, and 80 and over.

For the present analysis I selected those measures that best related to age at death and/or physical activity. The cut-off point for variables other than the physical activity measures was a correlation lower than 0.10 with age at death, either without education, or with education partially correlated. These 36 variables are listed and defined in Appendix 1. They reflect a broad range of social, psychological, and physical variables, which were included in the original work under the concept that the determinancy of longevity is extremely complex and variegated. The reader may refer to this material as the variables are considered in the analyses which follow.

Since the physical activity variables are the focus of our attention I will describe them here in some detail. Degree of physical exertion was assessed separately for on-job and off-job activity in accordance with the following common scale: (0) sedentary, (1) light, (2) moderate, (3) active, (4) very active. The assessments were also made within age decade groups: < age 20, 20–29, 30–39, 40–49, 50–59, and 60–69. In addition mean scores were calculated for each subject from available age decade scores.

All data collection was carried out by a single interviewer in the informant's home. The data collection instrument was an interview schedule that went through several pilot and pretest stages before substantive data collection began. Interviews were conducted with the survivor between 1 and 3 months after the death occurred. The major informant groups were 70% wives and 20% children.

Data analysis was conducted by zero-order and partial correlations, with age at death and physical activity as dependent variables. Stepwise multiple regression of age at death and physical activity yielded the variances accounted for by the predictors. Categorical variables were related to age at death and physical activity by one-way analysis of variance (ANOVA). Significance of difference in means was by the Duncan test. Details on the statistical procedures are contained in APPENDIX 2.

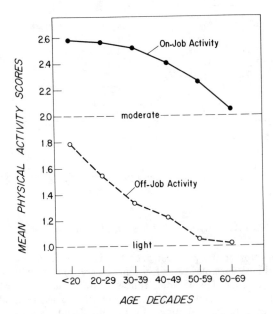

FIGURE 1. Mean scores by age decade of on-job and off-job physical activity.

RESULTS

Physical Activity

First I will present descriptive information on the physical activity variables according to FIGURE 1 and TABLE 1. There is a significant decrease in mean activity scores across age decades for both on-job and off-job measures. The age decrease is more marked for off-job activity. At all age decades, off-job activity is at a significantly lower level, with greater differences at the middle decades. From FIGURE 1 it is evident that off-job activity starts dropping off earlier in life, then levels off, while on-job activity stays fairly level then drops off later in life. On-job activity holds up better than off-job activity until the fourth decade because the physical levels are determined by the job. Off-job activity, on the other hand, is more subject to aging effects and changing life-styles related to age.

TABLE 2 shows whether the on-job variables are related to corresponding age decade off-job variables. In general, the two are unrelated. The only exception is at the oldest decade, 60–69, where the correlation is 0.16. This is

TABLE 1

ANOVA WITH REPEATED MEASURES FOR ON-JOB AND OFF-JOB PHYSICAL
ACTIVITY ACROSS AGE DECADES AND WITHIN AGE DECADES *

Age (yrs)	On-Job Activity Means	(n)	Off-Job Activity Means	(n)	F ratios within Age Decades
<20	2.58	(495)	1.79	(499)	125.0
20–29	2.56	(500)	1.54	(500)	247.7
30–39	2.52	(500)	1.33	(500)	378.3
40–49	2.43	(500)	1.22	(500)	408.8
50–59	2.25	(498)	1.06	(499)	404.7
60–69	2.04	(366)	1.02	(370)	382.4
F ratios across age decades	28.7		186.5		

* All F ratios significant at the 0.001 level.

probably related to the decrease in activity levels with age, and greater importance of aging effects in determining both on-job and off-job exertion levels.

Relationship of Illnesses with Physical Activity and Age at Death

The relationships of the physical activity measures to illnesses is shown in
TABLE 3. The illness variables refer to number of serious illnesses or operations
which occurred in each age decade. Illnesses were related to reduced on-job
activity only in the 50s and 60s decades. In off-job activity, illnesses were
related to reduced activity beginning with the 30s decade, with the effect growing stronger for each succeeding decade thereafter. The lower sensitivity of

TABLE 2

ZERO-ORDER CORRELATIONS OF ON-JOB PHYSICAL ACTIVITY VARIABLES WITH
CORRESPONDING OFF-JOB VARIABLES BY AGE DECADE

On-Job Activity Age Decade	(n)	Corresponding Age Decade Off-Job Variable
<20 years	(495)	−0.05
20–29	(500)	−0.03
30–39	(500)	−0.05
40–49	(500)	−0.03
50–59	(498)	0.04
60–69	(366)	0.16*
Mean on Job Score		0.01†

* p<0.001; all other r values were not significant at the 0.05 level
† This correlation relates standardized mean scores of on-job and off-job physical
activity. These scores are derived from means of the respective age-decade scores.

on-job activity to illness as compared to off-job again may be due to the salience of the job itself over individual factors.

In addition, TABLE 3 shows the relationship between the age decade illness scores and longevity. The correlations between the two increase with succeeding decades. Thus, illness in later years is more important for predicting longevity. This may be due to the fact that one is more vulnerable to serious illnesses in later years.

TABLE 3

ZERO-ORDER CORRELATIONS OF ILLNESS WITH PHYSICAL ACTIVITY VARIABLES WITHIN AGE DECADES, AND WITH AGE AT DEATH

Age Decade Illnesses	Corresponding Age Decade On-Job Activity Variable	Corresponding Age Decade Off-Job Activity Variable	Age at Death
<20 years	−0.06	0.03	−0.08*
20–29	0.00	−0.03	−0.18‡
30–39	−0.01	−0.08*	−0.22‡
40–49	0.00	−0.10*	−0.31‡
50–59	−0.14†	−0.20‡	−0.06‡
60–69	−0.20‡	−0.22‡	−0.55‡

* p<0.05.
† p<0.01.
‡ p<0.001.

Correlation of Physical Activity with Age at Death

TABLE 4 displays the degree to which the various physical activity variables are related to age at death. The correlations are controlled for education to help correct for the secular effect that may be involved. The effect of controlling this way is to reduce the age-at-death correlations of on-job activity and to increase the age-at-death correlations of off-job correlations. This is due to the secular decrease of on-job activity and increase of off-job activity over time. The secular effect is more marked in the on-job variables and is particularly evident before age 50, as shown by the greater shift in correlation in the on-job variables when partially correlating for education. For both on-job and off-job activity, the correlations with age at death are stronger in the older age decade measures.

The lifetime mean scores of physical activity highlight these findings. The correlation of the on-job score with age at death is 0.15, suggesting that a manual or blue collar occupation predicts longer life. This goes against most findings in the literature. However, when the correlation is controlled for education, it is reduced to 0.08, which is at least in the right direction away from a positive correlation. By contrast, off-job activity shows much less shift in correlation when the education level is controlled, going from 0.14 to 0.18. Here the direction of the shift is to stronger relationship with longevity. There-

TABLE 4

ZERO-ORDER CORRELATIONS OF PHYSICAL ACTIVITY VARIABLES WITH AGE AT
DEATH, AND PARTIAL CORRELATIONS CONTROLLING FOR EDUCATION
TO ADJUST FOR SECULARITY *

Age Decade	Partial r	r	Partial r	r
	On-Job Physical Activity		Off-Job Physical Activity	
<20	0.05	0.13‡	−0.03	−0.08
20–29	0.05	0.12‡	0.11†	0.06
30–39	−0.01	0.06	0.19§	0.16§
40–49	0.05	0.11‡	0.23§	0.20§
50–59	0.14†	0.19§	0.24§	0.22§
60–69	0.16†	0.22§	0.23§	0.22§
Mean score ¶	0.08†	0.15§	0.18§	0.14‡

* Since subjects died at same time, longer lived subjects were born earlier, and had
less education. Correlation between education and age at death was −0.21, which is
spurious because of the secular effect. Controlling for education helped to correct for
this effect.
　† p<0.05.
　‡ p<0.01.
　§ p<0.001.
　¶ Standardized mean score of age decade scores.

fore a truer picture of the longevity predictors may be surmised from the
partial correlations. In the succeeding analyses of this paper, therefore, all
predictors will in addition be displayed with the partial correlation.

If the zero-order partials were used, the on-job correlation to longevity
would have been as high (0.15) as the off-job correlation (0.14). This would
have given the erroneous impression that on-job and off-job activity are equally
important in a positive correlation with age at death. The first-order partials
give an entirely different picture. The on-job correlation is 0.08 and the off-job
correlation is considerably higher, 0.18, which clearly shows that off-job activity
is a better predictor of longevity. The partials for the 40–49 decade show even
more dramatically that off-job activity is a better predictor. Here the adjusted
correlation of on-job activity with longevity is nonsignificant (0.05), while the
adjusted correlation of off-job activity is 0.23.

The off-job correlations under age 20 show an interesting secular effect.
Here the unadjusted correlation shows a *negative* correlation with age at death
(−0.08). In other words, more off-job activity under age 20 is related to shorter
life. However, when the correlation is controlled for education, the correlation
is no longer significant at the 0.05 level (−0.03). Likewise, when the on-job
correlation with age at death is controlled for education, it also drops to a
nonsignificant level. So we conclude at the moment that neither more on-job
nor off-job activity in youth has anything to do with longevity. We will recon-
sider the importance of this variable within the context of regression analysis
below.

At the risk of repetition, further clarification of the indication for partial
correlations controlling for education may be useful. For illustration, let us take

the variable on-job physical activity, age 40–49. This variable applies to different epochs depending on the birth year of the subject. For example, for the subjects born between 1885 and 1895, it would apply to the period 1925 to 1935, for subjects of birth years 1895 to 1905, it would apply to the period 1935 to 1945, and so on. Because of the secular shift in on-job activity to lower levels of physical activity, those born later (and in the less long-lived group) would have less on-job activity. This would increase the correlation between more on-job activity 40–49 and longevity. TABLE 4 shows this actually happens. To correct for this secular contaminant, we should control the effect of birth year, but we can't do that since birth year parallels age at death, and you can't control for age at death when age at death is the dependent variable. So we use the next best variable, education, which is highly secular and gives us a handle on birth year.

Secular Variables as Longevity Correlates

TABLE 5 shows other correlates of longevity which prove to be sensitive to secularity. Both rural residence and native birth become less important as predictors of age at death when partially correlated for education. Both rural residence and foreign birth are obviously secular, since there has been a shift over time from rural to urban residence,[11] and from foreign to native birth.[12] First let us look at rural birth and longevity. Less education, the third variable, is statistically related both to rural birth and longer life. Therefore, when education is not controlled, the relationship between rural residence and longer life is greater than it should be. When education is controlled, the correlation between rural residence and longevity goes down. The same thing happens when the education level is controlled in the foreign birth–longer life correlation. Here too, education is inversely related to both foreign birth and longer life. When education is controlled in the foreign birth–longer life correlation, the correlation is lessened.

TABLE 5 also shows that occupational level and intelligence become more important with education controlled. I would argue that occupational level is a secular variable because of the shift that has taken place in the occupational structure toward higher level of skill. But I would be on thin ice indeed if I were to insist on a secular shift in intelligence. Rather, I would offer the following: Education is related both to intelligence ($r = 0.48$) and inversely to longer life (-0.21), the latter through the secular effect. As a result, the zero-

TABLE 5

CORRELATES OF AGE AT DEATH THAT CHANGE WHEN PARTIALLY CORRELATED
CONTROLLING FOR EDUCATION; PHYSICAL ACTIVITY VARIABLES NOT INCLUDED

	Partial r	r
Urban vs rural residence	0.24	0.28
Foreign vs native born	−0.20	−0.27
Occupational level	0.24	0.10*
Intelligence	0.20	0.07

* Significant at the 0.05 level; all others at the 0.001 level.

order correlation between intelligence and longer life is lower than is the case when the statistical effect of education is removed. Intelligence is not secular itself, but together with age-at-death is related to a third variable that is secular. The upshot is that a truer relationship between intelligence and age at death is given by the correlation of 0.20 rather than 0.07. This change occurs when the effect of the third variable is controlled.

In sum, the present test for secularity always involves controlling for a third variable (education). The converse, however, is not true: When a correlation changes with control of the third variable, it does not necessarily refer to a secular shift. It may only be an instance of two variables being related at least partly because they are related to a third variable. The only instance where the latter occurred, as above stated, was in the relation of intelligence to longevity where this could partly be ascribed to the fact that they were both related to education.

Variables More Strongly and Less Strongly Related to Longevity than Physical Exercise

In order to get at the relative position of physical exercise in the hierarchy of longevity predictors, one must identify those that are more important and less important than physical exercise. These data are presented in Tables 6 and 7. The reference physical activity variable was off-job activity, 40–49, since this had the highest correlation with age at death, and provided an optimal test for showing the importance of physical activity. Still, eight items were more important than the reference variable as based on the partial correlation (Table 6). These were, in order of decreasing correlation, fewer illnesses, younger age appearance, less smoking, less worried, rural residence and higher occupational level.[13, 14] If the off-job activity lifetime mean had been used as the reference variable, intelligence and foreign birth would have scored higher as longevity correlates (Appendix 1). If the on-job activity mean had been used as the reference, all of the variables would have scored higher (Appendix 1).

To return to the eight variables listed as more important than off-job activity, 40–49, please note that one has control only over smoking. Certainly one has less control over such things as age appearance or number of illnesses. However, the fact that off-job activity, 40–49, is ninth in importance gives us a sense of the importance of physical activity as compared to other factors. To complete the picture, Table 7 lists the items that are less important than the reference activity variable. Here we find a host of variables, 17 in all. In other words, off-job activity, 40–49, was 9th down in a total of 25 (Appendix 1, education not counted) or was ⅓ down in importance.

Regression Analysis of Longevity Predictors

The same variables were inserted into a multiple regression procedure (Table 8). Under this procedure, earlier entering variables usually sum up the variance (r^2) accounted for by later entering variables with which they are intercorrelated. Thus, the procedure produces a parsimonious set of predictors, or indices of predictors that do not get included, or do not get included at an

TABLE 6

VARIABLES MORE STRONGLY RELATED TO AGE AT DEATH THAN SELECTED
EXERCISE VARIABLES, BY ZERO-ORDER CORRELATION, AND PARTIAL
CORRELATIONS CONTROLLING FOR EDUCATION

	Partial r	Zero-Order r
1. Younger age appearance $\geq$ 40	0.47	0.46
2. Mean illnesses	-0.46	-0.47
3. Smoking $<$ 40	-0.29	-0.28
4. Smoking $\geq$ 40	-0.28	-0.30
5. Worried	-0.28	-0.30
6. Younger age appearance $<$ 40	0.25	0.25
7. Urban vs rural residence	0.24	0.28
8. Occupational level	0.24	0.10*
Off-job activity 40–49	0.23	0.20
Off-job activity mean *	0.18	0.14‡
On-job activity mean *	0.08†	0.15

* Standardized mean scores of age decade scores
‡ Significant at the 0.05 level.
‡ Significant at the 0.01 level; all others significant at the 0.001 level.

TABLE 7

VARIABLES LESS STRONGLY RELATED TO AGE AT DEATH THAN OFF-JOB PHYSICAL
ACTIVITY 40–49, BY ZERO-ORDER CORRELATIONS AND PARTIAL
CORRELATIONS CONTROLLING FOR EDUCATION

	Partial r	Zero-Order r
Off job activity 40–49	0.23	0.20
Foreign vs native born	-0.20	-0.27
Intelligence	0.20	0.07*
Mother's age at death	0.18	0.16
Activity compared to others	0.17	0.15
Conserved energy	0.16	0.17
Younger wife	0.15	0.18
Easily aggravated	-0.15	-0.12†
Diversional activity $<$ 65	-0.14	-0.15
Hazardous occupation	-0.14	-0.15
Catch colds easily	-0.14	-0.15
Age difference, oldest & youngest child	0.14	0.16
Married at older age	0.14	0.11†
Live dangerously	-0.12†	-0.11†
Drinking $\geq$ 40	-0.12†	-0.09*
Drinking $<$ 40	-0.11†	-0.07*
Trusting	-0.11†	-0.13†
Sense of humor	-0.09*	-0.11†

* Significant at the 0.05 level.
† Significant at the 0.01 level; all others significant at 0.001 level.

important level. The ten best predictors are those ten that account for most of the variance. Two procedures are shown, one with education partially correlated out before the first step (education forced in first) and another without such initial partial correlating. The differences in results reflect the effect of correcting, to some extent at least, for the secular error. In addition to the variance each predictor accounts for, TABLE 8, by way of comparison, also displays the zero-order correlations.

The ten best predictors together account for 44.2% of the variance after initial control for education. Since all of the 36 variables that entered the procedure accounted for 49.4% of the variance, the first ten account for 89.5% of this amount, indicating the efficiency with which these ten sum up

TABLE 8

TEN BEST PREDICTORS OF AGE AT DEATH BY STEPWISE MULTIPLE REGRESSION WITH AND WITHOUT INITIAL CONTROL FOR EDUCATION

| Step | Predictor | Education Controlled | | Education Not Controlled | | |
		r^2 Change (%)	r	Step	r^2 Change (%)	r
1	Younger age appearance ≥ 40	20.2%	0.47	2	9.8%	0.46
2	Illness mean	9.9%	-0.46	1	22.2%	-0.47
3	Smoking <40	4.3%	-0.29	>10		
4	Mother's age at death	1.8%	0.18	7	1.4%	0.16
5	Sense of humor	1.9%	-0.09*	5	2.0%	-0.11†
6	Urban vs rural residence	1.4%	0.24	8	1.1%	0.28
7	Intelligence	1.2%	0.20	>10		
8	Worried	1.1%	-0.28	6	1.4%	-0.30
9	Off-job activity 40–49	0.8%	0.23	9	1.1%	0.20
10	Off-job activity <20	1.6%	-0.03 (NS)	10	1.7%	-0.08*
>10	Smoking ≥ 40			3	4.3%	-0.28
>10	Foreign vs native born			4	2.9%	-0.27
Total r^2		44.2%			47.9%	

* Significant at the 0.05 level.
† Significant at the 0.01 level; unmarked r values are significant at the 0.01 level.

the predictive effects of the 36 combined. Please recall that these 36 were the best correlates of longevity out of the larger number of 200 variables that were investigated in the original work.

The three most important variables in the correlations are the same as in the regression: younger age appearance ≥ 40, fewer illnesses, and less smoking.[15] Mother's age at death [16, 17] and less sense of humor loom more important in the regression analysis than the zero-order correlations. Occupational level becomes less important to the point that it does not even appear in the first ten variables, though it has a correlation of 0.24 with longevity. This happened because its effect was summed up by earlier entering variables with which it is strongly correlated such as intelligence and off-job activity. Younger age appearance <40, whose correlation with longevity is 0.25, is not within the first ten either, again because its effect was summed up by the earlier entering variable, age appearance ≥ 40, with which it is strongly correlated. Rural residence maintains its modest level of importance both in the correlational and regression procedures.

Younger appearance, age 40 and over, and fewer illnesses were the two best predictors. However, since the correlation of age appearance was slightly higher than illness (0.47 vs 0.46), it nosed out illness, entering at step one. Since the two were strongly intercorrelated, the variable entering first "grabbed" the variance of the variable entering second. Thus, age appearance accounted for 20.2% of the variance, and illness 9.9%. The age appearance variance consists of its own variance and that part of the illness variance (as well as that of later entering variables) with which it has some redundancies.

This phenomenon is further highlighted by the second regression where education was not initially controlled. Here a reversal occurred: the zero-order correlation with illness was slightly higher than with age appearance (0.47 vs 0.46) so the former entered first and subsumed the variance of the latter. As a result, there was a reversal in the amount of variance they each accounted for, with illness accounting for 22.2% and age appearance accounting for 9.8%. These results underscore the following: One cannot conclude that a given variable is important in proportion to the variance it accounts for; but rather a given variable must be regarded as one of a group of variables that parsimoniously index an even larger number of measures.

Still another example was smoking $<$ age 40, which entered before smoking ≥ 40. It therefore subsumed the variance of the latter with which it was highly correlated, and as a result knocked it out of the first ten entries.

Off-job activity less than age 20, which entered 10th in the equation, is unusual in two ways. Its relationship with longevity is an inverse one, and the variance it accounts for (1.6%) is far out of proportion to its nonsignificant zero-order correlation (-0.03). What this means is that when the effects of previously entered predictors are removed (which is what happens in the stepwise procedure) the <20 off-job variable assumes an importance not evident from its poor zero-order correlation with longevity.

This finding was further investigated by the evolution of the partial r values in the stepwise procedure. The initial correlation of off-job activity <20, after education was controlled, was -0.03. After eight more variables were entered (refer to TABLE 8), the partial of off-job activity <20 had increased to -0.06 (evolution of partials not shown in TABLE 8). When off-job activity 40–49 entered in the ninth step, the partial r of off-job activity <20 suddenly jumped to -0.17. Thus, it appears that off-job 40–49 had been masking the importance of the inverse relationship between off-job activity <20 and longevity. Consequently, when the effect of off-job activity 40–49 was removed, the importance of more off-job activity <20 for predicting shorter life shone through, accounting for 1.6% of the variance in longevity. This was more than the variance accounted for individually by rural residence, intelligence, less worried, and off-job activity, 40–49.

It may very well be true that heavier off-job activity in youth is life shortening. But the reader should keep in mind the special circumstances, statistically speaking, from which this conclusion was derived. Please recall that the regression equation produces a parsimonious set of *indices* of longevity predictors, with accent on *indices*. In other words, if one wanted to predict longevity from a particular combination of variables, the "mix" would include "less physical activity under 20 years of age" accounting for a respectable amount of variance relative to other variables in the predictive set.

Please note that this "mix," as shown in TABLE 8 (in the regression with education controlled) shows more off-job activity age, 40–49, as accounting for a minuscule variance (0.8%). We know that in the real world this predictor is more important than appears in this regression equation. However, in the equation, its variance is summed up by the other variables, so we have to think that it is there but it's presence is indicated by other variables which index it. In this context, then, less activity <20, in combination with other variables, and in proportion to the indicated variances they respectively account for, yield a prediction of longevity.

A comparison with the regression without initial partially correlating for education shows the direction of the error introduced by the secular effect. Since partially correlating for education made foreign birth a less important correlate (reducing the correlation from 0.27 to 0.20) it did not enter within the first ten when education was initially controlled, though it entered fourth in the "secular" regression. Smoking ≥40 entered prior to smoking <40 and therefore knocked smoking <40 out of the first ten. Intelligence, which accounted for 1.2% of the variance in the regression with education initially controlled, did not appear at all in the "secular" regression. This was because the partial correlation of intelligence with age at death was 0.20, and when not controlled for education the correlation dropped to 0.07.

Correlates of Physical Activity

TABLE 9 shows the ten best correlates of physical activity. The criteria were the mean level of on-job and off-job activity over the decades. In order to check for the possibility of secular effects the procedures were run with and without partially correlating for age at death.

In the main, there were no marked differences when this was done. The only exception was foreign versus native birth. The correlation between this variable and on-job activity fell from −0.27 to −0.11 when age at death was partially correlated. In other words, the strong relationship between foreign birth and greater on-job physical activity was considerably weakened when corrected for secularity.

Note that both foreign birth and greater on-job activity are secular in that they were more prevalent in the earlier born who were by selection more long lived. The secular relationships of both to longer life therefore enhanced their statistical relationship. When age at death was controlled, the secular effect was removed and the correlation dropped. The true secular-free correlation between native birth and on-job activity can therefore be taken as −0.11.

In ranked order, the ten best correlates of on-job activity controlled for age at death were: less education, lower occupational level, rural residence, occupational hazard, lower intelligence, more activity compared to others, not conserved energy, and foreign birth. The correlations with off-job activity were not as high, and quite different from correlations with on-job activity. On the basis of the partial correlations, the notable differences were as follows: Higher education was related to lower on-job activity (0.36), but to higher off-job activity (0.19). Occupational level, urban residence, intelligence, and native birth followed the same pattern. Occupational hazard and drinking, which were among ten best correlates of on-job activity fell below the ten best correlates of off-job activity. Younger age appearance and less trusting were among the ten best correlates of off-job activity, but fell below the ten best of on-job activity.

Higher off-job activity, then, is related to very different life styles and social strata than is higher on-job activity. In summary, those involved in more off-job activity in ranked order of characteristics are generally more active than others, more intelligent, more educated, and of higher occupational level.

TABLE 9

TEN BEST CORRELATES OF ON-JOB ACTIVITY, BY PARTIAL r CONTROLLING
FOR AGE AT DEATH AND BY ZERO-ORDER r

	Partial r		Zero-Order r	
	On-Job Activity	Off-Job Activity	On-Job Activity	Off-Job Activity
Education	−0.36	0.19	−0.38	0.16
Occupational level	−0.32	0.15	−0.30	0.17
Urban vs rural residence	0.29	−0.08*	0.32	−0.04(NS)
Occupational hazard	0.21		0.18	
Intelligence	−0.20	0.25	−0.18	0.25
Activity compared to others	0.19	0.41	0.21	0.42
Drinking < 40	0.14†		0.12†	
Drinking ≥ 40	0.11†		0.09*	
Foreign vs native birth	−0.11	.0.13	−0.27 *	0.09 †
Conserve energy	−0.10*	−0.15	−0.08*	−0.12 †
Diversion < 65	−0.10*	0.16	−0.12†	0.18
Younger age appearance ≥ 40		0.11†		0.16
Trusting		−0.10*		−0.11†

* Significant at the 0.05 level.
† Significant at the 0.01 level; unmarked r values are significant at the 0.01 level.

Predictors of Physical Activity through Regression Analysis

TABLE 10 replicates TABLE 9 but using multiple regression analysis. With the on-job regression initially controlled for age at death, education comes in first since it has the highest correlation. Having done so, it subsumes some of the variance of variables with which it is associated, occupational level and intelligence. As a result, occupational level is lowered to the fourth step (whereas it ranked second in correlation), and intelligence is knocked below the tenth step. Less worried, fewer colds, and younger wife appear in the lower ranks of the ten variable on-job regression but fall below the ten best correlates shown in TABLE 9. The best predictors of on-job physical activity corrected for secularity (birth year) are in ranked order: less education, more activity compared to others, rural residence, lower occupational level, and greater occupational hazard. These five predictors account for 29.6% of the variance or 94.3% of the variance accounted for by the ten best predictors. The power of these five predictors to sum up the effects of all 20 variables entered into the procedure is shown by the fact that they account for 92.5% of the variance of all twenty.

TABLE 10

TEN BEST PREDICTORS OF ON-JOB AND OFF-JOB ACTIVITY BY VARIANCE (r^2)
ACCOUNTED FOR IN CRITERION, THROUGH STEPWISE MULTIPLE REGRESSION,
WITH AND WITHOUT INITIAL CONTROL FOR AGE AT DEATH *

	Age at Death Controlled		Age at Death Not Controlled	
	On-Job Activity	Off-Job Activity	On-Job Activity	Off-Job Activity
Education	13.0% †	0.5%	14.8%	0.7%
Activity compared to others	5.1	16.5	5.5	17.9
Urban vs rural residence	4.6	0.4†	4.6	0.4†
Occupational level	4.2 †		4.1 †	
Occupational hazard	2.7		2.6	
Worried	0.5†		0.6†	
Foreign vs native extraction	0.4†	1.0	0.4†	0.3
Drinking < 40	0.3		0.3	
Colds	0.3		0.3	
Younger wife	0.3	0.4	0.2	0.4
Intelligence		2.3		2.3
Diversion < 65		1.4		1.6
Trusting		0.9†		1.1†
Younger age appearance ≥ 40		0.3		0.6
Younger age appearance < 40		0.3		0.4
Total r^2	31.4	28.0	33.4	25.7

* Stepwise entry occurred in same order as magnitude of r^2.
† Inverse relationship with physical activity.

The best predictors of off-job physical activity corrected for secularity mirror the different life-styles of those who are high in off-job activity, just as do the correlations with off-job activity of TABLE 9. These predictors, in order, are more activity compared to others, greater intelligence, more hours of diversional activity under 65, and native birth. These four predictors account for 88.3% of the variance accounted for by the ten best predictors, and 83.1% of the variance accounted for by all 20 variables inserted into the procedure.

No remarkable differences between the regressions initially controlled and not initially controlled for birth year were found that may be ascribed to the secular effect, either for the on-job or off-job analyses. Please recall that in TABLE 9 the only secular difference in the correlations was between nativity and on-job activity. In the non-initially-controlled on-job regression (TABLE 10), the zero-order r of nativity was −0.27, but earlier entering variables associated with nativity subsumed enough of its variance to knock it out of the 10-variable equation.

Analyses of Categorical Variables

The final group of analyses have to do with categorical variables, and these are treated by ANOVA and the Duncan difference in means test. The results are displayed in TABLES 11 to 16.

Combinations of Light and Heavy On- and Off-Job Activity

TABLE 11 deals with longevity differences in four groups of individuals: (1) those whose on-job and off-job activity are both light (light–light); (2) those whose on-job activity is light but off-job is heavy, (light–heavy); (3) those whose on-job activity is heavy but off-job activity is light, (heavy–light); and (4) those whose on-job and off-job activity are both heavy, (heavy–heavy). "Light" and "heavy" were determined by dichotomizing the standardized physical activity scores at the mean. The aim was to find out which "mix" of activity was best for longevity. Also, to take into account the secular effect, the mean age at death of each group was covaried for education. The Duncan test specified which groups had significantly different means at the 0.05 level.

Based on the covaried means, the light–light group was less long-lived than the light–heavy and heavy–heavy groups. In addition, the heavy–light group was less long lived than the heavy–heavy group. The longevity differential in each instance was 2 years or more. Also there was no longevity difference between the light and heavy on-job if they were both heavy off-job. The findings all point to the special importance of greater off-job physical activity for more favorable longevity. This finding is consistent with previous findings regarding the greater relationship of off-job activity to age at death, and the differences in life-style characteristics between those who are high in off-job and those who are high in on-job activity.

I wondered whether a reduced level of off-job activity might be related to more illnesses,[18] and if so, this could explain, at least in part, the relationship to shorter life span. TABLE 11 shows the differences across the four groups with

TABLE 11

AGE AT DEATH AND ILLNESS DIFFERENCES IN PHYSICAL ACTIVITY GROUPS,*
BY ANOVA AND DUNCAN TEST,† AND COVARIED FOR EDUCATION

On-Job Activity	Off-Job Activity	(*n*)	Age at Death		Illnesses ‡	
			Covaried	Not Covaried	Covaried	Not Covaried
1. light	light	(142)	67.5	67.3	51.4	51.5
2. light	heavy	(110)	71.3	69.8	49.8	50.2
3. heavy	light	(136)	69.5	70.5	50.7	50.4
4. heavy	heavy	(111)	72.6	73.1	49.3	49.2
	F		5.016	5.339	3.562	3.480
	p		0.002	0.001	0.014	0.016
Duncan test †			1–2, 4 3–4	1–3, 4 2–4	1–2, 4	1–4

* The standardized on-job and off-job mean scores were dichotomized at the middle of the distributions into light and heavy.

† This test specifies which groups are significantly different at the 0.05 level, e.g., the shorthand designation 1–2, 4 signifies that group 1 is significantly different in longevity than groups 2 and 4. In this case group 1 has a younger age at death (67.5) than groups 2 and 4 (71.3 and 72.6, respectively).

‡ A standardized mean of age decade scores of number of serious illnesses.

respect to illness. Illness was measured by the standardized mean of the number of serious illnesses over the age decades. Looking at the covaried means, it is apparent that the light–light group has more illnesses than the light–heavy (group 1 vs group 2) and the heavy–heavy groups (group 1 vs group 4). Likewise, group 1 is less long lived (age at death 67.5) than both groups 2 and 4 (age at death 71.3 and 72.6). Thus, illness explains at least in part the age-at-death differences in these groups. The number of illnesses were the same for those who were light in off-job activity regardless of whether they were heavy or light in on-job activity (groups 1 and 3). These two groups were also the same with regard to age at death. There thus appears to be a three-way concordance between lighter off-job activity, shorter life, and more illnesses.

The only exception to this concordance are groups 3 and 4. Here, within the heavy on-job population, those light in off-job activity are more short lived than the heavy in off-job, but do not have more illnesses. For the heavy on-job population we may surmise that illness is not a factor in accounting for shorter life in those who are light in off-job. This may well be because greater on-job activity is not strongly related to longevity to begin with. However, illness was a factor in determining longevity within the light off-job population (groups 1 and 2).

The entire analysis was replicated without covarying for education to determine secular differences. Without the secular adjustment (we cannot say correction since it is unlikely that controlling for education completely corrects for the secular effect), longevity was reduced within the light off-job and heavy off-job populations when on-job activity was light rather than heavy. These findings make much less sense than the findings with covariation for education, since it suggests that the important predictor for longer life is heavier on-job physical activity. This is precisely the error that was introduced by the design that required that the earlier born (who were more in manual occupations) be longer lived.

Also note that the concordance between more illness and lighter off-job activity within the light on-job population did not hold in the unadjusted analysis; nor did this concordance hold between shorter life and this same group.

Longitudinal Change in Physical Activity and Illness

Another categorical variable that was investigated was a set of four groupings which defined longitudinal change in on-job and off-job activity occurring between the 20s and 40s decades. The aim was to find out whether change in physical activity had any effect on life span, and to pinpoint which type of change was important, whether off-job or on-job or whether from light to heavy or heavy to light. Another question was whether a particular change that was related to shorter life might be explained by concomitant change in illness across the two reference decades. Illness change was measured by subtracting the number of illnesses during the 20s from the number of illnesses during the 40s.

Age-at-death and illness differences in the groups exemplifying the various patterns of change are displayed for on-job and off-job activity in TABLES 12 and 13, respectively. For the group that was heavy in on-job activity during the 20s, those who shifted to light on-job activity during the 40s died 4.5 years earlier than those who did not so shift (66.6 vs 71.1 years). However, there was no differential in illness change between the two groups.

TABLE 12

AGE AT DEATH AND ILLNESS DIFFERENCES IN GROUPS SHOWING LONGITUDINAL
CHANGE IN ON-JOB ACTIVITY FROM THE 20s TO THE 40s DECADE, BY
ANOVA AND THE DUNCAN TEST, AND COVARIED FOR EDUCATION

| Change from 20s to 40s | (n) | Age at Death | | Differences in No. of Illnesses between 20s & 40s | |
		Covaried	Not Covaried	Covaried	Not Covaried
1. Stayed light	(194)	69.8	69.0	0.27	0.26
2. Light to heavy	(33)	70.7	70.6	0.46	0.45
3. Heavy to light	(62)	66.6	66.7	0.32	0.32
4. Stayed heavy	(211)	71.1	71.9	0.21	0.22
F		2.631	4.106	1.084	0.997
p		0.049	0.007	NS	NS
Duncan test †		3–4	1, 3–4	None	None

* To show change, on-job physical activity was dichotomized close to the mean into light (sedentary, light, moderate) and heavy (active and very active).
† See explanation TABLE 11.

TABLE 13

AGE AT DEATH AND ILLNESS DIFFERENCES IN GROUPS SHOWING LONGITUDINAL
CHANGE IN OFF-JOB ACTIVITY FROM THE 20s TO THE 40s DECADE BY
ANOVA AND THE DUNCAN TEST, AND COVARIED FOR EDUCATION

| Change from 20s to 40s * | (n) | Age at Death | | Differences in No. of Illnesses between 20s & 40s | |
		Covaried	Not Covaried	Covaried	Not Covaried
1. Stayed light	(245)	68.7	69.3	0.22	0.22
2. Light to heavy	(0)	—	—	—	—
3. Heavy to light	(73)	66.2	65.2	0.50	0.49
4. Stayed heavy	(182)	73.3	73.0	0.22	0.22
F		13.828	13.134	4.032	3.710
p		0.000	0.000	0.018	0.025
Duncan test †		1, 3–4	1–3, 4 3–4	3–1, 4	3–1, 4

* To show change, off-job physical activity was dichotomized close to the mean into light (sedentary & light) and heavy (moderate, active and very active).
† See explanation TABLE 11.

When education was not covaried, those who stayed heavy on-job lived longer than those who stayed light (71.9 years vs 69.0 years). This would have been a perplexing finding were it not for our insight that it was due to the secular contamination in the data.

For the covaried on-job data in TABLE 12, those in heavy activity who changed to light did not live as long (group 3, age at death 66.6 vs group 4, age at death 71.1). Those in light activity who changed to heavy showed no longevity change (group 1 vs group 2). In none of these instances were there any differentials in illness change across the decades.

We now go to TABLE 13 for the corresponding off-job data. Interestingly there were no cases who changed from light in the 20s to heavy in the 40s. The covaried age-at-death means show shorter life for those who started light and remained light (group 1, age at death 68.7 years) and longer life for those who started heavy and remained heavy (group 4, age at death 73.3 years). These longevity differences could not be ascribed to differences in illnesses across the decades. As in the on-job findings, those who stayed heavy lived longer than those who shifted from heavy to light (group 4 age at death 73.3 years vs group 3 age at death 66.2 years). But unlike the on-job findings, the longer lived group 4 did show less increase in illnesses. In addition, group 1 (stayed light off-job) had less increase in illnesses than group 3 (changed from heavy to light off-job), although there was no significant longevity differential between these two groups.

In sum, longitudinal shift from heavy to light on-job activity was not accompanied by shift to more illness, but the analogous shift in off-job activity was accompanied by shift to more illness. This is consonant with the finding in TABLE 3 regarding the greater sensitivity of off-job activity to illness.

Without covariation, those that stayed heavy in off-job activity across the decades (group 4, age at death 73.0 years) lived longer than those who reduced their off-job activity (group 3, age-at-death 65.2 years). This differential with respect to longer life was accompanied by less increase in illness across the decades. Please note these age-at-death differentials were similar to the on-job covaried age-at-death findings.

Religion

The next categorical variable dealt with was religion (TABLE 14). There were three major religious groupings: Catholic, Protestant, and Jewish. The relationships to on-job activity were as follows. Catholics had more on-job activity than Jews, but Protestants were not significantly different from Catholics and Jews in this respect. There was no change with secular correction, which suggests a stability over time in these relationships. The on-job activity means were also covaried for education (not shown in TABLE 14). With education controlled, the on-job activity differential between Catholics and Jews disappeared.

There were no relationships between religion and off-job activity. The findings were the same when the secular effect was corrected by controlling for age at death; nor did the findings change when education was controlled for.

In contrast to the paucity of findings with physical activity, religion showed a number of differences in longevity. When I adjusted for the secular effect by covarying education, Protestants were more long lived than either Catholics or

TABLE 14

Physical Activity and Age at Death Differences in Religion, by ANOVA and the Duncan Test, Physical Activity Means Covaried for Age at Death, and Age-at-Death Means Covaried for Education

	(n)	On-Job Activity*		Off-Job Activity*		Age at Death	
		Covaried for Age at Death	Not Covaried	Covaried for Age at Death	Not Covaried	Covaried for Education	Not Covaried
1. Catholic	(300)	50.5	50.4	50.1	50.0	68.4	68.8
2. Protestant	(109)	49.6	49.9	50.6	50.9	73.9	73.0
3. Jewish	(81)	48.0	48.1	48.7	48.6	70.0	70.2
F		2.682	2.205	1.209	1.446	9.437	5.346
p		NS	NS	NS	NS	0.000	0.005
Duncan test †		1–3	1–3	None	None	1, 3–2	1–2

* Standardized mean scores of age decade scores.
† See explanation, TABLE 11.

Jews (73.9 years vs 68.4 and 70.0 years). Also there was no significant longevity difference between Catholics and Jews. With no adjustment for education, the longevity differential between Protestants and Jews disappeared, but
the more favorable longevity of Protestants over Catholics was maintained
(73.0 years vs 68.8 years). It is interesting that with or without control for
education there was no longevity differential between Catholics and Jews. One
would have expected that without control for education Jews would have been
more long lived since they were better educated. However, please recall that
those of lower education were born earlier, and by selection lived longer. This
tended to neutralize the advantage of education for longevity in this instance.

In summary, it would appear that Catholic religion is associated with more
on-job physical activity as compared to the Jewish religion, and the Protestant
faith is associated with longer life as compared to Catholicism and Judaism.

Smoking

The question was asked: Are there any systematic relationships between
type of smoking, physical activity, and longevity? The findings are presented
in TABLE 15. There were three major smoking categories, nonsmokers, pipe
and/or cigar smokers, and cigarette smokers. With secular control, there were
no relationships between type of smoking and extent of either on-job or off-job
physical activity. However, cigarette smokers died earlier than either nonsmokers or pipe and cigar smokers. There were no significant age-at-death
differences between nonsmokers and pipe and cigar smokers.

With no secular control, pipe and cigar smokers were higher in on-job
activity than cigarette smokers and were also more long lived than cigarette
smokers (77.7 vs 65.8 years). This is a reflection of the fact that those born
earlier were more apt to be cigar and pipe smokers, while those born later (and
therefore in less long lived group) were more apt to be cigarette smokers, due
to the secular shift to cigarette smoking.

In summary, cigarette smokers were no different from other smoker types
in physical exercise but were shorter lived.

Drinking

The same questions regarding physical activity and longevity were raised
with the various drinking types (TABLE 16). There were five such categories:
teetotalers, beer drinkers, wine drinkers, hard liquor drinkers, and a final group
of eclectic drinkers who could not be categorized as being primarily in one of
the four preceding groups. Covarying for age at death, the hard liquor drinkers
had lower on-job activity than beer, wine and combination drinkers. Interestingly enough, the teetotalers were not significantly different in on-job activity
from any of the other four categories. When the on-job means were adjusted
for education (not shown in TABLE 16), only the combination drinkers were
more physically active on the job than the hard liquor drinkers.

Whether secularity was controlled or not, the hard liquor drinkers were less
active on the job than the wine and combination drinkers. However, there was
no significant difference between hard liquor and beer drinkers. The latter could
be explained by secular shift to more beer drinking and less on-job activity, or

TABLE 15

PHYSICAL ACTIVITY AND AGE AT DEATH DIFFERENCES IN SMOKING, BY ANOVA AND THE DUNCAN TEST, PHYSICAL ACTIVITY MEANS COVARIED FOR AGE AT DEATH, AND AGE-AT-DEATH MEANS COVARIED FOR EDUCATION

	(n)	On-Job Activity*		Off-Job Activity*		Age at Death	
		Covaried for Age at Death	Not Covaried	Covaried for Age at Death	Not Covaried	Covaried for Education	Not Covaried
1. None	(67)	48.8	49.5	50.8	51.4	75.8	75.8
2. Pipes, cigars	(122)	50.8	51.7	49.9	50.7	77.3	77.7
3. Cigarettes	(311)	49.8	49.3	49.8	49.3	65.9	65.8
F		1.255	3.421	0.370	2.113	66.166	71.096
p		NS	.033	NS	NS	0.000	0.000
Duncan test †		None	2–3	None	None	1, 2–3	1, 2–3

* Standardized mean scores of age decade scores.
† See explanation, TABLE 11.

TABLE 16

PHYSICAL ACTIVITY AND AGE AT DEATH DIFFERENCES IN DRINKING, BY ANOVA AND THE DUNCAN TEST, PHYSICAL ACTIVITY MEANS COVARIED FOR AGE AT DEATH, AND AGE-AT-DEATH MEANS COVARIED FOR EDUCATION

	(n)	On-Job Activity *		Off-Job Activity *		Age at Death	
		Covaried for Age at Death	Not Covaried	Covaried for Age at Death	Not Covaried	Covaried for Education	Not Covaried
1. Teetotal	(63)	49.3	50.1	50.1	50.4	73.6	73.0
2. Beer	(108)	50.8	50.3	49.8	49.3	65.5	65.6
3. Wine	(50)	51.7	52.4	49.8	50.4	74.9	76.0
4. Hard Liquor	(178)	48.3	48.2	50.8	50.7	69.6	69.2
5. Combinations	(101)	51.3	51.5	48.5	48.6	70.9	71.4
F		3.239	3.704	1.116	1.078	8.991	9.460
p		0.012	0.006	NS	NS	0.000	0.000
Duncan test †		2, 3, 5–4	4–3, 5	None	None	1–2, 4 2–3, 4, 5 3–4, 5	1–2, 4 2–3, 4 3–4, 5

* Standardized mean scores of age decade scores.
† See explanation, TABLE 11.

secular shift to less hard liquor and less on-job activity. This could account for absence of on-job differentials between hard liquor and beer drinkers when secularity was not controlled.

In contrast, there were no differences in off-job activity by type of drinker.

There were, however, definite differences in longevity by type of drinker. The teetotaler lived longer than the beer and hard liquor drinker (73.6 vs 65.5 and 69.6 years); and the wine, hard liquor, and combination drinkers lived longer than the beer drinkers (74.9, 69.6, and 70.9 vs 65.5 years). In addition, the wine drinker lived longer than the hard liquor and combination drinkers (74.9 vs 69.6 and 70.9 years). The beer drinkers, then, had the least favorable longevity, the hard liquor drinker had the next least favorable longevity and the teetotaler had the most favorable longevity.

In sum, the teetotaler and wine drinker, who lived the longest, were no different from the others in physical activity. On the other hand, the beer drinker with least favorable longevity had more on-job activity and poorer longevity than, for example, the combination drinker.

SUMMARY

By this time the reader must be weary of methodological discussions, as important as they are to the investigator. I therefore will confine this summary to substantive findings. However, I do hope that the reader has come to appreciate the importance of methodologic issues relative to substantive findings at the current state of the art of longevity prediction.

With detailed biographic data of 500 deaths, I considered the amount of physical exertion over the life cycle as it related to longevity in the context of other predictors of longevity. I considered physical activity separately in two areas: that occurring on-job, in the course of occupational pursuit, and that occurring off-job, i.e., in the residual area of one's life when not formally engaged in the pursuit of one's livelihood. I made this separation because higher exertion on the job was related to a manual or blue collar occupation, which was in turn related to lower social class life-styles and less favorable longevity. Indeed, the correlates of on- and off-job activity showed startlingly different characteristics. Higher education, occupational level, and intelligence went with higher off-job activity, and the inverse with higher on-job activity. In addition, those high in off-job physical exertion were more urban than those high in on-job activity. Since higher education, occupational level, and intelligence are also correlates of longevity, these differences help us to understand why higher off-job activity is much more related to longer life than higher on-job activity.

The special role of off-job activity in promoting longevity was further suggested by the following: Those in occupations requiring lighter physical exertion, but who indulged in heavier off-job physical activity, lived an average of 3.8 years longer than those light in both on- and off-job activity. In addition, those who were heavy in off-job both during their 20s and 40s lived 4.6 years longer than those who were light in off-job during both periods. Even more dramatic was the fact that those who stayed heavy during both periods lived 7.1 years longer than those who dropped from heavy in the 20s to light in the 40s.

Relative to other factors, physical exertion, specifically of the off-job type, was a better longevity predictor than about ⅔ of the variables considered. Off-job activity during the decade 40–49 was the best longevity predictor of any of the physical activity variables. Nevertheless, there were a number more important than this measure. Some of them in order of importance were: fewer illnesses, less smoking, and less worried. About as important were rural residence and higher occupational level.

When cigarette smokers were compared to nonsmokers and pipe/cigar smokers, they were found to be shorter lived (by 9.9 and 11.4 years, respectively), though no different in on- or off-job physical activity from the others. With respect to drinking, the teetotaler lived 8.1 years longer than the beer drinkers and 4.0 years longer than those who drank hard liquor. Again, there were no physical activity differences among these groups. Physical activity, then, was not involved in the smoking and drinking longevity differentials.

Finally, I ask the reader's indulgence for concluding with a methodological point. I must do this since it introduces an all-important next step in longevity prediction research. In any study of human subjects, differences in birth year may introduce a secular contaminant into the data. This is due to the differential impact of social and technologic change on the subjects of different birth year. Such birth year differences were present in this study and attempts were made to reduce the secular effect by statistical manipulations. However, it is important to carry out a secular-free design based on populations alike in birth year. Such a specific study has been proposed as a follow-up to the present investigation.

REFERENCES

1. GRUMAN, G. J. 1960. A history of ideas about the prolongation of life—The evaluation of prolongevity hypotheses to 1800. Trans. Amer. Philos. Soc. **56** (Part a).
2. EDDINGTON, D. W. 1972. Exercise and longevity: Evidence for a threshold age. J. Geront. **27:** 341–343.
3. ROSE, C. L. & B. BELL. 1971. Predicting longevity: Methodology and critique. D. C. Heath and Co. Lexington, Mass.
4. BELL, B., C. L. ROSE & A. DAMON. 1966. The Veterans Administration longitudinal study of healthy aging. Gerontologist **6:** 179–184.
5. BELL, B., C. L. ROSE & A. DAMON. 1972. The Normative Aging Study: An interdisciplinary and longitudinal study of health and aging. Aging and Human Devel. **3:** 5–17.
6. Metropolitan Life Insurance Co. 1938. College men long lived. Stat. Bull. **3**(8).
7. HAENSZEL, W., M. B. SHIMKIN & H. P. MILLER. 1956. Tobacco smoking patterns in the United States. Pub. Health Serv. Monograph No. 45, Pub. No. 463. Washington, D.C.
8. SPIEGELMAN, M. 1963. The changing democratic spectrum and its implications for health. Eugenics Q. **10:** 161–174.
9. COHEN, B. H. 1964. Family patterns of mortality and lifespan. Q. Rev. Biol. **39:** 130–181.
10. ROSE, C. L. & B. BELL. 1971. Predicting longevity: Methodology and critique. : 211–213. D. C. Heath and Co. Lexington, Mass.
11. THOMLINSON, R. 1965. Population dynamics, causes and consequences of world demographic change. : 132. Random House. New York, N.Y.
12. DUBLIN, L. I., A. J. LOTKA & M. SPIEGELMAN. 1949. Length of life. : 55. Ronald Press. New York, N.Y.
13. DUBLIN, L. I. & R. J. VANE. 1947. Occupational mortality experience of insured wage earners. Monthly Labor Rev. **64:** 1003.

14. GURALNICK, L. 1962. Mortality by occupation and industry among men 20–64
    years of age: U.S., 1950. Vital Statistics, Special Reports 3(2): 59–70.
15. HAMMOND, E. C. & D. HORN. 1958. Smoking and death rates—Report on 44
    months of follow-up on 187,783 men. Part I. Total mortality. J. Amer. Med.
    Assoc. 166: 1159–1172.
16. ZONNEVELD, R. J. & A. POLMAN. 1957. Hereditary factors in longevity. Acta
    Genet. Stat. Med. 7: 160–162.
17. WILSON, E. B. & C. R. DOERING. 1926. The "Elder Pierces". Proc. Nat. Acad.
    Sci. 12: 424–432.
18. PALMORE, E. 1971. Health practices, illness and longevity. In Prediction of life-
    span. E. Palmore & F. C. Jeffers, Eds. D. C. Heath and Co., Lexington, Mass.

APPENDIX 1

VARIABLES USED IN THE ANALYSIS OTHER THAN THE PHYSICAL ACTIVITY VARIABLES
LISTED IN ORDER OF DESCENDING PARTIAL CORRELATION WITH AGE AT DEATH,
CONTROLLING FOR EDUCATION

High Point of Variable	Definition	Partial r	Zero-Order r
1. T score total number of illnesses, mean	Number of serious illnesses, operations, or accidents (for illness variables within age decade, see TABLE 3)	−0.46	−0.47
2. Younger appearance, 40 and over	Score: 1, much older; 2, a little older; 3, looked his age; 4, a little younger; 5, much less younger	0.46	0.46
3. Less smoking before 40	Score: 1, very heavy, 2 or more packs of cigarettes, 7 or more pipes or cigars a day; 2, heavy, about 1 pack of cigarettes but less than 2 packs, 5–6 pipes, or 5–6 cigars a day; 3, moderate, about ½ pack of cigarettes, 3–4 pipes, or 3–4 cigars a day; 4, light, less than ½ pack, 1–2 pipes, or 1–2 cigars a day; 5, none, less than 1 cigarette, pipe, or cigar a day. The above are based on estimates of lifetime averages.	0.29	0.28
4. Less smoking, 40 and over	Same scoring as above.	0.29	0.30
5. Less worried	Score: 1, always; 2, usually; 3, rarely; 4, never.	0.28	0.30
6. Younger appearance under 40	Score: 1, much older; 2, a little older; 3, looked his age; 4, a little younger; 5, much less younger.	−0.25	0.25
7. Urban vs rural	Formula for score is $25(\Sigma XY - L)L$, where X = weight given to location in accordance with the following: 5, farm or village, 1,000 population; 4, town, 1,000 up to 10,000; 3, small city, 10,000 up to 100,000; 2, medium city, 100,000 up to 500,000; 1, large city, 500,000 and over; Y = years resided in each location; and L = age at death. Range of score is 00 to 99.	0.24	0.28
8. Occupational level	Score: 0, unskilled; 1, semi-skilled; 2, skilled; 3, white collar, clerical, sales; 4, semi-professional, proprietory; 5, professional.	0.24	0.10
9. Education	Score: 1, never attended school; 2, completed 4 grades; 3, completed 5–7 grades; 4, completed 8 grades; 5, entered high school, didn't graduate; 6, graduated high school; 7, some college, business school; 8, completed college; 9, beyond college.	—	−0.21

10.	Foreign vs native born	Score: 1, parents and son foreign born; 2, parents foreign born; son native born; 3, one of parents native and son native born; 4, both parents and son native born.	−0.20	−0.27
11.	Intelligence	Score: 1, far below average; 2, slightly above average; 3, average; 4, above average; 5, superior.	0.20	0.07
12.	Age at death of mother		0.18	0.16
13.	Less active than others	Score: 1, much more; 2, a little more; 3, same; 4, a little less; 5, much less.	−0.17	−0.15
14.	Conserved energy	Score: 1, always; 2, usually; 3, rarely; 4, never.	−0.16	−0.17
15.	Younger wife	Score: 1, spouse older by 10 or more years; 2, by 7–9 years; 3, by 4–6 years; 4, by 1–3 years; 5, same age; 6, spouse younger by 1–3 years; 7, by 4–6 years; 8, by 7–9 years; 9, by 10 or more years.	0.15	0.18
16.	Not easily aggravated	Score: 1, always; 2, usually; 3, rarely; 4, never.	0.15	0.12
17.	Greater age difference, oldest and youngest child		0.14	0.16
18.	More daily hours diversion before age 65		−0.14	−0.15
19.	No occupational hazard	Score: 1, very hazardous; 2, somewhat hazardous; 3, no hazard	−0.14	−0.15
20.	Not catch colds easily	Score: 1, yes; 2, no.	0.14	0.15
21.	Older age at first marriage		0.14	0.11
22.	Not lived dangerously	Score: 1, always; 2, usually; 3, rarely; 4, never.	0.12	0.11
23.	Less drinking, 40 and over	Amount of drinking is average daily drinking. One drink defined as jigger of hard liquor, cocktail, glass of wine, or 2 glasses of beer. Score: 1, very heavy, 5 or more drinks; 2, heavy, 3–4 drinks; 3, moderate, 1–2 drinks; 4, occasional, less than one drink; 5, none, teetotaler.	0.12	0.09
24.	Less drinking, under 40		0.11	0.07
25.	Less trusting	Score: 1, always trusting; 2, usually; 3, rarely; 4, never.	0.11	0.13
26.	Less sense of humor	Score: 1, always had sense of humor; 2, usually; 3, rarely; 4, never.	0.09	0.11

APPENDIX 1—Continued

Categorical Variables

27. Physical activity groups—TABLE 11.

28. Groups showing different patterns of longitudinal change in on-job physical activity—TABLE 12.

29. Groups showing different patterns of longitudinal change in off-job physical activity—TABLE 13.

30. Religious groups: 1, Catholic; 2, Protestant; 3, Jewish.

31. Smoker groups: 1, none; 2, pipes-cigars; 3, cigarettes.

32. Drinker groups: 1, teetotaler; 2, beer; 3, wine; 4, hard liquor; 5, combinations.

STATISTICAL PROCEDURES

The large variable set in this paper was dealt with by standard statistical methods. They are briefly described below.

Zero-Order Correlations: These involve the degree to which two variables are associated. The variables should be continuous and ordered. Mathematically, the correlation is the covariance of the two variables divided by the square root of the product of the variances. Variance is a measure of the dispersion of the data about the mean, and, mathematically, is the average squared deviation from the mean. Covariance is the average of the product of the individual deviations of the two variables from their respective means.

First-Order Correlations: These involve the degree to which two variables are associated, with the linear effect of a third variable removed and thereby controlled. They are useful for uncovering spurious relationships because of the fact that the two variables are both correlated with a third variable.

Stepwise Multiple Regression: This is used to isolate a subset of available predictor variables that will yield an optimal prediction equation with as few terms as possible. It is the best possible prediction of a dependent variable from a linear combination of independent variables. Independent variables are entered one by one on the basis of highest partial correlation with the dependent variable at that point. As each variable is entered, the effects of all previously entered variables have been controlled.

One-Way Analysis of Variance (ANOVA): This yields means and variances of an ordered dependent variable by groups of an independent categorical variable. An F ratio is used to determine whether there are significant differences among the group means. This test for equality among group means involves the ratio of the among-groups variance to the within-group variance. The among-groups variance is the weighted estimate of the population variance (sum of squared deviations of group means from grand mean, divided by the number of groups minus one). The within-group variance is the sum of the group variances divided by the number of individuals minus the number of groups. The level of statistical significance of the F ratio is dependent upon three factors: the value of the F ratio, the number of groups minus one, and the total number of individuals minus the number of groups.

Duncan Test for Difference of Means: This test performs a series of statistical tests on the significance of difference between each pair of means generated by an ANOVA. The Duncan test avoids the error of the t-test, which results from chance significant differences between a pair of means when there are more than two groups. For example, under the t-test, with 6 groups, or 15 pairs, the probability of a pair showing a significant difference at the 0.05 level on the basis of chance is 40%.

Analysis of Covariance: If an unmeasured third variable is believed to affect the relationship between an independent and dependent variable in an ANOVA, the effect on the dependent variable can be removed through analysis of covariance. This is done by regressing the dependent variable on the third variable. The regression formula yields a predicted score of the dependent variable for each individual. This is subtracted from the actual score of the dependent variable, giving a residualized score for each individual. This set of residualized scores becomes the scores of the dependent variable, and the ANOVA proceeds in the normal fashion.

Use of Software Packages to Carry Out Computer-Assisted Statistical Analysis: The Statistical Package for the Social Sciences (SPSS), designed by a group from the University of Chicago, provided the algorithms for the above procedures. This package is advantageous because it does not require extraneous programs for such tasks as handling missing observations, generating and recoding variables, and formatting the results of the statistical analysis on a print out.

A CRITIQUE OF SEVERAL EPIDEMIOLOGICAL STUDIES OF PHYSICAL ACTIVITY AND ITS RELATIONSHIP TO AGING, HEALTH, AND MORTALITY

K. S. Brown

Faculty of Mathematics
University of Waterloo
Waterloo, Ontario
N2L 3G1 Canada

Paul Milvy

Department of Community Medicine
Mount Sinai School of Medicine
New York, New York 10029

PREFACE

A word of explanation about the following and final paper in this session. One of the problems faced when soliciting papers for a conference is to assure scientific excellence. When a paper is submitted to a first-class scientific journal, it is, without exception, reviewed by one's colleagues, that is, by referees who are experts in the particular discipline. The paper is either published or not published, based on their opinion of its merit. This in general does not occur at a conference. The people who organize a conference endeavor to pick the best scientists and doctors of whom they are aware, and invite them to make a presentation. And they let it go at that. We thought in the very controversial area covered by this session where clearly there is a great deal of disagreement as to the virtues or vices of running (and even physical activity in general) in relationship to morbidity and mortality, that it might be a good idea to very carefully inform the authors of the papers at this session that we anticipated accurate and carefully conceived papers. We also suggested that explanatory appendices might be useful if they could help clarify the manner in which the investigator may or may not have handled his data. I mentioned this in my remarks opening this session. But we did not tell the authors that this final paper was intended as a critique of all the papers in this session with, I can assure you, the exception of the first paper. This final paper then is a critique of the manuscripts submitted for publication, which we received early on, before the start of the conference.

INTRODUCTION

In the first paper of this session, a number of the problems faced by the epidemiologist who wishes to establish the role of physical activity in the aging process or in the study of health were outlined. It was emphasized there that the definitive "experiment" in this area, that is, the clinical trial, is generally not practical because of the large sample sizes required, the lengthy duration of the study, the problem of dropouts and transfers to and from exercise groups possibly because of a number of health-related factors, and the possible intrusion of bias into such trials because blind or double-blind trials are not feasible.

Thus, in evaluating any study concerning the relationship between physical activity and health, the available evidence and study design must be appraised carefully with regard to the possible influence of self-selection; the presence of variables associated with both physical activity and health (confounding variables); the definition of both the "cause," physical activity, and the "effect," health status; the choice of control group; the appropriateness of any statistical technique used in the data analysis; and the validity of the conclusions. As well, an additional difficulty in assessing the effect of any variable (e.g., physical activity) on the aging process ought to be emphasized. Aging processes are generally considered to be progressive and irreversible and begin or accelerate at maturity in systems that undergo growth and development. Although many so-called risk factors may accelerate aging processes, other variables merely alter with age in a manner that suggests a relationship to the aging process. However, in the definition of an index of biological age, it is neither necessary nor sufficient to insist that an index correlates closely with chronological age.[1] Rather, it is required that abnormal levels of any such index predict increased morbidity or mortality at each age. Thus, in an attempt to show that physical activity affects aging processes it must be demonstrated that physical activity affects biological age and is not merely associated with an altered pattern of chronological age change.

Critical reviews of studies on physical activity and health have been published elsewhere,[2-4] but the purpose of the present paper is to comment on the papers presented in this session with regard to the above-mentioned factors.

CRITIQUES *

Goldman and Dill: A Physiological Profile of a Jogging Class: Young and Old, Male and Female

The authors report on a cross-sectional study of an entire cohort of joggers. Unfortunately, the lack of any control group, or of any preprogram measurements does not permit any evaluation of the relationship between the program and the health-related variables measured. Also, the dependent variable, $\dot{V}_{O_2 \, max}$, used as a measure of fitness is influenced by natural endowment and may not relate directly to the beneficial effects of habitual physical activity. Moreover, the authors do not mention confounding variables such as smoking and drinking habits or other life-style variables, and thus it is difficult to assess or generalize their findings. This, of course, represents a difficulty with most studies of this type.

With respect to the methodology employed, stepwise regression techniques were used to obtain a "reduced set" of variables that can predict $\dot{V}_{O_2 \, max}$. Based on this set, subjects were classified as to whether they are less fit or in a good state of fitness relative to the predicted value obtained from the reduced models. The authors comment on the difficulties of using such models since they are

---

* Authors' responses to these critiques may be found in the Addendum of this paper.

based on small sample sizes, because the R^2 values are small, and because the models may not be linear as assumed. Also, it should be noted that the stepwise procedure may not always produce an optimal subset of independent variables,[5] or there may be other sets that would predict $\dot{V}_{O_2 \, max}$ with the same degree of precision. In either case, subjects ranked "fit" might be predicted to be "unfit" under a different choice of model, and vice versa. More seriously, if the model chosen described the data adequately, then the positive or negative residuals will be due to *random* departures from the model and may not be related to fitness. Therefore such departures may not give a reasonable discrimination into the two fitness groups. Finally, had the psychological traits been analyzed in a 2×2 contingency table as shown (TABLE 1), the comparison of the "fit" and "unfit" in the sample would not have been based on a comparison of the groups to a reference population, the characteristics of which may not be similar to the one under study. That is, a more reasonable hypothesis to test would seem to be that the proportions of individuals with high levels of the psychological variable are the *same* in each "fitness" group (but not necessarily 0.5).

TABLE 1

2×2 CONTNGENCY TABLE ANALYSIS OF RELATIONSHIP BETWEEN FITNESS
AND A PSYCHOLOGICAL VARIABLE

| Fitness | Psychological Variable | |
	High	Low
High		
Low		

Leon and Blackburn: The Relationship of Physical Activity to Coronary Heart Disease and Life Expectancy

This paper represents a review, comparable to the first paper in the session, and covers similar ground; however, some points might be noted.

Reference is made to the populations in the Caucasus, and elsewhere, who have been reported to have significantly longer lifespan than other populations and who have some very old members. However, there is considerable doubt whether the relevant mortality data are reliable, and hence observations concerning that population should be regarded as unsubstantiated anecdotal evidence.[6] Related to this point is the statement that "much of the reduced work and cardiorespiratory capacity previously attributed to aging is actually the result of physical inactivity." In fact, as stated earlier, indices of aging are difficult to define and, unless reduced work and cardiorespiratory capacity can be shown to lead to a shortened lifespan, it is not justified to consider reduced work and cardiorespiratory capacity as representing a measure of aging processes. This, of course, is the crux of the problem, namely, whether physical inactivity reduces the lifespan, other parameters being equal.

Lastly, the final statement in their paper that exercise "should be carried out at least 2 to 4 times per week for 30 to 60 minutes a session" is unjustified since there is no evidence that such a precisely defined regimen would be beneficial to all members of the population, although it might be anticipated that it would be not harmful to the majority of the population.

Bassler: Marathon Running and Immunity to Atherosclerosis

This paper presents interesting anecdotal evidence regarding the relationship between marathon running and immunity to fatal atherosclerosis.† There are,

---

† Dr. J. E. Edwards of the Department of Pathology and Clinical Laboratories, Miller Division, United Hospitals, St. Paul, Minnesota, kindly consented to review the manuscript. His comments included the following:

"Actual interpretation of the material presented is open to question, as there is no clear documentation of the 200 reports that the author claims to have reviewed. In the actual material that he presents, there are certain fallacies, which I have taken up from the point of view of the attempts at pathologic documentation of his claims. My comments concerning these are considered below according to case numbers and corresponding figure numbers. From the material that will follow, it is apparent that, for Case 16, at least, there is good evidence of coronary atherosclerotic disease, while the author disclaims such a cause and, without scientific basis, explains away what should be accepted as a coronary death.

"In a general way, it is open to question as to whether atherosclerotic lesions developed to the point of showing fibrosis and calcification can resorb, and also it is peculiar that there is an implication that among marathon runners little coronary disease is present. This is contrary to findings in the general population and I would have been more inclined to believe the claims if there would have been more cases with some coronary atherosclerosis of some degree. To imply that atherosclerotic disease does not occur or is resorbed in the marathon runner just doesn't fit reality.

"*Case 1* (FIGURES 1 & 2): Lesion is that of atherosclerosis. An inflammatory reaction is not unusual.

"*Case 14* (FIGURES 3–6): FIGURE 3 is consistent with mild luminal narrowing from atherosclerosis. The legend of FIGURE 4 identifies this as the same vessel as in FIGURE 3 at higher magnification. The part of the vessel of FIGURE 3 that is shown in higher magnification is not identified. The process in FIGURE 4 is that of atherosclerosis. In FIGURE 5 the lumen is more than 50% narrowed by atherosclerosis. This degree of narrowing is consistent with significant atherosclerosis. For FIGURE 6, it is not indicated what part of the vessel in FIGURE 5 was enlarged to yield FIGURE 6. Atheroma shows vessels, a common phenomenon. It is not valid to conclude that the process of vessels being present is a sign of 'resorption.'

"*Case 16* (FIGURES 7–12): In FIGURE 7 the process is that of an organized thrombus in an atherosclerotic segment. It is wrong to imply that the 'new channels' resulted from running. They are simply part of the process of organization of a thrombus. FIGURE 8 is a picture of an organized thrombus. The vessels are not to be interpreted as a sign of 'resorption of fibrous plaque.' In regard to FIGURES 9 and 10, within myocardium, small vessels may show fibroelastic thickening of intima. The cause is unknown. Some are probably related to hypertension, others to old inflammation, among other causes. There is no established basis that such lesions result from smoking. In FIGURES 11 and 12, the ischemic microlesions may, in fact, be small infarcts related to demonstrated obstructive disease of the right coronary artery.

"The text relative to this case states, 'The vascular scar and recanalized artery may have been part of the increased collateral circulation, perhaps induced by the marathon training.' This statement makes a number of assumptions not supported by facts. Increased collateral circulation was not established. Even if it had been, the observed changes mentioned are common, every day situations. In organized coronary thrombi, vascular connective tissue is common, representing organiaztion of thrombi.

however, a number of points concerning the methodology and the presentation of the results that are open to serious criticisms.

For example the author claims that marathon running dictates a life-style that protects against fatal atherosclerosis (heart attack and stroke). However, it is not clear how it is possible to determine if it is the life-style that dictates marathon running or vice versa, or if some external factor (e.g., genetic disposition to large arteries, or a particular constitution type) tends to determine both the life-style and marathon running. That is, if, for example, nonsmokers are more liable to take up marathon running and these individuals develop less atherosclerosis (ASCVD), then the marathon running may have little to do with less ASCVD. On the other hand, if marathon running causes persons to quit smoking and subsequently develop less ASCVD, it is not clear that every individual who takes up marathon running will be affected similarly, since individuals who quit smoking after beginning to exercise may represent a subgroup which might have a lower probability of developing ASCVD in any case. The type of data presented do not allow this type of separation and therefore do not permit the examination of the effects of many variables undoubtedly confounded with any protective effect of marathon running.

To illustrate further the lack of quantitative documentation, the author claims in his "Methods" that more than 200 reports of deaths in marathoners (42-km-men) have been received and points out that, "many are duplicates. Most were below the 42-km threshold." His comment, "To date there have been no reports of fatal ASCVD, histologically proven, among 42-km-men," would have been more impressive had the total case load relevant to the hypothesis been provided. In the paper, only 22 selected cases, including Pheidippides are mentioned, and at least five of these were not 42-km-men.

With respect to the author's claim, it is of interest to estimate the number of deaths from ASCVD that would be expected in a cohort that generally does not smoke, is not obese, is well educated, young, and in an upper social class, and has no congenital heart disease, emphysema, bronchitis, or other disability that might preclude marathon training, but does not engage in marathon running. Such an examination of the 1975 American cohort of marathon finishers was presented earlier in this session [7] and suggests that, even if marathon running provided no direct protection, only one or two ischemic and related heart disease deaths per year would be expected in a cohort with a similar age structure and with similar relative weight and smoking characteristics as in the cohort of the marathon finishers.

Generally, the use of anecdotal reports and circular arguments detracts appreciably from this study. For example:

(1) Case 13: "ASCVD is a remote possibility in view of the normal stress test, no smoking, and the impressive number of 10-km runs."

(2) Case 17: "He had stopped running his usual 20 km per day; at the same time he markedly increased his fat intake."

(3) "The inflammatory reaction is less in the plaque of the 42-km-man than the 10-km-man in spite of the fact that the 42-km-man is twice the age of the 10-km-man. This difference is probably related to the content of UFAs (un-

---

Certain myocardial scars are highly vascular, a phenomenon that is common in the population. Such scars found in individuals dying suddenly of coronary origin are frequently misinterpreted in gross examination as acute infarcts, interpretations that are not borne out histologically as they simply are old vascular scars."

saturated fatty acids)." No information is provided as to how these men were matched or how this difference, based on a sample of size two, can be ascribed to the content of UFAs.

It is of course not possible, on the basis of the data provided, to dispute the claim that no fatal cases of ASCVD have been observed in 42-km-men. However, it should be stressed that without more precise information on the number of cases examined, and the number of cases expected in a similarly matched cohort of nonmarathon runners, the evidence provided does not justify the conclusion reached by the author.

A general point that relates to this study, and those of Rosenman *et al.* and Cooper and Meyer, is the validity of searching for deaths from one particular cause of death. That is, the evidence with regard to the relationship of physical activity to health would be more impressive in terms of a protective effect of physical activity if it were shown that an increased life expectancy was associated with marathon running or any other form a physical activity. In Dr. Bassler's paper, no information concerning the age at death of a marathon cohort has been provided, which would permit the testing of this hypothesis.

Noakes, Opie, Beck, McKechnie, Benchiniol, and Desser: Coronary Heart Disease in Marathon Runners

This paper has been presented in an attempt to refute the "Bassler Hypothesis." The six cases provide evidence that coronary arteriosclerotic heart disease may occur in marathon runners.‡ However, of the six cases only one

‡ Dr. Jose Meller, Director of Non-Invasive Laboratories, Mount Sinai Hospital, New York, New York, kindly commented upon the clinical findings and ECGs provided by Dr. Noakes, as follows:

"In case 1 the history is very suggestive of angina pectoris and acute myocardial infarction. It is disturbing that the patient died at 6:40 PM, in an intensive care unit, without any more information about the cause of death.

"Cases 2 and 6 have clear coronary artery disease, proven by angiography. Case 3 seems peculiar. It is difficult to recognize any coronary obstruction in the supplied figure; however, in reviewing the cineangiograms there is a significant left anterior descending coronary artery obstruction and an apical left ventricular aneurysm.

"Case 5 is equivocal. The patient was told of the diagnosis of mitral valve prolapse, subsequently not correlated by echocardiography. FIGURE 12 does not show a positive exercise test. Depression of the ST segments is seen (V5–V6), but it cannot be evaluated in the presence of a wandering baseline. As coronary angiography was not done on this patient, the diagnosis of coronary artery disease can be suspected only on the basis of a probable history and an abnormal electrocardiogram; however, if the patient did actually have mitral valve prolapse, the electrocardiographic findings then become more equivocal.

"In case 4 we see a markedly abnormal left ventriculogram with *diffused* asynergy (FIGURES 9a & b), as seen in cardiomyopathy. The degree of left ventricular dysfunction is out of proportion to the type of coronary artery obstruction reported (which I do not see in the supplied figure) and if it is present in cases like this we always assume it is only coincidental coronary artery disease.

"In summary, of the six patients, cases 1, 2, 3, and 6 seem to be patients with coronary artery disease, clinically, electrocardiographically, and/or angiographically. In case 4, the clinical and electrocardiographic findings suggest coronary artery disease; however, angiography showed coronary obstruction only in the distal branch of the right coronary artery, and with the available left ventriculogram pictures cardio-

involved death and no postmortem examination was performed. Technically then, these cases would not refute Bassler's claim that there have been no reports of fatal ASCVD, histologically proven, among 42-km-men. Nevertheless, the following statement should be noted:

". . . We conclude that the marathon runners studied were not immune to coronary heart disease, nor to coronary atherosclerosis and that high levels of physical fitness did not guarantee the absence of significant cardiovascular disease. In addition, the relationship of exercise and myocardial infarction was complex because two athletes developed myocardial infarction during marathon running in the absence of complete coronary artery occlusion. We stress that marathon runners, like other sportsmen, should be warned of the serious significance of the development of exertional symptoms.

"Our conclusions do not reflect on the possible value of exercise in the prevention of coronary heart disease. Rather we refute exaggerated claims that marathon running provides complete immunity from coronary heart disease."

Rosenman, Bawol, and Osherwitz: A 4-Year Prospective Study of the Relationship of Different Habitual Vocational Physical Activity to Risk and Incidence of Ischemic Heart Disease in Volunteer Male Federal Employees

This study represents a carefully analyzed prospective investigation of coronary heart disease (CHD) and coronary heart disease risk in relation to habitual vocational physical activity. The prospective study has the advantage that the supposed causes precede the supposed effects, but nevertheless it is unable to separate the effect of self-selection. Moreover, it is unable to assess the effects of changes in variables as measured originally in the study. Such changes (as opposed to absolute levels) might be important predictors of future CHD, and further might be expected to be more pronounced in "cases," and thus may help to discriminate between cases and controls.

This investigation presents an interesting example of confounding variables, namely, education and income. Education and income levels, as expected, are higher in the lower activity jobs, and thus the effect of activity level on CHD incidence will be confounded with the effects of income and education (i.e., socioeconomic status) and variables related to higher socioeconomic status (SES). For example, the authors note that the risk factors related to higher CHD incidence tend to increase from low to moderate to heavy physical activity groups, and from high to medium to low categories of SES. When SES is "controlled" by analysis of variance techniques, there does not appear to be any significant difference in CHD risk scores between the three physical activity groups.

With regard to the statistical treatment of the data, the authors use the coefficients from the multiple logistic model estimated from the Framingham data to compute CHD risk scores for their population. It should be noted that

myopathy seems a more likely diagnosis. Case 5 has a clinical history less suggestive of coronary artery disease, however, the electrocardiograms are consistent with such diagnosis. As coronary arteriography was not performed, the diagnosis of coronary artery disease seems possible, but not certain."

it is not necessarily justified to assume that these coefficients are relevant for this or any other population. Werko [8] emphasizes this point:

". . . considerations regarding the mode of selection of the populations for the Framingham Study thus lead to the conclusion that any result of this study is only applicable to that part of the population of the city of Framingham that has taken part in the study, i.e., at best a middle-class suburban population in a fairly good economic, social, and educational situation.

"Instead, research workers of all kinds have used the Framingham data as if it represented the male population not only in the USA, but in the whole Western industrialized part of the world."

In particular, the percentage of subjects with an abnormal ECG seems high, and the percentage of smokers seems low relative to the Framingham population.[9] Also, there has been no discussion concerning the goodness of fit of the multiple logistic models derived in the latter part of the paper, and while the major risk factors (age, blood pressure, serum cholesterol, and cigarette smoking) appear to distinguish cases from controls, no comparison to the Framingham models is provided. However, the use of these techniques illustrates the type of multivariate approach that must be followed if the complex associations between factors that elevate coronary heart disease risk are to be untangled, and the "essential" risk factors revealed.

In their conclusion, the authors emphasize that "the fundamental questions are whether physical conditioning significantly alters other risk factors for CHD, prolongs life, or reduces the incidence of primary or recurrent clinical CHD." This prospective study suggests that vocational physical activity in this population is not related to this increased risk of CHD. However, as the authors point out, whether purposeful exercise may be beneficial to certain subgroups of the population cannot be inferred from the data.

Cooper, Meyer, Blide, Pollock, and Gibbons: The Important Role of Fitness Determination and Stress Testing in Predicting Coronary Incidence

This paper presents a case-control study involving the matching at the individual level, of 27 males from the Cooper clinic, healthy when examined but who later experienced CHD, with 81 controls similar with regard to Framingham risk score but free of CHD at any examination. The matching appears to be carried out carefully, and assuming that the Framingham coefficients are relevant for this relatively select group of individuals (see comments in the previous critique and note that, in particular, the percentage smoking is low relative to the Framingham population [9] ought to provide each case with three matched controls. Since the major risk factors were controlled in this study, the chances are small that a nonmatched variable differed between cases and controls and accounted for the observed differences in both CHD incidence and levels of cardiorespiratory fitness and for presence or absence of stress test ECG abnormalities.

Unfortunately, with regard to the statistical analysis of the data, it seems that the authors have lost the pairing that they attempted to obtain. That is, after matching each case with three controls, cases and controls were pooled into two groups instead of analyzed retaining the matching (see, for example Miettinen [10]). It is not clear that this would alter any of the conclusions, but the data ought to be re-examined retaining the matching as there could be a marked increase in precision if case-control group to group variation were removed from experimental error under a matched type of analysis.

Karvonen: *Endurance Sport, Longevity, and Health*

This report examines the mortality pattern of athletes with regard to their increased longevity relative to the general population. Again, the choice of a suitable control group for athletes presents almost insurmountable difficulties. Thus, in the comparison of the best participants of the Oulu races of 1839–1950 and other champion skiers, with the general male population, it is important to emphasize that self-selection and influence of confounding variables may make such comparisons invalid. This follows because the general population includes the chronically ill and physically feeble or disabled who would not wish to or be able to ski competitively. Hence, the population of champion skiers presumably contains a much lower percentage of smokers and obese or hypertensive individuals than does the general population. In fact, the finding that heavy physical activity in lumbermen is not associated with increased life expectancy suggests that confounding variables, and not physical activity, may be responsible for the increase in the life expectancy of the skiers.

Reference is also made to the jogging habits of Finnish doctors with respect to their increased life expectancy. However, again, since many Finnish doctors have stopped smoking also, and since no information was given on the life expectancy of ex-smoking joggers compared with ex-smoking nonjoggers, it is not possible to separate the effect of taking up jogging from that of stopping smoking. Consequently, this paper provides additional confirmation of the *association* between physical activity and improved health, but provides no new information about the additional benefits of physical activity when other variables are controlled.

Kavanagh and Shephard: *The Effects of Continued Training on the Aging Process*

This study represents a cross-sectional examination of an entire volunteer cohort of elderly athletes. The authors mention a number of factors that may be confounded with any effects noted in their study (e.g., heavy use of dietary supplements, and vegetarian diets). However, they do not present any information on smoking habits or socioeconomic status, which would presumably be different in this group relative to the general population of this age, and would, therefore, be confounded with the observed effects of physical exercise. The absence of a suitably matched control group, and the above-mentioned confounding variables again make it impossible to determine whether exercise is responsible for the altered age pattern noted in certain of the variables. The authors comment on this self-selection phenomenon: "We have no proof that such differences as were demonstrated did not arise from either an initial process of self-selection or a subsequent selective attenuation of the athletic sample, men with problems such as hypertension ceasing to participate in competition." This statement and the effect of confounding variables would seem to invalidate the authors' earlier statement that their sample might indicate "the pattern of aging to be anticipated when middle-aged patients adhere faithfully to prescribed programs of progressive physical activity."

With regard to this pattern of aging, again the earlier definitional difficulties arise. The authors note that for this group the trends with chronological age seem slightly more favorable compared with the general population, but apart from the choice of the comparison group such chronological age-related changes may have little to do with biological aging in the sense that it affects the risk of death.

Rose and Cohen:
Relative Importance of Physical Activity for Longevity

This study illustrates some of the difficulties associated with measuring many of the variables involved in a study of the relationship between physical activity and aging processes. The dependent variable in the study, age at death, is probably the best measure of biological age, but in a retrospective study of this type a number of problems arise if such a variable is chosen. As the authors indicate, the presence of the secular effect (since longer-lived individuals were necessarily born earlier) presents difficulties in interpretation. For example, longer-lived individuals may not have been exposed in their formative years to certain deleterious life-style habits such as cigarette smoking, a habit that has increased until very recently. Thus, it is difficult to estimate the effects of such variables on life-span. Since there is also a strong secular component associated with education, the authors attempted to control for this secular effect by "controlling" educational differences by multiple regression and analysis of covariance techniques. (It should be mentioned that in the analysis of covariance, if the covariate differs significantly between levels of the categorical variable, to compare these levels at an average value of the covariate may be to compare them at a value that they would not normally attain [11]). Since the control of this secular component seems crucial to many of the conclusions reached, it would have been valuable to check the consistency of the results if some other measure of the secular effect (e.g., income or occupational level) had also been used.

This type of study does not permit the direct control of confounding variables, particularly of physiological variables that could not be measured. Attempts to control for some of these effects can be made by means of multiple regression techniques. Also, the effect of the self-selection of healthy individuals into occupations or leisure time activities involving physical activity could not be estimated.

Because of the research design, many of the variables that were considered were coded subjectively. For example, on- and off-job physical activity was coded 0 to 4 (sedentary to very active), sense of humor was coded 1 to 4 (always to never), and so forth. The interpretations of such codings, even when explained by a trained interviewer, may vary appreciably from subject to subject, thus lacking the consistency essential for valid statistical analyses. (For example, Leon and Blackburn indicate that there is a tendency for men to report less heavy physical work in their usual occupation following a heart attack.)

Also, such values are used as though they represent continuous quantitative measurements. For example, the coding of foreign to native born on a scale from 1 (if both parents and son are foreign born) to 4 (if both parents and son are native born) supposes a linear effect from low to high levels of the index (i.e., that differences between adjacent levels of the index are comparable). It is possible, however, that with some other arbitrary scaling (e.g., 1, 2, 6, 18) the results would be different. In fairness, it should be mentioned that there does not seem to be a generally accepted approach for handling such ordered variables when used as independent variables in regression analysis. However, when such variables are used as dependent variables (as in the regression of physical activity on the other variables in the data set) the assumption of the normality of errors becomes tenuous, and the calculated levels of significance may be meaningless. Similar considerations apply when assigning levels of significance to many of the correlation coefficients.

Further, the use of stepwise techniques by the authors deserves comment. With reference to stepwise regression techniques in which variables are entered (or deleted) one at a time into (or from) a regression equation on the basis of their correlation with the dependent variable (other variables in the model being controlled), Hocking[5] states, "It is unfortunate that many users have attached significance to the order of entry (or deletion) and assumed optimality of the resulting subset." Hocking also mentions examples where a variable may be the first to enter the model in a forward selection procedure, and the first to leave in a backward deletion procedure. Hence, it is unfortunate that the authors have suggested that the order in which variables enter the regression equations, and the proportion of explained variance ascribed to them, may be used to place the role of physical activity in proper perspective. In fact, under some other selection criterion, or with other variables entered in the model, the relative positions of the variables might change appreciably.

CONCLUSION

It is easier to criticize the studies of others than to produce definitive results of one's own. This is particularly true in much of epidemiological research where designed experiments are not feasible and thus any conclusion regarding cause and effect is tenuous due to problems of self-selection, confounding variables, and so on. However, as Keys[2] states, ". . . insistence on scientific purism and final 'proof' of cause and effect can lead to a degree of conservatism in which nothing is done. . . ." Further, there is no evidence that physical exercise, properly supervised, has harmful effects on health. More importantly, any effort to increase the level of participation might have considerable benefit because of the possible role that might be played by certain forms of physical activity in modifying the risk factor profile of an individual. It follows from this that the relevant investigations ought to be conducted using the best possible scientific principles and procedures, and that results should be reported with suitable emphasis on the limitations of the research design in order to prevent the dissemination of misinformation to the public. Unfortunately there has frequently been a certain amount of over-enthusiasm in presenting the results of such studies, whereas in fact at present there is no conclusive evidence that physical activity is beneficial to health, although there is suggestive evidence that this may be so.

ADDENDUM

The authors of the papers presented at this session were invited to comment on the preceding paper. Their comments are presented here.

Dr. Goldman:

The critique is technically correct; however, there are some points worthy of discussion. First of all, our goal was not to measure any health benefits of the classes. It is doubtful that a 30-minute exercise period, 4 days a week, for 8 weeks would yield meaningful differences when compared with a control group. This is especially true because our program was intended to be compatible with the actual ability of the subject. The confounding variables smoking and drinking will affect results, but our wide age range of participants precludes any objective treatment of these factors.

Using PRESS, a technique mentioned in Hocking's paper, we found our results turned out to be the same. I plan to do some cross-validation with some data we are presently collecting to test our models. Also, I have looked at categorizing "fit" and "unfit" by using models such as $\dot{V}_{O_2 \, max}$ versus age, $\dot{V}_{O_2 \, max}$ versus body fat, $\dot{V}_{O_2 \, max}$ versus RQ, and even $\dot{V}_{O_2 \, max}$ versus six other variables. The results agree extremely well but that really was expected because of the rather stable nature of R^2 values.

Dr. Bassler:

Brown and Milvy confirm again that "there have been no reports of fatal ASCVD, histologically proven, among 42-km-men."

I take serious exception to Noakes's call for a "moratorium" on my "public assertions," since each assertion usually follows a "false report." Noakes's own paper contains a fatality that originally appeared in the literature supported by detailed autopsy findings [12] when no autopsy had been performed.[13] He now presents this case with an EKG in which we see "no evidence of myocardial infarction." [14] His "moratorium" would allow false reports to be unchallenged.

Nonfatal cardiac events are not relevant to the "Bassler Hypothesis." Myocardial infarction may result from 44 different diseases, which are best identified at autopsy.[15] Edwards does a disservice to 42-km-men with his unpardonable conclusion that Noakes's cases are "atherosclerosis," since he neglects to identify the hazards of smoking, heat stress and dehydration. These hazards should be avoided by all runners, patients and nonpatients alike. Any investigator in the field of cardiac rehabilitation knows that abnormal angiograms are not unusual among 42-km-men. Patients have been finishing marathons since the mid-1960s; 43 ran in the Cardiac Division of the 1976 Honolulu Marathon; among them were cases of triple-vessel disease, infarction, and bypass grafts.[16] All developed ASCVD prior to becoming 42-km-men. It is estimated that 10,000 miles of endurance training will improve angiograms.[17] Noakes is premature in expecting improvement at lesser mileage.

Dr. Edwards violates basic forensic principle when he ascribes the death in case 16 to the right-coronary occlusion, since this lesion had been clinically inactive for 10 years. He betrays his lack of familiarity with current medical literature when he fails to recognize "smoker's small-vessel disease" (FIGURES 9 & 10). This may be the first report in humans. It had been previously produced in dogs.[18] My original observation has now been completely confirmed by Auerbach and co-workers who show that this small-vessel lesion is dose-related to smoking and unrelated to atherosclerosis.[19] Edwards is also unfamiliar with "ischemic microlesions" (FIGURES 11 & 12). Haerem recently found that these single-fiber lesions were present in 81% of cases of sudden death. This fits the history in case 16; infarction was not present.

Both Edwards and Noakes reject the concept of plaque resorption (FIGURES 6 & 8); however, regression of atherosclerosis has already been documented [20] under conditions far less demanding than marathon training. As long as 42-km-men appear to be immune to ASCVD, the burden of proof should be on those who question the value of this "protective" life-style.

Dr. Noakes:

The title of Dr. Bassler's paper and a number of his letters to journals (References 17 to 27 in our paper) have given the impression that because no marathon runner has yet been proven to die of fatal coronary atherosclerosis (a view that has now been seriously questioned by Dr. Edwards), then all marathon runners must be immune to coronary atherosclerosis. Intentionally or otherwise, this is the belief that has been conveyed to the marathon-running public.

The purpose of our paper was to refute this latter contention and to point out that Dr. Bassler's argument is epidemiologically untenable because coronary atherosclerosis may present as a variety of syndromes of which sudden death is only one.

To determine whether marathon running prevents coronary atherosclerosis, it would be necessary to investigate not only cases of sudden death, but also those of myocardial infarction and angina pectoris occurring in marathon runners.

Even then, such a study would be hard-pressed to prove, as has been pointed out by Brown and Milvy in their critique, that it was marathon running alone, and not some other factor, that was responsible for this protection.

We thank Dr. Meller for his careful review and constructive comments on our paper. We would like to deal with each of his comments separately.

Case 1. The patient died in a peripheral, nonteaching hospital. Despite contact with the Medical Superintendent of this hospital, we have been unable to obtain further details of this patient's illness.

We appreciate Dr. Meller's support for a diagnosis of acute myocardial ischaemia. In view of the man's age and the possibility of a genetic predisposition to the early development of coronary atherosclerosis, we investigated his children for lipid abnormalities. His daughter, aged 10, has a type 2B hyperlipidemia (cholesterol 375 mg%, triglycerides 271 mg%).

Case 4. We agree that Case 4 has only incidental coronary atherosclerosis and may suffer from cardiomyopathy. Indeed, the patient has a history of alcohol abuse.

The patient was included in the series because he had persisted in completing a marathon despite symptoms and because, despite his running, he was not totally immune to coronary atherosclerosis. We feel that the presence of such mild coronary artery disease, adds to our contention that marathon runners can develop myocardial infarction without coronary artery obstruction.

Case 5. This patient was included because he ran 20 miles in a competitive marathon despite symptoms, and because the diagnosis of myocardial infarction was not initially considered by the attending physician.

The question raised is whether or not this patient has mitral valve prolapse (Barlow's syndrome) as a cause for his myocardial infarction. That he suffered a transmural myocardial infarction during the marathon race is established by the appearance after the race and the subsequent evolution of diagnostic ECG and serum enzyme changes.

The diagnosis of mitral valve prolapse was made only by his personal physician who reported the characteristic auscultatory findings and found a compatible ECG (T-wave inversion in leads 2, 3, and AVF), three years earlier. This finding was not confirmed by three cardiologists who have examined the patient since myocardial infarction, nor was it corroborated by echocardiography. However, Barlow [21] believes that the auscultatory findings of mitral valve prolapse may disappear after myocardial damage and that echocardiography is often unable to confirm mitral valve prolapse even when loud non-ejection systolic clicks are present. But he has seen only one patient, a Black African, with a *transmural* myocardial infarction, normal coronary arteries and mitral valve prolapse.[22]

Thus we cannot exclude that this patient has or had mitral valve prolapse nor can we, without coronary angiographic evidence, prove that he has coronary artery disease. However, we interpret the exercise test as being positive and therefore highly suggestive.

Dr. Rosenman:

Perhaps we should have mentioned in our paper that we have justified our statistical treatment and the use of the Framingham coefficients.[23] Therefore, we do not believe that the comments made are entirely correct.

Dr. Cooper:

We appreciate the opportunity to respond to the review of Drs. Milvy and Brown.

Their comment regarding the relevance of Framingham coefficients for the population of the Cooper Clinic is addressed in a recently published report by Kannel and Gordon.[24] In their analysis, it was desired "to test the general applicability of the findings of the Framingham study on the relationship of major risk factors to coronary heart disease and death." With data from four other study populations used for comparison, the study showed that, "This analysis reinforces the conclusion that the results of the Framingham Study are widely generalizable to white middle-aged American men and can be used with confidence. . . . The results also provide further evidence of the utility of a multiple risk factor approach in predicting cardiovascular disease."

As to the discrepancy between cigarette smoking rates in Framingham and in the Dallas population, it should be remembered that the population selected for the case-control study reported was not representative and estimation of population rates should not be made from this sample.

In addition, a nationwide change in smoking habits occurring between the 1950s and the 1970s; some Framingham data were collected early in this period; our data are from the later period.

Although our paper was intended to present only preliminary results, deferring more detailed analysis to a later time, we are pleased to have this opportunity to report on several additional analyses:

(1) Using the procedure of Mantel and Haenszel [25] for matched studies, the difference observed between proportion of cases and controls with abnormal exercise ECGs is significant with p < 0.01, and when *abnormal or equivocal* exercise ECG's were considered, the test for difference of the proportions was significant with p < 0.005.

(2) The same procedure, when applied to the subset of controls for whom there was follow-up information and their corresponding cases, yields significant differences in treadmill performance time with p < 0.05 for the entire group, and p < 0.01 for men aged 50–59.

Drs. Kavanagh and Shephard:

Our initial reaction to the critique was that it overstated the obvious, and possibly did not call for comment. On reflection, however, we realize that a case should be made for those of us who have to deal with realities. The mathematician seeks a simple world where "treatments" such as physical activity can be rigidly allocated between test and control groups, with all other variables held constant. In such a setting, pragmatism is necessarily suspect; the equation must balance. Unfortunately, the populations we serve as physicians do not live in such a world. Inferences have to be drawn and treatments based on situations as they exist; all we can do is exercise considerable care in weighing the relative likelihood of truth and error in the conclusion we are drawing, being careful to distinguish between speculation and fact.

As we have clearly admitted in our article, it is conceivable that patients who undertake hard training in middle-age may have a different basis of initial selection and subsequent defection than those enrolling in the Masters Program. However, it is a reasonable working assumption that such factors as smoking habits and socioeconomic status are likely to be similar in any group of middle-aged men who carry through a program of hard endurance training. Our argument thus stands; the data "can be used to explore the *probable* response of the average person to a lengthy period of hard physical training." "By virtue of their average endowment and many years of regular endurance training, our sample *may* give some indication of the pattern of aging to be anticipated when middle-aged patients *adhere faithfully* to prescribed programs of *progressive physical activity.*"

Dr. Rose:

(1) Regarding the suggestions for using another handle in addition to education for controlling for secular effect, I did consider occupational level, but this did not turn out to be as good a candidate as education. Nonetheless, I replicated the correlations, partially correlating for occupation, and, as expected, the shift in *r* was not in the hypothesized direction, as occurred with the education partial. However, I did not include this detail in the final draft, which was already too long.

(2) In regard to the comment on the confounding effect of the omission of physiological (genetic) variables, it is true that such measures could not be

included given the design of the study, but variables were included that tapped or were related to these physical variables, such as frequency of illness, physical appearance, catching colds, and mother's longevity.

(3) In regard to the criticism of subjective coding, the rating of the physical activity variables was derived from detailed descriptions obtained from the informant. Examples: policeman, on foot all day, much walking or waving of arms; or policeman, at desk part-time and walking, doing detective work; age 18–25 carpenter, finish work, little physical lifting; up to age 20 active in sports most every day; age 35–50, fishing and some walking. Details on how ratings were derived are in the book *Predicting Longevity: Methodology & Critique*, pages 90–99. It is unreasonable to state categorically that such methods "lack consistency essential for valid statistical analysis."

(4) The criticism regarding use of parametric techniques is also unreasonable. It is true that the measures are not perfectly continuous, and don't completely satisfy parametric requirements, but I would challenge the critic to furnish a practical nonparametric procedure capable of doing the required multivariate job. The conversion of dichotomous variables such as foreign-native born into an ordered variable is also unjustifiably critized. Certainly this is preferable to inserting a dichotomous variable into the multiple regression or omitting the variable altogether. By the same token, it is preferable to use such imperfectly continuous measures as the dependent variable when needed rather than do nothing. A disservice is done to the reader when criticisms *sans* solutions are offered.

(5) The authors are criticized for using the order in which variables enter the regression equation and the proportion of explained variance ascribed to them as a way of placing the role of physical activity in proper perspective. The authors, however, clearly state the limitations of the stepwise procedure in this regard. They state in the first paragraph of the section "Regression Analysis of Longevity Predictors" that the earlier entering variables usually sum up the variances accounted for by later entering variables with which they are partially redundant. This produces a parsimonious set of predictors such that some do not get included, or do not get included at an important level. This indexing effect is frequently illustrated in subsequent pages of the paper. The regression equation is described as a parsimonious set of *indices* of predictors rather than of the predictors themselves. Therefore, a particular "mix" cannot be taken too literally. An example in TABLE 8 is the fact that off-job activity, age 40–49, accounts for a miniscule variance (0.8%). In the real world, and I quote from the text, this predictor is more important than appears in the regression equation, when its importance is summed up by other variables.

(6) In a general concluding statement, Brown and Milvy state that the evidence for physical activity being beneficial to health is suggestive, not conclusive. Again the reader should realize that this is true of most scientific findings. It is the nature of the beast that knowledge usually grows in slow increments rather than an accumulation of "suggestive" evidence.

REFERENCES

1. BROWN, K. S. & W. F. FORBES. 1976. Concerning the estimation of biological age. Gerontology **22:** 428–437.
2. KEYS, A. 1970. Physical activity and the epidemiology of coronary heart dis-

ease. *In* Physical Activity and Aging. Medicine and Sport. Vol. 4. Physical Activity and Aging. : 250–266. University Park Press. Baltimore, Md.

3. KEYS, A. 1975. Coronary heart disease—The global picture. Atherosclerosis **22:** 149–192.

4. TAYLOR, H. L., R. W. PARKIN, H. BLACKBURN & A. KEYS. 1966. Problems in the analysis of the relationship of coronary heart disease to physical activity or its lack, with special reference to sample size and occupational withdrawal. *In* Physical Activity in Health and Disease. K. Evang & K. L. Anderson, Eds. : 242–261.

5. HOCKING, R. R. 1976. The analysis and selection of variables in linear regression. Biometrics **32:** 1–49.

6. SCHENFELD, A. 1973. Longevity. J. Amer. Med. Assoc. **225:** 526.

7. MILVY, P. 1977. Statistical analysis of deaths from coronary heart disease anticipated in a cohort of marathon runners. Ann. N.Y. Acad. Sci. This volume.

8. WERKO, L. 1976. Risk factors and coronary heart disease—Facts or fancy? Amer. Heart J. **91:** 87–98.

9. KANNEL, W. B. & T. GORDON, Eds. 1973. The Framingham Study. An Epidemiological Investigation of Cardiovascular Disease. Section 28. U.S. Department of Health, Education and Welfare.

10. MIETTINEN, O. S. 1969. Individual matching with multiple controls in the case of all-or-none responses. Biometrics **25:** 339–355.

11. COX, D. R. 1958. Planning of Experiments. John Wiley & Sons, Inc., New York.

12. OPIE, L. H. 1975. N. Engl. J. Med. **293:** 941–942.

13. OPIE, L. H. 1976. N. Engl. J. Med. **294:** 1067.

14. SCAFF, J. H. 1976. N. Engl. J. Med. **295:** 105.

15. CHEITLIN, M. D., H. A. McALLISTER & C. M. DE CASTRO. 1975. Myocardial infarction without atherosclerosis. J. Amer. Med. Assoc. **231:** 951–959.

16. BASSLER, T. J. 1977. Br. Med. J. **1:** 229.

17. BASSLER, T. J. 1976. Is atheroma a reversible lesion?

18. AUERBACH, O., E. C. HAMMOND & L. GARFINKLE. 1971. Arch. Environ. Health **22:** 20–27.

19. AUERBACH, O., H. W. CARTER, L. GARFINKLE & E. C. HAMMOND. 1976. Cigarette smoking and coronary artery disease. Chest **70:** 697–705.

20. BASTA, L. L., C. WILLIAMS, J. M. KIOSCHOS & A. A. SPECTOR. 1976. Amer. J. Med. **61:** 420–423.

21. BARLOW, J. B. Personal communication.

22. CHESLER, E., R. E. MATISONN, J. B. LAKIER, W. A. POCOCK, I. W. PROMUND OBEL & J. B. BARLOW. 1976. Acute myocardial infarction with normal coronary arteries. A possible manifestation of the Billowing Mitral Leaflet Syndrome. Circulation **54:** 203–209.

23. BRAND, R. J., R. H. ROSENMAN, R. I. SCHOLTZ & M. FRIEDMAN. 1976. Multivariate prediction of coronary heart disease in the Western Collaborative Group Study compared to the findings of the Framingham study. Circulation **53**(2): 348–355.

24. KANNEL, W. B. & T. GORDON. 1976. The Framingham Study: An Epidemiological Investigation of Cardiovascular Disease. Section 31. April. U.S. Department of Health, Education, and Welfare.

25. MANTEL, N. & W. HAENSZEL. 1959. Statistical aspects of the analysis of data from retrospective studies of disease. J. Nat. Cancer Inst. **22** (4, April).

DISCUSSION

Paul Milvy, *Moderator*

Environmental Science Laboratory
Mount Sinai School of Medicine
New York, New York 10029

E. J. COLT (*St. Luke's Hospital, New York, N.Y.*): In any epidemiological study of activity and the heart, the alcohol consumption of the people should be mentioned. We all have read, and this may be apocryphal, that many of the Olympic runners ingest vast quantities of alcohol. I think that in future studies this should always be taken into account.

D. ADAMOVITCH (*Nassau County Medical Center, East Meadow, N.Y.*): Would any of the speakers care to comment on the mechanism of acute myocardial infarction during the marathon race since we do know it has happened?

T. D. NOAKES (*University of Cape Town, South Africa*): I mentioned yesterday that the normal heart can metabolize virtually any substrate, but, in the presence of ischemia, free fatty acids, ketone bodies, catecholamines are all deleterious. They have a deleterious effect at the myocardial cell level and it is possible that they are acting during the later phase of the marathon. In addition, you have hyperthermia and dehydration. But this is all just speculation. I think we must move away from the concept that myocardial infarction is necessarily always preceded by coronary thrombosis and we should move towards the concept that the myocardial cell itself may be important. Dr. Newsholme has given us most explicit diagrams of the ATP production and ATP supply, and one concept of myocardial infarction is that it results from a disparity between ATP supply and ATP demand, and I think that is what may have happened in our marathon runners. As I mentioned, I am not sure that the routine stress EKG can necessarily predict these problems.

R. HUGHSON (*McMaster University, Hamilton, Ont.*): I think there is one thing that was briefly alluded to in several of Dr. Bassler's slides. And that is the actual supply of oxygen to the working muscle cell. In the animal models, cardiac hypertrophy can be induced in a young animal in which the number of capillaries per muscle fiber is increased, whereas in the old animal the cardiac muscle fiber increases without an increase in the number of capillaries. Therefore, you get a great increase in the diffusion distance for oxygen. Now what's happening in the marathon runner? By encouraging someone to start exercising late in life, does hypertrophy of their heart occur without this concurrent increase in capillarization? If so, the interior of their heart muscle is possibly more susceptible to myocardial infarction. I think also that a question that I haven't heard raised here at all is, does exercise increase intracellular potassium? If you can believe Raab's work,* then by increasing intracellular potassium, you make the heart more resistant to infarction. What do we really know about these two phenomena?

---

* RAAB, W. 1969. Myocardial electrolyte derangement: Crucial feature of pluricausal, so-called coronary, heart disease (dysionic cardiopathy). Ann. N.Y. Acad. Sci. **147**(17): 627.

T. J. Bassler (*Centinela Valley Hospital, Inglewood, Calif.*): I can put your mind at rest about the capillary bed because we can take sections from the myocardium of the marathon runner of any age. The capillary bed is generous in a 70-year-old marathoner. I can show the sections to anybody without telling him the age, and if they say they are over 18 years old, then I'd assume that the runner wasn't doing enough mileage. The body is alive and the heart's alive and it changes almost every day.

W. P. Morgan (*University of Wisconsin, Madison, Wisc.*): I actually would like to direct this question to the entire panel, and in so doing, I would like to first respond to the first question that was asked by Dr. Colt because I think it's germaine, and it relates to the question I'm going to ask and nobody responded to it. First of all, I think this idea that the Olympic marathoner or the elite runner is a heavy drinker is a myth; and I think this is a myth for the following reasons. Number one, in our study of the elite runners, there were eight marathoners. Six of these runners did not, I repeat, did not consume hard liquor—six of the eight. One consumed an average of one drink per week, so we can say that seven did not drink liquor, and the last reported a weekly consumption of 18 ounces of hard liquor. If we look at the mean consumption then it's quite high. But, if we look at those runners individually, they are not drinkers. Four of the runners did not consume wine. The remaining four averaged 3 glasses per week with a range of one to five 6-ounce glasses. One of the runners abstained completely from beer, and the consumption in the remaining 7 averaged 9.7 bottles per week, that's 12-ounce bottles, with a range in those 7 of 1 to 30 bottles per week. The mean of 9.7 is as high as it is, then, as a result of 2 runners who reported consuming 24 and 30 bottles per week, respectively. So basically, we're talking about 2 beer drinkers in that group. Now it is of some interest that the runner who reported having 24 bottles per week also was the runner who consumed the largest amount of hard liquor, 18 ounces per week. (Laughter.) Now the net effect of that is that this individual becomes the yardstick for the marathon subculture in a sense, and that's where we get the emergence of this myth that marathoners, and the long distance runners generally, are heavy drinkers. In that elite group, that is not the case. When we look at all the other dietary factors in the elite runners, we see a very, very unique group of people, people who do not use aspirin at all or any analgesics, people who basically do not drink coffee. Those who drink coffee drink very, very small quantities, one or so cups per week. They do not drink tea, and so on. Dr. Bassler's slides depicting the typical kitchen of the marathoner was rather interesting, I thought. Now my question is this, the tacit assumption seems to be that when differences are shown that it's exercise per se that is responsible for this, and irrespective of our data with the elite runners, it's a very commonly accepted principle that individuals who become active in fitness programs or become interested in jogging, marathoning, or whatever, "get religion about health." There is a health consciousness that takes place, and this goes far, far beyond the running per se, and gets into a lot of other health-related variables.

Dr. Milvy has been the only one who has addressed that particular issue, and everyone has made the assumption that it's exercise per se, and I would like someone in the panel to respond to that because I don't think anyone has.

P. Milvy: It's an infinitely complicated problem not conducive of simple or totally satisfying solution.

J. H. Wilmore (*University of Arizona, Tucson, Ariz.*): I'm curious in light of Dr. Noake's presentation where actual myocardial damage was observed in the absence of total occlusion. This has always bothered me, this concept of false positive stress tests. I'm wondering if possibly we're looking at anatomical versus physiological factors. In other words, in what we call a false positive test, the myocardium is truly ischemic, and maybe this is something you're getting at with the data you have presented. Do you have any comments on that?

T. D. NOAKES: I think that that certainly is true. Again, we must look at the coronary arteries of the myocardium and see what's happening there.

B. ROSIN (*Torrance Memorial Hospital, Torrance, Calif.*): This is in defense of Dr. Bassler and is an attitude of cardiologists engaged in stimulating patients to participate in marathon-type activity. We recognize that every second person in this country is dying of cardiovascular disease and I think it's absurd to assert that anything is going to provide 100% immunity from coronary artery disease, whether it's marathon running or 10% fat diet or whatever. It's just a matter of time obviously, before we observe a myocardial infarction in a marathoner. But that still does not negate the fact that when we get individuals involved in rehabilitation programs and marathon-type activities that this is associated with life-style changes that do afford some significant protection from coronary artery disease.

D. ADAMOVITCH: Based on this series of papers, I think an article in last Sunday's *Newsday* is very apropos. It's entitled "Celibacy Wins the Race" and reads: "The secrets of long life were revealed in Athens yesterday by Dimitri Iordanidis, 98, after he had run 42 kilometers in 7 hours and 40 minutes in an annual marathon competition. You must give up sex, he said, adding that he gave it up at 85 years of age. Other necessities for long life include no smoking, no meat, no milk or butter, and lots of walking. He first took part in the marathon 2 years ago when he finished in 6 hours, 40 minutes. Of the hour's difference he said, 'I was younger then.' "

P. MILVY: The trick obviously is to be celibate and as Dr. Rose has shown in his paper (TABLES 7 & 10), to have a young wife. And I suspect that combining the two is a bit of a trick!

D. ZENMAN (*Newsday, Garden City, N.Y.*): I don't know if you're the proper one to address this to. How would you answer Dr. Peter Stainchrome in the book *You Can Increase Your Heart Power,* when he says "exercise is bosh, it will pay you no dividend in health. In fact, over-exertion is more likely to harm than help. If you are over 40, you are wise if they call you lazy."

P. MILVY: In the process of preparing the first paper of this session, I reviewed several hundred papers on physical activity and mortality with particular attention to physical activity and coronary heart disease. I reached the conclusion (and I think that Dr. Leon and many other epidemiologists have also reached this conclusion) that despite all of the tremendous problems of self-selection, of compounding variables, etc., etc., that confront the statistician and the epidemiologist, physical activity probably does confer a limited amount of protection from certain disease processes. Exactly how much is very, very difficult to estimate.

I am also aware of the fact that human epidemiological studies aside, for every animal study that demonstrates increased collaterals in exercising rats, for example, there is an equally valid study that seems to indicate that no additional proliferation of collaterals occurs. That's one side of the problem. I think it's also very clear that the opposite proposition that physical activity, intelligently pursued, is bad for you has infinitely less evidence to support it. In fact, I'm not sure that I came across any papers that indicate this at all. There were papers that indicated that it didn't do a bit of good for you, however one might define "good." But approximately twice as many papers conclude that it does help. Whether these conclusions are warranted, in view of the epidemiological problems of self-selection, confounding variables, and so forth that all the studies are confronted by, I leave for you to decide! Let me finally say that because this problem is so difficult to resolve, there is tendency to alter the entire discussion by maintaining that running adds "life to years" rather than "years to life." Quality rather than quantity. I'm a marathoner and it's the most wonderful thing one can imagine. It's exciting, it's fulfilling. It's all of the things we've ever asserted it to be. But that doesn't prove anything either, because the person who plays chess 4 nights a week would say the same of chess. Any hobby that you engage in is fulfilling but that's a self-fulfilling tautology, I suppose. Parenthetically, many chess players, certainly many of the Soviet chess players, train for chess matches by endurance swimming and endurance running. Bobby Fischer trained for his match against Spassky by endurance tennis and other relaxing exercises. The mind is part of the body. The two work together and have to be both handled with respect and care.

COMMENT: I just wanted to add one comment relative to the evidence that exercise is bad for you. I think this really comes from misunderstanding immediate risk versus the overall risk. There is perhaps a good deal of evidence that if one engages in unaccustomed, very vigorous activity that you are going to increase your risks of a heart attack immediately by the factor of perhaps 4, 5, or 6, and of course anyone who observes this says, therefore, exercise is bad for a person who is over 40. But what they fail to take account of, of course, is that although you may increase your risk for the 10 minutes while you are exercising, you may have diminished it more for the other 23 hours and 50 minutes a day, and therefore, you may end up better in a statistical sense over the course of the entire day. In addition this risk apparently only arises in those who exercise in an unwise fashion. Dr. Bill Haskell has recently carried out a very extensive survey of gymnasiums that are offering exercise programs. In the early days there did seem to be some evidence that the risk of going to those gymnasiums was greater than spending that same hour at home. But it's now reached the point, I believe, where you are actually safer off when you are in the gymnasium than you are sitting at home in an armchair reading a book.

G. SHEEHAN (*Red Bank, N.J.*): I find the problem of longevity and protection from coronary disease a fascinating one. It seems to me that we have to recognize that there are three races of men, and remember what Dr. Sheldon told us about ectomorphs, mesomorphs, and endomorphs, and recall Dr. Spain's classic study showing the predominance of endomesomorphs in the coronary group. If we look at it that way, we can see that we ectomorphs, now that we're free from the problem of bacterial invasion, can survive the dangers created by affluence and competition because we avoid both those problems. Most ectomorphs end up in academia or government, or are fortunate enough to practice medicine, where no matter how passive or ambivalent you are, you are able to make your buck. So we don't have the problem of affluence, which is the endomorphic tendency towards cholesterol and good living, or the competitive thing of the mesomorph. If we look at it that way then we can see why people who have studied athletes find that athletes live shorter, the same amount, or longer than the ordinary population. Polednak found among Harvard students, for instance, that football players die earlier than their classmates, and people like us would live longer. And we know that running is a white middle class intellectual sport with a disproportionate number of people who are in academic positions, and generally people who are parasites on society. Beyond that, if we all were put in a room together, we would pretty much look alike. Most of us would be ectomorphs. And it is those who will be most likely to live longer.

P. MILVY: Two quick comments. If we were all put in a room together, at least we would be able to see each other, whereas, the other group by virtue of the cigarette smoke, would probably not be able to see each other. This certainly distinguishes us as a group, George. In the same study that Dr. Sheehan referred to, the people who live the longest were the Phi Beta Kappas, presumably because they were put into a higher socioeconomic bracket either by virtue of birth, which gave them the necessary leisure to apply themselves fully to their studies, or by virtue of their Phi Beta Kappa status, which ultimately led to a well-paying job and a high, healthy standard of living. The mortality tables show that upper class men live longer on an average than upper middle class men.

And now, since we're running very far behind, would it be too much to ask that, instead of a short break in which we leave the conference room, we all stand up and jog in place?

OVERVIEW

Jack H. Wilmore

*University of Arizona
Tucson, Arizona 85721*

The 1970s will undoubtedly be remembered as the decade in which the female athlete emerged to assume her rightful position in the arena of athletics. While the female long distance runner has been a part of this far reaching movement, she is still limited to a considerable extent by the governing bodies of various national and international organizations. These groups have assumed the position that the female is sufficiently different from the male, and, consequently, she should not be allowed to compete in the longer distance races, i.e., greater than 1500 or 3000 meters. Only recently, outside the jurisdiction of these groups have females been permitted to participate in the longer distance races of marathon distance or longer. Is the female significantly different from the male relative to various physiological, biomechanical, medical, or psychosocial parameters, that would place her at a higher risk consequent to long distance running, or are the differences between the sexes relatively minor, which would then justify competition of the same intensity, duration and distance?

The format of this session on "Similarities and Dissimilarities among Men and Women Distance Runners," was established in an attempt to answer the above question. The topics of the following papers were selected to summarize information in those areas where at least limited evidence exists of a research nature, as opposed to those areas where there is little more than opinion and self-serving claims. While the following papers raise more questions than they answer, they at least form a small body of knowledge that lends valuable insight into an area which has previously been filled with many misconceptions and myths.

AEROBIC RESPONSES OF FEMALE DISTANCE RUNNERS TO SUBMAXIMAL AND MAXIMAL EXERCISE *

Jack Daniels

Physical Education Department
The University of Texas
Austin, Texas 78712

Gary Krahenbuhl

Arizona State University
Tempe, Arizona 85281

Carl Foster

Ball State University
Muncie, Indiana 47303

Jimmy Gilbert

National Aeronautics and Space Administration
Houston, Texas 77001

Sylvia Daniels

Lanier High School
Austin, Texas 78758

Introduction

That males outperform females in distance running has been readily observed for as long as performances have been recorded. Standards are about 10% slower for women in 1500- and 3000-meter races and nearly 25% slower over the marathon distance.

It has been suggested [1] that the female possesses an architecture less efficient for running. Pelvis width, obliquity of the femur, and length of the female leg and stride have all received attention as possible mechanical deficiencies.[2,3] These structural characteristics, however, may not accurately describe the accomplished female distance runner, who has been shown to possess a more masculine build with respect to hip width and leg length.[4-6]

Females in a wide variety of sports are generally reported as having more body fat than do males,[7] a factor that could harm performance in medium endurance events where the body weight is supported. Still, Wilmore and Brown [8] have found values as low as 6% among female distance runners. Another possibility is that females possess lower hemoglobin concentrations than do males,[9] resulting in a lower oxygen-carrying capacity of the blood.

In recent years the importance of the aerobic demands of running at submaximal speeds has received increased attention.[10,11] It appears that considerable individual differences may exist,[12] but whether the factor of running

* Supported in part by The Canadian Track and Field Association.

726

"efficiency," or economy, can be used to differentiate among nearly equal competitors is not at all clear.

Previous studies [13, 14] have explored male/female differences during either treadmill walking or work on a bicycle ergometer. On these tasks the absolute oxygen demands of work at submaximal loads are lower in females than in males, but this is basically a function of the lower average body weight of females. Also, since women possess a lower maximum aerobic power ($\dot{V}_{O_2 max}$),[9, 15] they are usually working at a higher percentage of their $\dot{V}_{O_2 max}$ during exercise involving a standard workload, and since blood lactate accumulation is determined largely by the percent $\dot{V}_{O_2 max}$ used during exercise,[16, 17] this disparity may contribute to sex differences in running performance.

Studies directly measuring sex differences in the aerobic demands of submaximal running have often been complicated by the difficulty of locating female subjects capable of submaximal runs at speeds that are more routine for male runners. If the aerobic demands of running can be shown not to differ between trained male and female runners, then the existing performance differences may be essentially just a function of differences in $\dot{V}_{O_2 max}$. The purpose of this study was to compare the aerobic demands of submaximal running in highly trained and talented male and female runners. Additionally, an attempt was made to explain differences that might be found to exist between men and women regarding $\dot{V}_{O_2}$ during submaximal running when the subjects either are not tested over, or are not capable of submaximal work over, a common range of speeds.

Methods and Procedures

The initial phase of this investigation involved 20 highly-trained runners (10 men and 10 women) who were tested during submaximal and maximal runs on a treadmill. The "submax" test session consisted of four 6–8-minute treadmill runs at approximately 202, 215, 241, and 268 m/min. Belt revolutions were counted to determine the exact pace and expired air was collected for the last 90 seconds of each run. The $\dot{V}_{O_2}$ calculated for each corresponding run was taken as representative of the aerobic demands of running at that speed.

The "max" test required the subjects to run on a treadmill with speed and/or grade increments added each minute. Speed was increased up to 10 mph, then 2% grade increments were added each minute until voluntary exhaustion. In each case, exhaustion was reached after 6 to 8 minutes of work. Consecutive 30- to 60-second expired gas samples were collected in meteorological balloons through a low resistance breathing valve and collection valve system,[18] starting at the end of the third minute of exercise. Gas samples were analyzed for CO_2 and O_2 content with a Lloyd Gallenkamp volumetric analyzer. The highest $\dot{V}_{O_2}$ reached during each run was considered $\dot{V}_{O_2 max}$.

To further examine the comparison of the aerobic demands of running between males and females and among a common group of runners when $\dot{V}_{O_2}/$ speed regression equations are derived from different speed ranges, an additional series of submaximal runs were completed by five male and five female runners. In this second series of tests the same procedures and methods as described above were employed except the speeds used ranged from 150 to 250 m/min. Five speeds, distributed approximately equally apart, were used and separate regression equations were calculated using the three slowest speeds, the middle three speeds, and the three fastest speeds.

In both phases of the investigation, the males and females were considered to be of comparable ability based on the average departure from current world records displayed by the two groups.

Results and Discussion

TABLE 1 presents the descriptive data for the 20 subjects used in phase 1 of the study. The men were clearly larger and had greater values for $\dot{V}_{O_2 max}$ (both in absolute terms and when expressed in ml/kg·min), $\dot{V}_E$, and O_2 pulse at $\dot{V}_{O_2 max}$. Maximum heart rates were higher among the women, but the difference was not significant ($p > 0.05$). These results are all as would be expected and are generally a function of the size difference between men and women. In regard to running performance, it appears that the greater $\dot{V}_{O_2 max}$ displayed by the male runners would give them a clear advantage in endurance events, a not surprising finding in light of the performance differences that do exist (19% difference in $\dot{V}_{O_2 max}$ in this study as opposed to the typical 10%– 25% difference generally noted in distance running performances between the sexes) and that a greater $\dot{V}_{O_2 max}$ by trained males is widely accepted.

The $\dot{V}_{O_2 submax}$ values from the phase 1 tests are presented in TABLE 2. Although the women were characterized by slightly greater $\dot{V}_{O_2 submax}$ values at the speeds used, none of the differences was significant. The women also showed somewhat greater variability in $\dot{V}_{O_2}$ at all speeds (the lowest and highest values were also recorded by females at all test speeds); the men were characterized by a tendency to become less variable as speed increased.

These findings strongly suggest that there are no sex differences in the aerobic demands of running when the range of speeds used is common to both groups of runners and when all subjects are similar in ability. Interestingly,

TABLE 1

DESCRIPTIVE DATA: TRAINED DISTANCE RUNNERS

Variable	Males ($n=10$) Mean	SD *	Females ($n=10$) Mean	SD
Height (cm)	179.3	6.1	166.2 ‡	4.7
Weight (kg)	65.7	5.6	52.1 ‡	3.7
6-site skin fold (mm) †	39.6	6.8	48.1 ‡	4.4
$\dot{V}_{O_2 max}$ (ml/kg·min)	73.7	5.1	59.6 ‡	4.4
$\dot{V}_E$ at $\dot{V}_{O_2 max}$	166.1	17.5	107.8 ‡	12.0
R at $\dot{V}_{O_2 max}$	1.11	0.07	1.08	0.03
Heart rate maximum	180.3	7.2	190.8	10.7
O_2/pulse (ml/beat)	26.9	2.7	16.3 ‡	1.7
Vent/O_2	34.3	3.4	34.7	3.0

* SD, standard deviation.
† Tricep, subscapular, suprailiac, umbilical, pectoral, mid-thigh (anterior).
‡ Significantly different from males ($p < 0.01$).

TABLE 2

COMPARISON OF MALE AND FEMALE DISTANCE RUNNERS ON THE AEROBIC DEMANDS
OF RUNNING AT FOUR SELECTED SUBMAXIMAL SPEEDS

Speed	$\dot{V}_{O_2}$* (ml/kg·min)	
(m/min)	Males ($n=10$)	Females ($n=10$)
202	36.2	38.0
	(32–39)	(31–42)
215	39.0	40.7
	(35–42)	(34–45)
241	44.6	46.0
	(41–47)	(40–50)
268	50.5	51.5
	(47–53)	(46–55)

* $\dot{V}_{O_2}$ values were calculated for common speeds from individual regression equations. Ranges are shown in parentheses below mean values.

the subject with the lowest $\dot{V}_{O_2 \, max}$ (a female) who would presumably be working at the greatest percent of her $\dot{V}_{O_2 \, max}$ at all submax speeds, recorded the lowest $\dot{V}_{O_2 \, submax}$ at every running speed. It appears that her ability to perform equally against other women with higher $\dot{V}_{O_2 \, max}$ is a function of her greater "efficiency" as demonstrated in the submax tests.

FIGURE 1 presents a plot of the $\dot{V}_{O_2}$ data collected at all submax speeds used in the first series of tests. Also shown are the combined linear and quadratic regression curves and the $\dot{V}_{O_2 \, max}$ mean values for the men and women. Although the linear regression equation proved very satisfactory in describing the relationship between running speed and $\dot{V}_{O_2}$, the second-order curve fit the data significantly better. Higher order polynomials were unsuccessful in reducing the deviation about the regression.

If the curvilinear relationship displayed is a function of higher speeds demanding increasingly greater energy, as the work represents a higher and higher fractional utilization of $\dot{V}_{O_2 \, max}$, then the women would show a greater $\dot{V}_{O_2}$ than the men at any given speed (which was only a nonsignificant tendency in the present study), based on the lower $\dot{V}_{O_2 \, max}$ of the women. It would seem an appropriate follow-up to the present work to compare males and females who have equal $\dot{V}_{O_2 \, max}$ values and who are equally well trained. This would eliminate the possibility that differences in fractional utilization may be a contributing factor.

The results of phase 2 of the investigation are summarized in FIGURE 2. Since there were again no differences between the male and female runners in $\dot{V}_{O_2}$ at any of the five submax speeds, the data were combined and used to construct three separate regression curves based on the three slowest speeds, the middle three speeds, and the three fastest speeds. If $\dot{V}_{O_2}$ values were calculated through extrapolation of one regression equation to determine the $\dot{V}_{O_2}$ related to a speed outside the confines of the data from which that particular curve was constructed (for example, 300 m/min running speed) then differences in the aerobic demands of running became evident. This was true whether men and women were compared or if either separate group or a combination of

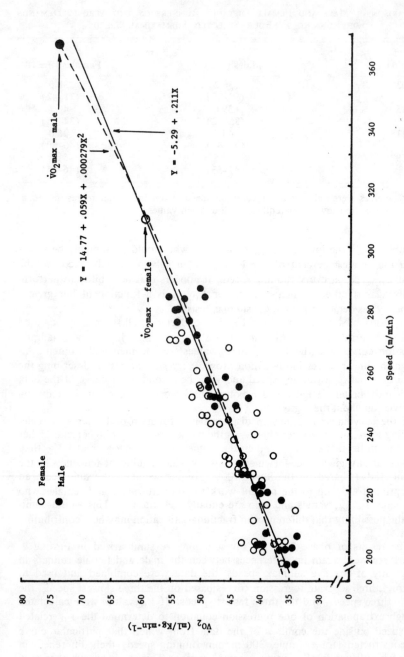

FIGURE 1. Linear and quadratic regression curves calculated from individual $\dot{V}_{O_2}$ and speed values for 20 runners. Also shown are mean $\dot{V}_{O_2max}$ values for 10 females and 10 males.

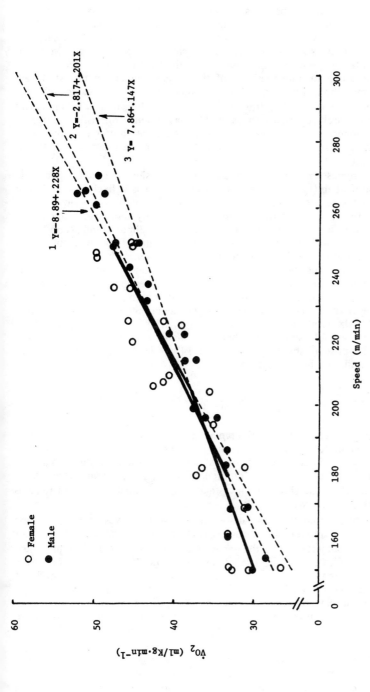

FIGURE 2. Linear regression curves calculated from $\dot{V}_{O_2 submax}$ values of five females and five males running at speeds (1) between 150 and 204 m/min, (2) between 178 and 225 m/min, and (3) between 204 and 250 m/min.

both was used in the comparisons. Also, this phenomenon was most evident when use of the slowest speeds was made. This could quite often lead to the mistaken conclusion that the aerobic demands of running differ between men and women since it is not unexpected that a slower range of speeds would be employed in testing women than those used with trained male runners.

It is interesting to note that two of the female runners in this study are sub-3-hour marathoners and both displayed very low $\dot{V}_{O_2\,\mathrm{submax}}$ values over the range of speeds at which they train most often, a finding that is in agreement with earlier research reported by Costill, Thomason, and Roberts.[10] Compared with other runners who competed more successfully at shorter distance races, however, the present marathon subjects did show a more rapid rise in $\dot{V}_{O_2}$ as speeds increased.

That the regression curve constructed from the slowest speeds appears to be much flatter than those calculated from higher speeds is likely a function of the difficulty the subjects had in running comfortably at the very slow speeds. There appeared to be a tendency to displace the body more vertically at the slower speeds, a finding that has been reported by Dillman [2] and Rapp,[19] and which may lead to a correspondingly greater expenditure of energy at the slower speeds. Once a more comfortable speed is reached (generally expressed by the subjects as being about 200 m/min and above) the changing workload appears to be more linearly related to changes in the aerobic demands of the work.

Although the slope of the regression curve describing all the present data appears steeper than that calculated from data describing young girls reported by Åstrand,[13] the regression equation calculated from his data ($y = 10.547 + 0.157x$) is remarkably similar to what was calculated from the three slowest speeds in the present study ($y = 7.86 + 0.147x$, FIGURE 2). The range of speeds was similar in the two instances.

Conclusions

(1) There appear to be no differences in the aerobic demands of running at submaximal speeds between males and females who are of relatively equal ability and fitness. That the effects of fractional utilization during submaximal running may produce measurable differences in $\dot{V}_{O_2\,\mathrm{submax}}$ at given speeds of running is not clear and should be investigated using trained males and females of both equal and widely different $\dot{V}_{O_2\,\mathrm{max}}$ values.

(2) It appears that the comparison of regression curves relating running speed and $\dot{V}_{O_2}$ for different speed ranges is clearly a hazardous practice. This is true whether subjects are of the same or opposite sex. The data presented in FIGURE 2 indicate that the use of speeds below 200 m/min produces a particularly flat regression curve and calculation of the energy demands of running at higher speeds based on data collected at very slow speeds would greatly underestimate the energy requirements of the faster running. A quadratic regression equation should be used when sufficient data are available. The following regression equations best fit the present data: $y = 14.77 + 0.059x + 0.000279x^2$, where $y = \dot{V}_{O_2}$ (ml/kg·min) and $x = $ speed (m/min), and $y = 83.74 + 2.798x + 0.014288x^2$, where $y = $ speed (m/min) and $x = \dot{V}_{O_2}$ (ml/kg·min).

(3) The differences in male and female running performances at middle

and long distance races are mainly attributable to differences in $\dot{V}_{O_2 \max}$. This being the case, and in the absence of other yet-to-be-detected sex differences that might be important particularly in marathon running, females of the caliber presently competing in middle distance races should be capable of marathon times in the range of 2 hours 20 minutes to 2 hours 30 minutes.

References

1. STANLEY, L. J. & C. E. BRUBAKR. 1973. Biomechanical and neuromuscular aspects of running. *In* Exercise and Sport Sciences Reviews. J. H. Wilmore, Ed. Vol. **1**: 189–216. Academic Press. New York, N.Y.
2. DILLMAN, C. J. 1975. Kinetic analyses of running. *In* Exercise and Sport Sciences Reviews. J. H. Wilmore & J. F. Koegh, Eds. Vol. 3. Academic Press. New York, N.Y.
3. OYSTER, N. & E. P. WOOTEN. 1971. The influence of selected anthropometric measures on the ability of college women to perform the 35-yard dash. Med. Sci. Sports. **3**: 130–134.
4. MALINA, R. M., A. B. HARPER, H. H. AVENT & D. E. CAMPBELL. 1971. Physique of female track and field athletes. Med. Sci. Sports **3**: 32–38.
5. SILLS, F. D. 1960. Anthropometry in relation to physical performance. *In* Science and Medicine of Exercise and Sports. W. R. Johnson, Ed. Harper. New York, N.Y.
6. TANNER, J. M. 1964. The Physique of the Olympic Athlete. Allen and Ulwin. London, England.
7. PLOWMAN, S. 1974. Physiological characteristics of female athletes. Res. Quart. **45**: 349–362.
8. WILMORE, J. H. & C. H. BROWN. 1974. Physiological profiles of women distance runners. Med. Sci. Sports **6**: 178–181.
9. ÅSTRAND, P.-O., T. E. CUDDY, B. SALTIN & J. STENBERG. 1964. Cardiac output during submaximal and maximal work. J. Appl. Physiol. **19**: 268–274.
10. COSTILL, D. L., H. THOMASON & E. ROBERTS. 1973. Fractional utilization of the aerobic capacity during distance running. Med. Sci. Sports **5**: 248–252.
11. DANIELS, J. & N. OLDRIDGE. 1971. Changes in oxygen consumption of young boys during growth and running training. Med. Sci. Sports **3**: 161–165.
12. DANIELS, J. 1974. Physiological characteristics of champion male athletes. Res. Quart. **45**: 342–348.
13. ÅSTRAND, P.-O. 1952. Experimental Studies of Physical Working Capacity in Relation to Sex and Age. Ejnar Munksgaard. Copenhagen, Denmark.
14. HERMANSEN, L. & K. L. ANDERSON. 1965. Aerobic work capacity in young Norwegian men and women. J. Appl. Physiol. **20**: 425–431.
15. SALTIN, B. & P.-O. ÅSTRAND. 1967. Maximum oxygen uptake in athletes. J. Appl. Physiol. **23**: 353–358.
16. COSTILL, D. L. 1970. Metabolic responses during distance running. J. Appl. Physiol. **28**: 251–255.
17. NAGLE, F., D. ROBINHOLD, E. HOWLEY, J. DANIELS, G. BAPTISTA & K. STOEDEFALKE. 1970. Lactic acid accumulation during running at submaximal aerobic demands. Med. Sci. Sports **2**: 182–186.
18. DANIELS, J. 1971. Portable respiratory gas collection equipment. J. Appl. Physiol. **31**: 164–167.
19. RAPP, K. E. 1963. Running velocity: body-rise and stride-length. Unpublished Master's Thesis. State University of Iowa. Ames, Iowa.

EFFECTS OF AN ENDURANCE TRAINING REGIMEN ON ASSESSMENT OF WORK CAPACITY IN PREPUBERTAL CHILDREN *

Louis Lussier and Elsworth R. Buskirk

Laboratory for Human Performance Research
The Pennsylvania State University
University Park, Pennsylvania 16802

Introduction

The effects of a physical conditioning regimen on prepubescent children were studied. The regimen involved running progressively longer distances over a period of 12 weeks. Most previous work involving physical conditioning of children has centered on subjects of pubescent ages (11 to 13 years) and older,[1-7] and only three studies were located dealing with children of prepubescent ages.[8-10] The latter data are summarized in TABLE 1: No effect of physical conditioning was found on the aerobic capacity of 8- to 11-year-olds in the first three studies listed in TABLE 1. The investigators in these three studies utilized interval training procedures. The duration of each exercise bout was short, but identifiable with how children play. Brief-bout interval training is probably closely related to the activity pattern that is normally exhibited by children. Brown *et al.*[1] were the only investigators to report significant increases in aerobic capacity with training. They trained prepubertal girls for cross-country running and utilized distance running, i.e., endurance training, but no control subjects participated in their study and their results could have been confounded by growth-induced changes. Growth during the prepubescent period can be assumed to be linear but growth remains a complicating factor in extended studies of physical conditioning in children. Short training programs have the advantage of minimizing the effect of growth because little growth occurs and any small changes that do occur can be identified with growth, particularly if a control group is employed. Thus, the effects of physical conditioning can be isolated as differences among those subjected to physical conditioning as compared to control subjects who engage in no organized physical activity.

Subjects and Methods

A group of 26 children (ages 8 to 12) volunteered and were divided into an exercise group and a control group. All were classified as stage I according to Tanner's standards for genitalia maturity and breast development. Bone age was determined from hand and wrist X rays taken with a General Electric Mobile 225 III X-ray Unit. The radiographs were taken at a focal length of 40 in. (1.15 m), 50 kV, 50 mA, 0.2 sec (10 mA·sec). A lead-lined elongated

* This work was supported by Research Grant AM08311 from the National Institute of Arthritis, Metabolism and Digestive Diseases.

734

TABLE 1

SUMMARY OF STUDIES IN THE LITERATURE DEALING WITH THE
PHYSICAL CONDITIONING OF PREPUBERTAL CHILDREN

Study	Sex	n	Duration (weeks)	Frequency (per week)	Duration of effort * (min)	$\dot{V}_{O_2max}$ $(ml \cdot kg^{-1} \cdot min^{-1})$
Bar Or and Zwiren [8]	M+F	92	9	2–4	1	−0.8
Stewart and Gutin [9]	M	24	8	4	1–3	−0.3
Mocellin and Wasmund [10]	M+F	53	7	1–2	3–6	—
Brown et al. [1]	F	12	12	4–5	> 15	≅ 11.5

* Duration of effort before resting. Several bouts per exercise session were employed by each investigator.

wooden pyramid was used to minimize radiation scatter. A developmental age was assigned to each of the 28 ossification centers using the Greulich and Pyle *Atlas* [11] and the mean age was calculated as described in Haas *et al.*[12] Because radiographs for bone age were taken at the time of the final testing, both physiological and chronological ages reported in TABLE 2 represent age at the end of the study. No significant differences between groups were found for either chronological or physiological age. Participation in organized physical activity outside the physical conditioning regimen was essentially the same for both groups. As indicated in TABLE 3, the number of girls in each group was unequal because of the small number of girls who volunteered to participate in the study.

After physical examination of the children, familiarization sessions were conducted for the various testing procedures. The children walked on a tread-

TABLE 2

AGE AND HABITUAL PHYSICAL ACTIVITY OF SUBJECTS
IN THE EXERCISE AND CONTROL GROUPS

Variable	Exercise Group $n=16$ Mean (±SD)* (Range)	Control Group $n=10$ Mean (±SD) (Range)	p
Chronological age, years	10.3 (1.2) (8–12)	10.5 (1.2) (8–12)	NS
Physiological age, years	9.6 (1.1) (7–11)	9.8 (1.1) (7–11)	NS
Hours of physical activity per week			
Fall season	4.6	3.0	
Winter season	4.4 †	4.3	

* Standard deviation.
† Excluding time spent in the physical conditioning program.

TABLE 3

SEX AND AGE DISTRIBUTION OF SUBJECTS
IN THE EXERCISE AND CONTROL GROUPS

	Exercise Group	Control Group
Sex		
Boys	11	9
Girls	5	1
Age groups *		
8–9 years	8 (10)	4 (5)
10–12 years	8 (6)	6 (5)

* In reference to chronological age. Physiological age groups are represented in parentheses.

mill at progressively increasing submaximal workloads (3 mph and 2.5% increments), and maximal effort was elicited through use of repeated 2.5-minute running workloads (modification of the procedure developed by Taylor et al.[13]). At least two sessions were required for these tests. Oxygen uptake, heart rate, blood pressure, and cardiac output were measured at submaximal workloads corresponding to 40%, 53%, 68% of $\dot{V}_{O_2 max}$, and oxygen uptake and heart rate during maximal effort. Collections of 45 to 60 seconds of expired air in Douglas bags were used to determine $\dot{V}_{O_2 max}$ and $\dot{V}_{CO_2}$. Analysis of O_2 concentration was accomplished using a Beckman Model E-2 paramagnetic analyzer; CO_2, with a Lira Model 300 infrared analyzer. Both analyzers were calibrated before each test with standardized gas mixtures. Gas volumes were measured with the use of a Parkinson Cowan gas meter and converted to STPD.

The CO_2 rebreathing method was utilized for cardiac output determination.[14, 15] End tidal and rebreathing bag CO_2 levels were analyzed using a Godart Capnograph Type KK infrared analyzer and the results were registered on a Brush Model Mark 280 recorder. Both the analyzer and recorder were calibrated with varying CO_2 concentrations prepared with a Gefag Type Eg 7382 gas mixer. The points from the rising curve were determined at 1-second intervals, as described initially by Jernerus et al.,[14] using a filtered output derived by analog signal processing of the original CO_2 input. The resulting filtered curve provided a reliable smoothed curve from which to calculate mixed venous CO_2 concentrations.[16] Leveling off of oxygen uptake was used where possible as the criteria to indicate that maximal oxygen uptake had been reached; not all subjects showed an oxygen uptake plateau, and leveling off of heart rate (HR) and inability to complete a workload (2.5 min) were also accepted as indicators of attaining maximal effort. Body densities as determined by underwater weighing,[17] skinfolds,[18] and anthropometry [19] were used to evaluate body composition and growth changes. Body composition measurements were repeated on both groups before and after the conditioning program. Student's paired t-test was used for within-group analysis. Only those differences shown to be significant when the exercise group was compared to the control group, were retained; a noncorrelated t-test was used for the between group analysis.

The conditioning program lasted 12 weeks, the children meeting four times per week, after school. The sessions were conducted in a large gymnasium and on a 200-meter indoor track. All sessions were supervised. Two sessions per week included continuous running for progressively longer periods of time, from 10 to 35 minutes over the 12-week program. The remainder of sessions were organized around running games and activities. A single session lasted 45 minutes. The distance covered per run was calculated knowing the track length and the number of laps run during a given training session. Intensity was evaluated from timed laps and by periodic verification of HR; the child was asked to stop suddenly and HR was counted using a stethoscope. A comparison was made with the target HR corresponding to 80% $\dot{V}_{O_2\,max}$ (about 185 bpm, 92% of HR_{max}).

Results

FIGURE 1 illustrates the running results for the overall program: The average cumulative distance totaled 94.5 km (or 58.4 miles), with a range from 63.3 to 126.0 km. The distance increments became quite large toward the end of the 12-week period. There occurred a drop in pace, which reached a low at the 8th week, but this was reversed during the last four weeks. The third curve presents distance per session and reflects both changes in pace and increases in duration of running at a given pace. The distance per session increased gradually throughout the 12-week conditioning period.

At monthly intervals, 10-minute run trials were conducted; FIGURE 2 shows the increased distances covered during successive trials (1.94, 2.13, 2.20 km) with paces of 188, 206, 213 m/min, respectively. The distances and paces were

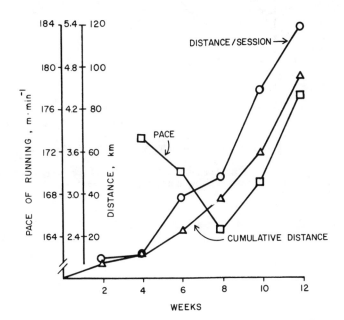

FIGURE 1. Mean pace, distance per session, and cumulative distance registered at 2-week intervals for those in the exercise group.

significantly different from each other (p < 0.5). In addition to these 10-minute trials, a treadmill test involving running for 2.5 minutes at near maximal workloads was performed following a 10-minute warmup. Maximal effort was not elicited in all children. Lower heart rates were recorded during the tests given at 1 and 2 months (196, 194.5), which were significantly different from HR_{max} (200).

FIGURE 3 shows oxygen uptake per kg body weight. A significant increase in aerobic capacity was evident by the third month of conditioning. The greatest increase in aerobic capacity appears to have taken place during the second month when the children were covering distances of 2.95 and 3.23 km per

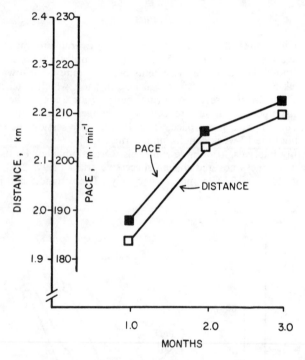

FIGURE 2. Monthly trials showing the average pace and the longest average distance covered in a 10-minute period by those in the exercise group.

session at paces of 165–170 m/min. HR_{max} and $\dot{V}_{E\,max}$ did not change significantly in either group nor did the control group show a change in $\dot{V}_{O_2\,max}$ (TABLES 4 & 5). Submaximal HR decreased significantly in the exercise group but not in the control group during performance of two standard workloads, one walking at 40% $\dot{V}_{O_2\,max}$ and one running at 80% $\dot{V}_{O_2\,max}$ (TABLE 5).

During submaximal workloads of 40%, 53%, and 68% of $\dot{V}_{O_2\,max}$, oxygen uptake, HR, cardiac output (Q), and blood pressure (BP) were measured (TABLE 6). With one exception, no differences were found; e.g., HR values were the same at all of the relative workloads except for a drop in the HR at

TABLE 4

EFFECT OF PARTICIPATION IN THE PHYSICAL CONDITIONING REGIMEN
ON AEROBIC CAPACITY ($\dot{V}_{O_2max}$) AND MAXIMAL PULMONARY VENTILATION ($\dot{V}_{Emax}$)

Variable	Group *	Mean Values ($\pm$SE)†		Δ	p
		Before	After		
$\dot{V}_{O_2max}$	E	1.76 (0.07)	1.96 (0.08)	0.20	NS
($l \cdot min^{-1}$)	C	1.83 (0.08)	1.96 (0.09)	0.09	
$\dot{V}_{O_2max}$	E	55.6 (2.07)	59.4 (2.28)	3.8	0.05
($ml \cdot kg^{-1} \cdot min^{-1}$)	C	53.1 (1.32)	53.9 (1.33)	0.8	
$\dot{V}_{Emax}$	E	54.18 (1.55)	61.50 (2.16)	7.32	NS
($l \cdot min^{-1}$)	C	55.70 (2.42)	57.9 (2.58)	2.21	

* E, exercise group, $n=12$; C, control group, $n=10$.
† Standard error.

the 40% workload in the exercise group after conditioning. BP changes were not significantly different at any workload (FIGURE 4). Oxygen uptake and ventilation were larger after conditioning at the 68% workload for the exercise group. Because of large individual variations in cardiac output, stroke volume, and arteriovenous oxygen difference, no significant differences in these variables were observed between groups that could be attributed to the conditioning program. It would appear that both an increased stroke volume and arterio-venous oxygen difference contributed to the increase in aerobic capacity.

The conditioning program was also without significant effect on the growth of these children: Increases in height, weight, and other anthropometric measurements were the same for both the exercise and control groups (TABLE 7). The suggested greater increase in body diameters and circumferences as well as in body density (TABLE 8) in the exercise group might suggest an increase

TABLE 5

EFFECT OF PARTICIPATION IN A PHYSICAL CONDITIONING REGIMEN
ON HEART RATE *

Variable	Group †	n	Mean Values ($\pm$SE)		Δ	p
			Before	After		
Submax HR at 40%	E	15	129.3 (1.96)	119.8 (1.85)	9.5	0.05
$\dot{V}_{O_2max}$ (walking)	C	10	126.2 (2.91)	126.7 (3.00)	0.5	
Submax HR at 80%	E	14	187.9 (2.41)	174.4 (2.75)	13.5	0.01
$\dot{V}_{O_2max}$ (running)	C	10	188.1 (2.43)	188.6 (1.86)	0.5	
HR_{max}	E	11	201.3 (1.87)	200.7 (2.12)	0.6	NS
	C	10	199.8 (2.43)	203.2 (2.17)	3.4	

* Heart rate (HR) in beats $\cdot min^{-1}$.
† E, exercise group; C, control group.

TABLE 6

EFFECT OF PARTICIPATION IN A PHYSICAL CONDITIONING REGIMEN ON CARDIAC OUTPUT ($\dot{Q}$), STROKE VOLUME (SV), ARTERIOVENOUS OXYGEN DIFFERENCE [$C(a\text{-}v)_{O_2}$], HEART RATE (HR), OXYGEN CONSUMPTION ($\dot{V}_{O_2}$), AND VENTILATION ($\dot{V}_E$)

Mean Values (±SE) — Workload (% $\dot{V}_{O_2max}$)

Variable	Group*	40%		53%		68%	
$\dot{Q}$ ($l \cdot min^{-1}$)	E	6.3 (0.2)	6.1 (0.3)	6.7 (0.2)	7.6 (0.4)	7.8 (0.3)	8.5 (0.3)
	C	6.7 (0.2)	6.7 (0.3)	7.6 (0.3)	8.0 (0.6)	8.5 (0.5)	9.4 (0.7)
SV (ml)	E	47.8 (1.4)	51.7 (2.8)	44.7 (1.4)	51.6 (2.3)	44.0 (2.0)	48.9 (1.7)
	C	53.1 (1.7)	52.9 (2.7)	50.8 (1.7)	53.5 (3.7)	49.0 (3.2)	54.9 (3.9)
HR* ($beats \cdot min^{-1}$)	E	129.3 (2.0)	119.8† (1.9)	148.0 (1.9)	148.0 (2.2)	173.5 (1.9)	174.8 (2.4)
	C	126.2 (2.9)	126.7 (3.0)	149.0 (2.6)	148.3 (2.4)	172.7 (1.4)	173.0 (1.4)
$C(a\text{-}v)_{O_2}$ ($ml \cdot 100\,ml^{-1}$)	E	11.8 (0.4)	11.0 (0.4)	13.9 (0.5)	13.3 (0.5)	15.4 (0.6)	16.0 (0.6)
	C	11.5 (0.3)	11.2 (0.3)	13.3 (0.5)	12.9 (0.4)	15.6 (0.5)	14.1 (0.6)
$\dot{V}_{O_2}$ ($l \cdot min^{-1}$)	E	0.73 (0.03)	0.67 (0.03)	0.91 (0.03)	1.04 (0.04)	1.16 (0.04)	1.35 (0.05)
	C	0.77 (0.03)	0.75 (0.03)	1.01 (0.04)	1.02 (0.06)	1.30 (0.06)	1.30 (0.07)
$\dot{V}_{O_2}$ ($ml \cdot kg^{-1} \cdot min^{-1}$)	E	22.7 (0.8)	20.2 (0.8)	28.6 (1.0)	30.9 (1.1)	36.3 (1.2)	40.3† (1.1)
	C	22.4 (0.9)	21.0 (0.9)	29.5 (1.1)	28.0 (1.5)	37.9 (1.0)	35.8 (1.6)
$\dot{V}_E$ ($l \cdot min^{-1}$)	E	17.5 (0.9)	18.5 (1.0)	20.9 (0.8)	27.0 (1.3)	28.2 (0.9)	35.4† (1.1)
	C	17.3 (0.9)	16.7 (1.0)	22.3 (1.2)	22.5 (1.2)	31.4 (2.0)	30.1 (1.6)

* E, exercise group, $n = 15$; C, control group, $n = 10$.
† Significant to the 0.05 level.

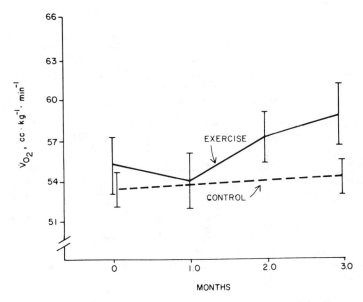

FIGURE 3. Change in aerobic capacity during the 3-month conditioning program. The control group was only tested at the beginning and end of the time period.

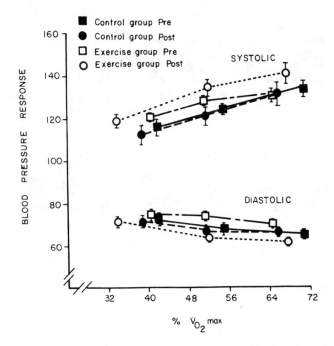

FIGURE 4. Blood pressure in relation to the relative workload expressed as a percentage of aerobic capacity.

TABLE 7

EFFECT OF PARTICIPATION IN A PHYSICAL CONDITIONING REGIMEN ON
ANTHROPOMETRIC MEASUREMENTS: HEIGHT, WEIGHT, DIAMETERS,
AND CIRCUMFERENCES

| Variable | Group * | Mean Values (±SE) | | | Δ | p |
		Before		After		
Height (cm)	E	138.7	(1.82)	141.1	(1.88)	2.4	
	C	140.2	(1.85)	140.0	(1.82)	1.8	NS
Weight (kg)	E	32.5	(1.30)	33.7	(1.38)	1.2	
	C	34.3	(2.18)	35.8	(2.34)	1.5	NS
Diameters, sum † (cm)	E	118.7	(1.44)	119.5	(1.23)	0.8	
	C	120.0	(2.31)	120.7	(2.43)	0.7	NS
Circumferences, sum † (cm)	E	455.7	(7.89)	463.7	(7.94)	8.0	
	C	467.3	(12.02)	471.5	(12.79)	4.2	NS

* E, exercise group, $n=16$; C, control group, $n=10$.
† Sum of 8 diameters and sum of 11 circumferences as described by Behnke.[19]

in lean body mass but the mean difference was not significant. Presumably a program longer than 12 weeks would be needed to show a measurable increase in fat-free weight or lean body mass.

The correlation coefficient between initial fitness expressed as $\dot{V}_{O_2 \, max}$ per kg body weight and total distance covered in the training program was $r = 0.5$ (FIGURE 5). The correlation coefficient between initial fitness and increase in fitness resulting from the program was essentially zero ($r = 0.05$) suggesting poor predictability from initial fitness of the effect of an endurance conditioning program on the aerobic capacity of prepubescent children.

TABLE 8

EFFECT OF PARTICIPATION IN A PHYSICAL CONDITIONING REGIMEN
ON BODY COMPOSITION AS REPRESENTED BY BODY DENSITY
AND SKINFOLD MEASUREMENTS

| Variable | Group * | n | Mean Values (±SE) | | | | Δ | p |
			Before		After			
Body density (g/cc)	E	12	1.053	(0.004)	1.055	(0.004)	0.002	
	C	7	1.057	(0.004)	1.057	(0.005)	0.006	NS
Skinfolds, sum † (mm)	E	16	88.1	(10.58)	85.7	(8.35)	2.4	
	C	10	86.4	(10.32)	85.1	(9.94)	1.3	NS

* E, exercise group; C, control group.
† Sum of 10 skinfolds as described by Allen et al.[18]

Discussion

Interval training has been used in most physical conditioning studies involving prepubescent children.[8-10] Repeated short bouts of high intensity effort with interspersed rest periods correspond to the observed habitual activity pattern of children, but very little effort has been made to quantify the intensity of their spurts of activity present throughout their games, sports, or spontaneous activity. Contrary to what is observed in adults, studies that have used this type of interval training have failed to show any improvement in aerobic capacity

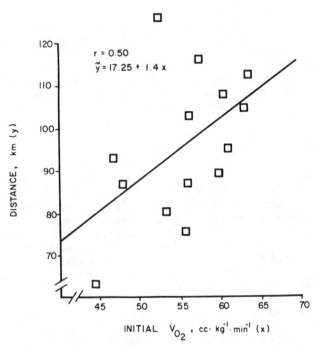

FIGURE 5. Initial aerobic capacity and total distance covered over the 12-week physical conditioning program.

of the children. More investigation is required to elucidate why this is so. Presumably their normal pattern of "interval" activity maintains their level of fitness at a reasonably high level.

Intensity of work should be monitored and quantified to provide an accurate accounting for study of training effects. Daniels and Oldridge[3] showed no increase in aerobic power in young track performers over 22 months of training, but no quantification of the intensity of workouts was mentioned, only yearly mileage. Brown et al.,[1] in contrast, showed substantial improvement in the aerobic capacity of young girls with training for cross-country running. The mean initial aerobic capacity of the youngest girls (8–9 years) was 36.6

$ml \cdot kg^{-1} \cdot min^{-1}$ and the mean for the older girls was 49 $ml \cdot kg^{-1} \cdot min^{-1}$. The mean increase in aerobic capacity for all of the girls was approximately 12 $ml \cdot kg^{-1} \cdot min^{-1}$. A control group would have been valuable in the study by Brown et al.[1] since Klissouras[6] has shown that changes in aerobic capacity are found in controls as well as exercising subjects. Nevertheless, the results of Brown et al.[1] indicate that increases in maximal oxygen uptake are produced by endurance work, particularly if the initial aerobic capacities are relatively low. Our results agree with this conclusion. The subjects of Brown et al.[1] covered greater distance per session, with more frequent training sessions, than the children in our study, which may partially explain the greater increase in aerobic capacity recorded in their runners.

Low initial fitness levels for young boys (11–13 years) have been noted.[4, 6, 7] Changes in aerobic capacity are more readily produced if the initial fitness level is low. The children in this study had relatively high aerobic capacities. The final aerobic capacity of those in the exercise group (59.4 $ml \cdot kg^{-1} \cdot min^{-1}$) is nearly equivalent to that of the subjects of Brown et al.[1] (60.3 $ml \cdot kg^{-1} \cdot min^{-1}$ for the 10–11-year-olds and 62.1 $ml \cdot kg^{-1} \cdot min^{-1}$ for 12–13-year-olds). Thus, the high initial aerobic capacity probably precluded large increases in fitness for those children who participated in this study.

Eriksson and Koch[20] showed that the increase in cardiac output associated with greater oxygen uptake at a given workload was due to an increase in stroke volume with little change in arteriovenous oxygen difference in response to physical conditioning. Their $\dot{V}_{O_2}$ values were 1.3 to 2 liters per minute higher than the values predicted from the regression equation calculated from our data, $\dot{Q} = 2.273 + 5.225 \ \dot{V}_{O_2}$. The stroke volumes measured in their subjects were 15 to 20 ml greater than those recorded here. Eriksson and Koch[20] used a dye dilution method whereas we used the CO_2 rebreathing method, and their subjects were about two years older than ours. The differences in technique and age of the subjects may be responsible for some of the variation noted. Our data agrees well with those of Bar Or et al.[15] who also used the CO_2 rebreathing method. Our results show that cardiac output and stroke volume increased moderately with time but that the increase in the exercise group was not greater than that observed in the control group. The coefficients of variation were found to vary from 12% to 15% and this variation was larger than the changes in cardiac output recorded (10% to 13% at the two highest workloads). Thus, there is the suggestion of a moderate increase in cardiac output during submaximal work with growth, but no effect attributable to physical conditioning.

The cumulative distance run during the training session over the 12-week period was the product of a number of factors including running efficiency, pace, motivation, and number of sessions attended, as well as health status and social interactions. Perhaps it is not surprising then that initial aerobic capacity explained only 25% of the variance in the cumulative distance covered during training. We had arbitrarily expected that those with high initial aerobic capacity would both run faster and farther during their training sessions. This was only partially true among the children studied.

The correlation between initial fitness and change in fitness was insignificantly different from zero ($r = 0.05$). The smallest increase in $\dot{V}_{O_2 \ max}$ was less than 1 $ml \cdot kg^{-1} \cdot min^{-1}$ in a child with an initial fitness of 53 $ml \cdot kg^{-1} \cdot min^{-1}$; on the other hand, the largest increase in $\dot{V}_{O_2 \ max}$ was 9.5 $ml \cdot kg^{-1} \cdot min^{-1}$ in a child whose initial fitness was 61 $ml \cdot kg^{-1} \cdot min^{-1}$. Both of these youngsters were high mileage runners compared to their colleagues and maintained fast paces. This difference in response to physical conditioning might be ascribed, in part, to the genetic makeup of each child, perhaps to an individual threshold for initiation of a training response as well as control of the magnitude of the response. In children as in adults, a training threshold must be reached to elicit changes in aerobic capacity. Habitual physical activity levels may alter both the threshold and the magnitude of the response, but the individual variation associated with genetic endowment is apparently predominant.

Further Comment

This study, as well as related ones, provide limited insight into the effects of physical conditioning on prepubertal children, and serious questions remain as to how intensity, duration, and frequency contribute to changes in aerobic capacity in them as compared to postpubescent children and adults. The role of genetic endowment needs further clarification as do the effects of growth. What interrelationships are there between physical activity, growth, and maturation? What effect will endurance training initiated during the period of early growth and development have on their cardiovascular physiology or on the rate of development of atherosclerosis and coronary heart disease? Are there special nutritional requirements for children who engage in endurance training regimens? Since children may be more heat intolerant, what are their environmental and physiological limitations for participation in long distance running? What effects attributable to chronic activity can be found by evaluation of weight-bearing joints? Such questions—and the list could be extensively increased—document the need for more knowledge before youngsters should be advised to participate on a mass basis in long distance training regimens and/or marathon competition.

Summary

The cardiovascular effects of a 12-week endurance training regimen were studied among normally active and healthy prepubertal children. Twenty-six 8- to 12-year-old children (20 boys and 6 girls) volunteered and 10 acted as control subjects. The training regimen consisted of distance running for progressively longer periods (from 10 to 35 min) 2 to 3 times per week, with 2 additional sessions per week devoted to running games. Those who were trained ran a cumulative average distance of 95.6 km (58.9 miles). Intensity of work was assessed from running pace and heart rate. The target workout intensity was 75% to 80% of aerobic capacity ($\dot{V}_{O_2 max}$). Growth and development accounted for increases in height, weight, body circumferences, and diameters, and fat-free body weight. Heart rate (HR) during submaximal workloads, both running and walking, decreased in the trained group ($p < 0.01$) and ($p < 0.05$). HR_{max} did not change, but $\dot{V}_{O_2 max}$ increased significantly (average 7%) in the trained group but not in the controls. No significant change attributable to training was found for submaximal cardiac output, stroke volume, or arteriovenous oxygen difference. The $\dot{V}_{O_2\,max}$ value before conditioning was a relatively poor predictor of the magnitude of improvement in functional capacity, but those with higher initial $\dot{V}_{O_2\,max}$ logged more cumulative training mileage. It was concluded that prepubertal children respond to an endurance training regimen by improving their running capacity, which is, to a limited extent, associated with increased aerobic capacity.

References

1. BROWN, C. H., J. R. HARROWER & M. F. DEETER. 1972. The effects of cross country running on preadolescent girls. Med. Sci. Sports. **4**(1): 1–5.

2. CUMMING, G. R., A. GOODWIN, G. BAGGLEY & J. ANTEL. 1967. Repeated measurements of aerobic capacity during a week of intensive training at a youth's track camp. Can. J. Physiol. Pharm. **67**(45): 805–811.

3. DANIELS, J. & N. OLDRIDGE. 1971. Changes in oxygen consumption of young boys during growth and running training. Med. Sci. Sports **3**(4): 161–165.

4. DOBELN, W. R. & B. O. ERIKSSON. 1972. Physical Training, maximal oxygen uptake and dimensions of oxygen transporting and metabolizing organs in boys 11–13 years of age. Acta Paediat. Scand. **72**(61): 653–660.

5. EKBLOM, B. 1969. Effect of physical training in adolescent boys. J. Appl. Physiol. **27**: 350–355.

6. KLISSOURAS, V. & G. WEBER. 1973. Training: Growth and heredity. *In* Pediatric Work Physiology. Proc. 4th Int. Symp. : 209–216. Wingate Institute, Israel.

7. KOCH, G. & B. O. ERIKSSON. 1973. Effect of physical training on pulmonary ventilation and gas exchange during submaximal and maximal work in boys aged 11–13 years. Scand. J. Clin. Lab. Invest. **31**: 88–94.

8. BAR OR, O. & L. D. ZWIREN. 1973. Physiological effects of frequency and content variation of physical education classes and of endurance conditioning on 9 to 10 year old girls and boys. *In* Pediatric Work Physiology. Proc. 4th Int. Symp. : 199–208. Wingate Institute, Israel.

9. STEWART, K. J. & B. GUTIN. 1976. Effects of physical training on cardiorespiratory fitness in children. Res. Quart. **47**(1): 110–120.

10. MOCELLIN, R. & U. WASMUND. 1973. Investigation of the influence of a running training program on the cardiovascular and motor performance capacity in 53 boys and girls of a second and third grade primary school class. *In* Pediatric Work Physiology. Proc. 4th Int. Symp. : 279–288. Wingate Institute, Israel.

11. GREULICH, W. W. & S. I. PYLE. 1966. Radiographic Atlas of Skeletal Development of the Hand & Wrist. 2nd ed. Stanford Univ. Press. Stanford, California.

12. HAAS, J. D., E. E. HUNT, JR. & E. R. BUSKIRK. 1971. Skeletal development of non-institutionalized children with low intelligence quotients. Amer. J. Phys. Anth. **35**(3): 455–466.

13. TAYLOR, H. L., E. R. BUSKIRK & A. HENSCHEL. 1958. Maximal oxygen uptake as an objective measure of cardiorespiratory performance. J. Appl. Physiol. **8**: 73–80.

14. JERNERUS, R., G. LUNDIN & D. THOMSON. 1963. Cardiac output in healthy subjects determined with a CO_2 rebreathing method. Acta Physiol. Scand. **59**: 390–399.

15. BAR OR, O., R. J. SHEPHARD & C. L. ALLEN. 1971. Cardiac output of 10–13 year old boys and girls during submaximal exercise. J. Appl. Physiol. **30**(2): 219–223.

16. FRANKLIN, B. A. 1976. Effects of a 12 week physical conditioning program on cardiorespiratory function, body composition and serum lipids of normal and obese middle-aged women. Ph.D. Thesis. The Pennsylvania State University, University Park, Pa.

17. AKERS, R. & E. R. BUSKIRK. 1969. An underwater weighing system utilizing "force cube" transducers. J. Appl. Physiol. **26**(5): 649–652.
18. ALLEN, T. H., M. T. PENG, K. T. CHEN, T. F. HUANG, C. CHANG & H. S. FANG. 1956. Prediction of total adiposity from skinfolds and the curvilinear relationship between external and internal adiposity. Metabolism. **5**: 346–352.
19. BEHNKE, A. 1961. Quantitative Assessment of body build. Amer. J. Physiol. **201**(6): 960–968.
20. ERIKSSON, B. O. & G. KOCH. 1973. Effect of physical training on hemodynamic response during submaximal and maximal exercise in 11–13 year old boys. Acta Physiol. Scand. **87**: 27–39.

PLASMA LIPOPROTEIN DISTRIBUTIONS IN MALE AND FEMALE RUNNERS *

Peter D. Wood, William L. Haskell, Michael P. Stern,
Steven Lewis, and Christopher Perry †

Stanford Heart Disease Prevention Program
Stanford University School of Medicine
Stanford, California 94305

In recent years there appears to have been a remarkable increase in the number of men, women, and children who regularly exercise by running or jogging. This is particularly true in northern California, as exemplified by the increase in size of the field for the annual 7.8-mile "Bay-to-Breakers" race in San Francisco from about 100 in 1963 to more than 5000 in 1976. It is clear that many of these new participants, particularly men in middle age, attribute health benefits, especially reduced risk of cardiovascular disease, to this form of increased aerobic activity. The Stanford Heart Disease Prevention Program advocates increased physical activity level as part of a hygienic life-style package for reduction of cardiovascular risk. We therefore decided to study cardiovascular risk factors, and in particular plasma lipids and lipoproteins, in groups of middle-aged male and female long distance runners in cross-sectional comparisons with control groups of people of similar age randomly selected from three northern California towns.

As this project started, considerable interest was developing in the possibility that relatively *high* concentrations of plasma high-density lipoprotein (HDL) cholesterol may be protective against coronary heart disease.[1] Certainly, higher levels of plasma HDL-cholesterol appear to be associated with relatively low prevalence of coronary heart disease in Hawaiian Japanese men,[2] in men of Evans County, Georgia,[3] and in the population of Framingham, Mass.[4] The quantitative distribution of total plasma cholesterol among the three major constituent lipoprotein classes within our runner and control groups therefore became of particular interest, since the effect of a program of increased physical activity upon plasma *total* cholesterol concentration has been the subject of conflicting reports,[5] even though the hypoglyceridemic effects of exercise are well established.[6-8] A few reports had appeared indicating that plasma HDL concentration may rise following increased physical activity level,[9, 10] and we had also noticed intensely-staining alpha bands (HDL) on agarose electrophoretograms of long distance runners, as compared to sedentary individuals. Reports of some of our findings in the male runners have appeared.[11, 12] The present report is concerned with measurement of concentrations of plasma lipids and lipoproteins, and of other risk factors for cardiovascular disease, among groups of dedicated male and female long distance runners, and comparisons with large control groups of relatively sedentary men and women.

* This work was supported by Contract NIH-2161-L and Grant HL 14174 from the National Heart, Lung and Blood Institute, National Institutes of Health, and by a grant from Best Foods, a Division of CPC International.
† Deceased October, 1976.

RUNNERS AND CONTROLS

Runners. For inclusion as a "runner" it was required that the individual had averaged at least 15 miles per week of running during the previous year, was not losing weight and was in active training at the time of the tests. Groups of 41 male runners, aged 35–59, and 43 female runners, aged 30–59, were examined (TABLE 1). Average miles run per week actually reported for the previous year were 37 ± 17 for men and 31 ± 15 for women (means $\pm$ standard deviations). All lived within 100 miles of Stanford University.

Controls. Control groups of men and women aged 35–59 were randomly selected from three northern California towns located within 90 miles of Stanford (Watsonville, Gilroy, and Tracy). They completed medical and behavioral examinations during the Fall of 1972 (response rate, 78% of those eligible to

TABLE 1

CHARACTERISTICS OF RUNNERS AND CONTROLS *

	Runners		Controls	
	Males	Females	Males	Females
Number	41	43	747 †	932 †
Age (years)				
Mean	45 ± 6.5	42 ± 8.4 ‡	47 ± 7.0	47 ± 7.0
Range	35–59	30–59	35–59	35–59
Blood pressure (mmHg)				
Mean systolic	123 ± 15.4 ‡	125 ± 15.0 ‡	133 ± 17.3	130 ± 21.1
Mean diastolic	72 ± 9.2 ‡	80 ± 9.1	84 ± 11.6	79 ± 10.9

* Mean $\pm$ standard deviations (SD).

† Randomly selected subsets of these larger groups were used for determinations of plasma lipoprotein cholesterol concentrations and treadmill performance.

‡ Mean for runners is significantly different (p <0.05) from appropriate control group.

participate).[13] Approximately 747 males and 932 females were included in the total groups (TABLE 1). The numbers of controls shown in other tables vary slightly as a result of a few missing values for some measurements. Randomly selected subsets of these total groups were used as controls for some measurements: 137 males and 85 females for graded treadmill testing (TABLE 2); and 145 males and 101 females for determinations of plasma HDL-cholesterol, low-density lipoprotein (LDL) cholesterol, and very-low-density lipoprotein (VLDL) cholesterol concentrations (TABLE 3). All of these control groups are believed to be reasonably representative of men and women aged 35–59 residing in northern California. A few moderately active men and women were included in the controls, but there is no doubt that they can be described as generally sedentary groups. It is recognized that the female runners were somewhat younger than the male runners or the female control group (TABLE 1).

TABLE 2

TREADMILL TEST RESPONSES *

	Runners		Controls	
	Males ($n=41$)	Females ($n=43$)	Males ($n=137$)	Females ($n=85$)
Duration of test (min)	16±3.0 †	13±2.8 †	9.4±1.9	6.7±2.0
Predicted maximum $\dot{V}_{O_2}$ (ml/kg·min)	58	45	39	32
Heart rate at 6 min (beats/min)	104±12.5 †	116±16.0 †	130±17.1	148±16.3
Systolic blood pressure at 6 min (mmHg)	162±22.2 †	156±19.7 †	183±24.3	175±24.4

* Means ± SD.

† Mean for runners is significantly different ($p < 0.05$) from appropriate control group.

METHODS

Resting systolic and diastolic blood pressures were measured using a standard mercury baummanometer with the cuff on the right arm and the subject sitting with the arm at heart level. Two measurements were recorded after the subject had been seated for several minutes and the second, taken about one minute after the first, was used for analysis. Venous blood was drawn in the morning into evacuated tubes containing 1 mg/ml disodium EDTA. Both

TABLE 3

PLASMA LIPID AND LIPOPROTEIN CHOLESTEROL CONCENTRATIONS, AND RATIO HDL-CHOLESTEROL/LDL-CHOLESTEROL, IN RUNNERS AND CONTROLS *

	Runners		Controls	
	Males ($n=41$)	Females ($n=43$)	Males ($n=743$ or 145 †)	Females ($n=934$ or 101 ‡)
Triglycerides (mg/100 ml)	70±24 §	56±19 §	146±105	123±89
Total cholesterol (mg/100 ml)	200±22 §	193±33 §	212±38	209±38
Cholesterol in (mg/100 ml):				
LDL	125±21 §	113±33 §	139±32	124±34
HDL	64±13 §	75±14 §	43±10	56±14
VLDL	11	7	28	28
Ratio HDL/LDL cholesterol	0.51	0.66	0.31	0.45

* Means ±SD.

† $n=145$ for LDL-, HDL-, and VLDL-cholesterol concentrations.

‡ $n=101$ for LDL-, HDL-, and VLDL-cholesterol concentrations.

§ Mean for runners is significantly d.•erent ($p < 0.05$) from appropriate control group.

runners and control subjects were asked by letter to fast overnight 12–16 hours before the test, and this was followed by an individual telephone call on the day before their visit. All participants were recumbent for not more than a few minutes during blood drawing. Both the runners and control subjects were requested not to exercise during the fasting period, so that they were not sampled immediately postexercise. Adherence to the requirements for abstinence from recent exercise, fasting, or both was checked by carefully questioning the participants at the time of their test; any nonfasting individuals were rescheduled. Plasma was prepared from blood within 2 hours and was kept at 4° C. Plasma total cholesterol and plasma triglyceride concentration were determined on the AutoAnalyzer I or II (Technicon Instruments Corp., Tarrytown, N.Y.) using a zeolite-mixture-treated isopropanol extract and following the procedures of the Lipid Research Clinic (LRC) program.[14] The instruments remained "standardized" according to LRC criteria[14] during all analyses. Determinations of plasma concentrations of cholesterol in HDL, LDL, and VLDL in the *runners* were performed using a combined ultracentrifugal and heparin-manganese precipitation method.[14] HDL accuracy was constantly monitored using a frozen plasma of known HDL-cholesterol concentration (Lipid Standardization Laboratory, Atlanta, Ga.) that appeared to be stable for at least 6 months. For the *control group*, HDL-cholesterol was again determined by the same heparin-manganese precipitation procedure, while LDL-cholesterol was estimated by the indirect method of Friedewald *et al.*[15] for all samples with triglyceride concentration less than 300 mg/100 ml. Control samples with triglyceride levels in excess of this value were subjected to the combined ultracentrifugal-precipitation procedure. Experience in our laboratory confirmed the findings of Friedewald *et al.* that the two procedures (ultracentrifugal-precipitation versus indirect) show good agreement, provided that the latter procedure is not used when triglyceride concentration is increased (in a comparison of 330 plasmas with triglyceride values of 250 mg/100 ml or less and an LDL-cholesterol range of 50–560 mg/100 ml, mean LDL-cholesterol findings of 145 mg/100 ml by the ultracentrifugal-precipitation method and 141 mg/100 ml by the indirect method were obtained, with a linear correlation coefficient of 0.962).

Percent body fat was determined for the *runners* by hydrostatic weighing;[16] detailed results for the male runners are contained in another report.[17] Body weight and height were recorded for all runners and control subjects, and relative weight was calculated for each individual as the ratio of actual to "ideal" weight. Ideal weight was considered to be the midpoint of the range of desirable weights for men 25 years of age and older and of medium build, according to the 1959 Metropolitan Life Insurance Company tables.

All runners, and random subsets of the male and female controls (Table 3), performed an ECG-monitored multistage treadmill exercise test, as described by Bruce *et al.*[18] A CM_5 bipolar ECG lead system was used, and brachial arterial blood pressure was measured by the indirect method at the end of each workload.

Questionnaires were administered to runners and controls that included enquiries about maximum body weight and weight at age 18, past and present cigarette smoking habits, frequency and amount of intake of alcoholic beverages, and dietary intake. The last item was not intended to be comprehensive, but rather was aimed at quantifying the total amounts of cholesterol and of saturated and polyunsaturated fat habitually consumed by participants.[19] The answers to questions about the frequency of ingestion and the usual portion size of all major food items containing significant amounts of these ingredients were key-punched directly from the questionnaire, and a computer program calculated the daily consumption of cholesterol and saturated and polyunsaturated fat for each participant, using the food composition data published by Fetcher et al.[20]

During the collection and processing of these data, constant efforts were made to ensure that the methods used were closely comparable for both runners and controls.

The statistical significance of the differences between the means for the lipid and lipoproteins, and for other measurements on the two groups was determined by the two-tailed Student's t-test, using the more conservative assumption that the variances of the groups were unequal.

RESULTS

As indicated in TABLE 1, the mean age of the 41 male runners was 45 while the mean age of the 747 male controls was 47. The 43 female runners (mean age 42) were somewhat younger than the 932 controls (mean age 47). Mean resting blood pressures were lower for runners than controls, except for diastolic pressures in women. Only two male runners and two female runners had blood pressures of 140/90 mmHg or above.

As anticipated, both male and female runners showed considerably greater cardiovascular fitness than their corresponding control groups, as measured during the Bruce multistage treadmill test (TABLE 2). Endurance to maximum effort during the test was greater for the runners, as was predicted maximum $\dot{V}_{O_2}$. Heart rate and systolic blood pressure at the 6-minute point during the test were considerably lower for runners than for controls. All of these differences were statistically significant ($p > 0.05$).

TABLE 3 shows mean plasma concentrations of triglycerides and of total cholesterol and cholesterol carried in the LDL, HDL, and VLDL lipoprotein fractions for runners and controls. Fasting plasma triglyceride concentrations were strikingly lower in the runners. Total cholesterol was lower in the runners—modestly so for men, more substantially for women. The distribution of the total cholesterol among the three major lipoprotein classes was different for runners compared to controls. For both sexes the LDL-cholesterol and the VLDL-cholesterol was lower in runners; however, the HDL-cholesterol was considerably *higher* (64 ± 13 vs 43 ± 10 mg/100 ml for men; 75 ± 14 vs 56 ± 14 mg/100 ml for women). The ratio of HDL-cholesterol/LDL-cholesterol was also markedly higher in the runners. The concentrations of plasma lipids and lipoproteins, and the HDL/LDL ratios, are shown as bar graphs in FIGURES 1–5. Differences between runners and controls were significant ($p < 0.05$) for both sexes for triglycerides, and for total, LDL-, and VLDL-cholesterol. Similar differences were seen when the runners and controls were divided into narrower age ranges (30–39 or 35–39; 40–49; 50–59). This is illustrated for plasma triglycerides in women (FIGURE 6), where no marked age trend is noted for the runners; and for plasma HDL-cholesterol in women (FIGURE 7), where a slight increase in concentration with age seems to occur for the runners.

Runners of both sexes were much leaner than controls (TABLE 4, FIGURE 8)

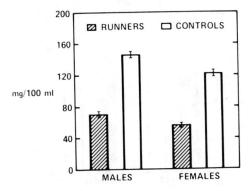

FIGURE 1. Plasma triglyceride concentrations [mean±standard error (SE)] for male and female runners and controls.

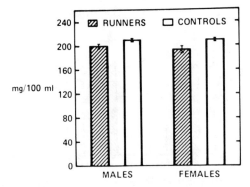

FIGURE 2. Plasma total cholesterol concentrations [mean±standard error (SE)] for male and female runners and controls.

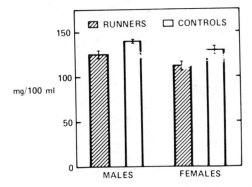

FIGURE 3. Plasma LDL-cholesterol concentrations [mean±standard error (SE)] for male and female runners and controls.

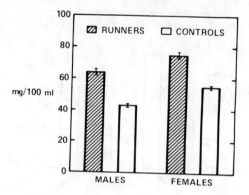

FIGURE 4. Plasma HDL-cholesterol concentrations [mean±standard error (SE)] for male and female runners and controls.

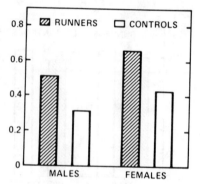

FIGURE 5. Ratio: plasma HDL-cholesterol concentration to LDL-cholesterol concentration for male and female runners and controls.

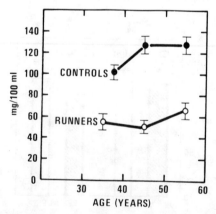

FIGURE 6. Plasma triglyceride concentrations for women runners and controls, by age [mean±standard error (SE)].

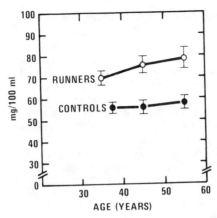

FIGURE 7. Plasma HDL-cholesterol concentrations for women runners and controls, by age [mean±standard error (SE)].

TABLE 4

BODY WEIGHT AND ADIPOSITY MEASURES IN RUNNERS AND CONTROLS *

	Runners		Controls	
	Males (n=41)	Females (n=43)	Males (n=747)	Females (n=932)
Present weight (kg)	71.0±7.0 †	57.6±6.6 †	81.1±12.7	66.3±13.9
Weight at age 18 (kg) (self-report)	68.1±8.3	57.5±6.5 †	68.5±10.7	54.8±8.4
Most ever weighed (kg) (self-report)	81.2±9.9 †	63.9±8.7 †	87.4±13.5	70.8±14.6
Relative Weight	1.02±0.08 †	1.04±0.08 †	1.22±0.17	1.25±0.25
Body fat (%)	13	21	—	—

* Mean values ±SD.
† Mean for runners is significantly different (p < 0.05) from appropriate control group.

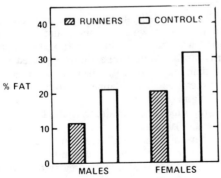

FIGURE 8. Body fat content (as percent of total body weight) by hydrostatic weighing for male and female runners and for control groups of relatively sedentary men [21] and women [22, 23] of similar age, as recorded in the literature.

as judged by mean relative weights. Low mean values for body fat content of the runners (13% for males; 21% for females) were recorded; these determinations were not made in this study for the control groups, but mean values of about 21% (males) [21] and of about 29%–35% (females) [22, 23] have been reported for groups of relatively sedentary middle-aged people. In addition, "present weight" for runners of both sexes was much closer to "weight at age 18," and further removed from "most ever weighed" than was the case for the corresponding control groups (TABLE 4).

The distribution of cigarette smokers of various degrees among runners and controls is shown in TABLE 5. All runners of both sexes were currently nonsmokers (compared with 57.5% of male controls and 68.0% of female controls). However, considerable proportions of both the runners (39% of males, 58.1% of females), and of the currently nonsmoking controls (54.0% of males, 19.7% of females) were ex-smokers.

TABLE 5

CIGARETTE SMOKING HABITS

	Runners		Controls	
	Males (n=41)	Females (n=43)	Males (n=747)	Females (n=932)
Current cigarettes/day				
0	100.0%	100.0%	57.5%	68.0%
1–10			7.6%	11.4%
11–20			16.8%	12.9%
21–30			8.7%	4.6%
31+			9.4%	3.1%
Ex-smokers *	39.0%	58.1%	54.0%	19.7%

* Percent of current nonsmokers who were formerly cigarette smokers.

Mean values for self-reported daily dietary intake of cholesterol, saturated fat, and polyunsaturated fat are shown for runners and controls in TABLE 6. Cholesterol intake reported was rather less in male runners, but rather more in female runners, than in controls. Male runners also appeared to eat relatively less polyunsaturated fat than male controls. Bearing in mind the somewhat insensitive nature of such recall data, there appeared to be no important dietary differences between runners and controls.

TABLE 7 contains self-reported data pertaining to the frequency and amount of alcohol consumption by the runners and controls. These data suggest that a smaller proportion of runners of either sex were nondrinkers, as compared to controls. Runners appeared to drink more frequently than controls. Wine consumption reported by runners was strikingly greater than that reported by controls; and among females, runners reported less beer drinking than controls. Differences in reported consumption of cocktails and mixed drinks were not seen.

TABLE 6

SELF-REPORTED DIETARY INTAKE OF CHOLESTEROL, SATURATED FAT AND
POLYUNSATURATAED FAT FOR RUNNERS AND CONTROLS *

	Runners		Controls	
	Males ($n=33$)	Females ($n=34$)	Males ($n=747$)	Females ($n=932$)
Cholesterol (mg/day)	523±223 †	520±175 †	623±273	452±223
Saturated fat (g/day)	40.4±16.7	34.6±12.6	43.4±18.9	31.6±14.2
Polyunsaturated fat (g/day)	8.0±5.2 †	8.9±4.9	10.0±6.1	9.3±6.1

* Mean values ± SD.
† Mean for runners is significantly different ($p < 0.05$) from appropriate control group.

DISCUSSION

Both male and female runners recruited for this study showed considerably greater cardiovascular fitness than controls of comparable age (TABLE 2), as was expected. The mean age, and the age distribution, for male runners and controls, were very comparable. Female runners were on average 5 years younger than control women; however, it seems unlikely that a difference of this magnitude would significantly affect the conclusions reached from the comparisons made for women.

TABLE 7

FREQUENCY AND AMOUNT OF SELF-REPORTED ALCOHOL INTAKE FOR
RUNNERS AND CONTROLS

	Runners		Controls	
	Males ($n=33$)	Females ($n=34$)	Males ($n=747$)	Females ($n=931$)
Frequency of drinking				
Daily	42.4%	44.1%	21.6%	25.6%
3–4 times/week	33.3%	23.5%	9.3%	7.1%
1–2 times/week	15.2%	11.8%	19.4%	17.4%
1–2 times/month	0	8.8%	15.6%	12.1%
Less than 1 time/month	9.1%	11.8%	34.2%	37.8%
Amount/week (mean ± SD)				
Number of bottles or cans of beer	2.45±3.1	1.21±2.3 *	2.55±7.6	2.94±7.5
Number of glasses of wine	6.52±10.3 *	5.76±5.3 *	1.18±3.7	1.80±5.9
Number of cocktails or mixed drinks	3.48±7.6	2.53±5.5	2.95±7.5	3.03±8.3

* Mean for runners is significantly different ($p < 0.05$) from appropriate control group.

The observation that fasting plasma triglyceride concentrations are lower in groups of very active people than in relatively sedentary groups has been made on several previous occasions. The present results are particularly striking in this respect, the runners showing less than one-half the concentration found in the sex-matched controls. This probably reflects the particularly high level of physical activity displayed by the runners. Mean female triglyceride levels were lower than male levels for both runners and controls, as would be anticipated from population studies.[24] The virtual absence from the running groups of individuals with even mildly elevated plasma triglyceride levels is indicated by the very low standard deviations for this measurement (TABLE 3). There was some indication that the known tendency of triglyceride level to increase with age is absent for the runners. This is suggested for women in FIGURE 6.

Previous studies on the possible association of relatively low plasma total cholesterol concentrations with vigorous exercise have given conflicting results.[5] Certainly, strikingly lower cholesterol levels (compared with sedentary controls) have seldom been reported. The present data, obtained with particular attention to methodological reliability, indicate that runners of each sex had a modestly, but significantly lower mean total cholesterol level than controls. As noted earlier, the manner in which the total cholesterol is carried by the three major groups of plasma lipoproteins has recently assumed considerable significance in relation to predicted risk of cardiovascular disease.[1, 2] FIGURE 9 shows diagrammatically the composition of the three major lipoprotein classes, VLDL, LDL, and HDL. The larger VLDL particles carry the majority of the total plasma triglyceride, but normally a relatively small proportion of the total cholesterol. It follows that the runners, with low levels of plasma triglyceride, have low concentrations (relative to controls) of VLDL. The LDL usually carry the majority of the total cholesterol. They also contain sizeable proportions of phospholipids and protein, and are intermediate in size between the VLDL and HDL lipoproteins. The small HDL carry the remainder of the cholesterol and large proportions of phospholipid and protein. As shown in TABLE 3, runners of each sex showed low concentrations of cholesterol in the larger VLDL, compared to controls. Of most interest was the distribution of the bulk of the cholesterol between the LDL and HDL: clearly, runners carry less cholesterol than controls in the LDL, but more in the HDL. These differences are shown clearly in FIGURES 3 and 4. The distribution of total cholesterol among the

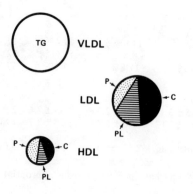

FIGURE 9. Diagrammatic representation of the chemical composition of the major plasma lipoprotein classes. The large VLDL contain triglyceride as the major constituent, with small proportions of cholesterol. LDL are intermediate in size and contain high proportions of cholesterol and phospholipids. The small HDL carry major proportions of cholesterol, phospholipids and protein. TG, triglycerides; C, cholesterol; PL, phospholipids; P, protein.

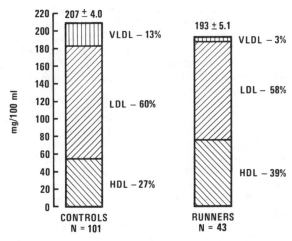

FIGURE 10. The distribution of total plasma cholesterol among the three major lipoprotein classes for women runners and controls. Total cholesterol levels are means±SE.

three component lipoproteins is shown for women runners and controls in bar graph form in FIGURE 10. The higher concentrations of cholesterol found in HDL in runners do not *necessarily* indicate that higher plasma concentrations of the total HDL macromolecules are present in runners compared to controls, although this is probably true. Some work in this area, relating to the degree of "saturation" of the HDL protein with cholesterol, has been reported.[25, 26] Further work on this area in these runners is in progress. An early report [10] in which plasma lipoprotein concentrations were measured by a quantitative electrophoretic method suggested that an exercise program resulted in increased levels of the total HDL macromolecules.

The present finding of marked differences between middle-aged runners and controls in respect to distribution of plasma cholesterol between LDL and HDL is of considerable interest in view of the increasing evidence that higher concentrations of LDL-cholesterol are atherogenic, whereas higher concentrations of HDL-cholesterol are possibly protective against atherogenesis. Certainly the epidemiological *associations* between low levels of plasma HDL-cholesterol and increased prevalence of coronary heart disease are clear for certain groups that have been studied.[1-4] It appears that male runners, and especially female runners, in middle age are in an advantageous position in this respect, as compared with controls. Rhoads *et al.*[2] have reported that the inverse relation of HDL-cholesterol to prevalence of coronary heart disease (in Hawaii Japanese men) was independent of LDL-cholesterol concentration. If this is generally true, the ratio of the HDL-cholesterol concentration to the LDL-cholesterol concentration should be a useful predictor of risk of heart disease. In fact, recent work [2, 4] suggests that this ratio should be considerably more powerful as a predictor than the traditional total cholesterol concentration. As shown in TABLE 3 and FIGURE 5, runners showed much higher ratios than controls. Women runners, for instance, showed a mean ratio over twice that observed for male controls (0.66 vs 0.31, respectively). In a number of women runners, and in a few male runners, HDL was the principal carrier of plasma cholesterol; i.e., the ratio HDL-cholesterol/LDL-cholesterol exceeded unity. This situation is very seldom found in adult populations, but is common in very young children, in relatively primitive peoples, and in certain animals (e.g., the rat) in which atherosclerosis almost never occurs. We therefore propose that in future prospective studies of cardiovascular disease this ratio be measured in addition to the usual determinations of total cholesterol and triglycerides.

The groups of runners studied here were, of course, different from the control groups in a number of respects in addition to their clearly greater physical activity level. Runners rather clearly had adopted a running "life-style package." Some further studies on these groups have started to indicate ways in which the runners were—and in some instances were not—different from the randomly selected controls. The runners were clearly leaner than controls (TABLE 4, FIGURE 8). Their present body weight was very close to that reported for age 18. Controls, on the other hand, were currently much heavier than they were at age 18. Runners were very close to "ideal weight," whereas controls averaged 22%–25% above ideal weight. The influence of leanness upon plasma lipid and lipoprotein concentrations, independent of physical activity level, is currently being investigated for these groups. Although not reported here in detail, it appears that approximately one-half of the difference in plasma triglyceride concentration between male runners and controls can be attributed to their leanness alone. Probably leanness contributes also to the relatively low mean blood pressures demonstrated by the runners. Mean diastolic pressure in women runners was an exception (TABLE 1), where there was no difference from controls.

None of the 84 runners studied here currently smoked cigarettes. This area of abstinence seems to be virtually absolute among dedicated runners—an observation that may have a message for scientists working in smoking control. The runners had clearly not been lifelong nonsmokers (TABLE 5); in fact very considerable proportions of runners and currently nonsmoking controls reported that they were ex-smokers. An analysis of smoking and nonsmoking controls indicated similar levels of plasma triglycerides and HDL-cholesterol, so that smoking alone does not seem to account for the observed differences in lipoprotein pattern.

It may be suggested that the runners' lipoprotein patterns could result from selection of a relatively hypocholesterolemic diet by a particularly health-conscious group. For this reason an attempt was made to evaluate certain self-reported dietary intake habits among runners and controls (TABLE 6). No difference was seen for estimates of daily intake of saturated fat. Male runners reported slightly *less* polyunsaturated fat intake. Male runners reported somewhat less, but female runners somewhat more, dietary cholesterol intake. From these data it would appear that runners are not particularly different from controls in their choice of "heart healthy" food. Three-day food records are available to us for runners and for a control group, and these more detailed data are in course of analysis.

Finally, alcohol intake habits were examined, since it has been reported that even moderate amounts of ethanol added to an ethanol-free diet result in some elevation of plasma triglycerides.[27] Thus, it might be thought that runners, embracing a healthy life-style in all its aspects, should be largely nondrinkers, or at least very light drinkers. The self-reported data in TABLE 7 seem to refute this contention. Apparently both male and female runners are more likely to be drinkers than are the controls, and they also drink more frequently. Although the intake of cocktails and mixed drinks by runners was not significantly different from controls, and female runners reported drinking less beer than female controls, it appeared that runners of each sex drink three to four times as much wine as controls. This habit is probably related to the generally higher socioeconomic status of the runners, which we noted but have not reported here. In any event, it seems clear that the favorable lipoprotein pattern of the runners, and in particular their remarkably low mean plasma triglyceride levels, cannot be attributed to their relatively modest alcohol intake, compared to controls. It might be postulated that moderate-to-generous drinking can proceed in runners without the increase in plasma triglyceride levels that would be anticipated for relatively sedentary groups. This finding may be of interest to scientists working in the alcoholism area.

In conclusion, it appears that the groups of male and female long distance runners studied here display remarkably low risk of cardiovascular disease by virtue of their advantageous plasma lipid and lipoprotein pattern, their leanness, their complete abstinence from cigarette smoking and their normal blood pressures. It seems that these and other desirable physiological and behavioral characteristics of runners are not necessarily accompanied by either a careful selection of low-cholesterol, low-saturated fat foods, or by lower-than-average alcohol intake.

SUMMARY

Recent studies have shown a consistent association between relatively *low* plasma concentrations of high-density lipoprotein (HDL) cholesterol and increased risk of coronary heart disease. A cross-sectional comparison was made of the distribution of plasma lipids and lipoproteins in groups of 41 male and 43 female long distance runners versus larger control groups matched for age and sex, randomly selected from northern California towns. The runners showed modestly lower total cholesterol concentrations, while their triglyceride levels were only 50% of control. HDL-cholesterol was *higher* in runners than controls (75 ± 14 vs 56 ± 14 mg/100 ml for women; 64 ± 13 vs 43 ± 10 for men), while low-density lipoprotein cholesterol was *lower* (113 ± 33 vs 124 ± 34 for women; 125 ± 21 vs 139 ± 32 for men). All differences were statistically significant ($p < 0.05$), and only partially attributable to known factors other than high physical activity level. Since the runners were predominantly normotensive, relatively lean, and exclusively nonsmokers, they appear to constitute a remarkably favored group with respect to risk of cardiovascular disease.

REFERENCES

1. MILLER, G. J. & N. E. MILLER. 1975. Plasma high-density lipoprotein concentration and development of ischaemic heart disease. Lancet **i:** 16–19.
2. RHOADS, G. G., G. L. GULBRANDSEN & A. KAGAN. 1976. Serum lipoproteins and coronary heart disease in a population study of Hawaii Japanese men. N. Engl. J. Med. **294:** 293–298.
3. TYROLER, G. A., C. G. HAMES, I. KRISHAN, S. HEYDEN, G. COOPER & J. C. CASSEL. 1975. Black-white differences in serum lipids and lipoproteins in Evans County. Prev. Med. **4:** 541–549.

4. CASTELLI, W. P., J. T. DOYLE, T. GORDON, C. HAMES, S. B. HULLEY, A. KAGAN, D. McGEE, W. J. VICIC & W. J. ZUKEL. 1975. HDL cholesterol levels (HDLC) in coronary heart disease (CHD): A cooperative lipoprotein phenotyping study. Circulation 52(Suppl. 2): 97.

5. HASKELL, W. L. & S. M. FOX, III. 1974. Physical activity in the prevention and therapy of cardiovascular disease. In Science and Medicine of Exercise and Sport. W. R. Johnson & E. R. Buskirk, Eds. 2nd edit. Harper and Row. New York, N.Y.

6. HOLLOSZY, J. O., J. S. SKINNER, G. TORO & T. K. CURETON. 1964. The effects of a six month program of endurance exercise on serum lipids of middle-aged men. Amer. J. Cardiol. 14: 753–760.

7. GOODE, R. C., J. B. FIRST BROOK & R. J. SHEPARD. 1966. Effects of exercise and a cholesterol-free diet on human serum lipids. Can. J. Physiol. Pharmacol. 44: 575–580.

8. OSCAI, L. B., J. A. PATTERSON, D. L. BOGARD, R. J. BECK & B. L. ROTHERMEL. 1972. Normalization of serum triglycerides and lipoprotein electrophoretic patterns by exercise. Amer. J. Cardiol. 30: 775–780.

9. HOFFMAN, A. A., W. R. NELSON & F. A. GOSS. 1967. Effects of an exercise program on plasma lipids of senior Air Force officers. Amer. J. Cardiol. 20: 516–524.

10. ALTEKRUSE, E. B. & J. H. WILMORE. 1973. Changes in blood chemistries following a controlled exercise program. J. Occup. Med. 15: 110–113.

11. WOOD, P. D., H. KLEIN, S. LEWIS & W. L. HASKELL. 1974. Plasma lipoprotein concentrations in middle-aged runners. Circulation 50(Suppl. 3): 115.

12. WOOD, P. D., W. HASKELL, H. KLEIN, S. LEWIS, M. P. STERN & J. W. FARQUHAR. 1976. The distribution of plasma lipoproteins in middle-aged male runners. Metabolism 25: 1249–1257.

13. WOOD, P., M. STERN, W. HASKELL, N. MACCOBY & J. FARQUHAR. 1974. Plasma lipid and lipoprotein concentrations in rural Californian communities. In Atherosclerosis III. Proceedings of the Third International Symposium. G. Schlettler & A. Weizel, Eds. : 837. Springer-Verlag. New York, N.Y.

14. LIPID RESEARCH CLINICS MANUAL OF LABORATORY OPERATIONS. Vol. 1. Lipid and Lipoprotein Analysis. 1974. HEW Publication No. NIH 75–628. U.S. Government Printing Office. Washington, D.C.

15. FRIEDEWALD, W. T., R. I. LEVY & D. S. FREDRICKSON. 1972. Estimation of the concentration of low-density lipoprotein cholesterol in plasma, without use of the preparative ultracentrifuge. Clin. Chem. 18: 499–502.

16. KATCH, F. I., E. D. MICHAEL & S. M. HORVATH. 1967. Estimation of body volume by underwater weighing: description of a simple method. J. Appl. Physiol. 23: 811–813.

17. LEWIS, S., W. L. HASKELL, H. KLEIN, J. HALPERN & P. D. WOOD. 1975. Prediction of body composition in habitually active middle-aged men. J. Appl. Physiol. 39: 221–225.

18. BRUCE, R. A., F. KUSUMI & D. HOSMER. 1973. Maximal oxygen intake and nomographic assessment of functional aerobic impairment in cardiovascular disease. Amer. Heart J. 85: 546–562.

19. STERN, M. P., J. W. FARQUHAR, N. MACCOBY & S. H. RUSSELL. 1976. Results of a two-year health education campaign on dietary behavior: the Stanford Three Community Study. Circulation 54: 826–833.

20. FETCHER, E. S., N. FOSTER, J. T. ANDERSON, F. GRANDE & A. KEYS. 1967. Quantitative estimation of diets to control serum cholesterol. Amer. J. Clin. Nutr. 20: 475–492.

21. BROZEK, J. & A. KEYS. 1951. The evaluation of leanness-fatness in man: norms and inter-relationships. Brit. J. Nutr. 5: 194–206.

22. YOUNG, C. M., J. BLONDIN, R. TENSUAN & J. H. FRYER. 1963. Body composition of "older" women. J. Amer. Dietet. Assoc. 43: 344–348.

23. POLLOCK, M. L., E. E. LAUGHRIDGE, B. COLEMAN, A. C. LINNERUD & A. JACKSON.

1975. Prediction of body density in young and middle-aged women. J. Appl. Physiol. **38:** 745–749.

24. WOOD, P. D. S., M. P. STERN, A. SILVERS, G. M. REAVEN & J. VON DER GROEBEN. 1972. Prevalence of plasma lipoprotein abnormalities in a free-living population of the Central Valley, California. Circulation **45:** 114–126.

25. BERG, K., A-L. BORRESON & G. DAHLEN. 1976. Serum-high-density-lipoprotein and atherosclerotic heart disease. Lancet **i:** 499–501.

26. ALBERS, J. J., P. W. WAHL, V. G. CABANA, W. R. HAZZARD & J. J. HOOVER. 1976. Quantitation of apolipoprotein A–I of human high density lipoprotein. Metabolism **25:** 633–644.

27. GINSBERG, H., J. OLEFSKY, J. W. FARQUHAR & G. M. REAVEN. 1975. Moderate ethanol ingestion and plasma triglyceride levels—a study in normal and hypertriglyceridemic persons. Ann. Intern. Med. **80:** 143–149.

BODY PHYSIQUE AND COMPOSITION OF THE FEMALE DISTANCE RUNNER

Jack H. Wilmore

Department of Physical Education
University of Arizona
Tucson, Arizona 85721

C. Harmon Brown

Student Health Services
California State University, Hayward
Hayward, California 94541

James A. Davis

National Athletic Health Institute
Inglewood, California 90301

Recently, it has been established unequivocally that exercise is a primary factor in both the control and alteration of body composition.[1] This has been demonstrated in the normal population [2] as well as in various athletic populations,[3] for males and females alike.[4] Within the domain of athletics, the male distance runner is among the leannest of all athletes,[5] with a distinct physique that is characterized as ectomesomorphic.[6] This leanness is undoubtedly the result of both a genetic predisposition to leanness and to the tremendous volume of running that appears necessary in training for distance running, e.g., running in excess of 100 miles per week.

Since females experience changes in body composition with endurance training programs similar to those found in males,[7] the question is raised as to how the male and female distance runners compare relative to body composition and physique. Is the female distance runner as lean as her male counterpart, or do the basic hormonal differences between the sexes dictate a greater amount of relative fat in the female as a result of higher estrogen levels? The latter would put the female at a distinct disadvantage in competition with males, as endurance performance has been closely linked to body composition; i.e., the greater the relative fat, the poorer the endurance performance.[8, 9] The purpose of the present study was to investigate the body composition and physique of the female distance runner to determine how she differs when compared to the male distance runner, female sprinters and middle distance runners, male and female athletes in various sports, and population norms for the average male and female of comparable age. In addition, the role of either or both reduced body weight and reduced body fat in menstrual irregularities was evaluated.

Experimental Design

World-class and national-caliber athletes were selected for participation in this study. The sample consisted of female distance runners ($n = 70$), female sprinters and middle distance runners ($n = 8$), and female shot put, discus, and

764

javelin throwers $(n = 9)$. In addition, 15 members of the University of California, Davis, women's swimming team were selected as a comparison group. The physical characteristics of the subjects are defined in TABLES 1 and 2. All tests were conducted during the competitive season for each group.

Body composition was assessed by the hydrostatic weighing technique.[10] Residual volume was assessed by the oxygen dilution technique [11] using closed-circuit spirometry. Residual volume measurements were taken out of water in a seated position similar to that posture assumed during the underwater weighing. The procedures used for the underwater weighing have been described previously.[12] A minimum of eight consecutive determinations were obtained for each subject. The representative underwater weight was selected on the basis of the highest weight if it was observed more than twice; the second highest weight if it was observed more than once, and if the first criterion was not met; or the third highest weight if neither the first nor the second criteria were met. The equation developed by Siri [13] was used to estimate relative fat from body density.

Body physique was assessed by the Heath-Carter modified somatotype method, using only anthropometric measurements to estimate each of the three components.[14] The first component, endomorphy, is estimated from the sum of the triceps, subscapular, and suprailiac skinfold thicknesses. The second component, mesomorphy, is assessed on the basis of two bone diameter (humerus and femur) and two circumference measurements (upper arm and calf), the latter two being corrected for the calf and triceps skinfold thicknesses. These two diameters and two corrected circumferences are evaluated relative to body height. The third component, ectomorphy, is assessed strictly on the basis of the ratio, height/$\sqrt[3]{\text{weight}}$. Somatotype was determined for approximately half of the sample of distance runners using only the anthropometric somatotype and not the combined photoscopic and anthropometric somatotype. The specific landmarks for each anthropometric measurement site have been described in detail in previous publications.[10, 15]

Results and Discussion

The body composition data for all groups is presented in TABLE 1 and the body physique data for 37 of the 70 distance runners is presented in TABLE 2. Since the procedure of estimating relative fat from body density is suspect in individuals who have not attained full growth and maturation, the sample of runners was divided into those 16 years of age and younger, and those who were 17 years of age and older. In the physically immature individual, where the density of the lean tissue is in a continual state of change, the conversion of body density to relative fat usually results in an overestimation of relative fat due to a lean tissue density that is actually lower than that assumed in the formula.[16]

TABLE 3 provides a summary of studies that have assessed the body composition in both normal males and females of the ages assessed in this study. TABLES 4 and 5 contain body composition values for male and female athletes respectively in various sports.

In comparison to the normal female population of similar age, the female distance runner is of average height, has a slightly lower total body weight, a lower fat weight, and a slightly higher lean body weight. This results in a considerably lower relative body fat in the distance runner when compared to

TABLE 1

BODY COMPOSITION OF THE VARIOUS FEMALE ATHLETES TESTED FOR THIS STUDY *

Group	n	Age (yrs)	Height (cm)	Weight (kg)	Lean Weight (kg)	Fat Weight (kg)	Relative Fat (%)
Distance Runners							
9–16 years	28	13.4±1.7	157.1±9.3	42.8±7.6	35.6±6.2	7.2±2.4	16.5±3.9 †
17–51 years	42	25.0±9.1	166.8±6.9	54.3±6.4	45.0±5.2	9.3±4.2	16.9±6.4
Total	70	20.2±9.3	162.9±9.2	49.7±8.9	41.3±7.2	8.4±3.7	16.8±5.5
Sprinters and Middle Distance Runners							
9–16 years	4	13.5±1.0	161.5±8.2	50.1±8.2	44.6±6.3	5.6±2.9	10.7±4.2 ‡
17–51 years	4	18.3±1.3	171.5±8.7	57.8±7.7	51.3±5.1	6.6±2.8	11.1±3.6
Total	8	15.9±2.7	166.5±9.3	54.0±8.4	47.9±6.4	6.1±2.7	10.9±3.6
Shot Put, Discus, and Javelin							
Throwers	9	18.8±3.0	173.9±6.9	80.8±21.1	58.9±9.6	21.8±12.2	27.0±8.4
Swimmers							
Sprinters	4	—	165.1±4.3	57.1±4.7	48.7±3.9	8.4±3.7	14.6±5.9
Middle distance	7	—	166.6±3.0	66.8±6.3	50.5±4.1	16.3±4.6	24.1±5.6
Distance	4	—	166.3±5.3	60.9±7.1	50.4±4.4	10.5±2.9	17.1±2.6

* Values represent means ± standard deviations.
† Body density of 1.061.
‡ Body density of 1.075.

TABLE 2

BODY PHYSIQUE OF THE FEMALE DISTANCE RUNNER *

Age Group	*n*	Endomorphy	Somatotype Mesomorphy	Ectomorphy
9–16	14	2.1±0.7	1.4±0.8	4.5±1.1
17–51	23	3.2±1.3	2.1±1.4	3.7±1.4
Total	37	2.8±1.2	1.9±1.2	4.0±1.3

* Values represent means ± standard deviations.

the average, by approximately 6 to 8 percentage points. The average female is approximately 12–13 cm shorter than the average male at full maturity, 16–19 kg lighter in total weight, 19–21 kg lighter in lean weight, 1–2 kg heavier in fat weight, and 8–11 percentage points greater in relative fat. When comparing the fully mature female distance runner with her male counterpart, the female is approximately 10 cm shorter, 13 kg lighter in total weight, 16 kg lighter in lean weight, 2 kg heavier in fat weight, and 6 to 7 percentage points greater in relative fat. Compared to the average male, the female distance runner is shorter, lighter in absolute, lean and fat weight, and is approximately the same in relative fat.

From the above, it would appear that the female distance runner is at a distinct disadvantage when compared to the male distance runner due to the additional fat she must carry during the run. From FIGURE 1, it is interesting to note that 7 of the 70 distance runners and 5 of the 8 middle distance runners

TABLE 3

BODY COMPOSITION VALUES IN NORMAL MALES AND FEMALES OF VARIOUS AGES

Group	*n*	Age (yrs)	Height (cm)	Weight (kg)	Relative Fat * (%)	Reference
Males	95	10.0	142.3	35.2	18.7	Wilmore and McNamara [16]
	66	9–12	—	—	22.3	Parízková [17]
	57	13–16	—	—	17.0	Parízková [17]
	48	17.0	178.6	72.1	10.9	Michael and Katch [18]
	133	22.0	177.3	75.6	14.6	Wilmore and Behnke [19]
	297	28.7	177.1	77.9	16.5	Wright and Wilmore [20]
	55	33.2	179.0	79.6	18.9	Wilmore, *et al.*[8]
Females	56	9–12	—	—	26.0	Parízková [17]
	31	9–13	151.9	45.7	23.2	Parízková and Roth [21]
	62	13–16	—	—	22.8	Parízková [17]
	128	21.4	164.9	58.6	25.7	Wilmore and Behnke [22]
	94	20.4	167.5	44.9	28.6	Young [23]
	64	19–23	165.9	58.4	21.9	Katch and Michael [24]
	50	20.2	165.0	55.5	22.9	Sloan, Burt, and Blyth [25]
	60	44.7	165.9	61.2	29.8	Pollock [26]

* Calculated from body density values using the equation of Siri.[13]

TABLE 4

BODY COMPOSITION VALUES IN MALE ATHLETES

Athletic Group or Sport	n	Age (yrs)	Height (cm)	Weight (kg)	Relative Fat (%)	Reference
Runners	10	22.5	177.4	64.5	6.3	Šprynarová and Pařízková [27]
	114	26.1	175.7	64.2	7.5	Costill et al. [5]
	11	40–49	180.7	71.6	11.2	Pollock et al. [28]
	5	50–59	174.7	67.2	10.9	
	6	60–69	175.7	67.1	11.3	
	3	70–75	175.6	66.8	13.6	
	45	47.2	176.5	70.7	13.2	Lewis et al. [29]
Track and Field *	9	21.3	180.6	71.6	3.7	Novak et al. [30]
	15	—	—	—	8.8	Forsyth and Sinning [31]
Discus	7	28.3	186.1	104.7	16.4	Fahey et al. [32]
	12	26.4	190.8	110.5	16.3	Wilmore [33]
Shot Put	5	27.0	188.2	112.5	16.5	Fahey et al. [32]
	2	22.0	191.6	126.2	19.6	Behnke and Wilmore [10]
Weight Lifters	14	24.9	166.4	77.2	9.8	Šprynarová and Pařízková [27]
Power	3	26.3	176.1	92.0	15.6	Fahey et al. [32]
Olympic	11	25.3	177.1	88.2	12.2	
Body Builders	2	29.0	172.4	83.1	8.4	
Wrestlers	2	26.0	177.8	81.8	9.8	Gale and Flynn [34]
	9	27.0	176.0	75.7	10.7	Pařízková [3]
	9	22.0	—	—	5.0	Sinning [35]
	37	19.6	174.6	74.8	8.8	Katch and Michael [36]
	94	15–18	172.3	66.3	6.9	

Swimmers *	13	21.8	182.3	79.1	8.5	Šprynarová and Parížková[27]
	7	20.6	182.9	78.9	5.0	Novak *et al.*[30]
Skiers	9	25.9	176.6	74.8	7.4	Šprynarová and Parížková[27]
Baseball players	10	20.8	182.7	83.3	14.2	Novak *et al.*[30]
	17	—	—	—	11.8	Forsyth and Sinning[31]
	16	27.4	183.1	88.0	12.6	Wilmore[33]
Football	16	20.3	184.9	96.4	13.8	Novak *et al.*[30]
	11			—	13.9	Forsyth and Sinning[31]
Defensive backs	15	17–23	178.3	77.3	11.5	Wickkiser and Kelly[37]
Offensive backs	15	17–23	179.7	79.8	12.4	
Linebackers	7	17–23	180.1	87.2	13.4	
Offensive linemen	13	17–23	186.0	99.2	19.1	
Defensive linemen	15	17–23	186.6	97.8	18.5	
Defensive backs	26	24.5	182.5	84.8	9.6	Wilmore *et al.*[38]
Offensive backs	40	24.7	183.8	90.7	9.4	
Linebackers	28	24.2	188.6	102.2	14.0	
Offensive line	38	24.7	193.0	112.6	15.6	
Defensive line	32	25.7	192.4	117.1	18.2	
Quarterbacks, Kickers	16	24.1	185.0	90.1	14.4	
Tennis	7	—	—	—	15.2	Forsyth and Sinning[31]
Gymnastics	7	20.3	178.5	69.2	4.6	Novak *et al.*[30]
Jockeys	21	30.9	158.2	50.3	14.1	Wilmore, unpublished data
Ice Hockey	12	26.3	180.3	86.7	15.1	Wilmore[33]
Basketball	15	26.8	193.6	91.2	9.7	

* Events not specified.

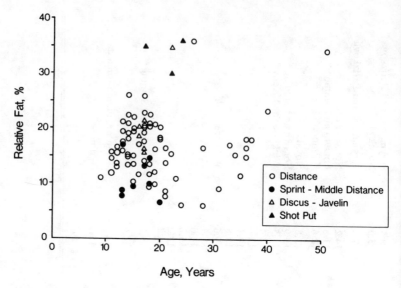

FIGURE 1. Relative body fat values for female track and field athletes.

TABLE 5

BODY COMPOSITION VALUES IN FEMALE ATHLETES

Athletic Group or Sport	n	Age (yrs)	Height (cm)	Weight (kg)	Relative Fat (%)	Reference
Runners	12	19.9	161.3 †	52.9 †	19.2 †	Malina *et al.*[39]
	11	32.4	169.4	57.2	15.2	Wilmore and Brown [40]
Sprinters	24	20.1	164.9 †	56.7 †	19.3 †	Malina *et al.*[39]
Jumpers & Hurdlers	11	20.3	165.9 †	59.0 †	20.7 †	
Discus & Javelin Throwers	10	21.1	168.1 †	71.0 †	25.0 †	
Shot-Putters	9	21.5	167.6 †	78.1 †	28.0 †	
Gymnasts	4	19.4	163.0	57.9	23.8	Conger and Macnab [41]
	14	20.0	158.5	51.1	15.5	Sinning and Lindberg [42]
	16	14.0	—	—	17.0	Parízková [3]
	8	23.0	—	—	11.0	
	7	23.0	—	—	9.6	Parízková and Poupa [43]
Basketball	21	19.1	169.1	62.6	20.8	Sinning [44]
	17	19.4	167.0	63.9	26.9	Conger and Macnab [41]
Volleyball	10	19.4	166.0	59.8	25.3	
Swimmers *	9	19.4	168.0	63.8	26.3	

* Events not specified.
† Estimated from a graphic plot of the data.

were below 10% relative fat. Two of the distance runners were only 6% fat, which is lower than the mean values reported in male distance runners.[5] These two runners were also the best performers of all 70 distance runners tested. In fact, nearly all of the distance runners and sprinters–middle distance runners below 10% fat were considered to be the elite or better runners. From this limited information, it would be tempting to conclude that females are at a disadvantage compared to males if they maintain relative body fats in excess of 10%. However, this must be considered pure speculation at this time until a more critical research design is implemented to validate this hypothesis.

From the above it is apparent that the distance runner is considerably leaner than the average population of similar age by 6 to 8 percentage points for males and females alike. It is impossible to determine from this study or from previous investigations whether this is the result of the intensive training programs required of distance runners where daily caloric expenditure is quite high (i.e., 1,000 to 2,000 kcal or more per workout), the result of genetic factors, or a combination of the two. From previous research it is well known that considerable alterations in body composition do occur with endurance training, i.e., decreased absolute and relative fat, and increased lean weight.[1, 2] Also, one of the subjects in this study who was assessed at 6% fat, took up running in high school to help her lose weight as she was considered obese. Over a period of several years, she lost over 40 pounds of weight as a result of her running program, established several national running records, and at one time held the best time in the world for the marathon. At the other extreme, the fatest subject tested in this study (35.8%) recently established the best time in the world for women in the 50-mile run (7:05:31) just shortly after being tested.

The potential genetic influence is, unfortunately, difficult to assess. Traditionally, distance runners have had a fairly characteristic somatotype (ectomesomorphic), and since somatotype is thought to change very little with age, indicating a probable genetic link, there must be a genetic component to distance running. There is also some evidence that muscle fiber type distribution by sport and event is genetically determined.[46] For the moment, it must be concluded that both genetic and environmental factors are operating to account for the lower fat values in distance runners. Identification of the primary factor must await longitudinal research of a more definitive nature.

When compared to other female athletes (TABLES 1 & 5), the female distance runner is of similar height, but has a lower total weight and relative body fat, except when compared to the gymnasts reported in previous studies,[3, 41–43] and the sprinters–middle distance runners reported in the present study have lower body fat values than the distance runners. The significance of this is not known at the present time. These lower values may be the result of a small sample size, or very low body fat may be a prerequisite for successful performance in the sport, since there is a high inverse correlation between body fat and physical performance where the body mass has to be moved either horizontally or vertically through space.[8, 9]

With regard to somatotypes, the female distance runner is predominantly an ectomorph with a moderately high endormorphic component. This finding is somewhat consistent with previous data for women middle distance runners,[6] although the middle distance runners had a lower rating in endomorphy and a higher rating in mesomorphy (TABLES 6 & 7). Male runners are predominantly ectomesomorphs,[6, 45] with moderately high readings in both ectomorphy and mesomorphy. The differences between the male and female distance runner

TABLE 6

SOMATOTYPE VALUES FOR MALE ATHLETES

Athletic Group or Sport	n	Age (yrs)	Height (cm)	Weight (kg)	Endo	Somatotype Meso	Ecto	Reference
Runners:								
Sprint	78	23.9	175.4	68.4	1.7	5.0	2.8	de Garay et al.[6]
Middle distance	41	22.9	177.3	65.0	1.5	4.2	3.6	
Long distance	34	25.3	171.9	59.8	1.4	4.1	3.6	
	19	—	174.4	60.8	2.7	4.2	4.3	Tanner[45]
Marathon	20	26.4	168.7	56.6	1.4	4.3	3.5	de Garay et al.[6]
	9	—	171.1	59.9	2.6	4.4	3.9	Tanner[45]
Track and Field:								
Jumpers	31	23.5	182.8	73.2	1.7	4.4	3.4	de Garay et al.[6]
Weight throwers	14	27.3	186.1	102.3	3.5	7.1	1.0	
Weight lifters	59	26.7	168.0	76.6	2.4	7.1	1.0	
Wrestlers	49	25.8	169.3	70.6	2.2	6.3	1.6	
	32	—	172.4	72.0	2.7	5.6	2.5	Tanner[45]
Swimmers	65	19.2	179.3	72.1	2.1	5.0	2.9	de Garay et al.[6]

in endomorphy and mesomorphy are undoubtedly truly sex-linked, as estrogen promotes fat accumulation and testosterone promotes growth of the lean tissue, i.e., predominantly the muscle mass.

The interactions of physical activity and the menstrual cycle have been of concern to sports physicians and coaches for many years. This interest has increased in recent years because of the greater number of women who are participating in intensive training programs, especially endurance activities. In earlier surveys of top-caliber women athletes, Erdelyi [47] and Zaharieva [48] found that 85% of the women had normal menstrual cycles, and only 7% to 9% had irregular or abnormal cycles. However, Erdelyi noted that those athletes who were in very strenuous or endurance sports tended to have irregular or absent menses during the competitive season. Menses generally returned to normal during the "off-season." As women have become more involved in year-round training programs, the incidence of menstrual irregularities has become more frequent. In a recent survey, Foreman [49] found that among a group of 47

TABLE 7

SOMATOTYPE VALUES FOR FEMALE ATHLETES*

Athletic Group or Sport	n	Age (yrs)	Height (cm)	Weight (kg)	Somatotype		
					Endo	Meso	Ecto
Runners:							
Sprint	28	20.7	165.0	56.8	2.7	3.9	2.9
Middle distance	18	20.0	166.9	54.3	2.0	3.3	3.7
Track and Field:							
Jumpers	12	21.5	169.4	56.4	2.2	3.3	3.7
Throwers	9	19.9	170.9	73.5	5.3	5.2	1.7
Swimmers	28	16.3	164.4	56.9	3.4	4.0	3.0

* Reference: de Garay *et al.*[6]

nationally ranked long distance runners, 19% had irregular menstrual periods, and 23% had severe oligomenorrhea or amenorrhea. Similarly, only one of seven cross-country skiers could be considered as having normal menstrual cycles, while two were amenorrheic. Conversations with coaches and athletes have affirmed that this is a common problem among women runners, as well as gymnasts, dancers and figure skaters.

The etiology of these menstrual changes has not been determined. While the "stress" of endurance training has been suggested as affecting the hypothalamic-pituitary-gonadal axis, no studies have been done to clarify this theory. Frisch and McArthur [50] have suggested that a minimal amount of relative body fat is necessary for the onset and maintenance of normal menstrual cycles, as young women who lose weight from a variety of causes are prone to amenorrhea. Further, these women resume menses once body weight (fat) is restored. In the present study, we have found that women long distance runners are quite lean compared to the average female. In previous studies of two groups of women distance runners, we found relative body fat of 15.2% and 11.7%, compared to a relative body fat of 23%–26% for the average young woman.[40, 51] Further, several women distance runners with scant or absent menses reported a return of menses when training was stopped and they gained a few pounds. The relationships between fat mass, training, and the menstrual cycle remain to be further clarified.

In conclusion, female distance runners can be classified as predominantly ectomorphs and lean compared to the normal female population, but on the average they are fatter and less muscular than male distance runners. However, it has also been observed that the better performing female distance runners are below 10% relative fat, approaching average values for male distance runners. It is probable that a lower relative fat facilitates the individual's running performance, thus fat reduction to absolute minimal levels would seem desirable. Whether these low values seen in the better female runners are determined genetically, by diet and intensive training, or by a combination of these remains to be seen. It is possible, however, that these low fat values may also be associated with menstrual irregularities, which are frequently reported in highly trained female athletes. Whether this is an undesirable consequence of reduced fat stores through intense training remains to be determined.

References

1. OSCAI, L. B. 1973. The role of exercise in weight control. *In* Exercise and Sport Sciences Reviews. J. H. Wilmore, Ed., Vol. 1: 103–123. Academic Press. New York, N.Y.

2. WILMORE, J. H. 1974. Physical exercise and body composition. *In* The Regulation of the Adipose Tissue Mass. J. Vague & J. Boyer, Eds., Excerpta Medica. Amsterdam, Netherlands.

3. PARÍZKOVÁ, J. 1973. Body composition and exercise during growth and development. *In* Physical Activity Growth and Development. G. L. Rarick, Ed., : 97–134. Academic Press. New York, N.Y.

4. WILMORE, J. H. 1975. Inferiority of female athletes: Myth or reality. J. Sports Med. **3**: 1–6.

5. COSTILL, D. L., R. BOWERS & W. F. KAMMER. 1970. Skinfold estimates of body fat among marathon runners. Med. Sci. Sports **2**: 93–95.

6. DE GARAY, A. L., L. LEVINE & J. E. L. CARTER. 1974. Genetic and Anthropological Studies of Olympic Athletes. Academic Press. New York, N.Y.

7. MOODY, D. L., J. H. WILMORE, R. H. GIRANDOLA & J. P. ROYCE. 1972. The effect of a jogging program on the body composition of normal and obese high school girls. Med. Sci. Sports **4**: 210–213.

8. WILMORE, J. H., J. ROYCE, R. N. GIRANDOLA, F. I. KATCH & V. L. KATCH. 1970. Body composition changes with a 10-week program of jogging. Med. Sci. Sports **2**: 113–117.

9. KIREILIS, R. W. & T. K. CURETON. 1947. The relationship of external fat to physical education activities and fitness tests. Res. Quart. **18**: 123–134.

10. BEHNKE, A. R. & J. H. WILMORE. 1974. Evaluation and Regulation of Body Build and Composition. Prentice-Hall. Englewood Cliffs, N.J.

11. WILMORE, J. H. 1969. A simplified technique for determination of residual lung volumes. J. Appl. Physiol. **27**: 96–100.

12. WILMORE, J. H. & A. R. BEHNKE. 1968. Predictability of lean body weight through anthropometric assessment in college men. J. Appl. Physiol. **25**: 349–355.

13. SIRI, W. E. 1965. Body composition from fluid spaces and density. Donner Laboratory of Medical Physics, University of California, Berkeley. Report. 19 March.

14. HEATH, B. H. AND J. E. L. CARTER. 1967. A modified somatotype method. Amer. J. Phys. Anthrop. **27:** 57–74.
15. CARTER, J. E. L. 1972. The Heath-Carter Somatotype Method. San Diego State University. San Diego, Calif.
16. WILMORE, J. H. & J. J. MCNAMARA. 1974. Prevalence of coronary heart disease risk factors in boys, 8–12 years of age. J. Pediat. **84:** 527–533.
17. PARÍZKOVÁ, J. 1961. Total body fat and skinfold thickness in children. Metabolism **10:** 794–807.
18. MICHAEL, E. D. JR. & F. I. KATCH. 1968. Prediction of body density from skinfold and girth measurements of 17-year-old boys. J. Appl. Physiol. **25:** 747–750.
19. WILMORE, J. H. & A. R. BEHNKE. 1969. An Anthropometric estimation of body density and lean body weight in young men. J. Appl. Physiol. **27:** 25–31.
20. WRIGHT, H. F. & J. H. WILMORE. 1974. Estimation of relative body fat and lean body weight in a United States Marine Corps population. Aerospace Med. **45:** 301–306.
21. PARÍZKOVÁ, J. & Z. ROTH. 1972. The assessment of depot fat in children from skinfold thickness measurements by Holtain (Tanner/Whitehouse) Caliper. Human Biol. **44:** 613–620.
22. WILMORE, J. H. & A. R. BEHNKE. 1970. An anthropometric estimation of body density and lean body weight in young women. Amer. J. Clin. Nutr. **23:** 267–274.
23. YOUNG, C. M. 1961. Body fatness in normal young women. N.Y. State J. Med. **61:** 1928–1931.
24. KATCH, F. I. & E. D. MICHAEL, JR. 1968. Prediction of body density from skinfold and girth measurements of college females. J. Appl. Physiol. **25:** 92–94.
25. SLOAN, A. W., J. J. BURT & C. S. BLYTH. 1962. Estimation of body fat in young women. J. Appl. Physiol. **17:** 967–970.
26. POLLOCK, M. L., E. E. LAUGHRIDGE, B. COLEMAN, A. C. LINNERUD & A. JACKSON. 1975. Prediction of body density in young and middle aged women. J. Appl. Physiol. **38:** 745–749.
27. ŠPRYNAROVÁ, S. & J. PARÍZKOVÁ. 1971. Functional capacity and body composition in top weight-lifters, swimmers, runners and skiers. Int. Z. Angew. Physiol. **29:** 184–194.
28. POLLOCK, M. L., H. S. MILLER, JR. & J. H. WILMORE. 1974. Physiological characteristics of champion American track athletes 40 to 75 years of age. J. Geront. **29:** 645–649.
29. LEWIS, S., W. L. HASKELL, H. KLEIN, J. HALPERN & P. D. WOOD. 1975. Prediction of body composition in habitually active middle-aged men. J. Appl. Physiol. **39:** 221–225.
30. NOVAK, L. P., R. E. HYATT & J. F. ALEXANDER. 1968. Body composition and physiologic function of athletes. J. Amer. Med. Assoc. **205:** 764–770.
31. FORSYTH, H. L. & W. E. SINNING. 1973. The anthropometric estimation of body density and lean body weight of male athletes. Med. Sci. Sport. **5:** 174–180.
32. FAHEY, T. D., L. AKKA & R. ROLPH. 1975. Body composition and $V_{O_2 max}$ of exceptional weight-trained athletes. J. Appl. Physiol. **39:** 559–561.
33. WILMORE, J. H. 1976. Body composition of national-caliber discus throwers, and professional baseball, ice hockey and basketball players. National Athletic Health Institute. Unpublished report.
34. GALE, J. B. & K. W. FLYNN. 1974. Maximal oxygen consumption and relative body fat of high-ability wrestlers. Med. Sci. Sports **6:** 232–234.
35. SINNING, W. E. 1974. Body composition assessment of college wrestlers. Med. Sci. Sports **6:** 139–145.
36. KATCH, F. I. & E. D. MICHAEL. 1971. Body composition of high school wrestlers according to age and wrestling weight category. Med. Sci. Sports **3:** 190–194.
37. WICKKISER, J. D. & J. M. KELLY. 1975. The body composition of a college football team. Med. Sci. Sports **7:** 199–202.

38. WILMORE, J. H., R. B. PARR, W. L. HASKELL, D. L. COSTILL, L. J. MILBURN & R. K. KERLAN. 1976. Athletic profile of professional football players. Phys. Sportsmed. 4: 45–54.

39. MALINA, R. M., A. B. HARPER, H. H. AVENT & D. E. CAMPBELL. 1971. Physique of female track and field athletes. Med. Sci. Sports 3: 32–38.

40. WILMORE, J. H. & C. H. BROWN. 1974. Physiological profiles of women distance runners. Med. Sci. Sports 6: 178–181.

41. CONGER, P. R. & R. B. J. MACNAB. 1967. Strength, body composition, and work capacity of participants and nonparticipants in women's intercollegiate sports. Res. Quart. 38: 184–192.

42. SINNING, W. E. & G. D. LINDBERG. 1972. Physical characteristics of college age women gymnasts. Res. Quart. 43: 226–234.

43. PARÍZKOVÁ, J. & D. POUPA. 1963. Some metabolic consequences of adaptation to muscular work. Brit. J. Nutr. 17: 341–345.

44. SINNING, W. E. 1973. Body composition, cardiovascular function, and rule changes in women's basketball. Res. Quart. 44: 313–321.

45. TANNER, J. M. 1964. The Physique of the Olympic Athlete. George Allen and Unwin, Ltd. London.

46. ERICKSON, B. O., P. D. GOLLNICK & B. SALTIN. 1972. Muscle metabolism and enzyme activities after training in boys 11–13 years old. Acta. Physiol. Scand. 87: 231–239.

47. ERDELYI, G. 1960. Gynecological survey of female athletes. Second National Conference on the Medical Aspects of Sports, American Medical Association, Washington, D.C. November 27.

48. ZAHARIEVA, E. 1965. Survey of sportswomen at the Tokyo Olympics. J. Sports Med. 5: 215–219.

49. FOREMAN, K. Unpublished survey. Seattle Pacific College, Seattle, Wash.

50. FRISCH, R. & J. MCARTHUR. 1974. Menstrual Cycles: Fatness as a determinant of minimum weight for height necessary for their maintenance or onset. Science 185: 949–951.

51. BROWN, C. H. & J. H. WILMORE. 1971. Physical and physiological profiles of champion women long-distance runners. Med. Sci. Sports 3: 1,h.

HEAT TOLERANCE OF
FEMALE DISTANCE RUNNERS *

B. L. Drinkwater, I. C. Kupprat,
J. E. Denton, and S. M. Horvath

*Institute of Environmental Stress
University of California, Santa Barbara
Santa Barbara, California 93106*

The thermoregulatory system of marathon runners is frequently challenged by the additive effects of metabolic heat production and environmental heat stress. Even on relatively cool days the rectal temperature of runners can reach 39° C within the first hour of the run and often exceeds 40° C by the end of the race.[1-4] The additional stress of a high ambient thermal load has long been recognized as one of the hazards of distance running. Since women have only recently been permitted or encouraged to compete in the marathon, very little is known about the response of female distance runners to a long-term submaximal effort in the heat.

A recent study [5] has shown that females with above average levels of aerobic power ($\dot{V}_{O_2 max}$) were better able to cope with acute exposure to submaximal work in the heat than women with an average $\dot{V}_{O_2 max}$ when both worked at the same $\% \dot{V}_{O_2 max}$. Although it was obvious that the less fit women were unable to maintain an adequate stroke volume, the specific mechanisms responsible for this difference in cardiovascular response could not be isolated. Since the aerobic power of female marathoners is among the highest ever recorded for women,[6] it was hoped that a comparison of their responses with those of a control group of women with an average $\dot{V}_{O_2 max}$ might clarify the role cardiovascular fitness plays in thermoregulation during an acute exposure to heat stress.

METHODS

Five women who had trained for and participated in the marathon were matched with a control group of five females on the basis of age and body surface area (BSA).† Every effort was made to match individuals as closely as possible on the basis of height and weight, but the lower body weights of the runners made it necessary to use BSA as the primary factor in matching for body size (TABLE 1). Prior to participation each subject was checked for cardiac or pulmonary abnormalities by a 12-lead electrocardiogram, a standard test of pulmonary function, and an exercise stress test. The latter, a modifica-

* This work was supported in part by the National Institutes of Health under Grants NIH ES–00849–4 and NIH AG–00021–7.

† The nature and purpose of the study and the risks involved were explained verbally and given on a written form to each subject prior to their voluntary consent to participate. The protocol and procedures for this study have been approved by the Committee on Activities Involving Human Subjects, of the University of California, Santa Barbara.

tion of Balke's multistage continuous treadmill test, was performed to the point of volitional fatigue in order to determine maximal aerobic power ($\dot{V}_{O_2 max}$).[7]

All experimental sessions took place between 0900–1200 to avoid problems related to circadian changes of body temperature. The subject arrived at the laboratory prior to 0800, had her height and nude weight recorded, inserted a rectal thermocouple to a depth of 12 cm, and donned a "bikini" style swimsuit, socks, and tennis shoes. She then entered an environmental chamber, 28° C, 16 Torr vapor pressure (RH 45%), where ECG electrodes (V_4 position) and seven copper-constantan skin thermocouples were attached. Skin temperatures were monitored at the following sites: (1) forehead, (2) upper arm, (3) tip of index finger, (4) thigh, (5) calf, (6) chest, and (7) abdomen. The subject then reclined in a semisitting position on a webbed cot while a Whitney mercury-in-silastic strain gauge was fitted over the belly of the right brachioradialus at a premeasured distance from the olecranon process. Approximately 5 minutes after the subject was seated, her blood pressure was recorded from the left arm by brachial auscultation. Immediately thereafter a 12-ml blood sample was taken from the antecubital vein and analyzed for hemoglobin (cyanmethemo-globin method), hematocrit (microhematocrit method), plasma protein (refractive index), plasma sodium and potassium (flame photometry), and plasma chloride (automatic silver chloride titration). After the subject had rested on the cot for 15 minutes, metabolic and temperature measurements were taken at 0–5 min and 10–15 min of this basal period. A PDP-12 laboratory computer, connected on-line to a paramagnetic oxygen analyzer (Servomex O.A. 137), an infrared CO_2 analyzer (Beckman LB-1), and a modified constant-flow dry gas meter(Parkinson-Cowan), provided minute-by-minute values for ventilatory volumes ($\dot{V}_E$), percent expired O_2 and CO_2, and oxygen consumption ($\dot{V}_{O_2}$). Temperatures were recorded on a multipoint recorder (Honeywell) connected to the computer and also printed once per minute. During the 6th and 16th minute of this period, cardiac output ($\dot{Q}$) was obtained by the modified ace-tylene rebreathing technique.[38] Measurements of forearm blood flow were taken from 7–10 minutes and 17–20 minutes using the standard Whitney tech-nique.[8]

After the basal measurements were completed, the subject remained on the cot and was wheeled into an adjacent chamber where ambient conditions were maintained at 48° C, 8.7 Torr vapor pressure (RH 10%). Her clothed weight ±10 g was recorded immediately, and she then returned to a semireclining position on a webbed lounge chair while her responses to the first 10 minutes in the chamber were monitored. All the measurements made during the basal period were repeated during this transient period.

At the end of 10 minutes, the subject was weighed and then moved to the treadmill where she began a 50-minute walk. The results of the preliminary stress test were used to adjust the slope and speed of the treadmill to elicit an oxygen uptake equivalent to ~30% $\dot{V}_{O_2 max}$. Metabolic, ECG, and temperature responses were recorded at minute intervals during 1–5, 20–25, and 40–45 minutes of work. Cardiac outputs were obtained during the 6th, 26th, and 46th minute. At the end of the work period, the subject was weighed and moved to the lounge chair for a 10-minute recovery period. Metabolic, ECG, and temperature responses were measured continuously while forearm blood flow was monitored during the first 3 and the last 2 minutes. Blood pressure was taken at the end of the 3rd minute and cardiac output following the 5th minute. Another 12-ml sample of venous blood was drawn during the 6th minute. After this recovery period, the subject was weighed and a second cycle of work-rest was begun if she was able to continue. The criteria for removal of the subject from the chamber were relatively conservative in order to minimize the possibility of heat illness. If (1) rectal temperature (T_{re}) $>39°$ C, (2) heart rate (HR) $\geq 90\%$ HR_{max}, or (3) nausea, headache, chills, or dizziness were noted, the subject was immediately removed from the chamber. Otherwise, the women left the chamber at the end of the second recovery period after a final clothed weight was recorded. Fluids were not replaced during the exposure. After the thermocouples were removed, the subject dried herself as thoroughly as possible and a final nude weight was taken.

Blood volume (BV) and percent body fat (% BF) were determined at least one week prior to or following the heat exposure. Blood volumes were obtained using the carbon monoxide technique.[9, 10] Body density was measured by the hydrostatic weighing procedure and the percent body fat calculated by the formula of Brŏzek *et al.*[11]

TABLE 1

PHYSICAL CHARACTERISTICS OF THE MARATHON RUNNERS ($n=5$)
AND CONTROL GROUP ($n=5$)

	Age (yrs)	Height (cm)	Weight (kg)	BSA * (m²)	$\dot{V}_{O_2 max}$ (ml/ kg·min)	% Body Fat
Marathoners						
Mean	28.6	162.3	49.8	1.51	56.3	12.5
SE †	5.5	2.8	4.1	0.07	5.8	2.0
Controls						
Mean	25.2	160.0	54.0	1.55	40.4	19.3
SE	6.1	3.4	4.9	0.08	2.3	2.2
Significance	NS	NS	NS	NS	$p<0.01$	$p<0.05$

* Body surface area.
† Standard error.

Plasma volume (PV) changes during the experiment were calculated according to the method of Dill and Costill[12] using both hemoglobin (Hb) and hematocrit (Hct) values from venous samples drawn during the *Basal* and *Recovery* periods.

Data were analyzed using a two-factor analysis of variance with repeated measures across measurement periods. Where significant interaction effects were observed, a test of simple main effects preceded the Newman-Keuls test of ordered means.[13] All tests of significance were made at $p < 0.05$.

RESULTS

As expected, the aerobic power of the runners was significantly higher than that of the control group (TABLE 1), ranging from a $\dot{V}_{O_2 max}$ of 43.0 ml/kg·min for the oldest runner (43 years) to 67.6 ml/kg·min for the current world record holder for the women's marathon. Although the runners had a lower % body fat, the calculated lean body mass (LBM) was the same for both groups, 43.6 kg. When vascular fluid volumes were expressed as a ratio to body weight, all were higher for the runners (TABLE 2). Only the mean corpuscular hemoglobin concentration did not discriminate between the athletes and the controls.

Basal Period

With the exception of heart rate (HR) and stroke index (SI), the responses of the marathon runners and the controls were similar while at rest in a thermoneutral environment (TABLE 3).

Transient Period

By the 8th minute of the transient period the HR for both groups had increased significantly over the basal rate, and by the 9th minute the rate was higher than during the first 3 minutes in the chamber ($p < 0.05$). Throughout this period the mean HR of the runners was lower ($p < 0.01$) than that of the controls (FIGURE 1a). Since SI for the marathon group remained higher ($p < 0.01$), cardiac index (CI) was the same for both groups (FIGURE 1a).

Mean skin temperature ($\bar{T}_{sk}$) also increased with time in the chamber and by the 8th minute was higher for both groups than during minutes 1–3. Since T_{re} showed the usual decrease noted during the early minutes of exposure to a hot environment, mean body temperature ($\bar{T}_b$) and body heat content (BHC) remained constant throughout the period. The slight decrease in forearm blood flow (FBF) was not a significant change from basal levels (FIGURE 2).

Work Period 1

During the first 50 minutes the runners were working at 159 kcal/m²·h, or 31% $\dot{V}_{O_2 max}$, and the controls at 134 kcal/m²·h, or 33% of their $\dot{V}_{O_2 max}$. The values T_{re}, $\bar{T}_{sk}$, and HR were lower for the athletes throughout the walk ($p < 0.05$) (FIGURE 3).

On the average, heart rates for runners were 18% lower than those of the control group, while their mean stroke volume (SV) was 32% higher. The resultant 17% greater $\dot{Q}$ for the athletes was not statistically significant, but it did account for the additional oxygen requirement at their higher absolute work loads.

The combined effect of work plus a high thermal load became evident as the walk progressed. The direction of change was the same for both groups with one exception. The values $\dot{V}_{O_2}$, $\dot{V}_E$(BTPS), HR, T_{re}, and $\bar{T}_b$ all increased significantly by the 20–25 minute measurement period $\dot{V}_E$(BTPS) continued to increase through 40–45 minute while $\dot{V}_{O_2}$ stabilized, resulting in a higher ventilatory equivalent (VE) toward the end of the walk. HR and T_{re} also continued to rise throughout the walk (FIGURE 3). However, the pattern of $\bar{T}_{sk}$ changes was different for each group (FIGURE 3). The runners' $\bar{T}_{sk}$ decreased

TABLE 2

BLOOD VOLUME (BV), PLASMA VOLUME (PV), RED BLOOD CELL VOLUME (RBCV), TOTAL HEMOGLOBIN (THb), AND MEAN CORPUSCULAR HEMOGLOBIN CONCENTRATION (MCHC)*

	Marathoners		Controls		
	Mean	SE	Mean	SE	p
Pre-exposure					
BV, ml/kg	103.8	9.8	76.3	4.3	<0.05
PV, ml/kg	67.8	6.8	50.3	2.9	<0.05
RBCV, ml/kg	36.0	3.8	25.9	1.6	<0.05
THb, g/kg	11.5	0.8	8.9	0.5	<0.05
MCHC, g/100 ml	0.330	0.02	0.344	0.01	NS
Recovery period 1					
ΔBV	−2.8%		−3.0%		
ΔPV	−2.9%		−5.8%		
ΔRBCV	−1.5%		+1.0%		
ΔMCHC	+1.5%		−1.0%		
Recovery period 2					
ΔBV	−7.2%				
ΔPV	−9.3%				
ΔRBC	−4.0%				
ΔMCHC	+4.0%				

* Pre-exposure values are expressed relative to body weight. Recovery values are shown as percent change from basal levels.

TABLE 3

CARDIOVASCULAR AND TEMPERATURE RESPONSES OF MARATHONERS AND CONTROLS DURING THE BASAL PERIOD, 28° C AND RH 45%

Measurement	Marathoners		Controls		
	Mean	SE	Mean	SE	p
$\dot{V}_E$(BTPS)	5.86	0.52	5.92	0.73	NS
$\dot{V}_{O_2}$, liters/min	0.20	0.01	0.21	0.02	NS
R	0.79	0.03	0.81	0.03	NS
HR, bpm	56.6	2.3	78.6	5.7	<0.01
CI, liters/min·m²	2.9	0.2	2.8	0.4	NS
SI, ml/beat·m²	51.9	3.5	35.2	4.4	<0.05
a-v O_2, ml/liter	44.6	1.8	51.6	7.8	NS
T_{re}, °C	36.78	0.1	37.12	0.2	NS
$\bar{T}_{sk}$, °C	33.7	0.3	33.4	0.4	NS
$\bar{T}_b$, °C	35.7	0.2	35.8	0.2	NS
FBF, ml/100 ml·min	2.44	0.92	2.43	0.62	NS
Hb, mM/liter	7.7	0.5	8.5	0.4	NS
Hct, %	39.9	1.2	41.2	0.9	NS
PP, g/100 ml	6.3	0.2	6.5	0.2	NS
SP, mmHg	96.0	5.3	101.2	6.0	NS
DP, mmHg	71.6	2.5	76.0	4.7	NS

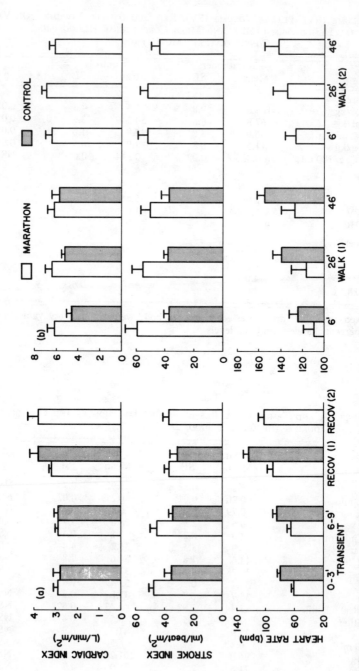

FIGURE 1. Circulatory responses of marathon (□) and control (■) groups during: (a) transient and recovery periods, (b) the 6th, 26th, and 46th minute of work (mean±SE).

significantly ($p < 0.05$) by 20–25 minute and then stabilized at 37.2° C. $\overline{T}_{sk}$ for the controls showed no significant change during the first 25 minutes of work and then increased ($p < 0.05$) by 40–45 minutes to 37.9° C.

Neither group was able to achieve a thermal balance. Although the runners were working at a higher absolute work load and producing more metabolic heat, their mean evaporative heat loss (E) of 226 kcal/m²·h was not significantly greater than that of the controls ($E = 189$ kcal/m²·h). Under these ambient conditions, the maximum evaporative heat loss (E_{max}) was calculated to be 295.9 kcal/m²·h for the runners and 288.2 kcal/m²·h for the controls, so that the observed rates were 76% and 66% of E_{max} for runners and controls, respectively. Calculation of heat storage by the standard heat balance equation

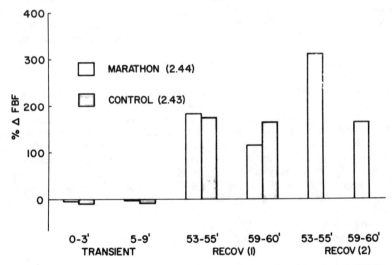

FIGURE 2. Percent change in forearm blood flow from basal levels (%ΔFBF) during transient and recovery periods. Numbers in parentheses represent basal means in ml/100 ml·min.

indicated that the runners were accumulating heat at a rate of 19.7 kcal/m²·h, or only 57% of the rate of the control group (34.4 kcal/m²·h). Changes in body heat content {BHC = [body wt (kg) × 0.83 × $\overline{T}_b$] ÷ BSA (m²)} from the onset of exercise through the 45th minute were 18 and 33 kcal/m²·h for runners and controls, respectively.

At the end of the first exercise period, the clothed weight of the marathoners had decreased by 1.2%; the controls, 0.9%. Two subjects in the control group failed to complete the full 50 minutes of work. The youngest subject, 13 years of age, was stopped at 46 minutes when her heart rate reached 172 bpm. The other subject, 34 years of age, was stopped when her T_{re} reached 39° C at 41 minutes. All other subjects completed the exercise period.

Recovery 1

For both groups, T_{re} and $\overline{T}_{sk}$ rose above the final values recorded during work, although the values for the runners remained lower (p < 0.01) than those of the controls (FIGURE 3). Mean heart rate for the marathon group was consistently below that of the control group (p < 0.01) by ~40 bpm (FIGURE 3). Neither SI nor CI differed significantly between the two groups, and both returned to levels comparable to those observed at the end of the transient period. Although neither systolic nor diastolic pressure (SP, DP) had risen significantly from the basal values (TABLE 3) for the runners (108/64) or controls (119/76), cardiac work had increased (p < 0.01) because of the multiplicative effect of the small increments in CI and SP.

Evaporative heat loss, calculated from prerecovery and postrecovery body weights, did not differ between groups. Both runners ($E = 296$ kcal/m²·h) and controls ($E = 235$ kcal/m²·h) had values far in excess of those required to account for the actual decrease in BHC. Drippage and transfer of sweat to the chair could not be accounted for and no doubt inflated calculated values for E.

Forearm blood flow increased significantly above that observed during the basal and transient periods, but there were no differences between groups (FIGURE 2). The mean decrease in plasma volume (PV) for the runners was 2.9%; for the controls, 5.8%. Since total plasma protein (PP) increased 8% and 9% for the marathon and control groups respectively, there was a net influx of protein into the vascular space. Based on plasma volume determinations obtained in a cool environment, this increase was on the order of 10.2 and 5.6 g protein for runners and controls, respectively. There were no differences between groups in recovery values for Hb, Hct, PP, or plasma electrolytes. The slight increases in Na^+ (+2%) and K^+ (+4.3%) observed during the recovery phase could be accounted for by hemoconcentration. Cl^- concentrations remained unchanged.

During the recovery period, T_{re} of two control subjects reached 39° C and they were removed from the chamber at the end of the period.

Work 2

Since only one member of the control group was able to continue into the second hour of work, no statistical comparisons between groups were possible. The control subject who did complete the second walk was 19 years of age and had the highest $\dot{V}_{O_2 max}$ in her group, 45.8 ml/kg·min. One of the five runners was stopped at the 46th minute of the walk when her T_{re} reached 39° C even though she had no other objective or subjective indications of distress.

The pattern of responses of the runners during this second work period was similar to that observed during work period 1 for HR, T_{re}, CI, and SI (FIGURES 1 & 3). The initial values for HR and T_{re} were at the same level as in the 40–45 minute interval of the preceding exercise period, and both increased further as work continued (p < 0.01). CI remained constant across time while SI decreased significantly (p < 0.01) by the 46th minute to 85% of the values recorded at 6 and 26 minutes. $\overline{T}_{sk}$ dropped 0.5° C from the final recovery value as the walk began and, after remaining constant during the first 5 minutes of exercise, increased to progressively higher values as work continued. By the

40–45 minute interval, $\overline{T}_{sk}$ was significantly ($p < 0.05$) higher than in any preceding period. As a result of the combined effect of T_{re} and $\overline{T}_{sk}$, T_b also increased significantly ($p < 0.01$) by the end of walk period 2. There were no changes in V_E or V_{O_2} during this period; both remained at the levels observed at the end of the preceding exercise period.

On the basis of prewalk and postwalk body weights, evaporative heat loss apparently increased to 270 kcal/m²·h, or 91% of E_{max}, during the second exercise period. However, inserting this value in the heat balance equation resulted in the anomaly of an apparent heat loss of −22.5 kcal/m²·h when body heat content actually increased by 10.7 kcal/m²·h. The discrepancy no doubt reflects drippage, which was calculated as ~12 kcal/m²·h by inserting storage $\{S = [\text{body wt (kg)} \times 0.83 \times \Delta T_b] \div \text{BSA (m}^2)\}$ into the heat balance equation. On the basis of these calculations, evaporative sweat loss was ~87% E_{max}.

Recovery 2

As in the first recovery period, T_{re} and $\overline{T}_{sk}$ rose to higher levels on cessation of work while HR, although decreasing, remained higher than in recovery 1 ($p < 0.05$) (FIGURE 3). Both T_{re} and $\overline{T}_{sk}$ were significantly higher than during the preceding recovery period ($p < 0.05$). Stroke index was maintained at the same level as in recovery period 1 with a slight elevation in cardiac index to meet an increase in metabolic rate from 0.24 to 0.29 liters of O_2 per minute (FIGURE 1a). $\dot{V}_{E\,(\text{BTPS})}$ was also elevated over the values recorded during the first recovery period. Again the calculated evaporative heat loss, 303 kcal/m²·h, exceeded that required to account for the decrease in body heat content and no doubt reflected a considerable increase in sweat loss due to dripping rather than evaporation. The subjects and their clothing were thoroughly wet by this time.

Forearm blood flow during the first 3 minutes of recovery was 65% higher than in the similar period during recovery period 1 but by the final 2 minutes had decreased to the same flow rate observed for the control group in the first recovery period. Neither systolic nor diastolic (112/67) blood pressure increased significantly over recovery period 1 values.

Changes in Hb, Hct, and PP all indicated hemoconcentration, calculated as a 9.3% decrease in plasma volume. Pre-experimental total plasma proteins (TPP), determined from the plasma volume figures obtained in a cool environment, were computed as 212.7 g. Correcting plasma volume for the 9.3% decrease noted in recovery period 2, TPP at the end of 2 hours of exercise were 222.7 g, a 5% increase or a net influx of 10.2 g protein into the vascular space. Increases in plasma electrolytes, Na⁺, K⁺, and Cl⁻, were minimal and within the range expected as a result of the hemoconcentration.

Based on the final nude weight, total body weight loss was 1.89 kg or 3.8% of the pretest weight.

DISCUSSION

If physical conditioning does confer some degree of protection against heat stress, one would expect to find that differences between trained and untrained subjects working in the heat would be found in the four classical signs of acclimation: (1) a lower heart rate, (2) an augmented sweating response, (3) a lower skin temperature, and (4) a decrease in internal temperature.[14, 15] Throughout the work and recovery periods, the female marathon runners did in fact have a lower HR, $\overline{T}_{sk}$, and T_{re} than the untrained controls. However, there was no difference in evaporative heat loss between the groups that could not be accounted for by the higher absolute work load of the runners. If the runners did benefit from an augmented sweat rate as a result of training, it was not evident during the first exercise period. However, the pattern of $\overline{T}_{sk}$ changes (FIGURE 3) starting at the 5th minute of work suggests that the onset of sweating occurred earlier in the period and at a lower T_{re} for the runners than for the controls. Even during the second walk period, $\overline{T}_{sk}$ for the runners was lower than that of the controls in walk period 1. Though the sweating threshold was not measured directly in this study, other investigators [16-18] have observed that trained men begin sweating at a lower T_{re} than untrained males. It seems likely that the same observation would apply to well-conditioned female athletes. Taken as a whole, the response of the marathon runners does suggest that their training regimens have provided them with some protection against the usual problems experienced by nonacclimatized subjects when working in a hot environment.

Previous studies of trained and untrained male subjects have been criticized because the two groups were not matched for body size and were assigned the same absolute work load in spite of wide differences in aerobic power.[19, 20] When these factors were taken into account in a recent study involving female athletes and nonathletes,[5] no differences were found between the two groups in rectal temperature, heart rate, mean skin temperature, or sweat rate when they walked at the same $\% \dot{V}_{O_2 max}$ in three ambient conditions: (1) 28° C, RH 45%, (2) 35° C, RH 65%, and (3) 48° C, RH 10%. However, in the hot dry environment (48° C) the nonathletes were unable to maintain an adequate cardiac output as stroke volume dropped precipitously during the final minutes of the first exercise period. While it was obvious that the women with higher levels of aerobic power were better prepared to cope with acute exposure to work in the heat, it was not possible to delineate the precise mechanisms responsible for this achievement. The greater disparity in cardiovascular fitness between marathon runners and controls in this study has emphasized other differences between the two groups that may clarify the role physical conditioning plays in the response of women working under heat stress.

Wyndham et al.[21] and Senay et al.[22] have suggested that expansion of plasma volume plays an important role in the early stages of the acclimatization process by stabilizing the central circulation. If so, individuals with larger than average plasma volumes might be expected to have fewer circulatory problems during an acute exposure to heat stress. This advantage should be evident in a lower heart rate and a higher stroke volume in spite of a shift in blood from the central to the peripheral circulation.[14, 23-25] The response of the marathon runners met these criteria. Not only was their mean plasma volume higher than that of the controls (TABLE 2), but when related to body weight (67.8 ml/kg) it was higher than that reported by Dill et al.[26] for highly trained middle distance runners (62.1 ml/kg). Not until the 46th minute of the second walk when their stroke index dropped to 44.2 ml/beat was there any indication of circulatory impairment in the marathon group. Even then they were able to maintain cardiac output by increasing their heart rate to 141.8 bpm, a level equivalent to 74% HR_{max}. At this point their cardiac reserve was still larger than that of the control group at the 46th minute of the first exercise period when their heart rate reached 82% HR_{max}.

Senay *et al.*[22] reported a 23% increase in pre-exposure plasma volume and total circulating protein by the 6th day of a 10-day acclimatization period with no marked changes during the final 4 days. Prior to any exposure to heat, mean plasma volume of the marathon group was 35% higher than that of the controls. If an expansion of plasma volume is an important factor in acclimatization,[21, 22] the larger initial volumes of the runners may have been a factor in their ability to maintain circulatory stability during the early stages of work under a high thermal load. Since resting values of plasma volume return to pre-exposure levels over an extended period of acclimatization,[21] it has been suggested that one of the benefits of acclimatization is the ability to increase plasma volume quickly upon re-exposure to heat stress by shifting protein into the vascular space.[22, 27] By the end of the first hour of work, the runners had gained an average of 10.2 g of plasma proteins compared to a 5.6-g increase for the controls. Since an influx of protein into the circulation would be accompanied by water and electrolytes, this may explain why the decrement in plasma volume after 1 hour of heat exposure was 50% greater for the controls (−5.8%) than for the runners (−2.9%). There was no additional increase in plasma protein during the second hour for the marathon group. It is interesting that the cessation of protein shift to the vascular volume was accompanied by a 6.7% decrement in plasma volume, a decrease greater than that of the control group during the first hour. Senay *et al.*[22] have also noted a stabilization of protein movement early in the exposure period and a net gain in pre-exposure protein levels of 31.8 g following 10 days of acclimatization. Initial levels of plasma proteins were 212.7 g for the runners and 176.5 g for the controls, a difference of 36.2 g prior to heat exposure. If the expansion of plasma volume and the ability to shift protein readily into the vascular space typify the acclimatized male,[22] the female marathon runners must be considered at least partially acclimatized to heat since their response fits the same pattern.

Two responses of the thermoregulatory system commonly reported as outcomes of the acclimatization process, a decrease in pre-exposure internal temperature and a lower threshold for the onset of sweating, have been observed for trained athletes and in men following a conditioning program.[16, 20, 28-30] Baum *et al.*[16] have suggested that a lower resting internal temperature would prolong performance since the length of time required to reach a dangerous level of body temperature would be increased. While the difference in basal rectal temperature between runners and controls ($\Delta T_{re} = 0.34$) was not significant, it is interesting to note that the only member of the control group who had a lower T_{re} than her "matched" runner was the woman who completed the full two hours in the heat. The 0.34 ΔT_{re} was also midway between the 0.2° C decrease following training[29] and the 0.5° C suggested by Givoni and Goldman[28] as representing the full effect of acclimatization on resting internal temperature. Since resting T_{re} may vary for women according to phases of the menstrual cycle, the expected difference between acclimatized and nonacclimatized females may be obscured at times. Nevertheless, it is interesting to note that the slope of the T_{re}/time relationship during walk period 1 is the same for both groups, lending credence to the hypothesis of Baum *et al.*[16]

Wyndham[31] suggests that the difference in resting T_{re} between acclimatized and unacclimatized males indicates a shift in set point and extends to the sweat-rate/core-temperature relationship. Acclimatized men not only begin sweating at a lower core temperature, but also increase their sweat rate beyond that of unacclimatized subjects.[14, 31, 32] The response of the sweating mechanism may represent the primary difference between the partial acclimatization resulting from physical conditioning in a neutral environment and the acclimatization achieved by exercise in the heat. Nadel *et al.*[17] concluded that fitness programs enhance sweat rate by training the sweat glands while standard acclimatization procedures reduce the zero central sweating drive and shift the sweating threshold to a lower internal temperature. However, most studies of the cross adaptation of acclimation to heat from physical training report just the opposite, a

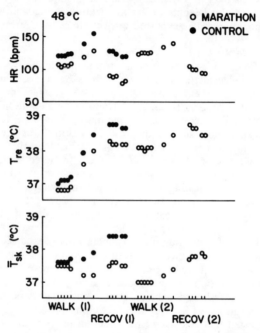

FIGURE 3. Heart rate (HR), rectal temperature (T_{re}), and mean skin temperature ($\overline{T}_{sk}$) of marathon ($\bigcirc$) and control ($\bullet$) groups during walk and recovery periods.

lowering of threshold for onset of sweating but no increase in sweat rate.[16, 20, 29, 33, 34] Acclimatizing to heat by exercising in a hot humid environment generally results in both an increase in the sensitivity and the capacity of the sweating mechanism,[14, 31, 32] suggesting that an external heat load is required to improve sweat gland function.[32] While design of this study did not permit a detailed examination of the sweating mechanisms, the lower $\overline{T}_{sk}$ of the runners from the 5th minute on does suggest that they benefited from an earlier onset of sweating (FIGURE 3). The lower $\overline{T}_{sk}$ may have attenuated the usual increase in compliance of the venous capacitance system observed during work in the heat and further improved the stability of the cardiovascular system.[35]

Since the two groups were working at different metabolic work loads, their ability to dissipate heat by evaporative cooling can only be compared in relative terms. Evaporative heat loss for the runners represented 86% of the total thermal load; for the controls, 79%. The resultant differences in heat storage plus higher initial levels of core temperature for the control group increased T_{re} for four control subjects to 39° C after one hour in the heat while that of the runners remained well below this level. It was not possible to compare total sweat production of the two groups because of varying work loads, and an occasional delay in obtaining the posttest nude weight. However, it is probable that the role of physical conditioning in augmenting sweat gland response would not be as apparent in a hot dry environment as in a hot humid condition since acclimation to dry heat does not necessarily increase sweat rate.[36] The role of physical conditioning in augmenting the sweat response requires further investigation. Part of the difficulty in resolving this question may lie in the definition of a "conditioned" subject. A 2–3 week training program, although it increases $\dot{V}_{O_2 max}$, does not represent the same level of conditioning exemplified by an endurance athlete whose training extends for months or years and may not have the same effect on sweat gland function.

Although the marathon runners were able to cope with short-term light work in a hot dry environment better than untrained women, this should not be interpreted as an indication they were fully heat acclimatized. As pointed out by Strydom *et al.*,[20] exposure periods longer than 2 hours are required to assess full acclimatization.

Direct comparison with men's performance under similar conditions is not possible since no males were included in this study. However, TABLE 4 presents data from previous studies in which the environment and activity levels were similar to those reported here. The primary difference between protocols is that water was available to the men but not to the women. The performance of the female marathon runners was not only equal to or better than that of the males, but was accomplished without the benefit of water replacement. These observations in addition to those reported earlier[5] emphasize again that aerobic power must be considered as an independent variable when male and female responses to work in hot environments are compared.

Marathon runners should not gain a false sense of security from these results. The work load was light, $\sim 30\%$ $\dot{V}_{O_2 max}$, compared to the 75%–80% $\dot{V}_{O_2 max}$ level observed during marathon runs.[37] Responses to heat stress are specific to the environmental conditions, the relative work load, the experimental protocol, and perhaps most importantly, individual variability. Any runner who anticipates having to race under high heat and/or humidity conditions would be wise to include heat acclimatization techniques in his/her training program for at least one week prior to the event.

ACKNOWLEDGMENTS

The authors gratefully acknowledge the assistance of David Brown, Kazuya Mayeda, Brigitte Hallier, Dorothy Batterton, and Tom Fuller for their help in this study. We are particularly appreciative of the technical assistance Nancy Cohen provided during the collection of the data.

TABLE 4

COMPARISON OF SELECTED RESPONSES TO WORK IN HOT DRY ENVIRONMENTS MADE IN THE PRESENT STUDY TO THOSE REPORTED PREVIOUSLY FOR MALES

Reference	n	Age (yrs)	$\dot{V}_{O_2\,max}$ (ml/kg·min)	T_{db} (°C)	T_{wb} (°C)	Activity	% $\dot{V}_{O_2\,max}$	Total Time (min)	T_{re} (°C)	$\overline{T}_{sk}$ (°C)	HR (bpm)	Forearm Blood Flow (ml/100 ml·min)
Wagner [39]	10♂	20.29	ND*	49.0	26.6	5.6 km/hr 0° grade	—	86†	38.4	37.1	142	7.95
Gisolfi [34]	6♂	21.0	52.2	48.9	26.7	5.6 km/hr 0° grade	—	74†	39.2	ND*	186	ND*
Greenleaf [19]	7♂	23.0	56.1	48.0	32.0	Bicycle	28%	76†	39.3	39.8	162	ND*
Shvartz [30]	14♂	23.5	ND*	50.0	28.0	5.6 km/hr 5° grade	—	<90†	39.2	39.1	180	ND*
Present study												
Marathoners	5♀	28.6	56.3	48.0	22.8	5.4 km/hr 2° grade	31%	99	38.5	37.4	142	8.24
Controls	5♀	25.2	40.4	48.0	22.8	5.0 km/hr 0° grade	33%	57	38.5	37.9	155	6.56

* ND, no data presented.
† Water replacement permitted.

REFERENCES

1. COSTILL, D. L., W. F. KAMMER & A. FISHER. 1970. Fluid ingestion during distance running. Arch. Environ. Health **21:** 520–525.
2. MARON, M. B., S. M. HORVATH & J. E. WILKERSON. 1975. Acute blood biochemical alterations in response to marathon running. Eur. J. Appl. Physiol. Occup. Physiol. **34:** 173–181.
3. MARON, M. B., J. A. WAGNER & S. M. HORVATH. 1977. Thermoregulatory responses during competitive marathon running. J. Appl. Physiol. **42.** In Press.
4. PUGH, L. G. C. E., J. L. CORBETT & R. H. JOHNSON. 1967. Rectal temperatures, weight loss, and sweat rates in marathon running. J. Appl. Physiol. **23:** 347–352.
5. DRINKWATER, B. L., J. E. DENTON, I. C. KUPPRAT, T. S. TALAG & S. M. HORVATH. 1976. Aerobic power as a factor in women's response to work in hot environments. J. Appl. Physiol. **41:** 815–821.
6. WILMORE, J. H. & C. H. BROWN. 1974. Physiological profiles of women distance runners. Med. Sci. Sports **6:** 178–181.
7. DRINKWATER, B. L. & S. M. HORVATH. 1971. Responses of young female track athletes to exercise. Med. Sci. Sports **3:** 56–62.
8. WHITNEY, R. J. 1953. The measurement of volume changes in human limbs. J. Physiol. (London) **121:** 1–27.
9. DAHMS, T. E. & S. M. HORVATH. 1974. Rapid, accurate technique for determination of carbon monoxide in blood. Clin. Chem. **20:** 533–537.
10. MYHRE, L. G., D. K. BROWN, F. G. HALL & D. B. DILL. 1968. The use of carbon monoxide and T-1824 for determining blood volume. Clin. Chem. **14:** 1197–1205.
11. BRŌZEK, J., F. GRANDE, J. T. ANDERSON & A. KEYS. 1963. Densitometric analysis of body composition: Revision of some quantitative assumptions. Ann. N.Y. Acad. Sci. **110:** 113–140.
12. DILL, D. B. & D. L. COSTILL. 1974. Calculation of percentage changes in volumes of blood, plasma, and red cells in dehydration. J. Appl. Physiol. **37:** 247–248.
13. WINER, B. J. 1971. Statistical Principles in Experimental Design. : 191–195. McGraw-Hill Book Co. New York, N.Y.
14. ROWELL, L. 1974. Human cardiovascular adjustments to exercise and thermal stress. Physiol. Rev. **54:** 75–159.
15. WYNDHAM, C. H. 1973. The physiology of exercise under heat stress. Ann. Rev. Physiol. **35:** 193–220.
16. BAUM, E., K. BRÜCK & H. P. SCHWENNICKE. 1976. Adaptive modifications of the thermoregulatory system of long-distance runners. J. Appl. Physiol. **40:** 404–410.
17. NADEL, E. R., K. B. PANDOLF, M. F. ROBERTS & J. A. J. STOLWIJK. 1974. Mechanisms of thermal acclimation to exercise and heat. J. Appl. Physiol. **37:** 515–520.
18. PIWONKA, R. W., S. ROBINSON, V. L. GAY & R. S. MANALIS. 1965. Preacclimatization of men to heat by training. J. Appl. Physiol. **20:** 379–384.
19. GREENLEAF, J. E., B. L. CASTLE & W. K. RUFF. 1972. Maximal oxygen uptake, sweating and tolerance to exercise in the heat. Int. J. Biometeorol. **16:** 375–387.
20. STRYDOM, N. B., C. H. WYNDHAM, C. G. WILLIAMS, J. F. MORRISON, G. A. G. BREDELL, A. J. S. BENADE & M. VONRAHDEN. 1966. Acclimatization to humid heat and the role of physical conditioning. J. Appl. Physiol. **21:** 636–642.
21. WYNDHAM, C. H., A. J. A. BENADE, C. G. WILLIAMS, N. B. STRYDOM, A. GOLDIN & A. J. A. HEYNS. 1968. Changes in central circulation and body fluid spaces during acclimatization to heat. J. Appl. Physiol. **25:** 586–593.
22. SENAY, L. C., D. MITCHELL & C. H. WYNDHAM. 1976. Acclimatization in a hot, humid environment: body fluid adjustments. J. Appl. Physiol. **40:** 786–796.

23. MacDougall, J. D., W. G. Reddan, C. R. Layton & J. A. Dempsey. 1974. Effects of metabolic hyperthermia on performance during heavy prolonged exercise. J. Appl. Physiol. **36:** 538–544.

24. Rowell, L. B., K. K. Kraning, II, J. W. Kennedy & T. O. Evans. 1967. Central circulatory responses to work in dry heat before and after acclimatization. J. Appl. Physiol. **22:** 509–518.

25. Rowell, L. B., H. J. Marx, R. A. Bruce, R. D. Conn & F. Kusumi. 1966. Reductions in cardiac output, central blood volume, and stroke volume with thermal stress in normal men during exercise. J. Clin. Invest. **45:** 1801–1816.

26. Dill, D. B., K. Braithwaite, W. C. Adams & E. M. Bernauer. 1974. Blood volume of middle-distance runners: Effect of 2,300-m altitude and comparison with non-athletes. Med. Sci. Sports **6:** 1–7.

27. Senay, L. C., Jr. 1975. Plasma volumes and constituents of heat-exposed men before and after acclimatization. J. Apply. Physiol. **38:** 570–575.

28. Givoni, B. & R. F. Goldman. 1973. Predicting effects of heat acclimatization on heart rate and rectal temperature. J. Appl. Physiol. **35:** 875–879.

29. Shvartz, E., A. Magazanik & Z. Glick. 1974. Thermal responses during training in a temperate climate. J. Appl. Physiol. **36:** 572–576.

30. Shvartz, E., E. Saar, N. Meyerstein & D. Benor. 1973. A comparison of three methods of acclimatization to dry heat. J. Appl. Physiol. **34:** 214–219.

31. Wyndham, C. H. 1967. Effect of acclimatization in the sweat rate/rectal temperature relationship. J. Appl. Physiol. **22:** 27–30.

32. Mitchell, D., L. C. Senay, C. H. Wyndham, A. J. van Rensburg, G. G. Rogers & N. B. Strydom. 1976. Acclimatization in a hot humid environment: Energy exchange, body temperature, and sweating. J. Appl. Physiol. **40:** 768–778.

33. Buskirk, E. R., P. F. Iampietro & D. E. Bass. 1958. Work performance after dehydration: Effects of physical conditioning and heat acclimation. J. Appl. Physiol. **12:** 189–194.

34. Gisolfi, C. 1973. Work tolerance derived from interval training. J. Appl. Physiol. **35:** 349–354.

35. Rowell, L. B., J. A. Murray, G. L. Brengelmann & K. K. Kraning. 1969. Human cardiovascular adjustments to rapid changes in skin temperature during exercise. Circ. Res. **24:** 711–724.

36. Robinson, S., E. S. Turrell, H. S. Belding & S. M. Horvath. 1943. Rapid acclimatization to work in hot climates. Amer. J. Physiol. **140:** 168–176.

37. Costill, D. L. 1970. Physiology of marathon running. J. Am. Med. Assoc. **221:** 1024–1029.

38. Simmons, R. & R. J. Shephard. 1971. Measurements of cardiac output in maximum exercise. Application of an acetylene rebreathing method to arm and leg exercise. Int. Z. Angew. Physiol. Einschl. Arbeitsphysiol. **29:** 159–172.

39. Wagner, J. A., S. Robinson, S. P. Tzankoff & R. P. Marino. 1972. Heat tolerance and acclimatization to work in the heat in relation to age. J. Appl. Physiol. **33:** 616–622.

BIOMECHANICAL COMPARISON OF MALE
AND FEMALE DISTANCE RUNNERS *

Richard C. Nelson, Christine M. Brooks, and Nancy L. Pike

Biomechanics Laboratory
Pennsylvania State University
University Park, Pennsylvania 16802

Interest in distance running among American girls and women has developed rapidly in recent years. This is evidenced by the increasing number of women participating in long distance races including the marathon. Many states have added girl's championships to their cross country and track and field programs as a consequence of the interest being generated in the high schools. Concurrent with these developments has been the revitalization of women's track and field and cross country teams in American colleges and universities.

The increase in women's running activities has stimulated many sport scientists to investigate the various aspects of female running performance. These research efforts have focused on the physiological, psychological, sociological, and to a lesser extent the biomechanical factors that influence performance. Studies [1,2] of body size and proportions of female distance runners have revealed them to be shorter, lighter, and leaner than other female track and field athletes and females from the normal population for comparable ages. However, very little information is available about the biomechanical features of female distance runners.

A direct outcome of the increased opportunities for women to participate under better coaching and improved training methods has been the marked improvement in their world record performances. The differences between male and female performances have been reduced steadily and this trend is expected to continue in the next few years. The current status of relative female performance in common running events can be seen in FIGURE 1. The male world records are represented by a value of 100 and the female records shown as percentages of the male record for the competitive events from 100 meters to the marathon. The female records are approximately 90% of the men's with the exception of the 5,000 meters and marathon. The latter two events are very new to women's competition, so the present differences will no doubt be reduced as greater numbers of female runners train for and compete in the events.

The vast majority of the research conducted to date on the biomechanics of running has involved male subjects. Research on female runners has been limited primarily to the study of sprinters such as the work of Hoffman.[3] Consequently, very little information is available on the biomechanics of female distance runners. This paucity of scientific data combined with the likelihood of increased emphasis on distance running among girls and women suggest that research directed toward a better understanding of the biomechanical aspects would be of both theoretical as well as practical significance.

* This work was partially supported by a grant from the U.S. Olympic Development Sub-Committee for Women's Athletics, Dr. Harmon Brown, Chairman.

The purpose of the present investigation was to obtain anthropometric and biomechanical data on the best American female distance runners. Such information would reflect the "state of the art" and provide a foundation upon which recommendations for future improvements could be made. A secondary but interrelated purpose was to compare these results with those of male runners of comparable ability, and thereby gain additional insight into female distance running performance.

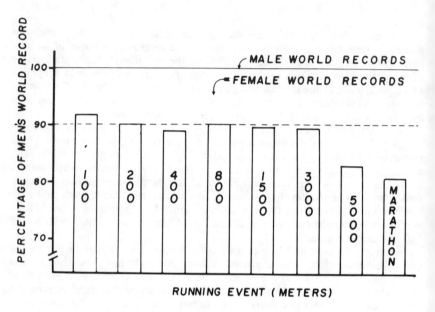

FIGURE 1. Comparison of male and female world records: 1976.

METHOD

Subjects

Three groups of distance runners were utilized in this investigation. The first consisted of 21 of the best American female runners (Elite Women) including a number of Olympians and national record holders. The second was comprised of a comparable group of 14 American male distance runners (Elite Men) who had participated in the study by Cavanagh and Pollock.[4] The third group consisted of 10 male runners from Penn State University (Penn State Men) who had participated in a longitudinal study previously reported by Nelson and Gregor.[5] A summary of the physical characteristics of the three groups is presented in TABLE 1.

Two male groups of runners who were similar in physical characteristics were included to provide for a more complete comparative analysis with the

TABLE 1

DESCRIPTIVE CHARACTERISTICS AND COMPARISON OF FEMALE AND MALE DISTANCE RUNNERS

Group	n	Ht (cm) Mean	SD*	Wt (kg) Mean	SD	LL (cm) Mean	SD	Relative Leg Length Mean	SD	Ponderal Index Mean	SD
U.S. Women	21	165.7	4.9	51.57	4.65	86.2	3.4	0.52	0.01	13.49	0.37
U.S. Men	14	178.0	6.7	63.12	5.72	94.3	4.0	0.53	0.01	13.54	0.34
Penn State Men	10	176.0	4.5	63.43	3.42						
Group comparisons (t values)†											
U.S. Women vs U.S. Men		6.23 ($p < 0.01$)		6.56 ($p < 0.01$)		6.39 ($p < 0.01$)		2.66 (NS)		0.39 (NS)	
U.S. Women vs Penn State Men		5.63 ($p < 0.01$)		7.13 ($p < 0.01$)							
Penn State Men vs U.S. Men		0.82 (NS)		0.08 (NS)							

* Standard deviation.
† Student's t-test.

elite women. The anthropometric comparisons were carried out using data from the elite men, which made possible the direct comparison of the top American male and female distance runners. Unfortunately, insufficient biomechanical data were available for the elite men and hence, it was necessary to incorporate results from the Penn State men in the biomechanical comparisons. Although these restrictions created less than ideal conditions for comparing male and female performers, the scarcity of such information on distance runners tended to override the inherent limitations.

Test Procedures

The data collection phase of the experiment was carried out in two parts. The first dealt with anthropometric measurements and the second with filming the runners at selected velocities. The physical measurements, which were limited to those presumed to be relevant to running technique, consisted of standing height (Ht), body weight (Wt), and leg length (LL), from which relative leg length (LL/Ht) and ponderal index (Ht/$\sqrt[3]{Wt}$) were calculated. The measurement procedures used were those recommended by Clauser *et al.*[6] It was anticipated that these data would aid in the interpretation of the biomechanical results.

Cinematographic and film analysis procedures were used to obtain the biomechanical data. The methods used to film the female runners were identical to those utilized with the Penn State Men and have been reported in detail by Nelson and Gregor.[5] Briefly, the procedures involve having the subject run at maximum velocity, and three predetermined paced velocities over a specified distance on a regular track. The velocities chosen covered a range of speeds from the marathon to sprint events. High-speed 16 mm films (150 frames/sec) were taken from which the biomechanical components were derived.

Film and Data Analysis Procedures

A Vanguard-Bendix film analysis system with paper tape output was utilized to obtain frame count, X and Y coordinate data from the film. These were used as input data for specially written computer programs that generated values for the specified biomechanical components of the running performance. These variables were: stride length (SL), stride rate (SR), time of support (TS), time of nonsupport (TNS), and stride time (ST). In addition, the actual running velocity was determined for each trial. The distance from the toe of one foot to the toe of the other foot at touchdown was used as a measure of SL. The number of steps per unit of time represented SR in steps per second. The elapsed time from takeoff of one foot to takeoff of the other foot indicated ST, which can also be calculated as the reciprocal of SR. The value for ST included TS, during which the foot was in contact with the ground, and TNS, when the runner was in flight.

These parameters were determined for each subject at each of the four velocities that were used in the calculation of interpolated values for the specific experimental velocities. These velocities were selected on the basis of the average speeds required for female world record paces in selected distance events. The seven velocities ranged from 15.86 ft/sec to 22.11 ft/sec spaced out at approximately 1 ft/sec intervals. Biomechanical parameters at each velocity for each subject were calculated from the basic data derived from the film analysis using a second order polynomial procedure. This resulted in interpolated data for all velocities, which could then be used for direct comparison of male and female runners.

In an attempt to compensate for individual differences in maximum speed, a second analysis was carried out in which relative velocities were utilized. These were based on 60%, 70%, 80%, and 90% of each runner's maximum velocity. The same method was used to calculate the interpolated values for these velocities as was used for the fixed velocities previously described. This

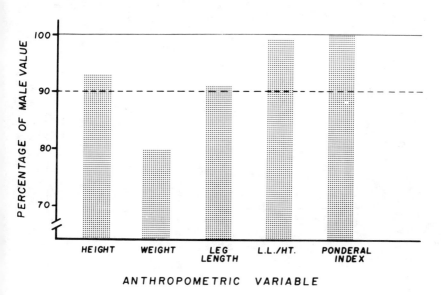

FIGURE 2. Comparison of physical characteristics of male and female distance runners.

procedure represented a somewhat unique approach to the study of running by linking the experimental velocities to each persons maximum level of performance.

RESULTS

Physical Characteristics

The results presented in TABLE 1 and FIGURE 2 reveal that the female runners were significantly (p < 0.01), shorter and lighter than both the elite and Penn State male athletes. They were also characterized by significantly shorter legs, but were similar in relative leg length and ponderal index when compared with the elite men. Although the two male groups differed in running achievement, they were similar in height and weight, which minimizes to some extent the limitations imposed by the fact that the best American female runners were compared with collegiate-level male runners. It is important to emphasize the absolute mean differences in height (12.3 cm), body weight (11.55 kg), and leg length (8.1 cm), which have a direct bearing on the biomechanical differences presented in the following section.

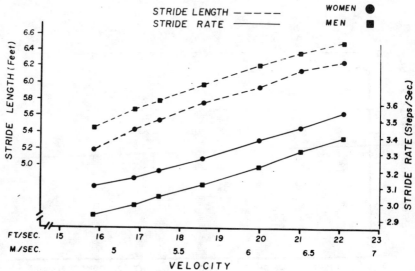

FIGURE 3. Male and female stride lengths and rates for selected absolute velocities.

Biomechanical Characteristics

The results for the biomechanical parameters are presented in two sections. The first contains the analysis for absolute velocities and the second for relative velocities.

The data for SL and SR presented in TABLES 2 and 4 and FIGURE 3 reveal that for absolute velocities the female runners had significantly shorter strides and higher stride rates. This consistent difference for both variables across all velocities can be seen in FIGURE 3 and is reinforced by the nonsignificant group × velocity interaction ($F = 0.01$) in TABLE 4. The mean SL for the female runners was 6.4 cm (2.5 in.) less than that for the males (96.5%). It is important to note that this percentage is higher than might be expected based on differences in height (92.5%) and leg length (91.1%).

As a consequence of their shorter strides female runners necessarily maintain higher stride rates. Their mean values were 0.14 steps/sec higher across all velocities (FIGURE 3). These results show clearly that for female runners to

TABLE 2

STRIDE LENGTH AND RATE AT SELECTED ABSOLUTE VELOCITIES

Velocity (ft/sec)	Stride Length (ft)				Relative Stride Length (SL/Ht)				Stride Rate (steps/sec)			
	Women		Men		Women		Men		Women		Men	
	Mean	SD	Mean	SD	Mean	SD	Mean	SD	Mean	SD	Mean	SD
22.11	6.29	0.320	6.51	0.204	1.18	0.084	1.13	0.048	3.55	0.238	3.41	0.107
21.06	6.16	0.317	6.38	0.219	1.15	0.062	1.11	0.050	3.46	0.214	3.31	0.110
19.97	6.01	0.367	6.22	0.218	1.12	0.056	1.08	0.049	3.36	0.243	3.22	0.108
18.62	5.79	0.419	6.00	0.193	1.08	0.061	1.03	0.045	3.25	0.281	3.11	0.098
17.50	5.59	0.428	5.79	0.163	1.04	0.062	1.00	0.040	3.17	0.289	3.03	0.086
16.88	5.46	0.417	5.66	0.151	1.02	0.060	0.98	0.037	3.12	0.282	2.98	0.081
15.86	5.24	0.380	5.44	0.165	0.98	0.055	0.94	0.037	3.05	0.254	2.92	0.079
Group means	5.79		6.00		1.08		1.04		3.28		3.14	

maintain the same velocity as their male counterparts they must maintain a higher tempo to offset the lesser absolute distance covered per stride.

The results for relative stride length (SL/Ht) are shown in FIGURE 4. In contrast to absolute SL the female runners have a significantly longer RSL than the male runners (104%). This indicates that even though they have shorter absolute SL they are covering a disproportionately greater distance per stride as compared to the men. The greater RSL and higher SR values for the females offer two compensatory mechanisms for overcoming their disadvantage imposed by their shorter stature.

The temporal components—time of support (TS), time of nonsupport (TNS), and time of support/stride time (TS/ST)—also reveal consistent differences between these groups. The patterns shown in FIGURE 5 and the results contained in TABLES 3 and 4 reveal that the female runners demonstrated lesser values for TS, greater TNS, and lower ratios of TS/ST. The greater absolute TNS is somewhat difficult to reconcile since they are covering less rather than more absolute distance per stride. When the TS/ST ratios are compared, the women show significantly lower values indicating they spent a smaller proportion of their stride time in contact with the ground, and conversely a greater proportion in flight.

The results derived from these data for absolute velocities can be summarized as follows. Female distance runners of national caliber differ significantly from their male counterparts in the biomechanical parameters investigated in this study. As a consequence of their lesser stature they necessarily take shorter absolute strides and therefore must maintain higher stride rates to maintain the same absolute velocities. Their longer relative stride lengths indicate that attempts to improve performance by emphasizing longer strides

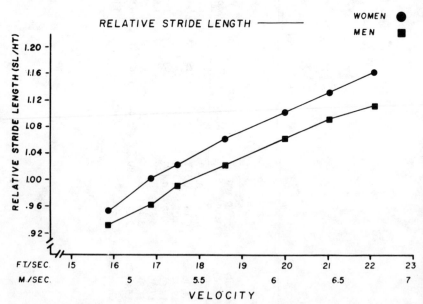

FIGURE 4. Male and female relative stride lengths for selected absolute velocities.

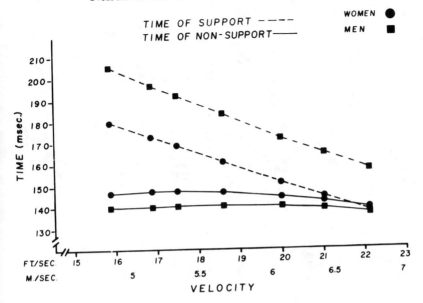

FIGURE 5. Times of support and nonsupport for male and female runners at selected absolute velocities.

appears ill advised. Other differences are observed when stride time is partitioned into contact and flight times. Here the female athletes have a disproportionately lower absolute contact time and a longer absolute flight time. In addition, their ratios of contact to stride time are less than those for the men. These results suggest that the running technique used by the females is not merely a "scaled down" version of the male model.

The results presented so far have been based on absolute running velocities which, from a practical standpoint, are the most important. However the biomechanical components under investigation change as velocity increases from a slow jog up to maximum velocity. Since the two groups of runners differ significantly in mean maximum running velocity (24.8 ft/sec vs 28.2 ft/sec; $p < 0.01$) it would be of interest to compare them at velocities that are relative to maximum for each individual. Biomechanical parameters were calculated for maximum and relative velocities of 60%, 70%, 80% and 90% of maximum velocity for this analysis. These results are presented in TABLES 5, 6, and 7.

Cursory examination of the group means for the biomechanical components for both absolute (TABLES 2 & 3) and relative velocities (TABLES 5 & 6) indicates that the values for women are quite similar while those for the men change considerably. This is most likely due to the fact the absolute velocity values for the females cover the same approximate portion of the velocity continuum because their maximum velocities are not too much greater than the top absolute experimental speed (22.11 ft/sec). In contrast, the male runners have considerably higher maximum velocities (mean 28.2 ft/sec), and consequently their relative speeds span a portion of the velocity continuum containing higher velocities.

TABLE 3

TEMPORAL COMPONENTS AT SELECTED ABSOLUTE VELOCITIES

Velocity (ft/sec)	Time of Support (sec)				Time of Nonsupport (sec)				Time of Support/Stride Time Ratio, TS/ST, (×100)			
	Women		Men		Women		Men		Women		Men	
	Mean	SD	Mean	SD	Mean	SD	Mean	SD	Mean	SD	Mean	SD
22.11	0.138	0.018	0.157	0.012	0.139	0.017	0.157	0.012	49.7	3.16	53.3	3.29
21.06	0.144	0.015	0.164	0.013	0.142	0.014	0.164	0.013	50.3	3.25	54.2	3.43
19.97	0.151	0.015	0.172	0.013	0.145	0.014	0.172	0.013	51.1	3.50	55.2	3.55
18.62	0.160	0.015	0.182	0.014	0.147	0.015	0.182	0.014	52.2	3.72	56.5	3.72
17.50	0.168	0.015	0.191	0.014	0.147	0.015	0.191	0.014	53.3	3.73	57.7	3.86
16.88	0.172	0.015	0.196	0.014	0.147	0.015	0.196	0.014	54.0	3.67	58.4	3.96
15.86	0.180	0.015	0.205	0.014	0.146	0.014	0.205	0.014	55.2	3.55	59.6	4.15
Group means	0.159		0.181		0.145		0.139		52.3		56.4	

When the absolute values for SL, RSL, and SR were adjusted to percentages of maximum velocity, the results showed a decrease for the females in comparison to the men. A similar analysis for TS, TNS, and TS/ST showed an opposite trend whereby the females showed an increase in these parameters relative to those of the men.

It is clear that basing biomechanical comparisons on velocities that are proportional to an individual's maximum speed does not eliminate the differences between male and female distance runners. Female values for the distance and rate components decreased while the temporal parameters increased in comparison with the men. These results are most likely due to the higher absolute velocities of the men at each relative velocity. In any case the concept of categorizing running velocity as a proportion of a persons maximum velocity

TABLE 4

SUMMARY OF ANALYSES OF VARIANCE FOR BIOMECHANICAL PARAMETERS
(ABSOLUTE VELOCITIES)

Biomechanical Parameter	F Ratios		
	Velocity	Group (Male-Female)	Group × Velocity Interaction
1. Stride length	40.51 *	17.54 *	0.01 (NS)
2. Relative stride length (SL/Ht)	398.25 *	6.50 *	285.50 *
3. Stride rate	22.03 *	19.00 *	0.00 (NS)
4. Time of support (TS)	37.52 *	106.51 *	0.08 (NS)
5. Time of nonsuppport	0.92 (NS)	7.72 *	0.17 (NS)
6. TS/ST †	11.15 *	67.16 *	0.06 (NS)

* Denotes significant F ratio ($p < 0.01$).
† Ratio, time of support to stride time.

offers a somewhat unique approach. Future research dealing with the physiological and biomechanical aspects of running may be enhanced by incorporating this concept of relative velocity.

DISCUSSION

This investigation represents one of the few attempts reported to date in which a direct comparison has been made between male and female distance runners on the basis of biomechanical parameters. Body proportion measures of height, weight, and leg length were also incorporated to aid in the interpretation of the results. The method employed to determine interpolated values for specific velocities made it possible to control for velocity and thereby permit a valid comparison of the two groups. This is of primary importance since most biomechanical factors are influenced by running velocity.

TABLE 5

STRIDE LENGTH AND RATE AT SELECTED RELATIVE VELOCITIES

Velocity (% of Maximum)	Stride Length (ft)				Relative Stride Length (SL/Ht)				Stride Rate (steps/sec)			
	Women		Men		Women		Men		Women		Men	
	Mean	SD	Mean	SD	Mean	SD	Mean	SD	Mean	SD	Mean	SD
Maximum	6.35	0.366	6.81	0.255	1.17	0.066	1.18	0.045	3.83	0.239	4.09	0.247
90	6.27	0.366	6.74	0.274	1.15	0.075	1.17	0.041	3.53	0.193	3.74	0.176
80	6.03	0.405	6.53	0.335	1.11	0.086	1.13	0.052	3.29	0.199	3.44	0.144
70	5.62	0.435	6.18	0.311	1.04	0.092	1.07	0.050	3.09	0.191	3.18	0.125
60	5.06	0.467	5.67	0.266	0.93	0.096	0.98	0.048	2.95	0.176	2.96	0.126
Group means	5.87		6.39		1.08		1.11		3.34		3.48	

TABLE 6

TEMPORAL COMPONENTS AT SELECTED RELATIVE VELOCITIES

Velocity (% of Maximum)	Time of Support (sec)				Time of Nonsupport (sec)				Ratio, TS/ST, Time of Support/Stride Time (×100)			
	Women		Men		Women		Men		Women		Men	
	Mean	SD	Mean	SD	Mean	SD	Mean	SD	Mean	SD	Mean	SD
Maximum	0.128	0.014	0.125	0.011	0.139	0.011	0.121	0.009	47.8	3.94	50.7	2.64
90%	0.143	0.018	0.139	0.013	0.145	0.012	0.130	0.007	49.5	4.47	51.5	3.11
80%	0.158	0.021	0.156	0.015	0.147	0.016	0.137	0.009	51.7	5.00	53.2	3.58
70%	0.174	0.019	0.176	0.016	0.147	0.016	0.140	0.011	54.2	4.69	55.6	3.87
60%	0.189	0.016	0.198	0.018	0.143	0.015	0.141	0.013	57.0	4.11	58.5	4.15
Group means	0.158		0.159		0.144		0.134		52.0		53.9	

The results for body proportion measures support previous studies (Eiben [1] and Malina *et al.*[2]) that indicate that female distance runners are lighter in weight and shorter of stature and leg length in comparison with male runners. The female runners in this study were significantly lighter (81.7%), shorter (93.1%) and had shorter legs (91.4%) than the male runners. Furthermore, they were unable to achieve similar maximum speeds (87.1%). As a consequence of these physical limitations, the females necessarily covered less distance per stride (96.5%) and performed at higher turnover rates (104%). However, their relative stride lengths (SL/Ht) exceeded those of the men (104%). With the male model as a reference, it appears that the females are "overstriding," which may be a means of compensating for their shorter stature (Figure 6).

TABLE 7

SUMMARY OF ANALYSES OF VARIANCE FOR BIOMECHANICAL PARAMETERS
(RELATIVE VELOCITIES)

Biomechanical Parameter	F Ratios		
	Velocity	Group (Male-Female)	Group × Velocity Interaction
1. Stride length	54.42 *	63.47 *	0.20 (NS)
2. Relative stride length (SL/Ht)	45.61 *	4.25 *	0.35 (NS)
3. Stride rate	120.50 *	18.73 *	1.87 (NS)
4. Time of support (TS)	63.53 *	0.02 (NS)	0.60 (NS)
5. Time of nonsuppport	3.38 *	21.1 *	1.55 (NS)
6. TS/ST †	18.40 *	6.22 *	0.14 (NS)

* Denotes significant F ratio ($p < 0.01$).
† Ratio, time of support to stride time.

It is interesting to note that if the females had in fact been similar to the men in relative stride length, their absolute stride length would thereby have been even shorter by approximately 4%. If this reduced stride length were subtracted from their absolute length it would result in a value of about 92.5% of the mean male stride length. This proportion is surprisingly similar to differences in height (93.1%) and leg length (91.4%) and further emphasizes the importance of body size to performance. Additional support of this point can be seen in the comparison of female and male world records at distances from 100 to 3000 meters (FIGURE 1). Female performances range from 89% to 91.7% of that of the males.

The results for the temporal factors revealed that the female runners were significantly different than the male competitors. It might have been expected that their distribution of TS and TNS would merely be a scaled down version of the male pattern with appropriate adjustment for differences in SR. This was not the case, however, as their TS was disproportionately short and the

TNS unaccountably long. The fact that they were in flight 4% longer than the men, but covered 4% less absolute distance during this time indicates clearly a different running pattern. It appears that the female runners takeoff at a higher angle and therefore greater vertical velocity, which would account for the greater flight time. The shorter contact time of the female runner lends further support to the preceding explanation. It would appear that the center of gravity of the women runners is not as far forward at takeoff. It is strongly recommended that future investigations concentrate on this aspect of female distance running.

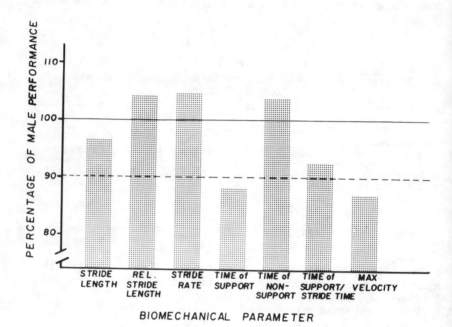

FIGURE 6. Summary of male–female comparisons for the biomechanical parameters.

SUMMARY AND CONCLUSION

In contrast with comparable male runners, the best American female distance runners are significantly shorter, lighter, have shorter legs, but are similar in relative leg length and ponderal index. In terms of biomechanical factors, the females had shorter strides, longer relative strides, higher stride rates, lesser times of support, and greater times of nonsupport. Furthermore these differences could not be completely accounted for by the differences in body size.

It is concluded that female distance runners differ significantly in running technique in comparison with their male counterparts.

ACKNOWLEDGMENTS

The authors wish to express their appreciation to Dr. Doris I. Miller, University of Washington, and Dr. Robert J. Gregor, UCLA, for their assistance during the filming phase of this investigation.

REFERENCES

1. EIBEN, O. G. 1972. The Physique of Women Athletes. The Hungarian Scientific Council for Physical Education. Budapest.
2. MALINA, R. M., A. B. HARPER, H. H. AVENT & D. E. CAMPBELL. 1971. Physique of female track and field athletes. Med. Sci. Sports 3(1): 32–38.
3. HOFFMAN, K. 1972. Stride length and frequency of female sprinters. Track Technique 48: 1522–1524.
4. CAVANAGH, P. R., M. L. POLLOCK & J. LANDA. 1977. A biomechanical comparison of elite and good runners. Ann. N.Y. Acad. Sci. This volume.
5. NELSON, R. C. & R. GREGOR. 1976. Biomechanics of distance running: A longitudinal study. Res. Q. 47(3): 417–428.
6. CLAUSER, C. E., P. E. TUCKER, J. T. McCONVILLE, E. CHURCHILL, L. L. LAUBACH & J. A. REARDON. 1972. Anthropometry of Air Force Women. National Technical Information Service Report. AMRL–TR–70–5.

SELF-PRECEPTIONS OF
FEMALE DISTANCE RUNNERS

Dorothy V. Harris and Susan E. Jennings

College of Health, Physical Education and Recreation
Pennsylvania State University
University Park, Pennsylvania 16802

In the 1970s society has been openly concerned with the concepts of masculinity and femininity; however, despite the ubiquitousness of the terminology and the frequency of measurements, precise descriptions or conceptual analyses of "masculinity" and "femininity" have only recently been attempted. The general point of view has been that masculinity included everything that males do and represent, or are supposed to do and are, while femininity is anything and everything that females are supposed to be and do. These generalized definitions, in addition to lacking clarity and specificity, also conceal a number of implicit assumptions whose implications need to be systematically investigated rather than taken for granted.

Integral to the concept of masculinity or femininity is biological gender. All human societies have accorded considerable significance to biological gender beyond the obvious physiological differences between being male and being female. Such things as standards for dress, behavior, legal rights and obligations, responsibilities and duties to family and society, and so on have been devised by all societies into generally polarized positions. These sex-role differentiations have generated sex-role stereotypes or normative expectations about the behavior males and females are expected to exhibit. While the etiology of these assumed differences is controversial, the belief that there are psychological differences between the sexes is widespread.

General agreement exists within society with regard to what men and women are like. The expected role of the female is to be passive, dependent, deferent, emotional, and concerned about what others think. The male, on the other hand, is expected to be active, independent, unemotional, assertive, rational, and autonomous. The expected behaviors are based on the assumption that what is masculine is not feminine and what is feminine is not masculine. This concept suggests that masculinity and femininity are bipolar opposites with most males falling at one end of a continuum on a cluster of attributes while the females fall at the opposite end. Overlap is not common and those who fall toward the opposite direction expected for their sex are viewed unfavorably.

Helmreich and Spence [1] contend that the relationship among the various components of masculinity and femininity, such as biological gender, sex-roles, sexual orientation, and especially psychological attributes of masculinity and femininity, and the adoption of conventional sex-roles is not as strong as has been traditionally assumed. The associations that have existed may be in process of breaking down. Patterns of sex-role differentiation are undergoing a change with greater latitude of behavior being allowed for both sexes.

Traditionally, sport has been the prerogative of the male and has served as a laboratory for the socialization of the boy into the man in society. At the same time, the behavioral and physical demands of strenuous and competitive

808

sport have been the antithesis of what femininity supposedly represents. The real fear of society has been that the participation of the female in such activities would masculinize her behavior. The general assumption has been that the female who found such experiences gratifying was not quite "normal," that there must be something wrong with her glands, and that she was trading off her feminine selfhood for such participation. And, indeed when bipolar behavior assessments were utilized, the athletic females did fall more toward the masculine end of the scale than those females who elected not to participate.

Helmreich and Spence have developed a new instrument to assess masculine–feminine components of behavior. While they have maintained the psychological aspects of masculinity and femininity, they have discarded a strictly bipolar model and structured an essentially dualistic notion. Their approach has been influenced by Bakan [2] who proposed that all living organisms are characterized by two fundamental modalities: a sense of *agency* and sense of *communion*. Agency demonstrates self-awareness and is manifested in self-assertion, self-expansion, and self-protection. Communion implies selflessness and concern for others. Both modalities are essential if society or the individual is to survive. Bakan further associated agency with masculinity and communion with femininity. Thus, according to Bakan, masculinity and femininity, in the sense of agency and communion, are two separate dimensions; however, the manifestation of one neither logically or psychologically precludes possession of the other.

The Helmreich and Spence instrument incorporates several notions. They first developed an instrument to measure masculinity and femininity by identifying a group of bipolar items such as dependent–independent, active–passive, and so on. All the items described psychological characteristics that both sexes believed differentiated the average male and female. In turn, these items had to differentiate the typical male and female when individuals were asked to rate themselves.

The next step involved dividing these items into separate masculinity and femininity scales where masculine attributes were those characteristics that were considered to be socially desirable in both sexes but were found to a greater degree among males. The feminine attributes were those that were socially desirable for both sexes but observed more often among females.

To determine the attributes that were socially desirable for each sex, Helmreich and Spence had subjects rate the attributes of the *ideal* man and woman. When items such as independent–dependent were polarized with a midpoint and the attributes of both the ideal male and female fell to the masculine side of the midpoint, they were considered "Masculine." Conversely, when the characteristics of the ideal male and female both fell to the feminine pole side of the midpoint, they were considered "Feminine."

The instrument developed utilizing this approach was called the Personal Attributes Questionnaire (PAQ). Two scores were generated, one on the Femininity scale, which indicated high femininity, and one on the Masculinity scale, which indicated high masculinity.

The next step involved finding the relationship between the two scales. Using several hundred subjects, Helmreich and Spence observed in both males and females a tendency for high masculine scores to be associated with high femininity and low scores on one scale to be related to low scores on the other scale. A bipolar conception would suggest that the sets of scores should be negatively related; that is, if one has a high masculine score the feminine score would be low. As indicated, this was not the case with those individuals sampled by Helmreich and Spence.

Additional data measuring social competence and self-esteem were generated by the Texas Social Behavior Inventory (TSBI) developed by Helmreich and Stapp.[3] When the data from the PAQ is correlated with that of the TSBI, masculinity correlated highly with self-esteem. This was observed among males where one would expect such a relationship; however, it was also observed among females. Femininity was modestly correlated with self-esteem (still highly significant) not only in women but in men as well.

Helmreich and Spence next devised a method of combining masculinity and femininity scores to understand how they jointly determined self-esteem. It was at this point that they developed a relatively simple classification scheme that was most useful to their overall concept of attributes. A 2 × 2 table as shown in TABLE 1 depicts the scheme.

Once a median is determined for masculinity and for femininity, each individual is classified according to his or her position relative to the median. At the lower right quadrant are those individuals who have scored above the me-

TABLE 1

SEX-ROLE CLASSIFICATION: PERSONAL ATTRIBUTES QUESTIONNAIRE *

Femininity	Masculinity	
	Below Median	Above Median
Below Median	Undifferentiated	Masculine
Above Median	Feminine	Androgynous

* After Helmreich & Spence.[1]

dian on both masculinity and femininity. Helmreich and Spence labeled these individuals *androgynous*. In the upper right quadrant are those individuals who scored high in masculinity and low in femininity. Males who corresponded to the typical male stereotype and females judged as cross-sex fell in this group and were labeled *masculine*. The lower left quadrant included those individuals who displayed the typical feminine attributes or those of a cross-sex male and were labeled *feminine*. Those who did not fall in any of the previous three categories, that is, they fell below the median on both masculinity and femininity were placed in the upper left quadrant in the 2 × 2 scheme and labeled *undifferentiated*.

After individuals were classified, Helmreich and Spence then determined the self-esteem score for each of the four groups. They found that the self-esteem of the undifferentiated was lowest, that of the feminine category next, followed by masculine, with the highest self-esteem being observed in the androgynous group. The differences between the means in the adjacent groups were great and significant. Females falling in the masculine classification did not perceive themselves as being less socially competent than the traditional female. Both males and females classified as androgynous displayed the higher self-esteem, those classified as masculine the next highest, those as feminine the next, with those classified as undifferentiated exhibiting the lowest self-esteem. This relationship held true for both males and females. Males and females did differ in the percentages that fell into each category. The college population had the same percentage of males and females classified as Androgynous, more males as Masculine and more females as Feminine and approximately the same as Undifferentiated. The high school population had a higher percentage of females classified as Androgynous, otherwise, they followed the same general pattern of the college population.

In summary, the Helmreich and Spence data suggested that masculinity and androgyny were both related to desirable characteristics and behaviors as well as self-esteem. These attributes provided the androgynous individual, either male or female, with behavioral advantages over those falling in other categories.

In an attempt to validate their findings, Helmreich and Spence selected unique populations of females where the existence or nonexistence of differences in the distribution of masculinity and femininity might support their theoretical proposition. Populations selected were female faculty members with a Ph.D. degree in science or engineering and female varsity athletes at the University of Texas. The percentages of the female scientists falling in the undifferentiated, feminine, masculine, and androgynous classifications were 8%, 23%, 23%, and 46%, respectively, while the female athletes were 20%, 10%, 31%, and 39%, respectively. These data also suggest that those females (both scientists and athletes) who succeed in areas of endeavor considered stereotypically masculine do not do this at the expense of their femininity. As a matter of fact, the data suggest that high-achieving women are more likely to possess both masculine and feminine attributes than their male counterparts without suffering any deficit in their femininity. On the contrary, they display significantly higher self-esteem than those females falling in other categories.

Method

The subjects of this study were female distance runners, most of whom were members of organized running groups. Initially, questionnaires were sent to a relatively small sample of runners who had been recognized nationally and/or internationally for their accomplishments in running. In turn, they provided additional names and addresses of runners who were contacted. Selected collegiate female cross country teams were also sent questionnaires. The Personal Attributes Questionnaire (PAQ), the Texas Social Behavior Inventory (TSBI), and the Work and Family Orientation Questionnaire (WOFO) were completed anonymously by all of the subjects. However, birthdate and years of running were requested.

The two groups analyzed in this study were determined by age; the scholastic group was composed of all runners 23 years of age or younger, the club group included those over 26 years of age.

The instruments were scored according to directions provided by Helmreich and analyzed by computer. It should be noted that the medians derived from the work Helmreich and Spence were used as the basis for classifying the subjects in this study.

TABLE 2

PAQ CLASSIFICATION OF RUNNERS *

| | Masculinity | | | |
| | Below Median | | Above Median | |
Femininity	n	% †	n	% †
	Undifferentiated		*Masculine*	
Below Median				
Total Sample	14	20.6	19	27.9
Club	7	20.6	12	35.3
Scholastic	7	20.6	7	20.6
	Feminine		*Androgynous*	
Above Median				
Total Sample	12	17.6	23	33.8
Club	5	14.7	10	29.4
Scholastic	7	20.6	13	38.2

* Club total $n=34$: Scholastic total $n=34$.
† Percentages are adjusted frequencies.

Results

The age range of the scholastic runners was 14–23 years and the age of the club runners was 26–59 years. The average number of years of training for the scholastic group was 3.6 while it was 5.2 years for the club group.

The results of the PAQ produced the sex-role classification shown in TABLE 2. The greatest percentage of the club runners were classified as masculine while the greatest percentage of the scholastic runners were classified as androgynous. The remaining scholastic runners were divided equally (20.6%) among the feminine, masculine, and undifferentiated classifications. The percentage of club runners classified as androgynous, undifferentiated, and feminine were 29.4%, 20.6%, and 14.7%, respectively.

As indicated in TABLE 3, the results follow the same pattern as those reported for female athletes and female scientists in the data presented by Helm-

TABLE 3

COMPARISON OF PAQ RESULTS WITH THE RESULTS OF HELMREICH AND SPENCE

| | Adjusted Frequencies | | | |
Subjects	Undifferentiated	Feminine	Masculine	Androgynous
Club runners	20.6%	14.7%	35.3%	29.4%
Scholastic runners	20.6%	20.6%	20.6%	38.2%
Female athletes *	20%	10%	31%	39%
Female scientists *	21%	39%	11%	29%

* Helmreich & Spence.[1]

reich and Spence. It should be noted that similar percentages of scholastic runners of this study and female athletes of the Helmreich and Spence study fell in the androgynous classification.

When the relationship of sex-role classification and self-esteem was examined among scholastic and club runners, the data corresponded with that reported by Helmreich and Spence with the exception of the fact that both scholastic and club runners classified as feminine displayed a lower self-esteem than the undifferentiated group. These data are presented in TABLE 4.

In the female college population analyzed by Helmreich and Spence, the undifferentiated group had the lowest self-esteem. All females classified as androgynous (both groups of runners and the female college group of Helmreich and Spence) exhibited the highest self-esteem scores. Those classified as masculine had the next highest self-esteem. Simple 1×4 analyses of variance showed that the main effect for these differences was significant, $F (28, 38) = 2.07$, probability at or beyond the 0.05 level. Tests of difference between all possible pairs of means were made by the Newman-Keuls test procedures for

TABLE 4

MEAN SELF-ESTEEEM SCORES FOR FOUR PAQ CLASSIFICATION

Subjects	Undifferentiated	Feminine	Masculine	Androygnous
Club runners ($n=34$)	34.1	30.8	43.2	44.4
Scholastic runner ($n=34$)	34.1	30.1	43.6	43.8
Total population * ($n=68$)	34.1	31.0	43.3	44.0

* One-way analysis of variance, p < 0.05.

unequal sample sizes. A conservative method and a 0.01 level of confidence were used to provide a more stringent test because of descrepancy of sample sizes.[4] All classifications were significantly different from each other beyond the 0.01 level except the comparison between Androgynous and Masculinity, which was not significant at a probability of less than the 0.01 level.

Further clarification of the interaction of the sex-role classification and the variables of the WOFO will be attempted in the near future. The preliminary work of Helmreich and Spence looking at the variables of the WOFO and PAQ categories suggest an interaction among the attributes measured by both instruments.

Discussion

It is encouraging to note that those females who are classified as androgynous and masculine also display the highest self-esteem. This was revealed in the analysis of Helmreich and Spence as well as among the runners who served as subjects in this study. Traditionally it has been assumed that those females who might perceive themselves as being more closely aligned with typical masculine behavior would have lower self-esteem.

Other investigators have also tested this assumption and reported similar findings. Snyder et al.[5] reported that their findings did not reveal negative associations between female sports participation and the two measures of self-identity. On the contrary, positive relationships emerged in the opposite direction. Snyder and his associates concluded that these findings raised serious doubts about the assumptions of the conflict being inherent in female athletes, which might produce a negative self-perception.

Monk [6] based her theoretical proposition on certain suppositions predicated by an extensive literature review. This review supported the notion that the traditional female role is incongurous with athleticism, that pursuing such traditionally masculine roles would serve as a source of conflict for the female athlete. Further, the role orientation of the female is generally culturally determined; that is, there appears to be little physiological basis for these differentiations. And finally, the literature supported the notion that the female role is less desirable than that of the male, both to males and females. According to the literature, the female's involvement should be a source of conflict by society's standards; this conflict should be reflected in her self-perception. However, Monk argued that since the involvement persisted among female athletes in spite of the negative sanction, there must be some source of positive feedback inherent in the participation, which tended to counteract the conflict. Monk reported that female athletes did exhibit a satisfaction with one's self to a greater extent than nonathletes. In addition, they were significantly more self-confident than nonathletes.

As Bardwick [7] indicated, contemporary society is allowing greater latitude for sex-role behavior with alternative roles becoming increasingly more observable. Females who have developed a sense of autonomy and a positive self-esteem may be better able to select their roles and enjoy a freedom of choice without experiencing conflict. Snyder et al. concluded that the intensity of the conflict between the roles of being a female and being an athlete seems to be disappearing. Based on the findings of Helmreich and Spence, Monk, Snyder et al., and this present study of distance runners, that would appear to be the case.

Summary

The concepts of masculinity and femininity were discussed, including the traditional models and a more recent theoretical position that exposed the replacement of the traditional bipolar model with a dualistic notion of masculinity and femininity. This dualistic approach emphasizes the value of individuals possessing both masculine and feminine psychological attributes, i.e., being androgynous.

The theoretical framework employed by Helmreich and Spence in devising the Personal Attributes Questionnaire (PAQ) was discussed. The PAQ was used in this study to classify female runners according to their sex-role (androgynous, masculine, feminine, or undifferentiated). Using the Texas Social Behavior Inventory (TSBI) designed by Helmreich and Spence to assess self-esteem, we found that there was a significant difference between the self-esteem of the subjects when classified by sex-role, with the androgynous subjects having the highest self-esteem. The results of this study were supportive of the work of Helmreich and Spence.

References

1. HELMREICH, R. & J. T. SPENCE. 1976. Sex roles and achievement. Paper presented at the North American Society for the Psychology of Sport and Physical Activity, Austin, Texas, May, 1976.
2. BAKAN, D. 1966. The Duality of Human Existence. Rand McNally, Chicago.
3. HELMREICH, R. & J. STAPP. 1974. Short forms of the Texas Social Behavior Inventory (TSBI), an objective measure of self-esteem. Bull. Psychonomic Soc. 4: 473–475.
4. WINER, B. J. 1971. Statistical Principles in Experimental Design. McGraw-Hill Book Co., New York, N.Y.
5. SNYDER, E. E., J. KIVLIN & E. E. SPREITZER. 1975. Females athletes: An analysis of subjective and objective role conflict. In Proceedings from the North American Society for the Psychology of Sport and Physical Activity. D. M. Landers, Pennsylvania State University. University Park, Pa.
6. MONK, S. V. 1976. An investigation of the self and ideal self profiles and the dissonance between them among field hockey players. Unpublished Masters thesis. Pennsylvania State University.
7. BARDWICK, J. 1971. Psychology of Women. Harper & Row, New York, N.Y.

DISCUSSION

Jack H. Wilmore, *Moderator*

Department of Physical Education
University of Arizona
Tucson, Arizona 85721

B. GUTIN (*Columbia University, New York, N.Y.*): Dr. Daniels, did you look at the relationship between the oxygen consumption at a given work load and performance within each sex? I don't believe you commented on that. I.e., were those runners who were more economical at a given work load (lower $\dot{V}_{O_2}$) also the better performers?

J. DANIELS (*University of Texas, Austin, Texas*): Unfortunately, we didn't look at that.

J. H. WILMORE: In terms of the athletes you tested, did you look at their training programs and the length of time they had been in training relative to differences between the male and female runners?

J. DANIELS: Most of the women in this study had been running for quite some time. Approximately 3 years was the least any of them had run, and some had run for 8 to 10 years. With regard to their training programs, we didn't analyze these critically, but I'm sure it was fairly intense for both groups considering the caliber of these athletes. I know there were girls in the study who trained 80 to 100 miles a week, and the male marathon runners were certainly equaling that.

H. DUVAL (*Indiana University, Bloomington, Ind.*): Dr. Lussier, did you test the control group only twice, before and after, while you tested the experimental group three times in addition to the before and after tests? Don't you think that would have an effect on your resulting $\dot{V}_{O_2 \, max}$ values?

L. LUSSIER (*Pennsylvania State University, University Park, Pa.*): Are you considering the possibility of habituation?

H. DUVAL: Yes, just repeating the test could influence your results. Your data indicates a decline in the second test, and this could counterbalance the experimental effect.

L. LUSSIER: This was something that bothered us also. Even though the work loads were either work loads they had started but not finished previously, or higher work loads, the heart rate was lower, and in certain instances the $\dot{V}_{O_2 \, max}$ was lower. The experimental group was tested twice during the 3-month conditioning program. This was used in place of a conditioning session. There is a possibility that some training effect could have taken place at that point. Although the heart rates were matched before and after for most of these children, and even though some of the control group managed higher work loads afterwards than they had previously, basically the $\dot{V}_{O_2}$ was identical. How much of an effect this would have we don't know. In some youngsters the conditioning program had absolutely no effect. The increase was less then 1.0 ml/kg·min. In other youngsters the increase was as much as 8 or 9 ml/kg·min, and this was not in the lower fitness children. These were those who had started with $\dot{V}_{O_2 \, max}$ values of 56–63 ml/kg·min. Thus, the effect of training or habituation as you have suggested, can not be quantified. It might have had a slight influence on the results.

816

A. S. LEON (*University of Minnesota, Minneapolis, Minn.*): Dr. Wood, we've just completed a study trying to determine whether you really need vigorous physical activity of that magnitude to change lipoprotein patterns. We took a group of obese male college students and put them on a treadmill walking program for 16 weeks. We found an increase in the HDL with a lowering of their LDL and VLDL, so that the HDL/LDL ratio was in the right direction. They also lost 4% of their body fat (about ten pounds) without changing their dietary habits, and had a reduction in their blood insulin and glucose levels with and without a challenge. It looks like you need only a brisk walking program to favorably modify coronary risk factors.

P. D. WOOD (*Stanford University, Palo Alto, Calif.*): I believe that is an extremely important finding and I'm glad to hear it because people keep asking me as to what level of activity they must pursue to gain relevant benefits from the exercise.

C. H. WYNDHAM (*Marshalltown, South Africa*): I'd like to congratulate Dr. Drinkwater on a most elegant presentation and a very beautiful paper. I believe this paper presented some of the clearest data I've seen of the marathon runner partially adapting to heat, particularly with reference to your plasma volume studies. I think these are very neat indeed. What one would like to see, and I'm sure you had this in mind, is to encourage these people to go through a full training regime to see how much further they can adapt. I'm sure this can be done. But clearly in terms of your plasma volume adaptation, it looks to me as though your runners have already made a very large proportion of the circulatory adaptation and probably what you would get in a more rigorous heat acclimatization would be a greater sweat gland adaptation.

B. L. DRINKWATER (*University of California, Santa Barbara, Calif.*): If I may comment on your comment, you'll find data in our written paper on the sweat mechanism, which I didn't have time to include in this presentation. As we have shown, it looks as if the marathoners have an earlier onset of sweating. We did do total sweat rate by prerun and postrun measurements. However, I am not comfortable with the controls' data, for sometimes they were in a rather precarious state at the end of the experiment and we had to keep them lying in a cool environment before we could get them to the scale. This makes it very difficult to have absolute accuracy when you have to divide sweat loss by time. A very gross calculation, however, showed only a 5% difference in total sweat rate per unit time for the two groups. However, I should also mention that in a hot dry environment Robinson and Horvath showed back in 1940 that the sweating mechanism is not stimulated to that extent. So yes, we hope to continue these studies and take a closer look at what happens when they do acclimatize to the heat.

P. B. RAVEN (*Institute for Aerobics Research, Dallas, Texas*): Dr. Drinkwater, were your subject groups matched in terms of the menstrual cycle and the possible difference in set point temperatures.

B. L. DRINKWATER: We attempted to do this. One of the things that we did with our pre-exposure bloods was to take a look at the estrogen and progesterone levels. We have been unable to find any relationship between those values and either rectal temperature, final rectal temperature, change in rectal temperature or sweat rate. Now that's not to say that the cycle does not have an effect on temperature. It certainly does. We know this because we've had a number of women take their temperatures prior to getting out of bed in the morning and we do see a rise in temperature during the luteal phase. What happens when they get out of bed and start moving may simply be that ordinary activities of the day override that influence, but we haven't been able to find a relationship there yet. As we get more and more data, not just on the marathoners, but on other women, we may find that picture changes.

D. S. KRONFELD (*University of Pennsylvania, Philadelphia, Pa.*): I would like to mention our field observations that seem to show a superior aspect of heat tolerance in women over men and ask the speaker and others like Dr. Wyndham if they have observed this themselves. I used to coach a crew of men and women on the Brisbane River in Australia under very hot and humid conditions. The men suffered very much from the tendency to hyperventilate, develop apnea, and grey out. We could control their breathing. Some excitable types seemed to be susceptible to this more than others. I thought that hyperventilation might be contributing to the problem in the heat as well as being a symptom of heat stroke. I coached about 30 girls over a period of 6 years and I never saw any of them do this sort of thing. I wondered whether this is a genuine phenomenon or just my chance observation that women might not suffer as much from hyperventilation contributing to greying out in the heat as do men.

B. L. DRINKWATER: We saw a lot of hyperventilation in the control group. We didn't see nearly as much in the marathoners. It might be that your women rowers were sitting and did not have to carry their body weight. Would you say that they were doing the same relative work load as the men?

D. S. KRONFELD: Yes, they were doing a lot of long distance work, and I think actually that they might work more than marathon runners because of the fact that the upper body as well as the lower body is involved.

B. L. DRINKWATER: All I can say is that we did see hyperventilation; extreme hyperventilation in our controls and some slight hyperventilation in the marathon runners who would probably be comparable to your oarswomen.

J. HEAD (*Atlanta Physical Fitness Institute, Atlanta, Ga.*): Dr. Harris, it's very refreshing to hear your presentation. Growing up during the time I did, I found women's sports were discouraged at the intercollegiate level. Also, there was little opportunity for young girls to participate in recreational sports. I can see now that research is changing the general attitude of people toward women in athletics. I appreciate what you've done.

D. V. HARRIS (*Pennsylvania State University, University Park, Pa.*): Thank you. I think we're going to find the trade-offs that have been assumed are not being made, that there is no trade-off in terms of one's femininity.

D. S. KRONFELD: Dr. Harris, androgynous and masculine sound very similar to me and I wondered if you would explain in more detail what you mean, i.e., how you discriminate between these two.

D. V. HARRIS: You ask males and females to define their concept of the ideal male and the ideal female. Anything that fell to the masculine side of the midpoint was considered masculine, and the same thing was true with behaviors that were considered typically feminine in a traditional sense but desirable both in males and in females. When any subject scored high on both of those then they were classified as androgynous. You have to be high, above the median, in both masculine and feminine characteristics to be androgynous, but only high above the median in masculine characteristics to be classified as masculine.

DIANE NYATT (*New York, N.Y.*): I'm the one who recently swam around Manhattan Island and I do a lot of long distance swimming. I wonder if the self-image and the self-esteem that an elete or world class athlete holds is different from a group of average women who are exercising but who are not successful athletes. In other words, I think that a woman who does very well, is in the limelight, and succeeds in what she does in athletics can go about what she does without any doubt, without any reservation and with the knowledge that no one will question her femininity.

D. V. HARRIS: Yes, you have to consider aspects such as motivations for running and whether the feedback becomes that intrinsic motivation in a hedonistic sense as opposed to extrinsic motivation. I think the rewards of recognition are probably relative to whatever one's position is in terms of their identity as an athlete. Having done quite a bit of research on self-perception, and the identity and the self-confidence of lesser known or unknown athletes, it appears that the same thing is operating; i.e., there is a relationship between a sense of, "I can do it," and the reinforcement of one's self-esteem at any level, and not just at the elite level.

P. MILVY: I would like to submit the following resolution. It's a resolution from the New York Academy of Sciences, Conference on the Marathon, to all member countries of the IAAF and all of the various committees of the IAAF, the United States Olympic Committee, and the Amateur Athletic Union of the United States. It reads, "Current research including that presented at this conference demonstrates that female athletes adapt to marathon training and benefit from it in virtually the same way male athletes do. There exists no pursuasive scientific or medical evidence, nor has any evidence been presented at this conference that long distance running, in particular, marathon running, is in any way contraindicated for the trained female athlete. Therefore, be it resolved that it is the considered judgement of the participants of this conference that a women's marathon event as well as other long distance races for women be included in the Olympics program forthwith."

(This resolution was passed unanimously by all those present.)

DEVELOPMENT OF THE MARATHON FROM PHEIDIPPIDES TO THE PRESENT, WITH STATISTICS OF SIGNIFICANT RACES

David E. Martin

College of Allied Health Sciences
Georgia State University
Atlanta, Georgia 30303

Herbert W. Benario

Emory University
Atlanta, Georgia 30322

Roger W. H. Gynn

Carpender's Park
Watford, Hertfordshire
WD1 5DR, England

INTRODUCTION

According to Webster (*Third New International Dictionary*) the word *marathon* as it relates to racing is either a footrace run on an open course, now usually 26 miles, 385 yards, or else a race of great length other than a footrace. The word originates from a city in Greece of the same name, where legend has it that an Athenian named Pheidippides ran from the battlefield of Marathon to Athens, a distance approximating 24 miles, to report victory over the Persians in a momentous battle fought in the year 490 B.C. As he gasped out the happy news upon his arrival in Athens, he fell dead from his exertions. The ancient evidence for this exploit is very slender indeed, and the man's name, in any case, was probably not Pheidippides.

Recorded history tells little of competitive long distance races specifically in the neighborhood of 25 miles until the Olympic Games in 1896 at Athens. There, the legend of Pheidippides was revived by a race called the marathon, 40 kilometers (24.85 miles) long, extending over a hopefully similar route, from Marathon Bridge to the Olympic Stadium. Since then, there has arisen a tremendous interest among civilized nations, in Europe and North America at first but now world-wide, in staging contests of similar length. Marathon running has developed a mystique and flavor all its own, at the local and international levels, adding to the desire for people of all ages and abilities to participate. Although races of longer distance are held annually in many parts of the world, the marathon distance of 26 miles 385 yards or thereabouts remains the king of distance running events.

The Olympic marathons have been described frequently,[1-5] and their excitement and intrigue sparked periodic surges of interest in distance running. Many of the details, however, concerning the initial development of marathon running as a sport (a period encompassing the years 1896–1910) are not generally known. These details are emphasized in this brief historical sketch, which describes the marathon during five time periods: (1) The era of Pheidippides, (2) the origin of the first modern Olympiad, (3) the period between the Olympic marathons at Athens (1896) and London (1908), (4) the era of professionalism in marathoning (1908–1909), and (5) continued development of the race into recent times. For good reason, the latter section is extremely cursory, since the number of races and runners during that 65-plus-year period increased so quickly and to such large proportions that only book-length coverage could adequately describe the events. Some compensation for this meager description is provided by the statistical summary of major races at the end of this presentation. Also, elsewhere in this volume, a more detailed glimpse of post-World War II marathon running is presented (by Lucas) and a history of women's participation in the marathon is outlined (by Kuscsik).

The Legend of Pheidippides

Our prime source is Herodotus, who lived approximately from 484 to 425 B.C., wrote his stupendous history in the last years of his life, and unquestionably was able to gain information from men, then advanced in age, who were alive at the time of the battle of Marathon. He tells us: [6] "And first, before they left the city, the generals sent off to Sparta a herald, one Philippides, who was by birth an Athenian, and by profession and practice a trained runner. This man, according to the account which he gave to the Athenians on his return, when he was near Mount Parthenium above Tegea, fell in with the god Pan, who called him by his name, and bade him ask the Athenians, 'Why they neglected him so entirely, when he was kindly disposed towards them, and had often helped them in times past, and would do so again in time to come?' . . . On the occasion of which we speak, when Philippides was sent by the Athenian generals, and, according to his own account, saw Pan on his journey, he reached Sparta on the very next day after quitting the city of Athens."

There are four important points in this narrative which merit special consideration: the runner's name, his profession, the distance he covered, and the absence of further information. Nothing is said about his return to Athens, his joining the army at Marathon, his participation in the battle, a subsequent run to Athens to carry the news, and the celebrated demise. All of this would have made precisely the kind of tale that Herodotus enjoyed so much; one cannot imagine him omitting such uplifting material, had he known it and had it happened. Clearly our hero did return to Athens to report that his mission was unsuccessful, but that is all of which we can be sure.

The distance is given by a later source [7] as 1240 stades; a *stade* is the length of the track in a stadium, and thus was not a precise measurement but one which varied from place to place. Nonetheless, it is generally estimated as about 200 yards; this will make a distance of 141 miles. If we raise the estimate of the stade to a furlong, the distance becomes 155 miles. Certainly one will not err very much by taking 150 miles as a round figure. We know that this distance is within reach of a trained runner within 24 hours; Herodotus informs us that the runner reached Sparta "on the very next day," which implies no more than 24 hours. But, even if we interpret it more loosely as "within two calendar days," it was still a stupendous achievement, for the terrain in the Peloponnesus is mountainous in the extreme. And he returned to Athens soon, if not immediately. Hence he would have covered some 300 miles in three or four days.

Ancient evidence leans toward recording the name as Philippides, although there is some manuscript evidence for Pheidippides. It is easier to explain corruption from the former to the latter than the reverse, for the real name means "the son of a lover of horses," and a later scribe may have considered that unworthy of a man who ranked as one of Athens' legendary heroes in subsequent ages.

Cornelius Nepos, a Roman historian of the first century B.C., in his life of the general Miltiades, who was chiefly responsible for the victory at Marathon, reports [8] that "the Athenians, distressed by this war so near and so great, in their own land, sought aid nowhere other than from the Lacedaemonians (Spartans) and sent Phidippus, a runner of that class known as hemerodromoi, to report how urgent was the need of aid." The hemerodromoi,[9, 10] men who ran for a day (or longer), were important in the life of early Greek cities, and even more important for the army, for they were generally the means of communication. And there is evidence that they could cover quite fantastic distances, although we cannot be at all certain of the time they required. One man covered 1000 stades (about 110 miles) in fifteen hours. (This compares favorably with an American record time [11] of 13:33:06 for 100 miles, set by Theodore Corbitt of New York. Corbitt averaged 8:08 per mile, while an approximation for the Greek would be 8:10 per mile.)

Pliny the Elder, a Roman polymath of the first century A.D., in his *Natural History,*[12] mentions Phidippides' great feat in a section on extraordinary distances covered by man; he speaks of a period of 2 days. For comparison, he points out that the longest distance covered by a human in 24 hours on horseback, with a constant change of horses along the way, was 200 Roman miles, about 180 English miles.

Lastly one may invoke the testimony of Pausanias, a Greek traveler of the second century A.D., who wrote a *Description of Greece:* [13] "Philippides was sent to Lacedaemon to tell that the Medes had landed, but came back reporting that the Lacedaemonians had deferred their march, for it was their custom not to march out to war before the moon was full. But Philippides said that Pan met him about Mount Parthenius, and told him that he wished the Athenians well and would come to Marathon to fight for them. So the god Pan has been honored for this message."

In the Latin authors, there are variant readings which offer Philippides for Phidippides; in the Greek authors the accepted reading is the former. This appears to us to be decisive, as it does to most classical scholars.

Two Greeks of the second century A.D. are the only sources for a run from Marathon to Athens. Lucian [14] gives the runner the name Philippides; Plutarch [15] mentions an entirely different runner, whose name may here continue in deserved obscurity.

The Origin of the First Modern Marathon: Athens, 1896

In 1889, Baron Pierre de Coubertin was commissioned by the French government to make a global study of physical culture and physical education in school systems. He found conflicts and strife, among individual sports and also among sporting interests, which were impeding the progress and success of physical education programs. He concluded that one means for resolving these difficulties would involve periodic international competition organized in a fashion similar to the ancient games at Olympia. His proposal to revive and introduce to the modern world the Olympic Games, announced on November 25, 1892 at the Sorbonne, was enthusiastically received. On June 16, 1894 an International Olympic Congress was convened to consider the logistics of such a revival.

An important figure in these meetings was Michel Breal, French linguist and historian; he was the one primarily responsible for recommending a distance race. Never before, during the Greek Olympiads, or even during the more recent English Olympics, begun in 1636, had an endurance running event been included. At the ancient festivals of Olympia, Nemea, Delphi, and Isthmia, the prime running competition was one stade, and there was a *diaulos,* down and back, of about 400 yards. The *dolichos* was the longest race, of varying distance in different stadia, but evidently nowhere longer than 24 stades, a little less than three miles, as at Olympia. Thus when Baron de Coubertin, accompanied by Breal, went to Athens to arrange the program, the discussion did not initially center upon a long distance event. Breal strongly recommended it, however, and penned a letter to the Baron saying: [1] "If the Organizing Committee of the Athens Olympics would be willing to revive the famous run of the Marathon soldier as part of the program of the Games, I would be glad to offer a prize for this new Marathon race." Coubertin delivered the letter to the Greeks, who, with their deep sense of history and national pride, accepted the idea at once. The prize would be a gold cup, and the long distance run, or marathon, would make its first appearance in any Olympic-style competition.

An authoritative description of the race is provided by Quercetani.[2] By race time, on April 10, 1896, emotions were very high, and for good reason. The Greeks had won nothing in the Games. The marathon was the final event, and there were several Greek entrants hoping to bring glory to their nation. Probably none of the runners had ever been the full race distance, and the legendary run was to be relived, most likely for the first time since 490 B.C. Twenty-five runners assembled on Marathon Bridge; the starter gave a few words, fired the gun, and the race was on.

The essence of the drama is that a native Greek, Spiridon Louis, postal messenger from the village of Marusi and veteran of many long military marches, finished seven minutes ahead of another countryman. The crowd at the ancient but refurbished Panathenaic Stadium, and the entire Greek nation, were thrilled almost beyond description. Louis averaged 7:12 per mile for the event, a tremendous feat considering the gravel road, the steady uphill grade for the first 30 km, and the warm temperatures. He did not reach the head of the pack of runners until km 32, where he ran with Australian Keith Flack until km 36. Louis took the lead and won, Flack later dropped out, and Haralambos Vasilakos (also recorded as Charilaos Vasilakos) was second. The marathon was born, and the virtual domination by the Greeks at the finish line (nine finished, eight from Greece) did more to vindicate the legend of Pheidippides and perpetuate the race for the future than any amount of published rhetoric.

Marathoning during the First Three Olympiads: 1896–1908

The United States was one of the nine nations in the Athens Olympics, and its participation was due in large measure to activities of athletes and officials from the Boston Athletic Association. Only one American entered the marathon, namely the 1500-meter silver medalist Arthur Blake. Although he had three days to recover, he dropped out at 14½ miles. The seed was planted, however, and the idea of the marathon returned to America with the Olympic participants. The first North American version was planned for the following spring, on Patriot's Day in Boston. No one could have predicted the eventual popularity of that event!

This was not to be the first organized competition in North American long distance foot racing, however. A most notable event of 19 miles was staged by the Canadians in Hamilton, Ontario on Thanksgiving Day, 1894.[16] A man named Marshall won it in 2 hours 14 minutes. The next year a man named Wood slashed four minutes from Marshall's time. This race eventually served as a proving ground for runners who were to run and win full-length marathons in the United States. The race is contested to this day, and thus is probably the oldest long distance footrace currently contested on an annual basis.

Also, this was not to be the first American marathon. Boston was preceded by seven months in its activities by the fall meeting of the New York City Knickerbocker Athletic Club at Columbia Oval on September 20, 1896. While regular track and field events were proceeding, 30 runners had gone by train to Stamford, Connecticut and began a 25-mile trek at 12:26 P.M. back to the track. A reporter for *The New York Times* covered the marathon race:[17] "For the first eight miles they plowed along through mud and slush, occasionally taking to a hard path by the side of the road . . .

"(John J.) McDermott kept the lead all the way from New Rochelle, but the miserable roads made it impossible for him to travel fast. Now and then he walked, but Hamilton Gray seemed to be unable in the last part of the road to get any nearer to him than 200 yards.

"The last part of the struggle was perhaps the hardest of all, although there was not a bit of mud in it. It was through Mount Vernon Avenue to the oval— a hill with a tremendous rise, and full of small projecting cobbles. It was almost enough to take the wind out of a fresh runner, not to mention one who was completing 25 miles, but both bicyclists and runners valiantly climbed to its top, where the cheers of the crowd were urging them on.

"Several events were being contested at 3:51 o'clock when from the gate came a wild shout: 'They're here!' 'They're coming!' The cry was taken up in the grand stand. Women who knew only that the first race of its kind ever held in this country was nearing a finish, waved their handkerchiefs and fairly screamed with excitement. Men dashed from their seats and down beside the track to get a look at the Americo-Marathon victor. There was a pandemonium of joy. Judges stopped their work; athletes found time to become spectators . . .

"And yet, when a bicycle rider and a pale-faced man came slowly in the gate nothing remarkable had been accomplished . . . [this remark appears incongruous to us; evidently the reporter was implying that McDermott's time of 3:25:55.6 was slow by Athens standards and hence set no new record for the distance].

"His failure to make a record, however, is not to his discredit, for the rain of the morning had filled many of the roads with mud, and the ground between Stamford and the oval is one of the many heart racking hills. There was still speed in the plucky winner, and as he circled the track, while the crowd was howling itself hoarse, he showed that, if anybody had tried to steal the laurel wreath from him when he had it in sight, he could have spurted to victory."

Hamilton Gray finished second in 3:28:27, to a tremendous ovation, and third place went to Louis Liebgold, in 3:36:58. Seven others crossed the finish line. Spectator interest in the marathon dominated over the other scheduled events. It gave a hint of the future, which would see crowds increasing in size and emotion to the point of unruliness, fighting, and even termination of the race in progress. Few sporting events were soon to grip the public's attention more than the marathon.

At the Boston Athletic Association Marathon Games, held on April 19, 1897, to honor the famous ride of Paul Revere in 1775, a 24.7-mile course extended from Metcalfe's Mill in Ashland to Boston's Irvington St. Oval. It was remarkably similar in topography to the Athens course, though about 250 meters short. Fifteen runners started, eight finished. John J. McDermott became the first two-time marathon victor with a time 6 minutes faster than the Athens victor, Spiridon Louis. Two other veterans of the New York marathon finished this race, and in fact the first seven of the total of eight finishers were from the New York area. Thousands of spectators witnessed the event, and the shorter races proceeding simultaneously at the Oval were again deemed secondary in importance.

The influence on the Boston Marathon of New York runners continued in 1898 and 1899. Twelve of the 21 starters in 1898 and six of the eleven finishers in 1899 were members of the Knickerbocker, St. George's, or Pastime Athletic Clubs of New York City. This dominance was short-lived, however, because in 1900 the Canadians from Hamilton literally stole the show at Boston. John J. Caffrey, William Sherring, and a runner named Hughson finished first, second, and third, all within a span of ten minutes, breaking the course record by more than 2 minutes. The fourth through eighth finishers were from the Boston area.

The Olympic Games were in Paris in 1900, and the majority of the American team was from the New York Athletic Club (as was the case in almost all other events). The drama of the chaotic Paris marathon has been often documented; with a twisting course, heat, and dust, no records were broken. Of the eight finishers, three were American. Ronald McDonald, 1898 Boston winner, finished eighth. This was one of the few Olympic contests which probably did little or nothing to enhance the spirit of marathon running.

The Boston Marathon continued its surge in popularity in numbers both of entrants and of spectators. The Canadians at Hamilton continued to develop, and their 19-mile Thanksgiving Day race became an annual classic. John Caffrey had won both events in 1900, and was again victorious at Boston in 1901, followed in second place by countryman William Davis. But New York was developing its talent as well, and a Yonkers native, Samuel A. Mellor, Jr., became the man to beat, as he won the Pan-American Exposition marathon at Buffalo on July 4, 1901, and the Boston Marathon and Hamilton race in 1902—a triple crown of sorts. The 1902 Boston event was a true spectacle—100,000 witnesses lining the streets made it the largest free sports show on earth.

Meanwhile, preparations were underway for America to host the Olympics in 1904, with St. Louis the venue. Thus, it is certain that thoughts of marathoning entered the minds of distance runners of the Midwest, notably in established clubs in St. Louis and Chicago. Details are somewhat obscure, as local city newspapers of that era have poor documentation of race activities, and some club records no longer exist. A 1914 fire completely wiped out the older records of the Missouri Athletic Club.

The American team had two marathon athletes from the Midwest, Sidney

Hatch of St. Louis and Albert Corey of Chicago. But there was great depth and superb quality from the East as well. The perennially good runner Thomas J. Hicks of Boston placed sixth, fifth, and second, respectively, in the 1900, 1901, and 1904 Boston Marathons. Fred Lorz finished fourth in 1905 and fifth in 1904 at the same race. Arthur Newton was fifth at the Paris Olympic Games. America was prepared to dominate, although several Greeks were hoping as well for a good finish.

The story of that fateful August afternoon in the scorching heat and suffocating dust of St. Louis is well known. The United States swept the first three places, in appropriately slow times, as well as sixth, seventh, eighth, eleventh, and thirteenth out of the 14 recorded finish times. It has been the only medal sweep by any nation in the marathon. Controversy at the victory stand resulted when dropout Fred Lorz entered the stadium after returning by car, and was mistaken as the winner. This certainly focused more attention on the marathon than would otherwise have occurred. Victorious Thomas J. Hicks was accorded a heroes welcome, but was so exhausted from the grueling ordeal that he doubtless was unable to appreciate the excitement of the moment.

Marathoning had nonetheless been introduced to the American Midwest, and the fine Olympic performances by Sidney Hatch of St. Louis and Albert Corey of Chicago sparked the beginnings of annual marathons in those cities. Sponsored by the local athletic clubs, they were very popular events during the next five years, a period which saw an unprecedented interest in marathon running perhaps unsurpassed until the recent era of the 1970s. Hatch won his native St. Louis race in 1906 and 1907, and one of his teammates, Joseph Forshaw, placed twelfth in the 1906 Athens Intermediary Games.

The 1906 Games were a sporting event of great importance which added a fresh new flavor to the entire international athletic movement and improved the image of the marathon. They were never given the title of "Olympic" since they were intended to be staged every 4 years in the middle of an Olympiad, in Athens.[18] They were scheduled as part of a compromise agreement between the Greeks, who desired a perpetual periodic Olympics in Athens, and Baron de Coubertin, who felt that shifting venues would enhance the international spirit of competition. It was agreed to have both, but the Intermediary Games were only held once, for the Baron's viewpoint convinced even the Greeks that his was the better choice.

The Paris and St. Louis Olympics had been staged concomitantly with world expositions, and were considered no more than a side show by many. The rumors of course-cutting along the complicated Parisian marathon route and the Lorz incident at St. Louis had given the event more infamy than fame. At Athens, the Games were the one and only event, and well-organized. The marathon was carefully planned, along a macadam route roughly paralleling the earlier course. The day (April 30) was very hot, and the Greeks were mobilized, counting 33 among the 53 starters. But serious training by runners from many nations eclipsed chances for a Greek victory. The winner was William Sherring, of Hamilton, Ontario, who finished in 2:51:23.6 for 41,860 meters (26 miles). Second place went to Sweden, third and twelfth to the USA, and fourth and fifth to Greece. This famous Athens course was not to see another competitive race for fifty years, when in 1955 a Marathon to Athens marathon was initiated on a biennial basis.

The London Olympics and the Rise of Professionalism

The 1908 Olympics proved a watershed in the marathon's popularity, and the finish of the race opposite the Royal Box in White City Stadium must rank as one of the most unusual and dramatic in all of sports. Its effects were felt directly for a year, and the story is now almost legendary. The course distance was unique—42,195 meters or 26.219 miles—simply to accommodate appropriate viewing from the Royal Box and still allow a start at Windsor Castle. Yet 16 years later it would be established as the official Olympic marathon distance.

It marked the first time that a professional athlete participated in the Olympics, namely the Onondaga Indian from Canada, Thomas J. Longboat. He had acquired tremendous stature as a distance runner: first ever to average less than six minutes per mile for the circa 25-mile distance (by winning the Boston race in 1907), three-time winner of the J. J. Ward Marathon in Toronto (1906, 15 miles in 1:31:10.4; 1907, 18 miles in 1:41:40; 1908, 19¼ miles in 1:59:29), and winner of some less prestigious events. Canada considered him a great hope, and despite protests, especially by Americans, he was allowed to compete.

John J. Hayes was the key figure in the American contingent, composed of other notables such as Sidney Hatch and Robert Forshaw. Of the European runners, Dorando Pietri of Italy appeared very promising. He had dropped from the Athens marathon in 1906 with stomach cramps, but redeemed himself later that year by winning the Paris and Turin marathons. He was also the 1907 Italian 20 km champion.

There were 56 starters on still another hot Olympic day, and among them the very finest of runners from many countries. The initial pace was fast, set by the British, who later faded, allowing the others to move into the lead. Tom Longboat never finished the race, and the last miles were mainly a battle between Charles Hefferon of South Africa, Dorando Pietri, and John Hayes. Hefferon, weakening, allowed Pietri to pass in the closing minutes, but this is not to say that Pietri was in fine shape. Upon reaching the track, he staggered, went the wrong way, fell, was assisted to his feet and set in the right direction around the stadium, which he did without much dispatch. He was assisted across the finish line, in spite of rules to the contrary, at which point he promptly collapsed, was carried off, and was disqualified. Hayes finished second, but was declared the winner; Hefferon came in third, and Forshaw fourth.

The assistance given to Pietri was primarily by Jack Andrew, the Honorary General Secretary of the Polytechnic Harriers. He reported, in the August, 1908 issue of *The Polytechnic Magazine*: [19] "As regard the actual finish, most of the reports of same are absolutely erroneous regards my assisting the winner —the doctor's instructions were emphatic, carrying them out caused disqualification; as the animated photographs show, I only caught Dorando as he was falling at the tape. What I did then I would do again under similar circumstances."

Sympathy aroused by the British for Pietri's efforts resulted, upon prompting by Sir Arthur Conan Doyle, in Queen Alexandra presenting him with a gold cup which was an exact replica of that awarded Hayes. The Americans, happy with their victorious first, third, and fourth places, strongly encouraged Hayes to go professional and sought to stage a rematch in New York. Longboat, anxious to restore his reputation, also became a target of the race promoters, and an entirely new era of marathon running had dawned.

In a 6-month period from November 1908 through April 1909, no fewer than eight professional marathons at the London Olympic distance were staged in the United States. They were primarily duels between two competitors, with Pietri involved in five of them, the first between him and Hayes in a rematch on November 25, 1908, designed, in Pietri's opinion, to show the world who indeed was the best. The race was extremely close, with Pietri winning by about 80 yards. Pietri's time was 2:44:20.4; Hayes followed with 2:45:05.2. The details of the race, as with most of the professional races, will scarcely be imaginable to current marathon runners. To run more than 260 laps on the indoor track in Madison Square Garden, amidst half-crazed spectators, most with great national pride, for stakes in the thousands of dollars is without equal in the annals of the event. *The New York Times* describes the flavor of this first Olympic rematch: [20]

"Long before the doors were opened for general admission, street hawkers with American and Italian flags were on hand ready for business, and the side streets were clogged. When the doors were opened the galleries filled swiftly, and until long after the time set for the spectators who occupied the choicer and more expensive seats, crowds flowed in steadily, at prices that varied from $1 for standing room in the galleries to $10 for arena box seats . . .

"The rivals took their places on the mark, with Hayes, who had won the toss for position, on the inside. . . . Dorando had a lead of two feet and the rail when they finished the first thirty-three yards at the chalk line marking the beginning and ending of the regular laps. Hayes dropped in just behind him, running in about the Italian's tracks, and then the earlier stages of the race settled down to the monotony of long-distance plugging. . . .

"Flags waved and partisans cheered until the big amphitheater trembled with sound, and through it all the rival runners plodded around the ten-laps-to-the-mile track, and inhaled the dust and tobacco smoke with which the hall reeked. . . .

"Finishing the twenty-fifth mile, Dorando (as he was popularly called) led by about four feet, in the next lap by ten feet, in the next by fifteen, and at that rate he steadily drew further and further away. When they finished the twenty-sixth mile, Dorando crossed the lap end mark while Hayes was just turning at the bend from which they had started, thirty-three yards back up the straight run on the north side of the track. . . .

"Then a riot was all but precipitated by thoughtless holders of arena box seats, who in the mistaken idea that the race was ended hurried from their boxes and on to the track when the racers still had two more laps to run. The track officials tried to warn the trespassers back, but there was no time for them to be at all gentle, for fierce partisans of the runners already were swarming on the course, eager to clear the way for the finish of the race. . . .

"Blows were struck, and sharp encounters followed, but a lane was cleared and Dorando, the winner, was challenged for all sorts of races, under all sorts of conditions, but his brother, who was his spokesman, would not announce any determination for the near future. Dorando, he said, had achieved all that he wished in beating Hayes, for he felt that his triumph confirmed the claim that he would have won the Marathon race in England at the Olympic games but for the interference of the officials. . . ."

Unfortunately, Dorando's victory spurred him to schedule another event on December 15, again in the Garden, this time against Thomas Longboat. Anxious to redeem his dropout performance in London, Longboat was well-trained and ready. Although the two remained together almost the entire race, with

Dorando usually leading, just after the 25th mile, Dorando [21] "relinquished the lead to Longboat. The latter, amid tumultuous applause, lengthened his stride and began to draw further ahead. Dorando kept pluckily at his task for three laps, when the Indian showed his real speed and began to leave the Italian behind. It was a frantic futile struggle for Dorando. He swerved as his legs weakened and then staggered and finally fell to the track exhausted.

"There was a glassy stare in Dorando's eyes as his brother and a trainer rushed to the track to help him to his feet. He was urged to make another effort, but was unable to stand, and fell back helpless in his brother's arms. He was too far gone to speak, and in response to the repeated urging simply shook his head. As he was carried to his dressing room he fainted, and was unconscious for some time. . . .

"The receipts of the race were $15,000, of which the contestants each received 25 percent, or $3,750."

A rematch was scheduled, at Dorando's request, but probably too soon to allow either runner to adequately recover. On January 2, 1909, only 18 days later, in Buffalo, Longboat again was victorious. Dorando led almost the entire distance, but at 18 miles and 2 laps he quit.

Still Dorando yearned for victory, and ran yet another race, this time 20 days later, on January 22 in Chicago, against Albert Corey, the Frenchman who had been residing for some years in the United States. Corey's feet were in bad condition by the end of the race, and Dorando won handily in 2:56:00.4. Happily, he took a few months rest but continued to train for a Marathon Derby in April 1909, which would match the best of the professionals for a $10,000 first prize.

Longboat staged another event,[22] this time against the Englishman Alfred Shrubb, on February 5, 1909. Shrubb led through 24 miles, or 240 laps, at Madison Square Garden, and at one point was nearly a mile ahead of Longboat. Exhaustion caused him to crack, however, and he collapsed at 24½ miles. Longboat passed him and won in 2:53:40.4. This was Shrubb's first marathon, and it was clearly a case of too fast an initial pace. Longboat was unphased by an eight lap deficit at 17 miles, and in fact was booed and hissed by the spectators for not picking up the pace in an overt attempt to catch up.

Professionalism had stirred the masses into participation as well as spectating, and marathons began to occur literally everywhere. The most unusual location was doubtless on the warship *Wyoming*,[23] lying in San Francisco harbor during December and waiting to be re-christened the *Cheyenne* on New Year's Day. On Christmas Day, however, eleven sailors began a 42,195-meter marathon with the rather onerous task of completing 355 laps on a 130-yard track outlined on the deck of the ship. Only two finished, the winner being J. P. White.

Probably the greatest geographical concentration of races in the history of the event—including the present day—occurred in the New York City area during the 4-month period beginning November 25, 1908—four professional races and five amateur events. In Yonkers, New York, on November 26, 1908, almost 150 starters left the Empire City track on a 26-mile loop through the city.[24] Five thousand people assembled in the stands at the start, but 20,000 were screaming wildly at the finish for their favorite, Samuel Mellor, Jr., 1902 Boston Champion. He finished second, however, the winner being Irish-American James Crowley, in a time of 2:49:16.4. The course was so foggy that at times the runners and officials on the track were invisible from the stands. Problems with the management in underestimating the size of the turnout caused the race to be declared over after only 20 finish times were recorded. One runner, Matthew Maloney, collapsed on the track.

Maloney recovered however, and on December 26, one month to the day, he led an unprecedented pack of 272 runners to a new record for 42,195 meters.[25] *The New York Evening Journal* sponsored the race, and Maloney ran from Rye to Columbus Circle in 2:36:26.2, averaging 5:58 per mile.

Subsequently, Maloney turned professional and staged a race at the 69th Regiment National Guard Armory on March 5, 1909, against the Irish professional champion Patrick White.[26] The crowds were rather thin for this match, evidence that the professional marathon craze was losing strength. The purse was large, however, $1,500 for the winner, $500 for the loser, and it was no small event for the contestants. White initiated a very fast pace, but, as usual, it was the slower, steadier pace that proved more effective. White quit at 19 miles 2½ laps, and Maloney finished strong at 2:57:23. It was his third victory in as many starts, since he had also won an amateur open race on the Madison Square Garden track on January 8 with a time of 2:54:45.4 over the Olympic distance.

The climax to the professional marathoning era came on April 3, 1909, in the New York Polo Grounds. Dorando, Hayes, Maloney, Shrubb, and Longboat appeared together for the first time in an outdoor track race. The race was called the Marathon Derby. A 5-lap-per-mile course was plotted on the grass and clay of the baseball field, and 25,000 spectators contributed to the winning purse. Heavy downpours the night previous had soaked the course, and the race was run mostly in a continuing rain.

The sentimental favorite was Hayes, but the bookmakers, operating freely in the stands, favored Longboat at 8 to 5 odds, Shrubb at 2 to 1, Dorando 3 to 1, Hayes 5 to 1, and Maloney 7 to 1. A sixth runner, from France, a restaurant waiter named Henri St. Yves, also entered the race. Virtually unknown, this little man, barely 5 feet tall, was given 40 to 1 odds, and his name will be forever etched in the annals of the marathon. He won the Marathon Derby.

As reported by *The New York Times*: [27] "It was a remarkable display. St. Yves had won the Edinburgh Marathon, beating Pat White and other good runners, but this performance was not good enough to entitle him to the same consideration before the race as that accorded to Longboat, Dorando, Shrubb, and Hayes. The majority of the spectators laughed in derision as the French runner took up the lead in the early part of the race, setting a heart-breaking pace (5:14 for the first mile), but ridicule turned to surprise as he killed off Longboat and Shrubb in succession (at 21 and 25 miles), and at the same time raced the three other contestants into such a state that they were unable to cause him the slightest worry or anxiety for the first twenty miles. . . ."

St. Yves won the race in 2:40:50.6. Second was Dorando in 2:45:37, followed by Hayes in 2:49:27 and Maloney in 2:50:29. Never again was such a spectacle seen in the ranks of professional marathon footracing. An era came to a close, and the marathon began to reassume its more normal status as an amateur participant sport.

The Marathon Assumes Maturity

While America was enjoying its series of professional marathon track races, involving European as well as North American athletes, the event was developing in Europe as well, but more on an amateur basis. The Intermediary Games of 1906 had sparked enthusiasm among many nations, and marathons were springing up everywhere. The Finns staged two such races four and five months after the Athens Games. Kaarlo Nieminen won both,[28] and later finished eleventh in the London Olympic marathon. The next year, a young 17-year-old Finn named Hannes Kolehmainen ran his first marathon, and in the next few years he, his older brother Viljami, and countless others reveled in the European marathon craze. It was only natural that this interest should lead to national championship races, especially to pick contenders for Olympic participation. Eventually, in 1934, an all-European championship meet was held, which is still contested periodically.

One annual European marathon stood out above the others, however, in those early days, and that began in 1909 at London. The Polytechnic Harriers devised a new course, still at the London Olympic distance of 42,195 meters, and advertised the race all over Europe. The influential newspaper *Sporting Life* put up a huge and exquisite sterling silver perpetual trophy on which the winner's name would be engraved. This trophy survived for more than 50 years "to encourage long distance running in Great Britain." [19] The race attracted 68 entries from seven nations. One of the Harriers, Fred Barrett, won the race, and that would happen on only a few more occasions. Initially, the annual character of the race was altered by the death of King Edward VIII in 1910 and by World War I from 1915 through 1918. But thereafter the "Poly" continued in unbroken sequence for more than 65 years, and ranks as the second oldest annual marathon, the oldest at the now standard Olympic distance.

The Stockholm Olympic marathon in 1912 was a gem of organizational perfection, with its well-marked out-and-back route, fluid replacement stations all along the course, and careful control over ministrations to the runners. Knowledge had been spreading around the world not only how best to run the marathon, but also how to manage the race. This was evidenced here in faster times and more participants.

The 1916 Games were scheduled for Berlin, but because of the war, and a policy of the Games being in the first year of an Olympiad, they were cancelled. The 1920 Games were originally scheduled for Budapest, but since Hungary was one of the defeated countries, it was not invited to participate, and Antwerp became the revised venue. The Antwerp marathon was the longest in Olympic history, measured incorrectly 2550 meters in excess of the distance at Stockholm. Yet the first three finish times were all faster than in any previous Games—well under 6 minutes per mile in pace. The Finns clearly made their mark as a nation to be reckoned with in distance running skills, a tradition continued to the present day. Hannes Kolehmainen won the gold medal, and Finns also placed fifth, ninth, and tenth.

1924 was a remarkable year for the marathon. Olympic officials had standardized the event distance as 42,195 meters, run at only one previous Olympiad (London). The Finns won the Olympic marathon in Paris, placing first and fourth; Albin Stenroos brought home the gold medal and capped another magnificent set of distance running performances for his tiny nation.

Boston Athletic Association officials, attempting to comply with the now standard Olympic marathon distance, had adjusted their course in time for their April run, 3 months prior to the Paris Olympic Games. Unfortunately, remeasurement a few years later revealed a 161 meter deficit.[29] The situation was remedied, but the Boston marathon at the 42,195 meter distance dates only from 1927. Even then this distance was not continued without a break, since road improvements along the course caused another inadvertent shortening during the years 1953 through 1956.

At Paris, one of the marathon's most distinguished personalities captured the bronze medal—Boston's own Clarence DeMar. In 1911 he won the Boston Marathon, and a year later took twelfth at the Olympics in Stockholm (2:50:46.6). He continued to compete, and improve, was victorious at Boston again in 1922, 1923, and 1924, medaled in Paris, maintained a very keen competitive edge for the next 6 years, and won at Boston in 1927, 1928, and 1930. He also placed 27th at the 1928 Olympics in Amsterdam (2:50:42). He was an early subject of medical research at the Harvard Fatigue Laboratory, in 1926 and 1928. While not as fast as in earlier years, he was a superb physical specimen. His 1927 Boston victory culminated a string of five consecutive wins in less than a year's time. He was a willing subject, and his many hours on the treadmill and bicycle provided some of the first detailed insights into the physiologic adaptations of man to endurance exercise.[30-33] He ran in at least 100 marathon-distance races; his performances at the Boston Marathon alone spanned 44 years, his last at the age of 66. He died in 1958 of metastatic rectal carcinoma. Autopsy [34] revealed some coronary atherosclerosis; however, the enlarged diameter of these arteries precluded supposition of any impaired coronary flow.

For Czechoslovakia, the 1924 Games stimulated the beginning of the third oldest annual marathon footrace, the international event at Kosice. Due primarily to the efforts of Mr. Vojtech Braun-Bulovsky [35] at a meeting of the East Slovakian-Subcarpathian district of the Czechoslovak AAU on August 19, 1924, an experimental 30-km race was organized. It was such a success that a full marathon was planned for October 28, 1924 on the road from Turna nad Bodvou eastward to Kosice. All runners were from Czechoslovakia. The next year, Hungary sent participants, and won the race, on a course that left Kosice and returned via the villages of Cana and Haniska. In 1926, an out-and-back course from Kosice to Sena was devised, and has been utilized ever since except for 1952, when a southbound point-to-point course was routed from Presov to Kosice. For years, it was a contest primarily of continental Europeans. In 1931, however, the year prior to the Los Angeles Olympic Games, the Argentine Juan Carlos Zabala sharpened his skills at international competition and brought the Kosice marathon to the attention of the world by cutting almost nine minutes off the course record. A year later he was victorious in the Los Angeles Coliseum.

The Kosice marathon was not held for 8 years during World War II, and in 1945, although the race was revived, difficulties with transportation, finance, and organization prevented foreign nations from participating. Sweden honored the race that year and organized one of its own, called the Marathon Race of Czechoslovak Liberty. But beginning in the following year, the Swedes, led by Karl Gosta Leandersson, and the Finns, collectively dominated the victory stand at Kosice for the next decade, winning eight out of eleven races between 1946 and 1956. The race continues to increase in entrants, nations represented, and quality of performance.

The period of the 1930s, centering about the 1936 Olympic Games in Berlin, also saw a new addition to the growing spirit of marathoning all over the world. Orientals firmly asserted themselves by winning both the gold and bronze medals in those Games. Four years previously, Norio Suzuki gave a hint of Japanese marathon skill by being the first to go under 2:30:00 (at Kashiwazaki on May

8, 1932 he finished in 2:29:20). Now, in 1936, Kitei Son lowered that mark by another 0.8 seconds—an Olympic record to stand until the performance of Emil Zatopek in 1952.

Growing political problems on the European continent during the 1930s, precipitating World War II in 1939, halted many periodic regional marathon championships. The British Commonwealth Games had been held in 1930, 1934, and 1938, but were discontinued until 1950. The European Championships began in 1934, were held in 1938, and then were halted until 1946 at Oslo.

Annual events did not fare as badly. The Polytechnic Harriers marathon continued throughout the war years, with courses redesigned to avoid city streets. The devastation of war never reached the United States, hence Boston had little difficulty in continuing its race. In 1935, at Yonkers, New York, an annual marathon race began, which continues to the present day. From 1938 until the late 1960s it was the site of the AAU championships. A tough and hilly course, it began and ended at the Empire City race track, where the Yonkers marathon races of 1908 and 1909 had been staged. The exact route has changed five times, always remaining at the standard Olympic distance, and has attracted good competition. It has the distinction of the longest string of victories by a single competitor among any of the major world marathons. John J. Kelley began this amazing feat in 1956, and continued for eight years through 1963. All were run at a pace below 2 hours, 30 minutes, which in itself had never been accomplished on the Yonkers course before his appearance.

This was the same John Kelley (born in 1931, a "Connecticut Yankee" English teacher from Groton) who won the Pan American Games marathon in 1959, the Boston Marathon in 1957 (runner-up many times), and placed 21st in the 1956 Olympic Games (2:43:40) and 19th in the 1960 Games (2:24:58). But it was not the same John Kelley, born in 1908, who won the Boston Marathon in 1935 and 1945, was second at Boston seven times, placed 18th in the 1936 Olympic Games (2:49:32.4), and who in 1975 ran his 45th Boston marathon. That was John A. Kelley, Bostonian, unrelated to John J., but nevertheless a close friend.

Following World War II, activities of life began to normalize, and with it came not only resumption of established earlier marathon competitions but also a flurry of new events. An annual race began at Otsu, Japan, on the island of Honshu, in 1946. A year later, the Asahi Shimbun Publishing Company sponsored a race at Kumamoto, changing venues around Japan until 1966, when it was permanently located at Fukuoka. In that year the Japanese Amateur Athletic Federation officially recognized the Asahi race as the International Open Marathon Championship. All three major annual Japanese marathons (the third started at Beppu in 1952) have been highly competitive, with winning times close to the world's best each year.

In Europe, a marathon began in 1947 in Holland, an out-and-back trip between Enschede and Haaksbergen. Although a biennial event, it remains a very popular race, the second oldest continuing on the Continent.

In America a race, later called the Culver City marathon, began in 1948 as part of the Los Angeles Coliseum Relays. That year, an outstanding French Canadian runner, Gerard Cote, added an unusual victory here to his already long and impressive list (four-time Boston winner, in 1940, 1943, 1944, and 1948; two-time Yonkers winner, in 1940 and 1943). Arriving at the Coliseum from Long Beach earlier than expected, he encountered locked gates and a hurdle race still in progress on the track. Nevertheless, he managed to enter the stadium and skirt the hurdles, win the race, light a huge cigar, and to the dismay of the health fanatics among the 70,000 witnessing sports fans, puffed his way around the track in a victory lap.

For many years the Culver City event has been termed by local officials as the "Western Hemisphere Marathon and National Marathon Championships." Controversy has often occurred among runners as to the true meaning of this title. In fact, the marathon does not determine the Champion for the Western Hemisphere, since no Pan-American agreement has designated it as such. On two occasions it established the AAU Senior Men's National Champion, and it has often been an AAU District Men's Championship race. Nevertheless, it is well established, and the third oldest marathon continuing in America.

During the 1950s at least six marathon races began which continue today. Two were mentioned earlier: Beppu (1952) and Marathon-to-Athens (1955). The Pan-American Games began in 1951 as a quadrennial event during the final year of each Olympiad, and a marathon race is an integral part of these Games. In 1957 a marathon began in Hungary on an out-and-back course from Szeged to Ferencszallas. For six consecutive years (1965–1971) its winner was the well known Hungarian Gyula Toth. In the United States, the Cherry Tree marathon began in New York City in 1959 on a course along the Harlem River. It continued through 1970 at that site, then was moved during 1971 and 1972 to Central Park. In 1973 the course was again relocated, to Nassau County, and renamed the Earth Day marathon. Since then, it has attracted very large numbers of participants.

A difficult and unusual marathon began in 1956 and consisted of a climb of more than 7700 feet virtually to the summit of Pike's Peak in Colorado. Although slightly longer than the standard distance, and run on a mountainous trail instead of paved surface, it has been a popular event for Americans to conquer—590 round trips have been recorded during its 21-year history. The idea of running up the peak actually dates to June 28, 1936 when a 13 mile footrace to the summit was staged, and won by Lou Wille in 3:24:35.

The 1950s saw the 2:20 barrier finally collapse. On June 13, 1953 Jim Peters finished the "Poly" at Windsor in 2:18:40.2. The barrier was broken twice more that year and once the next, but it was strictly a one-man show, for it was Peters on each occasion (2:19:22 at Enschede Sept. 12, 1953; 2:18:34.8 three weeks later at Turku Oct. 4, 1953; and 2:17:39.4 again at Windsor June 26, 1954). During 1955 no performance was under 2 hr, 20 min. However, in 1956 four different runners did it—all Finns and all in the same race, at Piek-samaki on Aug. 12 (Paavo Kotila, 2:18:04.8; Eino Oksanen, 2:18:51; Veikko Karvonen, 2:18:56.4; and Eino Pulkkinen, 2:19:27). During the last three years of the 1950s, the 2:20 mark was bettered only five more times—once in 1957, and twice each in 1958 and 1959.

In 1960, due principally to the Rome Olympic marathon, twelve sub-2:20 performances were recorded (five at the Rome race). Just as the 1930s marked the entry of Orientals into the forefront of marathoning, so the 1960s saw Africans begin to excel. Abebe Bikila of Ethiopia won the gold medal, and 25 seconds behind came Rhadi ben Abdesselem of Morocco in a now famous evening spectacle at Rome. Bikila in particular had a superb marathon career during the next several years, and became the only man to win an Olympic gold medal twice for the marathon when he was victorious in 1964 at Tokyo.

The decades of the 1960s saw tremendous global increase in interest in marathon running. More than three dozen races started in America alone. As a result, the number of top-level performances increased, and the world best time at the end of each year steadily improved (TABLE 1). Only bona fide 42,195-meter course distances were considered in compiling these data.

Two quite noteworthy facts are not evident in this tabulation. First, America, with its great upsurge in numbers of races, lagged behind in quality of performances. It was not until 1962 that an American ran below the 2:20 mark. Even then it was one lone runner, Leonard Edelen, once in 1962, twice in 1963, once in 1964, and once in 1965. Norman Higgins joined Edelen at the top level in 1965. Second, Japan became a truly dominating powerhouse for excellent performances. Their first such 2:20 performance was not until 1961 (only one) but they had 7 in 1962, 10 in 1963, 23 in 1964, 27 in 1965, and continued onward in similar fashion. The only nation approaching Japan with fast performances was perennially excellent Great Britain.

TABLE 1

IMPROVEMENT IN TOP-LEVEL MARATHON FINISH TIMES: 1960–1970

Year	Number of Sub- 2:20 Per- formances	World Best Time by Each Year's End	Time Set by	Date	Site
1960	12	2:15:16.2	Abebe Bikila	Sept. 10, 1960	Rome
1961	3	—	—	—	—
1962	11	—	—	—	—
1963	22	2:14:28	Leonard Edelen	June 15, 1963	Windsor
1964	47	2:12:11.2	Abebe Bikila	Oct. 21, 1964	Tokyo
1965	44	2:12:00	Morio Shigematsu	June 12, 1965	Windsor
1966	70	—	—	—	—
1967	58	2:09:36.4	Derek Clayton	Dec. 3, 1967	Fukuoka
1968	93	—	—	—	—
1969	82	2:08:33.6	Derek Clayton	May 30, 1969	Antwerp
1970	103	—	—	—	—

The period of the 1970s shows no apparent diminution of desire for people to run marathons. In fact the situation is the opposite—there is almost an epidemic of interest among almost all nations, age groups, and for both sexes. Age group records in America alone now extend from 5 to 84 for men, and from 5 to 61 for women.[36] TABLE 2 depicts this growth from several points of view: number of marathon races held in America, number of sub-3-hour marathon performances in America, 100th best world and American finish times, and 100th best all-time world and American finish times each year from 1969 through 1975. It is evident that both quality and quantity are on the increase.

An Olympic Games year often brings with it a surge of quality performances as athletes peak for this classic event. For the marathon, each Olympic event is in a real sense a homecoming, and the buildup to the 21st Olympiad Games in Montreal proved no exception. Runners at Fukuoka in December 1975

TABLE 2

GROWTH IN QUALITY AND QUANTITY OF MARATHON PARTICIPATION: 1969–1975

Year	Marathons Run in America *	American Performances Under 3 hr.*	100th Best Performance		100th Best All-Time Performance		Total World Sub-2:20 Performances †
			American *	World †	American *	World †	
1969	44	NA	2:36:17.0	NA ‡	NA	2:16:07.8	82
1970	73	812	2:34:39	2:20:11	2:25:14	2:15:31.2	103
1971	102	1120	2:29:08.6	2:19:14	2:23:46	2:15:15.8	142
1972	124	1428	2:27:11.8	2:18:18.4	2:22:46	2:14:47.8	173
1973	127	1721	2:29:53	2:19:42	2:22:00	2:14:28	161
1974	135	2450	2:27:12	2:18:11	2:20:21	2:13:59	214
1975	148	3005	2:24:22	2:17:45	NA	2:13:40	271

* Source: *Runner's World* Marathon Handbooks: 1970–1976. Mountain View, Calif.
† Compiled by Roger Gynn.
‡ NA, not available with accuracy.

delivered 29 sub-2:20 finish times to the officials. At the American Olympic Trials in May 1976, 69 runners started, all with sub-2:23 performances within the preceding year. Only three could qualify for the team, and 13 sub-2:20 times resulted in the ensuing battle for those berths. And then at Montreal, 25 additional sub-2:20 marks were added to the list, as a crowd of uncountable millions observed through television around the world. When it was over, the irony of the marathon was only too evident. Frank Shorter, in his bid to match Bikila's double gold medal record, took second place to a rising newcomer. And for who knows how long, the best performances in the two oldest continuous marathon races are now identical to the second—2:09:55.

Statistics from Significant Marathon Races

Among all track and field events, the marathon provides a double challenge to the statistician and others concerned with recording and evaluating the quality of performances. The first centers on course distance. Only since the Paris Olympics in 1924 has any internationally recognized standard marathon distance been established, namely, the dictionary-defined value of 26 miles, 385 yards (42,195 meters). Prior to that time, the distance usually ranged from about 24 to 27 miles. The 1908 London Olympic Marathon, however, the first at 42,195 meters, spawned a number of pre-1924 races at the now standard distance. The majority of marathon contests after 1924 have attempted to adhere to the Olympic standard, but there are exceptions for several reasons. Some courses were erroneously measured (Boston, 1924 through 1926, 1953 through 1956), others varied as a result of unplanned circumstances (Polytechnic, 1972), and still others elect to continue at a non-Olympic distance (Pikes Peak). For purposes of listings of performances, the 42,195 meter distance is considered standard, and no extrapolations are made for performances on longer or shorter courses.

The second challenge concerns accurate measurement of the course distance. No uniform set of measuring standards has been adopted at the international level. Many methods of measurement are employed by various authorities. The calibrated wheel (usually of bicycle-size) seems to be the method of choice in England, Canada, and the United States. The Kosice course has also been measured this way.

In recent years the Olympic Games, European Championships, and Commonwealth Games marathon courses have been wheel-measured. Japan has measured its courses using a 100-meter bamboo rule. However, once the measuring instrument has been determined, then the manner in which the course is measured on the specific selected route is important. Only recently has the Olympic Games marathon route been painted as a line 42,195 meters long on the road surface. In England, the Amateur Athletic Association rules demand measurement on the road one meter away from the left hand edge in the running direction. In the United States, the national AAU Committee on Standards has detailed written guidelines for "certification" of a marathon course as being the Olympic distance. Implicit among all of these measuring techniques is integrity of and meticulous care by the measuring personnel to ensure that whatever standard is used is employed with intent to measure fairly a course of exactly 42,195 meters. Provided that some form of official documentation is available to this effect, then the statistician has little recourse but to accept the course as *bona fide,* i.e., made with good faith and earnest intent. Recognized world lists have been prepared with these considerations in mind.[36, 37, 39]

Marathon times are affected considerably by environmental conditions. Shorter races are certainly not immune to these vicissitudes, but the long distance covered by marathon runners compounds the effects on performance. Weather is quite important, particularly temperature, humidity, and wind direction and velocity. Many marathons are run in cities having sizeable temperature extremes on any given day, making comparison of annual performances over a given course somewhat meaningless unless this information is available. It is in part for these reasons that a "world record" time has never been considered an appropriate label for the world fastest finish time.

Probably no two marathon courses are comparable in layout, in extreme contrast to regulation tracks, which now vary essentially only by the brand of artificial surface. Some courses have considerably more downhill than uphill terrain (Boston), others are essentially all uphill (Boone to Grandfather Mountain, N.C., rises gradually from 3266 to 4279 feet), and others are flat (Crowley, La.). One has an unpaved surface (Karl Marx Stadt, East Germany). Some are well above sea level and have performances significantly affected by altitude (Big Mountain to Salt Lake City, Utah, ranges from 4333 to 7500 feet; Manitou Springs to Pikes Peak, Colorado, and return involves a vertical climb of 7774 feet).

Nevertheless, without statistics on performances, there would be no basis for any objective assessment of their quality. Certain lay publications report annually the results of marathon races in North America;[36] some international coverage is provided in annual world lists.[36, 37] Results of major races prior to the most recent surge of interest in marathon running are difficult to acquire, often incomplete, and commonly fraught with errors. Some sources[36, 38] have elected to alter official finish times rounding tenths of seconds upward to the nearest second. It is the authors' opinion that such activity only adds to already existing confusion, and is most certainly not the prerogative of the statistician or the historian. Times officially recorded should remain as given; individual race directors should have the decision as to whether finish times will have accuracy recorded to tenths of seconds, unless internationally acceptable policy dictates otherwise. Since a world record is not currently recognized in the marathon, international rulings are not as well established concerning record-keeping as for the shorter distance events.

The statistics presented here (TABLES 3–17) were carefully researched for their accuracy, and are the first such compilation in scientific literature. No more comprehensive international coverage has appeared since the outdated summary by Gynn in 1972.[39] Exact dates, race sites, the winner, his nationality, and his finish time are provided for significant established races. Other information appears as available and appropriate, e.g., top three finishers for some major events, number of finishers, average pace per mile where the race had several different course distances, and annotations on course changes. Unique among marathon data is the profile of starters at the Kosice marathon, obtained from their race history[35] and official finish records.

Abbreviations for nationalities of all finishers conform to the system already used by Potts,[37] with certain exceptions of geopolitical origin (e.g., SOA refers to the Union of South Africa, which existed during the 1908 and 1912 Olympic Games; RSA refers to the present Republic of South Africa in the Potts system. Germany was a single nation in 1929 when Hans Hempel won at Kosice, hence

TABLE 3

OLYMPIC GAMES MARATHON

Date/Site	1st 3 Finishers	Nat.	Time	Pace	Distance (meters)	Finishers
Apr 10, 1896 Athens	Spiridon Louis	GRE	2:58:50	7:11.8	40,000	9
	Haralambos Vasilacos	GRE	3:06:03	7:29.2		
	Gyula Kellner	HUN	3:09:35	7:37.2		
Jul 19, 1900 Paris	Michael Theato	FRA	2:59:45	7:11.1	40,260	8
	Emile Champion	FRA	3:04:17	7:21.9		
	Ernst Fast	SWE	3:37:14	8:40.9		
Aug 30, 1904 St. Louis	Thomas Hicks	USA	3:28:53	8:24.3	40,000	14
	Albert Corey	USA	3:34:52	8:38.8		
	Arthur Newton	USA	3:47:33	9:09.4		
Jul 24, 1908 London	John Hayes	USA	2:55:18.4	6:41.2	42,195	27
	Charles Hefferon	SOA	2:56:06	6:43.0		
	Joseph Forshaw	USA	2:57:10.4	6:45.4		
Jul 14, 1912 Stockholm	Kenneth McArthur	SOA	2:36:54.8	6:16.9	40,200	34
	Christopher Gitsam	SOA	2:37:52	6:19.2		
	Gaston Strobino	USA	2:38:42.4	6:21.2		
Aug 22, 1920 Antwerp	Hannes Kolehmainen	FIN	2:32:35.8	5:44.7	42,750	33
	Yuriy Lossman	EST	2:32:48.6	5:45.2		
	Valerio Arri	ITA	2:36:32.8	5:53.6		
Jul 13, 1924 Paris	Albin Stenroos	FIN	2:41:22.6	6:09.3	42,195	30
	Romeo Bertini	ITA	2:47:19.6	6:22.9		
	Clarence DeMar	USA	2:48:14	6:25		
Aug 5, 1928 Amsterdam	Ahmed El Oufai	FRA	2:32:57	5:50	42,195	57
	Manuel Plaza	CHI	2:33:23	5:51.0		
	Martti Marttelin	FIN	2:35:02	5:54.8		
Aug 7, 1932 Los Angeles	Juan Carlos Zabala	ARG	2:31:36	5:46.9	42,195	20
	Sam Ferris	GBR	2:31:55	5:47.6		
	Armas Toivonen	FIN	2:32:12	5:48.3		
Aug 9, 1936 Berlin	Kitei Son	JAP	2:29:19.2	5:41.7	42,195	42
	Ernest Harper	GBR	2:31:23.2	5:46.4		
	Shoryu Nan	JAP	2:31:42	5:47.4		
Aug 7, 1948 London	Delfo Cabrera	ARG	2:34:51.6	5:54.4	42,195	30
	Tom Richards	GBR	2:35:07.6	5:55.0		
	Etienne Gailly	BEL	2:35:33.6	5:56.0		
Jul 27, 1952 Helsinki	Emil Zatopek	CSA	2:23:03.2	5:27.4	42,195	53
	Reinaldo Gorno	ARG	2:25:35	5:33.1		
	Gustaf Jansson	SWE	2:26:07	5:34.4		
Dec 1, 1956 Melbourne	Alain Mimoun	FRA	2:25:00	5:31.8	42,195	33
	Franjo Mihalic	YUG	2:26:32	5:35.3		
	Veikko Karvonen	FIN	2:27:47	5:38.2		
Sept 10, 1960 Rome	Abebe Bikila	ETH	2:15:16.2	5:09.5	42,195	62
	Rhadi Ben Abdesselem	MOR	2:15:41.6	5:10.5		
	Barry Magee	NZL	2:17:18.2	5:14.2		
Oct 21, 1964 Tokyo	Abebe Bikila	ETH	2:12:11.2	5:02.7	42,195	58
	Basil Healey	GBR	2:16:19.2	5:11.9		
	Kokichi Tsuburaya	JAP	2:16:22.8	5:12.1		
Oct 20, 1968 Mexico City	Mamo Wolde	ETH	2:20:26.4	5:21.4	42,195	57
	Kenji Kimihara	JAP	2:23:31	5:28.4		
	Mike Ryan	NZL	2:23:45	5:28.9		
Sep 10, 1972 Munich	Frank Shorter	USA	2:12:19.8	5:02.8	42,195	62
	Karel Lismont	BEL	2:14:31.8	5:07.8		
	Mamo Wolde	ETH	2:15:08.4	5:09.2		
Jul 31, 1976 Montreal	Waldemar Cierpinski	GDR	2:09:55	4:57.3	42,195	60
	Frank Shorter	USA	2:10:45.8	4:59.2		
	Karel Lismont	BEL	2:11:12.6	5:00.3		

TABLE 4

THE BOSTON MARATHON *

Date †	Winner	State or Country	Time	Distance (meters)	Pace (min/mile)
1897	John J. McDermott	NY	2:55:10	39,751	7:05.5
1898	Ronald J. McDonald	MA	2:42:00	39,751	6:33.5
1899	Lawrence J. Brignolia	MA	2:54:38	39,751	7:04.2
1900	James J. Caffrey	CAN-ONT	2:39:44.4	39,751	6:28.0
1901	James J. Caffrey	CAN-ONT	2:29:23.6	39,751	6:02.9
1902	Samuel A. Mellor, Jr.	NY	2:43:12	39,751	6:36.4
1903	John C. Lorden	MA	2:41:29.8	39,751	6:32.3
1904	Michael Spring	NY	2:38:04.4	39,751	6:24
1905	Fred Lorz	NY	2:38:25.4	39,751	6:24.8
1906	Timothy Ford	MA	2:45:45	39,751	6:42.6
1907	Thomas Longboat	CAN-ONT	2:24:24	39,751	5:50.8
1908 §	Thomas P. Morrissey	NY	2:25:43.2	39,751	5:54
1909	Henri Renaud	NH	2:53:36.8	39,751	7:01.7
1910	Fred L. Cameron	CAN-NS	2:28:52.4	39,751	6:01.6
1911	Clarence H. DeMar	MA	2:21:39.6	39,751	5:44.0
1912	Michael Ryan	NY	2:21:18.2	39,751	5:43.2
1913	Fritz Carlson	MN	2:25:14.8	39,751	5:52.7
1914 §	James Duffy	CAN-ONT	2:25:01.2	39,751	5:52.2
1915	Edouard Fabre	CAN-QUE	2:31:41.2	39,751	6:08.4
1916	Arthur V. Roth	MA	2:27:16.4	39,751	5:57.7
1917	Bill Kennedy	NY	2:28:37.2	39,751	6:01.0
1919	Carl W. A. Linder	MA	2:29:13.4	39,751	6:02.4
1920	Peter Trivoulidas	NY	2:29:31	39,751	6:03.1
1921	Frank Zuna	NJ	2:18:57.6	39,751	5:37.5
1922	Clarence H. DeMar	MA	2:18:10	39,751	5:35.6
1923	Clarence H. DeMar	MA	2:23:37.4	39,751	5:48.8
1924	Clarence H. DeMar	MA	2:29:40.2	42,034	5:44.0
1925	Charles L. Mellor	IL	2:33:00.6	42,034	5:51.7
1926	John C. Miles	CAN-NS	2:25:40.4	42,034	5:34.8
1927	Clarence H. DeMar	MA	2:40:22.2	42,195	6:07.2
1928	Clarence H. DeMar	MA	2:37:07.8	42,195	5:59.8
1929	John C. Miles	CAN-ONT	2:33:08.6	42,195	5:50.6
1930	Clarence H. DeMar	MA	2:34:48.2	42,195	5:54.5
1931 §	James P. Henigan	MA	2:46:45.8	42,195	6:21.8
1932	Paul de Bruyn	GER	2:33:36.4	42,195	5:51.7
1933	Leslie S. Pawson	RI	2:31:01.6	42,195	5:45.8
1934	Dave Komonen	CAN-ONT	2:32:53.8	42,195	5:50.1
1935	John A. Kelley	MA	2:32:07.4	42,195	5:48.3
1936	Ellison M. Brown	RI	2:33:40.8	42,195	5:51.9
1937	Walter Young	CAN-QUE	2:33:20	42,195	5:51.1
1938	Leslie S. Pawson	RI	2:35:34.8	42,195	5:56.2
1939	Ellison M. Brown	RI	2:28:51.8	42,195	5:40.8
1940	Gerard Cote	CAN-QUE	2:38:28.6	42,195	6:02.9
1941	Leslie S. Pawson	RI	2:30:38	42,195	5:44.9
1942	Bernard J. Smith	MA	2:26:51.2	42,195	5:36.2
1943 ‡	Gerard Cote	CAN-QUE	2:28:25	42,195	5:39.8
1944	Gerard Cote	CAN-QUE	2:31:50.4	42,195	5:47.7
1945	Jonn A. Kelley	MA	2:30:40.2	42,195	5:45.0
1946 §	Stylianos Kyriakides	GRE	2:29:27	42,195	5:42.2
1947	Yun Bok Suh	KOR	2:25:39	42,195	5:33.5
1948	Gerard Cote	CAN-QUE	2:31:02	42,195	5:45.8
1949	Karl G. Leandersson	SWE	2:31:50.8	42,195	5:47.7
1950	Kee Yong Ham	KOR	2:32:39	42,195	5:49.5
1951	Shigeki Tanaka	JAP	2:27:45	42,195	5:38.3
1952	Doroteo Flores	GUA	2:31:53	42,195	5:47.8
1953 §	Keizo Yamada	JAP	2:18:51	41,091	5:26.1
1954	Veikko Karvonen	FIN	2:20:39	41,091	5:30.9
1955	Hideo Hamamura	JAP	2:18:22	41,091	5:25.5
1956	Antti Viskari	FIN	2:14:14	41,091	5:15.8
1957 §	John J. Kelley	CT	2:20:05	42,195	5:20.8
1958	Franjo Mihalic	YUG	2:25:54	42,195	5:34.1
1959 §	Eino Oksanen	FIN	2:22:42	42,195	5:26.7
1960	Paavo Kotila	FIN	2:20:54	42,195	5:22.6
1961	Eino Oksanen	FIN	2:23:39	42,195	5:28.9
1962	Eino Oksanen	FIN	2:23:48	42,195	5:29.3

TABLE 4 (Continued)

Date †	Winner	State or Country	Time	Distance (meters)	Pace (min/mile)
1963	Aurele Vandendriessche	BEL	2:18:58	42,195	5:18.2
1964 §	Aurele Vandendriessche	BEL	2:19:59	42,195	5:20.5
1965	Morio Shigematsu	JAP	2:16:33	42,195	5:12.7
1966	Kenji Kimihara	JAP	2:17:11	42,195	5:14.1
1967	David McKenzie	NZL	2:15:45	42,195	5:10.8
1968	Ambrose Burfoot	CT	2:22:17	42,195	5:25.8
1969 ¶	Yoshiaki Unetani	JAP	2:13:49	42,195	5:06.4
1970 §	Ron Hill	GBR	2:10:30	42,195	4:58.8
1971	Alvaro Mejia	COL	2:18:45	42,195	5:17.7
1972 **	Olavi Suomalainen	FIN	2:15:39	42,195	5:10.6
1973 ††	Jon Anderson	OR	2:16:03	42,195	5:11.5
1974 ‡‡	Neil Cusack	EIR	2:13:39	42,195	5:06.0
1975 ¶	William Rodgers	MA	2:09:55	42,195	4:57.5
1976	Jack Fultz	DC	2:20:19	42,195	5:21.3
1977 ‡	Jerome Drayton	CAN-ONT	2:14:46	42,195	5:08.4

* Course has had three finish sites: 1897, Irvington St. Oval; 1898–1965, B. A. A. Clubhouse, Exeter St.; 1965 to present, Prudential Center. Several starting points have been used: 1897, Metcalfe's Mill, Ashland; 1898–1907, railroad bridge in Ashland; 1907–1924, Stevens Corner on Hopkinton Road; 1924–1965, various points closer to Hopkinton to accommodate for road shortenings; 1965 to present, Hopkinton town green.

† Event occurred on April 19 of each year except where noted by footnotes.

‡ April 18.

§ April 20.

¶ April 21.

** April 17.

†† April 16.

‡‡ April 15.

TABLE 5

POLYTECHNIC HARRIERS' MARATHON

Date	Winner	Nat.	Time	Course *
May 26, 1909	Fred Barrett	ENG	2:42:31	A
May 27, 1911	Henry Green	ENG	2:46:39	
May 18, 1912	Jim Corkery	CAN	2:36:55.4	
May 31, 1913	Alex Ahlgren	SWE	2:36:06.6	
Jun 20, 1914	Ahmed Djebella	FRA	2:46:30.8	
Jun 21, 1919	E. Woolston	ENG	2:52:30	
Jul 17, 1920	Bobby Mills	ENG	2:37:40.4	
Jul 16, 1921	Bobby Mills	ENG	2:51:41	
Jun 10, 1922	Bobby Mills	ENG	2:47:30.4	
Jun 16, 1923	Axel Jensen	DEN	2:40:46.8	
May 31, 1924	Duncan McL. Wright	SCO	2:53:17.4	
May 30, 1925	Sam Ferris	ENG	2:35:58.2	
May 29, 1926	Sam Ferris	ENG	2:42:24.2	
May 28, 1927	Sam Ferris	ENG	2:40:32	
May 26, 1928	Sam Ferris	ENG	2:41:02.2	
May 18, 1929	Sam Ferris	ENG	2:40:47.4	
May 31, 1930	S. Smith	ENG	2:42:24	
May 30, 1931	Sam Ferris	ENG	2:41:55	
May 28, 1932	Sam Ferris	ENG	2:35:31	
Jul 7, 1933	Sam Ferris	ENG	2:36:32.4	
Jun 2, 1934	Duncan McL. Wright	SCO	2:56:30	B
May 25, 1935	Bert Norris	ENG	2:48:37.8	
Jun 13, 1936	Bert Norris	ENG	2:35:20	
May 29, 1937	Bert Norris	ENG	2:48:40	
Jun 18, 1938	Henry Palme	SWE	2:42:00	C
Jun 17, 1939	Henry Palme	SWE	2:36:56	
Jun 15, 1940	Les Griffiths	ENG	2:43:41.6	D
Jun 21, 1941	G. Humphreys	ENG	3:12:00	E
Jun 20, 1942	Les Griffiths	ENG	2:48:45	
Jun 19, 1943	Les Griffiths	ENG	2:53:14	
Jun 17, 1944	Tom Richards	ENG	2:48:45	
Jun 16, 1945	Tom Richards	ENG	2:56:39	
Jun 15, 1946	Horace Oliver	ENG	2:38:12	F
Jun 14, 1947	Cecil Ballard	ENG	2:36:52.4	
Jun 19, 1948	Jack Holden	ENG	2:36:44.6	
Jun 18, 1949	Jack Holden	ENG	2:42:52	
Jun 17, 1950	Jack Holden	ENG	2:33:07	
Jun 16, 1951	Jim Peters	ENG	2:29:28	
Jun 14, 1952	Jim Peters	ENG	2:20:42.2	
Jun 13, 1953	Jim Peters	ENG	2:18:40.2	
Jun 26, 1954	Jim Peters	ENG	2:17:39.4	
Jun 18, 1955	Bob McKinnis	ENG	2:36:23	
Jun 6, 1956	Ron Clarke	ENG	2:20:15.8	
Jun 15, 1957	Eddie Kirkup	ENG	2:27:04.4	
Jun 28, 1958	Colin Kemball	ENG	2:22:27.4	
Jun 13, 1959	Dennis O'Gorman	ENG	2:25:11.2	
Jun 11, 1960	Arthur Keily	ENG	2:19:06	
Jun 10, 1961	Peter Wilkinson	ENG	2:20:25	
Jun 16, 1962	Ron Hill	ENG	2:20:59	
Jun 15, 1963	Leonard Edelen	USA	2:14:26	
Jun 13, 1964	Basil Heatley	ENG	2:13:55	
Jun 12, 1965	Morio Shigematsu	JAP	2:12:00	
Jun 11, 1966	Graham Taylor	ENG	2:19:04	
Jun 10, 1967	Fergus Murray	ENG	2:19:06	
Jun 15, 1968	Kenji Kimihara	JAP	2:15:15	
Jun 14, 1969	Phil Hampton	ENG	2:25:22	
Jun 13, 1970	Don Faircloth	ENG	2:18:15	
Jun 26, 1971	Phil Hampton	ENG	2:18:31	
Jul 1, 1972	Don Faircloth	ENG	2:31:52	
Aug 18, 1973	Bob Sercombe	ENG	2:19:48	G
Jun 15, 1974	Akio Usami	JAP	2:15:16	H
Sep 11, 1976	Bernie Plain	GBR	2:15:43	I
Jun 11, 1977	Ian Thompson	GBR	2:14:32	J

Courses *

* Courses: A, Windsor to Stamford Bridge, 42,195 m; B, Windsor to White City, 42,195 m; C, Windsor to Chiswick, 42,195 m; D, Windsor to Great Park, 42,195 m; E, Chiswick, 42,195 m; F, Windsor to Chiswick, 42,195 m; G, Course length erroneously 29 miles due to lead jeep going off the official course. H, Windsor, on local roads, course slightly less than 42,195 m; I, Windsor, on local roads, 42,195 m; J, Windsor Great Park, and local roads in Windsor. Race not held in 1975.

TABLE 6

KOSICE MARATHON

Date	Winner	Nat.	Time	Fin-ishers	Profile of Starters			
					Local	Foreign	Total	Nations
Oct. 28, 1924	Karoly Halla	CSR	3:01:35	7	8	0	8	1
Oct. 28, 1925	Pat Kiraly	HUN	2:41:55	11	15	5	20	2
Oct. 28, 1926	Hans Hempel	GER	2:57:02	24	30	6	36	4
Oct. 28, 1927	Jozsef Galambos	HUN	2:48:25.2	43	41	9	50	5
Oct. 28, 1928	Jozsef Galambos	HUN	2:55:45	22	32	8	40	4
Oct. 28, 1929	Hans Hempel	GER	2:51:31	30	32	6	38	4
Oct. 28, 1930	Istvan Zelenka	HUN	2:50:58.2	26	32	6	38	4
Oct. 28, 1931	Juan Carlos Zabala	ARG	2:33:19	27	27	9	36	4
Oct. 28, 1932	Jozsef Galambos	HUN	2:43:14.4	42	32	15	47	4
Oct. 28, 1933	Jozsef Galambos	HUN	2:37:53.2	31	24	9	33	3
Oct. 28, 1934	Josef Sulc	CSR	2:41:26.4	24	17	11	28	6
Oct. 28, 1935	Arturs Montmillers	LIT	2:44:57.2	26	14	21	35	6
Oct. 28, 1936	Gyorgy Balaban	AUT	2:41:08	30	25	17	42	6
Oct. 28, 1937	Desire Leriche	FRA	2:43:41.8	36	19	22	41	8
Oct. 28, 1945	Antonin Spiroch	CSR	2:47:21.8	29	36	0	36	1
Oct. 28, 1946	Mikko Hietanen	FIN	2:35:02.4	74	82	14	96	8
Oct. 28, 1947	Charles Heirendt	LUX	2:36:06	74	78	19	97	13
Oct. 28, 1948	Karl G. Leandersson	SWE	2:34:46.4	87	77	20	97	13
Oct. 23, 1949	Matti Urpalainen	FIN	2:33:45.6	77	66	30	91	10
Oct. 29, 1950	Karl G. Leandersson	SWE	2:31:20.2	91	78	25	103	10
Oct. 28, 1951	Jaroslav Strupp	CSA	2:41:07.8	69	75	0	75	1
Oct. 5, 1952	Erkki Puolakka	FIN	2:29:10	64	50	16	66	5
Oct. 18, 1953	Walter Bednar	CSA	2:53:32.8	41	62	0	62	1
Oct. 10, 1954	Erkki Puolakka	FIN	2:27:21	70	65	13	78	7
Oct. 16, 1955	Evert Nyberg	SWE	2:25:40	73	60	23	83	9
Oct. 7, 1956	Tomas Nilsson	SWE	2:22:05.4	72	47	28	75	9
Oct. 13, 1957	Ivan Filin	SOV	2:23:57.8	62	36	31	67	8
Oct. 12, 1958	Pavel Kantorek	CSA	2:29:37.2	64	53	18	71	10
Oct. 11, 1959	Sergey Popov	SOV	2:17:45.2	60	45	22	67	15
Oct. 9, 1960	Sam Hardicker	GBR	2:26:46.8	81	70	22	92	11
Oct. 12, 1961	Abebe Bikila	ETH	2:20:12	88	70	23	93	12
Oct. 7, 1962	Pavel Kantorek	CSA	2:28:29.8	78	66	20	86	11
Oct. 13, 1963	Leonard Edelen	USA	2:15:09.6	115	76	47	123	17
Aug. 8, 1964	Pavel Kantorek	CSA	2:25:55.4	95	83	18	101	11
Oct. 3, 1965	Aurele Vandendriessche	BEL	2:23:47	102	91	34	125	17
Oct. 2, 1966	Gyula Toth	HUN	2:19:11.2	121	81	50	131	16
Oct. 1, 1967	Nedo Farcic	YUG	2:20:53.8	120	71	54	125	17
Oct. 28, 1968	Vaclav Chudomel	CSR	2:26:28.4	113	120	0	120	1
Oct. 5, 1969	Demissie Wolde	ETH	2:15:37	98	57	47	104	14
Oct. 4, 1970	Mikhail Gorelov	SOV	2:16:26.2	261	197	81	278	15
Oct. 3, 1971	Gyula Toth	HUN	2:21:43.6	85	52	47	99	12
Oct. 8, 1972	John Farrington	AUS	2:17:34.4	104	58	54	112	17
Oct. 7, 1973	Vladimir Moiseyev	SOV	2:19:01.2	103	62	64	126	17
Oct. 6, 1974	Keith Angus	GBR	2:20:09	334	326	66	392	19
Oct. 5, 1975	Choi Chang-Soy	NKO	2:15:47.8	119	73	55	128	17
Oct. 3, 1976	Takeshi Sov	JAP	2:18:42.4					

TABLE 7

COMMONWEALTH GAMES MARATHON

Date/Site	1st 3 Finishers	Nat.	Time	Finishers
Aug 23, 1930 Hamilton	Duncan McL. Wrignt Sam Ferris John Miles	SCO ENG CAN	2:43:43 @ 880 yd.* @ 300 yd.*	10
Aug 11, 1934 London	Harold Webster Duncan McN. Robertson Duncan McL. Wright	CAN SCO SCO	2:40:36 2:45:08 2:56:20	11
Feb 12, 1938 Sydney	Johannes Coleman Arthur Norris Jackie Gibson	SOA ENG SOA	2:30:49.8 2:37:57 2:38:20	9
Feb. 11, 1950 Auckland	Jack Holden Sidney Luyt Jim Clark	ENG SOA NZL	2:32:57 2:37:02.2 2:39:26.4	14
Aug. 7, 1954 Vancouver	Joe McGhee Jack Mekler Johannes Barnard	SCO SOA SOA	2:39:36 2:40:57 2:51:49.8	6
Jul 24, 1958 Cardiff	Dave Power Johannes Barnard Peter Wilkinson	AUS SOA ENG	2:22:45.6 2:22:57.4 2:24:42	21
Nov 29, 1962 Perth	Brian Kilby Dave Power Rod Bonnella	ENG AUS AUS	2:21:17 2:22:15.4 2:24:07	12
Aug 11, 1966 Kingston	Jim Adler Bill Adcocks Mike Ryan	SCO ENG NZL	2:22:07.8 2:22:13 2:27:59	10
Jul 23, 1970 Edinburgh	Ron Hill Jim Adler Don Faircloth	ENG SCO ENG	2:09:28 2:12:04 2:12:19	24
Jan 31, 1974 Christchurch	Ian Thompson Jack Foster Richard Mabuza	ENG NZL SWA	2:09:12 2:11:18.6 2:12:54.4	23

* Official results only indicate the distance between runners at the time the winner finished.

TABLE 8

EUROPEAN CHAMPIONSHIP MARATHON

Date/Site	1st 3 Finishers	Nat.	Time	Finishers
Sep 9, 1934 Turin	Armas Toivonen Tore Enochsson Aurelio Genghini	FIN SWE ITA	2:52:29 2:54:35:6 2:55:03.4	8
Sep 4, 1938 Paris	Vaino Muinonen Squire Yarrow Henry Palme	FIN GBR SWE	2:37:28.8 2:39:03 2:42:13.6	14
Aug 22, 1946 Oslo *	Mikko Hietanen Vaino Muinonen Yuriy Punko	FIN FIN SOV	2:24:55 2:26:08 2:26:21	14
Aug 23, 1950 Brussels	Jack Holden Veikko Karvonen Fyedossey Vanin	GBR FIN SOV	2:32:13.2 2:32:45 2:33:47	18
Aug 25, 1954 Berne	Veikko Karvonen Boris Grishayev Ivan Filin	FIN SOV SOV	2:24:51.6 2:24:55.6 2:25:26.6	22
Aug 24, 1958 Stockholm	Sergey Popov Ivan Filin Fred Norris	SOV SOV GBR	2:15:17 2:20:50.6 2:21:15	22
Sep 16, 1962 Belgrade	Brian Kilby Aurele Vandendriessche Viktor Baikov	GBR BEL SOV	2:23:18.8 2:24:02 2:24:19.8	22
Sep 4, 1966 Budapest	Jim Hogan Aurele Vandendriessche Gyula Toth	GBR BEL HUN	2:20:04.6 2:21:43.6 2:22:02	26
Sep 21, 1969 Athens	Ron Hill Gaston Roelants Jim Adler	GBR BEL GBR	2:16:47.8 2:17:22.2 2:19:05.8	24
Aug 15 1971 Helsinki	Karel Lismont Trevor Wright Ron Hill	BEL GBR GBR	2:13:09 2:13:59.6 2:14:34.8	41
Sep 8, 1974 Rome	Ian Thompson Eckhard Lesse Gaston Roelants	GBR GDR BEL	2:13:18.8 2:14:57.4 2:16:29.6	22

* Course disance short, 40,200 meters.

TABLE 9

YONKERS MARATHON

Date	Winner	State or Country	Time
Nov 29, 1935	John A. Kelley	MA	2:38:43
Nov 8, 1936	Ned Porter	NJ	2:41:33
Nov 7, 1937	Pat Dengis	MD	2:42:50.2
Nov 6, 1938	Pat Dengis	MD	2:39:32.6
Nov 12, 1939	Pat Dengis	MD	2:33:45.2
Nov 10, 1940	Gerard Cote	CAN-QUE	2:34:06.2
Nov 9, 1941	Bernard Joseph Smith	MA	2:36.06.3
Nov 8, 1942	Fred A. McGlone	MA	2:37:54
Nov 7, 1943	Gerard Cote	CAN-QUE	2:38:35.3
Nov 12, 1944	Charles A. Robbins	MA-Navy	2:40:48.6
Nov 11, 1945	Charles A. Robbins	MA-Navy	2:37:14
Oct 27, 1946	Gerard Cote	CAN-QUE	2:47:53
Oct 26, 1947	Theodore Vogel	MA	2:40:11
May 15, 1949	Victor Dyrgall	NY	2:38:49.9
May 21, 1950	John A. Kelley	MA	2:45:55.3
May 27, 1951	Jesse Van Zant	MA	2:37:12
May 18, 1952	Victor Dyrgall	NY	2:38:28.4
May 17, 1953	Karl G. Leandersson	SWE	2:48:12
May 17, 1954	Theodore Corbitt	NY	2:46:13.9
May 22, 1955	Nick Costes	MA	2:31:12.4
Sep 30, 1956	John J. Kelley	MA	2:24:52
May 19, 1957	John J. Kelley	MA	2:24:55.2
May 18, 1958	John J. Kelley	MA	2:21:00.4
May 24, 1959	John J. Kelley	MA	2:21:54.4
May 22, 1960	John J. Kelley	MA	2:20:13.6
May 21, 1961	John J. Kelley	MA	2:26:33
May 13, 1962	John J. Kelley	MA	2:27:39.8
May 26, 1963	John J. Kelley	MA	2:25:17.6
May 24, 1964	Leonard Edelen	SD	2:24:25.6
May 16, 1965	Gar Williams	DC	2:33:50.6
May 15, 1966	Norman Higgins	CA	2:22:50.8
May 14, 1967	James McDonagh	NY	2:30:06.8
May 5, 1968	Gary Muhrcke	NY	2:32:41
May 18, 1969	Gary Muhrcke	NY	2:33:11
May 17, 1970	Bill Harvey	NY	2:31:10
May 16, 1971	Bill Harvey	NY	2:35:41
Jun 11, 1972	Max White	NJ	2:29:42.8
May 20, 1973	Norbert Sander	NY	2:25:56
Jun 2, 1974	Ron Wayne	OR	2:18:52.3
May 11, 1975	Marty Sudzina	PA	2:27:37.2
May 23, 1976	Ray Hall	NY	2:27:58
May 22, 1977	Peter Squires	NY	2:31:15

TABLE 10

OTSU MARATHON

Date	Site	Winner	Nat.	Time
1946	Osaka	Shinzo Koga	JAP	2:44:57
1947	Osaka	Shinzo Koga	JAP	2:43:17
1948	Osaka	Shinzo Koga	JAP	2:40:05
1949	Osaka	Saburo Yamada	JAP	2:40:32
1950	Osaka	Giichi Noda	JAP	2:37:25
May 6, 1951	Osaka	Tadashi Asai	JAP	2:32:41
May 4, 1952	Osaka	Yoshitaka Uchikawa	JAP	2:29:55.4
May 10, 1953	Osaka	Hinoshi Uwa	JAP	2:41:28
May 16, 1954	Osaka	Hideo Hamamura	JAP	2:27:56
May 8, 1955	Osaka	Kurao Hiroshima	JAP	2:26:32
May 5, 1956	Osaka	Yoshiaki Kawashima	JAP	2:27:45
May 3, 1957	Osaka	Kurao Hiroshima	JAP	2:31:30
May 11, 1958	Osaka	Takayuki Nakao	JAP	2:25:51
May 10, 1959	Osaka	Kurao Hiroshima	JAP	2:30:06
May 15, 1960	Osaka	Nobuyoshi Sadanaga	JAP	2:34:57
Jun 25, 1961	Osaka	Abebe Bikila	ETH	2:29:27
May 13, 1962	Osaka	Masayuki Nagata	JAP	2:27:37
May 12, 1963	Tokyo	Kenji Kimihara	JAP	2:20:24.8
Apr 12, 1964	Tokyo	Kenji Kimihara	JAP	2:17:11.4
May 9, 1965	Otsu	Abebe Bikila	ETH	2:22:55.8
Jun 5, 1966	Otsu	Yoshiro Mifune	JAP	2:26:01.6
May 14, 1967	Otsu	Yoshiro Mifune	JAP	2:25:53
Apr 14, 1968	Otsu	Akio Usami	JAP	2:13:49
May 11, 1969	Otsu	Kazuo Matsubara	JAP	2:22:44
Apr 12, 1970	Otsu	Bill Adcocks	GBR	2:13:46
Mar 21, 1971	Otsu	Yoshiaki Unetani	JAP	2:16:45.4
Mar 19, 1972	Otsu	Akio Usami	JAP	2:20:24
Mar 18, 1973	Otsu	Frank Shorter	USA	2:12:03
Apr 21, 1974	Otsu	Akio Usami	JAP	2:13:24
Apr 20, 1975	Otsu	Akio Usami	JAP	2:12:40
Apr 18, 1976	Otsu	Akio Usami	JAP	2:15:22
Apr 17, 1977	Otsu	Karel Lismont	BEL	2:14:08

TABLE 11

ASAHI-FUKUOKA INTERNATIONAL MARATHON

Date	Site	Top Finisher(s)	Nat.	Time
Dec 7. 1947	Kumamoto	Toshikazu Wada	JAP	2:45:45
Dec 5, 1948	Takamatsu	Saburo Yamada	JAP	2:37:25
Dec 4, 1949	Shizuoka	Shinzo Koga	JAP	2:40:26
Dec 10, 1950	Hiroshima	Shunji Koyanagi	JAP	2:30:47
Dec 9, 1951	Fukuoka	Hiroyoshi Haigo	JAP	2:30:13
Dec 7, 1952	Ube	Katsuo Nishida	JAP	2:27:59
Dec 6, 1953	Nagoya	Hideo Hamamura	JAP	2:27:26
Dec 5, 1954	Kamakura	Reinaldo Gorno	ARG	2:24:55
Dec 11, 1955	Fukuoka	Veikko Karvonen	FIN	2:23:16
Dec 9, 1956	Nagoya	Keizo Yamada	JAP	2:25:15
Dec 1, 1957	Fukuoka	Kurao Hiroshima	JAP	2:21:40
Dec 7, 1958	Utsunomiya	Nobuyoshi Sadanaga	JAP	2:24:01
Nov 8, 1959	Fukuoka	Kurao Hiroshima	JAP	2:29:34
Dec 4, 1960	Fukuoka	Barry Magee	NZL	2:19:04
Dec 3, 1961	Fukuoka	Pavel Kantorek	CSR	2:22:05
Dec 2, 1962	Fukuoka	Toru Terasawa	JAP	2:16:18.4
Oct 15, 1963	Tokyo	Jeff Julian	NZL	2:18:00.6
Dec 6, 1964	Fukuoka	Toru Terasawa	JAP	2:14:48.2
Oct 10, 1965	Fukuoka	Hidekuni Hiroshima	JAP	2:18:35.8
Nov 27, 1966	Fukuoka	Mike Ryan	NZL	2:14:04.6
		Hidekuni Hiroshima	JAP	2:14:05.2
		Hirokazu Okabe	JAP	2:15:09.2
Dec 3, 1967	Fukuoka	Derek Clayton	AUS	2:09:36.4
		Seiichiro Sasaki	JAP	2:11:17
		Dave McKenzie	NZL	2:12:25.8
Dec 8, 1968	Fukuoka	Bill Adcocks	GBR	2:10:47.8
		Yoshiaki Unetani	JAP	2:12:40.6
		Tadaaki Ueoka	JAP	2:13:37.6
Dec 7, 1969	Fukuoka	Jerome Drayton	CAN	2:11:12.8
		Ron Hill	GBR	2:11:54.4
		Hayami Tanimura	JAP	2:12:03.4
Dec 6, 1970	Fukuoka	Akio Usami	JAP	2:10:37.8
		Ken Moore	USA	2:11:35.8
		Yoshiaki Unetani	JAP	2:12:12
Dec 5, 1971	Fukuoka	Frank Shorter	USA	2:12:50.4
		Akio Usami	JAP	2:13:22.8
		Jack Foster	NZL	2:13:42.4
Dec 3, 1972	Fukuoka	Frank Shorter	USA	2:10:30
		John Farrington	AUS	2:12:00.4
		Kenichi Otsuki	JAP	2:14:00.6
Dec 2, 1973	Fukuoka	Frank Shorter	USA	2:11:45.0
		Brian Armstrong	CAN	2:13:43.4
		Eckhard Lesse	GDR	2:13:53.8
Dec 8, 1974	Fukuoka	Frank Shorter	USA	2:11:31
		Eckhard Lesse	GDR	2:12:02.4
		Pekka Paivarinta	FIN	2:13:09
Dec 7, 1975	Fukuoka	Jerome Drayton	CAN	2:10:08.4
		David Chettle	AUS	2:10:20
		Bill Rodgers	USA	2:11:26.4
Dec 5, 1976	Fukuoka	Jerome Drayton	CAN	2:12:35
		Ian Thompson	GBR	2:12:54.2
		Waldemar Cierpinski	GDR	2:14:56

TABLE 12

CULVER CITY MARATHON

Date	Winner	Country	Time
May 21, 1948	Gerald Cote	CAN	2:42:07
Nov 27, 1949	Robert Cons	USA	2:45:27
Jun 18, 1950	Mainhardt Bredt	USA (Alaska)	3:00:20
Jun 17, 1951	Lou Wen Ngua	CHN	2:45:10
Jun 16, 1952	Joseph Brooks	USA	2:50:37
Jun 27, 1953	Robert Cons	USA	2:46:30
Jun 20, 1954	Robert Cons	USA	2:32:46
Oct 1, 1955	Robert Cons	USA	2:37:21
Jul 21, 1956	Michael Allen	USA	2:40:49
Aug 3, 1957	Mal Robertson	USA	2:55:41
Sep 14, 1958	Michael Allen	USA	2:32:35.4
Dec 12, 1959	Thomas Ryan	USA	2:28:20
Dec 3, 1960	Robert Carman	USA	2:22:17
Dec 9, 1961	William R. Peck	USA	2:26:19
Dec 9, 1961	Peter McArdle	USA	2:17:11.4*
Dec 9, 1963	Norman Higgins	USA	2:19:33.4*
Jul 26, 1964	Peter McArdle	USA	2:27:01
Dec 11, 1965	Norman Higgins	USA	2:19:13
Dec 11, 1966	Mike Kimball	USA	2:27:10.4
Dec 10, 1967	James Freeman	USA	2:22:53.9
May 12, 1968	Robert Deines	USA	2:22:28
Dec 7, 1969	Thomas Heinonen	USA	2:24:43
Dec 6, 1970	Byron Lowry	USA	2:21:07.6
Dec 5, 1971	Bill Scobey	USA	2:15:21
Dec 3, 1972	Brian Armstrong	CAN	2:18:54
Dec 2, 1973	Reino Paukkoen	FIN	2:16:31.6
Dec 1, 1974	Mario Cuevas	MEX	2:18:08
Dec 7, 1975	Gary Tuttle	USA	2:17:27
Dec 5, 1976	Lionel Ortega	USA	2:18:19

* Course distance short of Olympic distance.

TABLE 13

PAN-AMERICAN GAMES MARATHON

Date/Site	1st 3 Finishers	Nat.	Time	Finishers
Mar 6, 1951 Buenos Aires	Delfo Cabrera Reinaldo Gorno Luis Velazquez	ARG ARG GUA	2:35:00.2 2:45:00 2:46:02.8	6
Mar 19, 1955 Mexico City	Doroteo Flores Oriesimo Rodriguez Luis Velazquez	GUA MEX GUA	2:59:09.2 3:02:25.6 3:05:25.2	6
Sep 2, 1959 Chicago	John J. Kelley Jim Green Gordon Dickson	USA USA CAN	2:27:54.2 2:32:16.9 2:36:18.6	8
May 4, 1963 Sao Paulo	Fidel Negrete Gordon McKenzie Pete McArdle	MEX USA USA	2:26:53.6 2:31:17.2 2:34:14	6
Aug 5, 1967 Winnipeg	Andy Boychuk Agustin Calle Alfredo Penaloza	CAN COL MEX	2:23:02.4 2:25:50.2 2:27:48.2	7
Aug 5, 1971 Cali	Frank Shorter Jose Gaspar Hernan Barreneche	USA MEX COL	2:22:40 2:26:30 2:27:19	11
Oct 20, 1975 Mexico City	Rigoberto Mendoza Chuck Smead Tom Howard	CUB USA CAN	2:25:02.8 2:25:31.6 2:25:45.4	8

TABLE 14

BEPPU MARATHON

Date	Winner	Time	Date	Winner	Time
Feb 1, 1953	Keizo Yamada	2:29:05	Feb 7, 1965	Toru Terasawa	2:14:38
Feb 7, 1954	Yoshitaka Uchikawa	2:34:48	Feb 13, 1966	Toru Terasawa	2:14:35
Feb 13, 1955	Katsuo Nishida	2:29:19	Feb 5, 1967	Kenji Kimahara	2:13:33.4
Feb 12, 1956	Kurao Hiroshima	2:26:24	Feb 4, 1968	Seiichiro Sasaki	2:13.23.8
Feb 10, 1957	Nobuyoshi Sadanaga	2:26:40	Feb 2, 1969	Tadaaki Ueoka	2:14:03.2
Feb 9, 1958	Kurao Kiroshima	2:25:16	Feb 8, 1970	Kenji Kimihara	2:17:12
Feb 8, 1959	Yoshitaki Tsuiji	2:23:40	Feb 7, 1971	Kenji Kimihara	2:16:52
Feb 14, 1960	Kazumi Watanabe	2:23:20	Feb 6, 1972	Yoshiro Mifune	2:19:10.4
Mar 12, 1961	Hiroshi Uwa	2:23:45	Feb 4, 1973	Kenji Kimihara	2:14:55.6
Feb 11, 1962	Hideaki Shishido	2:23:54	Feb 3, 1974	Yasunori Hamada	2:13:04.2
Feb 17, 1963	Toru Terasawa	2:15:15.8	Feb 2, 1975	Kenichi Ozawa	2:13:10.4
Feb 2, 1964	Toru Terasawa	2:17:48.6	Feb 1, 1976	Yukio Shigeraka	2:14:22.2

TABLE 15

MARATHON-TO-ATHENS MARATHON

Date	Winner	Nat.	Time
Oct 2, 1955	Veikko Karvonen	FIN	2:27:30
Oct 6, 1957	Franjo Mihalic	YUG	2:26:27.8
Oct 26,1959	Eino Oksanen	FIN	2:26:30
May 7, 1961	Abebe Bikila	ETH	2:23:44.6
May 19, 1963	Leonard Edelen	USA	2:23:06.8
May 21, 1965	Jozsef Suto	HUN	2:30:40.4
Apr 6,1967	Jurgen Busch	GDR	2:20:40
Apr 6, 1969	Bill Adcocks	GBR	2:11:07.2
Apr 6, 1971	Akio Usami	JAP	2:19:25
Apr 6, 1973	Colin Kirkham	GBR	2:16:45.4
Apr 9, 1975	Yuriy Laptyev	SOV	2:25:27

TABLE 16

PIKES PEAK MARATHON *

Date	Winner	State	Time	Finishers
Aug 10, 1956	Monte Wolford	CO	5:39:58	4
Aug 9, 1957	Monte Wolford	CO	5:15:53	9
Aug 8, 1958	Calvin Hansen	CO	4:29:40	8
Aug 7, 1959	Calvin Hansen	CO	4:20:18	13
Aug 14, 1960	Calvin Hansen	CO	4:14:25	12
Aug 13, 1961	Calvin Hansen	CO	4:07:15	12
Aug 19, 1962	Robert Mohler	KA	4:10:03	12
Aug 25, 1963	Jonn Rose	KA	4:01:22.8	15
Aug 23, 1964	Don Lakin	KA	4:03:33	13
Aug 22, 1965	John Rose	KA	3:53:57	14
Aug 21, 1966	Steve Gachupin	NM	3:52:04	14
Aug 20, 1967	Steve Gachupin	NM	3:50:05	28
Aug 4, 1968	Steve Gachupin	NM	3:50:05	22
Aug 10, 1969	Steve Gachupin	NM	3:44:50	19
Aug 16, 1970	Steve Gachupin	NM	3:45:54	25
Aug 15, 1971	Steve Gachupin	NM	3:46:26	32
Aug 13, 1972	Chuck Smead	CA	3:44:21	22
Aug 12, 1973	Richard Trujillo	CO	3:39:46	30
Aug 11, 1974	Richard Trujillo	CO	3:36:40	60
Aug 3, 1975	Richard Trujillo	CO	3:31:05	62
Aug 1, 1976	Richard Trujillo	CO	3:34:15	164

* Course is out and back, from Manitou Springs, Colorado, following the rugged Barr Trail in Pike National Forest. A vertical climb of 7774 ft. results in almost complete ascent of Pikes Peak (14,110 ft.). Length was 26 miles from 1956 through 1960, 26.8 miles from 1961 through 1975, and presently is 28 miles.

850

TABLE 17

KARL MARX STADT MARATHON *

Date	Winner	Nat.	Time
May 5, 1967	Jurgen Busch	GDR	2:16:09.2
May 19, 1968	Bill Adcocks	GBR	2:12:16.8
May 10, 1969	Tim Johnston	GBR	2:15:31.2
May 10, 1970	Jurgen Busch	GDR	2:14:41.2
May 1, 1971	Jurgen Busch	GDR	2:17:30.0
Apr 29, 1972	Eckhard Lesse	GDR	2:13:19.4
May 5, 1973	Eckhard Lesse	GDR	2:17:36.2
May 5, 1974	Gerald Umbach	GDR	2:15:59.8
May 3 ,1975	Eckhard Lesse	GDR	2:14:49.6
Apr 18, 1976	Waldemar Cierpinski	GDR	2:13:57.2

* Course is on an unpaved surface in a park, consisting of 8 laps each 5,228.6 meters long, with an additional 366.2 meters to total the full Olympic distance.

TABLE 18

NATIONAL ABBREVIATIONS

ARG	Argentina	ETH	Ethiopia	LIT	Lithuania
AUS	Australia	FIN	Finnland	LUX	Luxembourg
AUT	Austria	FRA	France	MEX	Mexico
BEL	Belgium	GBR	Great Britain	MOR	Morocco
CAN	Canada	GDR	German Democratic Republic	NKO	North Korea
CHI	Chile	GER	Germany	NZL	New Zealand
CHN	People's Republic of China	GFR	German Federal Republic	SCO	Scotland
COL	Colombia	GRE	Greece	SOA	South Africa
CSR	Czechoslovakia	GUA	Guatemala	SOV	Russia
CUB	Cuba	HUN	Hungary	SWA	Swaziland
EIR	Ireland	ITA	Italy	SWE	Sweden
ENG	England	JAP	Japan	USA	United States
EST	Estonia	KOR	Korea	YUG	Yugosalvia

GER indicates his nationality. Later races indicate the two German republics—GFR and GDR). A key to all abbreviations used herein is provided in TABLE 18.

References

1. MEZO, F. 1956. The modern Olympic games. Pannonia Press. Budapest, Hungary.
2. QUERCETANI, R. L. 1964. A World History of Track and Field Athletics, 1864–1964. Chap. **6:** 162–175. Oxford University Press. London, England.
3. HOPKINS, J. 1966. The Marathon. Stanley Paul and Company, Ltd. London, England.
4. ZUR MEGEDE, E. 1968. Die Geschichte der Olympischen Leichtathletik. Vols. 1 & 2. Bartels and Wernitz. Munich, West Germany.
5. KILLANIN, L. & J. RODDA. 1976. The Olympic Games. Book Club Associates. London, England.
6. HERODOTUS. Book **6:** 105–106. G. Rawlinson, Transl.
7. SOLINUS. Collectanea Rerum Memorabilium. Book **1:** 98.
8. CORNELIUS NEPOS. Miltiades. **4:** 3.

9. MATTHEWS, V. J. 1974. The hemerodromoi: Ultra long-distance running in antiquity. The Classical World **68:** 161–169.
10. KRENKEL, W. A. 1976. Cursores maiores minoresque. The Classical World **69:** 373–374.
11. HENDERSON, J. 1975. Marathon Handbook. World Publications. Mountain View, Calif.
12. CAIUS PLINIUS SECUNDUS. Historia naturalis. Book VII. Chap. **20:** 84.
13. PAUSANIAS. Description of Greece. J. G. Frazer, Transl. BOOK **1:** 28, 4.
14. LUCIANUS SAMOSATENSIS. A slip of the tongue in salutation. : 3.
15. PLUTARCHUS. Moralia. : 347c.
16. SULLIVAN, J. E. 1909. Marathon running. American Sports Publishing Company. New York, N.Y.
17. NEW YORK TIMES. 1896. Vol. XLVI. No. 14,067. Sep. **20:** 6.
18. BERLIOUX, M. 1976. Director, Comite International Olympique, Lausanne, Switzerland, personal communication.
19. WINTER, A. E. H. 1969. From the legend to the living. Benhill Press, Ltd. Rugeley, Staffordshire, England.
20. NEW YORK TIMES. 1908. **58**(18,569, Nov. 26): 1–2.
21. NEW YORK TIMES. 1908. **58**(18,589, Dec. 16): 1–2.
22. NEW YORK TIMES. 1909. **58**(18,641, Feb. 6): 1–2.
23. NEW YORK TIMES. 1909. **58**(18,606, Jan. 2): 7.
24. NEW YORK TIMES. 1908. **58**(18,570, Nov. 27): 7.
25. NEW YORK TIMES. 1908. **58**(18,600, Dec. 27): 1 (Pt. 4).
26. NEW YORK TIMES. 1909. **58**(18,669, Mar. 6): 5.
27. NEW YORK TIMES. 1909. **58**(18,698, Apr. 4): 1 (Pt. 7).
28. HANNUS, M. 1973. Finnish Running Secrets. World Publications. Mountain View, Calif.
29. NASON, J. 1966. The Story of the Boston Marathon. Boston Globe, Boston, Mass.
30. BOCK, A. V., C. VAN CAULAERT, D. B. DILL, A. FOLLING & L. M. HURXTHAL. 1928. Studies in muscular activity. III. Dynamical changes occurring in man at work. IV. The "steady state" and the respiratory quotient during work. J. Physiol. (London) **66:** 137–161, 162–174.
31. BOCK, A. V. 1963. The circulation of a marathoner. J. Sports Med. Phys. Fitness **3:** 80–86.
32. DILL, D. B., J. H. TALBOT & H. T. EDWARDS. 1930. Studies in muscular activity. VI. Response of several individuals to a fixed task. J. Physiol. (London) **69:** 267–305.
33. DILL, D. B. 1965. Marathoner DeMar: Physiological studies. J. Nat. Cancer Inst. **35:** 185–191.
34. CURREUS, J. H. & P. D. WHITE. 1961. Half a century of running: Clinical physiological and autopsy findings in the case of Clarence DeMar ("Mr. Marathon"). N. Engl. J. Med. **265:** 988–993.
35. BULOVSKY, V. 1960. Medzinarodny maraton mieru. Sport, nydavatel'stvo SUV CSTV. Bratislava, Czechoslovakia.
36. MARATHON HANDBOOK. 1976. Runner's World **11**(2): 21–73.
37. POTTS, D. R. 1976. ATFS annual 1975. Tafnews Press. Los Altos, Calif.
38. NELSON, B. 1975. Olympic track and field. Tafnews Press. Los Altos, Calif.
39. GYNN, R. 1972. International Marathon Statistics. 4th edit. Arena Publications, Ltd. London, England.

SIX-DAY PEDESTRIAN RACES

Thomas J. Osler

Mathematics Department
Glassboro State College
Glassboro, New Jersey 08028

Edward L. Dodd

Mathematics Department
Haddon Township High School
Westmont, New Jersey 08108

What are the limits of human endurance? This conference on the 26-mile marathon is in part a search for the extremes of human capabilities. To this end, it is well to review briefly a series of remarkable races that were staged a century ago and have now largely been forgotten. We refer to the six-day "go as you please" contests.

These races were so long that they make the present 26-miler look like a sprint for boys. The largest available hall would be rented for the contest and a track of from eight to perhaps twenty laps to the mile constructed. Starting on midnight Monday morning and continuing until midnight Saturday, the contestants would circle the track in an effort to log in the greatest possible mileage.

The "pedestrians" as they were called were free to run, walk, sleep, and eat at will, thus the term "go as you please." These were professional ventures, and the victorious pedestrian enjoyed not only international notoriety but financial security as well. When public enthusiasm for these contests was at its peak in 1879, the winner could expect twenty to thirty thousand dollars for his weeks work.

The following is a summary of the principal events in the history of the 6-day pedestrian contests:

1874—Weston's Three Failures. Edward Payson Weston, the "father of pedestrianism," was born March 15, 1839, at Providence, Rhode Island. He was a noted walker who had gained fame in 1861 by walking from Boston to Washington, 443 miles, to attend Lincoln's first inauguration. In 1867 he walked the 1,326 miles between Portland, Maine, and Chicago in 26 days to win $10,000. In 1874 he attempted to walk 500 miles in 6 days or 144 hours in New York City. This feat had been attempted by other pedestrians, but without success. Weston failed three times in 1874. In May he did 430 miles, in September 326 and in October 436. These trials took place at Barnum's Hippodrome, later to be known as Gilmore's Garden and Madison Square Garden in New York City.

December 14–19, 1874—The First 500 Miles. After three consecutive failures, Weston moved his trial to the Washington Street Rink in Newark, N.J. Here, in spite of underworld threats of sabotage, Weston managed 500 miles in six days less 26 minutes for the first time. He won $1,000 and a gold watch plus the title "Pedestrian Champion of the World."

O'Leary versus Weston. Daniel O'Leary, an Irish immigrant who developed his pedestrian art by selling bibles in Chicago, was Weston's major rival. In May of 1875 O'Leary walked 500 miles at the Rink in Chicago and thereby challenged Weston to a match race to decide the "World Champion." Each man put up $5,000 in a sweepstakes, for the week of November 15–20, 1875. O'Leary won with 501¼ miles to Weston's 450.

Weston Storms England. Early in the winter of 1876 Weston sailed for England to challenge the best British pedestrians. Although the British had a rich history of great pedestrian feats, they could find no champion who could match Weston's steps. In race after race he defeated all challengers. London went mad when he walked 501 miles at Agricultural Hall in six days. Weston was honored by men of great substance, and Sir John Drysdale Astley, a baronet and a member of Parliament, became his good friend. Astley agreed to back Weston against any man in the world.

O'Leary Follows Weston to Britain. In the fall of 1876, Daniel O'Leary, seeing Weston's great success in England, decided to follow. The British pedestrians had learned much by watching Weston's heels, and when O'Leary challenged them, he found stiff competition. He won his first two matches, but lost his next two to British rivals. Finally, O'Leary secured a match race with Weston, and the showdown was arranged for London, April 2–7, 1877. Once again, O'Leary triumphed with a new world record of 519 miles 1,585 yards to Weston's 510 miles.

Sir John Astley, who backed Weston, lost 20,000 pounds on the contest, but still presented Weston with a large purse of money for his efforts.

The Astley Belt (First and Second Contests). The time was ripe for an official world championship. Sir John Astley would be its sponsor. In January, 1878, Astley offered a belt valued at 100 pounds and $4,000 in prizes for the "Long Distance Challenge Championship of the World."

Weston failed to enter the first contest for the belt, and O'Leary won on March 18–24, 1878, with 520 miles 420 yards in London.

The second contest for the Astley Belt took place at Madison Square Garden in the Fall of 1878. Again O'Leary won with only 403 miles. His only opponent was John "The Lepper" Hughes who did an undistinguished 310 miles.

Charles Rowell—The British Champion. Sir John Astley and his friends were in search of a British pedestrian to win back the belt and world championship from the Americans. Their eyes fell on Charles Rowell, a lad of only 24 years, whose only claim as a pedestrian was a modest 9½-mile run in one hour. It is a tribute to Sir John's powers of observation that he could see Rowell's potential from so little evidence. Rowell was given support and time to train. He set sail for America in the winter of 1879 to vindicate British pedestrianism.

The Third Contest for the Astley Belt. On March 10–15, 1879, at Madison Square Garden, four men fought for the championship: Charles Rowell, Daniel O'Leary, John Ennis, and Charles Harriman (FIGURE 1). O'Leary, exhausted from too much racing, quit on the third day. There was a large crowd of Irish immigrants in the audience. They were fiercely partisan toward their countryman Ennis. When it became clear that the little Englishman Rowell might win, the atmosphere grew tense. Police reinforcements were called. Finally a drunken Irishman broke onto the track, but before he could strike Rowell, he was carried away by police. Ennis grasped Rowell's hand and warned the crowd that he would quit if any harm came to his British rival. Rowell won with 500 miles 180 yards. He went back to England a rich man, carrying $20,000 and the honor of World Champion.

The Fourth Contest—Weston Again Champion. Edward Payson Weston was 40 years old when the fourth Astley Belt contest took place in London on June 16–21, 1879. The bookmakers gave 10 to 1 odds against him. Nevertheless, the old walker had been watching Rowell. Rowell had proved that a good runner could beat a good walker. Weston found that he too could run. Rowell had to sit out the race with an injured heel. Weston started slowly, but assumed the lead on the fourth day. His pacing was magnificent. On the last day he recorded 7:39 for his 501st mile and 7:37 for his 526th. He won with a new world record of 550 miles.

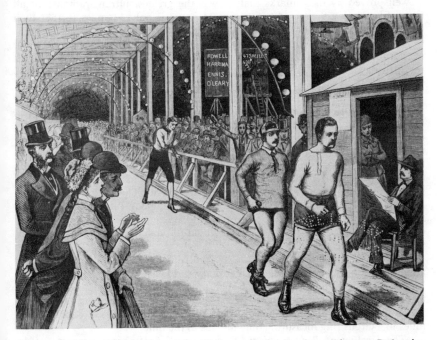

FIGURE 1. "New York City.—The third contest for the Long-Distance Pedestrian Championship of the World at Gilmore's Garden [Madison Square Garden], March 10th–15th.—View on the track on Saturday afternoon with Rowell, Ennis and Harriman walking together." (From *Leslie's Illustrated Weekly*, March 16, 1879.)

The Fifth and Last Astley Belt Contest. On September 22–28, 1879, at Madison Square Garden, Charles Rowell won back the championship belt from the Americans with 524 miles 77 yards. He won $30,000, the greatest prize ever given in a 6-day contest. Public interest had now reached its peak. Soon, however, they would lose interest in these contests.

Declining Public Interest. With Rowell's return to England, interest quickly dropped in these contests. On December 26–31, 1881, Patrick Fitzgerald set a new world record of 582 miles and 55 yards but won only $2,000. The management lost $2,000 on the contest.

Rowell's Magnificent Failure. Once again Charles Rowell returned to New York City. The week of February 27–March 4, 1882, was to see his final race.

He intended to make it memorable by establishing an unbreakable world record. He almost succeeded. His first three days saw the following:

$$
\begin{array}{ll}
100 \text{ miles} & -13:26:30 \\
200 \text{ miles} & -35:09:28 \\
300 \text{ miles} & -58:17:06 \\
24 \text{ hours*} & -150 \text{ miles } 395 \text{ yd.} \\
48 \text{ hours} & -258 \text{ miles } 220 \text{ yd.} \\
72 \text{ hours} & -353 \text{ miles } 220 \text{ yd.}
\end{array}
$$

Of these marks, only the 100 miles and 24 hours have been bettered today. Rowell proved by these marks that he was the greatest ultramarathoner of all time. Even today the world record for 24 hours is only 11 miles further than Rowell's 1882 mark, and Rowell faced another five days of running!

At the close of the third day, poor Rowell accidentally gulped down a cup of warm vinegar. His stomach became sick and he retired from the race on the fifth day. George Hazael won with a new world record of 600 miles 220 yards.

An Act of Barbarism. April 28–May 3, 1884, bore witness to a savage struggle at Madison Square Garden. On the morning of the last day of the race, Patrick Fitzgerald led Charles Rowell by 20 miles. Rowell had returned from retirement after his disappointing failure in 1882. Fitzgerald was all broken up, and Rowell was gaining quickly. By 7 AM Rowell was only 10 miles behind, and at noon, 4 miles. Again and again Fitzgerald's handlers forced the reluctant pedestrian back onto the track after momentary rests. Finally the Irishman's legs grew so stiff that he could not move. The race would be lost. In desperation his handlers had incisions made in poor Fitzgerald's thighs to relieve the stiffness. It worked, and Fitzgerald staggered to a new world record of 610 miles. Such scenes of barbarism would ultimately bring about the downfall of these contest.

Advancing the World Record. The year 1888 saw the final two successful attempts on the world record. On February 6–11, at Madison Square Garden, James Albert of Philadelphia did 621¾ miles, and on November 27–Dec. 2, George Littlewood of England did 623¾ miles at the same location. Littlewood was a man of unusual persistance, even among pedestrians. He once did 378 miles in a circus ring measuring only 38 laps to the mile.

The Decline of Pedestrianism. Promotion of 6-day races became a risky financial venture. Between 1891 and 1899 no such contests were seen in New York City. The public's attention was now attracted to long distance bicycle races. The wheelman soon gained a position of importance that the pedestrian never had.

In 1899 there was a modest revival of these races in New York City, but the contest often stopped before the 6 days were over because of lack of attendance.

The cities of Philadelphia, Columbus, St. Louis, and Pittsburgh saw revivals with only moderate success. By 1903 the sport was in a state of serious deterioration. One Philadelphia reporter wrote:

After the first twelve hours the expression go as you "please" became ridiculous, for no man if he retained his senses pleased to go anyway. That is where

---

* Actually 22 hours, 28 minutes, 25 seconds.

the trainers became valuable in forcing the poor, jaded, abused bodies to continue their suicidal work. . . . Imagine the brutality of standing there, eagerly, curiously watching the faces of the contestants pinched, drawn and lined with physical and mental ágony, and occasionally making cold blooded comments as to how badly a man's legs were swelled, or as to how much older he looked than a night before. . . . Prize fighting, football, wrestling and the like have been called dangerous sports. But the three played at one time would only represent a game of marbles in comparison with the six days "go as you please."

Weston Walks On. While the 6-day contests were taking their last breath, the incredible Edward Payson Weston was entertaining his greatest pedestrian ventures. Starting on his 70th birthday he walked from New York City to San Francisco, 3,900 miles, in 105 days. The next year he walked back from Los Angeles to New York, 3,600 miles in 77 days.

Weston had been an active competitor from 1861 to 1913, a full 52 years, in one of the most difficult sports on earth. How did he survive? He knew himself. He knew when to ease up, and when to let it all out. He was, in short, the champion's champion.

In 1927, his magnificent legs were replaced by a wheelchair. He had been struck by a cab. He died on May 13, 1929 at the age of 90.

The New York Times, on May 15, 1929 gave the grand old pedestrian a fitting eulogy:

He has gone at last on what one has called the "perfect walk," the walk for which solitude is essential, but in his pilgrimage across the earth he has led a multitude who will keep on walking till they too, come to the end of the road which is the longer for going on foot.

A BRIEF HISTORY OF MODERN TRENDS
IN MARATHON TRAINING

John Lucas

Department of Physical Education
Pennsylvania State University
University Park, Pennsylvania 16802

During the post-war decade 1946–1956, Emil Zatopek, the "Czechoslovakian Train" trained and competed a total of nearly 50,000 miles. Until someone else comes along to replace this record, it must remain the greatest concentration of running by anyone in the history of long-distance running. Make no mistake, in the world of sport during the first half of the 20th century, it was the athletes—men like Zatopek, rather than the athletics scientists—who were innovators, creators of new ideas, daring individuals risking unconventionality and possible physical danger. Zatopek represented an essential watershed in international distance running, and is thus far the single most important individual in modern long distance and marathon training.

Zatopek's use of Swedish "fartlek" training methods was a demonic innovation. The Scandinavians, a decade and more earlier, had evolved a method of alternate-speed running through the forests for 1 to 2 hours, accelerating, decelerating, running up-hill and down. It is an exhilarating, physiologically demanding, effective, but unscientific training regimen.[1] Zatopek, winner of all three distance races at the Helsinki Olympics, worked out a labyrinthian course through his own forest lands, frequently running a half-a-hundred repetitions of 400 meters. "At the same time Zatopek began to include 200 meter repetitions at nearly full speed in his workouts and by 1954 was using a complex training method—high repetitions of slow interval runs to develop the cardiorespiratory system and fast repetitions to improve metabolism."[2] Zatopek's biographer, Frantisek Kozik, gives a vivid description of extraordinary dedication and monumental physical pain: "He went at it like a madman."[3] A world cult had grown up about this five-medal Olympian. On the eve of his last Olympic competition, Zatopek toured India with his wife, Dana. In a Calcutta race in 1956, the "old man" of thirty-five easily won a 5-kilometer race from the Indian champion, Gulzara Singh. Touching Zatopek's shoes and sprinkling dust from the Czech's feet onto his own head, the Indian was overwhelmed as "Zatopek made him a present of his running shoes."[4]

Long-distance and marathon runners are a breed unto themselves.[5] Marathon runners usually emanate from a particular "school" of training.[6, 7] The Hungarian School of the 1950s demanded 2,000 training sessions over a 3-year period. Some of the running was long and slow; a great deal of it was hard and fast, with tortuous smaller and smaller rest intervals as the athletes plunged deeper into fatigue. Russian coaches, deeply influenced by Zatopek, devised a pseudo-fartlek method of running over the country for two hours with precise interval accelerations of 100, 200, 400, 800, and 1,200 meters. Bolotnikov, Filin, Vanin, Zhukov, and Kuts all were schooled this way. Ten days before Kuts won his two gold medals at the Melbourne Olympics in 1956, he warmed up 30 minutes, and then on grass ran 25 × 440 yards in 63–67 seconds, jogging 110 yards in 30 seconds after each.

In the United States during the mid-1950s, the two most influential marathon runners were John J. Kelley and Nicholas Costes. Both were Olympians, both successful Boston Marathon competitors, but different in temperament and, therefore, in training. Both ran twice a day; Kelley took long runs on grass and highway, interspersed with accelerations of indeterminate distances. The regimented Costes introduced massive interval training to American marathoning. He copied Zatopek, running hundreds of 220 or 440 sprints in a single week—a pioneer in hundred-mile-a-week running. A little later in the decade and half-way round the world, Arthur Lydiard began to influence Australian, New Zealand, and, eventually, the universal family of distance runners. His massive "marathon training" session laid the foundation for an eclectric 2 to 4 year training program incorporating fartlek, interval training, repetition runs, hill climbing, plus local, national, and international exposures. Lydiard influenced world champions Halberg, Snell, Ron Clark, sub-2:10 marathoner Derek Clayton, and a host of champions through the 1960s and to the present day. The orderliness, gradually demanding and therefore physiologically sound Lydiard approach gained acceptance all over the world.

The marathon gold medal at the 1956, 1960, 1964, and 1968 Olympic games were won by athletes from the African continent. The science of distance running, having gained a reluctant foothold with many athletes and coaches during this era, marked time for a while. The tough and single-minded 36-year old Algerian soldier, Alain Mimoun, finally shook off the Zatopek shadow and raced a warm 2 hours 25 minutes in the 1956 games. A harsh early life, a decade and a half of relentless running, characterized his background and that of the Black African marathon champions that were to follow him. Ethiopia's enigmatic Abebe Bikila parlayed a decade of harsh flat and hill training with one of the most fluid and efficient running styles ever seen to win both the Rome Olympic Marathon (2:15:16.2) and the Tokyo 42-kilometer race in 2:12:11.2. The African distance running "revolution" resulted in 1968 Mexico City victories in the 1,500 meters, 3,000 meter steeplechase, 5,000 and 10,000 meter runs, and culminated in another Ethiopian marathon victor— 34-year-old Mamo Wolde in 2:20:26.4.

The doctors and physiologists became more active after the mile-high Olympic Games of 1968. More attention was paid to Oregon's Bill Bowerman and his rhythm system of hard and easy runs. The pre-World War II controlled interval training of Woldemar Gerschler and Dr. Herbert Reindell,[8] giving rise to the successful coaching philosophy of Franz Stampfl, created mountains of research problems. Ironically, these beginnings of scientific marathon training owe a debt of gratitude to the coaching genius of America's Billie Hayes and the Indiana University school of runners during the 1930s and early 40s. Empiricism and the scientific thrust became uneasy companions after 1968. The coaching fraternity was slowly, ever so slowly, benefiting from the research of medical doctors, nutritionists, biomechanicians, and physiologists. At about this same time, popular or mass participation in distance and marathon training and running became not only an American but world phenomenon. Men and women in large numbers began running under 4 hours, and then 3½ hours. During the present decade, hundreds of men of all ages, and several dozen women have run a full marathon in under 3 hours. The guru of the over-40 marathoners, Jack Foster of New Zealand, consistently runs under 2 hours 20 minutes and finished among the elite top 20 in the Montreal marathon. They are all, possibly, in the forefront of a future significant health and preventive medicine movement.

In the briefest recapitulation of the major marathon training approaches of the 20-year period 1946–1966, one can see (1) the extensive use of fartlek, (2) the equally versatile interval training approach, (3) a demanding combination of fartlek and interval training, and (4) the elemental African commitment to running and more running. Emerging in the late 1960s was an approach that might be called "three-times-a-day compulsive training." Running 200 miles a week over extended periods of time is hazardous duty. Gerry Lindgren of the U.S.A. found it too difficult—although he ran a world-record 6 miles. David Colin Bedford of England stuck with it for several years, running a yet-to-be-broken 27:31.0 10 kilometers. His usual daily routine was 8 miles in the morning, 6 miles at noon, and a hard 16-miler in the afternoon, frequently at a 5½-minute-per-mile tempo.[9] The most successful three-workouts-a-day runner is the Olympic four-gold-medal winner from Finland, Lasse Viren. Less abrupt than Bedford, and therefore less prone to injury, Viren slowly builds up to the late afternoon 5-minute-per-mile tempo runs of 12–14 miles. His 30 miles a day, every day running, the result of a scientifically planned gradual adaptation to stress, must be considered a fifth major training approach for the marathon-distance runner.[10, 11]

Two more marathon runners must be mentioned. Both belong to that very select group that has run an accurately measured marathon in 2 hours 10 minutes or faster—an incredible average of under five minutes per mile. An even greater measure of athletic greatness is that both Frank Shorter and Waldemar Cierpinski won Olympic gold medals in the 1972 and 1976 games. Shorter's winning time in Munich of 2:12:19.7 was significantly improved by his 2:10:45 in finishing second to Cierpinski's Montreal race of 2:09:55. Both runners believe in fast tempo training. Both men have disciplined themselves to years of running, to the point where they are now able to run 125 miles a week, with most of it 4:45 to 5-minute-flat aerobic running for 12-, 15-, and 18-mile stints. For 5 years, American sport fans have been exposed to Shorter, the remarkable Yale graduate. He runs twice a day, seven days a week; his long afternoon affairs are hard sub-5-minute mile tempo runs for 70 and 80 minutes. Sometimes he has run a score of 440s under 60 seconds, with the briefest recovery period. America's greatest distance runner ever has indicated an interest in the Boston Marathon run of 1977. It would be his first. The stocky East German, Cierpinski, a 25-year-old ex-steeplechase runner from Halle is a product of the scientific school of physical training in the GDR. Only runners with proven speed and tenacity at 5 and 10 kilometers are "invited" to the marathon training camp. Very gradually the athletes build to 125 miles a week. Then intensity running begins—90% of the endurance runs at sub-5-minute mile tempo. "Interval work consisted mainly of ten to fifteen repetitions of 1,000 meters in 3:00 to 2:55 minutes with 4-to-6-minute jog recoveries."[12] This sixth form of training might be called, for lack of a better term, "the 125-minute marathon tempo training program." Probably before the Moscow Olympic Games of 1980, the experiment will have become a reality and the world will see a man sustain a 4:47 mile tempo for 26 miles 385 yards. I hope all of us here today can be witness to it.

References

1. Lucas, J. 1952. An analysis of American and Swedish long distance running and a suggested program for the American college track team. M.S. thesis. University of Southern California.
2. Karnikosh, O. 1973. The development of training methods in distance running. *In* How They Train. Fred Wilt, Ed. Vol. 2: 10. Track and Field News. Los Altos, Calif.
3. Kozik, F. 1954. Zatopek the Marathon Victor. : 129. Jean Layton, Transl. Artia Publishers. Prague, Czechoslovakia.
4. Run, run, and run—Zatopek. 1956. Sport and Pastime (Feb. 4) : 4.
5. Lucas, J. 1976. Forty kilometers and then some—A marathon history from Pheidippides to Will Rodgers. Amer. Med. Joggers Assoc. Newslett. (Parts 1 & 2, Summer & Fall); same article in 1976. J. Sport History 3(Summer): 120–138.
6. Lucas, J. 1969. Historical survey of middle and long distance running, or "Let's go back to school." Track and Field Q. Rev. (Dec.) : 31–37.
7. Freeman, W. H. 1975. Distance training methods, past and present. Track and Field Q. Rev. (Winter) : 4–11.
8. Sprecher, P. 1964. Visit with Dr. Woldemer Gerschler. *In* Run, Run, Run. Fred Wilt, Ed. : 150–152. Track and Field News. Los Altos, Calif.
9. Wilt, F. 1972. Training and performance profile of Dave Bedford. Scholastic Coach (Feb.) : 46.
10. Mitcheel, B. & F. Wilt. 1975. Lasse Viren's pre-Olympic training. Track Technique (March) : 1876.
11. Tschiene, P. 1974. Finnish middle distance "elasticity" training. Track Technique (Dec.) : 1850.
12. Kegel, K. 1975. Marathon training in East Germany. Track Technique (Dec.) : 1977.

THE HISTORY OF WOMEN'S PARTICIPATION IN THE MARATHON *

Nina Kuscsik

Huntington Station, New York 11746

National Women's Long Distance Running Committee
Amateur Athletic Union
Indianapolis, Indiana 46268

Women's Affairs Committee
New York Road Runners Club
New York, New York 10022

The year is 1976 and girls and women, ages 10 to 70, have become marathon runners. It is an exciting time to be a female long distance runner. Efforts for equal opportunities for women, and media exposure of the marathon runner to the world, have familiarized athletes and spectators alike with our event. National and international competition exists for us.

Since the marathon is an event that comes to the people, we and the public share a unique spontaniety: that of our reactions toward one another. And in only a few years that reaction has changed considerably. Spectators appreciate more our athletic abilities and have become less concerned that we are women.

Like our male counterparts, we sometimes wonder what cravings keep us out on the road. Prerace nerves and the fatigue that inevitably envelope us enroute have no sexual preference. Women, too, feel a tiredness that affects our whole psyche and we know intimately the words of Robert Frost, "but I have promises to keep and miles to go before I sleep." [1]

Indeed we love to run and we welcome the intensities of a lifetime that can be captured in the span of our race. We find there an admirable interdependence of our mental, emotional, and physical energies. We've concluded that marathon running is a truly human and healthy endeavor. This, however, is a very contemporary conclusion.

To find the initial efforts of women running the marathon, we have to search the yellowed pages of sport history. Only recently, however, did the jogging for fun and physical fitness craze, along with the concurrent feminist movement of the late 1960s, allow for the spectacular growth of women's participation in the marathon.

Early History, 1896–1960

I believe that women have been running prior to the time that men saw fit to record it. In the 19th century, Lewis Carroll, in his *Alice In Wonderland* fantasy, showed his understanding of the stamina of women when he included Alice in the famous caucus race. That race was somewhat of a long distance

---

* The editorial assistance of John Chodes is deeply appreciated.

run since its length was one-half hour, at which time everyone stopped and received prizes. Obviously, this was a participation event rather than a competitive one, and therefore in accord with the social attitudes of sport for women in that era.

Let's go back to the first marathon race. It was in the 1896 Olympics. It is alleged that a woman participated. Her name was "Melpomene." She was not allowed an official entry, but ran anyway. (Thus Melpomene became the first marathon runner to have her entry refused because of her sex.) She covered the 40 kilometers (the standard distance since 1924 is 42.195 kilometers) in around 4½ hours, accompanied by a bicycle escort. The Greek sportswriters felt that the Olympic Committee deserved to be reprimanded because it had been discourteous in refusing a lady's entry. They continued in their discourse, "We can assure those concerned that none of the participants would have had any objections." [2] I wonder about that. One must remember the article was written after all the Greek male runners completed the race well ahead of her.

Why Melpomene's assertiveness did not inspire other women is not known, but only sporadic attempts at marathon-type runs were made by women throughout the next 70 years.

In the 1920s, several women finished the 54-mile Comrades Marathon in South Africa and received as much acclaim as the winner. For centuries the Tarahumare Indian men and women of Mexico ran 50 or more miles a day in ball games and also used running as the safest and most efficient mode of transportation through the narrow mountain paths to other villages. Two teenage Tarahumare sisters wearing their customary long dresses were clocked in 4 hours and 56 minutes for 28.5 miles. And an undocumented report says that in the 1920s an emissary went to a Tarahumare chief to invite him to send runners to a marathon race in Kansas. When told that a marathon was a mere 26 miles, the chief ordered three girls to run it. [3]

The first 13-mile footrace ascending Pikes Peak (Colorado) was held in 1936 and two women ran in it. Then in 1959, 29-year-old Arlene Pieper ran the 26 miles up and down Pikes Peak in 9 hours, 16 minutes to become the first contemporary woman marathoner. [4]

The women I ran with pioneered the acceptance of women in the marathon in the late 1960s and early seventies, but we were not born yet when earlier distance running females were being ridiculed for their athletic aspirations. While tennis and swimming were acceptable for women in the early 1900s (there was women's lawn tennis in the 1900 Olympics), running was not. British women were called "brazen doxies" for their running habits and attire. [5]

In 1921, an international governing body for women's athletics,† the Feminine Sportive Federation Internationale (FSFI) was formed. It sponsored the first women's world championships in 1922. The longest race there was 1000 meters. After several international meets had taken place and performances improved consistently, a request was made to include women's athletics in the 1924 Olympics. The body that controls all athletic events in the Olympic games is the International Amateur Athletic Federation (IAAF). They turned down the request. Eventually an agreement was worked out providing dual control by the women's Federation and the IAAF, and five athletic events were included in the Games in 1928. The 800 meter was the longest running event.

† Athletics includes track and field, race walking, and long distance running.

I believe the result of that historic occasion set women's distance running back 50 years.

The 800-meter race itself was highly competitive, and although some of the entrants were not properly trained and collapsed enroute, the top six finished within 10 seconds of each other; the first three bettering the old world record.

Isn't the point of racing to reach one's limit at the finish line? When male runners collapsed enroute in the marathon, it was called drama, but when women reached this physiological level, it was labeled "frightful" and officials from several countries jumped on the IAAF to cancel the "frightful episode" from future Olympic games.[6]

Even though the leading United States woman 800-meter competitor had made the finals and set a new personal best, the United States was outspoken in the decision to cancel the future of the 800 meter. The sport-governing bodies in the U.S. had not encouraged women to run that distance and officials, therefore, felt justified in encouraging its cancellation.[7]

When the only distance event in the Olympics was lost, world interest waned. International meets were dominated by Britain and the Soviet Union.

Influence of Athletic Organizations

A brief overview of the involvement of athletic organizations and women physical educators in the "growth of athletics for women" in America from the early 1920s to the late 1930s is related to the problems women faced later in the 1960s.

The National Women's Collegiate and Scholastic Track Athletic Association was responsible for sending an American team to that first international championship for women in 1922. A report on that meet by the Association president, Harry Eaton Stewart, M.D., states "the longer runs—the 300 meter and 1,000 meters—have been used abroad for years with no recorded ill-effect. It is believed that they may be safely used by certain types of girls, but it might be thoroughly understood that they require a longer training period and repeated careful medical examinations if they are to be free from danger." [8]

Then, according to Daniel J. Ferris, Secretary-Treasurer of the Amateur Athletic Union (AAU) of the United States from 1927 to 1957, "When the Amateur Athletic Union took over control of women's track and field in 1922, it was decided that a 220-yard race be the longest event on the program. This proposal was made by the elderly leaders of women's physical training. Feeling that they were expressing the desires of all women's physical educators, the AAU went along with this line of thinking for several years to the detriment of distance running in the United States." [9]

The Women's Division of the National Amateur Athletics Federation (NAAF) went on record in 1929 as being opposed to the participation of women in the Olympic Games in 1932, and then in April 1930 petitioned M. le comte de Baillet-Latour, President of the International Olympic Committee to omit women's track and field events from the 1932 program. The Association believed that the Olympics "offered opportunity for exploitation and commercialization" for women and noted that Pierre de Coubertin, founder of the modern Olympic Games said at the 1928 Olympics, "As to the admission of women to the Games, I remain strongly against it. It was against my will that they were admitted to a growing number of competitions."

Many women's collegiate and physical education associations, including the Young Women's Christian Association adopted the resolution of the Women's Division of the NAAF—that programs of sports and games for women "shall (1) include every member of the group; (2) be broad and diversified; and (3) be adapted to the special need and abilities and capacities of the participant; with the emphasis upon participation rather than upon winning." [10]

This "new" philosophy for the place of sport in women's lives was spread nationally by physical educators.

So in 1936, Miss Helen Manley, supervisor of physical education for the University City, Michigan, public school system, said: "Athletics are now looked upon as educational, whereas formerly they were considered a form of amusement." "Let everyone play for enjoyment, not to specialize and win." And "I am against highly trained competition for women athletes. Women are not physically fit for the excitement and strain that this competition affords." She was of the opinion that fewer women would participate in the Olympics as time went on. [11]

In a 1901 article called "The Athletic Girl," I found this "new" philosophy expressed similarly: "The aim of athletics among women has been the establishment and maintenance of a high general standard of health and vigor, rather than some single brilliant achievement." [12]

1960 to Present—Women Athletes Begin to Exercise Their Rights and Talents in Long Distance Running

When the 800-meter was finally brought back to the Olympic games in 1960, distance running for women jumped in popularity. The United States was represented but found itself years behind other countries.

Avant-garde women around the country were starting a new trend in running by jumping into men's road races. They were labeled radicals for wanting to run over ¼ mile and the battle for women to be allowed to run longer distances emerged.

In 1961, when Julia Chase, a 19-year-old New England runner, participated in the Manchester, Connecticut, 5-mile road race, her entry was refused and she was told not to go through the finish line chute or she would be deprived of her amateur status. [13]

Women aspiring to run longer distances fought against many misbeliefs including one that running distance would make them musclebound. A few years before she ran her first road race, British runner and former record holder in the 800 meters, Chris McKenzie then living in the United States, decided to convince the local running officials they were wrong. She arrived at one of their monthly meeting wearing only a coat and a bikini. When the subject of muscles came up, she peeled off her coat and asked if she was too muscular. She was then given permission to run a longer distance, the ¼ mile.

Medical men who were runners began to speak out. In 1962, Dr. Charley Robbins predicted that since long distance running is primarily a test of heart and circulation, not brute muscular strength, the competition between men and women would become closer as the distances increased. [14]

Even before this, Dr. Ernst Van Aaken of West Germany had been accused of professional irresponsibility because of his beliefs in the inherent endurance and stamina of women.

In the early 1960s, two women from California, Lyn Carman and Merry Lepper, both in their early 20s, trained together and began to run unofficially in road races. In December 1963, they hid on the sidelines and then jumped in at the start of the Western Hemisphere Marathon in Culver City, California. A race official tried to push them off the road. Lyn punched him, asserting that she had every right to use the public streets for running. A sympathetic AAU official timed the women and Lyn went 20 miles while Merry finished the race in 3:37:07.[15, 16]

However, even as they were reaping benefits from their training, they were being warned by women physical educators who often held dual roles as AAU officials that running long distance was harmful and that they would not be able to bear children if they continued.[17]

A look at another marathon pioneer, Sara Berman of Massachusetts, shows her evolution. In 1961 Sara was 26 and a mother of two when her husband Larry, a distance runner himself, impressed upon her that the condition people are in by the time they reach thirty is most likely the condition they will stay in for the rest of their lives. So Sara learned to jog a mile, then more, until 8-mile workouts were routine. She soon saw that younger women were afraid of distance running, including the ½-mile distance, and she learned that the AAU of the United States was this country's governing body for women's running, but did not allow women to race any distance over a ½ mile.[18]

After taking time out to have her third child, Sara began attending the annual AAU Conventions and did a switch there from athlete to legislator. Under prodding from Sara and individuals from the Men's Long Distance Running Committee, the AAU Women's Committee gradually lengthened the distance that women could run. (A cross country distance was established in 1964 at 1½ miles, raised to 2, then 2½ until in 1968 a 5-mile limit was placed on women's competition.)

Faster than the AAU could establish limitations, women continued to exceed them. If the AAU Women's Committee would not sanction women's long distance running, women ran without their blessing and found they were none the worse.

Marathon Running

I believe that it was at the 1966 Boston Marathon that women's participation in the marathon took wings. Boston had long been one of the few major sporting events that anyone could enter; that is, anyone except a woman.

Roberta Gibb Bingay didn't know this. She did know that she loved to run. When she saw her first Boston Marathon in 1965, it had whet her appetite, for the men looked like they had a good thing going. So Roberta ran daily up to twenty miles and threw in some 5-hour runs. However, when she requested an application for the Boston race, she was refused one and was told that women couldn't run that far because they would get hurt.[19]

So she hid in the bushes in Hopkinton where the Boston Marathon begins, and she jumped into the mass of 415 runners to celebrate the joy of running. She finished the race in 3:21 beating ⅔ of the field. In taking some of the attention away from the male winner, she had an opportunity to explain herself.

She hoped that people would notice that she, a woman, was capable of this, and she hoped they would realize that if she was capable, many other women were also. Will Cloney, the marathon race director insisted at the time that Roberta Gibb Bingay did not run in *the* Boston Marathon; she merely covered the same route as the official race while it was in progress.[20]

However, Pandora's box had been opened. News of Roberta's run spread around the country. The Women's Running Committee became more paranoid about its sanctioning powers and declared itself an administration that controls all women runners, something like the Food and Drug Administration controls drugs.[21]

In 1967, Roberta returned to the Boston Marathon, starting again from the bushes. Another female, Kathrine Switzer, was there too. With an official number on her front, and a hood on her head, she started in the midst of the male runners. Her application was sent in without her full first name, and on the assumption that she was a male, a number was issued to her. When the press bus passed by several miles into the race, they noticed her.[22]

Will Cloney ran after her but couldn't catch her. Jock Semple, co-director tried to rip her number off, but Kathy's boyfriend intercepted and Jock landed on the curb. Roberta finished in 3:27 that year and Kathrine in 4:30. A few days later, Kathrine was thrown out of the AAU.

Her notification gave four reasons: She had run over the allowable distance for women; she ran with men; she fraudulently entered an AAU race; and she ran without a chaperone.[23]

A few weeks later, on May 6 in Toronto, Ontario, a 13-year-old Canadian girl, Maureen Wilton, ran a new world best ‡ of 3:15:22.8 topping by three minutes the previous world best by Mrs. M. McKenzie of New Zealand in 1964.[24]

Across the ocean, Dr. Van Aaken was seeing his beliefs become an actuality, when on September 16, 1967, Anni Pede-Erdkamp of West Germany, a follower of his and a mother of two, ran a marathon from Waldniel to Erdkamp in 3:07:26. Another world best. This one was to stand for three years.

The last few years of the 1960s were important to the running movement. Bowerman and Harris's *Jogging* book (1967) was in the bookstores, and Dr. Cooper's book *Aerobics* (1968) followed it. More and more men were attempting the marathon run. Women cashed in on the high that Roberta Gibb Bingay felt when she watched her first Boston Marathon. Sprinkles of the recently manifested feminist movement were felt by women runners as well as the spectators and the cries of "women's lib" were showered on women as they ran.

My first running race was the Boston Marathon in 1969. I came from a healthy 13-year athletic background of basketball, speed skating, and bicycle racing and consistently excelled in events requiring the most stamina. But I also listened and believed those who expressed the opinion that I was really too old to be doing that kid stuff. Finally, when I was 29 and a mother of three I decided that marathon running epitomized athletic achievement. So I applied my past training experiences to a running program and worked up to the marathon distance.

At the start at Boston I jumped in from behind the spectators, for the rumor

---

‡ Marathon records are not recognized by the IAAF because of the variability of race courses and conditions.

was that women would be stopped from running. This jumping in began to be a dangerous thing, for the number of runners increased each year (from 415 in 1966 to 887 in 1971) and when the gun went off there was little room to plant one's two feet on the road.

Sara Berman also ran the Boston Marathon for the first time in 1969 and began her string of three 1st place finishes at Boston, all unofficial.

Being unofficial at Boston had peculiar consequences. Our times were not recorded so we were required to do some detective work as we neared the finish line. We looked for the nearest male runner and got his number. Then we searched the race program until we found the name that corresponded to the number. After several months, every official finisher's time was listed in the running magazine, the *Long Distance Log*.§ We would search for this runner's name as if it was our own, for their time was the time we took for ourselves.

Most of the women engaged in this fabulous means of entertaining themselves in these years, had much in common. They were married, their husbands ran, some were mothers. Then another teenager emerged on the marathon scene when 16-year-old Caroline Walker ran a world's best of 3:02:53 in the Trail's End Marathon in Seaside, Oregon in February 1970. Her time averaged under 7 minutes per mile. A new plateau had been reached.

In retrospect we owe much to the Road Runners Club of America (RRCA) and one of its presidents, Vincent J. Chiappetta. That running club was organized in 1957 to promote long distance running and stood fast in its philosophy that if women were long distance runners, they deserved equal consideration with men at race time. With their persistence, more marathon race directors began accepting women in their races, unofficially of course. Arrangements were made for the first Road Runners Club of America National Women's Marathon Championship. Since it was "a club race" no AAU sanction was needed.

It was held in October 1970 along with an AAU men's marathon. On a cold rainy day, six women started and four finished. Sara Berman emerged as the champion.[25]

By the spring of 1971, the marathon record was being challenged at every race. If 3 hours separated the men from the boys, it would certainly put the female marathoner into a new class. Within a month the world best dropped to 3:01:42 run by Beth Bonner and then to 3:00:35 by the persistent Sara Berman. Our attention was turned from seeking official status to who would be the first woman to break the 3-hour barrier. We trained hard all that summer in preparation for our next meeting. It was to be at the New York City Marathon in September. I was one of the women who felt they were capable of a sub-3-hour marathon.

Beth Bonner and I ran neck and neck; she seemed to take the downhills faster, while the uphills in Central Park came more naturally to me (FIGURE 1). After 14 miles, she picked up the pace and I let her go. I lost sight of her, then saw her again at the 20 mile mark. The closer I came, the faster she went until we passed the finish line. She in 2:55:22 and I in 2:56:04. We became the fastest women marathoners in history.[26]

---

§ *Long Distance Log* is an official publication of the United States Track and Field Federation, published monthly 1957–1975, H. Browning Ross, Editor.

Later that year, under pressure from women runners,¶ the AAU women's hierarchy raised the legal limit to 10 miles. They also decided that selected women would be allowed to run marathons, upon approval of the National Chairman. Selected women were essentially those who had already run marathons, so in effect they went full circle and now approved what they did not allow.

Before 1971 was over the world best toppled again. Cheryl Bridges of California ran a 2:49:40 in Culver City.

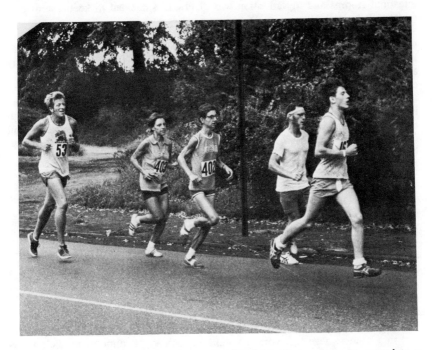

FIGURE 1. Beth Bonner and Nina Kuscsik (left), first women to complete a marathon in under three hours. New York City Marathon, September 19, 1971. (Photo courtesy of Walt Westerholm.)

The word of official status for women marathoners was spread by long distance runners. We determined that if women could be sanctioned for the marathon distance, then race directors could plan to run women's marathons along with the men's. Pat Tarnawsky contacted Will Cloney and on March 30, 1972, he announced that the forthcoming Boston Marathon in April would be the first official Boston Marathon for women.[27]

Eight women stood on the line that eventful day when 76 years after the marathon race was created, the women had one of their own. The women's

¶ Two women marathoners, Pat Tarnawsky and I attended the 1971 AAU Convention.

committee in sanctioning the race stipulated that the women either start at a different place or time than the men.[28]

This was easily enough arranged. We insisted that our newly found friend, Will Cloney, make a separate starting line for us. He extended the starting line over to the sidewalk. Then the women lined up wherever they chose and the race was on.

I was in the lead. After one hour of running time, I realized that I had the best chance of winning. As far as I could determine I should have been able to keep and expand my lead. I passed the half-way mark in 1:27. Then I felt intestinal cramps and my attention was diverted. I decided to keep running no matter what.

I remained unchallenged for the lead, even though my pace dropped. In my wildest fantasies I never thought I would be running through the streets of Boston with diarrhea! As I crossed the finish line, the winner in 3:10:21, my expression did not change. I was determined to find my warm-up outfit and cover up my source of embarrassment.

When the press and live media converged on me for an accounting of the race, I held back the true story. I decided that the press was not mature enough about women in sports to comprehend and broadcast this incident in a tasteful way. My only remark was "the race proved to me that I had guts" (no pun intended).

Overcoming Remaining Obstacles

Even after the widely publicized official status of women at the Boston Marathon, obstacles still had to be overcome.

The 1972 New York City Marathon was scheduled for October 1. Since its inception in 1970, this race had been organized by men and women for men and women. Now Fred Lebow, marathon director, was told by the AAU Women's Committee chairman, Pat Rico, that the women's section must be a separate event that must begin ten minutes before or after the men.[29] We said the race was separate if the women received separate prizes.

The outcome of the event has significance for two reasons. First it became the only event where the women voluntarily added 10 minutes to their times before they even started to run! When the gun went off for them to start, the watches started, but the women sat down behind the starting line and waited for the men's starting gun 10 minutes later.[30]

Second, this discrimination paved the way for a pending human rights lawsuit against the AAU for practicing discrimination in a public place.** On the West Coast of the United States, another lawsuit was also being prepared: The women there were required to produce medical certificates for a marathon race while the men were not.

I traveled to the AAU Convention prepared for a fight. However, at this point the Women's Committee realized it was fighting a losing battle. It not only raised the legal limit of women's running to the marathon distance; it defined that in long distance runs, men and women may start from the same

---

** Human Rights Laws of New York State (Executive Law Sec. 296 sub. 2) and New York City (Administrative Code Sec. BL–7.0 sub. 2).

starting line and from the same starting gun. As long as the women were scored separately and competed for separate prizes, they were considered as competing in a separate event.[31] From that point on, the AAU and women long distance runners have had fairly common goals.

National and International Competition

In October 1973, West Germany became the first country to hold a National Women's Marathon Championship. In the same month, the AAU agreed to legislation sponsored by women runners for the establishment of national championships for women in the marathon distance, and the first United States AAU National Marathon Championship for Women was scheduled for February 1974 in San Mateo, California.

TABLE 1

RESULTS OF THE UNITED STATES AAU WOMEN'S NATIONAL
MARATHON CHAMPIONSHIPS

1974	
Judy Ikenberry	2:55:17
Marilyn Paul	2:58:44
Peggy Lyman	2:58:55
Nina Kuscsik	3:04:11
Lucy Bunz	3:05:07
Marjorie Kaput	3:07:46
1975	
Kim Merritt	2:46:14.8
Miki Gorman	2:53:02.8
Gayle Barron	2:57:22
Joan Ullyot	2:58:30.8
Marilyn Bevans	2:59:19.8
Diane Barrett	3:01:41.4

By this time the world best stood at 2:46:36 run by Miki Gorman of California in the Culver City marathon in December 1973. By running remarkably at age 38, she put new hope into all the women runners who felt their careers were about to fade because of age. (Women felt the same excitement about Miki's performance when in October 1976, at age 41, she ran 2:39:11 in the New York City Marathon).

At that first National Marathon Championship there were 57 starters and 44 finishers. Judy Ikenberry of California was the winner in 2:55:17, and four women broke 3 hours. Mary Etta Boitano, a 10-year-old, ran 3:01:15 (TABLE 1).

The women's running scene has changed. Women now compete in many countries around the world. New marathon runners no longer compete with any consideration of women's rights, but for their own conglomerate of personal reasons.

1975 saw the world best topple three times: from 2:42:24 by Liane Winters of West German, to 2:40:15 by Christa Vahlensieck of the same country, and then to where it stands currently at 2:38:19 by Jacqueline Hansen of the United States (TABLE 2).

The Boston Marathon is now an international race for women (TABLE 3), and even with its qualifying standard of a 3:30 marathon run in the preceding 12 months, the number of starters grows each year. Only the New York City Marathon in 1976 surpassed it with 88 female starters.

In conclusion, our glory lies not only in our accomplishments but in our bright future. An Olympic Marathon for women looms as a reasonable goal. The United States and West Germany boast full national programs. Dr. Van Aaken was responsible for the two international marathons for women only. These events held in September 1974 and October 1976 are the only "women only" marathons to this date (FIGURE 2). Country competes against country for the team title. Eleven countries have participated (TABLE 4). West Germany won the first team title, and the United States the second.

Needed now is participation from even more countries. National programs must be established. We need area championships such as the Pan-American Games to be designated by the IAAF to include women's marathons.

Because we are still battling the misconception that women are physically unfit to run long distances, we need knowledgeable delegates to the International Amateur Athletic Federation to support the international and Olympic marathon concept for women. We need delegates to the International Women's Committee who will promote marathon running, and we need the International Medical Committee to certify to the International Olympic Committee that marathon running is not a detriment to the health of a young woman.

The New York Academy of Sciences Marathon Conference passed the following resolution. It should have far reaching consequences.

TABLE 2

PROGRESSION OF WOMEN'S WORLD BEST PERFORMANCES IN THE MARATHON

1964	3:18:—	Mrs. M. McKenzie, New Zealand
1967	3:15:22.8	Maureen Wilton, Canada
1967	3:07:26.2	Anni Pede-Erdkamp, West Germany
1970	3:02:53	Caroline Walker, USA
1971	3:01:42	Beth Bonner, USA
1971	3:00:35	Sara Berman, USA
1971	2:55:22	Beth Bonner, USA
1971	2:49:40	Cheryl Bridges, USA
1973	2:46:36	Miki Gorman, USA
1974	2:46:24	Chantal Langlace, France
1974	2:43:54	Jacqueline Hansen, USA
1975	2:42:24	Liane Winter, West Germany
1975	2:40:15	Christa Vahlensieck, West Germany
1975	2:38:19	Jacqueline Hansen, USA

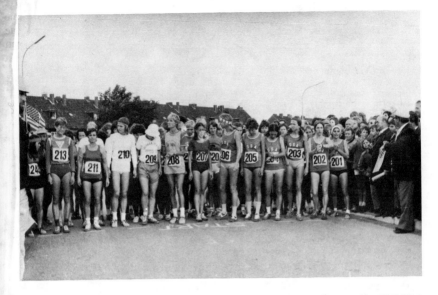

FIGURE 2. Start of the first international marathon for women only in Waldniel, West Germany, September 22, 1974. (Photo courtesy of Franz Leo Mal.)

To: All member countries of the IAAF
     IAAF Continental Associations
     IAAF Women's Committee
     IAAF Technical Committee
     IAAF Cross Country Committee
     IAAF Medical Committee
     IAAF Council
     United States Olympic Committee
     Amateur Athletic Union of the United States

RESOLUTION, which was passed unanimously by over 500 participants and attendees at the New York Academy of Sciences' "Conference on the Marathon: Physiological, Medical, Epidemiological, and Psychological Studies," held in New York City, October 25–28, 1976.

Whereas:

(1) Current research including that presented at this conference demonstrates that female athletes adapt to marathon training and benefit from it, in virtually the same ways male athletes do.
(2) There exists no persuasive scientific or medical evidence, nor has any evidence been presented at this conference that long distance running, in particular, marathon running, is in any way contraindicated for the trained female athlete.

THEREFORE BE IT RESOLVED: That it is the considered judgment of the participants of this conference that a women's marathon event as well as other long distance races for women be included in the Olympic program forthwith.

TABLE 3

PROGRESSION OF WOMEN'S PARTICIPATION IN THE BOSTON MARATHON

1966
Roberta Gibb Bingay, USA	3:21:40

1967
Roberta Gibb Bingay, USA	3:27:17
Kathrine Switzer, USA	4:20:02

1968
Roberta Gibb Bingay, USA	3.40:
Marjorie Fish, USA	4:45:

1969
Sara Berman, USA	3:22:46
Elaine Pederson, USA	3:43:
Nina Kuscsik, USA	3:46:

1970
Sara Berman, USA	3:05:07
Nina Kuscsik, USA	3:12:16
Sandra Zerrangi, USA	3:30:
Diane Fournier, USA	3:32:
Kathrine Switzer, USA	3:34:

1971
Sara Berman, USA	3:08:30
Nina Kuscsik, USA	3:09:00
Kathrine Switzer, USA	3:25:

1972
Nina Kuscsik, USA	3:10:21
Elaine Pederson, USA	3:20:35
Kathrine Switzer, USA	3:29:51
Pat Barrett, USA	3:40:29
Sara Berman, USA	3:48:30
Valerie Rogosheske, USA	4:29:32
Total: 8 women finished, all from USA	

1973
Jacqueline Hansen, USA	3:05:59
Nina Kuscsik, USA	3:06:30
Jenny Taylor, USA	3:16:30
Kathrine Switzer, USA	3:20:30
Sara Berman, USA	3:30:05
Gerda Reinke, West Germany	3:30:20
Total: 11 women finished, from USA and West Germany	

1974 (qualifying standards were established)
Miki Gorman, USA	2:47:11
Christa Kofferschlager, West Germany	2:53:00
Nina Kuscsik, USA	2:55:12
Manuela Preuss, West Germany	2:58:46
Kathrine Switzer, USA	3:01:39
Lydia Ritter, West Germany	3:05:18
Total: 20 women finished from USA, West Germany, and France	

TABLE 3—(*Continued*)

1975

Liane Winter, West Germany	2:42:24
Kathrine Switzer, USA	2:51:37
Gayle Barron, USA	2:54:11
Marilyn Bevans, USA	2:55:52
Merry Cushing, USA	2:56:57
Kathryn Loper, USA	2:59:10

Total: 28 women finished under 3:30 time limit, from West Germany, USA, Japan, and Canada

1976

Kim Merritt, USA	2:47:10
Miki Gorman, USA	2:52:27
Dorothy Doolittle, USA	2:56:26
Gayle Barron, USA	2:58:23
Nancy Kent, USA	3:00:53
Marilyn Bevans, USA	3:01:22

Total: 28 women finished under 3:30 time limit, from USA, Holland, Japan, and West Germany

TABLE 4

PROGRESS OF INTERNATIONAL WOMEN'S MARATHON IN WALDNIEL, WEST GERMANY

September 22, 1974

1. Liane Winter, West Germany	2:50:31.4
2. Chantal Langlace, France	2:51:45.2
3. C. Vahlensieck-Kofferschlager, West Germany	2:54:40.0
4. Manuela Preuss, West Germany	2:55:59.6
5. Jacqueline Hansen, USA	2:56:25.2
6. Joan Ullyot, USA	2:58:09.2

USA, West Germany, France, Holland, Sweden, Austria, and Italy participated; 40 women finished.

October 2, 1976

1. Christa Vahlensieck, West Germany	2:45:24.4
2. Kim Merritt, USA	2:47:11.2
3. Gayle Barron, USA	2:47:43.2
4. Claire Spouwen, Holland	2:47:50.4
5. Manuela Angenvoorth, West Germany	2:48:28.6
6. Sarolta Monspart, Hungary	2:51:23.0

USA, West Germany, France, Holland, Brazil, Hungary, Belgium, Switzerland, and Austria participated; 45 women finished.

References

1. LATHAM, E. ED. 1969. The Poetry of Robert Frost. Holt, Rinehart and Winston. New York, N.Y.
2. FÖLDES, E. 1964. Women at the Olympics. Report of the Fourth Summer Session of the International Olympic Academy. : 105, 113. Olympic, Greece.
3. SHRAKE, E. 1967. A lonely tribe of long-distance runners. Sports Illustrated. Vol. **26:** 56–60.
4. STACK, W. Personal communication.
5. POZZOLI, P. 1969. Doxies of the distances. Distance Running News **4**(No. 5): 22–26.
6. KILLANIN, L. & J. RODDA, Eds. 1976. The Olympic Games. MacMillan Publishing Company. New York, N.Y.
7. STEERS, F. L. 1928. Report of manager of women's track and field team. American Olympic Committee Report, 1928. American Olympic Committee. New York, N.Y.
8. STEWARD, H. E. 1923. International games for women, 1922, Paris. Spalding's Official Athletic Almanac. : 1–R.
9. FERRIS, D. 1976. Personal communication.
10. SEFTON, A. A. 1941. The Women's Division, National Amateur Athletic Federation. Stanford University Press. Stanford, Calif.
11. PELTER, B. 1936. Girl athletes told to shun cocktails and cigarettes. St. Louis Star-Times (December 2).
12. O'HAGAN, A. 1901. Athletic girl. Munsey **25:** 729–38.
13. CHASE, J. Personal communication.
14. ROSS, H. B., Ed. 1962. Long Distance Log **7** (No. 73): 26.
15. ROSS, H. B., Ed. 1964. Long Distance Log **9** (No. 98): 2.
16. CARMAN, B. 1964. Long Distance Log **9** (No. 103): 4.
17. CARMAN, L. Personal communication.
18. BERMAN, S. Personal communication.
19. BINGAY, R. G. Personal communication.
20. BROWN, G. S. 1966. A game girl in a man's game. Sports Illustrated **24:** 67.
21. MIRKIN, G. 1968. The fight to let women run. Distance Running News : 17.
22. THE NEW YORK TIMES. 1967. 2 girls don't have a lovely leg to stand on. (April 20): 55.
23. SWITZER, K. Personal communication.
24. ROSS, H. B., Ed. 1967. Long Distance Log **12** (No. 141): 16.
25. TARNAWSKY, P. 1971. What's this? Women welcome! Runner's World **6** (No. 1): 22, 23.
26. TARNAWSKY, P. 1971. Big day for the ladies. Runner's World. **6** (No. 6): 16, 17.
27. ASSOCIATED PRESS. 1972. Boston marathon adds a division for women. The New York Times (March 30): 50.
28. RICO, P. 1972. Written communication to Will Cloney (February 2).
29. RICO, P. 1972. Written communication to Fred Lebow (August 15).
30. ESKENAZI, G. 1972. In New York's marathon, they also run who only sit and wait. The New York Times (October 2): 39.
31. FOREMAN, K. 1972. Written communication (November 29).

AN OVERVIEW OF OVERUSE SYNDROMES IN DISTANCE RUNNERS

George A. Sheehan

Department of Electrocardiology and Stress Testing
Riverview Hospital
Red Bank, New Jersey 07701

When we hear the word athlete we immediately think of someone who is performing at his maximum, someone who has reached excellence in his chosen sport. And that is indeed the definition proposed by Professor C. T. Mervyn Davies of the London School of Hygiene and Tropical Medicine. The definition of an athlete, said Professor Davies, is someone who makes maximum use of his genetic endowment through training in his environment.

The athlete's formula for excellence therefore is genes plus training plus environment. And this formula, being the source of his excellence, is also the source of his "diseases of excellence," the varieties of overuse syndromes that we will deal with in this session.

The major part of athletic ability is inherent. It has been said that if you wish to be an Olympic champion or a world record holder you must choose your parents well. Roger Bannister said that about one person in a hundred is a motor genius, and added that the limiting factor in performance is the amount of training a person will accept. At that time the implication was that the limit would have to be something acceptable to a person's psyche and to his conception of how he should best live his life. Now it is apparent that the limitation is be the point of breakdown of the organism. Athletes, whether they are motor geniuses or not, simply multiply their training until disability occurs.

Studies show an astounding increase in training since World War II. Nowadays teen-age runners are training at distances unheard of for champion runners in 1930. Running 50 miles a week is now considered quite ordinary and some marathoners regularly run over 200 miles a week. Training includes anaerobic work as well, and this seems to have a special type of stress quite beyond the time and distance put into it.

Finally, the environment, which includes shoes, surfaces, meteorological conductions, diet, sleep, and other day-to-day activities, has contributed more and more into the stresses applied to the athlete. We must therefore take into account the entire milieu of the athlete as well as his training program and constitutional attributes in diagnosing and treating his illnesses.

All this is easily recognizable as the holistic approach to the patient that was urged upon us in medical school. We have gotten away from that approach. But nothing less than it will satisfy in treating the athlete. When he comes into your office you must begin at the beginning and try to know him and how he trains. You must not neglect looking at his shoes, finding what he wears in a race versus what he wears in practice, which side of the road he runs on, and whether he trains on hills or level ground.

These are all vital to the diagnosis and therefore to the treatment. Unless you consider all three aspects, genes, training, and environment, you will probably fail in the treatment of this patient.

But let us go back to the beginning:

These diseases of excellence always (if one can ever say always) begin with an inherent constitutional defect. "There is a crack in everything God made," said Emerson. When you run 100 miles a week you will find that crack. Whatever system breaks down, wherever the athlete begins to give way, there will be behind it some inherent weakness. This can be in any body system, but the musculoskeletal system can be seen as the prototype.

Analyze any runner with an overuse injury of the lower extremity and you will discover he has a structural problem, usually one of the following three:

(1) Biomechanically weak feet. This is usually a Morton's foot with the short big toe and the long second toe. This foot pronates abnormally due to laxity along the first metatarsal segment. Any other pronatory influence can do the same thing, however. The cavus foot is also at hazard.

(2) Leg length discrepancy. Shortening, usually of the nondominant leg, causes a variety of symptoms mainly referable to the low back and upper leg.

(3) Minor abnormalities of the lumbosacral area.

Now the runner with one or more of these constitutional problems superimposes them onto the effects of training. When you train, three things happen to your muscles; two are bad. Training establishes a strength/flexibility imbalance. The prime movers are overdeveloped and get tighter and less flexible. The antagonists become relatively weak. Eventually a muscle pulls. In a weak muscle this occurs in its belly. A strong muscle that pulls usually does so at its musculotendinous junction or at its bony attachment.

But overdeveloped prime movers and weak antagonists do more than pull muscles. They cause further pronation at foot-strike and thereby increase the tendency toward problems in the foot, leg, and knee. At the same time, they increase lordosis at the lumbar area creating low-back and sciatic difficulties.

Finally, the environment comes into play. Some shoes fail to handle impact or the pronatory influences. Slanted surfaces cause increased pronation. Running against traffic, for instance, will increase pronation in the right foot and cause symptoms. Therapeutic orthotics themselves cause difficulty because they overcorrect the inherent constitutional weakness.

At *Runners World* we conducted a poll and over 1000 responded to questions on injuries involving their running. Of the total, 60% said that they had been injured for a considerable length of time. Those injuries and their incidence are shown in TABLE 1. When we analyzed this by age, sex, mileage, and racing or nonracing participation we received the information in TABLE 2.

Unfortunately overuse syndromes in other systems have not been studied quite so closely and have not been so well documented. I know, however, from answering questions from runners over a period of 8 years that the other systems share in this phenomenon.

In the gastrointestinal system the runners' main complaints seem to be cramps, diarrhea, and retrostaltic symptoms. It is my impression that training brings to light underlying, previously asymptomatic tendencies and weaknesses much the same as it does in the musculoskeletal system.

So here we must consider lactase deficiency, gluten sensitivity, irritable colon, weak esophageal sphincter, diverticulitis, and ulcer susceptibility. Anyone of these diseases can be taken from a latent state to active illness by overracing or overtraining.

We know that the some systems have remarkably decreased blood flow during running. The splanchnic flow goes from 25% of the cardiac output at rest

TABLE 1

CHRONIC PROLONGED PROBLEMS REPORTED BY RUNNERS *

Knee	23.2%	Calf	7.0%
Shin	14.6%	Heel	7.0%
Achilles	12.4%	Ankle	6.7%
Forefoot	8.3%	Arch	4.2%
Hip	7.9%	Groin	2.2%
Thigh	7.5%		

* Results of a poll of over 1000 respondents of whom 60% reported prolonged injuries.

to about 3% with vigorous activity. Add dehydration and hypovolemia and you can see how the gastrointestinal system will be a frequent victim of the runners' urge to excellence.

Just so, we can see problems in every other system. The heart is certainly affected. Rhythm disturbances and abnormal EKGs abound. The excess parasympathetic tone leads to an alarming resting bradycardia, to Wenckeback heart block, and probably to Wolff-Parkinson-White patterns. The heart also

TABLE 2

ANALYSIS OF RUNNERS' INJURIES BY AGE, SEX, MILEAGE, AND OTHER FACTORS *

Variable	Injury Rate
Age	
< 19 years old	72%
> 40 years old	57%
Sex	
Female	90%
Male	60%
Mileage	
> 50 miles/wk	73%
< 25 miles/wk	34%
Years Running	
< 5	63%
5–9	52%
> 9	56%
Racing	
Yes	65%
No	27%
Surface	
No difference between hard surface and soft, but more minor problems with hard	

* Result of a poll of over 1000 respondents.

enlarges with the major increase being in end-diastolic volume. Resultant EKGs can sometimes bewilder the physician and wrongly cause him to terminate an athlete's career.

The respiratory system is not exempt. Exercise-induced asthma is a continuing mystery, but probably is due in part to faulty breathing mechanics and air-trapping.

And so it goes. I have seen people run themselves into an agitated depression, develop hematuria, be treated for anemia that appeared as training progresses. This last is a pseudoanemia due to an increase in blood volume that is proportionately more than the increase in hemoglobin.

Finally we are faced with the problems of staleness or exhaustion, the final indignity to the distance runner. Having found this sport and escaped injury, he finds his pursuit of excellence stymied by exhaustion. And he discovers that no one knows exactly what it is or what is the pathophysiology at its root. As yet we have no way of knowing when a runner is exactly at peak and therefore only a razor's edge from disaster.

In summary, the distance runner achieves excellence by making the most of his genetic endowment through training in his environment. This formula for greatness is also the cause of his diseases of excellence. The physician must take a holistic view of this illness and act accordingly.

FOOT TYPES AND THE INFLUENCE OF ENVIRONMENT ON THE FOOT OF THE LONG DISTANCE RUNNER

Richard O. Schuster

Department of Biomechanics
New York College of Podiatric Medicine
New York, New York 10035

FOOT TYPE

It is a recognized fact that some distance runners perform with less difficulty than others. For the most part, this appears to be related to the type of leg and foot structure the individual has inherited. It is also related to the bony relationships within the structure and the environment in which this foot structure functions.

Just as there are various normal body types, there are various normal foot types. These are the high arched feet (cavus), the low arched feet (planus), and the average feet, which are somewhere in between. Each foot type has slightly different functional characteristics that can be important to the runner.

The High Arched Foot

The high arched foot is usually a relatively rigid foot. Its joint ranges are usually less than average. It is usually associated with a tight calf muscle and usually has a tight long plantar ligament. It also has a relatively small weightbearing pattern. All this means that the foot is susceptible to a number of conditions including tendinitis, fasciitis, heel pains, pressure concentrations, and impact shock. The high arched foot type requires flexibility exercises, particularly for the short calf muscle. It functions best in a running shoe with a heel that is considerably thicker than the sole.

The high arched foot appears to serve the short distance runner better than the long distance runner.

The Low Arched Foot

The low arched foot is usually a relatively flexible foot. Its joint ranges are usually more than average. It has a relatively large weightbearing pattern, which means that impact shock and pressure areas are less of a problem.

The low arched foot appears to be somewhat less prone to injuries and serves the distance runner better than the sprinter.

Common Leg and Foot Imbalances

To be relatively free of difficulty, distance running requires ideal structural makeup. Ideal structure may be described in terms of Newtonian principles of equilibrium. Stated simply: Bony structures that are vertical should be perfectly vertical and those that are horizontal should be perfectly horizontal.

However, anthropologists agree that most individuals do not have ideal leg and foot structure and have not yet completely adapted to the function of bipedal walking and running.[1] Most—but not all—individuals carry within their structures bony slants and curves related to their evolutionary and fetal development. These may be tolerable under ordinary conditions but are not ideal for the extreme requirements of long distance running. Slants and curves in the bones of the leg and foot tend to tilt or unbalance the foot away from its parallel relationship to the ground. Under weight, these unbalanced feet may be forced down to the horizontal surface through the flattening process of abnormal pronation. The effect of this becomes particularly understandable when one realizes that a runner takes almost 1000 steps a mile and that the forces going through the foot and leg are sometimes equal to two and three times body weight.[2, 3] When all this is multiplied by as many as 26 miles or more, it can constitute serious depressing trauma to the running foot.

Once structural imbalances are recognized, much of the flattening process of abnormal pronation can be prevented.

There are three major types of leg and foot situations that can be recognized as imbalances. They involve the tibia (the long bone of the lower leg), the rearfoot, and the forefoot. These imbalances are usually situations where the lower end of one of these parts tilts toward the body midline. These are known as varus situations. (The opposite of varus situations are valgus situations, which are less common and will not be discussed.)

Varus Influence of the Tibia

This is a slant or bow of the tibia in which the lower part tilts toward the body midline. Ideally, the tibia should be straight. Varus influence may be noted by frontal observation.

Varus influence of the tibia is not an optimum situation for running since it places the running foot on the lateral side in the initial contact phase of the step. This foot may then go through an abnormal flattening process to make full contact.

Rearfoot Varus Foot Type

This is a torsion or curve in the heel (calcaneus) wherein the lower part of the heel slants toward the body midline. These variations can be recognized by having the individual lay face down on the table or kneel on a chair so that the back of the dependent heel may be observed. In the ideally normal foot, the rearfoot will rest in line with the leg, whereas the varus rearfoot will curve inward. A bisection line on the lower leg and heel will help to illustrate this deflection.

As with other varus situations, the varus heel tends to tilt the foot to the lateral side at the contact phase of the running step. Under weight, this foot may have to depress abnormally to reach the horizontal surface.

There is another serious problem relating to the varus type heel situation. The ideally normal heel can move inward and outward (invert and evert). In the varus heel, most, or all of the motion, is in the inward direction only. This means that the major amount of motion in the varus rearfoot type is inversion— a spraining type motion which does, in fact, encourage ankle sprains. Outward motion may have to come from other joints less adapted for this motion and may lead to a multiplicity of symptoms such as pains in the ankles, knees, groin, and hips.

Forefoot Varus Foot Type

This can be easily recognized by noting how the plane of the relaxed forefoot relates to the vertical axis of the heel while the individual is in the prone or kneeling position. In the ideal situation, the forefoot is perpendicular to the rearfoot.

When a varus attitude of the forefoot exists, the inner side of the forefoot is elevated. The effect of this on the function of the foot may be appreciated if one compares the foot to a tripod. If one leg of the tripod is shortened, the device will tilt toward the short side. The foot depresses on the varus side until the under surface of the foot is on the horizontal plane.

The Total Picture of Leg and Foot Imbalances

There is an accumulative aspect to imbalances of the leg and foot. While individual variations may be slight, the total influence on foot attitude may be significant. Also, since the depressions secondary to varus attitudes are not likely to be the same on both sides, there is always the possibility of one side depressing more than the other, thereby inviting symptoms of unilateral short leg. Thirdly, rotary situations occur when a foot depresses out of a varus attitude. These rotary situations involve the total leg. All these may become highly significant with the overuse of distance running. A suggestion of type and severity of imbalance may be obtained by noting shoe wear patterns.

It might be interesting to note that the average amount of imbalance per individual found among members of an eastern university track team was under 7 degrees per foot. In a comparison with a similar group of runner patients, the average amount of varus was over 11 degrees per foot. The implications are obvious.

One can obtain an approximate idea of total leg and foot imbalance by having the individual stand and placing the rearfoot in its neutral position. This is easily accomplished by placing the thumb and index fingers in the depressions just below and slightly in front of the inner and outer ankle prominences (the subtalar joint). Then maneuver the heel in and out until the joint under the fingers feels the same on both sides. This is neutral subtalar position. If leg and foot imbalances exist, part of the forefoot will come off the horizontal surface. The space under the elevated forefoot represents approximately the total amount of imbalance.

The Direction of Care for Leg and Foot Imbalances

The management of leg and foot imbalances consists of filling the space between the neutral foot and the horizontal surface. This can be accomplished in an oversimplified sense, by wedging or canting that part of the undersurface of the running shoe with soling material. A more practical approach is to place within the running shoe a foot formed insert that fills the gap between the neutral foot and the horizontal surface.

ENVIRONMENT

The foot environment of the runner is frequently a changing situation, which at times may be incompatible with the runner's structure.

Surface Hardness

Distance runners can appreciate the difference in accumulated impact shock between concrete surfaces and other surfaces. Concrete surfaces, of course, are the least desirable. Softer surfaces are generally preferred because they dampen impact shock. However, pot holes and other obstructions of softer surfaces can bring on problems.

There is now reason to believe that some stress fractures are due to accumulated impact shock which, of course, is more profound on the hard surfaces—this is in addition to the usual causes of stress fractures.

The problem of hard running surfaces can be managed by interposing soft inserts or soft-soled shoes between the foot and the hard surface.

Unusual soft running surfaces can also cause problems. Soft sand, for instance, can invite Achilles' tendinitis and other problems by allowing the heel to sink.

There are a few running shoes on the market that have unusually soft soles. While they have the advantage of absorbing shock, they have the disadvantage of permitting the foot to sink unevenly into the shoe—usually in a pronated manner.

Surface Friction

Low friction surfaces such as those that are wet or icy, are a major cause of muscle and ligament pulls. Of these, hamstring and groin pulls are the most common. In the case of groin pulls, the injury is usually not recognized until after the run.

Slanted Surfaces

The foot is an adapting mechanism. However, as already noted, some runners do not have the available range of motion in the foot to adapt to surfaces that slant the foot in an outward direction. This becomes a problem when running on beaches, banked tracks, and on the sides of crowned roads. The average road has a drainage slant of 7 to 9 degrees which is often more than some runners can adapt to. Running on such surfaces with an unaccommodating subtalar joint can force abnormal compensation.

Runners with unilateral imbalances will often find that one side of the road is more difficult to run on.

Problems related to slanted running surfaces can be helped with the use of balancing shoe wedges or inserts which put the foot in a more adaptable position.

Hill Running

Uphill running is particularly stressful to runners with short calf muscles, tight Achilles' tendons, tight plantar ligaments, and shin splints. Downhill running is particularly stressful to runners with knee problems. Balancing foot devices plus extra heel lifts are helpful in these situations.

Indoor Running

Running indoors is usually hard surface running. The effect of this has already been mentioned. A more serious aspect of indoor running is the fact that the runner may have to make as many as 36 turns a mile. This means that, in a sense, much of the indoor running is done in a slanted fashion, which interferes with the mechanism of normal running. Many indoor running facilities are alternating the direction of running traffic on a daily basis.

Width in Running Shoes

While there is a wide variety of widths of feet, most running shoes are available in only one width. This adds to the usual traumas of running. Fortunately, some manufacturers are beginning to produce running shoes in a variety of widths.

Heel Width

For several years, many running shoes have been made with heels narrower than the heels of the foot. At best, these heels are unstable and at worst they invite sprains and other problems. Fortunately, there is now a trend to make heels of running shoes at least as wide as the heels of the foot and in some cases even wider. However, narrow heeled shoes are still being sold.

Shoe Stiffness

There is a tendency for some running shoes to be made extremely stiff at the ball area. Some of these shoes require as much as 26 pounds of pressure to bend at the ball—the area that corresponds to the most flexible part of the foot. With the prolonged use of these shoes, runners frequently develop calf pains, which are relieved by loosening the sole with transverse cuts or by obtaining a shoe that bends easily at the ball.

Tread Design

Tread designs on soles of running shoes do not, as a rule, create problems, except when the design is rough and the sole is thin. Heavier runners are more likely to feel the roughness and the problem is easily solved by changing to a smoother or thicker soled shoe.

Running Shoes and the Large Runner

For heavy or otherwise large runners, some running shoes, on a comparative basis, are relatively skimpy—little more than the equivalent of bedroom slippers. For this reason, some large runners have found that work boots or other sturdy shoes are more suitable for their particular running needs.

Runners Nail

A frequent problem among runners is damaged toe nails due to pressure from the end of the shoe. This usually occurs to the longest toe or toes. Obviously, this can be caused by short shoes. However, from a shoefitting point of view, the outlook is not necessarily optimistic. Some feet tend to slide forward in even the best fitted shoes. The shoe stops its forward motion at contact and the foot continues forward some small distance after the shoe has stopped. The amount of forward slipping depends on a number of factors including the thickness of soft tissue on the undersurface of the foot. If an adequately fitting shoe does not reduce the occurrence of damaged toenails, the problem can usually be helped by making a one inch vertical cut in the leather strip over the first and second toes. Fortunately, most running shoes have a leather strip in this area.

Warmups

Patient files indicate that people who run in the morning have a higher incidence of injuries than those who run later in the day. Obviously, morning running requires more warmup time. Also, morning runners generalize that the need to get the day started takes away from warmup time.

Records also indicate that more people develop injuries in colder weather. There is now a trend to warm troublesome parts with heat applications for 10 to 15 minutes before a run.

Records also indicate that the large runner requires different warmups than the smaller runner. Big runners appear to do better with a walk that accelerates into a jog rather than the usual calisthenic warmups.

Leg Length Discrepancies

Records of running patients indicate that leg length discrepancies as small as $3/16$ of an inch, which would be ignored in an ordinary individual, may produce symptoms of leg shortness in runners. The long leg appears to show the effect of the added pounding, especially in the area of the knee. This problem can be easily managed by elevating the short leg with a lift on the outside or the inside of the shoe.

REFERENCES

1. KROGMAN, W. M. 1951. The Scars of Human Evolution. Sci. Amer. December.
2. SCHUSTER, R. O. 1976. Impact Loading in Running. 4th Annual Sports Medicine Seminar. California College of Podiatric Medicine, San Francisco.
3. MANN, R. 1975. American Academy of Orthopedic Surgery. 42nd Annual Conference, San Francisco, March.

A BIOMECHANICAL APPROACH TO RUNNING INJURIES

Steven I. Subotnick

19682 Hesperian Boulevard
Hayward, California 94541

INTRODUCTION

The foot is a marvelous structure designed to adapt to varying surfaces as well as to offer support and rigidity during jogging and running activities. The foot is responsible for accepting all of the rotations occurring from the hip down to the knee, leg, and foot. The foot must convert these rotations into meaningful forward motion. An injury anywhere in the lower extremity may originate at the foot. Long distance running injuries are often caused by a foot fault. An understanding of some basic principles helps the runner avoid these injuries.

BIOMECHANICS

The term biomechanics is now in vogue. This, simply, means the mechanics of function, in this case, the function of the lower extremity in running. The key term in Biomechanics is neutral position (FIGURES 1 & 2).[1-7] The neutral position is the situation that exists when the foot is stable. A neutral foot can support body weight, when both feet are on the ground, without the help of muscles or ligaments. In other words, the integrity of the bones and joints of the foot supports the weight of the body. Obviously, when the foot is neutral there is a normal arch, which is not too high or low. The foot is neither pronated (low-arched) or supinated (high-arched). The heel bone (calcaneus) is about perpendicular to the floor and parallel to the lower one-third of the leg. The metatarsal heads are resting on the ground and the plane of the metatarsal heads is perpendicular to the long axis of the calcaneus. In other words, when the calcaneus is straight up and down the foot is on the ground with a normal arch; the foot is neutral. Research using motion-analyzing films indicates that the foot must be neutral just prior to the time that the heel leaves the ground. When this situation does not exist, the muscles of the lower extremity work overtime, a stable propulsion is impossible, and there is an increased torque upon the leg, which results in overuse injury of the lower extremity.[8]

THE NEUTRAL FOOT

You can roughly tell what your neutral foot position is by planting your foot on the ground and externally rotating your leg, causing your knee cap to point outwards, until your calcaneus is about perpendicular to the floor and parallel to the lower one-third of your leg (FIGURE 1). This position may feel awkward but, you will notice that your arch appears much more normal.[3, 6-8]

FIGURE 1. Diagram of the bones of the normal (neutral) foot and leg. (After Subotnick.[37])

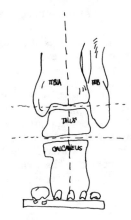

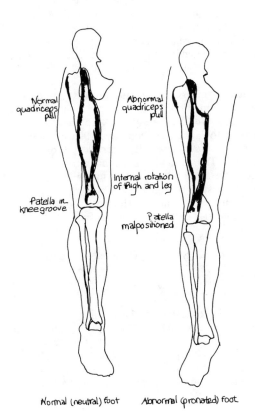

FIGURE 2. Diagram showing the neutral foot compared with the pronated foot. (After Subotnick.[37])

RELATIONSHIP BETWEEN THE FOOT AND LEG

The normal foot contacts the running surface on the outside of the heel, then quickly rolls inward (everts), to adapt to surface changes (FIGURE 2).[8, 9] This is called contact pronation. Contact pronation is normal for proper foot function. The foot is relatively unstable at heel contact to allow the foot to absorb stress.[4, 7] This is desirable. The foot must then quickly become more rigid (resupinate) to the extent that it is neutral prior to heel-off and rigid prior to toe-off. The foot is, thusly, a rigid lever at toe-off.[8]

Various structural abnormalities of the leg and foot result in prolonged pronation,[5, 7] in other words, if the foot never recovers from being relatively unstable at heel contact. The foot then never becomes a rigid lever at toe-off. Running is inefficient and overuse injury is more likely to occur.

OVERUSE INJURY

Overuse injuries include runner's knee, shin splints, stress fractures, Achilles' tendonitis, runner's heel bumps, heel spurs, arch fatigue, pain and cramps, neuromas, and boney deformity of the foot such as bunions and hammer-toes.[6, 7, 10-14] These injuries usually start off slowly and gradually increase in severity. They may be related to a sudden increase in mileage, a change in running terrain, improper shoes,[15] inflexibility of the body and mind, or faulty biomechanical structure.[16]

General preventative measures for the overuse syndrome depend upon proper training, proper conditioning, and proper biomechanical structure.[7]

Training should allow for hard–easy workout sessions on varying surfaces with shoes that provide for adequate shock absorbence. Train don't strain.[3]

Conditioning depends upon flexibility exercises before and even more important, after running. The muscles in the back of the thigh and leg (anti-gravity muscles) must be stretched. Muscles in the front of the thigh, leg and foot (gravity muscles) must be strengthened.[7, 17]

Biomechanical control is obtained through the use of functional foot orthotics made from a neutral cast of the athletes foot.[6, 7]

CARE OF SPECIFIC OVERUSE INJURIES

The Hip

Injuries about the hip, or even low back injuries, may be secondary to a limb length inequality (FIGURE 3).[18] The hip is prone to bursitis over the outside protruberance (greater trochanter), and at times the outside supportive tissue (iliotibial band) may snap. Ice and exercise may help this problem as well as limiting runs to level surfaces. Orthotics are sometimes helpful but usually resistant pain is in need of orthopedic consultation.[19]

The Thigh

Bursitis may be present between tendon bands deep in the thigh. These must be differentiated from tendon strains.[20] Pain is present with exercise and pressure. Treatment consists of limiting activity, ice massage ten minutes a day following activity, and evaluation by a medical practitioner with an interest in sports medicine.

Sciatica

Sciatica is a most disabling problem that results in pain radiating from the low back to the inside of the thigh down the leg. It is more pronounced with straight leg raises done while laying on the back. It appears to be aggravated by pronounced pronation of the foot and may be caused by a short leg syndrome.[18] There may be pain present beneath the muscles of the buttocks, which is aggravated by climbing or running up hills. Orthotics definitely help this problem as well as stretching exercises and back exercises.

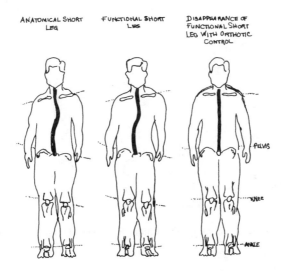

FIGURE 3. Limb length inequality. (After Subotnick.[37])

The Knee

Runner's knee plagues joggers and long distance runners as well as basketball players and jumpers. This syndrome is responsible for sidelining some of the most promising athletes.

Runner's knee may be any one, or a combination of factors: chondromalacia of the knee, patellar (knee cap) compression, patellar subluxation (FIGURE 4) or patellar tendonitis (jumper's knee). The syndrome may also include collateral ligament strain or snapping iliotibial bands. At times, even the cartilage of the knee joint itself (the meniscus) may be damaged.[7, 14, 19, 21–25]

Most runner's knee problems are related to improper foot function.[7, 14] As the foot abnormally pronates, and becomes excessively mobile with the arch flattening, the leg internally rotates. The thigh also internally rotates but, the foot is fixed on the ground and cannot turn in. This allows for an unstable patella and results in runner's knee.

Characteristically, there is a cracking sensation beneath the patella with excessive bending or flexion of the knee. Pain is present when walking up and down stairs, working the clutch of a car, or upon rising after sitting for a period of time. Hill running, especially downhill, aggravates the pain.

Treatment consists of exercises to build up and strengthen the muscles that stabilize the knee, the quadriceps and hamstrings. Straight leg raises and side leg raises, 20 times per leg, carried out twice a day, utilizing from a 2 to 5 pound weight, are helpful. Isometric exercises holding each contraction of these muscles for 20 seconds each are called quad sets and are of extreme benefit. The runner must avoid hills, and shoes should be in good repair. Foot orthotics are necessary. The main purpose of the foot orthotic is to provide stability at the knee by reducing independant rotation between the leg and foot,

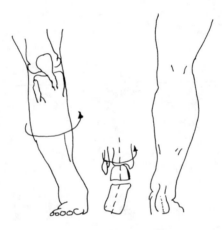

FIGURE 4. Lateral patellar subluxations compensating for tibial torsion. (After Subotnick.[37])

which occurs with excessive pronation. It appears as though orthotics encourage the runner to run more adducted. Thus, the foot and leg rotate inward and stabilize the knee cap. This provides for a straight line pull between the quadriceps, patella and patellar tendon.[7, 19]

Stress Fractures

Stress fractures are difficult to detect. They may not show up on initial X rays but will be present from 6 to 8 weeks following an injury. Persistent pain suggests stress fractures and activity must be limited. Medical supervision is suggested. An example of this is pain on the outside ankle bone that does not appear to be shin splints and does not respond to normal shin splint treatment. This may well be a stress fracture of the fibula and responds to rest for approximately 6 weeks. Stress fractures are also common in the metatarsal bones of the foot. They respond to resting the foot for 3 weeks following which the athlete may begin running again providing the foot is taped for an additional 3 weeks.[7]

The Leg

Three problems occur within the leg in regards to running. Shin splints, Achilles tendonitis and strains, and stress fractures.

Shin splints is a catch all term which encompasses inflammation of the bone (periostitis), inflammation of the muscle (myositis), or inflammation of the tendons (tendonitis).[7, 26]

The muscles in the front of the leg are more commonly involved with running on hard surfaces or hills. Weak muscles contribute to the problem. Overstriding aggravates this problem, which is called anterior shin splints. Anterior shin splints occurs with pain in the front of the leg at the beginning of the track season.

Treatment consists of exercising to strengthen the anterior muscles. In addition, the runner must stretch the Achilles' tendon. It is important to utilize ice following a running session on sore muscles for approximately 10 minutes. Workouts on softer surfaces help this problem. Foot orthotics as well as taping may be useful. Persistent or progressive swelling or pain is in need of immediate medical attention and may indicate a stress fracture or a tight muscle compartment.[27]

The muscles located on the inside of the leg are called the flexors and also include the posterior tibial tendon and muscles. They are prone to overuse injuries secondary to abnormal pronation of the foot. This is also a form of shin splints. Treatment consists of icing as well as foot orthotics. The results are quite good.

The Achilles' tendon may be injured secondary to improper flexibility exercises. Stretching is very important both before and after workouts. Hill running aggravates the problem of Achilles' tendonitis. Toe-dash runners should change their gait to a heel-foot-toe or foot-toe stride. Icing, stretching, and heel lifts are sometimes very effective in treating this problem.

Resistant and chronic tendonitis may be aggravated by abnormal heel roll which occurs with abnormal or excessive pronation of the foot. In these cases foot orthotics help. Persistent cases require the attention of a sports minded podiatrist or orthopedist.

When excessive swelling of the tendon sheath is present this may represent a tenosynovitis and is in need of medical attention. When excessive swelling of the tendon itself is present, this may represent a tendon strain or partial rupture, in which case, the tendon itself, has been injured and this requires immediate medical attention.

The Ankle

The ankle is involved with recurrent sprains as well as boney arthritis secondary to overuse.

Recurrent sprains suggest a need for stabilizing foot orthotics as well as taping before athletic events that occur on uneven surfaces or which involve excessive motion from side to side, such as football.[13, 28-30] Rehabilitative exercises to build up ankle flexibility and strength are very helpful. Limitations of ankle flexion secondary to boney spurs can be disabling and may require surgical intervention. Pain is usually present in the front of the ankle when this problem is involved.[7]

The Foot

A myriad of overuse injuries occur in the foot. The initial treatments of all foot injuries begin with establishing proper foot function with foot orthotics. Of course, a proper diagnosis must be arrived at. As with all injuries proper training and conditioning is outlined. Let us review the more common foot injuries.

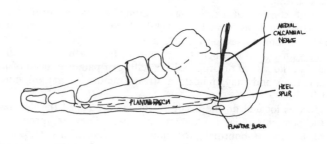

FIGURE 5. Heel spurs. (After Subotnick.[37])

Heel Spurs

Heel spurs (FIGURE 5) cause pain on the bottom of the foot where the arch meets the heel. An actual boney spur is present and this is noticed on X rays. This is often surrounded by soft tissue damage and bursitis. Orthotics as well as cortisone injections are helpful and usually resolve this problem. Low-dye taping and felt padding are helpful.[7] In resistant cases surgery may be indicated.

Heel Neuromas

Heel pain located in the center of the heel may be due to a heel bruise with secondary formation of a benign nerve enlargement. Treatment consists of injections of the traumatic neuroma as well as foot orthotics. A felt pad with an aperature may help. Surgery may be required, but usually no bone resection is necessary and recovery is rapid.[7]

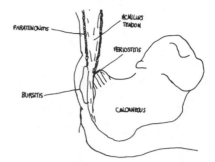

FIGURE 6. Retrocalcaneal exostosis (runner's bump). (After Subotnick.[37])

Runner's Bumps

Runner's bumps (retrocalcaneal exostosis) (FIGURES 6–8) occur beneath the Achilles' tendon on the outer back surface of the calcaneus.[31] This problem is aggravated by excessive heel roll at foot contact. Runners who are bow-legged or land excessively on the outside of their heel, are more prone to this problem. Foot orthotics with a rearfoot control help greatly with this problem. If bursitis is present, an injection of cortisone may handle the problem readily. Excessive boney projections may require surgical excision.

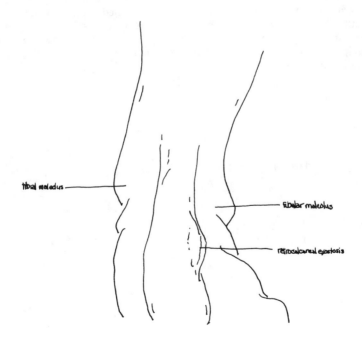

FIGURE 7. Retrocalcaneal exostosis, rear view. (After Subotnick.[37])

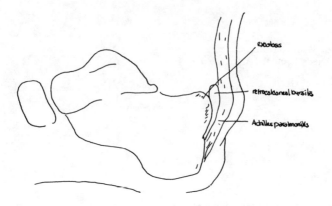

Arch Pain

Arch pain is often secondary to a fascia (FIGURE 9) or muscle strain, or a nerve entrapment. Pain more prevalent at toe-off suggests plantar fascial strain. Pain with pressure beneath the inner ankle bone, which radiates and is sharp, indicates nerve compression. This is called a tarsal tunnel syndrome (FIGURE 10). This may be accompanied by a tight muscle at the inner aspect of the arch. Taping, orthotics, and level-surface running at slow speeds appear to help. At times an injection of cortisone is necessary along with these other modalities.[7]

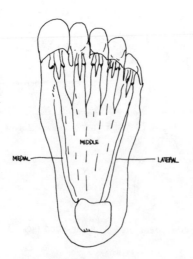

FIGURE 9. The plantar fascia. (After Subotnick.[37])

Bunions, Hammertoes, and Plantar Callouses

Boney deformity of the foot is either congenital or secondary to improper foot function. Foot function must be normal in order to help control these problems. These are problems that you should consult your podiatrist about.[32-36]

Shoes

Shoes are merely a covering for the foot. They protect the foot from the running surface, absorb shock, and grip the running surface. They do not, however, control abnormal pronation or offer any significant foot support. This has been amply demonstrated by motion analyzing films of runners.

A good training shoe should have two to three layers of various thicknesses and firmness of rubber, which provides resistance to wear, shock absorbance,

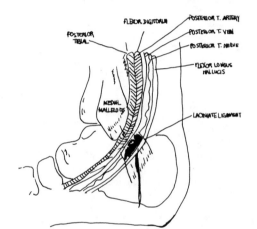

FIGURE 10. Tarsal tunnel syndrome. (After Subotnick.[37])

and stability. There must be ample room for the toes and a rounded toe box. The heel counter should be high enough to well grip the heel and prevent heel slippage. This also facilitates placing an orthotic within the shoe.

The running shoe must have an elevated heel of moderate degree. Attempts at running with a negative heel shoe have been disasterous. The role of the shoe should be thick, yet flexible at the junction of the ball of the foot to the toes. Nylon uppers are lighter and may be washed. Leather uppers can be stretched and water-proofed. Soles should be periodically repaired and a glue gun greatly helps in guarding against excessive shoe wear.[15]

SUMMARY

I have introduced the concept of controlling overuse syndromes by controlling the etiology. The etiology of most overuse syndromes is biomechanical deformity of the lower extremity as well as nonadherence to sound principles of training and conditioning. It is important to realize these factors to provide for many years of injury-free athletic involvement.

REFERENCES

1. ROOT, M. L., W. ORIEN, J. H. WEED & R. J. HUGHS. 1971. Biomechanical examination of the foot. *In* Clinical Biomechanics Corp. Vol. 1. Los Angeles, Calif.
2. SGARLATO, T. E. 1971. A Compendium of Podiatric Biomechanics. California College of Podiatric Medicine. San Francisco, Calif.
3. SUBOTNICK, S. I., Ed. 1975. Athlete's Feet. Runner's World Publications. Mountain View, Calif.
4. SUBOTNICK, S. I. 1971. The equinus deformity as it effects the forefoot. J. Amer. Pod. Assoc. **61:** 423–427.
5. SUBOTNICK, S. I. 1973. The flexible flatfoot. *In* Arch. Pod. Med. Foot Surg. **1(1):** 7–33.
6. SUBOTNICK, S. I. 1975. Orthotic foot control in the overuse syndrome. Phys. Sportsmed. 3(1): 75–79.
7. SUBOTNICK, S. I. 1975. The abuses of orthotics in sports medicine. Phys. Sportsmed. 3(7).
8. SUBOTNICK, S. I. 1974. The overuse syndrome of the foot and leg. Part II. Symposium, California College of Podiatric Medicine. San Francisco, Calif.
9. JAMES, S. L. & C. E. BRUBAKER. 1973. Biomechanics of running. Orthoped. Amer. 4(3): 605–616.
10. SYMPOSIUM ON SPORTS MEDICINE. 1969. American Academy of Orthopedic Surgeons. C. V. Mosby Co. St. Louis, Mo.
11. BRUBAKER, T. E. & S. L. JAMES. 1974. Injuries to runners. *In* Laboratory for Human Performance, University of Oregon.
12. CORRIGAN, A. B. & K. E. FITCH. 1972. Complications of jogging. Med. J. Austral. : 363.
13. O'DONOGHUE, D. H. 1975. Treatment of Injuries to Athletes. 2nd edit. W. B. Saunders Co. Philadelphia, Pa.
14. SHEEHAN, G. M. 1972. Chondromalacia in runners. Amer. College Sports Med. Newslett. 7(4).
15. SUBOTNICK, S. I. 1973. Shoes and injuries in shoes for runners. *In* Runner's World Booklet of the Month. Vol. **25:** 70–71.
16. SUBOTNICK, S. I. 1974. Morton's foot. Runner's World **94.**
17. DUVRIES, H. L. 1966. Physiology of Exercises for Physical Education and Athletics. William Brown & Co. St. Louis, Mo.
18. SUBOTNICK, S. I. 1974. Long legs, short legs. Runner's World **9:** 21–22.
19. JAMES, S. L. 1975. Personal communications.
20. CRAIG, T. T. 1973. Comments in sports medicine. J. Amer. Med. Assoc. **231:** 333.
21. BLAZINA, M. E., R. K. KERLAN, F. W. JOBE, V. S. CARTER & G. CARLSON. 1973. Jumper's knee. *In* Orthopedic Clinics of Northern America. Vol. 4 (3): 665–678.
22. KLINE, C. & F. L. ALMAN, JR. 1969. The Knee in Sports. Jenkins Publishing Co. The Premerton Press. Austin, Texas.
23. NICHOLAS, J. A. 1975. Injuries to the menisci of the knee. Orthoped. Clinic N. Amer. 4(3): 647–664.
24. O'DONOGHUE, D. H. 1975. Treatment of acute ligamentous injuries of the knee. *In* Orthoped. Clinic N. Amer. 4(3): 617–645.
25. SLOCUM, D. B., R. L. LARSON & S. L. JAMES. 1975. Late reconstruction procedures used to stabilize the knee. Orthoped. Clinic N. Amer. 4(3): 679–689.
26. JACKSON, D. W. & D. BAILEY. 1975. Shin splints in the young white: A nonspecific diagnosis. Phys. Sportsmed. 3(3): 45–51.

27. SUBOTNICK, S. I. 1975. Compartment syndromes in the lower extremities. J. Amer. Pod. Assoc. 65(4): 342–347.
28. CERNEY, J. P. A Complete Book of Athletic Taping Techniques. Parker Publishing Inc. West Nyack, N.Y.
29. JOHNSON & JOHNSON. 1958. Therapeutic Uses of Adhesive Tape. 2nd edit. New Brunswick, N.J.
30. NELLEN, J. W. 1968. Medicine and the Green Bay Packers. Upjohn Co.
31. SUBOTNICK, S. I. 1973. Why bumps grow. Runner's World : 24–30.
32. DUVRIES, H. L. 1964. Surgery of the Foot. C. V. Mosby Co. St. Louis, Mo.
33. GERBERT, J., et al. 1974. The Surgical Treatment of the Intractable Plantar Keratoma. : 247. Futura Publishing Co. Mt. Kisco, N.Y.
34. GERBERT, J., O. A. MERCADO & T. H. SOKOLOFF. 1975. The Surgical Treatment of the Hallux-Abducto-Valgus and Allied Deformities. : 140. Futura Publishing Co. Mt. Kisco, N.Y.
35. GERBERT, J., T. E. SGARLATO & S. I. SUBOTNICK. 1972. Preliminary study of a closing wedge osteotomy of the fifth metatarsal for correction of tailor's bunion deformity. J. Amer. Pod. Assoc. 62: 212–218.
36. SUBOTNICK, S. I. Observations of plantar callouses. Arch. Pod. Med. Foot Surg. 1(4): 329–337.
37. SUBOTNICK, S. I. 1975. Podiatric Sports Medicine. Futura Publishing Co. Mt. Kisco, N.Y.

ASSESSMENT OF CARDIAC FUNCTION IN MARATHON RUNNERS BY GRAPHIC NONINVASIVE TECHNIQUES

Samuel Zoneraich, Jai J. Rhee,
Olga Zoneraich, David Jordan, and
Jesse Appel

*State University of New York at Stony Brook
Clinical Campus at Queens Hospital Center
Jamaica, New York 11432*

The marathon runner's heart may simulate a diseased heart by exhibiting abnormal clinical findings, electrocardiographic abnormalities, and cardiac enlargement by X ray. Evidence gathered to date indicates the wide range of these findings in marathon runners. Radiologic documentation of an enlarged heart, however, is a poor indicator of the histologic and gross anatomic changes of the heart. The true significance of the electrocardiographic anomalies requires further clarification.

The purposes of this study were (1) to elucidate many of the common findings in marathon runners, (2) to assess their clinical value, (3) to report new and poorly recognized graphic findings, and (4) to explain the genesis of such abnormal graphic findings by employing a battery of noninvasive graphic techniques, such as echocardiogram, apexcardiogram, carotid pulse, electrocardiogram, vectorcardiogram, phonocardiogram, systolic time intervals, and treadmill stress testing.

SUBJECTS AND METHODS

Subjects

Twelve marathon runners participated as subjects in the study. The subjects had finished a marathon race in less than 3 hours. Testing was completed in the postabsorptive state on nonrunning days. The pretest characteristics of the subjects are presented in TABLE 1.

Data Collection

All data were collected in an air-conditioned laboratory (20°–21° C, 40%–50% relative humidity). Anthropometric data were obtained prior to the test run. Estimates of body fat were determined from three skinfold measures utilizing regression equations;[1] body surface area (BSA, m²) was calculated from a regression equation using standing height and body weight[2]; and resting heart rates and blood pressure were obtained.

The exercise tolerance test included a 5-minute warm-up and an 8–10 minute run (test run). For the warm-up all runners began walking a 4.83 kilometers per hour at 0% elevation. The speed was increased each minute by 1.61 km/hr. Following the warm-up, the treadmill speed was set at the approximate average marathon pace for each runner (range 13.7–16.1 km/hr). The elevation was 0%. At the end of each two minutes the elevation was increased by 2.5% until the runner voluntarily terminated the run.

Electrocardiograms were obtained from a single lead (V_5), and recorded with an 8-channel polygraph, and monitored continuously on a single channel oscilloscope. Exercise cardiograms were recorded for 5 seconds during each 30 seconds of the test. The shortest R-R intervals for each phase were used for calculating heart rates.[3]

Blood pressures were recorded utilizing an automatic cycling cuff pump, an electronic monitoring system, and a polygraph. During the last 5 seconds of each test stage, the cuff was inflated. Blood pressure measurement began as soon as the runner stepped off the treadmill. Systolic and diastolic pressures were read from the polygraph record. Estimated myocardial oxygen consumption ($M\dot{V}_{O_2}$) was calculated using a two-factor regression equation.[4]

TABLE 1

CHARACTERISTICS OF MARATHON RUNNERS

Variables	Mean	SD *
Age (yr)	38.7	10.12
Height (cm)	176.8	5.25
Weight (kg)	64.3	5.33
Systolic Blood pressure (mmHg)	123.5	3.91
Diastolic blood pressure (mmHg)	81.0	6.63
Heart rate (bpm)	50.6	5.10
Est. body fat (%)	5.5	1.60
Body surface area (m²)	1.80	.098
Training level (miles/wk)	75.8	16.8

* Standard deviation.

Pulmonary Function

Pulmonary function (TABLE 2) measures were obtained prior to the test run and during the test. At rest a milliliter respirometer was used. During the test, expired air was collected in 150–300 liter meteorological balloons during the last 60 seconds of each test stage. When the test stage was not completed by the runner, the collections were less than 60 seconds. Pulmonary ventilation ($\dot{V}_E$) (ATPS) was measured with a dry gas meter and corrected (BTPS) using a computer program.[5]

THE RESTING ELECTROCARDIOGRAM AND VECTORCARDIOGRAM

Twelve-lead electrocardiograms were recorded prior to the vectorcardiograms.

Frontal, horizontal, and right sagittal vectorcardiograms using the Frank lead system were recorded with a Hart Electronics PV–5 vectorcardiograph.

The cut-off frequency response used in this study was 100 Hz. The vector-cardiographic loops were interrupted at a rate of 500 times per second. In all tracings, the inscription was interrupted by the large end of the time dash. *Phonocardiograms, carotid pulses, apexcardiograms and electrocardiograms* were recorded with a Cambridge MCIV multichannel recorder. The phonocardiogram amplifier setting at the medium frequency range has a linear response from 250 to 1000 Hz. From 250 to 100 Hz, there is a decrease of 20 dB/octave. Cambridge Leatham microphones were used for sensing heart sounds (constant output 190 to 300 Hz and increases in sensitivity by 30 dB up to 1500 Hz). The microphone used for sensing heart sounds was placed at the mitral area. 1–665 Cambridge pulse transducers with a time constant of 3.5 seconds were used to record the apexcardiogram and carotid pulse (funnel shape pick-up). The paper speed was 100 mm/sec.

TABLE 2

MAXIMAL CARDIOPULMONARY CHARACTERISTICS IN MARATHON RUNNERS

Variables *	Mean	SD
$\dot{V}_E$ (BTPS) (liters/min.)	134.9	20.17
(liters/kg·min.)	2.10	.31
Systolic blood pressure	167.6	30.1
Diastolic blood pressure	74.9	10.61
Est. Myocardial $\dot{V}_{O_2}$ (ml/100 g LV)	34.9	5.46
Heart rate	177.2	9.13
	Cases/Total	
ECG ST depression > 1 mm		
> 0.08 msec	0/12	

* Abbreviations: $\dot{V}_E$, pulmonary ventilation; BTPS, body temperature pressure saturated; $\dot{V}_{O_2}$, oxygen consumption; LV, left ventricle.

Systolic Time Intervals

All subjects were placed in the left lateral decubitus. During held expiration, a 10-second simultaneous recording was made of the carotid pulse tracing, the phonocardiogram, and the electrocardiogram with a Cambridge multichannel MCIV recorder. The following variables were conventionally computed:

Electromechanical Systole Index (Q-S₂I): The time from the Q wave of the electrocardiogram to the aortic component of the second heart sound, corected for heart rate.

Left Ventricular Ejection Time Index (LVETI): Carotid upstroke to trough of carotid incisura, corrected for heart rate.

Pre-Ejection Period (PEP): Q-wave to leg of upstroke of the carotid pulse, corrected for pulse transmission time.

PEP/LVET: Ratio of pre-ejection period to the left ventricular ejection time.

Manual calculations of the systolic time intervals were read to the nearest 5 msec for 10 consecutive cycles. The rate-dependent raw values were corrected for heart rate and then averaged to obtain a representative value. Raw values that were not rate-dependent were directly averaged to obtain a representative value.

The results obtained by calculating the systolic time intervals in marathon runners were then compared with similar values obtained in this laboratory in a control group of 100 nonathletes.[6]

Echocardiograms

Echocardiograms were performed in the supine position in 12 marathon runners and 20 nonathletes matched for age, weight, and body surface area with an Ekoline 20 Echographic S.K.I. utilizing a 0.5-inch diameter 2.25 MHz transducer focused at 10 cm with a repetition rate of 1000 impulses/sec. The ultrasound transducer was placed in the fourth or fifth left intercostal space close to the sternum. The signal from the echograph was displayed and recorded on an Electronics for Medicine VR6 stripchart multichannel oscilloscopic recorder. Ultrasonic scans were obtained from apex to base and echocardiograms were recorded with rigid adherence to the technique and criteria previously established [7] and routinely employed in this laboratory.[8]

The following left and right ventricular dimensions were obtained:

(1) End-diastolic diameters (LVDd and RVDd), which are measured in centimeters as an internal antero-posterior axis or minor axis of the left and right ventricles at the time of the R-wave peak.

(2) Left ventricular end-systolic diameter (LVDs) is measured in centimeters as the shortest interval diameter during the same cardiac cycle.

(3) Left ventricular end-diastolic (LVEDV) and end-systolic volumes (LVESV) are calculated in milliliters by using the cubes of the diameter.

Left ventricular mass in grams (LV mass g) was calculated from the echocardiographic measurements by the method of Troy, Pombo and Rackley.[9]

(5) Stroke volume (SV) was measured in milliliters and calculated as end-diastolic ventricular volume minus end-systolic ventricular volume.

(6) Ejection fraction (EF) is expressed in percent and calculated as the ratio of stroke volume/to end-diastolic volume.

(7) The percent change in minor axis diameter ($\%\Delta D$) was calculated as $(LVDd - LVDs)/LVDd \times 100$ or $(RVDd - RVDs)/RVDd \times 100$.

(8) The aortic root diameter was measured from the anterior edge of the anterior aortic wall to the anterior edge of the posterior aortic wall at ventricular end-diastole. Five consecutive cycles were measured and the average value was utilized for analysis.

Results

Electrocardiography and Vectorcardiography

Electrocardiographic and vectorcardiographic abnormalities at rest were present in almost all marathon runners (TABLE 3). The most common abnormalities were sinus bradycardia, sinus arrhythmia, and ST-segment elevation greater than 1 mm. U waves was seen in all electrocardiograms. Wolff-Parkinson-White syndrome (WPW) was present in one case. Conduction disturbances were noted in five cases, including one case of first degree AV-block. Notched T waves were noted in two cases. In both cases, the vectorcardiograms revealed a semilunar pattern of the T wave (FIGURE 1), both limbs having a concave contour.

Three athletes met ECG criteria and one met VCG criteria for left ventricular hypertrophy (Sokolov and Lyon).[10] One had left ventricular hypertrophy by both methods, while all athletes failed to show right ventricular hypertrophy by either method. The treadmill exercise ECG was negative in all 12 athletes (TABLE 2), i.e., none had flat or down-sloping ST depression equaling or exceeding 1 mm (0.1 mV).

Echocardiography

The echocardiographic data obtained in all 12 athletes were evaluated both in raw form and corrected for weight and body surface area. No statistically significant differences were found in both sets of echocardiographic data. The results will be presented, therefore, in absolute form. FIGURES 2A and 2B illustrate the measurements of standard echocardiographic dimensions performed in two athletes. The results of echocardiographic measurements in 12 marathon runners and in 20 nonathletes are shown in TABLE 4. As seen in TABLE 4, when echographic measurements of the control group were compared with athletes, statistically significant differences were found in left ventricular end-diastolic and end-systolic dimensions. The left ventricular end-diastolic and end-systolic volumes, the stroke volume, the posterior left ventricular wall thickness, and the left ventricular mass were greater in marathon runners than in control subjects (p < 0.001). No statistically significant differences were found in values of ejection fraction and the percentage of internal diameter shortening.

TABLE 3

ELECTROCARDIOGRAPHIC AND VECTORCARDIOGRAPHIC ABNORMALITIES
IN MARATHON RUNNERS (CASES/TOTAL) *

Sinus arrhythmia and bradycardia			9/12
1° A-V block			1/12
IVCD			1/12
WPW			1/12
rSr' V_1			3/12
U wave			12/12

	ECG	VCG	Both ECG & VCG
LVH repolarization abnormalities	3/12	1/12	1/12
ST elevation > 1 mm	7/12	7/12	7/12
T wave notched	2/12	3/12	2/12

* Abbreviation: IVCD, intraventricular conduction delay; LVH, left ventricular hypertrophy; VCG, vectorcardiogram; WPW, Wolff-Parkinson-White syndrome.

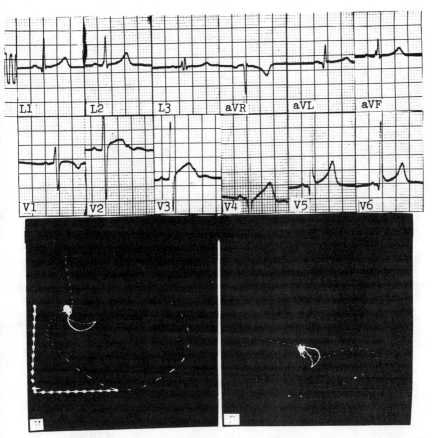

FIGURE 1. The ECG shows a markedly elevated S-T segment in L₁, V₅, and V₆. T wave shows notch on the descending limb (V₅–V₆). The vectorcardiogram shows increased anterior forces and a semilunar shaped T loop.

Right ventricular end-diastolic, aortic root, and left atrial dimensions were also increased in marathon runners compared with control subjects.

Phonocardiogram, Carotid Pulse, and Apexcardiogram

TABLE 5 includes the phonocardiographic findings. An apical short ejection systolic murmur was recorded in three athletes and S_3 was recorded in two. The carotid tracing (FIGURE 3) shows a bisferiens pulse in five marathon runners and the apexcardiogram (ACG) (FIGURE 4) showed a bifid systolic thrust in three. The A wave of ACG was normal.

X ray studies: The postero-anterior chest films (FIGURE 5) showed that four athletes had the cardiac diameters slightly enlarged or at the upper limits of normal.

TABLE 4

ECHOCARDIOGRAPHIC MEASUREMENTS IN MARATHON RUNNERS AND CONTROLS *

	Marathon Runners (n=12)	Controls (n=20)	p Values
LVDd (cm)	5.53±0.51	4.81±0.44	0.001
LVDs (cm)	3.63±0.49	3.22±0.42	0.02
PLVWT (cm)	1.0±0.2	0.7±0.1	0.001
LVEDV (ml)	172.69±48.33	113.57±30.41	0.001
LVESV (ml)	50.42±20.78	35.15±13.96	0.01
LV mass (g)	212.43±55.86	123.48±24.54	0.001
SV (ml)	122.27±32.80	78.42±20.44	0.001
EF (%)	71±7	69±7	N.S.
%ΔD	34.4±5.3	33.3±4.9	N.S.
RVDd (cm)	2.02±0.65	1.52±0.21	0.01
LA (cm)	3.57±0.39	2.94±0.35	0.001
Aortic root (cm)	3.05±0.28	2.69±0.43	0.03

* All data are reported as mean ± SD. LVDd, left ventricular end-diastolic dimension; LVDs, left ventricular end-systolic dimension; PLVWT, posterior left ventricular wall thickness; LVEDV, left ventricular end-diastolic volume; LVEDs, left ventricular end-systolic volume; LV mass, left ventricular mass; SV, stroke volume; EF, ejection fraction; %ΔD, % of internal diameter shortening; RVDd, right ventricular end-diastolic dimension; LA, left atrium.

TABLE 5

PHONOCARDIOGRAM, CAROTID PULSE AND APEXCARDIOGRAM IN MARATHON RUNNERS *

No.	S_1	S_3	S_4	Murmur	Carotid Pulse	ACG
1	N	–	–	–	Bifid	Bifid
2	weak	–	–	–	Bifid	N
3	N	+	–	–	N	Bifid
4	N	–	–	–	Bifid	N
5	N	–	–	Apical systolic murmur	Bifid	N
6	N	–	–	–	Bifid	Bifid
7	N	–	–	Apical systolic murmur	N	N
8	N	–	–	Apical systolic murmur	N	N
9	N	+	–	–	N	N
10	N	–	–	–	N	N
11	N	–	–	–	N	N
12	N	–	–	–	N	N

* Abbreviations: ACG, apexcardiogram; S, sound; N, normal.

Systolic Time Intervals

Total electromechanical interval and pre-ejection period (PEP) were increased in athletes compared with control subjects (TABLE 6) ($p < 0.05$). No statistically significant differences were found in the values of left ventricular ejection time index and PEP/LVET ratio for marathon runners when compared with nonathletes.

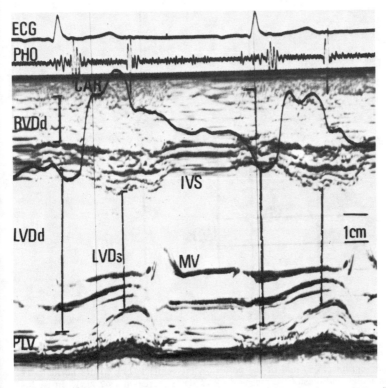

FIGURE 2A. Echocardiogram in a 47-year-old male marathon runner. The left ventricular end-diastolic dimension (LVEDd) is increased (6 cm) and left ventricular end-systolic dimension (LVEDs) is also increased (4.2 cm). The thickness of the interventricular septum (IVS) is slightly increased (1.2 cm), while the thickness of the posterior left ventricle (PLV) is normal. The right ventricular end-diastolic dimension (RVDd) is normal (1.8 cm.).

Pulmonary Function Tests

The pulmonary function measures showed that the marathon runners were comparable to national standard marathon runners (TABLE 2)[11] and professional soccer players[12] but below those values reported for normal university students.[13]

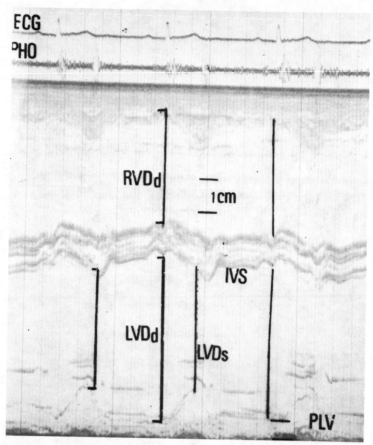

FIGURE 2B. Echocardiogram in a 30-year-old male marathon runner. The left ventricular end-diastolic dimension (LVDd) and left ventricular end-systolic dimension (LVDs) are normal, respectively, 5.3 and 3.7 cm. The thickness of the interventricular septum (IVS) and of the posterior left ventricle (PLV) are normal. The right ventricular end-diastolic dimension (RVDd) is increased (3.7 cm). In each of both examples, both the ejection fraction and percent internal diameter shortening are normal.

TABLE 6

SYSTOLIC TIME INTERVALS IN MARATHON RUNNERS *

Variable	Runners	Controls	Diff.	t	p Value
QS$_2$I	536.5±23.9	520.0±20.8	16.5	1.83	0.05
LVETI	409.2±16.9	417.0±19.4	−7.8	−0.06	ns
PEP	107±26.76	85.5±16.9	18.5	2.16	0.05
PEP/LVET	0.330±0.08	0.287±0.55	.43	0.01	ns

* Abbreviations: QS$_2$I, electromechanical systole index; LVETI, left ventricular ejection time index; PEP, pre-ejection period.

Discussion

Cardiac hypertrophy and dilatation commonly develop in well-conditioned athletes. Endurance athletes have been found to have various cardiac abnormalities usually associated with heart disease. In the past, the abnormalities were mostly limited to clinical EKG and radiologic abnormalities. The func-

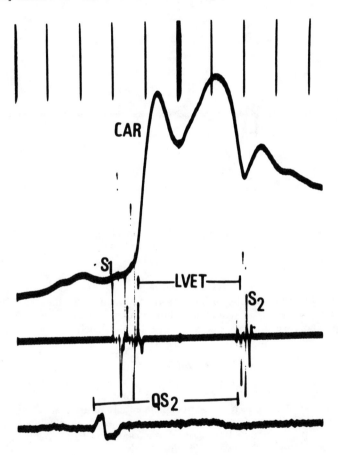

FIGURE 3. The carotid tracing shows a bisferiens contour. LVET, 320 msec; LVETI, 421 msec; CAR, carotid pulse; S_1, first heart sound; S_2, second heart sound; LVET, left ventricular ejection time; QS_2, electromechanical systole.

tional capacity of the hypertrophied left ventricle has been a controversial subject of intensive investigation. The newer noninvasive techniques such as echocardiography have provided sensitive means for assessing the size of cardiac cavities and myocardial wall thickness. Echocardiography and systolic time intervals have provided also reliable means for evaluation of left ventricular function. Other noninvasive graphic methods such as phonocardiography, apexcardiography, and carotid pulse tracings employed in our study added accuracy

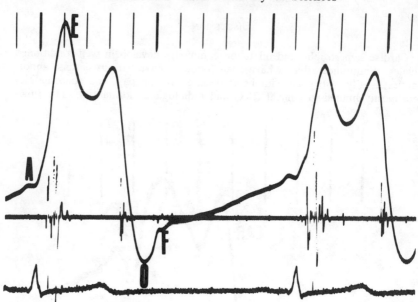

FIGURE 4. The apexcardiogram shows a bifid systolic thrust. (A) atrial wave; (E) ejection; (O) opening A-V valve; (RFW) rapid filling wave; (SFW) slow filling wave.

to the data obtained by physical examination and revealed newer and poorly recognized graphic findings of theoretical and practical significance. The vector-cardiogram revealed in some marathon runners, unusual concave semilunar shape of the T wave.

Echocardiographic Studies

The ultrasound data substantiated the presence of left ventricular hyper-trophy manifested by an increase in calculated left ventricular mass in marathon runners ($p < 0.001$). In the basal state these individuals exhibited normal left ventricular performance. Both, the left ventricular and right ventricular dimensions were significantly greater (TABLE 4) than those obtained in the control group. FIGURES 2A and 2B show that there was enlargement of the end-diastolic dimension of one of either ventricles in endurance athletes. The measures were significantly greater ($p < 0.001$) in marathon runners for left ventricular end-diastolic volumes and stroke volume. Careful recordings of the interventricular septum failed to demonstrate increased septal thickness previously reported by Roeske et al.[14] Gilbert et al.[15] reported that there was no significant difference in ventricular septal thickness between competitive runners and the control group. The end-diastolic thickness of the posterior left ventricular wall increased in our marathon runners and in those reported by others.[15] "Physio-logical hypertrophy" of the heart in the athlete [16] as detected by echocardiog-raphy is one of the results of adjustment to exercise.

A significant finding was also the relative enlargement of the aortic root and left atrial size, possibly resulting from volume overload. As compared with untrained normal persons of the same age, myocardial contractility of the marathon runners showed no significant statistical differences. The ejection fraction and percent fractional shortening in the marathon runners were not different from the control group. The formulae employed to calculate the indices of left ventricular myocardial contractility are reasonably accurate.[17-19]

Stack *et al.*[20] considered an individual to have abnormal left ventricular performance if the percent change in minor diameter ($\%\,\Delta D$) was less than 30%. In our group $\%\,\Delta D$ was 34.4 ± 5.3.

Some of the resting *electrocardiographic and vectorcardiographic* abnormalities present in our group of marathon runners require further clarification. It is important to recognize that factors other than ischemia can affect the ST segment.

The etiology of the *early repolarization syndrome*[21] (normal variant RS-T segment elevation) seen in 7 of 12 athletes remains a controversial topic. This syndrome is characterized by upward concave elevation of RS-T segment in the

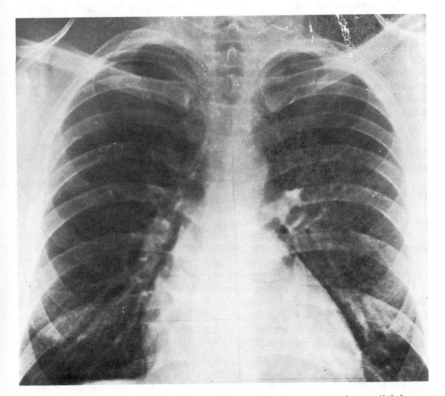

FIGURE 5. Chest X ray of a 24-year-old marathon runner showing a slightly enlarged cardiac silhouette. The cardiac diameters and ratios are, however, slightly above the upper limits of normal: transverse diameter, 15 cm; cardio-thoracic ratio, 52%; oblique diameter, 16.2; and angle of inclination, 30°.

precordial leads and rapid QRS transition in the precordial leads with counter-clockwise rotation. Less commonly found were tall R and T waves in the precordial leads and notched T waves documented in two cases.

The RS-T elevation was most commonly encountered in leads V_2 to V_5 and was most prominent in leads V_3 or in the transitional areas because the ST-T spatial vectors are relatively parallel with or slightly more anterior than the mean QRS and T vector.[22]

Because of this vector orientation, the repolarization vector often produces the most significant elevation in the precordial leads and is often associated with large T waves. Notched, upright T waves were present in two marathon runners.

A normal T wave in the adult is rarely notched.[23] When T waves are grossly notched, they should be regarded with suspicion, though these characteristics may sometimes occur in precordial leads as a normal variant.[24] Dressler et al.[25] felt that notching and inversion of T waves are closely related and indeed, have the same meaning, while inversion of T, points to a disturbance in the relative rapidity of the repolarization process in the subendocardial and subepicardial lamina of the myocardium. Notching of T wave is due to a disturbance similar in kind and different only in degree from that manifested in complete inversion of the T wave.

The vectorcardiographic display of the notched T waves (FIGURE 1) seem to follow a characteristic pattern in some marathon runners. The T loop has semilunar configuration, both limbs displaying a concave contour. Notched positive T waves in the electrocardiogram and the counterpart vectorcardiographic semilunar configuration recorded in our marathon runners are newer findings. Alike "labile" or "juvenile" T-wave patterns and "isolated T negative syndrome," those vectorcardiographic patterns of the T wave corresponds to the "early repolarization syndrome."

In a recent study,[26] electrocardiographically demonstrable left ventricular hypertrophy, as evidenced by high amplitude QRS voltage, was present in our study in 25%.

The vectorcardiogram revealed increased right ventricular forces in three of our marathon runners. This increase of anterior forces, did not fulfill all criteria of right ventricular hypertrophy.[27] Roeske et al.[14] reported a number of 18 athletes (43%) who met VCG criteria for right ventricular hypertrophy, as proven by the anterior and rightward location of more than 70% of the loop area in the horizontal plane.

The origin of the U wave found in all 12 marathon runners is unknown. It has been interpreted as corresponding with the after-potential[28] since the U wave occurs coincidental with the supernormal phase of ventricular excitability. The U-wave has also been attributed to the mechanical effect of ventricular distension during the early phase of rapid filling.[29] This explanation seems plausible in view of the existence of major right and left ventricular preloads, characterized by major diastolic filling in marathon runners.[30]

Phonocardiographic Studies

The phonocardiogram failed to document S_4 gallop or its counterpart, abnormal A waves in the apexcardiogram. On the other hand S_3 was recorded in two marathon runners. Short ejection systolic murmurs were recorded at the apical area in 3 individuals. The classical description of the athletic heart syndrome includes these findings, whereas, S_4 is less of a common finding.[31]

The double systolic apical impulse recorded in three runners (FIGURE 4) is one of the most interesting apexcardiographic findings, since, it is a clue to underlying cardiac abnormalities. Diseases which effect major right or ventricular preloads, characterized by major diastolic filling, result in sharp systolic upstroke and prominent late systolic waves. Valvular lesions such as aortic regurgitation, for example, which result in both augmented stroke output and left ventricular hypertrophy, can produce a bifid apex beat.[30]

Carotid Pulse Tracings

Pulses bisferiens recorded in five runners, is rarely found in normal subjects with very rapid ventricular ejection. It may be found in patients with pure aortic regurgitation and in mixed aortic regurgitation and aortic stenosis, when aortic regurgitation is the predominant lesion.[32]

As seen in FIGURE 3, the rapid ascending phase of the *carotid pulse* (percussion wave) is followed by a negative or downward dip. The tidal wave that follows and which forms a double peak with the percussion wave seems due to the summation of the still moving wave with multiple waves reflected from periphery. A review of the literature [33, 34] and our echocardiographic data showed that the hemodynamic load on the heart present in marathon runners is similar to that seen in patients with aortic or mitral regurgitation. The echocardiographic measurements of our marathon runners (TABLE 4) indicated a significant elevation of stroke volume even at rest. The left and right ventricular end-diastolic diameters and the left ventricular end-diastolic and end-systolic volumes are both increased. The left ventricular mass was significantly increased in our endurance athletes (212.43 ± 55.86 g) compared to the control group (123.48 ± 24.54 g) ($p < 0.001$). Of six marathon runners with abnormal carotid pulses and/or abnormal ACGs, three had increased left ventricular mass. The hemodynamic abnormalities and increased ventricular mass (TABLE 4) abnormalities found in the marathon runner's heart are responsible for the reduplicated apical impulse recorded by ACG and the bisferiens carotid pulse. The major response of the left ventricle to a significant load is dilatation and then hypertrophy, which is associated with an increase in cell size and length.[32] High "volume work" is tolerated reasonably well. Ejection fraction is maintained or even increased. The percentage of internal diameter shortening is not different from the control group (TABLE 4). But unlike aortic incompetence,[35] which requires with greater hypertrophy an increase in diastolic pressure, the endurance athlete's heart accommodates large volumes of blood without increase in pressure during diastole. Patients with aortic incompetence and prominent A waves on their ACGs usually have elevated left ventricular end-diastolic pressure (late stage of aortic incompetence).

The final filling and the final increase in end-diastolic fiber length and pressure of the left ventricle are obtained by atrial contraction. The stiffness (reduced distensibility) of the ventricular wall in a late stage interferes with passive ventricular filling. A strong atrial contraction is, therefore, required for proper ventricular filling (A wave).

In all of our marathon runners a prominent A wave on the ACG was conspicuously absent; no S_4, the counterpart of an enlarged A wave was recorded.

Thus, the *ACG* and *carotid pulse* reflect important hemodynamic changes taking place in the endurance athletes heart, as demonstrated by another non-invasive technique, echocardiography, and by cardiac catheterization.[31]

Left atrium and aortic root dimensions were larger in the marathon runners (TABLE 4). The hemodynamic load on the heart present in such individuals may account for those changes.

Systolic Time Intervals

In recent years, attention has been focused on the pre-ejection period (PEP) as a potential measure of intrinsic myocardial contractile performance. The major determinants of the duration of the PEP are the left ventricular end diastolic pressure (LVEDP), the aortic diastolic pressure and the rate of left ventricular pressure development (LV dp/dt) from onset of mechanical systole to the opening of the aortic valve.[36]

Increased PEP has been associated with increased myocardial dysfunction [37, 38] and decreased stroke volume.[39-41] Fardy,[42] Raab,[43] and Franks and Cureton [44] reported prolonged PEP with improved cardiovascular fitness. TABLE 6 shows that PEP was significantly prolonged in the marathon runners compared to sedentary individuals. This apparent paradox requires further elucidation. PEP is, in fact, a measure of overall left ventricular performance during iso-volumic systole and does not necessarily reflect the intrinsic contractile proper-ties of the left ventricle.

The ratio PEP/LVET found to be not significantly different in marathon runners compared to the control group has the advantage of including variations in both basic intervals, the PEP and LVET, and may reflect abnormality when neither measure is clearly beyond normal.[36] PEP/LVET has appeared to be a better indicator of ventricular performance. This ratio was correlated with left ventricular ejection fraction determined by quantitative angiography, left ventricular end-diastolic pressure, and left ventricular end-diastolic volume.[45] Our findings support this contention. Both the ejection fraction (TABLE 4) and the PEP/LVET ratio were not significantly different from the control group (TABLE 6).

Increased Q-S_2I (electromechanical systole index) found in our marathon runners, reflects increased stroke volume [39, 41] (TABLE 4).

Overall, cardiac evaluation by systolic time intervals seemed to be useful.

SUMMARY

The volume overload type of heart often observed in endurance athletes, may simulate a diseased heart.

We used a battery of noninvasive graphic techniques, i.e., echocardiogram, apexcardiogram, carotid pulse, electrocardiogram, vectorcardiogram, phono-cardiogram, systolic time intervals, and treadmill stress testing in 12 professional marathon runners, mean age 33.8 ± 11.1. Twenty nonathletes matched for age, height, sex, and weight served as a control group. Left ventricular (LV) end-diastolic dimension in marathon runners averaged 5.53 ± 0.5 cm compared to 4.81 ± 0.04 cm in nonathletes (p < 0.001), LV end-diastolic volume was 172.69 ± 43.3 ml compared to 113.57 ± 30.41 ml in nonathletes (p < 0.001), stroke volume was 122.27 ± 32.8 ml compared to 78.42 ± 20.44 ml in non-athletes ($p < 0.001$), the thickness of the posterior LV wall was 1.0 ± 0.2 cm compared to 0.7 ± 0.1 cm in nonathletes ($p < 0.001$), and LV mass was significantly increased, 212.43 ± 55.8 g compared to 123.48 ± 24.54 g in nonathletes ($p < 0.01$). Left atrium and aortic root were also relatively larger in athletes ($p < 0.01$). Right ventricular end-diastolic dimension was enlarged in marathon runners (2.02 ± 0.65 cm). No statistically significant differences were noted in ejection fraction, percentage of internal diameter shortening ($\%\Delta D$) and PEP/LVET. The carotid tracing had a bisferiens pulse in five marathon runners. The apexcardiogram showed a bifid systolic thrust in three and absence of abnormal A wave. These abnormalities were related to the overload type of heart as proven by echocardiogram. "Early repolarization syndrome" (abnormal RS-T segment elevation) and notched T waves in ECG had as counterpart a semilunar configuration in the VCG. Three athletes met ECG criteria and one met VCG criteria of LVH. The treadmill exercise ECG was negative in all 12 athletes. Biventricular enlargement and increased left ventricular mass are present in the marathon runner's heart. Myocardial contractility at rest was, however, not statistically different from nonathletes.

ACKNOWLEDGMENTS

The authors wish to thank Miss Ada Fantroy for her technical assistance, Mr. Fred Liebman for photography, Mrs. Karen L. Franklin for her secretarial assistance, and Mrs. Sherley Pozner for bibliographical assistance.

REFERENCES

1. BROZEK, J. *et al.* 1963. Densitometric analysis of body composition: Revision of some quantitative assessments. Ann. N.Y. Acad. Sci. **110:** 113–140.
2. DU BOIS, D. & E. F. DU BOIS. 1916. A formula to estimate the approximate surface area if height and weight be known. Arch. Int. Med. **17:** 863–871.
3. BLACKBURN, H., Ed. 1967. Measurement in Exercise Electrocardiography. Charles C Thomas, Publisher. Springfield, Ill.
4. HELLERSTEIN, H., *et al.* 1973. Principles of exercise prescription for normals and cardiac subjects in exercise testing and exercise training in coronary heart disease. J. Naughton & H. K. Hellerstein, Eds. : 150. Academic Press. New York, N.Y.
5. KEARNEY, J. T. & G. A. STULL. 1973. A fortron program for the reduction of open circuit data. Res. Q. **42:** 223–228.
6. ZONERAICH, S., O. ZONERAICH & J. RODENRYS. 1974. Computerized system for the noninvasive techniques. I. Its value for systolic time intervals. Amer. J. Cardiol. **33:** 643–649.
7. FEIGENBAUM, H. 1972. Echocardiography. Part **66:** 37. Lea and Febiger. Philadelphia, Pa.
8. ZONERAICH, S., O. ZONERAICH & J. J. RHEE. 1975. Echocardiographic findings in atrial flutter. Circulation **52:** 455–459.
9. TROY, B. L., J. POMBO & C. E. RACKLEY. 1972. Measurement of left ventricular wall thickness and mass by echocardiography. Circulation **45:** 602–611.
10. LIPMAN, B. S., E. MASSIE & R. E. KLEIGER. 1972. Clinical Scalar Electrocardiography. 6th edit. : 99. Yearbook Medical Publishers. Chicago, Ill.
11. FOX, E. L. & D. L. COSTILL. 1972. Estimated cardiorespiratory responses during marathon running. Arch. Environ. Health **24:** 316–324.

12. GETTMAN, L. R., M. L. POLLOCK & P. B. RAVEN. 1976. Physiological evaluation of an NASL professional soccer team. Med. Sci. Sports (Abstract) **8:** 67.

13. MCARDLE, W. D., F. I. KATCH & G. S. PECHAR. 1973. Comparison of continuous and discontinuous treadmill and bicycle ergometer test protocol for eliciting maximal oxygen intake. Med. Sci. Sports **5:** 156–160.

14. ROESKE, W. R., R. A. O'ROURKE, A. KLEIN, G. LEOPOLD & J. KARLINER. 1976. Non-invasive evaluation of ventricular hypertrophy in professional athletes. Circulation **53:** 286–292.

15. GILBERT, C., D. NUTTER, S. HEYMSFIELD, J. PERKINS & R. SCHLANT. 1975. The endurance athlete: Cardiac structure and function. Circulation (Suppl. 2): 115.

16. GRANDE, F. & H. L. TAYLOR. 1965. Adaptive changes in the heart, vessels and patterns of control under chronically high loads. *In* handbook of Physiology, Section 2. Circulation, Washington, D.C., Am. Physiol. Soc. p. 2615.

17. SEGAL, B. L., L. L. KONECKE, N. KAWAI, M. L. KOTLER & J. W. LINHART. 1974. Echocardiography. Current concepts and clinical application. Amer. J. Med. **57:** 267–283.

18. FEIGENBAUM, H. 1975. Evaluation of left ventricular function by echocardiography. Proc. N.Y. Cardiol. Soc., Dec. 4.

19. ZONERAICH, S., O. ZONERAICH & J. J. RHEE. In press. Left ventricular performance in diabetic patients without clinical heart disease evaluated with Systolic Time Intervals and Echocardiography. *In* Diabetes and the Heart. S. Zoneraich, Ed. Charles C Thomas, Publisher. Springfield, Ill.

20. STACK, R. S., C. C. LEE, B. P. REDDY, M. L. TAYLOR & A. M. WEISSLER. 1976. Left ventricular performance in coronary artery disease evaluated with systolic time intervals and echocardiography. Amer. J. Cardiol. **37:** 331–339.

21. KAMBARA, H. & J. PHILLIPS. 1976. Long term evaluation of early repolarization syndrome (Normal variant RS-T segment elevation). Amer. J. Cardiol. **38:** 157–161.

22. GRANT, R. P., E. H. ESTES & J. T. DOYLE. 1951. Spatial vector electrocardiography. The clinical characteristics of S-T and T vectors. Circulation **3:** 182–197.

23. BURCH, G. E. 1972. Primer of electrocardiography. 6th edit. : 154. Lea and Febiger. Philadelphia, Pa.

24. MARRIOTT, H. L. 1972. Practical electrocardiography. Williams and Wilkins, Balt. 5th Ed., p. 24.

25. DRESSLER, W., H. ROESLER & H. LACKNER. 1951. The significance of notched upright T-waves. Brit. Heart J. **13:** 496–502.

26. RASKOFF, W. J., S. GOLDMAN & K. COHN. 1976. The "Athletic Heart." Prevalence and physiological significance of left ventricular enlargement in distance runners. J. Amer. Med. Assoc. **236:** 158–162.

27. CHOU, T. C. & R. A. HELM. 1967. Clinical vectorcardiography. : 177. Grune and Stratton. New York, N.Y.

28. FRIEDBERG, C. K. 1966. Diseases of the Heart. : 44–45, 93, 627. W. B. Saunders, Philadelphia, Pa.

29. FERRERO, C. & J. P. DORET. 1954. Interpretation hemodynamique de l'onde U del' electrocardiogramme. Cardiologia **25:** 112–116.

30. BENCHIMOL, A. & K. B. DESSER. 1975. Clinical application of the apexcardiogram in non-invasive methods in Cardiology. S. Zoneraich, Ed. : 105–106. Charles C Thomas, Publisher. Springfield, Ill.

31. WENGER, N. K. & C. A. GILBERT. 1966. The athletes' heart. *In* The Heart. J. W. Hurst, Ed. : 1546–1548. McGraw Hill Book Company. New York, N.Y.

32. SCHLANT, R. C. 1966. Altered cardiovascular function of rheumatic heart disease and other acquired valvular disease. *In* The Heart. J. W. Hurst, Ed. : 808–814. McGraw-Hill Book Company. New York, N.Y.

33. DODGE, H. T. & W. A. BAXLEY. 1969. Left ventricular volume and mass in their significance in heart disease. Amer. J. Cardiol. **23:** 528–537.
34. GRANT, C., I. L. BUNNEL & D. G. GREENE. 1964. Angiographic observations on left ventricular function in man (Abstr.) Fed. Proc. **23:** 464.
35. MORGANROTH, J., B. J. MARON, W. L. HENRY & S. E. EPSTEIN. 1975. Comparative left ventricular dimensions in trained athletes. Ann. Int. Med. **82:** 521–524.
36. LEWIS, P. R., R. F. LEIGHTON, W. F. FORESTER & A. M. WEISSLER. 1974. *In* Systolic Time Intervals in Non-Invasive Cardiology. A. M. Weissler, Ed. : 301–368. Grune and Stratton, New York, N.Y.
37. HARRIS, W. S., C. D. SCHOENFELD & A. M. WEISSLER. 1967. Effects of adrenergic receptor activation and blockage on the Systolic preejection period, heart rate and arterial pressure in man. J. Clin. Invest. **46:** 1704–1714.
38. WHITSETT, T. L. & J. NAUGHTON. 1971. The effect of exercise on systolic time intervals in sedentary and active individuals and rehabilitated patients with heart disease. Amer. J. Cardiol. **27:** 352–358.
39. HARLEY, A. F., STARMER & J. C. GREENFELD. 1969. Pressure-flow studies in man. An evaluation of the duration of th phases of systole. Clin. Invest. **48:** 895–905.
40. AHMED, S. S., G. E. LEVINSON, C. J. SCHWARTZ & P. O. ETTINGER. 1972. Systolic time intervals as measures of the contractile state of the left ventricular myocardium in man. Circulation **46:** 559–571.
41. WEISSLER, A. M., W. S. HARRIS & C. D. SCHOENFELD. 1968. Systolic time intervals in heart failure in man. Circulation **37:** 149–159.
42. FARDY, P. S. Effects of soccer training and detraining upon selected cardiac and metabolic measures. Res. Q. **40:** 502–509.
43. RAAB, W. 1960. Degenerative heart disease from lack of exercise. Exercise and fitness. University of Illinois and Athletic Institute.
44. FRANKS, B. D. & T. R. CURETON. 1969. Effects of training on time components of the left ventricle. J. Sports Med. Phys. Fitness **9:** 80–83.
45. GARRARD, C. L., JR., A. M. WEISSLER & H. T. DODGE. 1970. The relationship of alterations in systolic time intervals to ejection fraction in patients with cardiac disease. Circulation **42:** 455–462.

THE ADRENAL EXHAUSTION SYNDROME:
AN ADRENAL DEFICIENCY *

F. G. Sulman, Y. Pfeifer, and E. Superstine

Bioclimatology Unit
Department of Applied Pharmacology
Medical Center
Hebrew University
Jerusalem, Israel

The "exhaustion syndrome" was recognized by our group in 1969 [1] as an adrenal medulla deficiency phenomenon. Further research showed that its detrimental effect is primarily due to adrenal medulla catecholamine deficiency; however, in most cases adrenal cortex hormones are also depleted, especially the androcorticosteroids (17-ketosteroids, 17-KS) and the glucocorticosteroids (17-hydroxysteroids, 17-OH). [2] This finding resulted from a study of urinary neurohormone excretion in persons exposed to permanent climatic heat stress. Such stress occurs mainly in tropic and subtropic regions where dry winds may blow during most parts of the year. It is, however, also common in countries where winds descend from high mountains, preserving their meteorological features of heat and dryness created by subsidence, which is defined as the slow downward motion of air panels over a large area usually combined with adiabatic (nonpermeable) warming up and drying of the subsiding air. As we have shown, people living in such an area suffer every year more and more from the effect of such winds, which create a state of permanent "perspiratio insensibilis." [3] This increased perspiration imposes heavy daily demands on the body's catecholamine secretion, which protects the body from "oversweating" by contracting skin blood vessels. Moreover, it demands constant 17-OH secretion to compensate for sodium loss, which may lead to hyperpotassemia. The demand on stress hormones, especially 17-KS, results in a typical decrease of 17-KS secretion during heat stress, a fact that may be explained by an adrenal shift from androcorticosteroid to glucocorticosteroid production.

In temperate zones, adrenal exhaustion is less frequent because the climate provides cold days at random the whole year round. Still, the demands of daily stress and aging induce adrenal exhaustion fairly often. [4]

Some hot dry winds of ill repute are the Santa Ana of Southern California, the Arizona desert winds, the Melbourne Northern winds, the Argentine Zonda, the Sirocco of the Mediterranean, the Maltesian Xlokk, the Khamsin and Sharkiye of the Arab countries, the Sharav of the Old Testament haunting Israel, and the Foehn of Switzerland, Germany, and Austria. They are notorious for causing depression and fatigue, culminating in exhaustion ("tropical lethargy"). There are also complaints of irritation, such as headaches, irritability, and exacerbation of respiratory ailments due to serotonin overproduction. [2] As the contradictory complaints of the millions of weather-sensitive patients do not allow proper diagnosis and treatment, we have differentiated the

* This work was supported by a grant from Mr. and Mrs. Herman Lane, New York.

918

complaints in 200 patients exposed to these winds by neurohormone urinalysis [2] (TABLE 1).

In an earlier paper [5] it was shown that in normal persons hot dry winds may cause increased sweat losses from 25% of the total fluid excretion under normal conditions, to up to 50%. The normal sodium chloride content of perspiration is 0.5%, so that the daily salt loss in the sweat may increase from 2 g to 4–5 g. This will naturally result in a smaller excretion of sodium in the urine and, in cases of dehydration, lead to a compensatory increased rate of potassium flow from the cells to the blood and urine. The flooding of the blood with potassium in extreme cases may explain the suffering and the typical ECG of cardiac patients from dry winds and the general adynamia noted by healthy people. The sodium loss activates aldosterone and glucocorticosteroid production in the

TABLE 1

URINALYSIS OF 200 PATIENTS SUFFERING FROM HEAT STRESS.
COMPARISON OF EXCRETIONS ON NORMAL DAYS AND HOT DAYS,
SHOWING TREND OF CHANGES

Parameters Studied	Excretion, per 24 hours	
	Normal Days	Heat Days
Epinephrine (μg)	1–4	0–1
Norepinephrine (μg)	10–50	0–20
17-KS female (mg)	8–12	6–8
male (mg)	12–18	8–10
17-OH female (mg)	2–3	3–4
male (mg)	3–4	4–5
Serotonin (μg)	0–50	51–100
5-HIAA (mg)	1–6	7–25
Histamine female (μg)	15–90	90–150
male (μg)	20–65	65–130
Thyroxine (μg)	10–20	21–37
Na^+ (mEq)	60–100	80–140
K^+ (mEq)	20–32	40–100
Creatinine (g)	1.5–2.5	3.0–4.0
Diuresis female (ml)	700–1,500	700–1,500
male (ml)	850–2,000	850–2,000

organism. Hence it is not surprising that 17-OH excretion rises on hot days. On the other hand, the chronic demand for catecholamines to prevent over-sweating may induce an exhaustion of the adrenal medulla in patients exposed continually to subtropical or tropical heat (tropical lethargy). This phenomenon is the topic of the present paper, and in addition it will be shown that it is also the cause underlying staleness of long distance runners, a condition not appreciated until now.

PATIENTS AND METHODS

In order to obtain a random population of weather-sensitive patients, the Hebrew University and the Israel Broadcasting Service issued a release in which people suffering from weather sensitivity were requested to apply to our Unit for proper examination and treatment. This appeal was answered at the time by about 200 patients eager to participate in this research. Today thousands of patients are under our permanent supervision and are relieved of their sufferings by specific preventive treatments (TABLES 1–3). The heat-sensitive patients include young students, soldiers, adults, elderly people, smokers, nonsmokers, drivers, immigrants from temperate and from hot zones, and people of varied ethnic origin subsisting on different diets. Recently we added 30 long distance runners to our supervision in order to establish norms for their neurohormone requirements and the relation of such to proper performance.

TABLE 2

THREE TYPES OF REACTIONS TO HEAT STRESS REVEALED BY NEUROHORMONE ANALYSIS

1. Irritation syndrome (serotonin hyperproduction). 43% of cases. Begins 1–2 days before arrival of heatwave because it is engendered by quickly moving air electricity.	Sleeplessness, irritability, tension, electrified hair, migraine, nausea, vomiting, scotoma, amblyopia, tinnitus, anorexia, edemata, palpitations, precordial pain, dyspnoe, rheumatic pains, flushes with sweat or chills, vasomotor rhinitis, conjunctivitis, laryngitis, tracheitis, vertigo, tremor, hyperperistalsis, polyuria or polakisuria.
2. Adrenal exhaustion syndrome (adrenal deficiency). 44% of cases. Increases every year.	Hypotension, fatigue, apathy, exhaustion, depression, confusion, ataxia, adynamia, hypoglycemic spells.
3. Intermittent hyperthyreosis. 13% of cases. Presents clinically a mixture of complaints listed in two types.	Tachycardia, sleeplessness, irritability, tension, nausea, vomiting, palpitations, precordial pain, dyspnoe, sweat, tremor, abdominal pain, diarrhea, polyuria, allergic reactions, reddening of skin, acne, increased appetite, weight loss, overactivity, fatigue, exhaustion, depression, adynamia, confusion, anxiety, alopecia.

Urine Collection

Every patient had to undergo a general physical examination. If he was found to be a typical weather-sensitive person, he was given a note containing directions for collecting and despatching his urine, reading as follows:

"All urine excreted during 24 hours should be collected in a jar containing two teaspoonsful (10 ml) 3 N hydrochloric acid. This preserving fluid (marked poison!) must be put into the receptacle jar *before* starting urine collection. During collection of urine, the patient should avoid eating bananas, avocados, tomatoes, pineapples, and guavas. The following drugs should be avoided: reserpine, methyldopa, pressor amines, tricyclic antidepressants, and monoamine-oxidase-(MAO)-blockers. Urine samples should be sent to the Department in 200 ml bottles specifying name of patient, quantity excreted during 24 hours and date of collection."

TABLE 3

RESULTS OF NEUROHORMONE URINALYSIS IN 200 PERSONS SUFFERING FROM HEAT STRESS IN RELATION TO THEIR CLINICAL COMPLAINTS ON HOT DAYS, COMPARED WITH NORMAL DAYS* THE QUANTITATIVE EVALUATION OF THE CHANGES FOUND BY URINALYSIS IS COMPILED IN TABLE 1, EVERY PATIENT SERVING AS HIS OWN CONTROL*

Group	Patients	Syndrome	Epinephrine, Norepineph-rine	17-KS, 17-OH	Serotonin, 5-HIAA	Histamine, T-4	Sodium, potassium	Percentage of cases
1	86	Irritation syndrome (serotonin hyper-production)	0	0	+	0	0	43%
2	88	Adrenal exhaustion syndrome (adrenal deficiency)	−	−	0	0	0	44%
3	26	Intermittent hyperthy-reosis	+	+	+	+	+	13%

* +, increase; −, decrease; 0, no change. The quantitative evaluation of the changes found by urinalysis is compiled in TABLE 1, every patient serving as his own control.

The long distance runners included 30 students under supervision of our University Sport Laboratory, who were considered fit for long distance training after physical examination, lung capacity determination, electrocardiogram (ECG), and blood pressure monitoring during exercise. These 30 students were asked to pass urine before and after running up to 5 km to allow a comparison between the pre-stress (ante) and the after-stress (post) neurohormone profile (TABLE 4). In these 30 students the only difference in urine collection was the immediate acidification of the urine *after* collection, the assay being evaluated per liter instead of per 24 hours' excretion.

Urinalysis

The following urine examinations were carried out: epinephrine, norepinephrine, 17-KS, 17-OHS, serotonin and its metabolite 5-hydroxyindoleacetic acid (5-HIAA), histamine, thyroxine, sodium, potassium, creatinine, and diuresis. Methods and results have been published by us.[2, 6]

Selection of Controls

The design of the study was double-blind throughout. Control values for neurohormone excretion of normal people are available in our Department from well over 1,000 persons. They show a daily epinephrine excretion of 1–4 μg/day and norepinephrine excretion of 25–50 μg/day. Similar values pertain to persons whose catecholamines are assayed in single urines and evaporated per liter urine. The standard values for other neurohormones are presented in TABLE 1. In the present study every weather-sensitive patient and every long distance runner had to serve as his own control. Urinalysis on normal days or before exercise yielded his normal neurohormone profile, whereas the changes due to heat or exercise were easily detected by comparison of the results of urinalyses. All figures were evaluated statistically by Student's t-test (p < 0.005). Completeness of urine collection was ascertained by the creatinine index in the 24 hours' urine.

RESULTS

Weather-Sensitive Patients

Urinalysis (TABLE 1) and clinical symptomatology (TABLE 2) allowed the climatic heat syndrome to be split up into 3 different groups (TABLE 3): "irritation syndrome" due to serotonin overproduction, 43% of cases;[7] "thyroid syndrome" due to intermittent hyperthyreosis, 13% of cases;[8] "adrenal exhaustion syndrome," 44% of cases.[9] The evaluation of the neurohormone profile in long distance runners presented greater difficulties because of three other interferences described in TABLE 5: influenza, dropping out before completing 5 km, and general lack of fitness.

Weather-sensitive patients may suffer from one or more of the following complaints of adrenal deficiency: hypotension, apathy, depression, fatigue, exhaustion, lack of concentration or confusion, ataxia or vertigo, and hypoglycemic spells, and they may also be prone to coronary insufficiency. The most typical complaint of this group is that its members suffer from climatic heat stress progressively more every year. This becomes especially evident in women, who react to it by chronic hypotension. We have shown in rats that the female is indeed more prone to heat stress exposure because of its lower level of androgenic stress hormones.[10, 11]

It is a well-known fact that weather-sensitive persons who have the chance of visiting a temperate climate during the hot periods of the year do not suffer from the typical progressive deficiency of adrenal activity, because there they encounter normal weather, which does not make any demands on their catecholamine, 17-KS, and 17-OH production. This gives them ample opportunity to restore the capacity of their adrenal gland. Urinalysis of such patients, at the brink of adrenal exhaustion, shows that they leave the tropics with subnormal hormone excretion and return with normal levels.

Comparison of catecholamine excretion in weather-sensitive patients showed the following fluctuations in patients suffering from the exhaustion syndrome. Their epinephrine excretion amounts to approximately 1 μg/day on normal days and falls to 0–0.9 μg/day on hot days; norepinephrine ranges at 15–50 μg/day on normal days, and 1–10 μg/day on hot days. Statistical evaluation ($n = 200$) yielded the following results:

Epinephrine, Mean Excretion ± Standard Error (SE):
   before heat spell: 1 ± 0.3 μg/day, $p < 0.005$;
   during heat spell: 0.4 ± 0.1 μg/day, $p < 0.005$;
   during heat spell on MAO blocker treatment: 0.9 ± 0.2 μg/day, $p < 0.005$.

Norepinephrine, Mean Excretion ± SE:
   before heat spell: 32 ± 5 μg/day, $p < 0.005$;
   during heat spell: 20 ± 3 μg/day, $p < 0.005$;
   during heat spell with MAO blocker treatment: 31 ± 4 μg/day, $p < 0.005$.
The 17-KS and 17-OH values showed less typical results.

Long Distance Runners

Different types of neurohormone reactions were found in healthy long distance runners. Thirty male students 20–25 years old, training for a long distance contest, had their urinary neurohormone levels tested before and after running 5,000 m at an embient temperature of 10°–15° C. The first 25 runners to reach the tape showed the following typical pattern of reaction (TABLE 4):

Stress Hormones, Average Decrease:
   17-KS: from 12.0 to 8.0 mg/liter;
   17-OH: from 3.8 to 2.5 mg/liter;
   5-HIAA: from 5.4 to 3.5 mg/liter.

Fight and Flight Hormones, Average Increase:
   Epinephrine: from 0.7 to 3.6 μg/liter;
   Norepinephrine: from 22 to 41 μg/liter.

TABLE 4

CHANGES OF URINARY NEUROHORMONE LEVELS IN 30 MALE LONG DISTANCE RUNNERS BEFORE (ante) AND AFTER (post) EXERCISE

Student	Age (yr)	Distance (km)		Epinephrine (µg/liter)	Norepinephrine (µg/liter)	17-OH (mg/liter)	17-KS (mg/liter)	5-HIAA (mg/liter)	Histamine (µg/liter)	Thyroxine (km) (µg/liter)
1	23	5	ante	0.9	13.4	3.2	10.0	4.2	26	10
			post	3.7	36.0	2.6	8.6	2.1	38	14
2	24	5	ante	0.7	15.8	3.1	10.0	5.5	44	10
			post	5.7	8.6*	2.7	11.1*	6.5*	41*	20
3	23	5	ante	0.0*	0.0*	3.6	20.5	3.1	40	12
			post	0.0*	0.0*	3.2	10.5	0.7	41	11*
4	25	5	ante	0.9	15.4	3.4	18.0	3.7	37	11
			post	4.0	41.5	2.6	15.0	3.0	80	20
5	23	5	ante	0.4	10.8	3.4	9.5	4.6	43	11
			post	3.7	37.6	3.0	6.5	2.8	67	16
6	25	5	ante	0.3	37.3	4.1	8.0	3.6	30	12
			post	2.7	38.5	2.8	5.3	3.2	40	19
7	24	5	ante	0.2	15.8	1.7	7.5	10.0	41	13
			post	0.8	57.0	1.6	7.0	5.3	52	14
8	25	5	ante	1.0	17.8	3.1	13.0	7.8	29	8
			post	2.4	35.0	2.4	10.0	5.1	51	14
9	21	5	ante	1.2	14.1	3.2	17.6	8.4	32	8
			post	3.5	28.3	2.1	11.9	7.6	57	13
10	22	5	ante	0.2	24.2	1.7	7.0	4.1	36	12
			post	0.8	52.0	1.0	6.6	3.8	58	24
11	21	3	ante	0.3	24.9	22.5	3.2	2.9	52	13
			post	0.9	53.0	10.5	2.6	1.7	53	14
12	22	2	ante	0.4	20.1	21.5	3.1	2.9	52	10
			post	0.8	42.1	21.0	2.8	1.0	42†	17
13	21	2	ante	1.8	19.7	22.0	2.8	5.8	30	8
			post	3.8	42.0	12.0	2.0	1.7	49	10
14	23	2	ante	0.4	18.4	12.3	2.1	2.7	40	9
			post	1.8	59.0	9.0	1.5	4.0†	9†	10

15	24	2	ante	0.3	16.3	12.5	3.8	8.0	40	12
			post	1.6	45.3	13.0†	3.1	10.0†	41	10†
16	23	2.5	ante	0.4	10.3	18.5	4.8	6.1	34	10
			post	1.7	29.4	12.0	4.0	8.1†	44	25
17	25	3.5	ante	0.5	19.5	19.0	3.1	3.8	28	8
			post	2.3	49.3	10.5	2.2	2.1	40	10
18	21	1	ante	0.8	44.3	10.0	2.4	4.5	31	9
			post	4.1	75.9	7.6	1.8	6.9†	39	17
19	24	2	ante	0.7	40.0	11.0	3.0	3.2	41	11
			post	3.9	59.9	9.5	2.6	1.8	64	18
20	20	2	ante	2.1	19.7	19.0	3.1	4.5	38	10
			post	0.3†	43.7	14.0	3.0	2.3	37	9†
21	25	5	ante	0.4	10.1	12.0	3.4	4.5	71	14
			post	3.1	24.3	15.5†	3.6†	2.3	93	19
22	24	5	ante	0.5	11.2	14.3	2.9	4.1	36	17
			post	4.1	23.4	11.4	2.0	2.1	38	19
23	25	5	ante	0.9	13.4	10.0	3.2	4.2	27	10
			post	3.8	36.0	8.7	2.5	2.3	38	14
24	23	5	ante	0.8	15.8	10.1	3.1	6.5	43	20
			post	0.7‡	9.7‡	11.1‡	3.7‡	7.6‡	40‡	12‡
25	22	5	ante	0.9	15.4	18.0	3.4	3.6	37	11
			post	4.1	41.6	15.1	2.7	3.0	70	21
26	25	5	ante	0.3	10.8	9.5	3.4	4.7	43	11
			post	3.7	36.6	10.5‡	3.1	4.9‡	57	17
27	24	5	ante	0.4	37.3	8.0	4.1	3.6	30	12
			post	2.7	38.6	5.3	2.8	3.2	41	19
28	23	5	ante	0.8	15.8	7.5	1.7	10.0	42	13
			post	1.6	57.6	7.1	1.6	5.3	52	17
29	22	5	ante	1.9	17.9	3.1	4.1	7.8	29	8
			post	3.5	35.6	2.4	2.4	5.1	51	14
30	25	5	ante	0.2	24.0	7.0	1.7	4.2	36	11
			post	6.8	52.1	6.6	1.0	3.6	58	22

* Anomalous finding caused by influenza infection.
† Anomalous finding, student did not complete 5 km.
‡ Anomalous finding, student was unfit.

Metabolic Hormones, Average Increase:
   T-4 (urinary): from 10 to 15 μg/liter;
   Histamine: from 30 to 42 μg/liter.
All changes were highly significant by Student's t-test.

THERAPY

Weather-sensitive patients can be treated at any time. Long-distance runners, however, can only be treated during their period of training, otherwise such treatment would be considered as illegal doping.

Treatment should consist of minidoses of monoamine oxidase blockers (MAO inhibitors). They allow better use of the adrenal catecholamine reserves and recuperation of the exhausted adrenal medulla. The efficacy of MAO inhibitor use is always based on an extremely low dosage, since we are dealing, essentially, with healthy persons without any psychogenic anamnesis or diagnosis. We start the patient on ¼ of a tablet (e.g., 2.5 mg isocarboxazid per day) of one of the accepted MAO blockers (FIGURE 1). Only rarely does the dosage have to be increased to ½–1 tablet per day, but never more. Placebos are used in every case, as they allow us to arrive at an unequivocal appraisal of the patient's requirements. Evaluation is facilitated by repeated neurohormone assays and use of special forms which the patient completes after taking the drug for a brief period.

After a long search for a MAO blocker with an immediate effect, we selected as the drug of choice, isocarboxazid (Marplan, Roche, FIGURE 1). This preparation is a MAO blocker which, without causing any excitement or tension in the patient as other MAO blockers or pressor amines are apt to do, brings about an elated mood within one hour, which completely changes the mental outlook of the patient. It is sufficient to give the patient ¼–½ tablet (2.5–5 mg) in the mornings to induce full work capacity. This treatment will normalize catecholamine production within 7 days (urine epinephrine rising from below 0.1 μg to 1–4 μg/day) without, however, unduly increasing the level of other biogenic amines, such as serotonin. Administration of ACTH is not necessary as 17-KS and 17-OH levels will automatically rise during treatment with MAO blockers. It is clear that protracted treatment with MAO blockers would be detrimental to the adrenal medulla, and could also precipitate the well-known hazards that every patient encounters when he takes MAO blockers for a prolonged time and inadvertently adds tyramine to his food intake by consuming cheese, beer, wine, or pressor amines.

The results of treatment were especially rewarding with regard to hypotension, which reverted to normal values, blood pressure, if low, rising by 10–20 mmHg. Ataxia or vertigo due to hypotension disappeared. Subjective complaints, such as fatigue, apathy, exhaustion, depression, confusion, and hypoglycemic spells were no longer reported. In nearly all cases the patients who were previously unable to pursue their work could now perform their duties without any difficulty and started to resume sport exercises as, e.g., long distance running.

Side reactions of the isocarboxazid therapy were very rare. They consisted mainly of sleeplessness and restlessness. These complaints disappeared when the patients were advised to take not more than ¼ dose of an MAO blocker

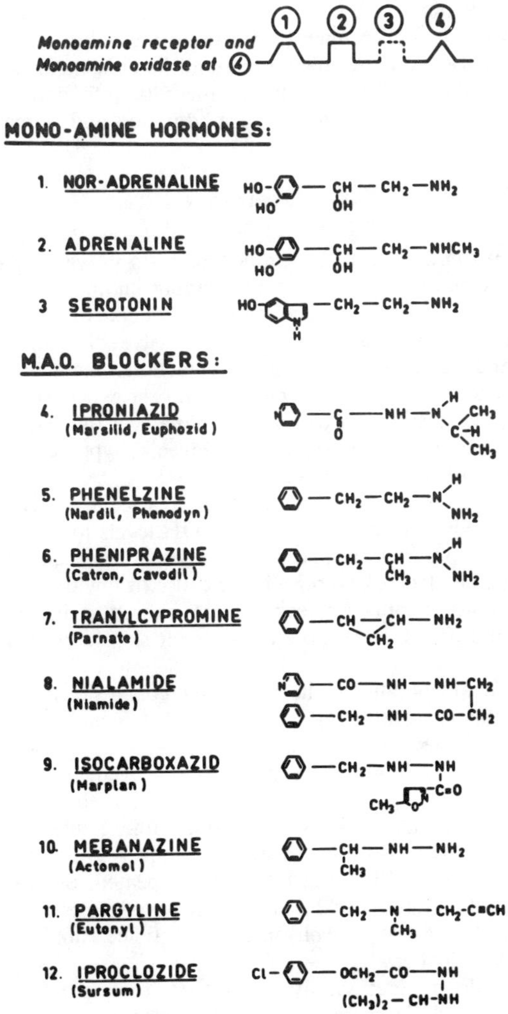

FIGURE 1. Synopsis of MAO-blockers and their mechanism of action by fitting into the receptor for catecholamines norepinethrine (1) and epinethrine (2) and serotonin (3). Compounds 7, 9, 10, and 11 are currently in use; compounds 4, 5, 6, and 8 have been withdrawn from the market. Compounds 7, 9, and 10 have an immediate effect, beginning 30–60 min after intake and lasting for 6–8 hours. Compound 12 is rarely used.

after breakfast. It is interesting to note that in this group there were also patients who preferred additional treatment with xanthine derivatives, such as caffeine, euphylline nicotinate (Hesotin), or xanthinone niacinate (Complamin). It is well known that such preparations mimic the action of catecholamines at the cyclic-3′,5′-AMP level. Amphetamine and its congeners are contraindicated since they force the debilitated adrenal medulla into complete atrophy and inactivity. Moreover they tend to produce addiction and, sometimes, psychosis.

Discussion

The different trends of catecholamine excretion in weather-sensitive patients and long distance runners are a most challenging finding because they show the difference between newcomers and veteran residents in the subtropics and tropics. As hot dry weather brings about passive dilation of the peripheral blood vessels and augments perspiration, catecholamine secretion becomes increased in order to contract the vessels and prevent excessive perspiration. This reaction is in contradistinction to the common view that wet heat may inhibit epinephrine secretion. Urinalysis clearly reveals hyposecretion of catecholamines as the cause of tropical lethargy.

Urinalysis also reveals that MAO-blocker treatment can restore the depleted epinephrine, norepinephrine, 17-KS, and 17-OH levels to normal values without affecting serotonin production. This finding would rule out the suspicion that tropical lethargy, i.e., lack of exercise is the cause of low urinary catecholamines.

In long distance runners catecholamine excretion increases considerably after exercise, and if it does not, the cause for it should be investigated (Table 4).

Perusal of Table 4 allows the following conclusions: Students 2 and 3 suffered from influenza on the day of exercise, yet because of insignificant fever reaction they were admitted to the 5-km training. The paradoxical reaction of their neurohormones is marked by an asterisk. Students 12, 14, 15, 16, 18, 20 dropped out after 1–2.5 km, probably because their neurohormone profile could not cope with the demands of a 5-km run. Students 21 and 24 were considered not fit for long-distance running, while No. 26 was regarded as not too severely hampered. When the tests were repeated, our assumption proved to be correct and the students 21 and 24 reverted to short-distance running, whereas student 26 was doing well on 5-km distance running after brief treatment with a MAO blocker.

Our findings do not necessarily imply that treatment with MAO blockers increases adrenal medulla output. It can, however, be assumed that better use of catecholamines, due to MAO blocker, allows the adrenal medulla to recuperate, an effect obtainable also by sending a patient for some months to a moderate climate. In any case the patients who had undergone the MAO blocker treatment with minidoses for 1–2 months were usually immune to heat-fatigue or long-distance-running staleness for a full year at least.

The beneficial effect of an MAO blocker like isocarboxazid on the adrenal medulla exhaustion syndrome finds its experimental backing in the observation by Randall and Bagdon (1959) who showed that the duration of its action *in vivo* may be as long as 20 days after a single dose.[12]

It is tempting to look for a teleological explanation of the typical pattern of neurohormone reactions in long distance runners. We have given pertinent interpretations to the typical changes encountered, which are compiled in TABLE 5.

SUMMARY

We have observed that people when exposed to extreme heat stress can suffer from depletion of epinephrine, norepinephrine, and adrenal corticosteroids. This was proven by daily urinalysis. Having ascertained that they were suffering especially from lack of monoamines, we found in them all the symptoms of catecholamine deficiency, i.e., hypotension, fatigue, exhaustion, apathy, depression, lack of concentration, confusion, hypoglycemic spells, and ataxia.

TABLE 5

MOOTED MECHANISMS OF NEUROHORMONE REACTIONS IN LONG DISTANCE RUNNERS

Hormone	Function	Reaction	Explanation
17-KS	Androgen metabolite	Decrease	Physical ability to cope with stress
17-OH	Cortisone metabolite	Decrease	Mobilization of sugar and sodium
5-HIAA	Serotonin metabolite	Decrease	Mental ability to cope with stress
Norepinephrine	Fight hormone	Increase	Improves circulation and mobilizes sugar
Epinephrine	Flight hormone	Increase	Improves heart action, circulation and sugar metabolism
Thyroxine Histamine	Metabolic hormones	Increase	Required for increased metabolism and heat production

The most typical complaint of such patients is that they suffer progressively more each year from "aging," exertion, or stress. Sport does not help them.

During heat spells or extreme effort, people have to secrete more catecholamines to cope with the demand and to contract their skin vessels in order to avoid excessive sweating. This repeated stress can induce adrenal medulla exhaustion with particularly low values of epinephrine. Norepinephrine follows suit, but it never reaches zero level (as epinephrine does) because of the extra adrenal production of norepinephrine as a sympathetic transmitter. The urinary excretion of 17-KS and 17-OH becomes sometimes reduced too.

Different results were obtained in long distance runners. Thirty male students, 20–25 years old, training for a long distance contest, had their urinary neurohormone levels tested before and after running 5,000 m at an ambient temperature of 10°–15° C. The runners to reach the tape showed decreases in the stress hormones 17-KS, 17-OH, and 5-HIAA; increases in the fight hormones epinephrine and norepinephrine; and increases in the metabolic hormones T-4 (urinary) and histamine. All changes were highly significant.

We have now been treating such patients for 10 years with minidoses of MAO blockers (1–10 mg/day). A low dosage of ¼–1 tablet/day completely cures the patients of their disability and adynamia, without any danger of a cheese tyramine reaction. Not every MAO blocker is suitable for this treatment: it has to be one with an immediate effect. We have singled out in particular the following preparations that produce relief within 30 minutes without producing any tolerance or addiction: isocarboxazid (Marplan, Roche) and mebanazine (Actomol, ICI). Replacement of the corticosteroids by anabolic hormones is rarely required.

REFERENCES

1. WELLER, C. P. & F. G. SULMAN. 1969. Effect of climatic heat stress on catecholamine excretion. Biometeorology (Suppl. to Int. J. Biometeorol.) 4(Pt. II): 30.
2. SULMAN, F. G., A. DANON, Y. PFEIFER, E. TAL & C. P. WELLER. 1970. Urinalysis of patients suffering from climatic heat stress (Sharav). Internat. J. Biometeorol. 14: 45–53.
3. SULMAN, F. G. 1976. Health, Weather, Climate. Karger Publications. Basel, Switzerland.
4. SULMAN, F. G. & E. SUPERSTINE. 1972. Aging and adrenal medulla exhaustion due to lack of monoamines and raised monoamine-oxidase levels. Lancet ii: 663.
5. SULMAN, F. G., N. HIRSCHMAN & Y. PFEIFER. 1964. Effect of hot, dry, desert winds (Sirocco, Sharav, Hamsin) on the metabolism of hormones and minerals. Proc. Lucknow Symposium on Arid Zones UNESCO : 89–95.
6. TAL, E. & F. G. SULMAN. 1972. Urinary thyroxine test. Lancet i: 1291.
7. DANON, A. & F. G. SULMAN. 1969. Ionizing effect of winds of ill repute on serotonin metabolism. Biometeorology (Suppl. to Int. J. Biometeorol.) 4(Pt. II): 135–136.
8. SULMAN, F. G., E. TAL, Y. PFEIFER & E. SUPERSTINE. 1975. Intermittent hyperthyreosis—A heat stress syndrome. Hormones Metabol. Res. 7: 424–428.
9. SULMAN, F. G., Y. PFEIFER & E. SUPERSTINE. 1973. Adrenal medullary exhaustion from tropical winds and its management. Isr. J. Med. Sci. 8: 1022–1027.
10. KOCH, Y., Y. PFEIFER & F. G. SULMAN. 1969. Effect of climatic heat stress on the development of rats. Int. J. Biometeorol. 13: 93.
11. WELLER, C. P., S. DIKSTEIN & F. G. SULMAN. 1969. The effect of heat stress on body development in rats. Biometeorology (Suppl. to Int. J. Biometeorol.) 4(Pt. II): 29.
12. RANDALL, L. O. & R. F. BAGDON. 1959. Pharmacology of isocarboxazid and other amine oxidase inhibitors. Ann. N.Y. Acad. Sci. 80: 626–642.

THE ATHLETE'S HEART SYNDROME:
A NEW PERSPECTIVE

Joel Morganroth *

*Hospital of the University of Pennsylvania
and Cardiovascular Section
University of Pennsylvania School of Medicine
Philadelphia, Pennsylvania 19104*

Barry J. Maron

*Cardiology Branch
National Heart, Lung and Blood Institute
National Institutes of Health
Bethesda, Maryland 20014*

Introduction

Over the past 70 years, physicians have studied the physiologic and anatomic consequences of prolonged strenuous exercise. The term "athlete's heart syndrome"[1] has been used to describe cardiac "abnormalities" (as detected by electrocardiograms, chest radiography, or physical examination) that are present in individuals who have either participated in competitive athletics for a number of years or have undergone prolonged physical training. Recently, the advances of diagnostic ultrasound[2, 3] have made it possible to more accurately define the structural and functional characteristics of the heart in trained athletes. The purpose of this communication is to comprehensively review the known features of the "athlete's heart" with particular emphasis on recent information provided by echocardiographic studies.

Radiographic Studies

Radiographic studies of the hearts of trained athletes (as well as electrocardiographic and echocardiographic studies that will be discussed below) have been performed on individuals competing in a variety of sports. Most of these studies have been made on athletes involved in strenuous prolonged exertion (i.e., endurance-type sports), such as marathon[4-10] and other long distance running,[2, 11-16] skiing,[14-16] rowing,[1, 12] swimming,[2, 12] and cycling.[17, 18] Most of these investigations were done under basal conditions before competition and during the peak of the athlete's training or career;[1-13, 16, 17] however, a few studies have been performed on former, but not totally deconditioned, athletes.[14, 15, 18]

One of the earliest observations made on the cardiac structure of athletes concerned the appearance of the heart on plane chest radiograph. Numerous

* Address for correspondence: 937 West Gates Pavilion, 3400 Spruce Street, Philadelphia, Pennsylvania 19104.

investigators have commented on the increased diastolic size [1, 10] (as determined by measurement of cardiothoracic ratio) or increased diastolic volume of the heart of athletes [13-16, 18] (as derived from the measured area of the heart shadow) either under basal conditions [14, 15, 18] or when related to maximal oxygen uptake.[13, 16] This finding of increased cardiac volume has, however, been refuted by others.[5, 12] Keys and Friedell [12] found no difference in diastolic heart volume between a group of trained athletes and untrained controls, although the athletes did show significantly greater heart volumes when the difference between diastolic and systolic volumes was calculated.

Electrocardiographic Studies

Numerous electrocardiographic findings believed to represent deviations from normal have been described in a number of studies on trained athletes.[1, 2-4, 6-11, 13, 16, 17, 19-27] It is accepted that the well-trained athlete has a relatively slow heart rate (usually 45–70 beats per minute), which is manifested as sinus bradycardia on the ECG.[2-4, 10, 14, 15, 17, 19, 25] Several arrhythmias have also been commonly observed in athletes, including sinus arrhythmia,[6, 9, 12, 26] second-degree atrioventricular block of the Wenckebach variety,[2, 6, 11, 18, 22] junctional rhythm,[1, 4, 6, 21, 25] and wandering atrial pacemaker.[1] Because these arrhythmias are usually abolished by exercise, they are believed to be due to enhanced vagal tone and suppression of the sinus or atrioventricular nodes. In addition, prolongation of the P-R interval (first-degree atrioventricular block) is relatively common in athletes (5% to 30% prevalence in the studies reviewed) and also is probably secondary to increased vagal tone. Lengthened QT_c intervals have also been reported in cyclists.[17]

Alterations in the P and QRS waves of the ECG, suggesting specific cardiac chamber enlargement, are also commonly observed in athletes. The presence of left or right atrial enlargement has been suggested by the findings of increased amplitude (>2.5 mm) [6, 8-10, 22] or duration (>0.11 second) [6, 10] of the P wave or notching of the P wave.[6, 25] Increased amplitude of the R or S waves in the standard or precordial leads, which frequently meet certain accepted ECG criteria for left [2-4, 6, 7, 9, 10, 16, 17, 20] or right [3, 4, 10, 17, 19, 20] ventricular hypertrophy, have been commonly described in athletes (17%–75% prevalence in the studies reviewed). These findings imply that the heart of the well-trained athlete manifests ventricular hypertrophy and perhaps also dilatation. However, it should be emphasized that there are difficulties in assessing the significance of the increased precordial voltages cited in these electrocardiographic studies and that the available ECG criteria for ventricular hypertrophy may not be strictly applicable to the ECG of trained athletes. For example, the criteria used for the ECG diagnoses of left or right ventricular hypertrophy differ among the various ECG studies, making it difficult to arrive at a uniform assessment of the data presented. Also, increased precordial voltages may be present in thin adult males who are not athletes and also in Blacks, where the increased voltages appear to be a racial variation in the ECG.[28] Nevertheless, autopsy studies of athletes who died accidently [29] or of noncardiac disease [30] have shown heart weights to be consistently greater than normal and, therefore, support the contention that hearts of athletes actually undergo an increase in mass due to physical training. Reindell et al.[29] found heart weights to be 350–540 grams (normal <350 g) in the 34 athletic subjects that he studied. Relatively minor conduction abnormalities such as intraventricular conduction defects, including notching, slurring, or prolongation of the QRS complex [4, 6, 7, 13, 17, 19] (in as many as 40%–50% of the subjects studied) and incomplete right bundle branch block have also been observed commonly in athletes.

ST segment changes present in the basal state may occur more commonly in the trained athlete than in the general population. These alterations, which may be present in as many as 10% of competitive athletes, consist of elevation of the J-junction (early repolarization) or true elevation of the ST segment; [1, 4, 6, 7, 13, 26] following exertion, these ST segment alterations usually return to the isoelectric baseline.[31-33] It should be noted that ST segment elevation (particularly the J-junctional variety) has been considered a variant of normal especially in nonathletic blacks without evidence of heart disease.[34-37] In addition, increased amplitude and broadening of the T waves in the standard and precordial leads [1, 4, 6, 8-10, 13, 17] and biphasic or negative T waves in precordial leads [4, 6-9, 17, 19, 23] are common findings in athletes studied in the basal state. Prominent U waves have also been described in the ECGs of athletes.[4, 10]

Echocardiographic Studies in Trained Athletes

The advent of echocardiography has permitted the detailed evaluation of the cardiac structural changes present in the trained athlete that was not possible with electrocardiography or chest roentgenography. We have recently studied by echocardiography 42 actively competing male college varsity athletes from the University of Maryland.[2] This study group included 15 swimmers, 15 long distance runners and 12 wrestlers. Each subject had participated in their athletic event for greater than 3 years and was training actively for more than 200 days per years. In addition, these athletes were identified by their coaches as being at the top of their competitive class. In addition, we have also studied 10 long distance runners and four shot-putters of world class caliber from the International Track Association (including two world recordholders). Athletes participating in these athletic events were selected in order to compare differences in the cardiac response to isotonic and isometric exercise. It has been suggested that athletes primarily participating in isotonic events (runners and swimmers) had cardiomegaly by chest radiograph whereas those athletes primarily participating in isometric events (wrestlers and shot-putters) usually showed peripheral muscular hypertrophy without obvious increase in cardiac size.[38-40]

Analysis of echocardiographic data on college runners and swimmers demonstrated that these athletes had increased left ventricular mass (FIGURE 1) compared to age- and sex-matched nonathlete controls, and that this increase in left ventricular mass was primarily due to increased left ventricular end diastolic volume (FIGURE 2) rather than increased ventricular septal and left ventricular free wall or septal thickness (FIGURE 3). The differences in echocardiographically determined cardiac dimensions between athletes and nonathletes were not accounted for on the basis of differences in body surface area or weight.

In comparing world class athletes participating in distance running with college distance runners, there was no statistical difference in echocardiographically determined cardiac dimensions (TABLE 1). Similar findings of increased cardiac mass in athletes due primarily to increased left ventricular internal dimension were reported by Roeske and co-workers [3] in ten professional basketball players studied by echocardiography. Furthermore,

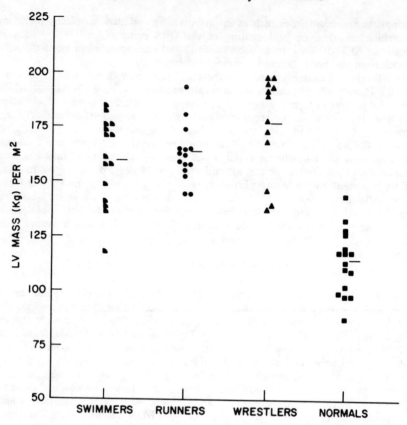

FIGURE 1. Echocardiographically measured left ventricular (LV) mass per body surface area in square meters in college athletes. Data on swimmers, runners, and wrestlers are statistically different from normals (p < 0.001).

Roeske *et al.*[3] found that right ventricular end diastolic volumes were also increased in basketball players compared to controls. Parameters of left ventricular function such as ejection fraction and mean circumferential fiber shortening (V_{cf}) have been reported as normal in athletes participating in isotonic sports.[2, 3]

An interesting contrast appears when athletes participating in isotonic exercise are compared to those participating in isometric sports. While college wrestlers and world class shot-putters (isometric exertion) had increased left ventricular mass of a similar degree as athletes participating in isotonic sports, the wrestlers and shot-putters had normal left ventricular end diastolic volumes but increased left ventricular wall thicknesses. Thus, the increase in left ventricular mass was accounted for solely by an increase in left ventricular wall thickness. In addition, there was no significant difference in echocardiographically determined cardiac dimensions between world class shot-putters and college wrestlers (TABLE 2).

Thus, these echocardiographic data clearly demonstrate that an increase in left ventricular mass may be present in highly trained athletes. The pattern of this "physiologic or adaptive" left ventricular hypertrophy, however, depends upon the nature of the athletic conditioning. Those athletes participating primarily in isotonic activity (of which the long distance runner may be considered the prime example) develop increased left ventricular mass almost solely on the basis of increased left ventricular end diastolic volume with insignificant to mild increase in left ventricular myocardial thickness. This contrasts with the

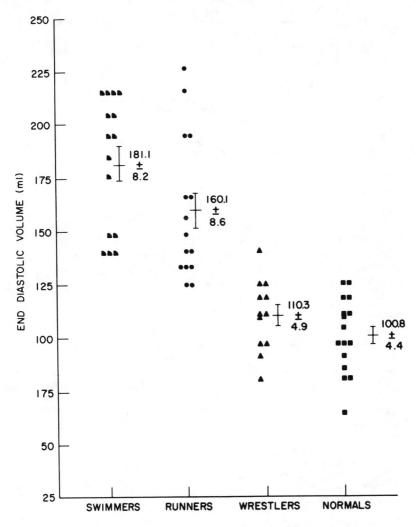

FIGURE 2. Echocardiographically measured left ventricular end diastolic volume in college athletes. Numbers represent mean values ±standard errors (SE). Data on swimmers and runners are statistically different from those of wrestlers and normal subjects (p < 0.001).

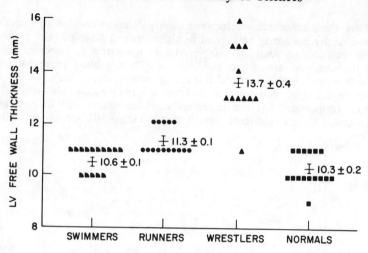

FIGURE 3. Echocadiographically measured left ventricular (LV) free wall thickness in college athletes. Numbers represent mean values ±SE. Data on wrestlers are statistically different from those of swimmers, runners, and normal subjects (p < 0.001).

structural changes seen in athletes participating primarily in isometric activity in which the increased left ventricular mass appears to be almost solely due to increased left ventricular wall thickness (TABLE 3).

Thus, "physiologic or adaptive" hypertrophy may be a common finding in professional and college athletes in which the repeated stress of training acts as a stimulus to alter cardiac dimensions, the nature of which depends upon the

TABLE 1

COMPARISON BETWEEN ECHOCARDIOGRAPHIC DATA IN COLLEGE RUNNERS AND WORLD CLASS RUNNERS *

	College Runners	World Class Runners
Number	15	10
LVIDd (left ventricular internal dimension at end diastole) (mm)	50–61	48–59
LVIDs (left ventricular internal dimension at end systole) (mm)	29–43	29–38
LVW (left ventricular posterior wall thickness at end diastole) (mm)	11–12	10–12
VS (ventricular septal thickness at end diastole) (mm)	10–12	10–12
LA (left atrial transverse dimension at end systole) (mm)	25–39	31–38
AO (aortic root transverse dimension at end systole) (mm)	24–30	23–30

* No statistically significant differences were found.

TABLE 2

COMPARISON BETWEEN ECHOCARDIOGRAPHIC DATA IN COLLEGE WRESTLERS
AND WORLD CLASS SHOT-PUTTERS *

	College Wrestlers	World Class Shot-Putters
Number	12	4
LVIDd (mm)	43–52	46–51
LVIDs (mm)	28–39	31–40
LVW (mm)	11–16	13–15
VS (mm)	10–15	13–15
LA (mm)	24–39	27–36
AO (mm)	21–32	23–29

* No statistically significant differences were found. For abbreviations see TABLE 1.

specific effort involved. The physical stress involved in isotonic activities produces an increase in cardiac output and a sustained hemodynamic burden for many hours each day while in training. This hemodynamic burden may be similar to that imposed in the diseased heart by a volume load on the left ventricle (e.g., aortic or mitral regurgitation); such patients characteristically develop an increase in left ventricular mass due to an increase in left ventricular end diastolic volume [41] (FIGURE 4). In contrast, those athletes who participate primarily in isometric activity develop "physiologic" left ventricular hypertrophy presumably due to the increase in systemic arterial pressure present during the stress of strenuous Valsalva maneuvers, which induces an increase in afterload upon the ventricle. The effect on the left ventricle of this stress is similar to that induced by pathologic conditions such as systemic hypertension or valvular aortic stenosis, in which the increase in left ventricular mass is due to increased ventricular thickening [41, 42] (FIGURE 4).

TABLE 3

COMPARISON OF CARDIAC ALTERATIONS OBSERVED IN ATHLETES PARTICIPATING
IN ENDURANCE (ISOTONIC) OR STRENGTH (ISOMETRIC) TRAINING *

	Endurance Training	Strength Training
Wall thickness	Normal	↑
End diastolic volume	↑	Normal
Mass	↑	↑

* In both groups there is an increase (↑) in left ventricular mass. In the endurance group, the increase in mass was due primarily to an increase in left ventricular end diastolic volume, whereas in the strength-training group, the increase in mass was due primarily to an increase in ventricular septal and free wall thickness.

Significance of Cardiac Alterations in Trained Athletes

Identification of increased cardiac mass in athletes (comparable to that seen in pathologic cardiac states) raises the question of the long-term significance of these changes. Increased cardiac mass in the trained athlete probably represents an adaptation to conditioning that is necessary to maintain optimal cardiac performance. However, these cardiac structural changes are probably not the only factors determining superior athletic performance. Although college athletes manifest consistently inferior competitive performances compared to world class athletes, these two groups of athletes nevertheless have similar cardiac dimensions as determined by echocardiography. It is, however, unclear whether differences in competitive performance in athletes are due to greater cardiac response

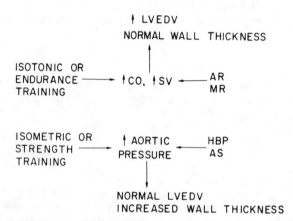

FIGURE 4. Schematic representation of the relation between isotonic and isometric training, resultant echocardiographically determined cardiac structural changes, and possible relationship of these changes to valvular heart disease or systemic hypertension. See text for details. Abbreviations: ↑CO, increase in cardiac output; ↑SV, increase in stroke volume; ↑Aortic pressure, increase in mean aortic pressure; ↑LVEDV, increased left ventricular end diastolic volume; AR, aortic valvular regurgitation; MR, mitral valvular regurgitation; HBP, systemic hypertension; AS, aortic valvular stenosis.

to maximal exertion or to differences in peripheral circulatory adaptations (such as decreased arterial resistance or increased oxygen extraction), noncardiovascular mechanisms (such as greater muscle strength, enhanced aerobic or anaerobic sources of energy production), or psychological factors. Finally, it is possible that the echocardiographically determined differences in cardiac dimensions in athletes compared to nonathlete controls are not entirely the result of prolonged physical training but rather are influenced substantially by genetic factors that predispose such individuals to become athletes initially.

Finally, further echocardiographic studies are needed to determine the long-term significance of the cardiac structural changes present in trained athletes, i.e., whether the cardiac hypertrophy will regress after active training ceases, and whether it will ultimately be harmful to the athlete. Electrocardiographic and radiographic studies on former endurance athletes suggest that cardiac structural changes in athletes may not regress entirely after termination of active competition. For example, Pyörölä[14] has demonstrated that 61 former champion endurance athletes, when compared to 54 nonathlete controls, had larger maximal QRS vectors, larger heart volumes determined by chest roentgenography, and slower heart rates. Finally, although cardiac function has been shown to be normal in athletes by echocardiography, sufficient data is not currently available to determine whether continued athletic participation at high levels of intense effort for decades will, in effect, be deleterious to the cardiovascular system.

Summary

Although earlier electrocardiographic and roentgenographic studies suggested that the heart of trained athletes differed from that of nonathletes, little was known of the cardiac dimensions of the athlete's heart until the advent of echocardiography. Echocardiographic studies have demonstrated that trained athletes may have increased left ventricular mass and that the structural change accounting for this increase is related to the type of physical conditioning. Athletes participating primarily in isotonic exercise have an increase in left ventricular end-diastolic volume with little or no increase in left ventricular wall thickness whereas those athletes participating primarily in isometric exercise have an increase in left ventricular wall thickness associated with normal left ventricular end-diastolic volume. Comparisons between echocardiographically determined cardiac changes in college and world class athletes were made, and the electrocardiographic and chest roentgenographic changes present in the athlete's heart syndrome were reviewed.

References

1. GOTT, P. H., H. A. ROSELLE & R. S. CRAMPTON. 1968. The athletic heart syndrome. Arch. Intern. Med. 122: 340.
2. MORGANROTH, J., B. J. MARON, W. L. HENRY & S. E. EPSTEIN. 1975. Comparative left ventricular dimensions in trained athletes. Ann. Int. Med. 82: 521.
3. ROESKE, W. R., R. A. O'ROURKE, A. KLEIN, G. LEOPOLD & J. S. KARLINER. 1976. Noninvasive evaluation of ventricular hypertrophy in professional athletes. Circulation 53: 286.
4. SMITH, W. G., K. J. CULLEN & I. O. THORBURN. 1964. Electrocardiograms of marathon runners in 1962 Commonwealth Games: Brit. Heart J. 26: 469.
5. GORDON, B., S. A. LEVINE & A. WILMAERS. 1924. Observations on a group of marathon runners. Arch. Intern. Med. 33: 425.
6. NAKAMOTO, K. 1969. Electrocardiograms of 25 marathon runners before and after 100 meter dash. Japan. Circ. J. 33: 105.
7. VENERANDO, A. & V. RULLI. 1964. Frequency morphology and meaning of the electrocardiographic anomalies found in Olympic marathon runners and walkers. J. Sports. Med. Phys. Fitness 4: 135.
8. MCKECHNIE, J. K., W. P. LEARY & S. M. JOUBERT. 1967. Some electrocardiographic and biochemical changes recorded in marathon runners. S. Afr. Med. J. 41(Suppl., S. Afr. J. Lab. Clin. Med.): 722.
9. HÄNTZSCHEL, K. & K. DOHRN. 1966. The electrocardiogram before and after a marathon-race. J. Sports Med. Phys. Fitness 6: 28.

10. BECKNER, G. L. & T. WINSOR. 1954. Cardiovascular adaptations to prolonged physical effort. Circulation **9:** 835.

11. GRIMBY, G. & B. SALTIN. 1964. Daily running causing Wenckebach heart block. Lancet **ii:** 962.

12. KEYS, A. & H. FRIEDELL. 1938. Size and stroke of the heart in young men in relation to athletic activity. Science **88:** 456.

13. GRIMBY, G. & B. SALTIN. 1966. Physiological analysis of physically well-trained middle-aged and old athletes. Acta Med. Scand. **179:** 513.

14. PYÖRÄLÄ, K., M. J. KARVONEN, P. TASKINEN, J. TAKKUNEN, H. KYRÖNSEPPÄ & H. PELTOKALLIO. 1967. Cardiovascular study on former endurance athletes. Amer. J. Cardiol. **20:** 191.

15. PYÖRÄLÄ, K., M. KARVONEN, P. TASKINEN, J. TAKKUNEN & H. KYRÖNSEPPÄ. 1967. Cardiovascular studies on former endurance athletes. *In* Physical Activity and the Heart. M. Karvonen & A. J. Barry, Eds. : 301. Charles C Thomas, Publisher. Springfield, Ill.

16. SALTIN, B. & G. GRIMBY. 1968. Physiological analysis of middle-aged and old former athletes. Circulation **38:** 1104.

17. VAN GANSE, W., L. VERSEE, W. EYLENBOSCH & K. VUYLSTEEK. 1970. The electrocardiogram of athletes: Comparison with untrained subjects. Brit. Heart J. **32:** 160.

18. HOLMGREN A. & T. STRANDELL. 1959. The relationship between heart volume, total hemoglobin and physical working capacity in former athletes. Acta Med. Scand. **163:** 149.

19. BESWICK, F. W. & R. C. JORDAN. 1961. Cardiological observations at the sixth British Empire and Commonwealth Games. Brit. Heart J. **23:** 113.

20. ARSTILA, M. & A. KOIVIKKO. 1964. Electrocardiographic and vectorcardiographic signs of left and right ventricular hypertrophy in endurance athletes. J. Sports Med. Phys. Fitness **4:** 166.

21. SHAMROTH, L. & E. JOKL. 1969. Marked sinus and A-V nodal bradycardia with interference-dissociation in an athlete. J. Sports Med. Phys. Fitness **9:** 128.

22. SARGIN, O., C. ALP, C. TANSI & L. KARACA. 1970. Wenckebach phenomenon with nodal and ventricular escape in marathon runners. Chest **57:** 102.

23. ROSE, K. D. 1969. Relationship of cardiac problems to athletic participation. J. Amer. Med. Assoc. **208:** 2319.

24. LICHTMAN, J., R. A. O'ROURKE, A. KLEIN & J. S. KARLINER. 1973. Electrocardiogram of the athlete. Arch. Intern. Med. **132:** 763.

25. KLEMOLA, E. 1951. Electrocardiographic observations on 650 Finnish athletes. Ann. Med. Fenn. **40:** 121.

26. HUNT, B. P. E. 1963. Electrocardiographic study of 20 champion swimmers before and after 110 yard sprint swimming competition. Canad. Med. Assoc. J. **88:** 1251.

27. CULLEN, K. J. & R. COLLIN. 1964. Daily running causing Wenckebach heart block. Lancet **ii:** 729.

28. MASICA, D., B. J. MARON & L. J. KROVETZ. 1972. Racial variations in the childhood electrocardiogram. Amer. Heart J. **84:** 153.

29. REINDELL, H., K. MUSSHOFF & H. KLEPZIG. 1956. Regulative und myogene dilatation des herzens. Fortschr. Geb. Rontgenstr. Nuklearmed. **85:** 385.

30. CURRENS, J. H. & P. D. WHITE. 1961. Half a century of running: Clinical, physiologic, and autopsy findings in the case of Clarence de Mar ("Mr. Marathon"). N. Engl. J. Med. **265:** 988.

31. WASSERBURGER, R. H., W. J. ALT & C. J. LLOYD. 1961. The normal RS-T segment elevation variant. Amer. J. Cardiol. **7:** 184.

32. GOLDMAN, M. J. 1953. RS-T segment elevation in mid and left precordial leads as a normal variant. Amer. Heart J. **46:** 817.

33. CHELTON, L. G. & H. B. BURCHELL. 1955. Unusual RT segment deviations in electrocardiograms of normal persons. Amer. J. Med. Sci. **230:** 54.

34. GRUSIN, H. 1954. Peculiarities of the African's electrocardiogram and the changes observed in serial studies. Circulation 9: 860.
35. THOMAS, J., E. HARRIS & G. LASSITER. 1960. Observations on the T wave and ST segment changes in the precordial electrocardiogram of 320 young Negro adults. Amer. J. Cardiol. 5: 468.
36. POWELL, S. J. 1959. Unexplained electrocardiograms in the African. Brit. Heart J. 21: 263.
37. WALKER, A. R. P. & B. F. WALKER. 1969. The bearing of race, sex, age and nutritional state on the precordial electrocardiograms of young South African Bantu and Caucasian subjects. Amer. Heart J. 77: 441.
38. MOREHOUSE, L. E. & A. T. MILLER. 1967. Physiology of Exercise. 5th edit. : 286–287. St. Louis, Mo.
39. FRICK, M. H., A. KONTTINEN & H. S. SARAJAS. 1963. Effects of physical training on the circulation at rest and during exercise. Amer. J. Cardiol. 12: 142.
40. SJOSTRAND, T. 1953. Volume and distribution of blood and their significance in regulating the circulation. Physiol. Rev. 33: 202.
41. GRANT, C., I. L. BUNNELL & D. G. GREENE. 1964. Angiographic observations on left ventricular function in man (abstract). Fed. Proc. 23: 464.
42. DODGE, H. T. & W. A. BOXLEY. 1969. Left ventricular volume and mass and their significance in heart disease. Amer. J. Cardiol. 23: 528–537.

MYOGLOBINURIA IN MARATHON RUNNERS: POSSIBLE RELATIONSHIP TO CARBOHYDRATE AND LIPID METABOLISM

William J. Bank

Department of Neurology
Hospital of the University of Pennsylvania
Philadelphia, Pennsylvania 19104

The limitations of human endurance have long intrigued the physiologist, biochemist, and clinician as well as the athlete. Often the warnings of such a limit are exceeded under the stress of competition. To the clinician, myoglobinuria, manifest as a dark discoloration of urine, is often an early clue to serious muscle destruction. In the past two decades, several specific inborn errors of metabolism have been detected that present with exercise intolerance and myoglobinuria. It is hoped that by reviewing these well-understood but rare disorders that we can clarify the normal and pathologic processes in individuals undergoing long periods of exercise.

Myoglobinuria

Myoglobin is the normal constituent of human skeletal muscle and readily leaks into plasma during any form of acute muscle destruction. This was first recognized during crush injuries in World War II and has since been associated with a wide variety of causes.[1, 2] Myoglobinemia is cleared by the renal tubule resulting in myoglobinuria. The passage of this pigment through the kidney is apparently directly toxic to the renal tubule and may result in acute renal failure. As renal function diminishes, urinary output will decrease and possibly cease for hours or days. The hazard to the patient is a direct consequence of renal dysfunction with buildup of life-threatening metabolites in the body.

It is assumed that during muscle injury, the integrity of the muscle sarcolemma is disrupted resulting in leakage of intracellular constituents including myoglobin. This phenomenon has been associated with many drugs but, in fact, the cause of muscle injury may have been coma with subsequent crush injuries of limbs.[3] Seizures and hyperthermia have also been implicated as contributing factors in myoglobinuria.[4, 5]

Marathon Runners and Myoglobinuria. Exercise intolerance with muscle destruction has also been seen in normal individuals after extreme exertion, especially if physical conditioning has been poor.[6-8] Recently, we have seen several cases of marathon runners who are presumably well-conditioned but had pigmenturia and renal failure as a consequence of a strenuous race. Of particular interest are several cases of runners who are incapacitated or did poorly after high carbohydrate loading.

Case No. 1. A 34-year-old physician who had been jogging for 4 years gradually progressed to long distance running at marathons. He ran in the Boston Marathon in 1974 quite uneventfully. In training for the 1975 Marathon, he regularly underwent a carbohydrate-loading diet that caused him no

942

discomfort while training. That year he ran his fastest marathon in a time of 2 hours and 40 minutes. Although he felt well during the race, several hours thereafter he noted dark urine and rapidly became acutely ill with mental confusion, nausea, and general weakness. Acute renal failure with myoglobinuria was diagnosed and intensive medical management was necessary for renal failure for 8 days. The patient then recovered full renal function spontaneously with no recurrent myoglobinuria. He has again taken up running but no long distances. He also has discontinued the carbohydrate-loading diet.

Case No. 2. A 22-year-old college student had been a competitive runner in high school and was a mile-runner on his college track team. In addition, he had developed as a cross-country runner and undertaken the marathon. He had successfully competed at 9 or 10 miles without discomfort. When he underwent a high carbohydrate loading diet as part of his training, he noted that he "tied up" frequently and much sooner than usual. On several occasions he had dark urine that was identified as myoglobin. His myoglobinuria was always transient and did not result in decreased or altered renal function. He has subsequently discontinued the high carbohydrate diet and long distance running. He is, however, successful and symptom-free at the mile.

Metabolic Disorders Resulting in Myoglobinuria

Several distinct and well-recognized metabolic disorders have been identified that present as exercise intolerance and myoglobinuria. In 1959, Brian Mc-Ardle[9] described a patient who was generally well, and not weak. When he exercised beyond a specific limit, his muscles became firm and tender and difficult to contract. Many patients with a similar disorder describe a distinct exercise limit that they cannot exceed. Early warnings are tightness in muscles that become severe and painful with uncontrolled cramping if exercise persists. Frequently this results in pigmenturia after several hours and has been associated with renal failure. McArdle's patient was quite limited in his ability to do anaerobic exercise and developed a painful contracture of the forearm after one minute of ischemic exercise. Such patients subsequently were also shown not to produce the normal rise in venous lactate after ischemic exercise. The definitive diagnosis in such patients was made by muscle biopsy, which showed an abnormal accumulation of muscle glycogen and complete absence of muscle phosphorylase, the enzyme necessary for glycogen degradation (FIGURE 1). In the absence of this enzyme, muscle glycogen is unavailable for anaerobic glycolysis and lactate cannot be produced. The patient with McArdle's disease is therefore not incapacitated until voluntary effort and metabolic demands exceed energy derived from aerobic metabolism. The inability to generate ATP from endogenous muscle glycogen presumably impairs the energy-dependent relaxing factors of striated muscle. This results in a contracture and eventual muscle breakdown resulting in myoglobinuria. This contracture has been likened to *in vivo* rigor mortis. It is noteworthy that many patients with proven myophosphorylase deficiency were able to perform vigorous athletics when younger and insidiously developed exercise intolerance in the second and third decades.

More recently, several patients have been described who have the identical clinical syndrome of exercise intolerance, contracture, and subsequent myoglobinuria.[10, 11] These patients have had normal muscle phosphorylase concentration although glycogen content is again elevated. The enzyme absent in these

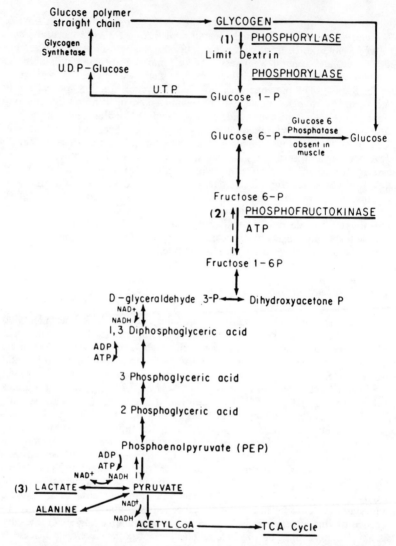

FIGURE 1. Pathways of glycogen metabolism. Absence of phosphorylase (1) or phosphofructokinase (2) result in glycogen storage in muscle and inability to produce lactate (3).

cases is phosphofructokinase (PFK), which also is required to metabolize glucose via the anaerobic pathway (FIGURE 1).

We have recently investigated two brothers who had exercise-related myoglobinuria resulting in renal failure. Both brothers had a normal venous lactate rise after ischemic exercise with no contracture. Examination of their muscles showed normal glycogen content, and phosphorylase and phosphofructokinase were present. These patients had an unusual response to dietary studies, including a 72-hour fast. Although both patients were symptom-free after a 72-hour fast, there were traces of myoglobin in urine and creatine phosphokinase (CPK) had risen markedly in the plasma. These findings both indicate muscle breakdown. In addition, plasma triglycerides, which were already elevated, continued to rise during fasting. Subsequent tests with fat loading showed that both patients handled lipids abnormally and their free fatty acids (FFA) remained markedly elevated and resulted in hypertriglyceridemia (FIGURE 2). Muscle showed no structural abnormality or lipid deposits. In both brothers, carnitine palmityl transferase (CPT), an enzyme necessary for incorporation of free fatty acids in mitochondria, was absent in muscle.[12] This deficiency prevented beta-oxidation of free fatty acids in muscle and resulted in an increase of plasma

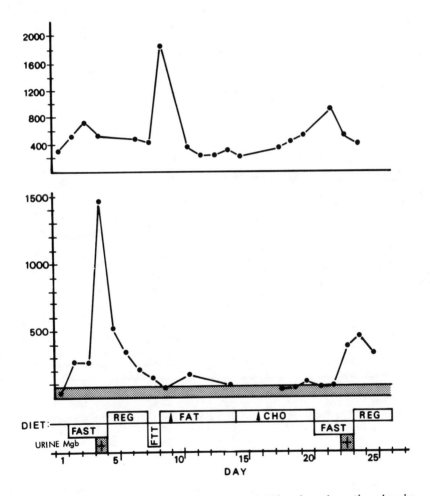

FIGURE 2. Plasma triglycerides, in mg per 100 ml (Above), and creatine phosphokinase in international units per liter (Below). During a 72-hour fast, plasma triglycerides and muscle enzymes (creatine phosphokinase) rose, and urinary myoglobin (Mgb) was detected. Triglycerides after a fat tolerance test (FTT) were markedly elevated. (From Bank et al.[12] By permission of The New England Journal of Medicine.)

free fatty acids with subsequent excessive formation of triglycerides (FIGURE 3). These patients did not have exercise intolerance as seen in phosphorylase or PFK deficiency, but both developed myoglobinuria after periods of vigorous exercise coincident with fasting or poor diet.

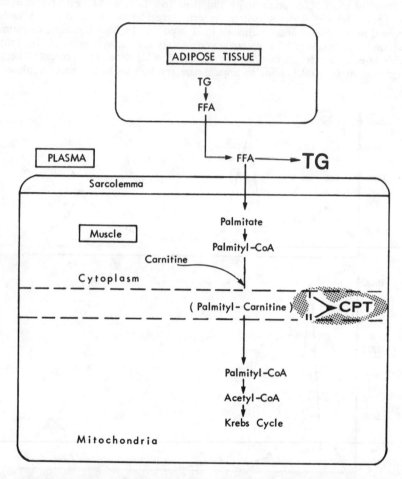

FIGURE 3. Lipid metabolism in muscle in absence of carnitine palmityl transferase (CPT). CPT enables long-chain fatty acids to enter muscle mitochondria and be oxidized. In the absence of muscle CPT, unused free fatty acids (FFA) result in high plasma triglycerides (TG). (From Bank *et al.*[12] By permission of *The New England Journal of Medicine.*)

Fatty acid oxidation in man at rest and on regular diet provides more than 50% of the energy required by muscle and accounts for a substantial percentage of body utilization of fatty acids and ketones.[13] Long-chain fatty acids are predominantly mobilized from fat cells during fasting and oxidized within mitochondria.[14] Fatty acids cross the mitochondrial membrane only as esters of carnitine and cannot be utilized via the Kreb's cycle in the absence of carnitine palmityl transferase (CPT). During normal activity and diet, patients lacking CPT could therefore utilize muscle glycogen or glucose and tolerate moderate exercise. After unusual exercise, especially with some degree of fasting, glycogen storage was rapidly depleted and long-chain fatty acids could not enter muscle mitochondria to serve as a source of energy. Presumably the lack of energy again disrupted the sarcolemmal integrity resulting in myoglobinuria.

Discussion

It is of interest that both runners described were superior athletes who were well-conditioned and in no way fit into the categories of glycogen or lipid storage disease. When they significantly altered their dietary intake during extremes of exercise, however, they had very similar consequences. Individuals lacking CPT also were symptom-free except during extreme exercise and especially if they had fasted. The high carbohydrate loading currently in vogue among runners may predispose certain individuals to the hazards of myoglobinuria. High carbohydrate loading is generally achieved by deliberately depleting muscle glycogen with a vigorous run lasting 90 minutes or more. For several subsequent days, a low-carbohydrate diet is continued during which exercise is maintained. This is followed by a period of rest for several days with high-carbohydrate meals. This has been shown to increase muscle glycogen content with the intent of prolonging or improving muscle endurance.[15] While many such "loaders" show dramatic improvement as did Case No. 1, others have been severely hampered by leg cramps and inordinate fatigue. A similar phenomenon has long been recognized in horses, known as "tying up."[16] This is frequently seen in horses after a period of rest and high carbohydrate meal. In work animals this was known as "Monday morning disease" because of the weekend rest during which the animals were heavily fed. The exact nature of this condition has never been clarified.

While we do not know of a specific abnormality in the cases described, we have good evidence that there is a critical threshold beyond which human skeletal muscle cannot normally function. Measurements on marathon runners have shown that muscle fiber type[17] and enzyme content[18] reflect the adaptation of muscle in such individuals. Variations in muscle glycogen in human subjects during rest or moderate exercise are small; however, during heavy exercise, even in the well-conditioned athlete, glycogen stores are rapidly depleted.[19] It seems clear that muscle glycogen utilization is a significant limiting factor in prolonged exercise. At the extremes of exercise such as at 80%–90% of maximal oxygen uptake for 100–200 minutes, the depletion of glycogen is well-correlated with the exhaustion point of the individual.[20] The usual signs of functional limitation such as fatigue, pain and cramps are ignored during the heat of competition. Subsequent depletion of critical biochemical substrates results in disruption of the muscle sarcolemma, and myoglobinemia may occur. The well-conditioned athlete may be especially vulnerable when diet and critical substrates required by muscle are significantly altered. As our understanding of glycogen and lipid metabolism of normal muscle improves, we should be better able to control and recognize the limitations of normal human muscle function. It is important to recall that myoglobinuria, regardless of the cause, may have serious renal consequences and in fact be life-threatening if it is not recognized and treated.

Acknowledgment

The author is indebted to Dr. G. A. Sheehan for description of Case No. 1.

References

1. BYWATERS, E. G. L., G. E. DELORY, C. REMINGTON & J. SMILES. 1941. Myo-hemoglobin in urine of air raid casualties with crushing injury. Biochem. J. 35: 1164–1168.
2. PENN, A. S., L. P. ROWLAND & D. W. FRASER. 1972. Drugs, coma, and myoglobinuria. Arch. Neurol. 26: 336–343.
3. ROWLAND, L. P. & A. S. PENN. 1972. Myoglobinuria. Med. Clin. N. Amer. 56: 1233–1256.
4. DIAMOND, I. & T. I. AQUILO. 1965. Myoglobinuria following unilateral status epilepticus and epsilateral rhabdomyolysis. N. Engl. J. Med. 272: 834–837.
5. WILSON, R. D., D. L. TRABER, C. R. AARON & L. L. PRIANO. 1971. Malignant hyperpyrexia. South. Med. J. 64: 411–414.
6. SMITH, R. S. 1968. Exertional rhabdomyolysis in Naval officer candidates. Arch. Int. Med. 121: 313–316.
7. GELLER, S. A. 1973. Extreme exertion rhabdomyolysis. Human Pathol. 4: 241–250.
8. DEMOS, M. A., E. L. GITIN & L. J. KAGAN. 1974. Exercise myoglobinuria and acute exertional rhabdomyolysis. Arch. Int. Med. 134: 669–673.
9. MCARDLE, B. 1951. Myopathy due to a defect in muscle glycogen breakdown. Clin. Sci. 10: 13–33.
10. TARUI, S., G. AKUNO, Y. IKURA, *et al.* 1965. Phosphofructokinase deficiency in skeletal muscle: A new type of glycogenosis. Biochim. Biophys. Res. Commun. 19: 517–523.
11. LAYZER, R. B., L. P. ROWLAND & H. M. RANNEY. 1967. Muscle phosphofructokinase deficiency. Arch. Neurol. 17: 512–523.
12. BANK, W. J., S. DiMAURO, E. BONILLA, D. CAPUZZI & L. P. ROWLAND. 1975. A disorder of muscle lipid metabolism and myoglobinuria: Absence of carnitine palmityl transferase. N. Engl. J. Med. 292: 443–449.
13. KAYHILL, G. F., JR., M. G. HERRERRA & P. MORGAN, *et al.* 1966. Hormone-fuel interrelationships during fasting. J. Clin. Invest. 45: 1751–1769.
14. HOPPEL, C. L. & R. J. TOMEC. 1972. Carnitine palmityl transferase: Location of two enzymatic activities in rat liver mitochondria. J. Biol. Chem. 247: 832–841.
15. BERGSTROM, J., L. HERMANSEN & E. HULTMAN, *et al.* 1967. Diet, muscle glycogen and physical performance. Acta Physiol. Scand. 71: 140–150.
16. HAMMEL, E. Personal communication.
17. COSTILL, D. L., W. J. FINK & M. L. POLLOCK. 1976. Muscle fiber composition and enzyme activities of elite distance runners. Med. Sci. Sports 8: 96–100.
18. HOLLOSZY, J. O. 1975. Adaptation of skeletal muscle to endurance exercise. Med. Sci. Sports 7: 155–164.
19. HULTMAN, E., J. BERGSTROM & A. E. ROCH-NORLUND. 1971. Glycogen storage in human skeletal muscle. Adv. Exp. Med. Biol. 11: 273–288.
20. SALTIN, B. & J. KARLSSON. 1971. Muscle glycogen utilization during work of different intensities. Adv. Exp. Med. Biol. 11: 289–299.

DISCUSSION

George Sheehan, *Moderator*

Riverview Hospital
Red Bank, New Jersey 07701

G. SHEEHAN: As a preliminary comment, what we've seen here indicates that the use of butazolidine and cortisone shots in a problem that is primarily biomechanical is to live in the dark ages, and perhaps if nothing more will come out of our section of the conference it will be an understanding of the necessity of looking at the basic biomechanical problems in the runner.

L. D. LUTTER (*St. Paul, Minn.*): If we're then looking at a group of people who we can get to be 70 years old with good cardiopulmonary function but haven't the structural ability to walk to the mailbox, I think we haven't solved all of our problems. The question that I'm raising is something that all of us dealing with muscoloskeletal problems both have to ask ourselves and are asked, which is: is there any increase in degenerative arthrosis particularly of knees, hips, and spine in individuals who are running for 20 years' time? Are we truly going to wear out?

R. O. SCHUSTER (*N.Y. College of Podiatric Medicine, New York, N.Y.*): I've been worrying and wondering about this myself and I haven't had records on these people long enough. But I certainly don't get the impression that this happens. I can't tell you it won't happen but I haven't seen it.

S. I. SUBOTNICK (*California College of Podiatric Medicine, Hayward, Calif.*): Studies in European literature suggest that using a joint or running increases the synovial pumping mechanism whereby activity allows the synovial fluid to nourish the subchondral bone and chrondral bone more so than it would in an inactive person. Instead of degenerative arthritis especially in the hips, this leads to increased healthiness or state of well-being of the hip joints and/or knee joints. That's one thing to consider.

Point number two is, doing proper stretching exercises, you will have a greater range of motion in all your major joints. This also leads to less incidence of arthritis.

R. HANLON (*Providence College, R.I.*): Dr. Schuster, I think you made mention of the fact that you thought it was appropriate for a runner to have a build-up heel. If a runner, a young runner especially, is jogging 80 or 90 miles a week with a build-up heel, he is immobilizing the tendon to an extent. If he then puts his race shoes on and runs a race on an indoor track, all the stress is on that right leg on the outside. Now, under competition, a high anxiety situation, he is putting undue stress in an area that, in my way of thinking as a layman, hasn't been developed. I just wonder how you would reconcile this with your training with a build-up heel.

R. O. SCHUSTER: I certainly should have told you the whole story. It is very important that these people do stretching exercises. We insist that they do stretching exercises, and that they do them several times a day. I am not at all upset about relaxing that calf muscle when they are running, if stretching it at all other times.

My ideas about heels anyway are a little bit heretical. I do feel that we are getting to a high heel even in our street shoes for very good develop-

949

mental physiological reasons; and this is no contradiction, I do feel it's good for us to stretch, for athletes especially. You know these people come into the office and you can say, "Hey, you haven't been running lately, have you?" He says, "How, do you know?" "Well you've got total range of dorsiflexion in the foot." They loosen up. When they're running they tighten up.

R. STEINMULLER (*Albert Einstein College of Medicine, The Bronx, N.Y.*): How much can you alter these inbalances or correct them by exercise of the foot and calf, etc.? If so, to what degree then should you approach the problem by attempting to alter the architecture through exercise versus compensating for it with orthotics. Related to the last question, also, what about the use of so-called negative heel shoes for continuous daily wear to help stretch the Achilles?

S. I. SUBOTNICK: First of all if you're going to be involved with sports medicine, you have to have a holistic view of the athlete and treat the total athlete, and all of us who treat our patients do a complete muscle test on them for strength and flexibility and range of motion. All of our athletes are put on a flexibility and strengthening program depending on what their problem is, and certainly if you have somebody with a tight posterior muscle group this will cause midstance pronation, the same if you have a true equinous problem, and you could put them on stretching exercises and that may take care of the problem.

After they have been on a good flexibility program, then we may need a more permanent rigid sophisticated support and this will be an indication for it.

As far as the negative heel shoe goes I did a study which will be published, a one-year study where I gave 50 *Roots* shoes away to my patients. Thirty percent of the patients within 2 weeks returned all the shoes to me, even though they cost $40.

The rest of the people use the shoe as an exercise device. The negative heel shoe is not for walking in my approximation. It is an exercise device to be used 3 to 4 hours a day after running, just to stand in it and cause a static stretch. It's good for standing, but in my approximation it is not good for running. Furthermore we did a study where we used a negative heel shoe for running: We all put them on, it was a tennis shoe, and we all went out for our normal 6-mile run; we went one block, came back, threw the shoes away, and put on our normal elevated heel shoes. You can't run in those.

H. W. RYDER (*Cincinnati, Ohio*): I have a question for Dr. Subotnick. In runners who are developing early signs of stress fractures in the metatarsal shafts, is there any treatment that he can recommend to keep the runner running while preventing the biomechanical inbalance that's producing the fracture?

S. I. SUBOTNICK: If somebody has a stress fracture and they come into your office, you know they have a stress fracture. You don't have to X-ray them. They have dorsal edema and they have classic symptoms and you can see it's a stress fracture. The only other differential is extensor tendinitis. It doesn't matter; you treat it the same way. I tape them and put a strap on the foot. I put a felt pad in and I tape them up well and I tell them to use common sense. If it hurts, don't run. If it doesn't hurt, run. Stay on a soft surface. Now you don't have to go to a doctor to know if it hurts don't run. That's my approach. At the same time I evaluate them biomechanically and I start in with the processes of making them a functional soft orthoses, which I usually can get made quickly enough to give to them within a week. But I make a temporary support then and there. And they can run.

QUESTION: I'd like further information on the hip cross-over in women. How frequent is it? How does it cause injuries and loss of efficiency? Is there a way to self-diagnose it, and can it be corrected with improved technique?

S. I. SUBOTNICK: It depends on how wide your pelvis is. If you have a wide pelvis you are going to cross over. You can tell if you have a cross-over or not just by running in the sand and seeing what your foot placements are like or just watching how you put your foot down when you're running, or have somebody run behind you, they can tell. The more you cross over the greater stress can be placed on that leg because it causes you whole leg to be imbalanced, and then you have to pronate more just to get your foot on the ground.

QUESTION: Is there a ratio of height to pelvic width that might let you know if you had a tendency to do this?

S. I. SUBOTNICK: There may be but I don't have the statistics.

QUESTION: What would be the ideal distance between your feet in running?

S. I. SUBOTNICK: Well, Steidler is the only one who did any work on that and if you look at his textbook he has some figures. Whether they are relative or accurate enough, I don't know. I haven't done the work on that myself.

A. N. ROSENBERG (*Princeton University, Princeton, N.J.*): So far you have discussed the "perfect" runner. But most people who come into an office like yours will not be perfect runners and will have a very different form then a perfect form. I wonder what compensations should the podiatrist take for people with different form just because they run differently.

S. I. SUBOTNICK: I think there are a couple of things that I should point out. Number one is that the general population that comes to a doctor's office has significant biomechanical deformity because this is a walking population and there has to be a lot wrong or they wouldn't be coming in. When an athlete comes into your office, by and large he has good structure and he has very little wrong with him, biomechanically. The less he has wrong the harder he is going to be to treat and usually the more serious is the complaint. In other words, the runner with very little wrong structurally who has a bad knee problem is a real problem because you don't have much to work with. And I see this all the time. It's easy to treat a runner who has bad structure because just a little correction and they're on their way. But many of the runners don't have much wrong so you don't have much to work with. So it's not that much deformity that we're working with in the first place.

A. N. ROSENBERG: What do you do with the runners form?

S. I. SUBOTNICK: Well, an orthotic is going to change the angle of gait. When you change the angle of gait that's going to change the form.

QUESTION: Dr. Sheehan, when you mentioned the incidence of injuries in long distance runners you did not mention low back problems.

G. SHEEHAN: I think the problem there is that most runners don't realize the problem is in the low back because their symptoms are sciatic. They get pain in the buttocks or thigh, or even, as we've seen, numb feet at about fifteen miles, which is sciatic. So that's the reason why they don't report that. I think sciatica is quite frequent.

COMMENT: I would like to say that we see a lot of incidence in this group of low back pain. We have had excellent results with yoga exercises and stretching exercises, and I personally have had the same problem and have used those exercises very well.

S. I. SUBOTNICK: In our community any patient with low back pain is referred to my office to have them checked out for leg length discrepancy. Especially a runner. If a runner has a little bit wrong with leg length discrepancy it can cause low back pain, whereas in a walking population or sedentary population it takes quite a bit of change to make a difference. Biomechnically it's a total different game when you're talking about athletes. So little is wrong in the first place.

P. MILVY (Mt. Sinai School of Medicine, New York, N.Y.): I had warned yesterday about using anecdotal evidence as scientific evidence, so this is more in the nature of feedback to the physician. About one year ago I started doing stretching exercises and 2 weeks later while jogging very easily I incurred a hamstring injury. In subsequent weeks I mentioned this to a number of friends and I heard incident after incident of people shortly after doing stretching exercises while jogging easily, whatever, getting injuries. This is a statistic that you should take note of.

R. O. SCHUSTER: I'd like to make a comment about this. I wanted to make it before but I missed the opportunity. I think most runners who stretch do so too vigorously. The individual who runs is competitive and he gets competitive with himself and stretches to beat all fury and tears himself apart. A lot of people go out and run in the morning and this is the worst time to run. They have no patience with stretching.

P. CAVANAGH (Pennsylvania State University, University Park, Pa.): I just want to make one comment about this cross-over and point out that I'm not sure, but I don't think it's just specific to women. Many of the athletes that we've looked at including some of the elite athletes had quite marked cross-over.

G. SHEEHAN: I must say I'm delighted with the interest shown. It confirms what we've been finding at Runners World that people are much more interested in participation than performance. We always think of lowering our times a few seconds, but it's when we get injured that we really know what we want to do, which is to keep running.

The musculoskeletal injuries are perhaps a little more obvious, and of practical interest, but the extent of pathological changes due to this overuse on the other systems of the body propose much more difficult and possibly more serious problems.

C. G. CLARK (Princeton Medical Center, Princeton, N.J.): I heard a lot about the difference between the elite and the better runners. My question is what, as we're getting older, what makes a difference between the 20-year-old runner and the runners that are over 40? What happens physiologically that people do slow down?

J. MORGANROTH (University of Pennsylvania, Philadelphia, Pa.): The type of information we need in order to answer that question really results if we take a group of individuals who have increase in left ventricular mass such as the individuals we've studied a couple of years ago. Unfortunately it is hard to find such individuals who are willing to stop their athletic activity so that we can study them over a period of several months to find out how fast or how soon, if at all, their changes regress. And of course we would like to have longitudinal studies like there have been with electrocardiographic studies in younger individuals, and then there are those sorts of noninvasive studies are followed up 20 years later during the slow-down period. But I don't know of any specific data that can, from my cardiac functional characteristic or physiologic basis, answer that.

J. P. LISS (*St. Francis Hospital, Hartford, Ct.*): With the use of echocardiography now and the ubiquity of the mitral valve prolapse syndrome I've noted that no one has made a comment in relationship to this, especially because of the propensity of the particular syndrome with arrhythmias and the occasional sudden death, I would like to know if either of you have seen that, and two, if they do have arrhythmias what do you suggest if they are long distance runners?

J. MORGANROTH: Well, the prevalence of mitral valve prolapse by echocardiography is settling down from an initial range of 3% to 20% to around 6% in the population, with females over males of about 7 to 1. We've studied 58 college people, 42 of whom were athletes and all of them were men, and 14 individuals from outside. You would expect that we could see one or two prolapses. We didn't. There is only one other study that was published, and it didn't report any mitral valve prolapse either. I'm sure it will come up. I've not heard of or seen a case of a competitive athlete with mitral valve prolapse after that particular issue came up. But I'm sure it will and then one will have to deal with that in a problem as one would with any idiopathic arrhythmia that occurs in active individuals.

H. GALBO (*University of Copenhagen, Copenhagen, Denmark*): Is the shape of the left ventricle the same in trained and untrained individuals? In other words do you apply the same formula when you calculate ventricular mass in trained and untrained individuals?

S. ZONERAICH (*Queens Hospital Center, Jamaica, N.Y.*): As far as my work goes we apply the formulas and we try to correct certain things for heart rate, and of course in athletes, as we've shown before, we have an average rate of around 50 and so on, but the application at rest and the formulas are the same. We have more special formulas for trained than for untrained unfortunately. Your question is very well taken.

G. SHEEHAN: I think the import of Dr. Sulman's paper may be a return to the consideration of the adrenal medulla in that we have been mainly emphasizing the adrenal cortex, at least in the theories of training.

P. G. HANSON (*University of Wisconsin, Madison, Wisc.*): Just going back to the question of the adrenal cortex, have you made any attempts to try to stimulate some of these athletes? Do they have a responsive cortex? Is there any explanation that we should look for?

F. G. SULMAN (*Hebrew University Medical Center, Jerusalem, Israel*): The explanation is very simple. You can stimulate them surely by excitation. We did it in some cases. But this is only the beginning to show that they really are involved.

D. THOMASHOW: A common pathway of many of these things may turn out to be prostaglandin. Have you done any work, or do you know of any work regarding prostaglandins in this syndrome in athletes?

F. G. SULMAN: No, we have not yet included the prostaglandins. It is very difficult to assess prostaglandins from urine, and in these cases we would have had the problem of taking it from the blood, which would have complicated the whole procedure. Everything was done from the urine.

H. GALBO: First, I find it very difficult to say anything about the secretion rate of hormones from concentrations measured in the urine. Second, I find that your suggestion of MAO inhibitors to improve performance could be due to a placebo effect.

F. G. SULMAN: You are very wrong in stating this because the MAO blockers that we give are always controlled with the effect we have immediately a rise in the adrenal artery. But there is one thing: I would never give an MAO blocker to a long distance runner; then we would run into the problem of illegal doping. So, we are dealing with two different problems. One is the normal person who needs such a treatment in order to recover his adrenal gland, and the other is the athletic long distance runner who should never be given a drug, but he should be advised what to do on the basis of these findings.

Our examinations have been now taken all over the world for assessing the neurohormone level of the patient, and there is no better way then that obtained during a 24-hour urine collection, which gives you the complete picture of one day. If you would do it from the blood you would make the big mistake of getting just the picture of one moment, which will never give you the results. In addition to that, as we are assessing the stress hormones, we would get even the reaction of the stress by putting in the needle. So with all these things in mind we have developed a method of the urine examination that has been accepted now all over the world.

QUESTION: Don't you think that your findings could be predicted on broad biological grounds, meaning that you're not intended to run long distances in hot climates, and there is probably some evidence to show that the Black African is a better sprinter rather than a long distance runner. Therefore you would expect the findings that you predicted?

F. G. SULMAN: I think that's a very good question because here we have a good proof what happened in Mexico where under high temperatures the results were not as good as in Canada. That is one point. The second point is that an African with his black skin is of course exposed to much more heat accumulation in his body. The third point is that Africans if they are in the cold climate do very well, and if they are in a hot climate they do very poorly. So we can surely state that once people tried to carry out sports in a hot climate they start from a very bad, not suitable set point of all their body strength and body hormones, which brings them from the very beginning into an adverse position.

G. SHEEHAN: Dr. Sulman, given your studies and speaking as a runner, could I get an assessment of my adrenalin and noradrenalin as an indication that I have reached the exhaustion stage and should not train that day for a suitable period of time? Would a 24-hour urine on a runner really indicate his protein in that area of staleness?

F. G. SULMAN: This is a very important aspect. The first examinations done on rather sensitive people were done on the 24-hour urine. But the examinations in the long distance runners were done just before and after returning from the run. That means there was a difference of approximately one hour in between. So I would suggest that if examinations in long distance runners are done they should be done according to this principle of avoiding the urine before and immediately after that. Still very many other problems come in when one tries to assess it. We should compare it with creatinine excretion in the same experiments that we did. It should also be done on the basis of evaluation of serotonins, which we could not do. Serotonin requires large amounts of urine. Such a runner normally produces 100 ml of urine, or

200 ml before and after, not more. This is not enough. Then you have reason to introduce microexaminations, which we have not yet introduced.

P. MILVY: With regards to the last question, do you think that we should suggest to the wonderful Black African long distance runners that they take up sprinting?

F. G. SULMAN: Well, that's a difficult question. I think that everybody should be assessed for his possibility in his best ability to cope with the stress, and if you find out what he can do then we can really help him and advise him. But I would not put this into a general rule and say you must do that because you come from such a climate. Truly one thing is clear, that the hot climate brings down our adrenal ability to cope with such a stress.

QUESTION: Dr. Bank, how do you think your patients get any myocardial metabolism? My second question is more cynical rather than theoretical. We had eight patients who had had acute renal failure. They want to know whether they can go back to running. Two of them have already done so. If you had a fasting stress test on them and you measured CPK, do you think this would isolate some people who may produce myoglobinuria? I'd appreciate your comments.

W. J. BANK (*University of Pennsylvania, Philadelphia, Pa.*): The first one that started the cardium was congestion. There was clinically no abnormality in their myocardium, and as a model, if you will, the phosphorylase deficiency is an isolated specific enzyme deficiency in muscle. The phosphorylase is normal in liver and it's been clearly measured in some individuals. The two patients with the transfer insufficiency are the only ones published today, and we don't know about their cardium, but I have no reason to suspect that that would be abnormal.

The point of screening tests is a very difficult one. I think every runner who has pigmenturia has to be cautioned about that hazard because they simply don't know they're in trouble until the damage is done. Cramps, in the sense that I suspect most athletes have them, aren't a significant clue or most people would stop running half-way through a race. But I think the ones who get pigmenturia should clearly be looked at. If you did the stress test, if you starved them or exercised them and the CPK went up, that would certainly indicate that more studies should be done. If it were normal I would not take it as a safe indication that you were home-free either.

W. NEWKIRK (*New York, N.Y.*): Dr. Bank, if an otherwise normal athlete runs or trains with an injured muscle, would he get darkening of the urine?

W. J. BANK: That's entirely possible. The trouble, when you say injured muscle, is that I think generally it's a subjective thing. A muscle that hurts is called an injured muscle. For me an injured muscle is one that is literally damaged. I might just add that in the past pigmenturia was sort of discounted, not so much in athletes although even there in football players it was always thought to be hematuria, and it was from kidney trauma or something vague like that. I think that anybody who has what is thought to be blood in the urine may well have myoglobin in the urine and not blood. That's a clinical distinction that has to be made.

D. THOMASHOW: Dr. Bank, do you attempt to treat your patients in any way? In the wake of the last Olympics we've been faced with numerous charges that Eastern European runners used any number of drugs to prolong their efforts. Do you know of any way and did you treat the patients? Do you know of any way to improve fatty acid metabolism?

W. J. BANK: The only treatment really was suggested because they didn't even have exercise intolerance unless they starved. For example, if they didn't eat and went out on a long hike they got in trouble. If they ate and had an adequate glucose level they had no symptoms.

D. THOMASHOW: How did you find them?

W. J. BANK: Because of the renal failure. In other words, they presented with renal failure that was subsequently recognized to be due to myoglobin, and then it went backwards from them. The other question about drugs is a difficult one. There are certainly drugs that can facilitate release of free fatty acids, but I don't know of anything that can increase utilization of it.

D. S. KRONFELD (University of Pennsylvania, Philadelphia, Pa.): I'd like to present two unusual points of view which relate to carbohydrate loading. I'm still unconvinced that it's going in the right direction. I think that it is potentially dangerous, as Dr. Bank has pointed out. One is the anthropological point of view that when the chimp came out of the trees 3 to 5 million years ago and started to chase, he was running on a diet of raw meat, and that was for 5 million years; and about 10,000 years ago we learned how to cook and started to eat those cereal grains that started to sweep across the Middle East after the Ice Age. It is hard for me to see how an animal, and man is still an animal, that adapted to a very low carbohydrate, high meat, and high fat diet for 5 million years suddenly in 10,000 years becomes a great glucose burner. I still am in the direction of thinking that we should be using nutritional strategies that favor fatty acid oxidation and a long exhaustive work, and my thinking in that direction comes from studies of comparative nutrition. Carbohydrate loading in horses has the classical myoglobinuria syndrome. It also does it in racing dogs, and in our studies of racing dogs we found that by feeding less carbohydrates we can avoid that syndrome. In fact there are major benefits from the persistent feeding for many months of low carbohydrate, high fat, and high protein diets. I think it's a pity that the people interested in diet in humans have never persisted with diets of this kind. The final point concerns vitamin E and selenium. Although man seems to have a lower requirement than most species, there are some horses, by no means all, that respond; or let's put it the other way, you can protect them against myoglobinuria by giving injections of vitamin E and selenium. I have had experience with this: a horse of my own that would get this condition in various degrees of severity, and I could prevent this with a vitamin E and selenium injection for 4 months, and then it would wear off and would need another one. I wonder whether vitamin E and selenium are being looked at in human athletes in this regard?

W. J. BANK: Of the last point I have no experience at all. But the animal anecdotes are fascinating. In the horse it's what's described as a "tying up" syndrome. It was well recognized when horses were more prevalent. It occurred when the horse was put in the stall for the weekend, where he was standing still, resting, and presumably eating a lot; then when he got up that Monday morning he would tie up. So it seems to be a factor that had to do with both inactivity and diet.

N. RUDE-FIELD (New York, N.Y.): Dr. Bank, can you tell me if there is a relationship between muscle destruction and fasting, and if so at what point in long-term fasting would this occur?

W. J. BANK: You're talking about long-term fasting and not just the trial of 72 hours. What happens with normal fasting is that there is a compensatory use of endogenous fat. Within 24 hours endogenous fats from lipids are free for use, and what I showed here was that these people could not respond to that normal stimulus. What happens in a long-term fast, which in the normal well-nourished individual is a matter of as much as 80 days of fasting, is that you get to a point of protein wasting; namely, the body finally is out of carbohydrates and particularly fats and then consumes protein as polypeptides. It's at that point that muscle would go and that's the life-threatening stage of criminal fasting. But I don't think it's significant in how you mean it. That's literally end-stage starvation.

B. GUTIN (*Columbia University, New York, N.Y.*): With respect to the question of whether we should be eating fat and protein and carbohydrates, we've heard all three at this meeting, and I'm wondering whether there is a distinction that could be made with respect to short-term and long-term ingestion of these. In other words maybe over the long term protein would be better, and over the short term before one stressful event something else might be better.

W. J. BANK: I think so, and I don't have any personal experience with this. But the analogy would be that, yes, you definitely can increase endogenous glycogen by loading, and yes, the more glycogen you have the more you will endure. But if you go beyond that you will deplete that glycogen, and when it's gone it's gone no matter how much you had. If you do an endurance exercise that exceeds the stored glycogen, then it's gone, and what you then resort to is fats.

G. SHEEHAN: If I can make a final comment, and perhaps Dr. Bank may respond, Paul Slovick did this study with a questionnaire and a number of people who loaded had trouble, but no one who partially loaded had trouble. In other words, the ones who avoided the depletion phase and only used carbohydrate loading had no trouble. The eight or nine who reported difficulty, including one practiced marathoner who had to stop at 8 miles, went through the routine procedure. So it seems that what we've learned from Dr. Bank is the possibility that it's the depletion phase that is the dangerous thing.

W. J. BANK: I think that's a fair statement. If I could just put in a last plug for my own interest. If any of you, and I'm a clinician not involved in marathon running, have runners with recurret pigmenturia, I would be very eager to hear about that and help if I can.

EFFECT OF CHRONIC EXERCISE ON THE PERSONALITY OF ADULTS

A. H. Ismail and R. John Young

*Department of Physical Education for Men
Purdue University
West Lafayette, Indiana 47907*

Recent evidence pertaining to the physiological, biochemical, and psychological status of "normal" middle-aged men indicated that distinct personality differences existed between trained and untrained individuals. Further, the data suggested that participation in a 4-month physical conditioning program influenced not only physiological parameters but also personality characteristics, particularly those dealing with emotional stability.[1-4] These findings were based on univariate and multivariate analyses of personality data collected using the Cattell 16 PF Questionnaire [5] and the Eysenck Personality Inventory.[6]

Research in the areas of animal and human endocrinology has provided evidence for the relationship between serum levels of several compounds and specific behavioral patterns. The compounds moset frequently associated with emotional conditions are corticosteroids,[7] catecholamines,[8] glucose,[4, 9, 10] cholesterol,[4, 11-13] and more recently, androgens.[14]

Personality characteristics such as competitiveness and aggression,[15] extraversion,[13] and feelings of depression and fear [12] have been shown to be associated with elevated cholesterol levels. The emotional conditions associated with high cholesterol levels may have cardiodynamic effects probably mediated by the catecholamines.[13] Catecholamines have been observed to be liberated in a variety of stress states [16-18] and to reflect the intensity of emotional reactions.[19, 20] Increased concentrations of circulating catecholamines have been found in patients with essential hypertension [21-23] and in the urine [24] and plasma [25] of patients recovering from myocardial infarction.

Although sex hormones primarily influence sexual behavior, a clear role of testosterone has been established in aggression [26-28] and social behavior.[14] Various stressful situations, in both animals and humans, have been shown to deplete testosterone secretion. These include surgical stress,[29] climate,[30] shock avoidance,[31] and psychological stress.[32] Further, recent evidence has related elevated testosterone in males to the increased incidence of coronary heart disease [33] possibly due to the hypocholesterolemic effect of estrogen.[34, 35]

Most studies designed to demonstrate the relationship of these compounds to human personality characteristics have used as subjects mental patients with extreme manifestations of psychosis,[36] depression,[37] schizophrenia,[15] and anxiety.[13, 20] Surprisingly, the nature of these relationships in the "normal" population has hitherto been relatively unexamined. Thus, an attempt was made to investigate, in a multivariate fashion, the relationships between selected biochemical compounds and personality characteristics before and after a long-term exercise program. Specifically, the purpose of the study was to determine the effect of an exercise program on the relationships identified.

958

Subjects

The subjects were selected from 90 Purdue University faculty and staff members and local businessmen, 21 to 61 years of age, who volunteered to participate in a 4-month physical fitness program. Passing a physical examination by their family physician was considered a prerequisite for acceptance into the program. Complete data were obtained on 58 men who had at least 60% attendance in the program.

Physical Fitness Program

The physical fitness program consisted of three 90-minute sessions each week for 4 months. At each session subjects took part in: jogging for warm-up (10 minutes maximum), progressive calisthenics (25 minutes maximum), progressive running (25 minutes maximum), and self-selected recreational activities (30 minutes maximum). Attendance was recorded at each meeting and the running and calisthenics were progressively intensified during the 4-month period. Whereas the distance run varied according to the ability of the individual, it was between ½ and 5 miles. The recreational activities provided were basketball, volleyball, squash, handball, and swimming.

Physical Fitness Assessment

To provide evidence as to the difference between data before and after the physical fitness program, relevant physiological data were collected and physical fitness scores, based on the regression equation of Ismail *et al.*,[38] were obtained for each subject before and after the program. The regression equation is as follows:

-1.33   (submaximal exercise pulse rate)
4.88   (percent lean body weight)
2.50   (maximal oxygen uptake ml/kg lean body weight)
-119.02   (submaximal minute volume ventilation/kg body weight)
-1.36   (resting diastolic blood pressure)
1.31   (resting pulse pressure)
61.90   (constant).

The protocol for assessing physical fitness consisted of a 10-minute bed rest in the supine position during which electrodes were attached to the subject's chest to permit accurate monitoring, via an electrocardiogram, of the subject's heart rate during exercise. At the end of the 10-minute rest, heart rate and systolic and diastolic blood pressures were recorded.

The subject then walked on a treadmill for 10 minutes at 3 mph (a distance of ½ mile) with the grade being increased by 2 degrees every 2 minutes to a maximum of 8 degrees. During the last 30 seconds of the walk a submaximal respiratory gas sample and heart rate were collected.

Without stopping, the subject then commenced running at a speed of 6 mph with the grade being increased each 2 minutes from zero to a maximum of 10 degrees if exercise was not terminated beforehand. The heart rate was continuously monitored and the subject indicated when he wanted to terminate the run whereupon the expired air and heart rate were collected. Submaximal and maximal $\dot{V}_{O_2}$ were determined using Beckman O_2 and CO_2 analyzers. The percentage of O_2 and CO_2 obtained were applied to a nomogram [39] to obtain the the true O_2 percentage. Oxygen consumption in liters was then calculated using the true O_2 percentage and the expired air volume (STPD). This volume was converted into liters per minute and divided by lean body weight in kilograms to obtain the desired unit of measurement.

In the postprogram test subjects performed a second run during which a new maximum was attained. The same measures were taken at the end of the second run as were collected at the end of the first.

VARIABLES

Preprogram and postprogram data were collected on the following variables:

Biochemical

Four biochemical variables were selected because of their previously documented relationship to certain personality characteristics: [4, 9, 11–13, 31]

Serum glucose, determined by the procedure of Hultman [40] as modified by Dubowski [41] using reagents obtained from Hycel, Inc., Houston, Texas.

Serum cholesterol, determined by the Hycel direct serum method, Hycel, Inc., Houston, Texas.

Serum testosterone, determined by an adaptation of the radioimmunoassay technique described by Chen et al. [42] using reagents supplied by Wien Laboratories, Inc., Succasunna, N.J.

Free catecholamines (epinephrine and norepinephrine), determined from a 24 hour urine sample using ion-exchange resin columns supplied by Bio-Rad Laboratories, Richmond, Calif.

Venous blood samples were drawn, following a 10-minute bed rest, from the antecubital vein using a standard plain Vacutainer system. Two 10-ml Vacutainers of blood were extracted and allowed to stand for 15 minutes after which they were centrifuged and the serum extracted. All samples were obtained between the hours of 07:00 and 10:00, stored at $-20°$ C and assayed within 2 months from the time of collection. For consistency, the acidified 24-hour urine sample was collected on a Sunday. A 50-ml aliquot was stored at $-20°$ C and analyzed within 2 months from the time of collection.

Personality

Data were collected on the following personality factors using the Cattell 16 PF questionnaire (16 PF), Form A (1970):

(A)   Reserved versus sociable and outgoing.
(B)   Low intelligence versus high intelligence.
(C)   Emotional instability versus emotional stability.
(E)   Mild and submissive versus dominant and aggressive.
(F)   Serious versus enthusiastic.

(G)   Expedient versus conscientious.
(H)   Shy and timid versus adventurous and uninhibited.
(I)   Tough-minded versus tender-minded.
(L)   Trusting versus suspicious.
(M)   Practical and conventional versus imaginative and bohemian.
(N)   Naive versus shrewd.
(O)   Secure versus insecure.
(Q_1)   Conservative versus experimenting.
(Q_2)   Group-dependent versus self-sufficient.
(Q_3)   Uncontrolled versus socially precise.
(Q_4)   Composed versus tense.

In addition, the following variables were determined using the Eysenck Personality Inventory (EPI), Form A (1963):

Introversion versus extraversion (EXT).
Stability versus neuroticism (NEUR).
Conformity scale (LIE).

One variable was determined by using the Multiple Affect Adjective Check List: [43]

Anxiety Scale (MAACL-A)—"In General" Form.

Statistical Analysis

As a preliminary step, factor analysis was used to reduce the psychometrical data from 20 personality variables to 10. Then the canonical correlation technique was used to determine the relationships between psychometric assessments of certain personality characteristics and selected biochemical compounds. Using this technique we determined the maximum correlations between linear functions of the biochemical (p) and personality (q) sets of variables, before and after the physical fitness program. The correlation coefficient is expressed as $\sqrt{\lambda_i}$.[44, 45] In this study the canonical relationships are presented in terms of (λ_i) and may be considered as the squared product moment correlation between the ith linear compounds of the p and q sets. As suggested by Pillai and Dotson,[46] two criteria were used for testing the relationship between p and q sets, namely, the largest root and the summation of roots [47] criteria.

RESULTS

The means and standard errors of the selected physiological variables are presented in TABLE 1 to illustrate the improvement in the physical condition of the subjects. The increase in physical fitness score and the decrease in maximal heart rate from preprogram to postprogram tests were significant at the 0.01 level. For interest, the preprogram and postprogram means and standard errors of the four biochemical and ten personality variables are presented in TABLE 2.

Preprogram Results

The canonical correlations, the percent of total possible variance and the weights associated with each correlation between the biochemical (p) and the

TABLE 1

NORMATIVE DATA OF SELECTED PHYSIOLOGICAL VARIABLES BEFORE AND AFTER THE PHYSICAL FITNESS PROGRAM

	Preprogram Test		Postprogram Test		
Variable	Mean	SE *	Mean	SE	t
1. Age (yr)	43.24	1.29	43.57	1.29	—
2. Height (cm)	179.53	.94	179.53	.94	—
3. Weight (kg)	80.22	1.76	79.92	1.70	0.12
4. % Lean (body wt)	81.45	.72	81.94	.73	0.42
5. Systolic blood pressure (mmHg)	127.22	1.91	126.10	1.71	0.44
6. Diastolic blood pressure (mmHg)	82.40	1.51	81.98	1.38	0.20
7. Maximal heart rate (per minute)	171.47	1.51	165.45	1.44	2.88†
8. Maximum $\dot{V}_{O_2}$ (ml/kg·min)	41.94	1.14	44.14	1.10	1.39
9. Physical fitness score	337.84	7.12	368.67	6.33	3.12*

* Standard error.
† With 57 d.f., t=2.68 is needed to be significant at the 0.01 level.

TABLE 2

NORMATIVE DATA OF THE BIOCHEMICAL AND SELECTED PERSONALITY VARIABLES BEFORE AND AFTER THE PHYSICAL FITNESS PROGRAM

	Preprogram Test		Postprogram Test	
Variable	Mean	SE	Mean	SE
Biochemical				
1. Glucose (mg %)	97.90	2.15	92.22	2.13
2. Cholesterol (mg %)	206.38	4.80	197.95	5.50
3. Testosterone (ng/100 ml	645.79	31.76	674.62	30.66
4. Catecholamnies (μg/24 hr)	41.55	2.02	40.91	1.98
Personality				
1. Factor C	6.35	0.27	6.66	0.27
2. Factor E	5.74	0.24	5.50	0.23
3. Factor G	6.33	0.26	6.21	0.25
4. Factor M	6.93	0.25	6.71	0.22
5. Factor N	5.97	0.25	5.81	0.22
6. Factor O	4.36	0.24	4.21	0.27
7. Factor Q_4	4.83	0.29	4.90	0.29
8. Extraversion (EXT)	10.33	0.45	9.93	0.49
9. Neuroticism (NEUR)	6.36	0.64	6.17	0.66
10. Conformity (LIE)	2.93	0.21	3.03	0.22

personality (q) sets of variables are presented in Table 3. The relationship between the p and q sets was significant at the 0.01 level using the largest root and the summation of roots criteria.

The relative weights associated with the first canonical correlation indicated that the majority of the variance between the biochemical and personality sets was due to the relationships between testosterone and glucose and the personality variables: neuroticism, factor E (submissive vs aggressive), and factor

TABLE 3

CANONICAL CORRELATION ANALYSIS BETWEEN FOUR BIOCHEMICAL
AND TEN PERSONALITY VARIABLES AT THE PREPROGRAM TEST

No.	Variables	I	II	III	IV
Biochemical					
1.	Glucose (mg %)	0.43	−0.65	−0.64	−0.28
2.	Cholesterol (mg %)	−0.31	−0.60	−0.82	−0.02
3.	Testosterone (ng/100 ml)	0.92	−0.08	0.39	0.19
4.	Catecholamines (µg/24 hr)	−0.04	−0.10	−0.35	−0.96
Personality					
1.	Factor C	0.59	0.37	−0.71	0.20
2.	Factor E	0.73	−0.08	0.36	0.06
3.	Factor G	−0.05	0.72	−0.33	−0.50
4.	Factor M	0.20	0.36	0.04	0.25
5.	Factor N	0.19	−0.11	0.14	−0.34
6.	Factor O	−0.05	0.38	0.04	0.15
7.	Factor Q_4	0.20	0.58	−0.51	1.23
8.	Extraversion (EXT)	−0.34	0.02	0.24	0.43
9.	Neuroticism (NEUR)	1.01	−0.48	−0.07	−0.89
10.	Conformity (LIE)	0.37	0.55	0.77	0.12
	Canonical correlations	0.71	0.46	0.33	0.27

Total related variance accounted for: 1.7654, out of a possible 4.0.
Percent of total possible variance accounted for: 44.13%

Test Criterion *	Observed Value	Level of Significance	
		0.05	0.01
O_4	0.7054 †	0.4452	0.5021
V^4	1.7654 †	0.9400	1.0488

* $m=2.5, n=21.0$.　　　　　　　† Significant at the 0.01 level.

C (emotional instability vs emotional stability). Examination of the univariate correlation matrix to ascertain the direction of the relationships revealed that the pattern in this correlation indicates that individuals with high serum testosterone and glucose concentrations tend to be neurotic and aggressive.

The second canonical correlation indicated that the majority of the variance between the two sets was due to the relationships between glucose and cholesterol and factor G (expedient vs conscientious), factor Q_4 (composed vs tense), and the conformity and neuroticism scales of the EPI. The pattern in this case suggests that high serum levels of glucose and cholesterol are related to low superego strength, tension, nonconformity, and emotional instability. The data suggest that individuals with hyperglycemia and hypercholesterolemia are likely to be fickle, self-indulgent, disregarding of rules, undependable, and lacking a drive to do one's best.

The third canonical correlation is similar to the second canonical and the weights indicated that the majority of the variance between the two sets was due to the relationships between serum cholesterol and glucose and the conformity scale of the EPI, factor C (emotional instability vs emotional stability) and factor Q_4 (composed vs tense). This pattern indicated that hypercholesterolemia and hyperglycemia are related to nonconformity, emotional instability, and tension. Individuals therefore who are high on cholesterol and glucose are likely to be emotionally unstable and nonconformist. This canonical differs from the second canonical in terms of superego strength.

The fourth canonical correlation indicated that the majority of the variance between the two sets was due to the relationships between urinary catecholamine excretion and factor Q_4 (composed vs tense), neuroticism, and factor G (expedient vs conscientious). This canonical showed that a high catecholamine excretion rate is related to neuroticism and tension.

At the preprogram test, 44.13% of the total possible variance was accounted for by all four roots.

Postprogram Results

The canonical correlations, the percent of possible variance, and the weights associated with each correlation between the biochemical (p) and the personality (q) sets of variables are presented in TABLE 4. The relationships between the sets were found to be significant at the 0.01 level using the largest root and the summation of roots criteria.

The canonical correlations found at the postprogram test were slightly different from those found at the preprogram test. Initially, glucose was the compound implicated most frequently in the four canonicals. During the final testing period, glucose was replaced by catecholamine excretion in this respect.

In the first canonical correlation the relative weights indicated that the majority of the variance between the biochemical and personality sets was due to the relationships between urinary catecholamine excretion and serum testosterone concentration and the following personality variables: factor O (secure vs insecure), neuroticism, and factor M (conventional vs bohemian). In this instance, a high catecholamine excretion rate when combined with a high serum testosterone level is related to neurotic aggression and unconventionality. Both preprogram and postprogram canonicals illustrate the relationship of catecholamine excretion to those personality traits characterizing neuroticism.

The second canonical correlation illustrated the relationships between serum cholesterol concentration and catecholamine excretion and factor G (expedient vs conscientious), factor M (conventional vs bohemian), and the extraversion scale of the EPI. The pattern observed in this correlation suggests that hypercholesterolemia and a high catecholamine excretion rate are related to low superego strength, unconventionality, and extraversion.

The third canonical correlation revealed that the relationships were between serum testosterone and catecholamine excretion and neuroticism, factor O (secure vs insecure), and the LIE scale of the EPI. This canonical supports the univariate correlation matrix and factor analytic structure in which high levels of testosterone and glucose are related to neuroticism and aggression. The same pattern was observed finally except for the shift to catecholamine excretion over glucose in the relationship.

The fourth canonical correlation indicated that the majority of the variance between the two sets was due to the relationships between serum glucose concentration and factor C (emotional instability vs emotional stability) and

TABLE 4

CANONICAL CORRELATION ANALYSIS BETWEEN FOUR BIOCHEMICAL
AND TEN PERSONALITY VARIABLES AT THE POSTPROGRAM TEST

No.	Variables	I	II	III	IV
Biochemical					
1.	Glucose (mg %)	−0.21	0.17	−0.25	−0.93
2.	Cholesterol (mg %)	0.27	0.96	−0.19	0.17
3.	Testosterone (ng/100 ml)	−0.43	0.08	−0.88	0.26
4.	Catecholamines (μg/24 hr)	0.78	−0.48	−0.43	−0.13
Personality					
1.	Factor C	−0.28	−0.19	−0.12	0.85
2.	Factor E	0.20	−0.12	0.02	−0.42
3.	Factor G	−0.17	−0.81	0.25	−0.34
4.	Factor M	0.55	−0.76	−0.36	−0.03
5.	Factor N	−0.20	0.47	0.12	−0.13
6.	Factor O	1.24	0.06	−0.50	−0.32
7.	Factor Q_4	−0.52	0.13	0.24	−0.30
8.	Extraversion (EXT)	−0.39	0.65	−0.14	0.71
9.	Neuroticism (NEUR)	−0.78	−0.46	−0.58	0.24
10	Conformity (LIE)	0.38	0.02	0.50	0.47
Canonical correlations		0.51	0.47	0.43	0.23

Total related variance accounted for: 1.6373, out of a possible 4.0.
Percent of total possible variance accounted for: 40.93%.

Test Criterion *	Observed Value	Level of Significance	
		0.05	0.01
O_4	0.5136 †	0.4452	0.5021
V^4	1.6373 †	0.9400	1.0488

* $m=2.5$, $n=21.0$.   † Significant at the 0.01 level.

extraversion. In this instance, hypoglycemia was related to emotional stability and extraversion.

At the postprogram test, 40.93% of the total possible variance was accounted for by the four roots.

DISCUSSION

This study has sought to determine the relationships between certain psychometrically assessed personality characteristics and selected biochemical compounds before and after a physical fitness program. The subjects were observed to undergo beneficial physiological changes (TABLE 1), since at the postprogram test they exhibited more efficient cardiovascular performance particularly at maximal performance.

The canonical correlation results confirmed that the selected biochemical compounds were, in fact, related to personality characteristics, which supports Eysenck's proposition.[48] Comparison of the initial with the final results show that subtle changes occurred in these relationships—possibly as a result of the exercise program. Initially, individuals with high serum testosterone and glucose concentrations tended to be neurotic and aggressive. Aggression has been linked with testosterone secretion [26-28] and glucose with neuroticism.[4, 49] Stanaway and Hullin [49] have suggested that the relationship between glucose and neuroticism may be due to the actions of epinephrine and the sympathetic nervous system in stimulating the release of glucose from the liver by the breakdown of glycogen.

Preprogram hypercholesterolemia and hyperglycemia were found to be correlated with self-indulgence and low superego strength. In contrast, at the postprogram test hypercholesterolemia was associated with catecholamine excretion. Serum lipids have been shown to be related to several personality traits.[4, 12, 15, 17] Young and Ismail [4] found that hypercholesterolemia was associated with extraversion and obesity at the beginning of the physical fitness program, but not at the end. In this study serum cholesterol and glucose were implicated with emotional stability and conformity initially, but cholesterol appeared to be related to testosterone and a lack of physical fitness at the end of the program. Although cholesterol did not decrease significantly from preprogram to postprogram tests, its relationship to other measures was altered possibly as a result of the conditioning program.

Urinary catecholamine excretion rate was found to be related to neuroticism and tension—especially at the postprogram test. This finding supports the catecholamine hypothesis of affective disorders, proposed by Schildkraut,[20] which is based largely on studies of urinary metabolites of catecholamines. The hypothesis implies that some, if not all, depressions are associated with a deficiency of catecholamines, particularly norepinephrine, at functionally important adrenergic receptor sites in the brain.

Despite the conspicuous improvement in the physical fitness condition of the subjects, the relationships between the biochemical and personality variables did not change markedly over the 4-month period. Since the organism is always in a dynamic state of homestasis the slightly altered relationships between the two domains (observed at the postprogram test) may reflect such a mechanism. It would seem reasonable to speculate that a considerably longer and intensified period of regular (habitual) exercise is necessary to cause a dramatic change in personality parameters. Such a change would be the result of a significant alteration in body chemistry since physiological, biochemical, and personality domains are inextricably interrelated.

REFERENCES

1. ISMAIL, A. H. & L. E. TRACHTMAN. 1973. Jogging the imagination. Psychol. Today 6: 78–81.
2. ISMAIL, A. H. & R. J. YOUNG. 1973. The effect of chronic exercise on the per-

sonality of middle-aged men using univariate and multivariate approaches. J. Human Ergol. **2:** 45–54.

3. ISMAIL, A. H. & R. J. YOUNG. 1976 Influence of physical fitness on second and third order personality factors using orthogonal and oblique rotations. J. Clin. Physchol. **32:** 268–272.

4. YOUNG, R. J. & A. H. ISMAIL. 1975. The relationship between anthropometric-physiological, biochemical and personality variables before and after a four month conditioning program for midle-aged men. J. Sports Med. Phys. Fitness. **16**(4): 267–276.

5. CATTELL, R. B., H. W. EBER & M. M. TATSUOKA. 1970. Handbook for the Sixteen Personality Factor Questionnaire (16 PF) in Clinical, Educational, Industrial and Research Psychology. Institute for Personality and Ability Testing. Champaign, Ill.

6. EYSENCK, H. J. & B. G. EYSENCK. 1963. Manual for the Eysenck Personality Inventory. San Diego, Calif. Educational and Industrial Testing Service.

7. MASON, J. W. 1968. A review of psychoendocrine research on the pituitary-adrenal cortical system. Psychosomatic Med. **30:** 576–607.

8. MASON, J. W. 1968. A review of the psychoendocrine research in the sympathetic-adrenal medullary system. Psychosomatic Med. **30:** 631–653.

9. HEANMAN, G., J .B. MARTINEZ & S. POLONSKI DE PANTOLINI. 1970. Psychological aspects of the insulin-dependent diabetic. Excepta Medica Foundation **209:** 180.

10. KOCH, M. F. & G. D.MOLNAR. 1974. Psychiatric aspects of patients with unstable diabetes mellitus. Psychosomatic Med. **36.**

11. JENKINS, C. D., C. G. HAMES, S. J. ZYZANSKI, R. H. ROSENMAN & M. FRIENDMAN. 1969. Psychological traits and serum lipids. Psychosomatic Med. **31:** 115–128.

12. RAHE, R. H., R. T. RUBIN, E. K. E. GUNDERSON & R. J. ARTHUR. 1971. Psychologic correlates of serum cholesterol in man: A longitudinal study. Psychosomatic Med. **33:** 399–401.

13. SLOANE, R. B., A. HABITS, M. B. EVESON & R. W. PAYNE. 1961. Some behavioral and other correlates of cholesterol metabolism. J. Psychomaitc Res. **5:** 183–190.

14. ROSE, R. M., T. P. GORDON & I. S. Berstein. 1972. Plasma testosterone levels in the male rhesus: Influence of sexual and social stimuli. Science **178:** 643–645.

15. SLETTEN, I. W., J. A. NILSEN, R. C. YOUNG, & J. T. ANDERSON. 1964. Blood lipids and behavior in mental-hospital patients. Psychosomatic Med. **26:**261–266.

16. EULER, U. S. v. 1974. Sympato-adrenal activity in physical exercise. Med. Sci. Sports **6:** 165–173.

17. KONZETT, H., H. HORTNAGL & H. WINKLER. 1971. On the urinary output of vasopressin, epinephrine and norepinephrine during different stress situations. Psychoparmacologia **21:** 247–256.

18. RAO, L. N. & H. V. BHATT. 1972. Stress response during surgery and anesthesia. Internat. Suprg. **57:** 294–298

19. FRANKENHAEUSER, M. 1970. Catecholamines and behavior. Brain. Res. **24:** 552–553.

20. SCHILDKRAUT, J. J. 1965. The catecholamine hypothesis of affective disorders: A review of supporting evidence. Amer. J. Psychiat. **122:** 509–522.

21. AXELROD, J. & R. WEINSHILBOUM. 1972. Catecholamines. N. Engl. J. Med. **287:** 237–242.

22. Engleman, K., B. PORTNOY & A. SJOERDSMAN. 1970. Plasma catecholamine concentrations in patients with hypertension. Circ. Res. **26:** 141–145.

23. WARTMAN, R. J., C. CHOU & C. ROSE. 1970. Catecholamines and neurologic diseases. N. Engl. J. Med. **282:** 45–46.

24. GHOSE, J. C., S. CHATTERJEE & S. SIRCAR. 1972. Urinary excretion of catecholamines in acute myocardial infarction. Journal of the Indiana Medical Association. **58:** 280–283.

25. VIDEBAEK, J., N. J. CHRISTENSEN & B. STERNDORFF. 1972. Serial determinations of plasma catecholamines in myocardial infarction. Circulation 46: 846–855.
26. LEE, C. T. W. GRIFFO. 1973. Early androgenization and aggression phermone in inbred mice. Hormones and Behavior 4: 181–189.
27. PAYNE, A. P. & H. H. SWANSON. 1972. The effect of sex hormones on the aggressive behavior of the female golden hamster (Mesocricetus Auratus Waterhouse). Animal Behavior 20: 782–787.
28. PERSKY, H., K. D. SMITH & G. K. BASU. 1971. Relation of psychologic measures of aggression and hostility to testosterone production in man. Psychosomatic Med. 33: 265–277.
29. CARSTENSEN, H., N. TERNER, L. THOREN & L. WIDE. 1972. Testosterone luteinizing hormone and growth hormone in blood following surgical trauma. Acta Chirurgica Scand. 138: 1–5.
30. BRIGGS, M. H. & M. BRIGGS. 1972. Testosterone and the tropics. Lancet ii: 1374.
31. MASON, J. W., W. W. TOLSON, J. A. ROBINSON, J. V. BRADY, G. A. TOLLIVER & T. A. JOHNSON. 1968. Urinary androsterone, etiocholanolone, and dyhydroepiaandrosterone response to 72-hr. avoidance sessions in the monkey. Psychosomatic Med. 30: 710–720.
32. KREUZ, L. E., R. M. ROSE & J. R. JENNING. 1972. Suppression of plasma testosterone levels and psychological stress. Archives of General Psychiatry. 26: 479–482.
33. MORSE, W. I., R. A. HARKNESS, K. S. HOQUE, A. H. ISMAIL & M. NICKERSON. 1968. Sex hormone metabolism and serum lipids in male survivors of myocardial infarction. J. Atherosclerosis Res. 8: 869–884.
34. FURHAM, R. H. 1968. Are gonadal hormones (estrogen and androgens) of significance in the development of ischemic heart disease? Ann. N.Y. Acad. Sci. 149: 822–833.
35. KASE, N. 1974. Editorial: Estrogens and the Menopause. J. Amer. Med. Assoc. 227: 318–319.
36. PERSKY, H., M. ZUCKERMAN & G. C. CURTIS. 1968. Endocrine function in emotionally disturbed and normal men. J. Nervous Mental Dis. 146: 488–497.
37. JAKOBSON, T., M. BLUMENTHAL, H. HAGMAN & E. HEINKKINEN. 1969. The diurnal variations of urinary and plasma 17-Hydroxycortiocosteroid (17-OHCS) levels and the plasma 17-OHCS response to lysine-8-vasopress in depressive patients. J. Psychosomatic Res. 13: 363–375.
38. ISMAIL, A. H., H. B. FALLS & D. F. MacLEOD. 1965. Development of a criterion for physical fitness tests from factor analysis results. J. Appl. Physiol. 20: 991–999.
39. CONSOLAZIO, C. F., R. E. JOHNSON & L. C. PECORA. 1963. Physiological Measurements of Metabolic Functions in Man. McGraw-Hill Book Company, Inc. New York, N.Y.
40. HULTMAN, E. 1959. Rapid specific method for determination of aldosaccharides in body fluids. Nature 183: 108–109.
41. DUBOWSKI ,K. M. 1962. On O-toluidine method for body fluid glucose determination. Clin. Chem. 8: 215–235.
42. CHEN, J., E. ZORN, M. HALLBERG & R. WEILAND. 1971. Antibodies to testosterone-3-bovine serum albumin, applied to assay of serum 17B–OL androgens. Clin. Chem. 17: 581–584.
43. ZUCKERMAN, M. & B. LUBIN. 1965. Manual for the multiple effect adjective check list. Educational and Industrial Testing Service. San Diego, Calif.
44. COOLEY, W. W. & P. R. LOHNES. 1962. Multivariate Procedures for Behavioral Science. John Wiley & Sons, Inc. New York, N.Y.
45. MORRISON, D. F. 1967. Multivariate Statistical Methods. McGraw-Hill Book Company. New York, N.Y.
46. PILLAI, K. S. & C. O. DOTSON. 1969. Power comparisons of tests of two multi-

variate hypotheses based on individual characteristic roots. Ann. Inst. Math.
   21: 49–66.
47. PILLAI, K. S.   1960. Statistical Tables for Tests of Multivariate Hypotheses.
   Statistical Center, University of the Philippines. Manila.
48. EYSENCK, J. J.   1964. Experiment in Motivation. : 290–291. Pergamon Press.
   London.
49. STANAWAY, R .G. & R. P. HULLIN.   1973. The relationship of exercise response
   to Personality. Psychological Med. **3:** 343–349.
50. KAISER, H. F.   1958. The varimax criterion for analytic rotation in factor
   analysis. Psychometrika **23:** 187–200.

RUNNING, PSYCHOLOGY, AND CULTURE

Ernst Jokl

University of Kentucky Medical School
Lexington, Kentucky 40506

With my eldest son, who is 11, I go to a track at the foot of Parliament Hill in London on most Sunday mornings. We both belong to a North London athletics club. We find ourselves changing in a room which frequently contains a mixture of schoolboys, undergraduates, building laborers, clerks, teachers and lawyers ranging in age from 10 to 75. I am glad this is so, though I would not be stupid enough to say that all the uneasy suspicions between men of different generations and classes are thereby removed.

Social communication is made easier, and not only with others—between myself and my son too. Through doing athletics together, my son has a kind of induction to manhood and I a kind of fulfilment of fatherhood. I have a second chance of realizing, through him, some failed ambitions, and I can experience the joy of fashioning him, if only to a slight extent, in my own image. This is one of the meanings, or needs of parenthood. Together we can grow up and maintain our affection through a common enterprise. We do not need to talk or to be self-consciously father and son. We get up early on a summer morning, run over Hampstead Heath and through Ken Wood. We learn the rudimentary art of running, hurdling and throwing the javelin. We can feel cool air on our cheeks, sustain our limbs in a rhythm of effort, and later feel the glow of a really deserved relaxation. I realize there will be a time when we shall not want to do this, but for the moment it is a breathtaking projection of idealism—of the individual who is utterly dependent on his own fragile resources but also inescapably linked by invisible threads to his own flesh and blood and hence to mankind.

Peter Townsend [1]

Allegorical Connotations of "Work" and "Rest"

The biblical story of the expulsion of Adam and Eve from the Paradise conveys the divine injunction that "mankind is to earn its bread by the sweat of its brow." Work, we are told, was to be punishment for man's transgression of the law. Contrariwise, rest was considered a reward. God himself rested after He had created the world: and He sanctified the Sabbath.

While to the scientific inquirer exercise and recovery are ubiquitous physiological events, the terms work and rest have assumed anthropological connotations of their own: the one carries a curse, the other a blessing.

Though the acceptance of the working day has marked the beginning of all civilization, it was left to Western Society to declare work a virtue. "Ora et labora" has been a leitmotiv of the Catholic Church during one of its most dynamic periods. Leopold van Ranke, the historian, once remarked that the conversion of the Germans to Christianity in the 8th century led to their habit of rising early in the morning to attend mass instead of sleeping until noon as had been their custom before. It was also thus that they got used to regular labor.

970

Work as Slavery

Whatever virtue may be attached to work in its various forms, to many it remained a curse. It is little more than a hundred years ago that the abolition of child labor in England initiated one of the greatest social revolutions in the history of mankind, a revolution which brought to an end an epoch in which work had all too often been identical with slavery (FIGURES 1 & 2). The following excerpts from the evidence given before the Committee on Factory Children's Labor in 1831 in England affords a glimpse into a world that—one is happy to say—has now virtually disappeared.

Question: At what time in the morning, in the brisk time, did these girls go to the mills?

Answer: In the brisk time, for about six weeks, they have gone at 3 o'clock in the morning and ended at 10, or nearly half past, at night.

Question: What intervals were allowed for rest or refreshment during those nineteen hours of work?

Answer: Breakfast, a quarter of an hour, and dinner half an hour, and drinking a quarter of an hour.

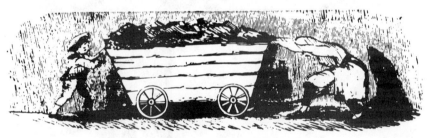

FIGURE 1. Children dragging a coal truck.

Question: Was any of that time taken up in cleaning the machinery?

Answer: They generally had to do what they call dry down: sometimes this took the whole of the time at breakfast or drinking; and they were to get their breakfast and dinner as they could; if not, it was brought home.

Question: Had you not great difficulty in awakening your children to this excessive labor?

Answer: Yes, in the early time we had to take them up asleep and shake them, when we got them on the floor to dress them, before we could get them off to their work; but not so in the common hours. . . .

Question: What was the length of time they could be in bed during those long hours?

Answer: It was near 11 o'clock before we could get them into bed after getting a little victuals, and then at morning my mistress used to stay up all night, for fear that we could not get them ready for the time; sometimes we have gone to bed, and one of us generally awoke.

Question: At what time did you get them up in the morning?

Answer: In general me and my mistress got up at 2 o'clock to dress them.

Question: So that they had not above four hours' sleep at this time? The common hours of labor were from 6 in the morning till half past eight at night?

Answer: Yes.

Question: With the same intervals for food?
Answer: Just the same.
Question: Were the children excessively fatigued by this labor?
Answer: Many time; we have cried often when we have given them little vic-
          tualing we had to give them; we had to shake them, and they have
          fallen to sleep with the victuals in their mouths many a time.

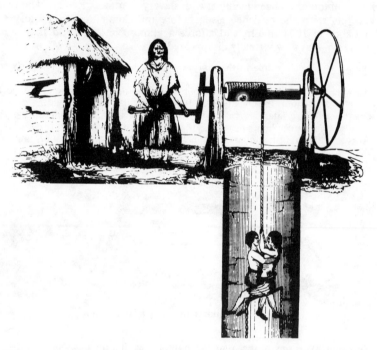

FIGURE 2. Children being lowered into a mine shaft. With the invention of machinery, a horde of workless, starving vagrants had flocked from the countryside into the towns. Children were driven by the poverty of their parents into factories and mines. Child-slaves, orphaned and friendless, were supplied in droves by the work-houses to employers. Children of ten, of seven, of five and even of three, spent twelve hours at a time in the darkness of the mines. Lord Shaftsbury was among the most active proponents of reforms. "Never," he said in a parliamentary debate on child labour in the House of Commons, "have I seen such a display of selfishness, frigidity to every human sentiment, such ready and happy self-delusion." In 1859, children of less than ten as well as girls and women were excluded altogether from the mines. But it was not until 1875 that boy chimney sweepers were prohibited. The seventies saw compulsory free education established throughout Great Britain and thus a bar-rier was interposed between children and the factories. In the same decade the first kindergartens were introduced. The Society for the Prevention of Cruelty to Children, founded in 1872, took the initiative in promulgating progressive social legislation.

To understand why, during the past decades, sport has become one of the major leisure pursuits of mankind, it must be realized that the concepts of both leisure and sport have only recently assumed their present meaning. The idea that time for leisure would be available to the common man sounded revolu-tionary not so long ago when the worker, unless he was working, rested to recuperate from and gather new strength for work. The boys and girls who slaved in coal mines and textile mills around the middle of the 19th century had neither the time nor the strength to play. Their as well as their elders' situation was incomparably worse than that which had prevailed during the preceding millennium in the relatively stable, predominantly rural village environment throughout Western Europe.

Veblen and Russell on Leisure

In 1899, Thorstein Veblen, the American sociologist, published a book *The Theory of the Leisure Class* in which he argued that from primitive times to modern days most societies have supported a leisure class. Veblen defined leisure as the "non-productive consumption of time," and leisure people as "propertied non-industrial consumers." These people were not lazy or unemployed. On the contrary, they were usually in government, war, sport, or devout observances. They lived upon the productive work of others and signified their position in society by their "conspicuous wealth" and their "conspicuous consumption," phrases which have won their place in economic and social literature. In the United States of America, Veblen detected his leisure class chiefly in the Southern States where slavery existed until the Civil War and where a planter aristocracy lived a fairly leisured existence based upon slave and later cheap labor.

Thirty years ago, the case for leisure for the common man was summarized by Bertrand Russell in an essay entitled *In Praise of Idleness*.[2] Russell asserted that there is far too much work done in the world, that immense harm is caused by the belief that work is virtuous, and that what needs to be preached in modern industrial countries is quite different from what had always been preached. From the beginning of civilization until the Industrial Revolution, he said, a man could as a rule produce by hard work little more than was required for the subsistence of himself and his family, although his wife worked at least as hard as he did, and his children added their labor as soon as they were old enough to do so. Modern technique, he foresaw, would make an end to a time in which leisure was the prerogative of a small privileged class. Leisure would become a right evenly distributed throughout the community. The morality of work, he wrote, is the morality of slaves, and the modern world has no need for slavery. Athenian slave owners, he pointed out, employed part of their leisure in making a permanent contribution to civilization, which would have been impossible under just economic systems. Leisure is essential to civilization and in former times leisure for the few was only rendered possible by the labors of the many. But their labors were valuable, not because work is good, but because leisure is good.

In America, Russell observed, men often work long hours even when they are already well off; in fact, some of them dislike leisure not only for themselves but also for their sons. Oddly enough, they do not mind their wives and daughters having no work at all. The snobbish admiration of uselessness, which in an aristocratic society once extended to both sexes, is, under a plutocracy, confined to women; this, however, does not make it more in agreement with common sense.

The wise use of leisure is a product of civilization and education. A man who has worked long hours all his life is likely to feel bored if he suddenly becomes idle. But without a considerable amount of leisure a man is cut off from many of the best things. For thousands of years, the rich have preached the dignity of labor while taking care themselves to remain undignified in this respect. The notion that the desirable activities are only those that bring a profit has made everything topsy-turvy. We think too much of production and too little of consumption.

Russell recommended that education should provide tastes that would enable a man to use leisure intelligently. In the past there was a small leisure class and a large working class. The leisure class enjoyed advantages for which there was no basis in social justice, though it invented theories to justify these privileges. However, it did contribute nearly the whole of what we call civilization. It cultivated the arts and discovered the sciences; it wrote the books, invented the philosophies, and refined social relations.* Even the liberation of the oppressed has frequently been inaugurated from above. Without the leisure class mankind would never have emerged from barbarism.

It is of great interest to note that as late as the early 1930s Russell did not refer to the sports movement as an activity that did or would play a part in the leisure pursuits of the masses. Actually, none of the sociologists born during the Victorian period foresaw this development. Russell's prediction that leisure would cause the masses to acquaint themselves with philosophy, the arts, and literature has certainly not become true. Nor has George Bernard Shaw been right in saying that art would refine the people's "sense of character and conduct, of justice and sympathy, their self-knowledge, self-control, precision of action, and considerateness, and make them intolerant of baseness, cruelty, injustice, and intellectual superficiality or vulgarity."

The Discrepancy between the Social and Cultural Roles of Sport

Maheu, who considers sport and physical education training "human disciplines with a social function and a role in the formation and full development of the personality," has pointed out that the roots of sport and culture are identical in that both spring from leisure, from the availability of spare time and unspent energy. However, if we take culture in the sense of any of its current forms of expression, there are today no demonstrable contacts between it and sport. Though the modern sports movement has gained widespread *social* acceptance, there have been hardly any worthwhile *cultural* works with sport as their basis. In philosophy, literature, the theater, painting, sculpture, and music, and even the cinema, there are no artistic counterpoints to the struggles and dramas of athletics, no symphonies, songs, and ballets, no preludes or meditations that reflect or deepen the concept of the balanced mastery of body and soul, which, we are sure, sport is able to establish. Contests in literature, music, and sculpture, which Coubertin wanted to be integrated with the Olympic Games, have yielded lamentably mediocre results and they were dropped from the program since 1956. All this adds up to the "astounding, dismaying, infuriating and even, to be frank, scandalous situation in which sport, otherwise triumphant, is excluded from what I shall not call culture but culture's modes of expression." [5]

---

* Professor Ely Devons of the London School of Economics said in 1963 that the chief task of English universities today is that of making provision for an "intellectual" leisured class." [3]

The Concept of Culture

Sigmund Freud wrote in 1902 that all culture, all civilization, is based on the repression of natural instincts; that mankind achieves culture only by pushing under its strongest emotional drives; and that this repression breeds tension, which in turn leads to outbursts of violence, war, and crime. Other possibilities of canalizing these tensions did not occur to him, so as they did not occur to Russell with his exaggerated belief in the "intelligence of the masses." In any event, neither of these two great thinkers took cognizance of the sports and physical education movement, which began to grow up during their lifetime.

The German word "Kultur," that Freud used is not synonymous with either of the two English terms "culture" or "civilization." Actually, the English term "culture" has two different connotations. Anthropologists and sociologists apply it to describe a type of society indentifiable by its technical, religious, moral, economic, social, and artistic peculiarities. Thus, we speak of Polynesian, South American, or Scandinavian cultures. But the word "culture" has also a second sense—the sense in which one speaks of a "cultured person," or a Minister of Culture, or a cultural counsellor at an embassy; of someone cultivated in literature, art, languages, history, and so forth, and of course manners; a sense that is allied to the concept of excellence. It was of this last sense of culture that a hundred years ago Matthew Arnold was thinking when he defined culture as "acquainting ourselves with the best that has been said and done in the world." †

Sir Charles Snow has said that what previously was looked upon as "culture" has now become "two cultures"; one which is scientifically orientated; while the other complies with the criteria of humanistic tradition. However, Lord Hailsham, Minister of Science in England, has recently emphasized that it is impossible to draw a line between "the sciences" and "the humanities." "My Department," he explained, "had to discuss the question whether anthropology was a science, and we were told by the Treasury that physical anthropology was a science and social anthropology was an art." Dr. Magnus Pyke, looking from a different angle upon the same problem, arrived at the following conclusion: "If we wish to reflect upon the relationship between a man and a woman, we can turn for enlightenment either to Romeo and Juliet of the humanists or to the Kinsey Report of Science." ‡

Maheu on the Nature of Sports in Technological Societies

According to Maheu, in most societies in which the modern sports movement has taken root, "culture" has remained a prerogative of a minority. "It is one of the major aberrations of our culture," he writes, "that many forms in which it expresses itself lie beyond the reach of the workers and the peasants." Sport on the other hand has attained its firmest grip upon the

---

† As to his own compatriots, Arnold saw them divided into three kinds: the upper classes "with their blood sports and drink and playing cards," whom he called "barbarians;" the middle class, "caring for nothing but moral rectitude and money," who were to him "Philistines;" and the "populace" which was "brutalized by illiteracy and poverty."

‡ Compare also the editorial article in Reference 4.

classes that are—or were—the least privileged. Sport thus represents a form of social elevation as well as an advance towards a status of greater equality and freedom. This is one of the reasons why sport has become a mass movement; but also why sport has so far remained separate from culture pursuits. The categorical significance of the newly emerging science and philosophy of sport lies in the fact that it represents a new effort of bridging the gap between intellectualism and those areas of life that are shared by all. The science of sport is derived from lived as well as reflected human existence.

It is too early to assess the influence that this new development will exert upon society. Current humanistic theory does not yet admit that the body may be of equal dignity with the heart, the mind, and the soul. Contemporary thinking is still permeated by medieval philosophical teachings to the effect that the body represents the animal part of man that must be kept under.

The 17th-century English Nonconformist preacher John Bunyan, author of *Pilgrim's Progress*, thought that dancing and playing hockey or tipcat on the village green were sins. Once, after hearing a sermon against games and dancing, he nevertheless yielded to temptation:

> I shook the sermon out of my mind and to my old custom of sports and gaming I returned with great delight. But the same day as I was in the midst of a game of cat and having struck it one blow from the hole, just as I was about to strike it a second time, a voice did suddenly dart from heaven into my soul, which said "Wilt thou leave thy sins and go to Heaven or have thy sins and go to Hell?" At this I was put in an exceeding maze; wherefore, leaving my cat upon the ground, I looked up to heaven and was as if I had with the eyes of my understanding seen the Lord Jesus looking down upon me, as being hotly displeased with me, and as if he did threaten me with some grievous punishment for those and other ungodly practices.

In our civilization the body still ranks low in the scale of values. In Western societies the body has for centuries been assailed on two fronts: it was anathematized as sinful and it was made a target for contempt. Religious ethics, contemporary literature, the utilitarian ideology of mechanization, and absolute scientific positivism, all have the disparagement of the body in common. Maheu stresses the contrast between the respect for the body, which prevailed in antiquity and to a lesser extent still prevailed in the Renaissance, with the contempt for the body that characterizes the intellectual climate in our time.

In current literature, the body, if treated at all, is considered synonymous with sex. But of all bodily manifestations, sex is of least relevance to the physical phenomena with which sport is concerned; while those bodily manifestations of sport to which specific human significance attaches are looked upon by scientists as if they were equivalents of the kinetic performances of machines. Such an attitude is all the more anachronous since machines tend to render the body useless, turn it into an automaton.

> Machines are taking over more and more what the body used to do and science, that essential and determining factor in modern civilization, is perhaps the most deadly enemy of any humanism of the body; for in the final count the whole teaching of science is that the body is merely a machine and can be improved by means which practically deny its humanity.

With the advent of the industrial age the sociological status of the "populace" has undergone a change. Illiteracy and extreme poverty have virtually gone; child labor has gone. In terms of social justice a lot has been gained, though at a cost that was altogether unforeseen. Freud's view was vindicated, as those of us who have witnessed events in Europe between 1933 and 1945 know only too well. The new status of the "masses," characterized by the mechanization of transport, by the emergence of a white collar class of workers by the bureaucratization of life and by the automatization of production has repressed natural instincts to an extent that is without parallel in the history of mankind.

Homo faber had become *Homo sedentarius*. However, the ancient curse allegedly imposed upon work seems to have remained in force, even though the biblical injunction that mankind is to earn its bread by the sweat of its brow no longer applies in industrial societies. The physical stress of labor has been largely eliminated by the introduction of machines. As a result of this development, man's "sense of movement" and with it its natural relationship to his body have deteriorated. Fundamental instincts and emotional outlets that physical exercise in its various forms has afforded in the past are no longer available. In 1961 two American physicians, H. Kraus and W. Raab, wrote a book entitled *Hypokinetic Disease* in which a new category of health hazards is described, hazards due to the lack of exercise in our technological world.[6]

The Contemporary Scene in the United States

Because of the magnitude of the problem, Presidents Eisenhower and Kennedy made public statements on the need to adopt measures to counteract the increasing trend toward unfitness in the United States. Evidently, universal affluence is not an unmixed blessing. The great potentialities of sport and physical education as reintegrating influences upon life have so far not been fully utilized. A recent American survey assessed the leisure activities of people over 15 years of age on a given weekday: 57% watched television, 38% visited with friends or relatives, 33% worked around the yard or garden, 27% perused newspapers, 18% read books, 17% went for pleasure driving, 14% listened to records, 11% attended meetings or other organizational activities, 10% were engaged in special hobbies like wood-working or knitting; and 8% had gone out for dinner. Sport was not among the ten most frequent leisure activities. The U.S. Opinion Research Corporation Study, in which information was obtained from a national probability sample of 5021 persons, revealed that in the age group 15–19 not more than one quarter had indulged in sport on a given day.

In a recent American book entitled *Time, Work and Leisure* it was stated that two-thirds of college-educated women and more than four-fifths of women who never attended college were engaged in no sport whatsoever. Of the minority who did participate in sport, as few as 13.5% and 6.4%, respectively, included swimming in their activity schedule. Only about 10% of women practiced systematically golf, tennis, bowling, basketball, softball, or volleyball; while even fewer indulged regularly in ice skating, skiing, or tobogganing in winter and fishing and boating in the summer.[7]

Though the number of people who watch sporting events is much greater than that of those who participate, the amount of money spent in the United States for television repairs alone is much greater than that spent on all spectator sports, including baseball, basketball, and football.

To place all these facts into perspective, it is also necessary to remember that the United States produces many of the world's best performers in several of the chief branches of athletics. Because of the favorable nutritional, health, and other environmental conditions that characterize the economic status of the people in the United States as well as in all other technologically advanced countries, their potential physical performance capacity has greatly benefited. This is shown by the acceleration of their growth during the past hundred years. However, the transformation of performance-potential into performance presupposes sustained application, efforts, and continuous training.

Plessner on Fragmentation of Labor

Helmut Plessner has pointed out [8] that the traditional pilgrimage to Mecca which until not so long ago necessitated several weeks of walking, can now be undertaken by plane within hours or minutes. The result is that "the pilgrim arrives at the Holy Shrine in advance of his mind." Similarly, modern labor no longer conveys the sense of satisfaction that once came with the completion of a meaningful task. Work on assembly lines in factories is repetitive, sense-less, and boring. The occupational situation of the majority of white collar workers is frustrating. The worker as a human being has become anonymous. Fragmentation of labor and depersonalization of the laborer engender powerful inner tensions.

There is another aspect to consider: the general lack of recognizability of success and achievement of the individual worker. The progressive specialization of the production process presupposes acquaintance with the specific nature of the occupational activities that are demanded, an acquaintance that nobody is able to obtain in fields of employment other than his own. We know little of what the next person is doing, how well he is accomplishing his task and how successful he is in his career. Then there is the fact that the industrial world depends upon science. Not only the learned professions but at an ever growing rate also the crafts and other vocations now demand highly differentiated, intellectualized, and organized preparation, often over many years.

All of this seems to impose on man a morbid alienation. And it is interesting to note here how one man tried to deal with this condition:

> In 1964, the City of Prague held a ceremony to pay tribute to Franz Kafka, its great son. Eighty-year-old Max Brod delivered an eulogy in which he referred to Kafka as "one of the twentieth century's earliest chroniclers of the alienation and loneliness of man in industrial society." At the same time, Brod said, Kafka "was a lover of life and passionately interested in sport. Like the theatre, sport enabled him to express his joyful nature."

Sport is indeed capable of establishing a new balance vis-à-vis the in-equalities that are caused by the steadily progressing transformation of society. Like art, sport washes away from the soul the dust of everyday life. Sport renders possible the expression and the satisfaction of many desires that the modern world awakens as well as represses; desires for recreation and social contact, for aggression and play, for self-assuredness and hero worship. True, athletics and sport are not the only means to attain such satisfaction; but they would seem to be among the most readily accessible and the most rewarding.

Marathon Running

Marathon running as it is now developing in the United States as a branch of the "sports-for-all movement" exemplifies the issue. The following is an entry I made into my diary on December 19, 1975. It refers to details known only to those who have adopted the "third culture," in addition to the "first and second" of which Sir Charles Snow wrote in his essay lamenting the schism that has developed between the natural sciences and the humanities.

During the past week I was in Honolulu. The occasion was the yearly Marathon race preceded by a 3-day meeting organized by the American Medical Joggers Association (AMJA) whose president is Dr. Ronald Lawrence. Dr. Tom Bassler is Editor of an interesting circular letter which he sends out from time to time on behalf of the AMJA. Dr. Jack Scaff of Honolulu was in charge of the scientific sessions as well as of the Marathon race.

To begin with a few remarks on the race, which is now an event of genuine importance for the entire State of Hawaii. It has become clear that practically everybody can learn to run 26 miles, the length of a marathon course. Until a few years ago we did not know this. Physicians did not consider the far-reaching implications of this ubiquitously present but mostly undeveloped source of happiness and enhanced self-esteem. Participants in the 1975 Honolulu race included children as young as 8, boys and girls, adolescents, adults of all shapes and colors, as well as men and women up to the age of 82. Special awards were offered for various age groups, for family teams, for father-and-son, mother-and-daughter, and other entries. Furthermore, 15 "heart patients" presented themselves at the start and finished the race, several among them with documented clinical histories of previous myocardial infarctions. The "cardiac marathoners" wore special shirts ornamented with a flaming heart design. They had trained over several months under the supervision of Dr. Scaff, Dr. Morris, and Dr. Wagner of the staff of a prestigious private clinic engaged in group practice in Honolulu. These physicians routinely test each patient who wishes to join their exercise groups, monitoring pulse rates, EKG, and blood pressure on a treadmill. A demonstration of the procedure was given to us at the Honolulu YMCA by Dr. Morris.

About 750 persons had registered for the 26-mile race. Some had sent their entry forms beforehand, others presented themselves the day before the event at the Honolulu Municipal Park, which served as headquarters. The park also proved to be a suitable place for the victory ceremony after the marathon when prizes and certificates were handed to each runner who had completed the course.

The starting line for the race was alongside a small Public Garden situated next to the Aloha Tower in the Honolulu harbor region. Runners, coaches, helpers, friends, and admirers assembled between 5 and 6:30 A.M. It was pitch dark when Peter and I arrived at the scene. The assembled crowd radiated an atmosphere of excitement, of good natured tension and of a special kind of comradeship. Everybody seemed to feel that he belonged to a tightly knit community possessed by great self-discipline and a high level of physical fitness, both of which are beyond the reach of "ordinary" people who are "ordinary" because unlike the marathoners, they do not have the energy to train themselves day after day over months.

When at 6:25 A.M. the starter speaking through a bullhorn requested everybody to line up for the race I distinctly perceived the feeling of pride shared by the runners as they got ready for the ordeal. Among the participants were several of Olympic caliber. Four of the best women marathoners in the world had entered the race including Jacqueline Hansen, the all time record holder who looked pretty, dignified, and self-assured. Her best time, 2:38:99, is faster than that of the winner in the men's Olympic Marathon in 1924.

All runners were expertly dressed, their shoes carefully chosen, shoulders, legs, and feet rubbed with vaseline to protect against the sunlight. Many competitors take various kinds of tablets or drinks or "food supplements," vitamin pills, and other harmless nutritive "aids." Marathon runners constitute a community of faith of their own, some of them adhering to innocuous superstitions. For example, one physician who ran his 15th marathon recommended drinking moderate amounts of a special brand of beer before and during the event. Others believe that wheat germ oil, or large amounts of vitamin C are helpful. Many follow special eating schedules such as the "carbohydrate loading" diet which is at present popular because of reports of favorable results obtained in muscle biopsy studies conducted by well-known American, Swedish, and Danish investigators. However, it is by no means proven that it helps. Frank Shorter who won the Olympic marathon in Munich told me that he never heard of "carbohydrate loading" and that he ate his usual steak and eggs breakfast on the morning before his 1972 victory.

The fact that no evidence is available for any of the above-mentioned rituals does not impress the faithful. They point out that their procedures are of advantage to them, adding that "school medicine" has always been hostile to innovations. One of the best women marathon runners is a medical doctor holding a Harvard University degree. She is an admirer of a German physician–coach who holds that long distance running prevents and possibly cures cancer. He derives his ideas for the discovery by Professor Otto Warburg that malignant tumor cells, unlike normal cells, can exist without oxygen. They ferment sugar and prefer this source of energy even if oxygen is available, the "Pasteur effect," as Warburg called it. The German physician–coach writes that people get cancer because their bodies do not receive sufficient O_2. Since running improves the O_2 supply of the tissues, he argues that cells which otherwise would switch to fermentation and become cancerous will not do so in those who run. He reported on a group of old long distance runners who had trained for several years under his supervision. They are free of malignancies, and their good health, he believes, is due to the fact that they run. He discounts the possibility that they are able to run at their age because they are healthy.

Back to the race. The first part of the Honolulu Marathon course led through downtown, from there towards Diamond Head and back to the park. It was a warm and humid day. Clouds afforded a measure of protection against the sun. But the atmosphere was tropical. The men's winning time of 2:17:00 was remarkable, considering the circumstances. All participants had, of course, been jogging a great deal during the preceding months. Their staying power was excellent provided they were able to keep their body temperature down and had sufficient strength in legs and feet. This is an important observation because of the almost exclusive concern in exercise laboratories in the United States today with oxygen transport. But oxygen transport did not turn out to be a crux with most of the Honolulu marathoners.

The need for fluid intake in all endurance events is now generally recognized. Excellent arrangements were made at Honolulu for supply of drinks throughout the race. One boy of 19 refused to drink on the course. He finished in good time (2:56) but in poor condition, dehydrated, confused, cold, sweating, and vomiting. One hour after completing the race he had a seizure and was sent by ambulance to the hospital where he promptly recovered following intravenous replenishment of his body liquids.

All in all, the condition of most of the runners at the finishing line was good, reflecting their superior cardiorespiratory status. Only a handful were too pooped to pop after the race. The majority just walked from the finishing line to the water-and-coke counter set up nearby, happy, proud, and nicely tired. "Feet trouble" was a common complaint, much of it, no doubt, avoidable. A podiatrist addressed the medical meeting and gave good advice. Many runners reported that "their undercarriage had folded up during the last 6–10 miles."

Here we are confronted by a problem that has been neglected by exercise physiologists. Its ergometric as well as its biomechanical aspects deserve to be studied. What does happen to a hip joint after 4 hours of continuous "normal functioning?" How does skeletal muscle respond to prolonged uninterrupted activity such as marathon running? I do not know and I think nobody else does.

The AMJA group is an excellent clinical laboratory for the investigation of a variety of problems of sports medicine. Experiences with long distance runners open up new vistas for research in nutrition, pharmacology, psychology, psychiatry, geriatrics, and other medical specialties. The fact that unusual questions are raised by the group's medical members is interesting. E.g., I find Dr. Ron Lawrence's exploration of "osteopuncture"—as distinct from acupuncture—worthwhile. He reports his method's usefulness in the treatment of painful joint and muscle conditions. Dr. Lawrence places needle electrodes through small bore holes into bone and applies low grade electric current. Dr. Tom Bassler holds that every person who can run the 26 mile course thus demonstrates a distinctly favorable cardiac status and will not be afflicted by the manifestations of the ischemic myocardial diseases as long as he keeps in training. The determination with which AMJA physicians insisted upon the clarification of a report published in 1975 in the *New England Medical Journal* by Dr. Opie alleging that seemingly healthy men died during marathon races is admirable. The AMJA physicians' enquiry led to a complete withdrawal of the statement on which the original *Journal* report had rested.

I listened with interest to the jogging psychiatrist from San Diego who told us in Honolulu that his life had dramatically changed for the better 2 years ago when he took up running and thus got rid of bad habits of eating and drinking. He now formulates theories that reflect the nature and scope of his experiences. Several of his patients accompanied him on this trip to Honolulu and, like himself, ran the marathon. I enjoyed listening to an ophthalmologist from San Diego who spoke on a phenomenon discovered 10 years ago in my laboratory in Lexington that intraocular pressure decreases during exercise. Another fine contribution was made by a neurologist from Albuquerque who discussed autonomic adjustment to exercise, with special reference to successful results in the treatment of migraine.

The Honolulu week was a memorable event. It was conducted throughout in a fair spirit and in a good natured atmosphere of togetherness. The AMJA has shown that running is the best kind of psychotherapy. Running is of course much more—how much more, the AMJA will, I am sure, find out.

Recognizability and Communication

The universal recognizability of success and failure in sport is an essential element of communication and thus a means of advancement of freedom. Outside of sport, the range within which workers can move about without restraint and project their personality has become steadily decreasing with the uniformization of their environment. The trend towards restriction of freedom of self-projection has progressed pari passu with all recent material achievements. Press, radio, television, movies, organized traveling, and mass fabrication of goods reduce the scope of private existence to a minimum. In this calamitous situation sport offers possibilities for display of the self, which life otherwise does not render feasible. This statement applies chiefly to the active participants in athletics, but within limits also to the much greater numbers of spectators who identify themselves with the spectacle that takes place before their eyes.

Empathy and Catharsis

Like the art connoisseur, Maheu says, the spectator at a sporting contest is linked with the object of the event by a "current of sympathetic participation." In the theater as well as in the stadium an intense empathy develops between spectator and performer. "Spectator sports," Maheu writes, "are the true theater of our day." Sport, because it involves a particular facet of contest-play, is able to release and, in the Aristotelian sense, to purge the emotions of the spectator just as effectively as any work of art in general and the theater in particular. In reference to this close link generating a current of understanding and support from nameless crowds of watchers and listeners to the individual taking the sporting stage and "expanding himself," Maheu says that it takes us back to the very start of the theater of antiquity, the theater of Greece. Like culture and the arts in general, sport exteriorizes the feelings and emotions of the player and by empathy causes the spectator to experience "catharsis," the purification of the soul of which Aristotle has written long ago.

Lewis Mumford [9] has pointed out that sport presents three main elements: the spectacle, the competition, and the personalities of the gladiators. The spectacle itself introduces the esthetic element, so often lacking in the "paleotechnic industrial environment" itself. The race is run or the game is played within a frame of spectators, tightly massed: the movements of this mass, their cries, their songs, and their cheers, are a constant accompaniment of the spectacle: they play, in effect, the part of the Greek chorus in the new machine-drama, announcing what is about to occur and underlining the events of the contest. Through his place in the chorus, the spectator finds special release: he is now at one with a primitive undifferentiated group; he feels relieved from the passive role of taking orders and automatically filling them, of conforming by means of a reduced "I" to a magnified "it." In the sports arena the sports spectator has the illusion of being completely mobilized and utilized. Moreover, the spectacle itself is one of the richest satisfactions for the esthetic sense that the machine civilization offers to those that have no key to any other form of culture: the spectator knows the style of his favorite contestant in the way that the painter knows the characteristic line or palette of his master and he reacts to the bowler, the pitcher, the punter, the server, or the air ace, with a view not only to his success in scoring but to the esthetic spectacle itself. This point has been stressed in bull-fighting; but of course it applies to every form of sport.

Changing Leisure Patterns Reflected in Art

The profound changes that the Industrial Revolution has introduced into the leisure pattern of society are reflected in the artistic styles, techniques, subjects, and interpretations of the past four or five centuries. Jan Steen's picture of "The Skittle Players" mirrors the relaxed informality of rural recreation around 1650 (FIGURE 3). Gustave Courbet's portrait "Les Demoiselles au bord de la Seine" painted in 1856, still emanates the quiet and idyllical spirit of leisure at its best, (FIGURE 4). Less than a century later, artists began to give us images of a different world. In 1950, Pablo Picasso presented his own version of Courbet's "Les Demoiselles" of 1856: He showed the two young girls fragmented, like pieces of a jigsaw puzzle which defy all efforts toward in-

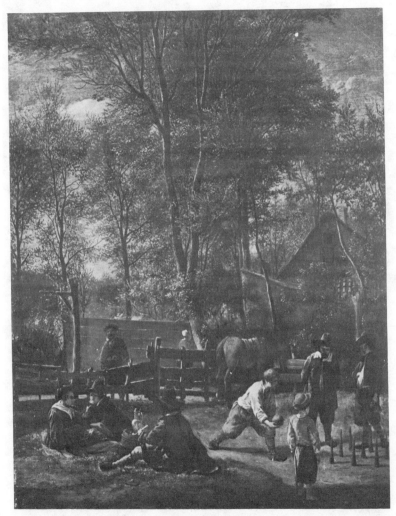

Figure 3. Jan Steen's (1626–1679) painting, *The Skittle Players* (13 × 10½ in.), (National Gallery, London), completed in 1652, is one of a series of pictures in which the artist depicts the manners and morals of the peasantry of the time, their way of life and all the gaiety and drollery that went with it. "The ideal moment," Hegel wrote over a century ago, "consists precisely in this carefree license. This is the Sunday of life, leveling all before it and doing away with what is evil. Men endowed with so much good humor cannot be mean and vile at heart."

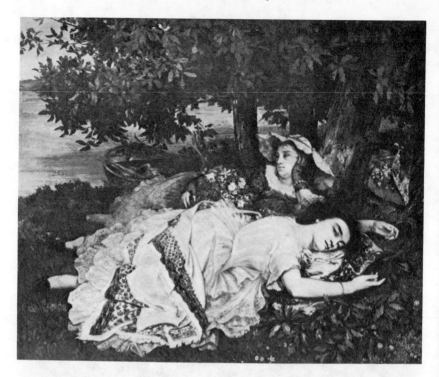

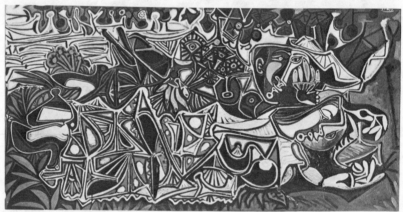

FIGURE 4. Gustave Courbet's (1819–1877) *Les Demoiselles au Bord de la Seine* (top), (Petit Palais, Paris, 173×205 cm) and Pablo Picasso's (1881–1975) *Les Demoiselles au Bord de la Seine after Courbet* (bottom), (Öffentliche Kunstsammlung, Basel, 100×200 cm). The latter was painted as a replica of Courbet's work in a deliberately fragmented technique which Picasso cultivated between 1945 and 1950. It allegorizes a trend that pervaded and continues to pervade contemporary civilization. Though esthetically marking a decline of standards that seemed to be firmly established during the preceding centuries, the artistic significance of Picasso's work lies in the fact that it expresses intelligently and sensitively a development which for better or worse characterizes the social climate of his time.

tegration into normal human beings. The fundamental incongruity between technology and human nature was allegorized in 1914 by the German painter George Scholz in a composition *Flesh and Iron* (FIGURE 5). In this picture the artist expressed his feeling of the incommensurability of the two women being placed in juxtaposition to a machine.

George Tooker, an exponent of the U.S. "Sharp Focus School" of the post-World War II period, uses a carefully realistic technique to allegorize the artificiality, drabness, and depersonalization of life in the "megalopolis," which calls for an entirely new approach to the problem of leisure time activities and recreation (FIGURE 6).

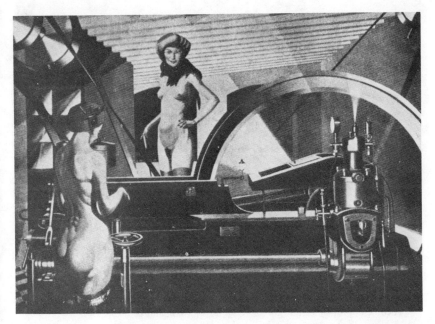

FIGURE 5. The fundamental incongruity between technology and human nature was allegorized by the German artist Georg Scholz (1896–1942) in his composition *Flesh and Iron*.

A sense of total dissolution of form and content in art is conveyed in "abstract painting" with its disregard of tradition, its totalitarian claims for recognition and its intolerance of criticism. Hans Hoffmann's picture *Emerald Isle* was recently described as the "work of an old master in modern art" (FIGURE 7). Ortega y Gasset has appropriately spoken of the new style that it represents as being indicative of "dehumanization of art." [10]

This is how the philosopher Houston Smith of the Massachusetts Institute of Technology expressed himself on the subject:

> As long as reality was conceived as a great chain of being—a hierarchy of worth descending from God as its crown through angels, men, animals, and plants to inanimate objects at the base—it could be reasonably argued that great art should attend to great subjects: Scenes from the Gospels, major battles or

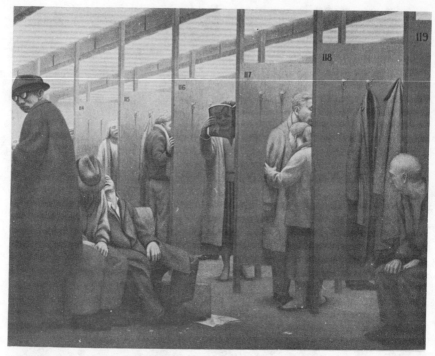

FIGURE 6. George Tooker (born 1920), an exponent of the U.S. "Sharp Focus School" of the post-World War II period uses in his painting *Megalopolis* a carefully realistic technique to emphasize the artificiality, drabness and depersonalization of life in the Big City.

distinguished lords or ladies. With cubism and surrealism, the distinction between trivial and important disappears. Alarm clocks, driftwood, pieces of broken glass become appropriate subjects for the most monumental paintings.

The British Broadcasting Corporation's weekly journal *The Listener* included in its issue of March 24, 1977 the following statement by G. Reichardt, entitled "The Art of Despair."

In the majority of modern literary and pictorial artists whom the critical establishment's weakness for extremes has rendered fashionable, what we see is a cult of infantilism and a virtual abandonment of all sophistication and contrivance, based on the very naive principle that the best way to demonstrate the utter futility of human life is to adopt the most rudimentary, even kindergarten, forms of expression in art. The Theatre of the Absurd patently belongs to this category of neotenic regressiveness, but even more so the boringly simplistic paintings of Johns and Rothko and the pictorial litter-bins of Rauschenberg."

Desmond Morris has written a book entitled *The Biology of Art*,[11] which deals with "paintings" by apes, among them a "water color" by a chimpanzee called Congo (FIGURE 8). The following is a quotation from Morris's concluding chapter:

Today picture-making has turned full cycle and is back almost where it began before ape-man became man-hunter. Now, at last the ape and the modern man have much the same interest in producing pictures, and it might even be argued that the modern human artist has little more reason for painting a picture than does a chimpanzee. As we have seen, the outcome of this is that contemporary human picture-makers and ape picture-makers produce startlingly similar results.

Evidently, the path along which 20th-century art has traveled towards dehumanization has reached its self-chosen goal.

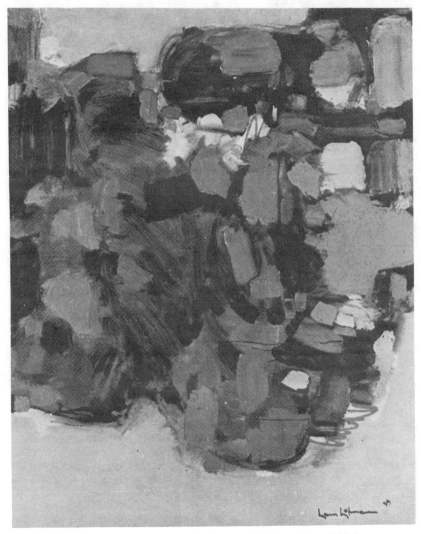

FIGURE 7. Hans Hofmann's (born 1908) picture *Emerald Isle*.

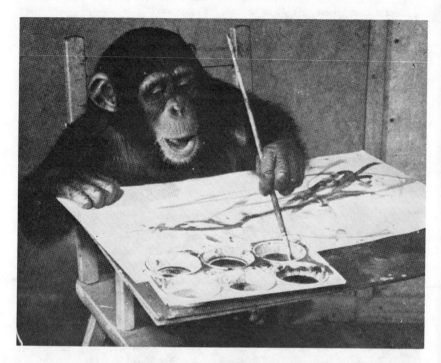

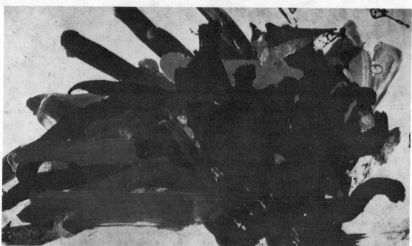

FIGURE 8. Desmond Morris has written a book entitled *The Biology of Art*, which deals with "paintings" by apes (top), among them the "water color" (middle) by a chimpanzee named Congo. (From Morris.[11])

Sherrington on Meaningful Images

A penetrating comment on the issue under reference is contained in Sir Charles Sherrington's book *Man on his Nature*.[12] The human mind, Sherrington said, can fathom the external world only in meaningful images. When Socrates spoke of his desire to "go to the other world" to see there "an earthly love, or wife, or son and conversing with them," he remarked that he would be infinitely delighted to be able to talk to Odysseus and to the leaders of the Trojan expedition. "To imagine Paradise," Sherrington observed, "a lofty mind thus invokes its favorite pursuit from earth and custom of earth's social creature, man. Mind's earthliness innately shapes all it does, perhaps most so when it tries to be unearthly."

The 16th-century painter Hieronymus Bosch was greatly interested about the "Evil One" and about "transmundane demons" (FIGURE 9). Yet his vision could achieve nothing to the purpose beyond contriving ugly hybrids from familiar shapes of terrestrial creation. Nor could the noble imagination of Dante transcend the limits of actual experience: when the poet traveled the Inferno, Purgatory, and Paradise "he still walked Italy, the Italy he loved and grieved for."

Esthetic Evaluation of Human Movements

One of the great cultural attributes of sport is that it creates beauty. The esthetic value of human movements engendered in sport is synonymous with that which emanates from art at its best. Maheu believes that the beauty which sport begets "is immanent in the very act which creates it." The two, he thinks, are inseparable from the fleeting moment. He therefore conceives a contrast between the beauty of sport and the beauty of art. "Art expresses itself through signs, through stylization, not of things, not of body or of living creatures."

Art places a distance between the object and the creation of beauty. For Maheu, signs and symbols are the substance of art; while the substance of sport is the living body itself. Sport belongs wholly to the present; the actor merging completely with the action.§ The same synonymity, he feels, is not possible in art whose objects are connected with the finished work by a relationship of meaning, a relationship that is arbitrary, removed from natural contacts. This characterization, Maheu holds, applies alike to the man of letters and the writer who do not work with emotions or ideas or passions but with words; to the painter who works with colors and light effects which represent or can represent other things or objects; though for him the sign is all important. Even in sculpture and in music, he says, it is the sign that counts.

> Between the creator and the object he creates is fixed that distance which liberates art and endows it with its quality of eternity. Sport consists wholly of action; art, on the contrary, by its employment of the sign which freed it from the object and from life, moves into eternity. Thus, sport and art face in opposite directions.

§ S. Wenkart is in agreement with Maheu's viewpoint: "In the transition from subject to object there is a complete elimination of schisms, and an existential experience of oneness."[13]

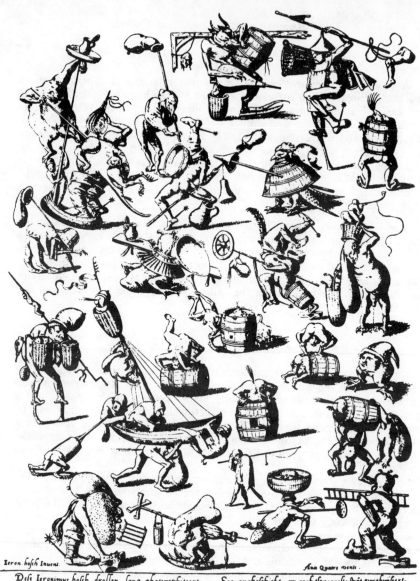

FIGURE 9. Hieronymous Bosch (1450–1516) transposed the well-nigh demoniacal eloquence of the popular preachers of his time into the language of art. He created visual equivalents of written or spoken homilies, gave striking forms to proverbs and a prodigious actuality to abstractions. However, Bosch never reversed this order of transforming abstractions into readily identifiable scenes. Nowhere did he try to present reality as mere arrays of lines and colors. Many of Bosch's pictures engender an atmosphere of enigmatic unreality. Still, everything remains recognizable. Even where he transcends the boundaries of our everyday world, he never becomes "inhuman," to use the term which Ortega y Gasset has introduced in his critical interpretation of contemporary art.

990

Maheu concludes that sport cannot as yet give us what we are offered by artistic expression and culture, namely, a meaning that enables us to transcend the temporary, to transcend all that is ephemeral and to discover something that is of eternal value. But he is confident that one day sport will cross the threshold and that a true element of culture will emerge from it.

Are we in fact justified in thus separating the esthetic manifestations of sport from those of the arts? Is the beauty that is derived from ice skating and dancing, from gymnastics and water diving, from soccer, hockey, and horseback riding categorically different from that of, say, music and the stage? Is it true that only in sport the beauty that the performer's action begets is immanent in the very act that creates it? I believe that the answer to these questions is in the negative. The esthetic implications of the acts that engender beauty in sport are fundamentally the same as the acts that engender beauty in music and on the stage. They all belong to the present, so as Maheu has rightly pointed out in respect of sport. Like the performing athlete, the performing musician and the performing actor merge completely with their action. Esthetics in sport and esthetics in music and on the stage also have the same double character in that on the one hand they appeal but for a "fleeting moment": while on the other their performances can be rendered permanent: in music through staff notation, in literature through the written word; in sport through graphic symbolization, e.g., in choreography. Also, of course, through photography and the film and the latter's use in television. All these forms of esthetic revelation can therefore be reflected upon and repeated; all of them thus attain a quality of the "external."

Motor Notation

Though the development of systems of notation of movements in sport is not as far advanced as that of notation of music and literature, sufficient progress has already been made in the symbolization of the dance, of calisthenics, of gymnastics, and of other activities to justify the statement that sport has crossed the threshold of which Maheu has spoken; and that for this reason alone it moves towards the emergence of a new and dynamic cultural force.

The British mathematician H. Levy has stated the problem in its categorical relevance:

> Science has a dual history. It is the tale of the birth of men with great powers of abstraction, and it is the story of the evolution of languages peculiarly adapted to these abstractions. Our heritage from Newton would have been a much poorer thing but for the differential calculus, as our indebtedness to Einstein is enriched by the tensor notation. What does the development of organic chemistry not owe to the interlocking of Dalton's atomic theory with the synthetic possibilities suggested by graphical formulae? Notation is indeed the very lifeblood of science.
>
> Without a musical notation how could the great masters have left a permanent record of their creations, or even conceived detailed and elaborate symphonies? Thought and experience have ever striven for a language rich in expression as an adequate channel for communication; and so in music a notational scheme for precise tonic description was inevitable, and once achieved the way was open for a magnificent outburst of musical art on a grand scale.
>
> He would be bold who would deny the possibility of a similar advance in the art and science of movement, once the kinetics of bodily limbs have been suitably notated.

The fact that no universal system of motor notation has yet been accepted greatly retards the establishment of sport and physical education as a cultural force. In the absence of such a system it is impossible to develop tradition, to formulate concise esthetic criteria, to rely upon a sufficiently wide range of didactic variants and to engender a sense of historical continuity. Dame Margot Fonteyn, the British ballerina, has expressed her concern over "the distressing realism of some of the more contemporary ballets," adding that dancers today do not "assimilate their great heritage from the past." [14]

The validity of this view is shown by the influence that the perfection of staff notation has exerted upon the cultural impact of music upon society—without it musicians would have been unable to "assimilate the great heritage from the past"; without it the works of Bach and Haydn, Mozart and Beethoven, Schubert, Schumann and Brahms would have been lost. It is insufficiently realized that it took several centuries to evolve the present five-line pattern of musical staff notation; and that its perfection is due to the combined intellectual, didactic, and artistic efforts of a small number of exceptionally able musicians. During his youth Johann Sebastian Bach still had to study keyboard, vocal and instrumental music that was notated on seven lines, like the Buxheimer Orgelbuch; or on six lines like the Lute Book of Vincenzo Capirola; or on four lines, the standard version of transcription of many Gregorian chants since the 12th century. The five-line pattern of musical staff notation as it is now used was generally accepted only during the second half of the 17th century, largely as a result of Bach's determination. As yet, sport and physical education have at their disposal no means of graphic communication comparable in conciseness and broad applicability to that available in music.

To work out a universal system of motor notation represents, I think, the most important single challenge to the science of sport and physical education of our time.

Acquisition of Skill as Prerequisite of Communication

The problem of the acquisition of skill assumes a significance of its own in that the enhanced performance capacity that is established through training reveals itself as a prerequisite for the mediation of a certain kind of human experience and for the conveyance of particular categories of introspective and social values.

Eva Bosakova, the Czechoslovakian athlete, has given a description of the years of preparation which preceded her Olympic victories in the gymnastic contest on the balancing beam in 1956 and 1960. When she was 15 years old her father, himself an outstanding gymnast, began to supervise her training:

> He prescribed daily 30-minute periods of work on the beam during which it was necessary to remain on the apparatus constantly in action, walking, hopping, turning, and again walking without rest. I spent hundreds of hours and uncounted kilometers walking and running on the beam.

After some time the beam became her favorite gymnastic event.

> I constantly searched for new methods, elements, and dynamic combinations for my exercises. In the process I gained complete confidence, accustomed myself to unfamiliar movements and lost all fear of falling. Each individual exercise

period lasted more than one hour. During this time I went through my whole routine five to seven times. Afterwards I worked on individual elements of the exercises and their connections, selected passages and their combinations. At the height of my career, it took me from about six to eight months to acquire mastery of a new exercise such as those prescribed for the Olympic Games.

It is thus that skill is acquired. Sustained practice of precisely designed sequences of movements establishes advanced levels of control, of differentiation, and of precision of motor acts such as are beyond the integrative control of the untrained.

Keyboard Music

The area of human skills in which didactic techniques are most advanced is keyboard music. As an example I refer to the role of the "study" or of the étude, defined in Grove's *Dictionary of Music and Musicians* as a class of musical composition of extremely varied scope and design, whose chief object is the cultivation of the powers of execution.

Facility to play on the keyboard is achieved by practicing technical exercises, such as scales and arpeggios, by each hand separately, consequently by both hands in unison. Up to the middle of the 18th century such technical exercises were taught in a dry and unattractive form. In Voltaire's Candide, which was published in 1759, the "Illustrissimo Lord Pococurante" complained that "music nowadays is merely the art of executing difficulties and in the end that which is only difficult ceases to please." Important attempts to improve this kind of shortcoming were made by Domenico Scarlatti and by Johann Sebastian Bach whose Notenbüchlein for his wife Anna Magdalena and his son Friedemann have ever since been used by music teachers. Moreover, Bach in seeking to establish the perfect relationship of the tempered scales, produced 48 preludes and fuges that, besides being inherently beautiful, have remained the classical touchstone of piano pedagogy. More than a century later Chopin, who always limbered up for his own concerts by playing from Bach's *Well-Tempered Clavichord,* presented a series of "field maps of the territory he felt had to be explored in order to enlarge the range of piano technique.[15] In almost every one of them he dealt with technical problems involved in the new kind of music he was composing. Each étude was designed as an exercise to overcome specific difficulties of execution. The study in thirds (Opus 25, No. 6) and the tremendous one in octaves (Opus 25, No. 10) reveal their teaching purposes at a glance (FIGURE 10). Even such a passionate outburst as the "revolutionary" étude (Opus 10, No. 12) is essentially a technical study of the very highest order for the left hand.

These études initiated a world-wide advancement of piano technique, so as 150 years before Chopin, Bach had caused an advancement of musical technique in its entirety. The cellist Pablo Casals said once that he played Bach "so as pianists play Chopin." In setting forth technical problems, both Bach and Chopin created music of great esthetic values, thus providing the motivation without which nobody can be induced to spend the necessary time practicing. The best of Chopin's études are among the finest compositions for the piano. It has been truly said that he who can play Chopin's études can play anything in modern piano literature.

The history of the musical study represents a model of educational me-

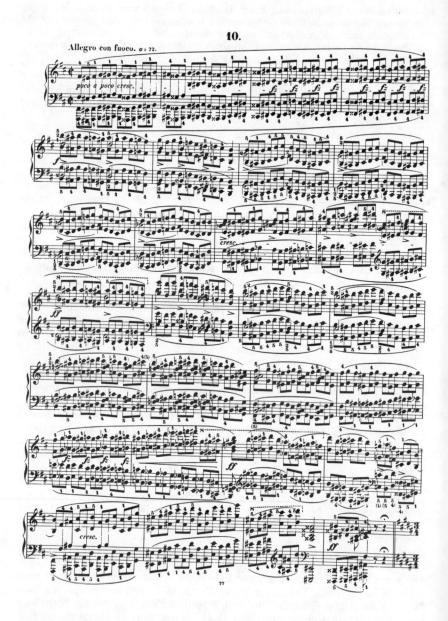

FIGURE 10. First page of Chopin's Study in Octaves, Opus 25, No. 10.

thodology pertaining to the acquisition of skills of all kinds. The time will come when it will serve as a didactic guide for the development of gymnastics and physical training.

Education in all human pursuits that aspire at the attainment of excellence of performance demands that the pupil spends a great amount of time practicing. Track champions devote four to five hours per day to their training. In a comprehensive study of Sweden's best girl swimmers, Astrand *et al.* found that performances differed in accordance with the volume of training: those girls who swam 60,000 meters per week achieved significantly better results than others who swam 10,000 meters. The former also developed a more pronounced adaptive enlargement of their hearts and a greater capacity to absorb oxygen.

Ruskin's Law

Ninety years ago John Ruskin, the British art critic, made a statement whose validity extends beyond the field to which it was meant to apply:

> If we were to be asked abruptly, and required to answer briefly what qualities chiefly distinguished great artists from feeble artists, we should answer, I suppose, first, their sensibility and tenderness; secondly, their imagination; and thirdly, their industry. Some of us might, perhaps, doubt the justice of attaching so much importance to this last character, because we have all known clever men who were indolent, and dull men who were industrious. But though you may have known clever men who were indolent, you never knew a "great" man who was so; and, during such investigation as I have been able to give to the lives of the artists whose works are in all points noblest, no fact ever looms so large upon me—no law remains so steadfast in the universality of its application—as the fact and law that they are all great workers. Nothing concerning all great workers is a matter of more astonishment than the quantity they have accomplished in the given length of their life; and when I hear a young man spoken of, as giving promise of high genius, the first question I ask about him is always— Does he work?

Ruskin's law is equally valid in sport. J. M. Tanner has identified a number of anthropometric characteristics of successful participants in a variety of athletic contests. H. Reindell of Freiburg, Germany, has described discongruities of patterns of cardiovascular adaptation between Olympic long distance cyclists and weight-lifters. In my own laboratory, diverse personality features were found to distinguish successful basketball players from outstanding swimmers. There is overwhelming evidence showing that each kind of athletic performance has its own specific psychological structure. At the same time, the history of every champion athlete reveals the determining role played in his career by intensive, sustained training. Intensive, sustained training is an indispensable prerequisite for athletic as well as artistic success. Without it, the full potentialities of neuromotor skill cannot unfold themselves.

Sport as a Creator of Myths

Like the arts, sport is a creator of myths and imagery. Athletic champions of the past appear in retrospect greater than their heirs do at present, even though the evidence proves the contrary conclusion to be justified. In the mind of those of us who competed many years ago in athletic contests, the memory of our triumphs remains vivid and may even shine brighter as time passes on.

The desire to create myths in sport often overrules scientific considerations. In 1957 a group of eminent American physicians met at Peter Bent Brigham Hospital in Massachusetts to discuss medical observations made during the Boston marathon race. A psychiatrist proclaimed that "death may be the vague ultimate aim of marathon runners"; that those athletes "always run to the point of utter exhaustion and into collapse" like the King's messengers of old who took pride in sacrificing themselves for their master. He went on quoting from Robert Browning's poem, "Incident of the French Camp," which describes how a runner brought news from a distant battle to Napoleon. No sooner was the message delivered than he perished:

> "You're wounded!" "Nay," the soldier's pride
> Touched to the quick, he said:
> "I'm kill'd Sire" And the chief beside
> Smiling the boy fell dead.

"One always sees in these messengers a moment of exaltation," the psychiatrist continued, "when they have finally won through and delivered the news; then it seems to be an almost inexorable destiny for them to drop dead—anything but death would be a dull, sudden, anticlimax."

In conclusion he alluded to the mythological story of Icarus, "that high flyer who soared upward until he nearly reached the sun in spite of the warning of his father Daedalus".

> Alas! The sun's heat melted the waxen wings, and he plummeted into the seas. This rise to triumph followed almost at once by the fall to death may bear some kinship to the kind of drama that seems to unfold in the ancient messenger or the marathon runner.

The learned audience at Peter Bent Brigham Hospital received this imaginative effort of phantasy on the part of the psychiatrist with considerable appreciation. The *New England Journal of Medicine* referred to it in an editorial article entitled "Icarus Complex." The fact that nobody has ever died from marathon running was completely lost behind the allegorical clouds raised by the inspired myth.

Of course mythology was allegorization; symbolic allusion and simile have at times been interwoven with fruitful scientific theorizing—but fruitful only if the iron rules of interplay of imagination and verification were observed. Paul Ehrlich invoked the medieval symbol of the "magic bullet" while he demonstrated the capacity of selected chemical compounds to combine with specific pathogenic microorganisms. Freud introduced terms like "Oedipus complex" in an effort to identify certain psychological constellations that, he held, characterize the *conditio humana;* and from the colorless world of Hades of ancient Hellas he enticed into the light of the 20th century the shadows of Agamemnon, Electra, and Orestes.

All creative human endeavors—including the natural sciences and the arts —have engendered their own mythology.[16] Insofar as sport has shown itself possessed by powers of a like kind, it has revealed equivalent creative potentialities.

Sport is one of the avenues of mankind's never ceasing strive for excellence.

Its uniqueness lies in the intimacy between the physical happenings of our bodies and their repercussions in our minds; as well as in the general recognizability of the social and esthetic values that sport engenders. Sport evokes experiences that are exclusively human and independent of the changing forms, patterns, and customs of a civilization that involves profoundly modifying components of our environment. The anthropological relevance of this differential interrelationship has been shown by Erwin Straus in his essay, "The Upright Posture," [17] which, as he puts it, reflects the unchangeable and prearranged material framework of human existence, in contrast to the changeability of the world around us. The concern of physical culture with the cultivation and improvement of the individual's own motor resources relates to both the body and the mind from which it originates. "The ethics of sport," Maheu writes, "proclaim the dignity of the body and deny that there can be any possible comparison between the machine that is the human body and a machine fashioned by man, or even any comparison, as Jean Prevost has said, between the skill and strength of an animal and the skill and strength of a man."

Poetic Interpretation of Sport and Play

The phenomenological meaning of the terms sport, play, and game has changed in the course of time. For centuries poets have given metaphoric expression to their awareness that sport contains elements of experiences that are absent in ordinary life.

In his *Fairie Queen*, Edmund Spenser dwelt upon the problem of unpredictability or, as he preferred to call it, "mutability" in play.

> What man that sees the ever-whirling wheel
> Of Change, the which all mortal things doth sway,
> But that thereby doth find, and plainly feel,
> How Mutability in them doth play
> Her cruel sports, to many men's decay?

In Shakespeare's *Othello*, Iago refers to his general's love for Desdemona:

> She is sport for Jove.

Play can remove the pressure of anxiety and in doing so alter the sense of time. In *A Midsummer Night's Dream*, Theseus asks:

> Is there no play to ease the anguish of a torturing hour?

The quality of the exceptional, of the festive, and of the enjoyable that is attached to sport at its best, is revealed in the following lines spoken by the prince in *Henry IV:*

> If all the year were playing holidays,
> To sport would be as tedious as to work;
> But when they seldom come, they wish'd for come.

Play's combination of reality and phantasy creates an enclave whose boundaries are delineated against the drab territory in which daily life takes its course. Also, play's appeal is universal and independent of time and place.

Cassius: How many ages hence
Shall this our lofty scene be acted o'er?
In states unborn and accents yet unknown?
Brutus: How many times shall Caesar bleed in sport?

In his *Tale of a Tub*, Ben Jonson speaks of the sports of love:

Come, my Celia, let us prove
while we can the sports of love.

The same metaphor appears in John Milton's "Lycidus":

Alas! What boots it with uncessant care
To tend the homely, slighted, shepherd's trade,
And strictly meditate the thankless Muse?
Were it not better done, as others use,
To sport with Amaryllis in the shade,
Or with the tangles of Neaera's hair.

And more lately in a poem by Robert Bridges:

I heard a linnet courting
His lady in the spring;
His mates were idly sporting,
Nor stayed to hear him sing
His song of love—
I fear my speech distorting
His tender love.
I heard a linnet courting.

Jane Austen refers in *Pride and Prejudice* to the unpredictability of the continuous interplay between man and his neighbors.

For what do we live but to make sport of our neighbors
and laugh at them in our turn

while the following four lines appear in Matthew Arnold's *Empedocles on Etna*:

Nature, with equal mind
Sees all her sons at play,
Sees man control the wind,
The wind sweeps man away.

Concluding Remarks

In many ways the humanistic and sociological functions of sport as leisure are synonymous with those of art. Both sport and art are means of modifying and enriching man's experiences.¶

In his lecture "On Actors and Acting," Max Reinhardt said that the immortality of the theater is derived from the eternal longing of the human mind to be transformed. This statement equally applies to sport. We all, Reinhardt wrote, carry in us the capacity of experiencing every conceivable emotion.

¶ "The purpose of the universe is play. The artists know that play and art and creation are different names for the same thing—a thing that is sweats and agonies and ecstasies. The artists who know more than anyone else about play which is art, which is creation, must be the leaders and guides." Don Marquis.

Nothing human is foreign to us. If it were different, we would be unable to understand each other, in life as well as in art which renders possible the projection of latent feelings and moods and thoughts in their concealed diversity. All this is true also for sport as a medium of communication of unlimited range and appeal; perhaps even more so than for art, whose appeal is more selective. Thus Max Reinhardt's dictum that immortality has been bestowed upon the theater because of the ever present desire of the human mind to be transformed applies still more ubiquitously to play and game and sport.

I am inclined to believe that in all technological societies, sport represents the strongest remaining link between man and nature. Sherrington said that our bodies are the one part of nature of which we have "direct" knowledge. One may well add that there are grades of such direct knowledge, and that the improvement of physical efficiency that accompanies training facilitates its acquisition.

In his *Notebooks 1935–1942*,[18] Albert Camus wrote that "the body, a true path to culture, teaches us where our limits lie." Camus knew of course that these limits are not fixed and that game and play and exercise can extend them. Of his student days, Camus spoke as follows: "Sport was the main occupation of all of us, and continued to be mine for a long time. That is where I had my only lessons in ethics. . . ." In his novel *LaChute,* the main character of the story faithfully reflects the writer's personal attitude when he says: [19]

> "I was really sincere and enthusiastic during the period when I played games, and also in the army when I acted in plays which we put on for enjoyment. . . . Even today the stadium crammed full of spectators for a Sunday match, and the theater which I love with unequalled intensity, are the only places in the world where I feel innocent." [19]

The body had taught Camus not only "where his limits lay" but also how he could vary and extend his limits.

The sedentary life of the ordinary city dweller of today renders the acquisition of deep "knowledge of nature" almost impossible. Susan Langer has pointed out that most town people have no notion of the earth's productivity; they do not know the sunrise and rarely notice when the sun sets. Ask them what phase the moon is in or when the tide in the harbor is high, and likely as not they cannot answer. Seed time and harvest are nothing to them. The power of nature is not felt by them as a reality. Realities are to them the motors that run elevators and cars; or the steady feed of water and gas through the mains, and of electricity over the wires; or the crates of foodstuffs that arrive by night; or the concrete and brick, bright steel, and dingy woodwork that take the place of earth and waterside and sheltering roof for them. Nature as man has always known it, he knows no more.

Scope and nature of the transformation which sport at its best can bring about has been revealed in neurological case studies of Olympic champions who reached the summit of achievement though they were afflicted with major physical handicaps. Harold Connally, who had suffered a birth injury that caused his left arm to remain withered, broke the world record for the hammer throw. The Hungarian crack pistol shot Karoly Takasc lost his dominant right arm in an accident, but won gold medals at the 1948 and 1952 Olympic Games, holding the weapon in his left hand. The Danish equestrienne Lis Hartel, whose muscular power remained critically reduced after an attack of poliomyelitis, proved herself the best woman rider in the Olympic dressage contests in Finland in 1952, and in Sweden in 1956.

The human brain can use any part of the motor system to convert abstractions into concrete movements. This fact was alluded to by the 18th-century German poet Gotthold Ephraim Lessing, who wrote in his drama *Emilia Galotti* that "Raphael would have become an immortal painter even if he had been born without arms."

The exclusively human power of converting abstractions into movements enables sport to mediate exceptional experiences so profound as to alter a person's life. Until recently such transformation had been thought to be possible only along ethical and esthetic lines: the New Testament account of the conversion of St. Paul is a case in point. In Johann Sebastian Bach's *B-minor Mass*, ritual, text, and music combine to convey the idea of the transubstantiation of the bread and of the wine. The Greek dramatists stressed the transforming power of "catharsis," the reverberation in the mind of the onlooker of the happenings on the stage. In lyrical poetry, literary allegory tells of reality undergoing magic change: in Heinrich Heine's *Dichterliebe* tears turn into flowers, and sighs into a chorus of nightingales.

To these imaginative categories of transformation we can now add that which may take place as subjective counterpart of superb accomplishments in athletics. Acquisition of skill, e.g., in the instances quoted of hammer throw, pistol shooting and horse riding can engender extraordinary experiences that may change a person's life, so as religious or artistic experiences have been known to do. The three great athletes who persevered even though they were handicapped challenged their fate by mobilizing resources of their own. They prevailed because they acted where others lose themselves in self-pity and despair.

The French poet Paul Valery wrote that all human cultures and religious and metaphysical systems are "play," in that they represent but potentialities of conceptual thinking, sketches of a power of the mind that can be projected into reality. But they can also be withdrawn; every culture is mortal as the study of history has taught. The culture of sport, however, is projected primarily into ourselves. Its universal reverberation is derived therefrom. It can thus be explained that once again the Olympic ideal appeals today to all people, so as it appealed long ago to the people of Greece at the height of Hellenistic civilization. Sport renders accessible to us mobilization of elements of which other cultural manifestations do not partake. Sport as leisure enables man to discover and develop cultural resources that are hidden in himself.

References

1. TOWNSEND, P. 1963. The man inside: Idealism and athletics. The Listener (London, June 27).
2. RUSSELL, B. 1935. In Praise of Idleness. George Allen & Unwin Ltd. London.
3. DEVONS, E. 1963. The Listener (14 March).
4. Editorial. 1963. The "art" and "science" of medicine. J. Amer. Med. Assoc. (13 April).
5. MAHEU, R. 1962. Sport and Culture. UNESCO Internat. J. Adult Youth Ed. 14(4).
6. KRAUS, H. & W. RAAB. 1961. Hypokinetic Disease. Charles C Thomas, Publisher. Springfield, Ill.

7. DeGrazia, S. 1962. Time, Work and Leisure. Twentieth Century Fund. New York, N.Y.
8. Plessner, H. 1956. Die Funktion des Sports in der industriellen Gesellschaft. Wissenschaft und Weltbild (December).
9. Mumford, L. 1940. The Culture of Cities. Secker & Warburg. London.
10. Ortega y Gasset. 1956. The Dehumanization of Art. Doubleday. Garden City, N.Y.
11. Morris, D. 1962. The Biology of Art. Methuen, London.
12. Sherrington, C. 1940. Man on his Nature. Cambridge University Press. Cambridge, England.
13. Wenkart, S. 1963. The meaning of sports for contemporary man. J. Existential Psychiat. 3 (12, Spring): 397–405.
14. Guest, I. 1960. The Dancer's Heritage. Pelikan. New York, N.Y.
15. Brockway, W. & H. Weinstock. 1937. Men of Music. New York, N.Y.
16. Dawe, P. G. M. 1963. Mind and machine. The Listener (17 October): 591.
17. Straus, E. 1952. The upright posture. Psychiat. Quart. 26: 529.
18. Camus, A. 1963. Notebooks 1935–1942. Alfred A. Knopf. New York, N.Y.
19. Cruickshank, J. 1959. Albert Camus and the Revolt of Literature. Oxford University Press. Oxford, England.
20. Jokl, E. 1961. Über den Aufbau der menschlichen Leistung. Theorie und Praxis der Körperkultur (11/12).
21. Kerr, W. 1962. The Decline of Pleasure. Sinmon & Schuster. New York, N.Y.

LONG DISTANCE RUNNING AS MEDITATION

David Shainberg

Postgraduate Center for Mental Health
New York, New York 10016

The word "meditation" means: consider, study, plan, exercise the mental faculties. The root "med" means measure, also "to care for." Other connections include the word "mode," which is defined as "tune or melody." And, interestingly enough, "plan," one of the definitions of meditate, is defined as "a diagram exhibiting the relative position and size of the parts of a thing." All of these meanings together convey that meditation is an action of attention, an awareness and concern for what is actually occurring in body and mind; seeing the position of actions in relationship to each other and the world. So meditation is not a behavior projected to the future, it is not getting ready for something else, it is not an attempt to improve anything, it is not a tranquilizer. It is not becoming. It is an acknowledgment of what is now. It hears the tune; it is the observation of parts in terms of the whole. And meditation is more that is undefinable: it acts in silence when the brain, thought-movements, and plans cease.

Long distance running as meditation has a particular place in our world because it provides a special opportunity to understand the action of time, our relationship in space and movement. These relationships are distorted in our technological society. We have rockets that travel millions of miles in short times and machines that do things at the push of a button. We unconsciously come to think that space can be traversed at rocket speed and that the time of life moves with the same rhythm as these machines.

My meditation begins with awakening from sleep. I know certain inattention has occurred while I slept. I feel a distance between my thoughts and the tensions of my body. The drowsiness complicates the uncertainty of what happened during my night of unconsciousness. The disconnection is apparent when my attention is drawn to it. Simultaneously, there is awareness that I am going to run. My first act of meditation is when I acknowledge this inattention. It is no exaggeration, I think, to say that the meeting between attention and inattention is the first step of the run. My impulse to run may, in part, be also a return to that memory of yesterday's pleasure; but when my running is that memory, I am thinking of myself as a machine that I want to recycle. I see this, but I am also aware that seeing the inattention of my night leads to my wanting to see the way things are today. From the moment I begin to dress, especially when I put on my track shoes, I feel like I am slipping into the comfortable realness of my body. I observe the movements of my legs and arms, my neck and my fingers that I did not watch during the night or during the early parts of the morning prior to dressing.

Aristotle observed that nature is like a runner, in that it goes, he said, from nonbeing to being and back. When we run, we discover the sense in which nature is present in our bodies. Each morning there is a discovery of the texture and sinews of my muscles; the first steps of the run assert the presence of my connection to the rest of the matter of the universe. In one sense, as I run, it is clear that my body is mechanically organized and performs the functions of my run in a similar manner each day. I depend on the actualities of nature. The movements of running come along together, one after another once I go out there and run. I recognize my coordination each day and feel a kind of respect for the way it works together without my doing anything that puts it together.

But each day the run has a different context. The weather is different, the day before was different, the distance is different because I may be intending to go further and therefore what comes before the half-way point will be different, a different anticipation of what the new distance will demand; I wonder what the end stages will be after having come a little bit further than before. Although my body appears to be the same as yesterday, it is in fact quite different and its difference partakes of the almost infinite number of variations in this new day's run.

Within this newness of the run, there is a memory of old runs. This memory retains an idea of yesterday's experience, and when the memory appears, it seems to have the intention of blocking out the changing present in which my brain is on the run as part of my body. My brain is connected to all parts of my body through my nerves, blood vessels, and heart. It is also connected to a world I feel to be outside my body through what I see, what I hear, feel on my skin, and receive through my pressure receptors. This brain, however, seeks order, which is to say, a relationship between all these connections. One important function of this brain is thought. It is a material process of a material organ and it is composed of memories. Thought as memory functions in my brain as a separate action and does not seem to remain connected to any unity of the relationship of all these connections of body and brain and world. I am aware that my brain is seeking a kind of order when my memories appear, but I feel forced to perceive fragments of thought sequences that have nothing to do with the present run. My brain has all kinds of knowledge of what was good about yesterday or what would be good in tomorrow's experience if I could get it to be like something in last year's pleasure. My brain repeats these thoughts while I am running as if thought would give me the longed-for sanctuary I crave while on the run. Despite the fact that there are an infinite number of details to face every minute, my brain persists in this habit of going over old situations. In a way, the brain operates during the run as it does in dreams, where the incomplete events of the day are reworked. On the run, puzzles from other parts of life tend to appear. The past invades the present, and attention to the run is shifted to what has been.

The rhythm of thought is different from the rhythm of the run. The incompleteness of the run is evident in each step, but the brain, in the form of thought, seems desperate to search for conclusions. My memory of the remnants of each thought creates a kind of residue of continuity. Out of the little bits of each thought that are similar to bits before, my brain consolidates an identity, an "I" or "me" who now I unwittingly feel is the runner. I begin to feel there is this one permanent "thing" that is persistent through all the changes of the run. On one occasion, for example, I began the run feeling stiff and it seemed to take longer than usual to loosen up. I began to wonder if something was wrong. I noticed about six miles later, already quite flexible, I still seemed to see myself as I did at the beginning; I was wondering if I could make it through to the end of the run. The early set of observations had become an image of myself for that day and I did not appreciate that the image was no longer the runner of that day.

As the opening minutes of the run evolve, thought lags. There is this wanting, longing—call it what you will—to go on thinking about that problem I was concerned with when I woke up: "Wait, just a minute, I want to understand why she said that last night. What did she mean? It doesn't seem possible she could be so cruel about this matter." As I go on running, imagination keeps building on these ideas, working them back and forth as if my brain were not on the run and were free from this hill I am on. But I break out in a sweat, my body is moving, there are definite pains in my legs. Now the pains are not there. I was so absorbed in my legs only a moment ago and now I am into a completely different event. Yet when I was so worried about those pains, they seemed to be all there was in the world.

Some days when it is very humid, I develop a certain weakness in my knees and legs. I feel that I can't go on; I feel the weather is weighing me down, I am sweating more than usual, and my legs feel they will not hold me enough to get up this next incline. There is a sensation of a big hole at the bottom of my stomach and my brain does not bring me the air I need in this hole. I am complaining about running today and I feel afraid. Finally I stop. I walk. Suddenly I realize a silence. The connection of all these parts is not clear, but when I stop, the anxious grabbing is no longer there.

This event is so different from my life. I often feel I have a second-hand existence: I think a lot, I have a lot of ideas, and I make up a lot of reasons why things are the way they are. I have my schedule and my plans about how things should go. I try to make life fit my plans. I arrange to spend my time mostly with people who support me and I mostly live comfortably, finding easy ways to go from one place to another as well as pleasant entertainments in the places I go. I read a lot of books that offer me even more ideas about life. It seems like I live as if I am over there in a television set where things are made so clear, where a moment is replayed and ordered smoothly in a frame, without the heat and the sweat of the road, the sun, and the hills. Instant replay, slow motion even define the event on television so I can grasp it without seeing the complexity of velocity in relationship.

In this context, I am reminded of last year's New York Marathon. When Tom Fleming came across the finish line, he looked light, full of energy, and centered. After twenty-six miles, he was in tune. It was a thrilling sight. Standing next to me, a woman with her six-year-old son noticed television cameras were present. She said to her child, "See, you can see this on TV later." What was real did not have the meaning that TV had—perhaps it was too vibrant, changing, and alive. When it was boxed, framed, and limited, it could be comprehended.

Sometimes I cannot help myself, but there is some problem which will have its way. This problem is completely absorbing. I find, for example, that I am thinking of my early life, my relationship with my mother when I was an infant, my fears in that relationship. It is best when I watch all of these different, flashing thoughts. At these times, there is nothing to do: what is is what is. During such runs, I have discovered patterns in my relationship to my brother, my father, my children, my wife, and my mother. The whole panorama goes by and I often feel a deeper acceptance after having been able to run and be with the whole movement without judgment or choice. I simply recognize all of this is what makes up my being for the day.

On other occasions, I get caught in one of my thoughts. It becomes a localized focus of concern that is the opposite of the flowing connectedness of the above. Say I have an argument with someone. I hope they will call me today and I will be able to tell them something that will even the score. I will win by putting them down. This vindictive pattern is persistent. I am desperate about being ahead of this person. I can't stand the thought that he is putting me down. One thought leads to another each time this sequence recurs; it is all tied up with my image of myself. I feel ridiculed and weakened by his words. It is really uncomfortable the way it is so self-absorbing. But at some point inside each sequence, suddenly I am aware that I have been playing a tape recorder while running. The inhale–exhale momentum of the run captures my attention and I see I am fragmented inside the circles of these repetitious thoughts. I see that the thoughts are hold-backs that go over and over my weakness without completing the problems they pose. When this insight strikes me, there is a change. I see that my body is different from the insubstantiality of this brain. I feel I have discovered myself as a small and petty creature at play in a mud house when there is a vast world of connections outside in the fresh air. It seemed as if I began the run, but it is soon apparent that it is not "I" that began, but the whole: both the "I" and the coordinated body and mind. Before the run, I was sitting in my chair or I was walking, but I was certainly more than all those thoughts I was thinking when I did those things.

I feel kind of frightened to discover how naive and petty I am, somewhat like a drug addict, identifying with myself as a separate and isolated person, thinking about myself as something unconnected to others. I see what has happened: I was caught up in a process of hope. Very subtly, "I," as all my images of myself, came into being. "I" hope to conclude the sequence of thoughts in a pleasurable way that would make "me" feel good. As this hope burgeons, it calls the "me" more and more into its web and consciousness becomes a focus. "I" wanted desperately to work out the different trials and errors, pain and solutions of my thoughts. When the demands of the run saw this edge of inattention, it was apparent the run was a different and more substantial present.

One of the most interesting parts of this meditation is that it points up the deceptiveness of the content of thought. Every day I come there really believing in my thinking. Thought is like an old friend to me. I depend on its taking me seriously and I take it seriously. It happens something like this: As I run, I think about a problem. For example, I really want to understand how to get even with this guy that puts me down. As I go over the details of how he did what he did and how I am going to strike back in my way, I note a suspiciously obsessive character to my meanderings. It is obvious that my thought movement is not toward a resolution of the problem at hand. It is an indulgence. Feeling weak on the run, I am living out my weakness in my worry over my weak feeling with him. My thought never goes forward beyond a certain point of the things it is considering. I begin to see my so-called interest in the problem is not serious.

The run is present and thought is a smoke screen that avoids what is happening here with the run. I have been deceived by this old friend who pretended to be interested, but was really protecting my brain from dealing with the uncertainty I feel right now.

Meanwhile, there is duration. It has concrete mements which I feel as a metabolism of time; it is not a time of past, present, into future. Each minute is an attention. It is, however, not what I had been calling time as schedules, memories, or how long it will take me to get from here to the next turn. It shifts and becomes only particular events of step by step. I find each step to be immensely selective. I am sweating. This hill is hard. I find going down the hill is even harder because I am not in control of my own momentum. I feel drawn forward faster than I want to go. I am aware of the tension in my arms. I drop them and let them hang. At the beginning, there was a small hill and I am breathing a bit hard with an awareness that it is beginning, but now there is a leveling in both the land and in my breathing. I see everything is in relationship and nothing can be taken as an absolute: no thought, no breath, no tension, no pain is the definition of this run now or ever; each moment I think I know the run, something new appears to show me I do not know. It shows me that what I thought I knew about the run was part of what just happened and is over now.

At certain points, some memory of a previous second is retained and I want to continue with it. There is a secret delight in what just happened when I felt that step-by-step. Very quietly and subtly, the memory of that joy becomes a hook in me. I look at what happened just a minute ago; how can I keep it; I want to get back there now. I was there looking directly at the step-by-step. Now I will look directly at the step-by-step. Except that now I am looking at myself looking at the step-by-step. I am in a tangle of trying to get back to where I was. I am trying. So if that is the case and I cannot get back there now, maybe I can figure out how I got out of the awareness of each step, and I will be able to avoid losing that pleasure when I am lucky enough to be there again. I want to have that good time again and I don't want to have the pain of losing it again.

As I get more tangled, I see all of this is a lesson in how *not* to learn. There is something about running that is a unique opportunity for meditation. I *never* run according to what I know. I cannot ever run according to a plan I have arranged from accumulated information of what to do to have the perfect run. A good run is when I am present in each moment. I learn by watching what happens each moment. When I tried to hold on to that good moment of the step-by-step, I was not in the step-by-step. I was trying. If I were "successful" and saw what happened when I got into this "trying," then I would have information about running and getting out of the run. But if I tried to use that information, I would run with an idea of the right way to run. Any event on the run would be compared with that idea and my action would be modified to fit the concept. I would be running with attention to the ideas and not to the run. It would not be possible to learn what was happening right there in the moment. I see I have only the possibility of learning by watching the run now when the action is happening and the facts are created. The whole of the run, the body-brain-space-time event in relationship is irreversible biological process in action. The whole fits together. It is not something I "do" as it happens according to a movement of its own. When I am in the run, I see the changes go continually into new forms. A breath now is a breath on this road, and each new breath is different. This time has a particular feel and if I get into one of those attempts to retain a moment, I learn about my grabbing at time. But more deeply, I learn I am alone and I cannot go back to the beginning of a run or back to the stage before the step-by-step went sour. I can't fix it to make this now sweeter.

The time of the run is irreversible, like my life. It is as uncertain as when

I will die. There is something about this irreversibility that conflicts with the way I live when I am not running. Here I see these unfolding moments and I see how alone I am, knowing I cannot depend on the authority of anyone to see or look for me. The whole body-brain-time-space continuum changes and I must look at it. But outside the run, in my family, my profession, in society, I lose my attention to the particularity of my moment. My attention gets blurred in coordinating with others. I wonder if I don't use all the others to protect me from that aloneness of my daily change and the inevitable fact of my death and the death of those I love.

Yet another feature of the danger I unconsciously find in the irreversibility of the run is the way it contradicts my particular dependency on the mechanical. I come to expect things to go smoothly. My car has a cycle that repeats itself endlessly and easily when I press the accelerator. If something goes wrong with it, it stops; then I take it to a mechanic who fixes the particular defective part of the cycle and I comfortably watch the car again take up its repetitive habit. The job to be done is that the car is to carry me from place to place and the moving parts of each phase of the cycle are to go together to accomplish this task. When I got out of the step-by-step of my run, I looked for the particular piece of the motion that was out of kilter. I would fix it and re-establish the right rhythm to return me to the proper running order. But machines I can turn back and forth with the same results endlessly: they follow simple cause and effect. My life is not only irreversible, but it also does not show this simplicity of one-to-one relationships. I learned quickly on the run that I could not say "Hey, wait a minute. Let me start over, fix this breath, get it right from the beginning." It is not possible to change the breath without changing the whole.

It feels so hard somewhere about two miles from the end. Two miles is a measure. Everything is so different when I have a goal. Each step has no goal. But can I make it? If I don't make it, what then? Am I asking can I make it to my own death? Seems such a silly question, of course I will make it to that goal. Everyone does. Am I asking can I make it to my own death "perfectly?" Or "successfully?" Why has it become so important to get to that goal? The absurdity of this is ironic. I made it perfectly to the line I drew as an appropriate end. On my tombstone, they will put: Here lies David Shainberg, he was perfect and successful in getting here. I see this joke and laugh to myself. That laugh is what meditation is all about. As I run on with my laugh, a wave of relaxation comes over me. I don't have to push myself, I can stop wherever and whenever I feel like stopping; but then there is a new wave of doubt (I am not laughing anymore): Can I really go on with this effortless feeling? If I do not set up these efforts, these arbitrary pushes of myself, will I ever get to any of my goals. I am afraid nothing will happen to me, I will lose touch with reality, which at this moment seems to need to be grabbed rather than depended upon to support me. I push to hold, then again that laugh, and I see "how pushy" I am—and then life comes into each step and I am back with my legs into the run.

But here another very tricky aspect of this game called "end-watching" comes into the foreground. It always creeps up in one form or another, and the further I go, the sooner it appears. I center on the end of the run that is a distance I have set myself for the day or I can see it up ahead, or in my mind's eye. It may be no more than the top of a hill beyond which I cannot see, but it becomes a mechanical fixation. Or it is an image of the pleasure of being finished and out of this agony of having to breathe within the rhythm of the run. I will be out of having to be without "me." I sometimes begin spontaneously and unwittingly to concentrate on the end of some measured segment which I have taken to be important. It is like a magnet around which I orient. "I" will have "me" again.

Sometimes I play a game here: I remind myself that there are people who run twice as far as I do; this points up the arbitrary nature of my measurements. This also undercuts any self-pity that I have worked so hard for such a long distance.

These last stages have certain specific characteristics which the end watching obscures. The actual transitions of the end call for new expenditures of energy. These new expenditures are now after the earlier periods when the rhythm of body and mind were accommodating each other. The end-watching thoughts are about a place that is actually still over two miles away and, as with the other thoughts along the run, they block my attention to the step-by-step. As I see this end-watching maneuver, there is a change in the whole way of the run. These end moments of giving more energy are suddenly experiences of coordinated running. I accept each step as hard-earned space and I am alone and secure, knowing I have a kind of strength and dependability. Running those last miles is an experience in which I know how far I have come and what it means to my whole body.

Then another dilemma may turn up; all was going smoothly for a moment, or at least so it seemed, but now I am wildly thinking about many things. The run had become a hypnotic state. I was attentive to the actions of my body or my brain until suddenly I am aware of this wild kind of randomness to the sequences of my thought. When I reflect, I see: I really am finding myself just coming out of this trance into this disorder. It is now the spasm of a disordered mind that had been trapped by its routine. The automaticity of the running had become a narcotic and blunted my attention. Then the wild disorder of thought came on. This is a dangerous part of the meditation of running. It is a danger of all forms of meditation that can produce a dulling of the mind into mechanical, robotlike behavior, a false tranquility without making the mind sensitive, alert, and fresh the way running-as-meditation can. When I see this fragmentation of my thought as it emerges from the trance, I am brought up short. I am inattentive and so attentive when I see it, and then my mind is sensitive to all my movements again. With this awareness, I feel a new connection to the place in which I am running. I see the trees and the light and shadows. In the quiet of my mind I hear the birds and then see the movements of the other runners. My body wants to do the run. It is not a wish or a thought and it does not feel like "me" or "I" want to do the run. But my body pulls itself together; it moves, orders, and dominates the run. At these points, I do not tend to get hooked on thoughts or the desire to find that old pleasure from another time. Metaphors come and go for the run. They point beyond themselves, suggesting more ordering in the thought content; then they give up and go on to new contents and new forms.

This order strikes me as particularly different from the machine world with which I came into the run. I had a vague, unconscious sense that I could push a button to get things done. Now I discover something that shifts and changes according to new information. There is no switch that I flip to get this body to work together. The run has its own path and its own specific ways that are not standardized and all the same, the way the food in the supermarket or the clothes in the department store are. I discover new experiences and new energy as the run unfolds. It isn't something that is prepared and finished from the beginning.

As the experience goes on, I find that I do not want it to be over. I live a kind of death on the run as I give up my thoughts of "I" and "me." And I cease to desire to have everything be easy at every moment and I accept that this is work and effort. I lose my continuity and I pay attention to my steps. Attention for a moment became a trance, but when I saw that trance, there was a different condition. I see all this without choice and now I do not feel I am hypnotized. I don't want the run to end. The meditation of the run, however, turns up again to show me that my not wanting it to end is holding my breath— I simply can't run if I don't let go of each breath. It shows me again that everything keeps moving on the run, and the end is another one of those facts.

A PYSCHOLOGICAL STUDY OF 100 MARATHONERS USING THE MYERS-BRIGGS TYPE INDICATOR AND DEMOGRAPHIC DATA

Teresa Clitsome and Thaddeus Kostrubala

Department of Mental Health
Mercy Hospital and Medical Center
San Diego, California 92103

The majority of research conducted to date on marathon runners has focused on the physiological aspects of the marathoner, specifically in terms of abilities and disabilities. A review of literature revealed that few avenues of investigation have been concerned with the psychological aspects of a "marathoner." Personality characteristics have been investigated with regard to athletic subgroups.[1, 2] However, there is still a considerable lack of information specifically regarding the psyche of the marathon runner.

Investigators such as Husman[3] and Morgan[4] studied college distance runners, however. Husman used projectives such as the Thematic Apperception Test and Sentence Completion Test, among other psychometric tools.[3] Morgan used the Eysenck Personality Inventory (EPI) and found cross-country runners to be significantly more introverted than other groups of athletes.[5] In addition, Morgan and Costill[6] measured nine marathon runners in terms of their level of introversion–extraversion, neuroticism–stability, anxiety, and depression using the EPI, the IPAT 8-Parallel-Form Anxiety Battery (Form A), and the Depression Adjective Check List (DACL) (Form A). Morgan and Costill concluded that these nine marathoners should not be considered "necessarily representative of marathon runners in general, . . . [as] more research should be performed prior to advancing such generalizations."[6]

To the knowledge of the investigators, no one to date has conducted a large-scale study of marathoners ($n = 100$ or more) focusing specifically on personality type without inclusion of psychopathology. Further, no one has ever used the Myers-Briggs Type Indicator (Form F) in describing personality traits of marathon runners as representing a select populace.[7]

Typology

Probably the earliest and best-known classification of men into types was set forth by the Greek physician Hippocrates.[8] His division of men into sanguine, phlegmatic, choleric, and melancholic types was in terms of a disease-oriented basis. Even though this method was not considered particularly scientific, it did illustrate that men then, as now, tried to classify people into various categories merely from a physical basis. Other theorists such as Freud, Kretschmer, Sheldon, Spranger, and so forth, continued from that point to incorporate the psychological aspects in addition to the physiological aspects as associated with personality type.[8]

There have been some objections to the theories of type in general.[8] These objections have usually been based on misconceptions regarding the objectives.

Typology does not insist on the existence of isolable personality categories, but only of dominant trends within some personalities. Further, it is the combination of these various parts (traits) of a person into wholes which exemplifies the concept of type.[9] For the purpose of this investigation, type has been defined as, "not a static, but a dynamic concept which denotes the consequences of developing one's preferred ways of using his or her mind."[10]

Carl Jung incorporated typology as part of his system of analytical psychology. He suggested that the personality of an individual could move in either of two different directions, depending on whether the conscious mind was expressed during serious tension or rational thinking.[11] The dominant modality indicated whether the individual was a thinking or an emotional type. Further, the thinking type was depicted as the introvert, and the emotional type was seen as the extravert.[11]

The extraverted personality was directed toward people, toward the objective, nonreflective world and a life centered on action.[8, 11] The introverted personality moved in the opposite mode to one of quiet, one free from people, and centered on subjective experiences such as meditation, i.e., more personal and subjective.[8, 11] But as a precaution it should be understood that introversion is not the same as egocentrism, peculiarity, and unsociableness. According to Eysenck, "Jung certainly did not equate introversion with incipient neurosis as Freud apparently did, nor did Jung believe that lack of sociability is necessarily a mark of introversion."[12]

Further division of extraverts and introverts was based on how the intellectual functions express themselves. This was explained by viewing an individual's libido in terms of rational or irrational forms.[6] If rational, for example, he or she may have been dominated by thinking or feeling; and if irrational, he or she may have been dominated by sensation or intuition. So on the basis of one of these modalities exhibiting dominance, Jung divided both the extravert and introvert into four aspects of type: thinking, feeling, sensation, and intuition.[11] Jung's theory assumed that if a person was to function well, he must have a well-developed system for perception (either sensing or intuition) and a well-developed system for making decisions or judgments (either thinking or feeling).[10, 11] In conjunction, then, all these preferences combined to form 16 possible personality types, each containing four basic preferences. It was in an attempt to measure these preferences that the Myers-Briggs Type Indicator was developed (FIGURE 1).

Overview of Myers-Briggs Type Indicator

The Myers-Briggs Type Indicator (MBTI), Form F, was the psychological test employed in the present study. It developed over a 20-year period and was first published by the Educational Testing Service in 1962. In his critique of the MBTI, Sundberg related that the reliability figures were "comparable to those of leading personality inventories."[13] Over 75,000 individuals have been measured in terms of personality type using the MBTI.

The instrument was developed specifically to implement Carl Jung's theory of type: "The gist of the theory is that much apparently random variation in human behavior is actually quite orderly and consistent being due to certain basic differences in the way people prefer to use perception and judgment."[10] Further, the aim of the MBTI was "to ascertain from self-report of easily reported reactions people's basic preferences in regard to perception and judgment, so that the effects of the preferences and their combinations may be established by research and put to practical use." [14] Following are the basic definitions of preferences as measured by the MBTI. An understanding of these definitions becomes essential in accurately interpreting the data presented in this investigation.

Extraversion (E): "a direction of interest and attention to the outer world of objects, people, and action." [14]

Introversion (I): "a direction of interest to the inner world of ideas and contemplation." [14]

Sensing (S): "a preference for looking at the immediate, the real world, the tangible, the solid facts of experience." [14]

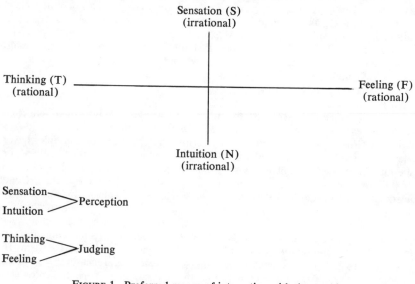

FIGURE 1. Preferred means of interacting with the world.

Intuition (N): "a preference for seeing the possibilities, meanings, and relationships of experience, often with only a passing interest in the facts themselves." [14]

Thinking (T): "a rational process used in decision-making and a preference for making decisions objectively, impersonally analyzing the facts and ordering them in terms of antecedents and consequences, materially oriented and following logical principles." [14]

Feeling (F): "a rational process used in decision-making that is decided by a valuing process, weighing the importance of alternatives to oneself, or others; oriented toward working with or studying people." [14]

Judging (J): "a preference for living in a planned, decided orderly way, aiming to regulate life and control it." [14]

Perception (P): "a preference to live in a flexible, spontaneous way, aiming to understand life and adapt to it." [14]

Purpose

The purpose of the present investigation was to assess the personality type of marathon runners. More specifically, it was the intent of the investigators to: (1) describe the personality type of male and female marathoners using the Myers-Briggs Type Indicator (MBTI), Form F; (2) describe basic demographic characteristics of marathoners; and (3) discover if marathon runners exhibit a predictable personality type.

Procedure

Names of potential subjects for this investigation were secured from an official list of those who had completed the Mission Bay Marathon in San Diego, Calif., the Palos Verdes Marathon in Palos Verdes, Calif., and/or were a member of one or all of the following running clubs: San Diego Track Club, San Diego Marathon Clinic,[15] and the Honolulu Marathon Clinic. A prerequisite of potential participants was the completion of at least one marathon and a minimum age of 18.

All potential subjects ($n = 125$) were contacted by telephone or in person. All subjects contacted agreed to participate. The testing materials (MBTI, Demographic Questionnaire) were mailed to each potential subject during January and February 1976, with instructions to complete and return the materials as soon as possible. One hundred ($n = 100$) of the original 125 potential subjects returned the completed test materials within three months. These, then, comprised the subject populace studied in this investigation. Anonymity of the participants was respected.

Results

A total of 100 marathon runners (83 males, 17 females) participated in the present study. All of the subjects completed a demographic questionnaire including information such as: age, number of marathons completed, number of years they have been running, number of miles per week they trained, and their level of education. All subjects also completed the MBTI indicating their preferences in terms of Extraversion versus Introversion, Sensing versus Intuition, Thinking versus Feeling, and Judging versus Perception.

Personality preferences for both male and female marathon runners ($n = 100$) revealed the following frequencies: 54 were classified as Extraverted and 46, Introverted; 54, Sensing, and 46, Intuitive; 57, Thinking, and 43, Feeling; 44, Judging, and 56, Perceptive. Specifically, male marathon runners ($n = 83$) demonstrated the following preferences: 46 were Extraverted and 37, Introverted; 47, Sensing, and 36, Intuitive; 48, Thinking, and 35, Feeling; 35, Judging, and 48, Perceptive. Female marathon runners ($n = 17$) revealed the following preferences: 8 were Extraverted and 9, Introverted; 7, Sensing, and 10, Intuitive; 9, Thinking, and 8, Feeling; 9, Judging, and 8, Perceptive (TABLE 1).

Chi-square comparisons of the above frequencies of preference for the entire marathoners ($n = 100$) as well as male versus female subgroups revealed no significant difference between Extraversion and Introversion, Sensing and Intuition, Thinking and Feeling, and Judging and Perception. More specifically, a comparison of Extraversion versus Introversion revealed a ratio of approximately one to one (1:1), as did the comparison of Sensing versus Intuition. The general population reveals Extraversion versus Introversion and Sensing versus Intuition in a ratio of approximately three to one (3:1).[16] A comparison of these two ratios indicates that approximately twice as many marathoners (2:1) were Introverted as opposed to Extraverted. In addition, approximately twice (2:1) as many marathoners were sensing as opposed to intuitive when compared with the general population.

Frequency distributions of 16 possible personality types were also recorded for male and female runners combined, as well as male and female marathoners separately. Male and female marathoners combined revealed a maximum frequency of 16 for ISTJ types and a minimum frequency of 2 for INTP types. Male marathoners revealed a maximum frequency of 15 for ISTJ types and a minimum of 1 for INTP types. Female marathoners revealed a maximum

TABLE 1

FREQUENCY AND MEAN SCORE COMPARISONS FOR PERSONALITY TYPES OF MALE AND FEMALE MARATHON RUNNERS

Personality Type	Male Marathoners			Female Marathoners			Male and Female Marathoners		
	n	Mean Score	SD *	n	Mean Score	SD	n	Mean Score	SD
A. Extravert	46	24.74	15.54	8	22.75	12.07	54	24.44	14.99
B. Introvert	37	14.78	12.59	9	20.11	11.19	46	15.83	12.39
C. Sensing	47	24.79	16.91	7	18.71	12.30	54	24.00	16.41
D. Intuitive	36	22.28	14.98	10	25.20	14.41	46	22.91	14.74
E. Thinking	48	18.33	14.55	9	23.44	14.17	57	19.14	14.49
F. Feeling	35	20.51	14.02	8	22.38	13.23	43	20.86	13.74
G. Judging	35	23.49	16.44	9	21.00	9.27	44	22.98	15.19
H. Perceptive	48	24.33	15.62	8	23.00	14.74	56	24.14	15.37

* Standard deviation.

frequency of 3 for ESTJ and a minimum or zero frequency for INFJ, ISFP, and ESTP types. Again, chi-squares revealed no specific personality type as having a significantly greater frequency than any of the other types within this sample (TABLES 2, 3 & 4).

The range in age for male marathoners was 18 to 57 years, and for females the range was 18 to 45 years. The mean age for both males and females combined was 32.96 years. The mean age for male marathoners only was 33.46 years. The mean age for female marathoners only was 30.53 years. Critical Ratios ($\overline{Z}$-tests) were performed comparing age and personality type. Female extraverts were found to be significantly younger than male extraverts with $\overline{Z} = 3.24$ at the level of $p < 0.01$ (TABLES 5 & 6).

The number of marathons completed for male marathoners only revealed a range of 1 to 36 and for females a range of 1 to 17. The mean number of marathons completed for both male and female marathoners was 5.3. Male marathoners only revealed a mean of 5.78, and female marathoners revealed a

TABLE 2

FREQUENCY DISTRIBUTION OF TYPES FOR MALE AND FEMALE MARATHON RUNNERS
($n=100$)

	Sensing (S)		Intuition (N)	
	Thinking (T)	Feeling (F)	Feeling (F)	Thinking (T)
Introverted (I)				
Judging (J)	ISTJ 16	ISFJ 7	INFJ 4	INTJ 5
Perception (P)	ISTP 7	ISFP 4	INFP 9	INTP 2
Extraverted (E)				
Perception (P)	ESTP 3	ESFP 3	ENFP 7	ENTP 9
Judging (J)	ESTJ 11	ESFJ 3	ENFJ 5	ENTJ 5

mean of 2.94. Z-tests revealed that male marathoners had completed significantly more marathons than female marathoners with $\overline{Z} = 1.98$ at the level of $p < 0.05$ (TABLES 5 & 6).

The number of years male marathoners had been running revealed a range of 1 to 27 years, and female marathoners revealed a range of 1 to 13 years. The mean number of years both male and female subgroups had been running

TABLE 3

FREQUENCY DISTRIBUTION OF TYPES FOR MALE MARATHON RUNNERS
($n=83$)

	Sensing (S)		Intuition (N)	
	Thinking (T)	Feeling (F)	Feeling (F)	Thinking (T)
Introverted (I)				
Judging (J)	ISTJ 15	ISFJ 6	INFJ 4	INTJ 3
Perception (P)	ISTP 6	ISFP 4	INFP 7	INTP 1
Extraverted (E)				
Perception (P)	ESTP 3	ESFP 2	ENFP 5	ENTP 7
Judging (J)	ESTJ 8	ESFJ 3	ENFJ 4	ENTJ 5

TABLE 4

FREQUENCY DISTRIBUTION OF TYPES FOR FEMALE MARATHON RUNNERS
($n = 17$)

	Sensing (S)		Intuition (N)	
	Thinking (T)	Feeling (F)	Feeling (F)	Thinking (T)
Introverted (I)				
Judging (J)	ISTJ 1	ISFJ 1	INFJ	INTJ 2
Perception (P)	ISTP 1	ISFP	INFP 2	INTP 1
Extraverted (E)				
Perception (P)	ESTP	ESFP 1	ENFP 2	ENTP 2
Judging (J)	ESTJ 3	ESFJ	ENFJ 1	ENTJ

was 5.51. Individually, male marathoners indicated a mean of 5.87, and female marathoners indicated a mean of 3.76. In comparison, male marathoners had been running significantly longer than female marathoners with $\overline{Z} = 1.87$ at the level of $p < 0.05$ (see TABLES 5 & 6).

No significant difference was evidenced in comparing personality type and the number of miles per week each type ran. No significant difference was evidenced in comparing mileage per week between male and female marathoners. The mean number of miles per week that male marathoners ran was 51.59, and for females the mean was 43.0. Both subgroups of male and female marathoners combined revealed a mean of 50.13 miles per week. The range in number of miles per week for male marathoners was 15 to 140, and for females the range was 25 to 120 (TABLES 5 & 6).

TABLE 5

PRESENTATION OF DEMOGRAPHIC DATA FOR MALE AND FEMALE MARATHON RUNNERS

Group	n	Age		No. of Marathons Completed		No. of Years Running		No. of Miles per Week in Training	
		Mean	SD	Mean	SD	Mean	SD	Mean	SD
A. Males	83	33.46	11.09	5.78	7.86	5.87	5.60	51.59	25.97
B. Females	17	30.53	7.37	2.94	4.56	3.76	3.79	43.00	25.17
C. Males and females	100	32.96	10.56	5.30	7.46	5.51	5.37	50.13	25.90

TABLE 6

DEMOGRAPHIC DATA FOR MINIMUM AND MAXIMUM AGE,
NUMBER OF MARATHONS COMPLETED, NUMBER OF YEARS JOGGING,
AND NUMBER OF MILES PER WEEK IN TRAINING FOR MALE AND FEMALE
MARATHON RUNNERS

Group	n	Age Min	Age Max	No. of Marathons Completed Min	No. of Marathons Completed Max	No. of Years Running Min	No. of Years Running Max	No. of Miles per Week in Training Min	No. of Miles per Week in Training Max
A. Males	83	18	57	1	36	1	27	15	140
B. Females	17	18	45	1	17	1	13	25	120

Of the entire group of marathoners, 91% had at least one year of college education or better. Of the male marathoners, 93% revealed one year of college or better as compared with 82% of the female marathoners. The national average (1975) in education for the same age group and level of education revealed 42% of males and 30% of females had had one year of college or better. In comparison, male marathoners and female marathoners were significantly more educated than the average populace in the United States (TABLE 7).

Discussion

In pursuit of the elusive goal of understanding the nature of man, we have developed an appreciation for the value of the abnormal, the unusual, the unique. For example, in medicine we have increased our understanding of natural cardiovascular functioning by research into cardiovascular pathology.

A review of investigations in any field concerned with the study of man reveals the polarities of normal and abnormal; further, the study of either polarity increases the understanding of its opposite. For example, an understanding of the psychology, physiology, and sociocultural factors of schizophrenics provides both a stimulus to and a contrast with "normals" in our population.

TABLE 7

FREQUENCY OF EDUCATIONAL LEVELS OF MALE AND FEMALE MARATHONERS

Group	n	High School	College	Graduate School	Doctorate
A. Males	83	6	47	14	16
B. Females	17	3	10	3	1
C. Males and females	100	9	57	17	17

When investigating a population that is unique, specifically because it lacks a particular disease common to other populations, we study every possible factor of that population. In so doing, we attempt to isolate any significant differences in these factors, whether psychological, hereditary, cultural, dietary, or environmental. We are becoming increasingly aware of the interconnection of all factors, regardless of whether our concern is with the specific presence or the specific absence of a particular disease.

The group of 100 marathoners investigated in this study is just such a distinct and unique population. There is as yet no complete definition of a marathoner. The most basic description of such an individual is one who has successfully run a distance of 26 miles, 385 yards in an official, public event called a marathon.

However, this individual has other characteristics that attract the attention of those who measure his performance. These characteristics relate to factors such as age, sex, weight, training mileage, percentage of body fat, potential immunity to certain diseases, and so forth. The data currently accumulated permits the construction of a physical profile of the "typical" marathoner.

Investigators in this study have attempted to begin the construction of a psychological profile of the marathoner. The Myers-Briggs Type Indicator (Form F) was employed, a psychological test that specifically delineates personality type, excluding psychopathology. Further, this test evolved from the work of Myers and Briggs in their attempt to assess the validity of C. G. Jung's theory of personality type.

In addition to this measurement, the investigators collected physical and demographic data as a check on their subject population as well as to provide future investigators with a potential comparison group.

The demographic information collected reveals that the typical marathoner is approximately 33 years old, has completed five marathons, has been running for 5½ years, and runs approximately 50 miles per week training distance. In addition, the typical marathoner is better educated than the general population— 93% of the male marathoners and 82% of the female marathoners studied had completed at least one or more years of college education. The 1975 national average for the same age group was 42% for males and 30% for females. This indicates that marathoners as a group have achieved a higher level of education than the general population in the United States.

An examination of the MBTI results indicated that of the 100 marathoners tested, 54 were Extraverts and 46 were Introverts, a ratio of approximately 1:1. According to studies accumulated by the Center for Application of Psychological Type, the usual distribution of Extraverts/Introverts in the general population (U.S.A.) is 3:1. Thus, marathoners differ from the general population in a tendency toward introversion by a ratio of approximately 2:1.

A study of the personality types reflected in the combination of preferences comprising the 16 possible personality types reveals an unusual uniformity. This uniformity is demonstrated explicitly in that no statistical difference was revealed between Extraversion/Introversion, Sensing/Intuition, Thinking/Feeling, and Judging/Perceiving.

Summary

One hundred marathoners (83 males, 17 females) were given the Myers-Briggs Type Indicator (MBTI) and a demographic questionnaire. The resulting data was subjected to computerized statistical analysis using standard deviation, mean, chi-square, and $\bar{Z}$-test. The findings revealed that these marathoners were 33 years of age, had run five marathons, had been running 5½ years, trained 50 miles per week, and had a 91% chance of having one or more years of college education. Additionally, the findings revealed these marathoners to be more introverted and sensing when compared with the general population, and did not show any statistical difference between individuals within the group regarding variables examined by the MBTI.

Acknowledgments

We thank Kathleen Ahner for her valuable time and editorial assistance. Raymond G. Murphy performed the statistical analysis.

References

1. COSTILL, D. L. 1968. What research tells the coach about distance running. American Association for Health, Physical Education, and Recreation. Washington, D.C.
2. MORGAN, W. P., Ed. 1970. Contemporary Readings in Sport Psychology. Charles C Thomas, Publisher. Springfield, Ill.
3. HUSMAN, B. F. 1955. Aggression in boxers and wrestlers as measured by projective techniques. Res. Quart. 26: 421–425.
4. MORGAN, W. P. 1968. Extraversion-Neuroticism and Athletic Performance. 15th Annual Meeting of the American College of Sports Medicine, University Park, Pa.
5. MORGAN, W. P. 1974. Selected psychological considerations in sport. Res. Quart. 45(4): 374.
6. MORGAN, W. P. & D. L. COSTILL. 1972. Psychological characteristics of the marathon runner. J. Sports Med. 12: 42–46.
7. MCCAULLEY, M. H. Director, Center for Applications of Psychological Type Personal Communication. Gainesville, Fla.
8. BONNER, H. 1961. Psychology of Personality. The Ronald Press Co. New York, N.Y.
9. CLITSOME, T. 1975. A Comparison of Intensive Care Unit and General Staff Nurses' Personality Types, Job Satisfaction, and Job Turnover. 1st National Conference on the Uses of the Myers-Briggs Type Indicator, University of Florida, Gainesville, Fla.
10. MYERS, I. B. 1962. The Myers-Briggs Type Indicator. Educational Testing Service. Princeton, N.J.
11. JUNG, C. G. 1933. Psychological Types. Harcourt, Brace, and World. New York, N.Y.
12. EYSENCK, H. J. 1947. Dimensions of Personality. Routledge. London.
13. BUROS, O. K., Ed. 1970. Personality Tests and Reviews. Olympus Publishing Co. Highland Park, N.J.
14. MCCAULLEY, M. H. 1974. The Myers-Briggs Type Indicator and the Teaching Process. Paper presented at the 1974 Annual Meeting of American Educational Research Association, Session 20.24, Chicago, Ill.
15. KOSTRUBALA, T. L. 1976. The Joy of Running. J. B. Lippincott Co. New York, N.Y.
16. MCCAULLEY, M. H. Personal communication.

A PSYCHOLOGICAL STUDY OF 50 SUB-3-HOUR MARATHONERS

Austin Gontang, Teresa Clitsome, and Thaddeus Kostrubala

Department of Mental Health
Mercy Hospital and Medical Center
San Diego, California 92103

Introduction

Very little research has been done on the psychological characteristics of sub-3-hour marathoners. In 1969 there were 812 sub-3-hour marathoners in the United States. During that same year there were fewer than 40 marathons sponsored in the United States. Six years later there were more sub-3-hour finishers in a single marathon than in the 40 marathons of 1969: 850 men and 7 women completed the 1975 Boston in under 3 hours. Current U.S. figures on sub-3-hour marathoners list more than 3,050 men and 17 women for 1975,[1] an increase of 375% over the last six years.

A review of literature reveals an increase in research concerning the psychological effects of physical activity.[2-8] While numerous popular books [9-13] have been published recently on the psychological aspects of running and jogging, little research has been conducted on the psychology of the marathoner, a rapidly increasing population. Morgan and Costill [14] were forerunners in this area with their investigation of the psychological characteristics of selected marathon runners ($n = 9$); however, they concluded their study by indicating the need for additional research on marathoners prior to advancing valid generalizations. The study by Clitsome and Kostrubala [15] of 100 marathoners regarding personality type contributes to this area of investigation, as does the more recent work by Morgan.[16]

Purpose

The scope of this study was limited to an investigation of personality type as measured by the Myers-Briggs Type Indicator (MBTI), Form F, and focused by a selected group of sub-3-hour marathoners. In addition, basic demographic data was collected for each participant ($n = 50$). It was the intent of the investigators to assess whether or not there was a relationship between personality type and sub-3-hour marathoning.

Methods

The subjects of this study were sub-3-hour marathoners. They were selected at the following events: (1) Avenue of the Giants Marathon (May 2, 1976) in Mendocino County, California; (2) Palos Verdes Marathon (June 12, 1976) in Los Angeles, California; and (3) The National AAU One Hour Run (June 23, 1976) in San Diego, California. Sub-3-hour marathoners were contacted personally by the investigators at these events. Potential subjects ($n = 75$) who agreed to participate in the investigation were given a packet containing the MBTI and a demographic questionnaire. Of the initial 75 potential subjects, 62 returned the test materials. Since the number of potential females ($n = 2$) was insufficient to insure validity, this study was limited to the first 50 male participants who returned the testing material. A prerequisite for all potential subjects was the completion of at least one sub-3-hour marathon and a minimum age of 18. Anonymity of participants was respected. Results were made available to all participants.

The Myers-Briggs Type Indicator

The psychological test used in this study was the MBTI; it determines an individual's personality type in terms of four basic preferences. These preferences are: extraversion–introversion, sensing–intuition, thinking–feeling, and judging–perceiving.[15, 17] These qualities are defined in a previous paper of this volume.[15]

The MBTI is based on the Jungian theory of personality type.[19] Briefly, the theory states that "much apparently random variation in human behavior is actually quite orderly and consistent, being caused by certain basic differences in mental functioning."[17] These basic differences concern the way in which an individual prefers to deal with his environment—using either perception or judgment. Together, these preferences constitute a substantial portion of the individual's total mental activity as well as govern one's outer behavior to a significant degree; by definition one's perception determines one's awareness in a situation and one's judgment determines one's action in that situation.[17]

In the area of perception there are two distinct and contrasting methods of perceiving. The first is sensing, by which one obtains direct information by using the five senses; the second process is intuition, by which one perceives indirectly via the unconscious and its accompanying ideas, associations, and so forth. Such unconscious contributions are evident in situations attributed to a "hunch" or a "woman's intuition," as well as in creative art and scientific discovery.[17] For example, Kekulé, while researching the molecular structure of benzene, dreamed of a snake with its tail in its mouth. He interpreted this dream to mean that the molecular structure of benzene was a closed carbon ring. Similarly, Nobel Prize winner Maria Mayer made her discovery concerning the constituents of the atomic nucleus in an intuitive flash of insight triggered by a colleague's remark.[20] While each individual utilizes both types of perception, from infancy on he will show a preference for one type.

The judging process operates in a similar manner. The individual utilizes one of two contrasting and distinct methods of judging. The first of these is thinking, which is a rational thought process aimed at impersonal decision making. The second is feeling, which is also a rational thought process, but which relies upon an individual's value system in the decision-making process. An individual who indicates a preference for thinking focuses on an analysis of the facts and adhering to logical principles; an individual who prefers feeling focuses on "weighing the importance of alternatives" to himself or others.[18]

Depending upon whether one prefers to use perception or judgment when dealing with one's environment determines one's inclination toward extraversion or introversion.

TABLE 1

FREQUENCY AND MEAN SCORE COMPARISONS FOR PERSONALITY TYPES
OF SUB-3-HOUR MARATHONERS

| Personality Type | n | Sub-3-Hour Marathoners | |
		Mean Score	SD *
Extravert	16	15.00	14.53
Introvert	34	20.24	13.23
Sensing	28	24.50	19.34
Intuitive	22	20.73	10.98
Thinking	27	19.67	13.32
Feeling	23	21.83	15.90
Judging	35	25.60	14.09
Perceiving	15	22.47	19.15

* Standard deviation.

Results

The MBTI indicated the personality preferences of the sub-3-hour marathoners in terms of extraversion versus introversion, sensing versus intuition, thinking versus feeling, and judging versus perceiving. The frequencies, means and standard deviations for these preferences are presented in TABLE 1. A chi-square (χ^2) test was made on the frequencies of these preferences. A χ^2 value of 6.48 between extraversion and introversion was significant ($p < 0.01$). A χ^2 value of 8.0 between judging and perceiving was significant ($p < 0.005$). These results are summarized in TABLE 2.

TABLE 2

CHI-SQUARE COMPARISON OF FREQUENCIES FOR SUB-3-HOUR MARATHONERS

Personality Type	Frequency	χ^2
Extravert	16	
Introvert	34	6.48 *
Sensing	28	
Intuitive	22	0.72
Thinking	27	
Feeling	23	0.32
Judging	35	
Perceiving	15	8.00 †

* p <0.01 significance.
† p <0.005 significance.

The frequency distribution of the sixteen possible personality types for the 50 sub-3-hour marathoners is represented in FIGURE 1. The chi-square test of frequencies for all 16 types revealed a χ^2 value of 63.28, which was significant at the 0.000005 level. Sub-3-hour marathoners showed a maximum frequency of 13 for the ISTJ types and a minimum or zero frequency for the ISTP and ESTP personality types. The next greatest frequency for a particular type was 8 for ISFJ.

Demographic data for the 50 sub-3-hour marathoners included: age, height, weight, years running, age began running, number of marathons before first sub-3-hour marathon, total number of marathons, time of first sub-3-hour marathon, time of best sub-3-hour marathon, average miles/week, number of days running per week, and average pace. Summation of this data is included in TABLE 3. In our investigation, 7 of the 50 marathoners would be considered

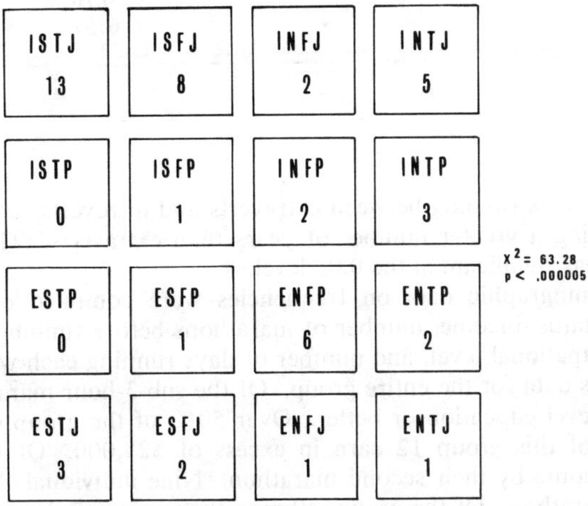

ISTJ 13	ISFJ 8	INFJ 2	INTJ 5
ISTP 0	ISFP 1	INFP 2	INTP 3
ESTP 0	ESFP 1	ENFP 6	ENTP 2
ESTJ 3	ESFJ 2	ENFJ 1	ENTJ 1

$\chi^2 = 63.28$
$p < .000005$

FIGURE 1. The frequency distribution of the 16 personality types for the 50 sub-3-hour marathoners. The observed frequencies in this sample of sub-3-hour marathoners deviate most significantly from the expected population frequencies. (I) introverted; (E) extraverted; (S) sensing; (N) intuitive; (J) judging; (P) perceiving; (T) thinking; (F) feeling.

world class, i.e., under 2 hours, 30 minutes. Two of these seven were under 2:23. The range of best marathon performance was 2:20:01 to 2:50:40 (mean 2:45:23; SD † 10:59). The range of the first sub-3-hour marathon was 2:24:06 to 2:59:40 (mean 2:53:08; SD 7:06). The range for total marathons was 1 to 50 (mean 11.14; SD 11.52). The number of miles per week ranged from 40 to 140 miles (mean 76.14; SD 23.49). Critical ratios ($\overline{Z}$-tests) performed on the preferences indicated significance in extraversion–introversion and judging–perceiving. The tests were used to compare number of years running, age began running, time of best marathon, and average number of miles run each week. The only observed statistically significant value involved

† Standard deviation.

TABLE 3

GENERAL CHARACTERISTICS OF 50 SUB-3-HOUR MARATHONERS

Characteristics	Mean	SD
Age	32.90	7.84
Height (cm)	176.99	5.49
Weight (kg)	65.68	5.45
Years running	8.88	5.75
Age began running	22.62	9.65
No. marathons before first sub-3-hour	2.16	1.78
Total no. marathons	11.14	11.52
Time of first sub-3-hour marathon	2:53:08	7:06
Time of best sub-3-hour marathon	2:45:23	10:59
Average miles/week run	76.14	23.49
No. days/week run	6.78	0.46
Average pace	6:57	:37

the number of years running between extraverts and introverts, where introverts had been running a greater number of years than extraverts. The observed $\bar{Z}$ value of 1.97 was significant at the 0.05 level.

Further demographic data on frequencies were compiled on educational level, marital status, income, number of marathons before running a sub-3-hour marathon, occupational level, and number of days running each week. TABLE 4 summarizes this data for the entire group. Of the sub-3-hour marathoners, 96% had a college level education or better. Over 50% of the group earns $15,000 or more, and of this group 12 earn in excess of $25,000. Of the group, 34 had broken 3 hours by their second marathon. Nine individuals broke 3 hours in their first marathon. Of the group, 40 marathoners run 7 days a week, 9 run 6 days a week, and 1 runs 5 days a week. The occupational categories are described as follows: low blue collar, unskilled labor; low white collar, clerical or technical; high blue collar, skilled labor or trade; high white collar, nondoctoral professional with specialized degrees or training; professional, doctoral degree; and student, high school, college, or graduate school.

The 50 sub-3-hour marathoners were compared with 83 male marathoners from the study by Clitsome and Kostrubala[15] in the following categories: age, number of marathons, number of years running, and number of miles run per week. The results are compiled in TABLE 5. All factors except age were significant at the 0.01 level.

A comparison of frequencies in educational level and occupational level was made between sub-3-hour marathoners and the male marathoners from the Clitsome and Kostrubala study.[15] Comparing the two groups by percentages, the sub-3-hour marathoners had twice as many men who were in or had completed graduate school. The slower marathoners had 5% more doctorates and 8% more on the college level of education. With regard to occupation, sub-3-hour marathoners had over 20% more men in high white collar occupations than marathoners. These results are summarized in TABLE 6.

Discussion

This investigation has attempted to delineate some of the demographic and personality characteristics of sub-3-hour marathon runners. This particular group was chosen arbitrarily from the ranks of athletes who participate in this particular race.

TABLE 4

FREQUENCY TABLE OF DEMOGRAPHIC DATA OF 50 SUB-3-HOUR MARATHONERS

	N=50
Educational level	
High school	2
College	24
Graduate school	17
M.D., Ph.D., J.D.	7
Marital status	
Single	23
Married	23
Widowed	0
Divorced	3
Separated	1
Income ($\times 1,000$)	
0–4	7
4–9	5
9–12	5
12–15	7
15–20	11
20–25	3
25 plus	12
No. marathons before first sub-3-hour	
0	9
1	11
2	14
3	6
4	3
5	3
6	4
Occupation	
Student	7
Professional	8
High white collar	29
Low white collar	4
High blue collar	1
Low blue collar	1
No. days/week run	
5	1
6	9
7	40

TABLE 5

A COMPARISON OF 50 SUB-3-HOUR MARATHONERS WITH 83 MARATHONERS

Factor	Sub-3-Hour Marathoners ($n=50$)		Marathoners * ($n=83$)		
	Mean	SD	Mean	SD	$\bar{Z}$-Value
Age	32.90	7.84	33.46	11.09	0.36
Number of marathons	11.14	11.52	5.78	7.86	3.04 †
Number of years running	8.88	5.75	5.86	5.60	2.94 †
Number of miles/week	76.14	23.49	51.59	25.97	5.58 †

* Data from Clitsome & Kostrubala.[15]
† p < 0.01.

The first qualifying factor for this group relates to time and distance: in order to complete a sub-3-hour marathon, the runner must average a 6:50-mile over a distance of 26 miles, 385 yards. At this rate his completion time will be 2:59:09.

At the moment when the 6:50-paced marathoner crosses the finish line, the 7-minute-per-mile runner will be one half mile behind him; for the 8- and 9-minute-per-mile runners the figures are 4 and 6 miles behind, respectively.

From the data collected in this study, the investigators constructed the following profile of a sub-3-hour marathoner. Demographically he is approximately 33 years old. He has run about 11 marathons and has been running for almost 9 years; he maintains an average running distance of 76 miles per

TABLE 6

A COMPARISON OF FREQUENCIES BETWEEN 50 SUB-3-HOUR MARATHONERS AND 83 MALE MARATHONERS WITH REGARD TO EDUCATIONAL LEVEL AND OCCUPATION

	Sub-3-Hour Marathoners ($n=50$)	Marathoners * ($n=83$)
Educational level		
High school	2	6
College	24	47
Graduate school	17	14
Doctorate	7	16
Occupation		
Low blue collar	1	2
Low white collar	4	7
High blue collar	1	9
High white collar	29	31
Professional	8	15
Student	7	19

* Data from Clitsome & Kostrubala.[15]

week. A striking finding is that he ran his first sub-3-hour marathon in his second marathon attempt.

A closer examination reveals that in all likelihood he is at least a college graduate who earns a mean income of $13,000 annually.

An examination of the data obtained from the Myers-Briggs Type Indicator (Form F) reveals that there are twice as many introverts as extraverts among this population. An examination of the study by Clitsome and Kostrubala of 100 marathoners [15] reveals that their marathoner is as likely to be introverted as to be extraverted. In addition, their study reveals that among the general population of nonmarathoners, the ratio of extraverts to introverts is 3 to 1. It therefore appears that marathoners are distinctly different from the general, nonmarathoning population, and that these differences are accentuated in this particular sub-3-hour marathon population. A valid assessment of whether this tendency toward introversion among marathoners existed prior to marathon running or whether it is related to the psychologic effects of training cannot be determined from within the scope of this study. Certainly the marathoner's level of educational achievement was established prior to his first marathon.

An analysis of the data obtained from use of the MBTI test along with information presented in the *MBTI Manual* describing the complete spectrum of possible personality types indicates that the sub-3-hour marathoner will more likely be an ISTJ type or an ISFJ type than any of the other 16 possible personality types. The *MBTI Manual* describes these types as follows: "He is the most thorough of all the types, painstaking, systematic, hard-working, and patient with detail and routine. His extreme perseverance tends to stabilize everything with which he is connected. He does not enter into things impulsively, but once in, he is very hard to distract, discourage or stop. He does not quit unless experience convinces him he is wrong." [17]

It is extremely interesting to note that a psychologic measurement such as the MBTI, with all the difficulties inherent to its development and refinement, so accurately reflects the common observations about marathoners. The MBTI is a specific derivative of C. G. Jung's theory of personality type and was developed as such to test his theory for consistent validity and use. This may indicate that the most useful and accurate theoretic framework for further investigation in this area is Jungian.

Summary

A group of 50 sub-3-hour marathoners were studied using the Myers-Briggs Type Indicator, Form F, (MBTI) and demographic data. Their mean age was 32.9. The mean for the number of marathons run was 11.14 and for the number of years running was 8.88. The mean for the number of miles run per week was 76.14. The results of the MBTI revealed that there were twice as many introverts as there were extraverts and twice as many judging types as there were perceiving types. The predominant personality type was ISTJ. Of the sub-3-hour marathoners, 96% had a college level education or better. From the previous study of Clitsome and Kostrubala,[15] it appears that marathoners are distinctly different from the general, nonmarathoning population, and that these differences are accentuated in this particular sub-3-hour marathon population.

Acknowledgments

Special thanks and appreciation go to Kathleen Ahner for her invaluable assistance and helpful criticism in the preparation of this study, and to Raymond G. Murphy who assisted in computing the statistics and the analysis of data.

References

1. THE 1976 MARATHON HANDBOOK. World Publications. Mountain View, Calif.
2. LAYMAN, E. M. 1974. *In* Exercise and Sports Science Reviews. Vol. 2. Academic Press. New York, N.Y.
3. JOHNSON, W. R. & E. R. BUSKIRK, Eds. 1974. Science and Medicine of Exercise and Sport. 2nd edit. Harper & Row. New York, N.Y.
4. HARRIS, D. V. 1973. Involvement in Sport. Lea & Febiger. Philadelphia, Pa.
5. CRATTY, B. J. 1968. Psychology and Physical Activity. Prentice-Hall. Englewood Cliffs, N.J.
6. MORGAN, W. P. 1969. Physical fitness and emotional health: A review. Amer. Corr. Ther. J. **3:** 124–127.
7. MORGAN, E. P., Ed. 1970. Contemporary Readings in Sports Psychology. Charles C Thomas, Publisher. Springfield, Ill.
8. STEVENSON, C. L. 1975. Socialization effect of participation in sport: A critical review of the research. Res. Quart. **46:** 287–301.
9. GLASSER, W. 1976. Positive Addiction. Harper & Row. New York, N.Y.
10. HENDERSON, J. 1976. The Long Run Solution. World Publications. Mountain View, Calif.
11. KOSTRUBALA, T. 1976. The Joy of Running. J. B. Lippincott Co. Philadelphia, Pa.
12. ROHÉ, F. 1974. The Zen of Running. Random House. New York, N.Y.
13. SPINO, M. 1976. Beyond Jogging. Celestial Arts. Millbrae, Calif.
14. MORGAN, W. P. & D. L. COSTILL. 1972. Psychological characteristics of the marathon runner. J. Sports Med. **12:** 42–46.
15. CLITSOME, T. & T. KOSTRUBALA. 1977. Ann. N.Y. Acad. Sci. This volume.
16. MORGAN, W. P. 1977. Ann. N.Y. Acad. Sci. This volume.
17. MYERS, I. B. 1962. The Myers-Briggs Type Indicator. Educational Testing Service. Princeton, N.J.
18. MCCAULLEY, M. H. 1974. The Myers-Briggs Type Indicator and the Teaching Learning Process. Unpublished paper presented at the 1974 Annual Meeting of American Educational Research Association, Session 20.24. Chicago, Ill.
19. JUNG, C. G. 1971. Psychological Types. Princeton University Press. Princeton, N.J.
20. JUNG, C. G., M. L. VON FRANZ, J. L. HENDERSON, J. JACOBI & A. JAFFE. 1964. Man and His Symbols. Doubleday & Co., Inc. Garden City, N.Y.

DEPRESSION FOLLOWING MYOCARDIAL INFARCTION: THE EFFECTS OF DISTANCE RUNNING

Terence Kavanagh, Roy J. Shephard,
J. A. Tuck, and S. Qureshi

Toronto Rehabilitation Centre
Toronto, Ontario
M4G 1R7 Canada

Department of Preventive Medicine and Biostatistics
University of Toronto
Toronto, Ontario
M5S 1A1 Canada

A previous report from our laboratories [1] noted a high incidence of depression (as measured by the D scale of the Minnesota Multiphasic Personality Inventory) in patients examined 16 to 18 months following myocardial infarction. The severely depressed patients apparently formed a distinct population group, demonstrating also the so-called neurotic triad (hysteria, hypochondriasis, and psychasthenia). A 4-year follow-up has now been completed on 44 of the more depressed patients who have been participating in an exercise-based rehabilitation program; the findings form the basis of the present report.

METHODS

Subjects. The subjects were 44 depressed "postcoronary" patients who had a very high "D" score (STEN ≥ 70) on the Minnesota Multiphasic Personality Inventory (MMPI) * when examined 16–18 months following myocardial infarction. Over the 4-year period 1972–1976, they continued to participate in the exercise rehabilitation program offered by the Toronto Rehabilitation Centre.[2] This provided personally-prescribed and progressive long slow distance jogging, individual patients advancing as far and as fast as their clinical condition and enthusiasm allowed.

Personality Testing. The MMPI tests were completed in 1972 and in 1976 under the immediate supervision of a professional psychologist. All subjects satisfied the validity checks (scales Q, L, F, and K) on both occasions that the test was completed, and the results reported have been adjusted for K scores.

Laboratory Tests. All subjects performed a standard battery of laboratory tests at regular intervals. The figures cited in this report were obtained concurrently with the initial and the final personality measurements. Data include height, weight, and skinfold readings taken by standard anthropometric techniques,[3] aerobic power as predicted from a multistage bicycle ergometer test carried to 75% of maximum oxygen intake,[4, 5] blood pressures at rest, and during exercise (standard sphygmomanometer cuff estimates), and depression of the ST segment of the exercise electrocardiogram (data obtained at a fixed exercise heart rate, averaged over 16 complexes by analogue computer).

---

* The Psychological Corporation, 304 East 45th St., New York, N.Y. 10017.

Results

Personality Scores. Standardized D scores for the 44 depressed patients showed a highly significant (p < 0.001) improvement over the 4-year study, from an average of 80 to 72 units. There were also statistically significant decreases in the scores relating to hysteria (Hy), hypochondriasis (Hs), and psychasthenia (Pt). Nevertheless, 22 of the 44 still had a D score more than 2 SD† above the population average (≥70 units). In 27 of the 44 men, the crude D score decreased by 2 units or more. The average changes in raw scores for this group (TABLE 1) were D, 6.4 ± 4.7 units; Hs, 3.8 ± 4.6; Hy, 4.9 ± 4.8; and Pt, 3.9 ± 5.2. Other changes in those whose depression lessened included significant decrements in scores for schizophrenia (2.9 ± 6.0) and social introversion (3.7 ± 6.5).

Ten patients showed only marginal changes of D score, but in seven the D score increased by two or more units. Where depression worsened, there was a significant increment of scores for hysteria, with insignificant increments on the hypochondriasis, psychasthenia, and social introversion scales.

Changes in the D scores were analyzed with regard to the effects of medication (TABLE 2). Of the group, 31 were not receiving medication likely to induce depression. Their D score diminished from 28.9 to 26.0, a change of 2.9 ± 6.8 units over the 4 years. In 13 cases treated by propranolol ("Inderal"), the change was somewhat larger, from 29.1 to 25.6 units. In the improved group four patients were taking propranolol at the time of the first test; three of these were on the same dosage 4 years later, and the fourth was taken off the drug in the interim. Five other individuals who were not on the medication initially were taking substantial dosages at the time of the final assessment. Of the seven patients who deteriorated in mood, one was on the same dosage for the duration of the study, and another was placed on propranolol a year prior to the final test. The group who showed no change in mood contained two subjects who ceased taking the drug subsequent to the first assessment (TABLE 3).

Changes in D scores were related to compliance with the prescribed exercise, compliance being defined as attendance at a minimum of 60% of available exercise sessions (TABLE 4). The decrease was substantial (3.97 ± 6.39 units) in those meeting their prescription, whereas those who failed to comply showed virtually no change of D scores.

The 50th percentile of masculinity/femininity (Mf) scores for normal men lies at 20.6 units, higher scores reflecting a more feminine personality tendency. All of the postcoronary patients had high scores on the masculinity/femininity axis. This might have been anticipated from earlier research linking heavy smoking with feminine personality traits in the male and masculine traits in the female;[6, 7] however, another explanation is the effect of education and cultural variables on this particular MMPI trait.

Physiological Changes. Physiological responses to the four additional years of rehabilitation are summarized in TABLE 5. There was a substantial increase of body weight; while this could be attributed in part to a gain of lean mass, there was also a small increase of skinfold thickness over the period of observation.

The aerobic power, as predicted by the oxygen scale of the Åstrand nomo-

† Standard deviations.

Table 1

4-Year Follow-Up of MMPI Scores in Postcoronary Patients with High Initial D Scores *

	Hypochondriasis (Hs)	Depression (D)	Hysteria (Hy)	Psychodyslepsia (Pd)	Masc/Fem (Mf)	Paranoia (Pa)	Psychasthenia (Pt)	Schizophrenia (Sc)	Megalomania (Ma)	Social Introversion (Si)
All cases (n=44)										
1972	18.2±4.5	29.0±3.6	25.1±4.6	22.5±5.2	28.6±4.3	9.8±3.3	30.6±6.1	26.7±7.8	19.0±4.1	33.5±8.4
1976	16.0±4.6	25.9±5.2	22.5±4.5	21.5±5.2	28.1±4.9	9.6±3.4	28.6±5.8	25.1±6.9	18.3±3.2	32.7±9.2
Δ	−2.2±4.9 †	−3.1±6.0 †	−2.6±4.9 †	−1.0±4.4	−0.5±3.0	−0.2±3.2	−2.1±5.7 †	−1.6±5.6	−0.7±3.5	−0.8±8.0
Improved (n=27)										
1972	18.4±4.0	29.5±3.8	25.7±4.2	22.5±4.6	30.0±4.1	9.7±3.2	30.7±6.1	26.7±8.1	19.3±4.4	34.3±8.2
1976	14.6±4.3	23.1±3.7	20.7±5.7	21.1±5.0	29.7±5.0	8.9±3.1	26.7±3.8	23.8±5.7	18.4±3.1	30.6±7.1
Δ	−3.8±4.6 †	−6.4±4.7 †	−5.0±4.8 †	−1.4±4.4	−0.3±3.0	−0.8±2.7	−4.0±5.2 †	−2.9±6.0 †	−0.9±3.5	−3.7±6.5 †
No change (n=10)										
1972	19.8±4.9	28.1±3.1	26.3±4.8	22.7±6.6	24.6±2.8	11.2±3.8	30.0±6.9	27.2±9.0	18.0±3.4	31.7±8.7
1976	19.5±3.5	28.3±2.9	24.2±5.3	20.6±5.7	23.7±3.1	10.1±3.4	31.3±8.1	26.9±8.5	17.9±1.9	33.3±12.6
Δ	−0.3±3.8	−0.2±0.9	−2.1±4.3	−2.1±4.0	−0.9±2.7	−1.1±2.5	+1.3±4.5	−0.3±3.6	−0.1±2.9	+1.6±5.4
Worse (n=7)										
1972	15.3±5.0	28.0±3.1	21.1±3.3	22.3±5.9	28.7±3.7	8.0±2.6	31.1±6.0	26.1±5.5	19.3±5.0	33.1±9.5
1976	16.4±4.8	33.3±4.0	24.0±3.1	24.0±5.4	28.3±3.0	11.1±3.8	32.0±6.7	28.1±8.1	18.1±5.4	39.9±8.2
Δ	+1.1±5.2	+5.3±3.2 †	+2.9±2.9 †	+1.7±4.5	−0.4±3.6	+3.1±4.3	−0.9±7.2	+2.0±5.5	−1.2±5.3	+6.8±11.0

* Values are presented as raw scores for each of the major personality scales. Mean±standard deviation (SD).

† Significant differences (p <0.05) between initial and final measurements.

1031

TABLE 2

INFLUENCE OF DRUG THERAPY ON "D" SCORES OF POSTCORONARY PATIENTS *

	Initial D Score	Final D Score	Δ
No drug treatment ($n=31$)	28.9±3.7 (80)	26.0±5.5 (72)	2.9±6.8
Propranolol ($n=13$)	29.1±3.1 (80)	25.6±4.6 (71)	3.5±4.1

* Initial observations made 16–18 months after infarction, final observations made 4 years later. STEN scores are shown in parenthesis.

gram, showed a substantial continuing gain, to the point where normal standards for the sedentary population [5, 8] were being approached. None of these reactions differed markedly between those with decreased and those with increased D scores.

The resting blood pressure changed but little in those patients whose depression was reduced, but in the men whose D scores increased there was a significant fall of resting systolic pressures, accompanied by an insignificant rise of the diastolic readings. During exercise, both groups of patients showed an augmentation of systolic pressures at the 75% loading, with insignificant changes in diastolic pressures.

The ST segmental depression at 75% of maximum oxygen intake showed no change in the men with lowered D scores; in contrast, among the group where D scores increased the negative ST voltage was significantly augmented over the period of observation.

TABLE 3

RELATIONSHIP BETWEEN TAKING OF PROPRANOLOL AND MMPI EVALUATIONS

	Taking medication at:		
	Both Tests	Initial Test Only	Final Test Only
Decreased D Score ($n=9$)	3	1	5
Increased D Score ($n=2$)	1	0	1
Unchanged D Score ($n=2$)	0	2	0

TABLE 4

RELATIONSHIP BETWEEN EXERCISE COMPLIANCE AND CHANGES
IN MMPI DEPRESSION SCORES *

	Initial Score	Final Score	Δ
Subjects complying with prescribed exercise	29.2±3.6	25.3±5.5	3.97±6.39
Subjects not complying with prescribed exercise	27.1±4.5	27.1±2.3	0.0±4.0

* Initial data obtained 16–18 months after infarction, final scores obtained 4 years later.

TABLE 5

A COMPARISON OF PHYSIOLOGICAL RESPONSES BETWEEN PATIENTS SHOWING
A DECREASE IN THEIR D SCORE ON THE MMPI ($n=25$)* AND THOSE SHOWING
AN INCREASE ($n=6$)† ‡

	D Score Diminished			D Score Increased		
	Initial	Final	Δ	Initial	Final	Δ
Age (yr)	51.4			47.2		
	±7.9			±5.3		
Height (cm)	172.3			171.0		
	±8.7			±4.3		
Weight (kg)	73.4	76.3	+2.9	71.7	72.9	+1.3
	±8.6	±7.9	±3.9	±7.3	±7.7	±2.5
Excess weight (kg)	6.4	9.3	+2.9	5.4	6.6	+1.2
	±7.1	±6.4	±3.1	±6.9	±6.7	±2.5
Average skinfold (mm)	14.5	15.3	+0.8	13.5	14.1	+0.6
	±4.6	±5.7	±4.7	±3.9	±4.2	±1.3
Aerobic power						
(liter/min STPD)	1.99	2.47	+0.5	1.75	2.11	+0.36
	±0.46	±0.76	±0.5	±0.27	±0.51	±0.51
(ml/kg·min STPD)	26.3	32.1	+5.8	25.0	29.8	+4.8
	±6.2	±9.1	±6.7	±4.4	±8.4	±6.7
Blood pressure, at rest						
Systolic (mm Hg)	131.8	131.4	−0.4	136.7	121.0	−15.7
	±15.4	±15.7	±18.1	±10.3	±14.6	±14.2
Diastolic (mm Hg)	87.9	88.5	+0.6	76.7	80.0	+3.3
	±10.7	±8.8	±8.9	±8.2	±8.9	±12.1
Blood pressure (75% load)						
Systolic (mm Hg)	167.1	179.2	+12.1	165.0	182.2	+17.2
	±26.0	±27.6	±24.0	±17.6	±19.4	±15.6
Diastolic (mm Hg)	99.6	98.3	−1.3	95.0	96.7	+1.7
	±8.1	±11.3	±8.5	±5.5	±8.2	±9.8
ST depression (75% load)	−0.10	−0.10	0.0	−0.03	−0.07	−0.04
(mV)	±0.12	±0.14	±0.15	±0.05	±0.07	±0.04

* Data incomplete for 3 patients.
† Data incomplete for 1 patient.
‡ Ten patients showed no change in D scores.

DISCUSSION

Depression and Infarction. The present data confirm observations from our own [1] and other laboratories [9-19] in showing a substantial and persistent depression among a segment of the "postcoronary" population. Theoretically, no more than 2.5% of people should attain a score of more than 70 units on the D scale of the MMPI, yet 44 of 100 cases showed such a result 16 to 18 months after infarction, and 22 of this group still had a score of over 70 units 5½ years after the critical episode. The results of such objective testing stand in marked contrast with responses to superficial questioning.[1] Many of the patients deny depression,[1, 20, 21] to the point where it may be overlooked by both the family physician [21] and the specialist in cardiology.[22]

In a previous article,[1] we referred to the popularly held opinion that MMPI scores reflected inherent personality characteristics rather than a mood state engendered by immediate problems, and we discussed how far the very high D scores of the infarct victim could be attributed to his basic personality. The Napoleonic physician Corvisart [23] wrote "repeated depressing emotions . . . may be the origin of refractory disorders of the heart." Brozek *et al.*[24] also noted high hypochondriasis scores in subjects who subsequently developed infarction. On the other hand, Ostfeld *et al.*[25] found no initial differences of MMPI scores between normal individuals and those who later sustained infarctions. A second possible variable is the act of volunteering for an exercise-based program. Volunteers may demonstrate certain psychological peculiarities,[26] and although they did not comment on this specific point, Naughton *et al.*[10] recorded high D, Hy, and Hs scores in sedentary "controls," who volunteered for physiological and psychological testing. However, the postcoronary patient is typically inhibited from physical activity by his depression,[27, 28] and it is thus hard to imagine that an exercise program selectively attracted patients with a high depression score. A third consideration is age. The postcoronary victim is inevitably middle-aged, and it is well recognized that there are small increments of D score as a person becomes older; however, it is inconceivable that aging could produce a large population with D scores averaging three standard deviations greater than the mean values for young adults. Thus while it seems likely that the depression arose subsequent to infarction, we still cannot exclude the possibility that it is a preinfarct life-style trait in a coronary vulnerable individual.

Another possible explanation is that the depression is a side-effect of drugs used in the treatment of hypertension and dysrhythmias. Compounds such as rauwolfia, guanethidine, and propranolol can all produce effects of this type. Some 30% of our depressed patients were receiving propranolol at some time or other during the 4-year study, but scores for this subgroup (STEN average 80 units) were similar to those not receiving drugs. Furthermore, analysis of the time intervals over which the drug was taken show that in only two patients could the variation in D scores reflect medication induced mood change.

Other factors contributing to depression include inappropriate and inadequate explanations from the attending physician [29] and interaction with tense, over-anxious wives.[11, 20, 30] However, the main reasons for depression are almost certainly the patient's own anxiety, lack of confidence and fear of sudden death.[22]

Factors Modifying Depression. Although this segment of our postcoronary population has remained seriously depressed, nevertheless D scores have improved significantly over the 4 years of rehabilitation. We must now assess how far this change can be attributed to the exercise program and other forms of treatment that have been administered to our patients.

Some authors have held that the postcoronary patient shows an inevitable improvement with time, as both he and his spouse adapt to the problems created by the infarct.[30] Furthermore, it could be argued that by selecting patients who were initially very depressed, we increased our chances of seeing a reversion towards the mean.[31, 32] A number of workers have now demonstrated a reduction of depression coincident with participation in an exercise program,[10, 15, 18, 21, 33] but in the one experiment that included control subjects [10] the decrease of depression score was not significantly enhanced by the training process. McPherson *et al.*[32] suggested that many of the observed benefits might accrue from group support rather than from the exercise per se.

Nevertheless, it is a matter of common experience that exercise makes a person "feel good." [34] It thus seems logical that compliance with an exercise prescription should help the recovery of a depressed patient. Our data (TABLE 4) apparently supports such a contention, although we cannot entirely exclude the possibility that a worsening of clinical condition was responsible for both an increase of depression and noncompliance with the prescribed exercise.

From the practical viewpoint it seems that the mere act of complying with the exercise program is effective in alleviating depression. Interestingly, however, two patients who made the most gains (D, 39 to 16; D, 33 to 24) were taking mood elevators, diazepam and chlorpromazine. The main objection to many of the antidepressants has been their liability to provoke dysrhythmias and sudden death;[19] however, there seems a potential to explore the further use of such medication in the treatment of the severely depressed postcoronary patient. Whereas propranolol is reputed to have a depressant effect, this may be outweighed in the postcoronary patient by its ability to suppress angina and dysrhythmias and to allow for greater participation in our exercise program; nine of the 27 patients who improved their D score were taking the drug at the end of the study as compared with five at the start.

The physiological data gave little guide as to which patients would succeed in reducing their D scores over the course of rehabilitation. There were substantial gains of aerobic power, both among those whose D scores decreased and also among those in whom depression became greater; indeed the increment of maximum oxygen intake was only marginally smaller in the second subgroup. The resting systolic pressure was more labile in those whose depression increased, possibly indicating a more anxious personality. Of greater clinical significance, there was no change of ST segmental depression or ST segmental sagging in those whose D scores increased. This supports the idea of an association between depression and a progression of the coronary vascular disease.

Other Facets of Personality. We have not commented previously on MMPI scores in our patients other than those for hypochondriasis, hysteria, depression, psychasthenia, and hypomania. The high masculinity/femininity scores for all of the group at first glance appears paradoxical, since coronary artery disease is a sex-linked phenomenon and one might anticipate that the more "masculine" men would be at greater risk. Using the Cattell Test we have found in previous studies an association between feminine personality traits and heavy cigarette smoking in the male,[6, 7] and certainly such smoking is well recognized as a major risk factor for coronary disease. A second intriguing possibility is that one factor leading to myocardial infarction was the discrepancy between the personality of the individual and the demands placed upon him in fulfilling the male sex-role. A further explanation is that emasculation is a reaction to changes forced upon the patient by his heart attack. It should be noted, however, that the group Mf score showed remarkably little change over the 4-year period, irrespective of compliance with the program, alteration in mood, or medication. Possibly the explanation lies in the effects of a superior education on cultural values and interpretation of which vocational and avocational activities are socially acceptable for men as well as women, e.g., ballet, poetry, art, and so forth. Many of the patients are from the white-collar ranks, and it might be fruitful to investigate this aspect further.

There was a significant decrease in scores for social introversion (-3.7 ± 6.1) and schizoid traits (-2.9 ± 6.0). This could reflect the beneficial effect of group interaction, even though the only overt reason for attending the classes, and indeed the only active "therapeutic" procedure carried out by all subjects was endurance-type training.

Summary

A proportion of postcoronary patients seen 16 to 18 months after infarction are seriously depressed (high D score on Minnesota Multiphasic Personality Inventory). A follow-up of 44 such depressed patients showed a significant ($p < 0.001$) decrease of standardized D scores, from 80 to 72 units over 4 years of exercise-based rehabilitation. There were associated decreases in scores for hysteria, hypochondriasis, and psychasthenia.

A decrease of D score was associated with exercise compliance. An increase of D score was associated with a significant ($p < 0.05$) worsening of ST segmental sagging, suggesting that progression of the disease process had contributed to the increase of depression. All of the patients had high (feminine) scores on the masculinity/femininity scale of the MMPI test. This finding was unrelated to the daily running distance or medication; it could represent a "feminine" personality, or be a typical response in a well-educated white collar group. Evidence of successful group interaction may be indicated by reduction in scores for social introversion and schizophrenic traits.

References

1. Kavanagh, T., R. J. Shephard & J. A. Tuck. 1975. Depression after myocardial infarction. Canad. Med. Assoc. J. **113**: 23–27.
2. Kavanagh, T. & R. J. Shephard. 1973. The importance of physical activity in post-coronary rehabilitation—A special review. Ann. Phys. Med. **52**(6): 304–313.
3. Weiner, J. S. & J. A. Lourie. 1969. Human Biology: A guide to field methods. Blackwell Scientific. Oxford, England.
4. Andersen, K. L., R. J. Shephard, H. Denolin, E. Varnauskas & R. Masironi. 1971. Fundamentals of Exercise Testing. World Health Organization. Geneva.
5. Shephard, R. J. 1977. Endurance Fitness. 2nd edit. University of Toronto Press. Toronto, Canada.
6. Rode, A., R. Ross & R. J. Shephard. 1972. Smoking withdrawal programme. Personality and cardio-respiratory fitness. Amer. Med. Assoc. Arch. Environ. Health **24**: 27–36.

7. SHEPHARD, R. J., A. RODE & R. ROSS. 1973. Reinforcement of a smoking withdrawal programme. The role of the physiologist and the psychologist. Canad. J. Publ. Health **64**(Suppl.): 41–51.

8. BAILEY, D. A., R. J. SHEPHARD, R. L. MIRWALD & G. A. MCBRIDE. 1974. Current levels of Canadian cardio-respiratory fitness. Canad. Med. Assoc. J. **111**: 25–30.

9. BENDIEN, J. & J. GROEN. 1963. A psychological statistical study of neuroticism and extroversion in patients with myocardial infarction. J. Psychosomat. Res. **7**: 11–14.

10. NAUGHTON, J., J. G. BRUHN & M. T. LATEGOLA. 1968. Effects of physical training on physiologic and behavioral characteristics of cardiac patients. Arch. Phys. Med. Rehab. **49**: 131–137.

11. RUSKIN, H. D., L. L. STEIN, I. M. SHELSKY & M. A. BAILEY. 1970. MMPI: Comparison between patients with coronary heart disease and their spouses together with other demographic data. Scand. J. Rehab. Med. **2–3**: 99–104.

12. KEEGAN, D. L. 1973. The coronary patient: A psycho-social glimpse. Canad. Fam. Phys. **19**(3): 66–68.

13. KLEIN, H. P. & O. A. PARSONS. 1968. Self-Description of Patients with Coronary Disease. Perceptual and Motor Skills. Southern Universities Press. Birmingham, Ala.

14. MILLER, C. K. 1965. Psycho-physiological correlates of coronary artery disease. Psychosomat. Med. **27**: 257–265.

15. VERWOERDT, A. & R. H. DOVENMUEHLE. 1964. Heart disease and depression. Geriatrics **18**: 856–864.

16. JENKINS, C. D. 1971. Psychologic and social precursors of coronary heart disease. N. Engl. J. Med. **284**: 307–317.

17. PARKES, C. M., B. BENJAMIN & R. G. FITZGERALD. 1969. A broken heart. A statistical study of increased mortality among widowers. Brit. Med. J. **i**: 740–743.

18. FRIEDMAN, E. H. & H. K. HELLERSTEIN. 1973. Influence of Psychosocial factors on coronary risk and adaptation to a physical fitness evaluation programme. *In* Exercise Testing and Exercise Training in Coronary Heart Disease. J. P. Naughton & H. K. Hellerstein, Eds. Academic Press. New York, N.Y.

19. HACKETT, T. P. & N. H. CASSEM. 1973. Psychological adaptation to convalescence in myocardial infarction patients. *In* Exercise Testing and Exercise Training in Coronary Heart Disease. J. P. Naughton & H. K. Hellerstein, Eds. Academic Press. New York, N.Y.

20. DOBSON, M., A. E. TATTERSFIELD, M. W. ADLER & M. W. MCNICOL. 1971. Attitudes and long-term adjustment of patients surviving cardiac arrest. Brit. Med. J. **iii**: 207–212.

21. BRUHN, J. G. 1973. Obtaining and interpreting psychosocial data in studies of coronary heart disease. *In* Exercise Testing and Exercise Training in Coronary Heart Disease. J. P. Naughton & H. K. Hellerstein, Eds. Academic Press. New York, N.Y.

22. FISHER, S. 1970. International survey on the psychological aspects of cardiac rehabilitation. Scand. J. Rehab. Med. **2–3**: 71–77.

23. CORVISART. 1806. Essai sur les Maladies du Coeur et des gros Vaisseaux. Paris, Cited by L. F. Bishop & P. Reichert. 1971. Psychosomatics **12**: 412–415.

24. BROZEK, J., A. KEYS & H. BLACKBURN. 1966. Personality differences between potential coronary and non-coronary subjects. Ann. N.Y. Acad. Sci. **134**: 1057.

25. OSTFELD, A. M., B. Z. LEBOVITS, R. B. SHEKELLE & O. PAUL. 1964. A prospective study of the relationship between personality and coronary heart disease. J. Chron. Dis. **17**: 265.

26. SHEPHARD, R. J. & M. KEMP. Unpublished report. U.K. Chemical Defence Establishment, Porton Down, U.K.

27. GELFAND, D. 1960. Factors relating to unsuccessful vocational adjustment of cardiac patients. Pennsylvania Office of Vocational Rehabilitation.

28. Return to work after myocardial infarction (Editorial). 1971. Lancet (Sept. 11): 591.
29. HINOHARA, S. 1970. Psychological aspects in rehabilitation of coronary heart disease. Scand. J. Rehab. Med. 2–3: 53–59.
30. SKELTON, M. & J. DOMINIAN. 1973. Psychological stress in wives of patients with myocardial infarction. Brit. Med. J. ii: 101–103.
31. DOTSON, C. O. 1973. Analysis of change. Exercise Sport Sci. Rev. 1: 393–420.
32. MCPHERSON, B. D., A. PAIVIO & M. S. YUHASZ. 1967. Psychological effects of an exercise program for post-infarct and normal adult men. J. Sports Med. 7: 95–102.
33. GRODEN, B. M. & R. I. F. BROWN. 1970. Differential psychological effects of early and late mobilization after myocardial infarction. Scand. J. Rehab. Med. 2–3: 60–64.
34. MORGAN, W. P., J. A. ROBERTS & A. D. FEINERMAN. 1971. Psychologic effect of acute physical activity. Arch. Phys. Med. Rehab. 52: 422–426.

DISCUSSION

Thaddeus Kostrubala, *Moderator*

Mercy Hospital and Medical Center
San Diego, California 92103

R. H. RAHE (*Naval Health Research Center, San Diego, Calif.*): I would like to try to perhaps stimulate the discussion on the psychological aspects of sport by having us consider the level of exercise versus the psychology or what goes through your mind, both in training and in high level performance. Again, my specialty is swimming, but I believe Dr. Jokl's table or figure indicates that swimmers in fact train harder than runners and that if you were to observe the training, you would see that swimmers do about 7 hours a day at 85% to 90% of maximal performance. Maybe you can't do that with a land sport because of the risk of injury and a lot of the other things we saw in Dr. Jokl's graph. But the point I want to make for discussion is this: at a low level of training your mind is free to have all kinds of input, whether it be meditation, thoughts about what happened to you today, what will happen tomorrow, and so forth. At a high level of training you are dealing with a very severe input of painful stimuli and your mind simply can't think of much else except how to get through this and why you ever got yourself into it and, in fact, promising yourself that you will never do it again—until you are out of the pool or out of the race and can recover, and then you say that was kind of fun. There is a level of physical output, very casual, even to the point of being a very pleasant kind of meditation experience. But in certain sports such as swimming, I suggest that in high level performance you use all coping abilities just to forget the pain so you can carry on and perform.

D. SHAINBERG (*Post-Graduate Center for Mental Health, New York, N.Y.*): I don't have much to say about this, except insofar as I've talked to many of the marathoners and everyone described something similar to this, where they say that in the later stages of the marathon, especially after 17 or 18 miles, that sense of the glass bubble drops around them and they just grab it and lose touch, and they are only responding to the event that you're talking about. I think your point could be looked at from another angle; if you ran into a snake in the woods, you're not going to stop and think about the snake; you're going to respond automatically. The event is going to be complete and total, and I think that what you're saying carries the thing I'm saying a little bit further. It really raises the question of what is the function of thought. If the organism is not thinking when it's involved in this task—this physical task—then why do we think at all and what do we use thought for? I agree with you that in these kinds of stressful events there isn't thought, you tend to just deal with the immediate transitions of biological phenomena, and in that way thought is not necessary because thought is always old.

A. H. ISMAIL (*Purdue University, West Lafayette, Ind.*): I have nothing to add to this, except that I know from experience that you completely zero in your own work, or your own effort is not true. I find that the mind is always like a computer. We are always assessing what we have been in, not only physiologically or biochemically, and always assessing what it is going to do next. Is he going to speed up, is he going to stop, is he going to reduce, is he going to catch up? We are always processing this kind of data; the human machine is going on, and I don't think that the marathoner is just running in a vacuum. He is always collecting information and the fascination about this information is that it is always changing; this is not static information. Thus, he is actually even "thinking" in the time of his agony. Actually, just running in a blank is completely inaccurate because we are not robots, we are always assessing, we are always evaluating, we are making decisions, although they are minor decisions—still they are decisions.

T. KOSTRUBALA: I would like to add one thing to this. Your question really reflects a basic research question in the whole area of study of the effects of exercise or running and the personality. It is very difficult to assess the psychological effects of what happens without explicitly measuring the degree of effort the individual is expending. If he's at 50% of his maximum cardic output or 80% or 90%, I think we have a different kind of phenomenon. The second aspect that we have to deal with is the amount of time; is it just for 10 minutes, 30, 50, 60, 2 hours, and so forth, and my hunch is that at certain points in time we obliterate functions of the left cortex, the logical, sequential, ordering function of the mind which drives us to the point of where we again allow the right cortex to come into play. The next question you bring up is the definition of pain. Pain is a uniquely subjective experience. It cannot be quantified externally. It is defined only by the individual. The interpretation of that subjective event called pain produces one of the most fruitful areas of understanding of the human psyche.

A. N. ROSENBERG (*Princeton University, Princeton, N.J.*): My reaction to the swimming question was that running is qualitatively different from swimming in the sense that a swimmer will often go down the same lane repeatedly. A marathoner generally won't use the same road more than twice, once in each direction. I think that the fact that one is travelling to different places has a lot to do with the mentality of the runner as opposed to the mentality of a swimmer. Could you comment on that?

T. KOSTRUBALA: The prime sensorial input of the swimmer is different from that of the runner. The swimmer is surrounded by water. We saw from Dr. Jokl's brief reference to the fact that immersed in fluid, his heart is in a different state, he's floating. His visual perceptions are limited because of the medium that he's in. If it is true that man is the greatest long distance land animal on our planet—that is, that man can run down any other land animal—this indicates that there may be a biological or evolutionary pattern or archetype which resonates to very deep levels of our unconscious. That's what happens with the runner. The other possibility is that perhaps at one time we were in water, and it may be this quality that the swimmer attempts to recapture.

D. E. MARTIN (*Atlanta, Ga.*): I would like to ask something on a bit of a different note. Yesterday we heard the commentary as to what perhaps the fastest women's marathon time might be in the future. We haven't yet heard an estimate of what the best men's marathon time might be for the future. Professor Jokl has gained international acclaim for his "Jokl-grams" where he projects such information. This being a marathon conference, do you know whether or not he has prepared such information regarding marathon times?

T. KOSTRUBALA: I do not know. My personal prediction is that a male will run a marathon in two hours by the year 2000.

J. W. FARIS (*University of Wisconsin, Madison, Wis.*): I would like to ask Dr. Ismail to comment on Morgan's ideas that running is effective in the alleviation of mood states such as anxiety and depressive affects, but that longer lasting characteristics such as perhaps a paranoid personality would not be ammenable to change by any amount of running. I'm wondering about how that relates to your ideas of the change in personality type; for example, an obsessive person who runs around the track at the same speed every day falls apart when he stops.

A. H. ISMAIL: I'm very glad you asked this question because most of us here—hoping I'm wrong—are interested in how to reduce time, how to go through this training before others, but we haven't actually addressed ourselves fully to what running has done to our personality; and everyone rumors that if you run this, you will drop dead, and we address ourselves only to perfection or improving the time rather than to the question of "what has the running done to me?" We are a highly tensed society who are actually on the verge of neuroticism, and we are climbing walls, and somehow there is an actual medicine called running, exercising, and jogging. We have to take advantage of this, and we've discovered that people who are involved in exercise do so continuously, regularly—everyone according to his ability, according to his capacity. They move from neuroticism to stability. Actually, they keep their hair loose and become less tense, more secure. We have found this to be true. I have already demonstrated that this is not only a psychometric approach, but biochemical as well.

D. SHAINBERG: I'd like to respond to that briefly. I think one of the differences between the paranoid personality and the depressive personality relates to organization. Without going into the biochemistry of it, the depressive personality is much more suspicious about this own thought processes; if you use the model that I wrote about here, during the process of the run there may be a greater willingness to drop into the physiological rhythms. However, in the paranoid personality the use of thought or perception is much more reactive and much more an organizational phenomena to hold perception together, so that in the process of the run—again, using the model that I have here—there is less likelihood of a willingness to drop away thought or perception because the dangers of disorganization are much greater.

D. BROWN (*Halcon International, Inc., New York, N.Y.*): I'm both a runner and swimmer in competition. I have a number of observations to make. In the first place, I am really impressed with the problem you have here in organizing a considerable amount of data and in using many complicated statistical methods. We use them in our business too. However, I am a single individual and I can attest to the facts. I began running and swimming when I was about 49 years old; I'm now 59. A remarkable peace of mind has accompanied the very heavy exercise, I think there was a considerable change in my psychological situation, which may have been due to the accumulated chemical changes. I haven't the faintest idea. I just work my tail off and run as hard as I can, and what I try to do is win. The other thing I've observed is that as runners and swimmers approach maximum speed, the differences between them diminishes. In swimming the power increases with the cube of your speed, while in running I think it's something between the second power and the first power. So it's very, very difficult to get your speed up very high as you swim; that's why the swimmer flattens out closer to his maximum speed, as he can really feel the force of the water against him as he increases his speed.

D. S. KRONFELD (*University of Pennsylvania, Philadelphia, Pa.*): I have been interested in the relationship between metabolism and psychological behavioral events as an avocation in sport and as a vocation in nutrition. I would like to bounce off Dr. Ismail and Dr. Shainberg the parallel between eating and exercising and the tranquility followed by both; maybe you've had a similar sort of metabolic event taking place. It seems to me that this is a pretty close parallel and it's not all due to change, and I feel a bit like one of the previous discussants, that in light exercise perhaps your mind can wander, whereas in really exhaustive exercise your attention focuses on what you're doing; when you've got all these metabolic factors working its more likely that afterwards you'll get into a physiological/psychological state conducive to reflection, tranquility, and meditation.

A. H. ISMAIL: I would like to address myself to this point from a biochemical point of view. During the first 7 or 8 minutes of exercise you are actually relying on serum glucose, and after that you begin to rely on the adipose tissues and insulin. You are going to go on a high, steady state relying on fatty acids, and then the glucose goes to the central nervous system, because the central nervous system is nourished by glucose alone. This explains why after a good run you may feel physically exhausted but mentally alert, and what is actually occurring is this kind of experience.

T. KOSTRUBALA: I would like to add that I think Dr. Ismail and I have a basic disagreement at this point: I do not see the brain solely as a computer. There is an illogical or alogical aspect to our psyche, and I think it is this area that is stimulated with certain states of exercise.

L. JANSEN (*St. Lawrence College, Bronxville, N.Y.*): I would like to ask you as a psychiatrist what you feel the cultural factors are in making people—especially automobile drivers—so incredibly hostile, both verbally and physically, towards runners.

D. KOSTRUBALA: Well, I don't know how much I have to indict myself; my friends all know that I have a tendency to "wing out" while running. First of all, I totally agree with you. We are dealing with this kind of phenomenon when we run, and as we're out there doing this "odd" behavior we are identifying ourselves to the culture around us as being significantly different. Now of course, the question is why do they identify us as a threat? Why do they try to run us down? Why have they run some down? In an informal discussion with Tom Bassler about deaths of runners, he said yes, there are deaths of runners, and it's quite clear as far as he could determine—although it can't be proven—that in cases of runners hit by automobiles it did not appear to be an accidental death. So what are we dealing with here? What kind of forces are we messing with? At times when I get into the meditative state which we talked about, I sometimes have the feeling that a basic hostility exists between the world of the machine and the world of man, and that by running with very little equipment, running along finding my body and my soul, somehow those machines don't like me. Those fellows inside those machines don't like me, and there is a fusion of mutual hostility at that point.

M. POTTER (*Hunter College, New York, N.Y.*): In listening to Dr.

Shainberg's meditation I thought of a proverb that some of the Japanese have in the sense that nothing we do is really reasoned. Reason is really the defense we use after the fact. You've run your race neurologically before you start it and are therefore able to get into that state. I think that by the time you stop your daily activities and the neurotransmitter blockage that you've built up all this time stops working normally, you have plenty of chance to stop and recycle, and in that recycling time you are then going into various biochemical states. In the recycling of neurotransmitter substance we go through a morphine state, and I've often wondered as this occurs whether we're not just hitting it really nice when we run at the right time. The other factor is that when we're running we have the opportunity to work on the negative neurotransmitter system, which shuts off, allowing us to develop concentration on certain things.

P. MILVY (*Mt. Sinai School of Medicine, New York, N.Y.*): Dr. Clitsome, I have a couple of questions I would like to ask. I was not sure what your controls were initially, and then you showed them at the end and I understand. You're looking at a 4-year period, and the people who have not complied with what their god or doctor wanted them to do over those 4 years might be disappointed with themselves, might become depressed at the fact that, "here my doctor wants me to go out and jog every day, and I'm not able to, I'm not motivated enough" to do whatever it might be, and there may be continued depression or even an increased depression. A prior question relates to the infarct: after an infarct some of you will be depressed, and obviously as you learn to live with the infarct you will be less depressed as the 4 years proceed. Dr. Clitsome, you had mentioned that this group in Florida stated that there was a 3 to 1 ratio between extraverts and introverts, respectively, in the general population, and in the marathon population that ratio is 1 to 1. I would like to know what you would find if you looked at a subpopulation, for example, if the Florida group has a subpopulation of college people? Also, on Dr. Gontang's paper the lists of characteristics such as perseverence, willingness to defer gratification, and so forth ideally fits the college student who is willing to grind away at night to eventually get his B.S. or Ph.D. or whatever he pursues. Since 90% of your runners did indeed have more than one year of college, marathoners by and large are much more educated than nonmarathoners. In other words, I'm asking the whole question of self-selection as presented yesterday.

A. GONTANG (*Mercy Hospital, San Diego, Calif.*): I think that's exactly what we're trying to examine—the self-selection process of sub-3-hour marathoners; and in regards to college and sub-3-hour marathoners, approximately 10 or 11 of the group that I studied were actually still in college.

P. MILVY: Would they look any different than a group of college students who don't run marathons?

T. CLITSOME: What we did was to use information that accumulates. We did compare them with college level students at the University of Florida itself. But for the purposes of this paper we had to limit it in terms of relating to the data base of 75,000, but we also related it just to college level education as well. Regarding self-selection, that was one of the most interesting aspects of the study: it indicates peoples' preferences. In other words, it indicates peoples' choices, so that no matter what a person would select it would always represent his preference.

S. VERNON (*Willimantic, Conn.*): I would like to make some comments.

Concerning the incredible hostility of motorists, I think we should remember that motorists pass each other while driving, and a motorist who has been passed when he really didn't anticipate it may turn at the next light and curse the motorist who passed him. Now, if he sees someone on the road who is no longer dependent upon a mode of transportation which he has become addicted to, and if he feels sadistic—recognizing in this introversive marathoner a certain kind of weakness—it may be that the sadistic, aggressive motorist whose self-esteem has been injured might be taking a cheap shot. In response to this behavior, I feel that a threatened marathoner should take evasive action; on the other hand, if—without making his evasive action clear —he makes some threatening but nonphysical gesture, such as showing his teeth, he may show that he's not a good subject for a cheap shot, and that the odds may not be what the motorist thinks they are. Anoher thing I'd like to mention—not being a marathoner myself—is that marathoners seem to have an incredible tolerance to the inhalation of car exhaust fumes. I have been on streets where there has been a lot of exhaust and can't even walk along that street. I wonder what breed of people these marathoners are who can run along a road, and if the exhaust fumes from cars are heavy, they continue regardless.

T. KOSTRUBALA: Yes sir, I would agree that as a breed marathoners are noticeably persistent.

S. VERNON: Absolutely. I'll say that many times over, and it's part of the neatness, part of the introversion, part of the nonaggressiveness, part of the fact that you're seeking a noncontact sport, and part of the fact that you're planning to punish yourself as much as possible and not punish another person while you are doing it, unlike a variety of other contact sports. I think that if you want to improve the duration of your life you do three things right: One is to exercise right, another is to rest right, and the third is proper nutrition. I didn't hear anything mentioned about developing skills to in achieving rest, though, and I do think marathoners should develop relaxation skills in addition to their other disciplines. I would like to note the caloric value of swimming and running; running uses twice as many calories. Thus, when you begin to compare the two sports they are not identical. Now, there is one more thing that some people are waiting to hear: while you've dissected and completely analyzed the scientific, objective things that happen in the marathoner's metabolism, no one as yet has correlated these with the phenomenon of second wind. Why don't people talk about second wind any more? Thank you very much.

COMMENT: I would like to direct this comment and question to Dr. Kavanagh. The people whom you're dealing with have a lot of training to do before they can achieve anything like the maximum level of fitness for their particular age group. I have been concerned from time to time about the negative conclusions that were based on short periods—3 or 4 months—of an activity program. I'm sure that the investigators were very aware of the pitfalls in studying this, and in reaching premature conclusions. I wonder if you would care to comment in general about your own reaction to this, and in particular in relation to your own studies. If you could have a greater compliance and a higher training effect, would the results be even better?

T. KAVANAGH: Let me review a period in the late 1960s, when our first study used relaxation and randomly assigned one group to relaxation therapy classes and the other group to exercise classes. At the end of the year we found that the psychological and physiological gains were not that spectacular, but they were present and they were present equally in both groups. The study was continued for an additional year, but instead of having the exercise group continue the exercises they had been accustomed to, we decided to accelerate them and began them in very violent training—namely, jogging up to an hour—and that's when we came to this endurance training. It also suggested to us that you don't really get very much gain to speak of in less than a year, and it takes two to obtain anything worthwhile. So, in the sense in which we operate, we don't expect great improvement that's easily measurable in less than one year, preferably two. The men operate at about 60% to 70% of their potential, and we prefer that they work out five times per week, and we would like them to do a work out which is individually prescribed for a period from 30 to 60 minutes. But the compliance is dependent to a large degree upon the degree of expectation that you have. We have, in a way, said right from the beginning: you will come to the center as little as possible; we will really try to educate you while you are there, and then we will give you a work out that you will do on your own. If we cannot get you to do it on your own, then we are not going to be very successful. But we wanted you to come as little as possible, so we began it at once per week. That's the only expectation we had. Since we knew we would be going for 2 years anyway, we knew that it was reasonable to expect that, and it worked very well.

D. GOLDBERG (*University of Toronto, Toronto, Ont.*): I would like to ask a personality question on introversion and perseverence. Have there been any studies which have examined other sports involving long-term training with delayed success in which people were examined for introversion and perseverence, such as swimming, gymnastics, noncontact sports?

T. KOSTRUBALA: As far as I know, no such study has been done.

M. POTTER (*University of Florida, Gainesville, Fla.*): I would like to ask two questions regarding your study of the marathoner. I noticed that most of the people with whom you work are really inexperienced runners—they are really short-term types. As far as the marathon is concerned, I consider someone who has been running for less than 5 years inexperienced. I'm wondering if you have studied and recorded changes in the personality after running for 3 and 5 years. You now have a lifetime situation going on there. In viewing your slide on perseverence, I can see that the difference between the 50 sub-3-hour marathoners and the over 3-hour or general population marathoners is just a matter of setting a goal. The other point relates to the masculinity/femininity ratio you have. In the sexual development of the over-40 male there is the beginning of feminization in the sexual role as a natural tendency of male menopause. I notice that all of your population is in that group, so you should have a higher femininity rate. I wonder how we would compare that with, for example, untrained males or same personality type males in the college level, but for example in a younger group.

T. KAVANAGH: These particular figures are age-match controlled. In other words, they are considerably higher than those of the general population.

P. MILVY: Dr. Kavanagh, I have a really difficult question. I've heard the "nagging wife syndrome" mentioned a few times during the course of this conference. What would happen if you made a real effort—presumably these wives don't jog—to get them to jog with their husbands, get them out on the track until 10 o'clock at the "Y" and just see what happens. I think it would be therapeutic for their hearts as well as perhaps for their "hearts."

T. KAVANAGH: I agree with you. The only thing we have found is that females who have had heart attacks—and therefore have an impetus to train—have not taken as readily to jogging as to other forms of activity.

P. MILVY: I'm referring to healthy wives jogging with their unhealthy husbands.

T. KAVANAGH: We would like to think that we could do that, but I expect it would be very difficult.

P. MILVY: I would like to conclude simply by saying that while I've often heard psychiatrists say that life is only one walk around the block, I prefer to think that it's quite a few jogs around the reservoir. Thank you.

Author Index

(Italicized page numbers refer to comments in Discussions)

1047

Subject Index

Waldniel, West Germany
first international marathon for women
  only. *See* Marathon races
Walker, Carolina. *See* Women marathon
  runners, famous
Water
  consumption, 185
  content of skeletal muscle. *See* Skeletal
    muscle
  loss from blood plasma. *See* Blood
    plasma
  transcapillary movement
    and exercise, 186–187
Weather-sensitive patients . *See* Heat
  stress—patients suffering from
Weight
  body weight and adiposity. *See* Run-
    ners
  lean body weight. *See* Body composi-
    tion
  loss in distance runners, *143*
  of smokers. *See* Smokers
  of track competitors. *See* Track com-
    petitors, aging
Weston, Edward Payson. *See* Pedestrian
  racers, famous; Pedestrian races
Wettedness of skin. *See* Sweating rate
Wheat germ oil. *See* Energy substrates
White, Pat. *See* Marathon races, professional
Wind, hot dry
  effect on body, 918
WOFO. *See* Work and Family Orientation Questionnaire
Women
  aerobic capacity prediction. *See* Aer-
    obic capacity
  femininity. *See* Femininity
  menstrual cycle. *See* Menstrual cycle
  pelvic width and hip cross-over. *See*
    Pelvic width
  physiological statistics, *552, 553, 554*
  self-esteem. *See* Female self-esteem
  training in old. *See* Aerobic capacity—
    improvement in old women after
    training
Women athletes
  body composition, *770,* 771
  self-esteem. *See* Female self-esteem
  somatotype values, 771, 773, *773*
Women distance runners, 811
  acclimatization
    basal rectal temperature, 787
    heart rate and body temperature,
      786
    to heat, 787

aerobic capacity, 726–729, 732–733
aerobic demands of running, 726–729,
  732–733
aerobic power, 727
body composition, 765, *766,* 771
body fat values, 767, *770,* 771
difference from male counterparts,
  726
efficiency of running, 726–727, 729
fractional utilization of aerobic capacity, 729, 733
heat tolerance, 777–780, 783–789
  aerobic power, 786
  methodology in chamber for study,
    779
  physical conditioning, 785–786
  role of cardiovascular fitness, 777
menstrual cycle
  oligomenorrhea or amenorrhea, 773
physique, 765, 767
plasma volume, 784
  expansion, 786
  hemoconcentrations, 785
  total proteins, 785
selected responses, cf. males in other
  studies, 789, *790*
self-perception, 808–815
somatotype
  ectomorphy, 774
submaximum aerobic capacity, 728,
  732
sweating response, 786
  evaporative sweat loss, 785
  onset of sweating, 787
  threshold, 786
  zero central drive, 788
temperature regulation
  blood pressure, 778
  body heat content, 783
  cardiac index, 780
  evaporative heat loss, 783
  forearm blood flow, 780
  heart rate and stroke index, 780
  heat storage, 783
  mean skin temperature and rectal
    temperature, 780
  role of cardiovascular fitness, 777
Women long distance runners. *See also*
  Aeken, Ernst van
  and athletic organizations. *See* Athletic
    organizations' influence on wom-
    en's long distance running
  difference from male counterparts, 725
Women marathon runners, 979. *See also*
  Aaken, Ernst van; Marathon
  races; Olympic Games Marathon;
  Olympic program